PATHOLOGY OF
THE LUNGS

SECOND EDITION

ELSEVIER CD-ROM LICENCE AGREEMENT

PATHOLOGY OF
THE LUNGS

SECOND EDITION

Bryan Corrin MD FRCPath
Emeritus Professor of Thoracic Pathology
National Heart and Lung Institute
Imperial College School of Medicine
and
Honorary Consultant Histopathologist
Royal Brompton Hospital
London, UK

Andrew G. Nicholson DM FRCPath
Consultant Histopathologist
Department of Histopathology
Royal Brompton Hospital
and
Professor of Respiratory Pathology
National Heart and Lung Institute
Imperial College School of Medicine
London, UK

Contributor:
Margaret M. Burke MB FRCPath
Consultant Histopathologist
Harefield Hospital
Harefield, Middlesex, UK

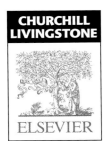

CHURCHILL
LIVINGSTONE

ELSEVIER

© 2006, Elsevier Limited. All rights reserved.

First edition 1999
Second edition 2006

The right of Bryan Corrin and Andrew G. Nicholson to be identified as authors of this work has been asserted by them in accordance with the Copyright, Designs and Patents Act 1988

ISBN 0 443 07476 3

EAN 978 0 443 07476 9

British Library Cataloguing in Publication Data
A catalogue record for this book is available from the British Library

Library of Congress Cataloging in Publication Data
A catalog record for this book is available from the Library of Congress

Commissioning Editor: Michael Houston
Project Development Manager: Hilary Hewitt
Project Manager: Glenys Norquay
Design Direction: Erik Bigland
Illustration Manager: Mick Ruddy
Marketing Manager (UK): Leontine Treur
Marketing Manager (US): Ethel Cathers

Last digit is the print number: 9 8 7 6 5 4 3 2 1

Printed in China

CONTENTS

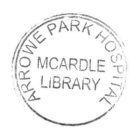

PREFACE

This book is aimed primarily at the practising diagnostic histopathologist. However, the clinical, functional and radiological consequences of the structural changes described are not neglected and the resultant clinicopathological correlation should be of interest to thoracic clinicians, radiologists and surgeons as well as general histopathologists. The intention has been to cover lung disease in as comprehensive yet succinct a manner as possible.

There are now two authors but close collaboration has minimised repetition and avoided the delays that often render obsolete parts of some multi-author works. Indeed the opportunity has been taken to update both text and references at the latest possible point in the production schedule. It is also hoped that this close collaboration will have resulted in uniformity of style and a proper balance between chapters. The text is about 100 pages longer than the first edition, mainly due to increased illustration and referencing.

We thank our medical colleagues at the Brompton and Harefield hospitals, in particular Margaret Burke who revised the transplantation chapter, and David Hansell, who provided many radiographic images and took time to show us what they represent. We also thank the many pathologists who have provided illustrations or referred cases that expanded our knowledge of lung pathology. We are also indebted to our laboratory and secretarial staff for their unstinting support and help, in particular Richard Florio, David Butcher, Ann Dewar, Anne-Marie Campbell, Shehnaaz Ghazali, Nathalie Goodwill, Matthew Pynegar, James Croud, Anthony Phillips, and Christian Archer, and also the many staff at Elsevier for their excellent support, notably Michael Houston, Hilary Hewitt, Lyn Taylor and Glenys Norquay.

BC thanks his wife Sheila for her support and is pleased to acknowledge the debt he owes to his teachers, in particular Winston Evans, who first steered him towards a career in pathology, Hugh Cameron, Colin Campbell, Herbert Spencer and Averill Liebow.

AGN gratefully acknowledges several pathologists in particular - Tom Colby, Bill Travis, Elisabeth Brambilla, and Bryan himself - for providing friendship and tutelage in the art of pulmonary pathology over the years. However, his biggest thank you goes to family and friends outside medicine who keep his life in perspective – Jimmy, Betty, Iain, Caroline, James, Tess and Robbie Nicholson (who will no doubt be the first to read this book), Simon and Marion Pennington, Blair Cameron, and William Johnson amongst many - and lastly but most of all, Francesca for her love and support.

Bryan Corrin and Andrew G. Nicholson
London

1

The structure of the normal lungs

ANATOMY OF THE LUNGS AND AIRWAYS

Soon after entering the thorax, the trachea divides to form two main bronchi, one to each lung. The right main bronchus follows more closely the direction of the trachea and because it branches earlier, is only half the length of the left. The right main bronchus is wider than the left and carries 55% of each breath. It enters the lung behind the right pulmonary artery and is said to be 'eparterial' whereas the left main bronchus crosses behind the left pulmonary artery to enter the lung below it and is therefore said to be 'hyparterial' (Fig. 1.1 and see Fig. 10.10, p. 481 and Fig. 10.11, p. 482).

The two lungs, enclosed within the visceral pleura, fill their respective pleural cavities. Tissue is reduced to a minimum in the interests of gas exchange. At mid-inspiration over 80% of lung volume is air, 10% is blood, 3% comprises conductive airways and blood vessels and only 3% is alveolar tissue. The normal combined weight of the lungs averages 850 g in men and 750 g in women. Lung weights in children are given in Table 1.1.[1]

The lungs abut the mediastinum medially, rest on the diaphragm below, and elsewhere are enclosed by the rib cage. On their medial surface, the main broncho-vascular structures connect the hilum of the lung with the mediastinum and here the visceral pleura is reflected off the lung to become the parietal pleura. The pleura is described in more detail in Chapter 13.

Oblique fissures divide the lungs into upper and lower lobes and on the right, a transverse fissure separates off a middle lobe. The main bronchi divide in a corresponding manner to give five lobar bronchi. The next division supplies the lung segments, of which there are 19, a segment being the smallest bronchopulmonary unit that can be distinguished and excised separately by a surgeon. The airways branch repeatedly and there may be as many as 23 divisions before alveoli furthest from the trachea are reached, as opposed to alveoli nearer the hilum of the lung, which are reached after as few as eight divisions. The pattern of branching is one of asymmetrical dichotomy, meaning that each airway has two branches that often differ in diameter or length.

The airways of the first four generations are individually named and the pathologist must be familiar with the

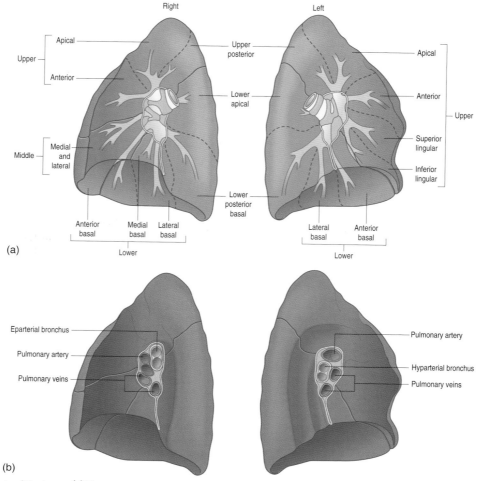

Figure 1.1 Medial aspects of the lungs. (a) The arrangement and nomenclature of the lobes and their segments. (b) The positions of the main bronchi, arteries and veins at the hila.

terminology of the 19 lung segments and their bronchi so that lesions can be localised accurately and the pathological findings correlated with those of radiologists and surgeons. Figure 1.2 illustrates the trachea, main, lobar and segmental bronchi diagrammatically, using an internationally recommended nomenclature.[2] A plastic cast of the proximal airways coloured according to the lung segments is shown in Figure 1.3. It will be noted that the following anatomical features are common to the two lungs:

- each upper lobe has apical, anterior and posterior segments
- each lower lobe has an apical segment and anterior, lateral and posterior basal segments.

The two lungs differ in the following respects:

- After giving off the upper lobe bronchus, the right main bronchus continues through a lower (intermediate) part to supply the middle and lower lobes, whereas the left main bronchus continues as the left lower lobe bronchus.
- The right lung has a middle lobe served by a branch of the lower (intermediate) part of the main bronchus, whereas the lingula of the left lung, which is the homologue of the

right middle lobe, is served by a lingular division of the upper lobe bronchus, the other branch of which is known as the upper or superior division.
- The two segments of the right middle lobe are medial and lateral whereas the two segments of the lingula are superior and inferior.
- The right lower lobe has an extra segment, known as the medial or cardiac segment.

Beyond the segmental bronchi, individual airways are unnamed but a distinction is drawn between bronchi, which have glands and cartilage in their wall, and bronchioles, which do not. Transition from bronchus to bronchiole takes place in airways approximately 1 mm in diameter. The first orders of bronchioles, which are known as membranous bronchioles, are purely conductive. The bronchioles comprising the last order of purely conductive airways are known as terminal bronchioles, despite them leading into further orders of bronchioles. These further bronchioles have alveoli opening directly off them and are known as respiratory bronchioles; they both conduct gas and participate in gas exchange. Such airways form what is termed a transitional zone between the purely conductive

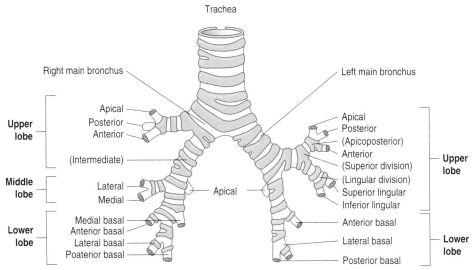

Figure 1.2 Nomenclature of the main, lobar and segmental bronchi. Beyond the segmental bronchi individual airways are unnamed.

Table 1.1 Lung weights in children[1]			
Age	Body length (cm)	Right lung (g)	Left lung (g)
Birth–3 days	49	21	18
3–7 days	49	24	22
1–3 weeks	52	29	26
3–5 weeks	52	31	27
5–7 weeks	53	32	28
7–9 weeks	55	32	29
3 months	56	35	30
4 months	59	37	33
5 months	61	38	35
6 months	62	42	39
7 months	65	49	41
8 months	65	52	45
9 months	67	53	47
10 months	69	54	51
11 months	70	59	53
12 months	73	64	57
14 months	74	66	60
16 months	77	72	64
18 months	78	72	65
20 months	79	83	74
22 months	82	80	75
24 months	84	88	76
3 years	88	89	77
4 years	99	90	85
5 years	106	107	104
6 years	109	121	122
7 years	113	130	123
8 years	119	150	140
9 years	125	174	152
10 years	130	177	166
11 years	135	201	190

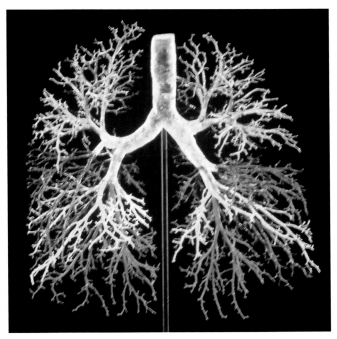

Figure 1.3 Posterior view of a plastic cast of the proximal airways with individual segments distinguished by colour.

walls. Numerical data appertaining to individual orders (generations) of airways are shown in Table 1.2.[3]

The lung substance is divided into primary and secondary lobules. The primary lobule is that portion of the lung supplied by one respiratory bronchiole but it is seldom referred to today and the unqualified term lobule generally equates to the secondary lung lobule. The secondary lobule is a portion of lung surrounded by fibrous septa that are visible on the cut surface of the lung (Figs. 1.4, 1.5) and through the visceral pleura, particularly when their contained lymphatics are outlined by

airways and the alveoli. It comprises about three generations of respiratory bronchioles and two to nine generations of alveolar ducts, the last of which terminate in alveolar sacs; all these structures have increasing numbers of alveoli opening off their

Table 1.2   The Weibel model of the bronchial tree[3]

Number of branches	Generation	Diameter (mm)	Length (mm)	Structure
1	0	18.0	120.0	trachea
2	1	12.2	47.6	B
4	2	8.3	19.0	B
8	3	5.6	7.6	B
16	4	4.5	12.7	B
32	5	3.5	10.7	B
64	6	2.8	9.0	B
128	7	2.3	7.6	B
256	8	1.86	6.4	B
512	9	1.54	5.4	MB
1024	10	1.30	4.6	MB
2048	11	1.09	3.9	MB
4096	12	0.95	3.3	MB
8192	13	0.82	2.7	MB
16 384	14	0.74	2.3	MB
32 768	15	0.66	2.0	MB
65 536	16	0.60	1.65	TB
131 072	17	0.54	1.41	RB
262 144	18	0.50	1.17	RB
524 288	19	0.47	0.99	RB
1 048 576	20	0.45	0.83	AD
2 097 152	21	0.43	0.70	AD
4 194 304	22	0.41	0.59	AD
8 388 608	23	0.41	0.50	AD

B, bronchi; MB, membranous bronchioles; TB, terminal bronchioles; RB, respiratory bronchioles; AD, alveolar ducts. The data are based on a combination of morphometry and assumption.

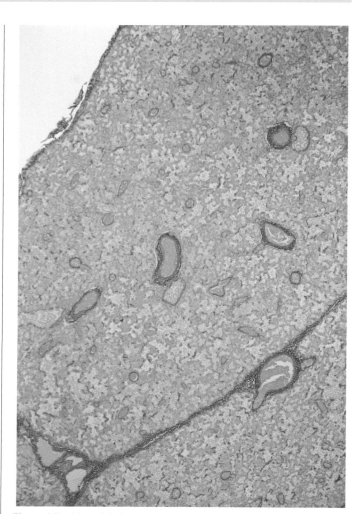

Figure 1.5   A lung lobule demarcated by the pleura and interlobular septa, which are stained red in this elastin van Gieson preparation, as are the periarterial cuffs of connective tissue. The arteries (and poorly stained accompanying airways) mark the centres of the lung acini while the veins are situated in the interlobular septa.

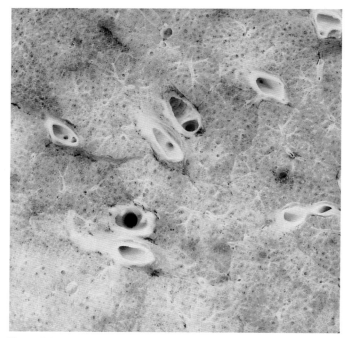

Figure 1.4   Poorly demarcated fibrous septa incompletely separate the lung lobules. The pulmonary arteries accompany the airways in the centres of the lung acini whereas the pulmonary veins are situated at the periphery of the lung lobules in the interlobular septa.

dust or tumour (Fig. 1.6). However, the fibrous septa that demarcate the secondary lobules are unevenly developed. They are quite well represented laterally in the lower lobes (where they appear radiologically as Kerley B lines when thickened by interstitial oedema), but are poorly represented medially and deep in the lungs. The lobules they demarcate are polyhedral. In the adult lung, each lobule measures 1–2 cm across and is in turn made up of 3–10 acini, an acinus being that portion of the lung supplied by one terminal bronchiole. The volume of a lobule is approximately 2 ml and that of an acinus approximately 0.2 ml. An acinus is 0.5–1 cm long,[4] so that the bronchi and purely conductive bronchioles make up all but this length of the total gas pathway. Each acinus contains about 2000 alveoli and it is estimated that the two lungs together contain about 300 million alveoli.[5] The edges of adjacent acini interdigitate without any intervening septa and it is impossible to detect where one acinus ends and the next begins, either with the

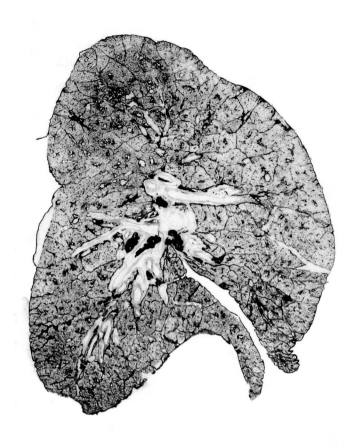

Figure 1.6 A Gough–Wentworth paper-mounted whole lung section of a city-dweller's lung in which the interlobular septa and centriacinar structures are particularly well seen because of dust in the lymphatics.

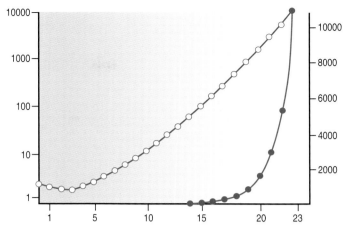

Figure 1.7 Summed cross-sectional area (cm²) plotted against airway generation. Logarithmic scale on the left (open circles), linear scale on the right (solid circles). Note the striking increase in total cross-sectional area of the peripheral airways. The arithmetic plot is often duplicated in mirror image fashion to illustrate a classic trumpet-shaped concept of the increasing airway cross-sectional area in the paired lungs. (Weibel's data redrawn from Horsfield K. The relation between structure and function in the airways of the lung. Respiratory Medicine 1974; 68:145–160. With permission from Elsevier Ltd.[3,7])

naked eye or the microscope. However, in adult lungs, the centres of the acini are generally 'tattooed' with carbon for it is here that lymphatics commence and dust-laden cells accumulate in what Macklin termed 'dust sumps' (Fig. 1.6).[6]

Each generation of airways is shorter than its predecessor and whereas individual members of each generation are narrower than their parents, beyond the segmental bronchi the summed cross-sectional area for each generation progressively increases logarithmically (Fig. 1.7),[3,7] and at the periphery, resistance to airflow is negligible. Because of this, gas flow velocity falls rapidly in the respiratory bronchioles and gas mixing in the last few airways is largely by diffusion. Diffusion across tissue is less efficient than in the gas phase but at the surface of the alveolar walls, gas transfer is maximised as the inspired gas is spread over an area of about 70 m².[8] There is therefore considerable reserve in the conductive capacity of the peripheral airways, large numbers of which may be obliterated before there is any appreciable shortness of breath; for this reason the finer airways have been termed the 'silent area of the lung'.

Lambert's canals are tubular communications approximately 30 μm diameter that connect terminal and respiratory bronchioles with adjacent peribronchiolar alveoli, thus bypassing the main pathway.[9] They represent accessory air inlets to, or outlets

from the more distant alveoli. In coal miners, these canals and their associated alveoli are early sites of dust cell accumulation, while in fibrotic lung disease, cuboidal bronchiolar epithelial cells often extend through them to line the peribronchiolar alveoli, a metaplastic process that is often termed alveolar bronchiolisation or Lambertosis (Figs 1.8 and 3.37A, p. 118).

To what extent the 30 μm diameter Lambert's canals provide collateral circulation is uncertain. They appear to offer a better anatomical pathway than the 2–13 μm diameter pores of Kohn, described below, but may be less effective than certain interconnecting respiratory bronchioles that measure 120 μm in diameter[10] and the 200 μm diameter interacinar and 80–150 μm diameter intersegmental connections that have been demonstrated using injection techniques[11] and corrosion casts,[12] respectively.

The two main pulmonary arteries arise from the bifurcation of the pulmonary trunk shortly after its origin from the right ventricle and divide to follow the lobar bronchi. Segmental and subsegmental pulmonary arteries continue alongside their corresponding airways and in the periphery of the lungs most small pulmonary arteries enter an acinus with the terminal bronchiole and are thus found at the centre of the acinus (Figs 1.9, 1.10). As well as these axial vessels there are also small supernumerary branches which do not accompany airways.[13] The pulmonary arteries divide to supply the pulmonary capillaries, which form a meshwork situated in the alveolar walls, regrouping at the periphery of the acinus to form pulmonary veins. In the periphery of the lung, the pulmonary veins run in the interlobular septa and are thus separate from the artery and airway in the centre of the acinus (Figs 1.5, 1.9), but they take up a position alongside the artery and bronchus proximal to the entry of these structures into the lung lobule.

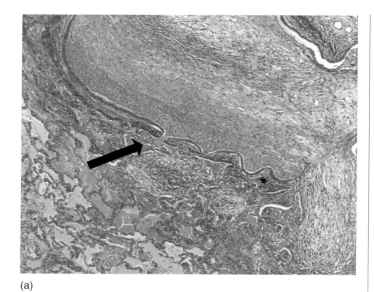

(a)

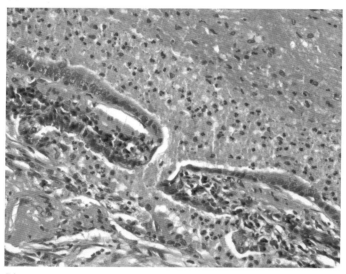

(b)

Figure 1.8 Canal of Lambert (in a case of organising pneumonia). (a) The canal (arrow) provides a direct connection between bronchiole and alveolus. (b) Fibrinopurulent debris tracks directly between airway and alveolus.

MICROSCOPY OF THE AIRWAYS

The bronchial wall consists of a thin mucosa and a more substantial submucosal coat, outside which there is the peribronchial sheath of loose connective tissue that also surrounds the accompanying pulmonary artery. The mucosa consists of respiratory epithelium resting on a basement membrane and beneath that a supportive connective tissue layer rich in elastin fibres. There is no clear boundary between the mucosa and the submucosa but muscle, glands and cartilage are conventionally regarded as belonging to the submucosal coat (Fig. 1.11).

In the extrapulmonary bronchi and trachea the cartilage forms irregular, sometimes branching, rings that are incomplete

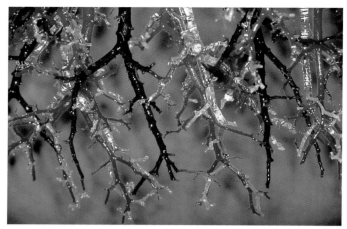

Figure 1.9 A plastic cast showing that the pulmonary arteries (red) accompany the airways (white), and that pulmonary veins (blue) are separate.

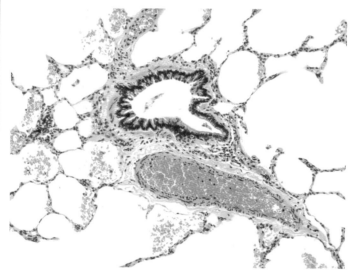

Figure 1.10 Bronchioles and pulmonary arteries lie alongside each other in the centres of the lung acini, sharing a connective tissue sheath.

dorsally, the gaps being bridged by smooth muscle. In intrapulmonary bronchi the intercartilaginous gaps are more numerous and haphazardly distributed but in large bronchi the cartilage plates are numerous enough to be found in any cross section. In small bronchi, the cartilage is less abundant and may be missed in some sections. Airways that completely lack cartilage and glands are termed bronchioles.

Smooth muscle, present only in the dorsal intercartilaginous gaps of the trachea, completely encircles the intrapulmonary bronchi, internal to the cartilage. It comprises two sets of fibres that wind around the bronchial tree as opposing spirals, thereby appearing incomplete in individual cross sections. The arrangement is such that as the muscle contracts, the airway both shortens and constricts. The muscle forms a more complete ring in the membranous bronchioles than in bronchi or respiratory bronchioles. When respiratory bronchioles are encountered in longitudinal section, the muscle is seen only as small knobs

smokers and asthmatics.[16] Transverse ridges are also evident in the bronchial mucosa; these lack elastin fibres and probably represent folds produced by muscular shortening of the airways.

Around the pulmonary arteries and to a lesser extent the airways, there is a wide sheath of loose connective tissue (Fig. 1.10). This connects with the visceral pleura at the hilum and distally with the delicate connective tissue of the respiratory bronchioles and the alveolar interstitium and through the latter with the interlobular septa and the visceral pleura. The periarterial sheath carries nerves and lymphatic vessels and is expanded considerably in oedema, acting as an interstitial sump for extravascular fluid and thus protecting against this spilling over into the alveoli.

The epithelium of the main airways is pseudostratified, meaning that all its cells rest on the basement membrane, but not all reach the airway lumen (Figs 1.13, 1.14). Most epithelial cells are columnar and ciliated but these are interspersed with mucous cells, finely granulated neuroendocrine cells, basal cells, brush cells, nerve terminals and migratory lymphocytes and mast cells.[17–19] The airway epithelium decreases in height distally, becoming cuboidal in the bronchioles. The mucous cells decrease in number as the bronchioles are approached and in these small airways Clara[20] and serous[21] cells are found among the ciliated cells.[22] Major histocompatibility antigens of both class I (HLA-A, B and C) and II (HLA-DR) are expressed by bronchial, bronchiolar and alveolar epithelium.[23] All airway epithelial cells express cytokeratin 19, while the basal cells also express cytokeratin 17.[24] In contrast to pleural mesothelium, cytokeratins 5 and 6 are not expressed by airway epithelium or its malignant derivatives, this providing a useful point of distinction between pulmonary adenocarcinoma and epithelioid mesotheliomas (see p. 710).[25]

In the main airways, there is a surface layer of mucus supported by an aqueous hypophase (Fig. 1.15). More distally, the bronchial mucus layer is discontinuous.[26] In the smaller bronchioles there is a continuous surface layer similar to that lining the alveoli (see below).[27]

The thickness of the surface layer is of considerable importance. In its proximal movement, the surface layer is constantly being added to by airway secretions, yet this material has all to be accommodated on a progressively reducing surface area (Fig. 1.7). Despite losses through evaporation and clearance being faster proximally (Fig. 1.16),[28] the larger airways would be occluded by the bronchial secretions were these not concentrated by an epithelial ion exchange mechanism. This vital function is under the control of an epithelial transmembrane regulator, faults in which underlie the development of cystic fibrosis (see p. 65). The same control mechanism operates in reverse in panting dogs to facilitate heat loss. The thickness of the aqueous hypophase is also of crucial importance to ciliary function (see below).

The various epithelial cells are held together by desmosomes, gap junctions and near the lumen by terminal bars that prevent excessive fluid movement across the epithelium.[29] However, irritants such as tobacco smoke, sulphur dioxide and mast cell mediators render the terminal bar permeable to particulate markers placed in the lumen.[30–32]

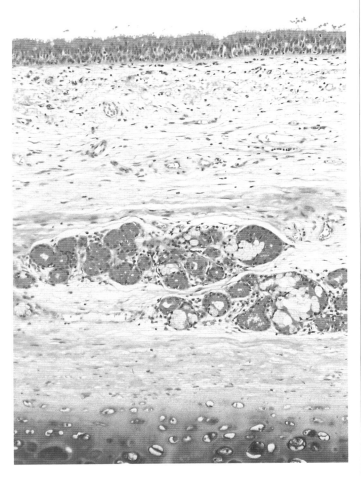

Figure 1.11 Normal bronchus, showing surface epithelium resting on elastin-rich connective tissue (these elements constituting the mucosa, see also Fig. 1.12), beneath which are the submucosal glands and cartilage. The glands are of mixed seromucous type. The apparent absence of submucosal muscle at this point is attributable to its double spiral arrangement.

between the mouths of the numerous alveoli that open off these airways.

If the trachea and main bronchi are opened from the front, longitudinal mucosal corrugations or ridges are evident on the posterior wall.[14] Most of those in the trachea pass into the right main bronchus but there are an equal number in the left main bronchus where they commence anew beyond the carina. In the trachea and main bronchi, the ridges are limited to the membranous parts but distal to the lobar bronchi the ridges are distributed all around the walls of the airways. They represent longitudinal bundles of elastin fibres situated in the subepithelial mucosal lamina propria (Fig. 1.12). Although the bundles become progressively thinner they persist throughout the bronchial tree and link up with spiral elastin fibres described in the alveolar ducts[15] and with the elastic tissue of the alveolar walls. They are thought to contribute to elastic recoil during expiration and are more prominent in men, older subjects,

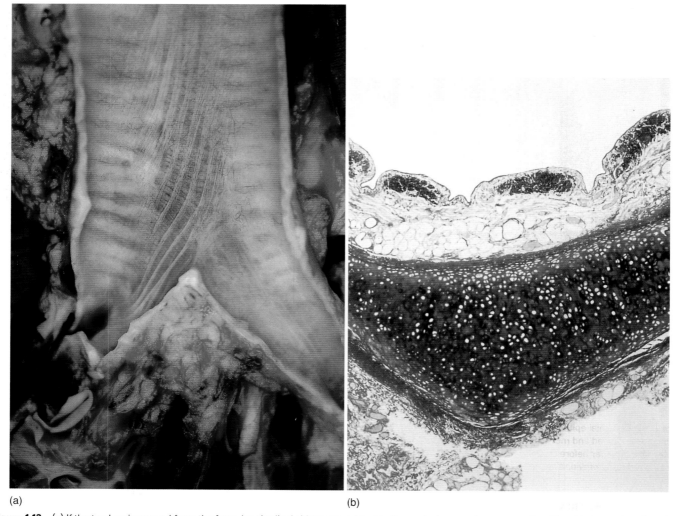

(a)   (b)

Figure 1.12 (a) If the trachea is opened from the front, longitudinal ridges are evident in the posterior membranous portion. The ridges continue into the right main bronchus while others commence in the left main bronchus. (b) Microscopy shows that the ridges consist of longitudinal bands of elastic tissue staining black (top). Together with the surface epithelium, not evident in this preparation, this elastin-rich connective tissue constitutes the bronchial mucosa. The bronchial cartilage is also darkly stained but the intervening submucosal glands and muscle are poorly stained. (Elastin van Gieson stain.)

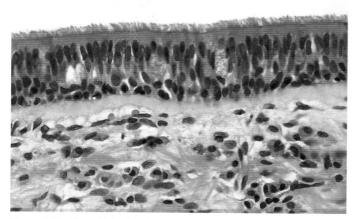

Figure 1.13 Bronchial epithelium composed of pseudostratified columnar ciliated cells interspersed with occasional mucus-secreting (goblet) cells.

The epithelial cells rest on a basement membrane that consists of three layers, a lamina lucida, which makes contact with overlying epithelial cells, a lamina densa and a lamina reticularis. The last of these consists of fine fibrillary collagen and is only present in adults. It is not considered to be part of the 'true' basement membrane but it is this layer that is thickened in asthma and, to a lesser extent, a variety of other airway diseases. The laminae lucida and densa comprise the 'true' basement membrane. They each measure 50 nm in thickness, well below the resolution of the light microscope. They are made up of type IV collagen, laminin and fibronectin. They have a negative charge, due to sulphate and carboxyl moieties, which partly contributes to their permeability. This is relatively high; the basement membrane is therefore a poor barrier to the movement of macromolecules and even cells.

Surface epithelial cells are replaced only slowly, less than 1% being in division at any one time, although the mitotic index

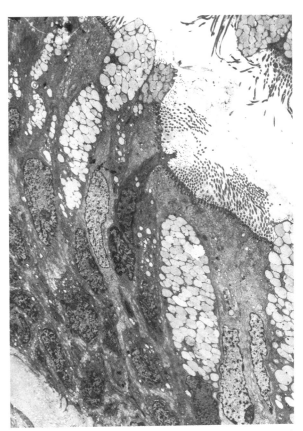

Figure 1.14 Bronchial epithelium. Transmission electron micrograph showing basal, ciliated and mucous cells. The electron-lucent mucus granules fuse together before discharge. Most of the surface is formed of ciliated cells. (Figure provided by Mrs D Bowes, Midhurst, UK.)

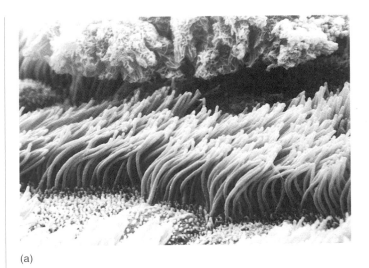

(a)

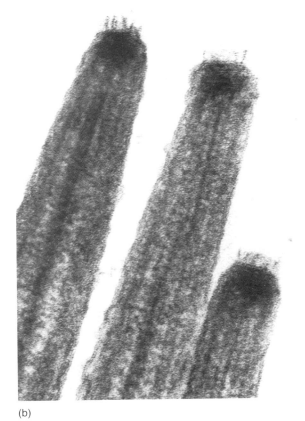

(b)

Figure 1.15 (a) Scanning electron micrograph of the bronchial surface showing mucus (top) resting on the tips of the cilia. The cilia beat in an aqueous hypophase. (b) High power transmission electron microscopy shows that the tips of the cilia are equipped with hooklets. (Figure provided by Professor PK Jeffery, Brompton, UK.)

increases in response to various forms of injury.[33] The role of the basal cell as the sole progenitor has been questioned following recognition that other non-ciliated cells, notably the mucus and Clara cells, have an important stem cell function.[33,34]

Approximately 10 000 l of air are inhaled each day and considerable amounts of potentially harmful environmental agents escape the filtering action of the nose to reach the lower respiratory tract. The respiratory epithelium provides the first line of defence against these.[35] It does this in three ways:

- by providing an intact surface barrier comparable to the skin and the epithelium of the alimentary tract
- by secreting an array of substances that act against physical and biological agents
- by coordinating secretory and ciliary function so that there is effective mucociliary clearance.

The morphology and function of the individual epithelial cells will now be considered in turn.

Ciliated cells

Ciliated cells possess numerous mitochondria and two types of surface projection: stubby microvilli about 0.4 µm in length and long slender cilia up to 6 µm in length. There are 200–300 cilia per cell, each beating at about 20 times/s. The rate at which the cilia beat falls with temperature[36] and the upper respiratory tract plays an important role in warming and moistening the inspired air. The ciliary beat consists of a straight-armed effective stroke followed by a curling return stroke.[37] Ciliated cells are arranged in groups within which the cilia beat in a coordinated fashion,

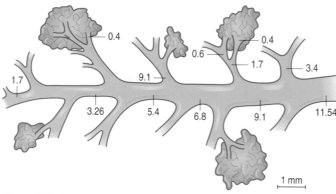

Figure 1.16 Velocity of mucus transport in the airways of a rat. The figures indicate the velocity of transport in mm/min at a particular site at 37°C. From left to right the velocity increases 7-fold. (Redrawn from Iravani J and van As A. Mucous transport in tracheobronchial tree of normal and bronchitic rats. The Journal of Pathology.[28] Copyright Pathological Society of Great Britain and Ireland. Reproduced with permission. Permission granted by John Wiley & Sons Ltd on behalf of PathSoc.)

probably governed by contact with the overlying mucus. The beating appears to be spontaneous. It is independent of nervous control and persists for several hours after death.

The cilia beat in a low viscosity layer beneath the surface mucus and move the overlying mucus only by their tips, which possess minute terminal hooklets (Fig. 1.15).[38] The depth of the aqueous hypophase is crucial to ciliary action: too much and the mucus is lifted off the tips of the cilia, too little and the cilia become clogged by mucus. The periciliary fluid is thought to derive from the airway epithelial cells under the control of the transmembrane regulator referred to above. The cell surface available for fluid transport is greatly increased by its microvilli, which are akin to the brush border of the intestinal epithelium.

The fine structure of cilia has become of medical importance with the recognition of the ciliary dyskinesia syndromes (see p. 63). Cilia have an axial central pair of microtubules with an outer ring of nine double microtubules (9 + 2 structure) (see Fig. 2.42a, p. 64). Small dynein side arms extend from one doublet towards the next and spokes connect each doublet with the central microtubules. All the microtubules fuse together near the tip, while near the cell, the central pair disappear and the doublets become triploid and fuse together as a cylinder which extends into the cytoplasm as the ciliary basal body. Cilia beat when the microtubules, powered by adenosine triphosphate elaborated in the dynein arms, slide past each other.

Basal cells

Basal cells are found particularly in the large airways but although they diminish in number peripherally, they reach down as far as the bronchioles. They have only sparse cytoplasm, which often contains bundles of cytokeratin tonofilaments that lead into prominent hemidesmosomes.[39] The basal cell was formerly thought to be the main stem cell of the airways but with the recognition that Clara and mucous cells are important in this respect[33,40,41] this view has had to be modified. Although they continue to be recognised as progenitor cells,[42]

adhesion of the columnar cells to the basement membrane is now thought to be an additional major function of basal cells.[43,44]

Mucous cells

Mucous cells[19] vary in appearance with a cycle of secretory activity that culminates in the discharge of mucus into the airways. Devoid of mucus, they are slender and possess abundant endoplasmic reticulum and well-developed Golgi apparatus. As they synthesise mucus, electron-lucent mucus granules accumulate, enlarge and fuse together to produce a large secretion vacuole that distends the apical cell cytoplasm, giving the mature cell its characteristic wine glass or goblet shape. Discharge takes place by further fusion involving the secretion vacuole and apical cell membranes.

Mucins are high molecular weight glycoproteins in which oligosaccharide sidechains are attached to an elongated protein core. The mucus granules of the surface mucous cells contain an acidic mucin, with sialic acid or sulphate groups at the end of the oligosaccharide side chains of the peptide core. The amount and viscoelasticity of the mucus are important to airway clearance and the chemical structure of the mucus probably influences its physical properties and hence the ease with which it is cleared by ciliary activity or coughing. Out of the nine different mucin genes identified in human tissues, seven are expressed in the respiratory tract, namely: MUC1 – MUC4, MUC5AC, MUC5B and MUC7.[45,46] While MUC5B and MUC7 expression is predominantly restricted to cells of the submucosal glands,[47] MUC2 and MUC5AC mucins are located more in the surface epithelium.[48] The predominant components of respiratory mucus are MUC5AC and MUC5B,[49] and these are upregulated by various stimuli such as air pollutants or bacteria and also in asthma and cystic fibrosis.[50,51] The actual number of mucous cells increases in response to irritation. This also induces inflammation and although the viscosity of mucus is primarily dependent on its glycoprotein content, it is markedly augmented by DNA released from effete inflammatory cells. It is impossible to state at exactly what point goblet cell hyperplasia begins, as numbers vary dependent on the site of the biopsy, but a crude figure is more than three per ten cells at any point in the respiratory tract.

Apart from the mucus secreted by mucous cells in the surface epithelium and submucosal glands (see below), non-secretory cells such as the ciliated cells have a thin mucoid glycocalyx forming the outer part of their cell membrane. This differs chemically from the main mucous lining and is probably formed by the cell of which it forms the outermost part. The glycocalyx of the cilia differs chemically from that of the microvilli on the same cell, while in the alveolus, different lining cells have chemically different forms of glycocalyx.[52]

Submucosal glands

The submucosal glands far exceed the secretory elements of the surface epithelium in cell mass and are the major source of bronchial secretion. They are situated between the muscle coat and the cartilage (Fig. 1.11) and between individual cartilage plates, their ducts piercing the muscle coat and mucosa to reach the lumen. They are mixed seromucous glands and the secretory acini are arranged so that the serous secretion has to pass through the mucus tubules.[53] The two secretions are therefore well mixed before they reach the bronchial lumen. Serous and mucous cells both have abundant rough endoplasmic reticulum and Golgi apparatus but the secretory granules of the serous cells are electron-dense, small and discrete, whereas mucus granules are electron-lucent, large and confluent (Fig. 1.17). The serous granules often show zonal variations in their fine structure implying a variety of secretory products. The mucous cells contain large amounts of both acid and neutral glycoprotein, while the serous cell granules contain smaller amounts of these glycoproteins[52,54] together with lysozyme,[55] lactoferrin[54] and a small molecular weight antiprotease specific to the airways.[56] The demonstration of carbonic anhydrase in serous cells implicates them in the production of a watery non-viscous secretion that could facilitate transport of the more viscous mucus secreted downstream.[53] The serous cells are also the major site of the secretory component of IgA[57–59] and of epithelial peroxidase.[60]

Collecting-duct cells are devoid of secretory granules but often have the characteristics of oncocytes, their cytoplasm being packed with numerous mitochondria. The oncocytes increase in number with age and may form metaplastic nodules (Fig. 1.18).[61] A fluid regulating role has been suggested for them but similar cells present in several other organs are considered to be degenerative. Glandular secretion is assisted by myo-epithelial cells, which are situated between the secretory and duct lining cells and the basement membrane. Neuroendocrine cells similar to those in the surface epithelium are also found in this situation, while unmyelinated nerve axons are observed in close association with serous, mucus, collecting-duct and myoepithelial cells.[62]

Neuroendocrine cells

Neuroendocrine cells, which are also known as Kultschitsky-type cells, Feyrter cells and APUD cells are found in the basal layer of the surface epithelium and in the bronchial glands.[62,63] In the surface epithelium they occur singly and in groups, the latter known as neuroepithelial bodies.[64,65] Single neuroendocrine cells are basally situated but send a thin cytoplasmic process to the surface. They are found throughout the airways from the main bronchi to the bronchioles but are only rarely found in the terminal bronchioles and alveoli.[66,67] Neuroendocrine bodies extend from the basement membrane to the surface. They are found particularly at airway bifurcations and have sensory neuronal connections[65,68–71] but are less numerous in man than in many laboratory animals.[67] Adjacent capillaries have a fenestrated endothelium, as found in many endocrine organs.

Neuroendocrine cells are characterised by numerous small granules, 70–150 nm diameter, consisting of a round electron-dense central core separated from an outer membrane by a clear halo (Fig. 1.19). In the fetus, two other morphological varieties of granule have been described.[64] The granules are scattered

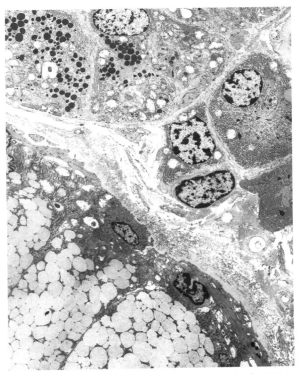

Figure 1.17 Bronchial gland composed of serous cells (top) which have discrete electron-dense granules and mucous cells (bottom) in which the secretory granules are electron-lucent and fuse together before discharge. In close proximity to the serous cells is a group of plasma cells (centre right). Immunoglobulin A is produced by plasma cells that lie close to the bronchial glands: it passes through the serous cells to reach the lumen and in so doing acquires its secretory component which is synthesised by the serous cells. (Transmission electron micrograph reproduced with permission from Bowes D, Corrin B. Ultrastructural immunocytochemical localization of lysozyme in human bronchial glands. Thorax 1977; 32:163–170.[55] With permission from the British Medical Association.)

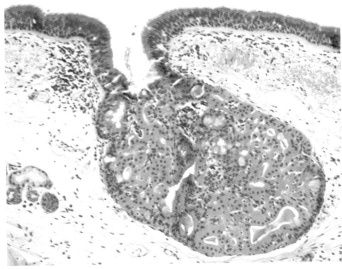

Figure 1.18 A seromucinous gland shows oncocytic metaplasia.

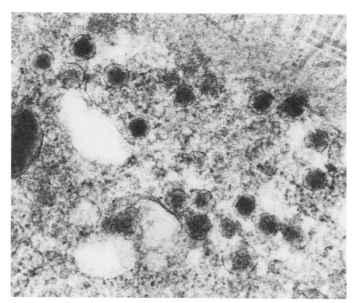

Figure 1.19 Bronchial neuroendocrine cell granules consist of a dense central core separated from an investing membrane by a thin electron-lucent zone. (Transmission electron micrograph provided by Miss A Dewar, Brompton, UK.)

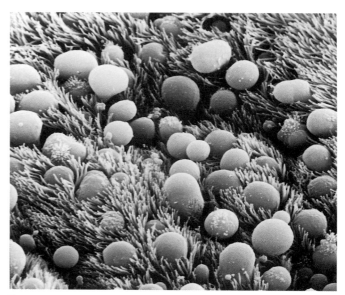

Figure 1.20 Terminal bronchiole showing non-ciliated Clara cells protruding above the adjacent cilia. (Scanning electron micrograph provided by Professor PK Jeffery, Brompton, UK.)

throughout the cytoplasm, but are often concentrated near the basal cell membrane. The neuroendocrine cells only occasionally display argyrophilia or formaldehyde-induced fluorescence but these reactions, indicative of biogenic amines, may be enhanced by prior incubation with precursor substances such as 5-hydroxytryptophan and dihydroxyphenylalanine.[72] Immunohistochemistry shows that both single neuroendocrine cells and neuroendocrine bodies may contain L-amino acid decarboxylase[73] and 5-hydroxytryptamine,[74] general neuro-endocrine markers such as neurone specific enolase,[75] chromogranin A,[67,76] synaptophysin[77] and neural cell adhesion molecule (CD56)[78] and peptides such as human bombesin (gastrin-releasing peptide),[67,79–82] calcitonin,[67,80,83,84] leu-encephalin,[80] substance P,[85] guanine nucleotide-binding protein[86] and adreno-corticotrophic hormone.[81] Chromogranin, a constituent of the granules and CD56 are probably the most sensitive and specific immunocytochemical markers.[67,78,87,88]

The main function of the pulmonary neuroendocrine system in man is thought to concern the control of growth and development of the lungs *in utero* and thereafter the regulation of pulmonary regeneration and repair. Neuroendocrine cells are more numerous in the fetal than the adult lung and one of their products, human bombesin, has trophic properties in regard to the other cells. Hyperplasia of neuroendocrine cells has been described during epithelial repair,[89–91] following asbestos exposure[92] and in pulmonary fibrosis,[93] infantile bronchopulmonary dysplasia,[94] pulmonary arterial disease,[95] bronchiectasis associated with tumourlets[81] and bronchi bearing carcinomas of all cell types.[96] Neuroendocrine cell hyperplasia also plays a role in the development of carcinoids and is thus regarded as a pre-neoplastic condition.

A subsidiary function of the neuroendocrine cells, which appears to be better developed in lower species, concerns the pulmonary response to hypoxia. Animal experiments have demonstrated that neuroendocrine cells increase in number and degranulate in hypoxic conditions, suggesting a chemoreceptor function.[97–100] In the case of the neuroepithelial bodies this function is modulated by intrapulmonary axon reflexes.[101] However, the relevance of these observations to man is uncertain.

Clara cells

These cells are named after the Austrian histologist Max Clara who provided a detailed description of them in 1937.[20] They are most numerous in the terminal bronchioles where they protrude above the ciliated cells (Fig. 1.20). The region immediately above the nucleus contains many large mitochondria with unusually sparse cristae. The apical portion is notable for a rich smooth endoplasmic reticulum network and, immediately beneath the luminal cell membrane, small electron-dense secretory granules of about 500 nm diameter. The granules are angulated in man, but round in many species. There is considerable species variation in the internal structure of Clara cells. The nature of the secretory product of the Clara cell and its precise mode of secretion are uncertain, but the major constituent of the granules is a 10-kDa protein (CC10) that inhibits several inflammatory cytokines and is therefore thought to be important in modulating bronchiolar inflammation; mice that are deficient in this protein are more susceptible to the damaging effects of hyperoxia.[102] Cytochrome P-450-dependent mixed-function oxidase activity[103] and an airway specific antiprotease that may be important in protecting the lung against emphysema[56] have also been identified in Clara cells. Mixed-function oxidases are involved in metabolising many environmental chemicals, including carcinogens that require catalytic activation. Intracellular levels of glutathione are important in protecting the Clara cells from injury by reactive intermediates produced by the metabolism of xenobiotics such as 3-methylindole, trichloroethylene and naphthylamine.[104–106] Clara cell secretion of endothelin, a powerful bronchoconstrictor and vasoconstrictor, has also been demonstrated.[107] The Clara cell also has stem-cell potentiality and in response to irritation gives rise to both ciliated and mucous cells.[40,104,108]

Brush cells

Brush cells occur infrequently at all levels of the airways from the trachea to the alveoli where they have been called type III pneumocytes.[109] They have a brush border of closely packed stubby microvilli up to 2 μm in length, the axial filaments of which continue into the cell without ending in a terminal web. A resemblance to intestinal cells has led to a belief that they are concerned in fluid absorption, although a chemoreceptor function is also suggested.[110]

MICROSCOPY OF THE ALVEOLAR TISSUE

Beyond the terminal bronchioles, which constitute the last of the purely conductive airways, alveoli are found in progressively increasing numbers through three orders of respiratory bronchioles and two to nine orders of alveolar ducts (Figs 1.21, 1.22).[111] The walls of the alveolar ducts consist only of a thin spiral band of collagen and elastin, between which are the mouths of the alveoli, also arranged in a spiral fashion.[15] The arrangement is like the coils of a spring, lengthening in inspiration and closing up in expiration. The alveolar openings usually have four straight sides while the alveolar walls consist of flat pentagonal or hexagonal plates arranged as a polyhedron. The alveoli are thus like boxes with one open side:[112] were the alveoli spherical, their walls would stretch on inspiration and the alveolar capillaries would close. The alveolar duct system and the polyhedral shape of the alveoli act together like a concertina and seem well designed to permit changes in volume without alterations in surface area.

The human adult lungs contain about 300–500 million alveoli,[5,113] each measuring about 250 μm in diameter when expanded, although gravitational forces result in them being bigger in the upper than the lower parts of the lung.[114] The size of the alveoli and the surface tension of their lining layer are the major determinants of distensibility and hence elastic recoil of the lungs; tissue components such as elastin and collagen contribute to a lesser degree.[115] The Laplace equation indicates that the collapsing force acting on the lungs is proportional to alveolar surface tension and inversely proportional to alveolar size. Surface tension is reduced and expansion of the lung thereby facilitated, by certain lipids, collectively known as pulmonary surfactant, that are secreted by alveolar lining cells (see below).

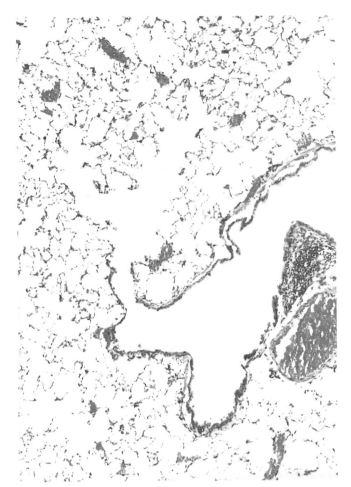

Figure 1.21 A terminal bronchiole dividing into alveolated respiratory bronchioles, this representing the termination of the purely conductive membranous bronchioles, the commencement of the transitional zone of the lung and the apex of a pulmonary acinus. A pulmonary artery is seen alongside the bronchiole. Artery and bronchiole are of roughly the same calibre. Between them is a lymphoreticular aggregate, this marking the point at which lymphatics commence.

Small holes, the pores of Kohn, are found in the alveolar walls of many species, including man (Fig. 1.23). Their diameter ranges from 2 to 13 μm and there are from 1 to 7 in each alveolus. The pores are absent at birth and only develop after the first year of life. For this reason, some argue that they are abnormal and represent the beginnings of emphysema. Others believe that they are normal and provide collateral ventilation, although perfusion fixation, which preserves the alveolar lining layer demonstrates that the pores are normally plugged by this layer.[116] In pneumonia, however, threads of fibrin can sometimes be seen passing through the pores from one alveolus to another. Transmission electron microscopy shows the edge of the pores to be lined by an intact epithelium.

Under the light microscope the alveolar wall is evidently rich in blood capillaries but it is not generally clear whether cells bordering the capillaries are endothelial, epithelial or

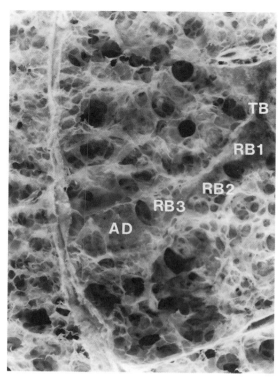

Figure 1.22 The cut surface of part of a lung lobule, showing some of the branches of an acinus. TB, terminal bronchiole; RB 1, 2 and 3, successive orders of respiratory bronchioles; AD, alveolar duct. The fibrous septa that border the lobule are also seen. (Reproduced from Heard and Izukawa.[111])

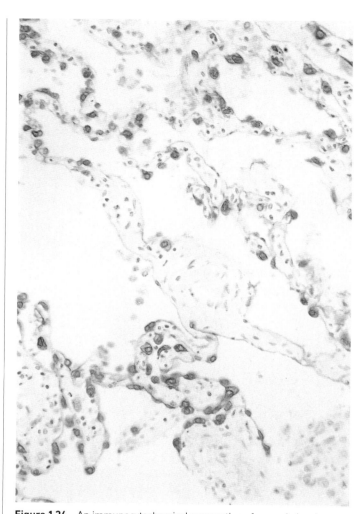

Figure 1.24 An immunocytochemical preparation of normal alveolar tissue shows that epithelial cells are plentiful but by light microscopy it is not apparent that the epithelial lining is complete. Immunoperoxidase for cytokeratin.

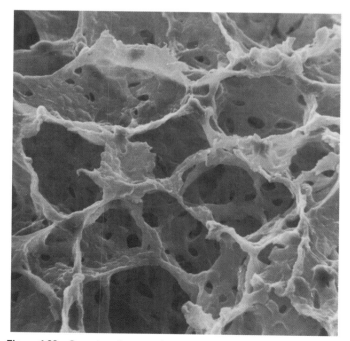

Figure 1.23 Scanning electron micrograph of normal mouse lung. The small holes in the alveolar walls are the pores of Kohn. (Figure provided by the late Professor BE Heard, Brompton, UK.)

interstitial. Cytokeratin immunocytochemistry shows that epithelial cells are plentiful but by light microscopy the alveolar epithelium appears to be incomplete (Fig. 1.24). It was not until 1953 that electron microscopy clarified an age-old dispute concerning the nature of the alveolar lining layer, showing that a complete simple epithelium extends throughout all alveoli (Figs 1.25, 1.26).[117] It is continuous with that of the airways. The lining epithelium is separated from the underlying connective tissue by a supportive basement membrane.

On one side of the alveolar wall the capillary is closely applied to the alveolar epithelium. Here the endothelial and epithelial basement membrane fuse and the air/blood barrier is at its thinnest, about 0.15 μm. On the opposite side of the alveolar wall, interstitial tissue separates endothelium from epithelium; this is known as the thick side of the air/blood barrier (Figs 1.25, 1.26). The alveolar epithelium, interstitium and capillary endothelium constitute about 30%, 40% and 30%, respectively of the air/blood barrier.[118]

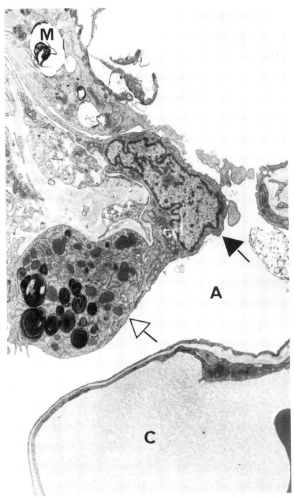

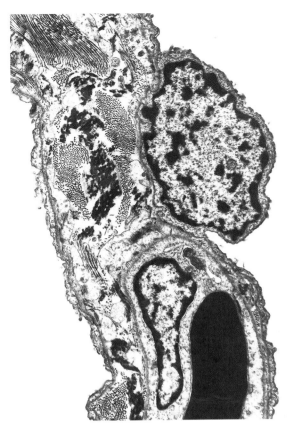

Figure 1.26 Alveolar wall with the nuclear portion of a type I cell and the thin part of the air/blood barrier on the right hand side. The interstitium contains bundles of collagen surrounding very electron-dense elastin. (Transmission electron micrograph provided by Miss A Dewar, Brompton, UK.)

Figure 1.25 Parts of two alveolar walls, the lower showing the thin portion of the air/blood barrier. The upper alveolar wall is lined by the nucleated portion of a type I cell (solid arrow) and a type II (open arrow) cell, the former partly covered by an alveolar macrophage (M). A, air space; C, capillary lumen. (Transmission electron micrograph provided by Mrs D Bowes, Midhurst, UK.)

The alveolar epithelium consists of two principal cell types, variously known as: I and II, respectively. These will now be considered.

Type I alveolar epithelial cells

These cells have few cytoplasmic organelles but are remarkable for their attenuated cytoplasm, which extends long distances from the nuclear zone of the cell (Figs 1.25, 1.26) and may even penetrate the alveolar wall so that one cell contributes to the lining of more than one alveolus.[119] They each cover up to 5000 μm^2 of the alveolar surface yet generally measure no more than 0.2 μm in thickness.[120] Their function is to provide a complete but thin covering, preventing fluid loss but facilitating rapid gas exchange. Type I cells are connected to each other and to type II cells by tight junctions and the alveolar epithelium

provides the major barrier to fluid movement into and out of the alveolus. Nevertheless, a variety of proteins known as aquaporins that facilitate water transport across epithelia have been identified in the cell membrane of type I alveolar cells.[121] Following large volume alveolar lavage for lipoproteinosis (see p. 318) it has been found that about 53% of the residual fluid is absorbed within 1 h.[122] Numerous small pinocytotic vesicles are seen within the type I cells and macromolecules are absorbed from the alveolus by this route.[123] Very fine particles reach the interstitium from the alveolar lumen by the same vesicular transport mechanism.[124,125] Such absorption is probably important in sensitising the host to inhaled antigens but as a clearance pathway the alveolar epithelium is of trifling importance compared with the alveolar macrophages. The long thin cytoplasmic processes of the type I epithelial cells are extremely sensitive to damage by various injurious agents. Together with the capillary endothelium these cells represent the component of the lung most vulnerable to damage (see Ch. 4).

Type II alveolar epithelial cells

These cells are taller and twice as numerous as the type I cells but they cover only 7% of the alveolar surface.[120] They usually occupy the corners of alveoli and often all but the apex of the cell is covered by neighbouring type I cells. The free surface has blunt microvilli and the cytoplasm includes mitochondria, endoplasmic reticulum, Golgi apparatus and characteristic osmiophilic lamellar structures, which represent the secretory vacuoles of pulmonary surfactant (Figs 1.27, 1.28). These appear in fetal life at the time when surfactant can first be identified and an extra-uterine existence first becomes possible. Their role in surfactant secretion has been established by experimental ultrastructural autoradiography, tracing the incorporation of surfactant precursors in a sequential fashion through secretory organelles and into the lamellar structures.[126–129] Cell separation techniques enabling pure type II cell suspensions to be studied *in vitro* support the role of these cells as secretors of surfactant.[130] Lysosomal enzymes identified in the lamellar structures are derived from multivesicular bodies which fuse with them.[131,132] One of these hydrolases, phosphatidic acid phosphatase, controls an essential step in surfactant synthesis.[133] Further vesicles and multivesicular bodies located immediately beneath the cell membrane are concerned in the secretion of certain surfactant-specific proteins, which are described below.[134]

After injury, there are found occasional alveolar epithelial cells that possess features of both type I and type II cells (see Fig. 4.10, p. 135). These are flattened squamoid cells, but they have the surface microvilli and osmiophilic lamellar inclusions of the type found in type II alveolar epithelial cells. Such intermediate cell forms are explained by labelling experiments which indicate that the type II cells are the stem cells from which type I cells differentiate.[135,136] The type II cell is therefore not only

the source of surfactant but the progenitor cell from which the alveolar wall is relined after injury to the more delicate type I cell. With chronic damage, type II cells multiply, but do not differentiate and the alveolar wall becomes lined by a cuboidal epithelium recognisable with the light microscope (see Fig. 4.8, p. 134). Animal studies have shown that in the normal lung the turnover time of type II cells is 25 days and transformation of type II to type I cells takes two days.[136] In the developing lung a similar mechanism operates: undifferentiated cells rich in glycogen first differentiate into type II cells and these then transform into type I cells.[137]

Pulmonary surfactant[138–140]

The tendency of the lung to contract is due partly to its elastic framework but largely to the surface tension at the alveolar air–liquid interface. Pattle reasoned from Laplace's law that if the alveolar lining film had the surface tension of serum, the small radius of the alveolus would mean that the power required to expand the newborn's lungs would far exceed the force of even an adult's respiratory muscles and concluded that the surface tension in the alveoli must be considerably less than that of an aqueous film. He went on to squeeze the fluid from mature and immature animal lungs and noted that whereas the bubbles in the foam derived from mature animals were stable, those from fetal lungs lacked stability. This led to a series of experiments, from which it is now known that an extracellular layer that has the surface-tension-reducing properties necessary to permit expansion of the lung covers the alveolar epithelium and lines the alveolus.[141] In immersion fixed tissue, surfactant is represented by irregular fragments of osmiophilic material

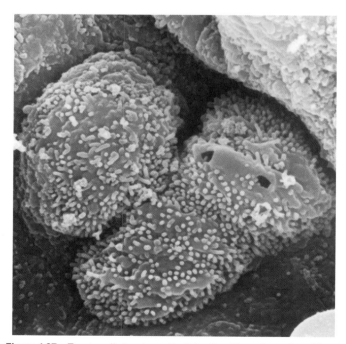

Figure 1.27 Two type II alveolar epithelial cells with surface microvilli and two surface pits through which surfactant has been secreted from vacuoles within the cytoplasm. (Scanning electron micrograph provided by Dr JHL Watson, Detroit, USA.)

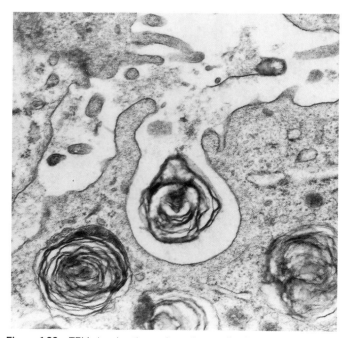

Figure 1.28 TEM showing the surface of a type II cell showing microvilli and a surfactant-secreting vacuole discharging its lamellar body.

apparently floating free in the alveolar lumen but perfusion fixation shows that it is smooth and continuous.[142] The lining is relatively thick in the corners of the alveoli and thin over the lateral extensions of the type I cells. It is biphasic and consists of an aqueous hypophase and a thin surface layer of osmiophilic lattice-work material derived from the lamellar inclusions of type II cells via intermediate tubular myelin (Fig. 1.29).

The biophysical properties of the lining layer are largely due to a series of phospholipids that are notable for their high content of saturated fatty acids, in particular palmitic acid (Box 1.1). Dipalmitoyl-phosphatidylcholine is the surfactant component, which is predominantly responsible for the reduction of alveolar surface tension. It includes a small fraction of surfactant-specific proteins, upon which the surface activity is also dependent;[143] some of them also promote phagocytosis and are thus important in lung defence (Table 1.3).[144,145] These proteins (surfactant apoproteins A–D)[51] also play a role in some congenital disorders through gene mutations and subsequent deficiencies. The lining layer also contains antioxidants that are probably important in protecting the lung against inhaled pollutants.[146]

Some spent surfactant is removed by alveolar macrophages,[147] but most is taken up again by type II cells to be first degraded and then re-used in surfactant synthesis.[148–151]

Alveolar interstitium

The interstitium of the lung is its connective tissue framework. It is abundant around the airways and arteries in the centres of the lobules and around the veins at their periphery where it forms the interlobular septa. At the alveolar level these two main connective tissue locations are connected by fine ramifications that make up the alveolar interstitium. On the thin side of the air/blood barrier, this consists of only the fused epithelial and endothelial basement membranes whereas on the thick side it also comprises all the intervening elements – collagen and elastin fibres, fibroblasts, myofibroblasts, pericytes, histiocytes, mast cells and scanty nerves and nerve terminals (Fig. 1.26).

The myofibroblasts are notable, in that their myofibrils are oriented perpendicular to the plane of the alveolar wall and are attached to dense insertion points on the epithelial or endothelial cell membrane.[152] The myofibroblasts therefore span the interstitium and appear to restrict its compliance. It is also suggested that they control perfusion of the alveoli and counteract

Table 1.3	Surfactant-specific proteins		
	Molecular weight (kDa)	Surface activity	Main functions
A	26–38	None	Promotes phagocytosis Regulates surfactant secretion
B	9	High	Optimises surface activity
C	4	Very high	Optimises surface activity
D	43	None	Promotes phagocytosis Regulates surfactant secretion

Surfactant apoproteins A and D are hydrophilic and act as opsonins. They also promote the unwinding of the lamellar bodies and are thereby involved indirectly in lowering alveolar surface activity, which in conjunction with surfactant phospholipids is the prime function of the hydrophobic apoproteins B and C.

Box 1.1 Surfactant composition	
• Saturated phosphatidylcholine	50%
• Unsaturated phosphatidylcholine	17%
• Phosphatidylglycerol	7%
• Phosphatidylethanolamine	4%
• Phosphatidylinositol	2%
• Sphingomyelin	2%
• Other phospholipids	3%
• Other lipids	5%
• Serum proteins	8%
• Surfactant-specific proteins	2%

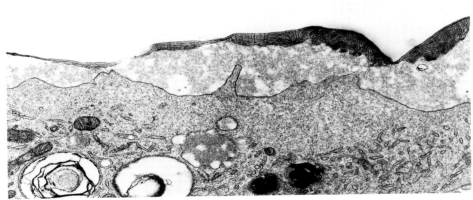

Figure 1.29   Alveolar epithelium covered by a biphasic lining layer. The osmiophilic lattice-work material represents surfactant resting on an aqueous hypophase. (Transmission electron micrograph provided by Mrs D Bowes, Midhurst, UK.)

capillary distending pressure.[153,154] Pericytes are sparse but also appear to control perfusion for they too contain myofilaments and are closely applied to capillaries. They also show many pinocytotic vesicles and have long processes that are intimately related to the basement membranes.[155]

Further interstitial cells include mast cells, which are considered later (see p. 28) and a form of histiocyte intermediate between blood monocytes and alveolar macrophages.[156–159] The lymphoid elements of the lung, including Langerhans and dendritic reticular cells, are dealt with separately (see p. 27).

Lymphatics are not found in alveolar walls. From the alveoli, interstitial fluid drains to the more abundant connective tissue in the two main connective tissue locations mentioned above, which is where the lymphatics commence (see below).

Alveolar macrophages

These cells are the lung's principal means of ridding the alveoli of inhaled exogenous particles and endogenous detritus. Increased numbers are found in smokers[160] and those exposed to dust and as a non-specific reaction accompanying many lung diseases.

The ultimate source of alveolar macrophages is the bone marrow but the immediate origin is the population of pulmonary interstitial cells referred to above.[156,161,162] In disease states marked by an increase in alveolar macrophages, poorly differentiated interstitial cells are increased in number and are occasionally seen breaking through the alveolar epithelium, or interposed between the alveolar epithelium and its basement membrane.[163] Kinetic studies show that most monocytes destined to become alveolar macrophages pass quickly into the alveoli but that a minority first divide in the interstitium.[156,161,164] Maturation of monocytes into macrophages involves cytoplasmic enlargement, loss of myeloperoxidase and the development of lysosomes more characteristic of mature macrophages. When demand is brisk many immature macrophages with scanty lysosomes are found in the alveolar lumen.[165] Mitoses are occasionally observed amongst macrophages free in the alveolar space[166] and there is evidence that proliferation in this site is the main mechanism by which alveolar macrophage numbers are maintained.[167] The number of alveolar macrophages may therefore increase by both enhanced migration from the interstitium and division of cells which have already gained the alveolar lumen. Phagocytes lining the hepatic sinusoids may enter the circulation and utilise this transpulmonary route as an excretory mechanism.[168] Phenotypically distinct subsets of alveolar macrophages reflecting the functional maturity of the cells can be recognised with appropriate antibodies and separated by density-gradient centrifugation.[169–171]

The normal sojourn of macrophages in the alveolus is 7 days,[164] the vast majority being drawn to the terminal bronchiole along with the alveolar lining film and hence to the pharynx to be swallowed or expectorated. Up to five million macrophages leave the lungs by this route every hour.[172] Respiratory movements appear to promote the movement of alveolar macrophages, for these cells tend to accumulate in alveoli bordering the relatively fixed bronchovascular structures at the centres of the lung acini.[6] Re-entry of macrophages into the interstitium takes place principally at this site.[173,174] It is estimated that 8700 alveolar macrophages reach the hilar lymph nodes daily in the normal guinea pig.[175] This interstitial translocation of macrophages is thought to be critical to antigen presentation and the induction of lung immunity.[174] It is also important in the development of dust-induced lung disease.

Although of similar origin to macrophages in other sites, the alveolar macrophage differs from the peritoneal macrophage in having an aerobic rather than anaerobic metabolism.[176] Nonspecific esterase is an ectoenzyme prominent on the surface of alveolar macrophages and in this position may be important in controlling the behaviour of these cells in relation to others or in the response of the macrophage to factors released by other cells, such as lymphokines.[177] Lymphokines to which the alveolar macrophage responds include a macrophage fusion factor which induces the formation of multinucleate giant cells[178] and macrophage aggregation, migration and inhibition factors.[179] Alveolar macrophages or their immediate precursors in the interstitial tissues interact with pulmonary lymphocytes in a reciprocal manner. As well as responding to lymphokines released by antigen-stimulated T lymphocytes, they are important in presenting antigen to lymphocytes and are aided in this by the presence of immunoglobulin and complement receptors on their surface.[177] Furthermore, alveolar macrophages appear to modulate the expression of immune reactions in the lung for in differing circumstances they appear to either enhance or suppress the proliferation, differentiation and function of antigen-stimulated lymphocytes.[180]

The alveolar macrophages are normally situated within the alveolar lining film, but are floated off into the alveolar lumen during immersion fixation. They are irregular in outline and have prominent pseudopodial cytoplasmic extensions (Fig. 1.30). The cytoplasm contains many dense bodies rich in lysosomal enzymes (Fig. 1.31).[131,132] Phagosomal vacuoles and multiloculated phagolysosomes are also numerous.

The alveolar macrophage is avidly phagocytic[124,125,181] (Fig. 1.32) and represents an important defence mechanism against inhaled bacteria. It also provides the major means of clearing the alveolus of inhaled dust. In smokers, the phagolysosomal inclusions are more plentiful and pleomorphic and contain characteristic 'tar bodies' or minute kaolinite crystals (Fig. 1.33).[182] Lung lining material is a chemotactant for alveolar macrophages[183] and the phagocytic action of alveolar macrophages is potentiated by the surfactant-associated proteins SP-A and SP-D.[144,184] Conversely, alveolar macrophages provide one means of removing spent surfactant.[147]

Phagocytosis involves a process of membrane fusion concerning first the cell membrane and then those of the phagosome and lysosomes. In addition to acid hydrolases, alveolar macrophages contain catalase and a peroxidase distinct from myeloperoxidase, but which in the presence of iodide and peroxide has similar antibacterial properties.[185,186] Superoxide production by alveolar macrophages is characterised by a burst in oxygen consumption and glycogenolysis that is stimulated by

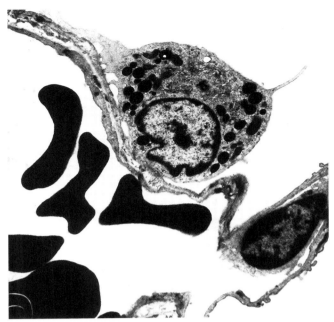

Figure 1.30 An alveolar macrophage with prominent lysosomal dense bodies and pseudopodia is seen close to the alveolar wall. (Transmission electron micrograph provided by Professor PK Jeffery, Brompton, UK.)

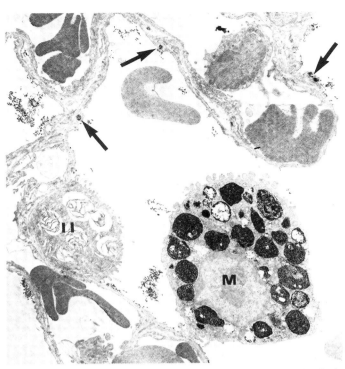

Figure 1.32 Unstained electron micrograph of rat lung injected with finely divided electron dense tracer particles via the trachea. Numerous large phagosomes are evident in an alveolar macrophage (M) but are scanty and minute in the alveolar epithelium (arrows). II, type II pneumocyte. (Reproduced with permission from Corrin B. Phagocytic potential of pulmonary alveolar epithelium with particular reference to surfactant metabolism. Thorax 1970; 25:110–115.[124] With permission from the British Medical Association.)

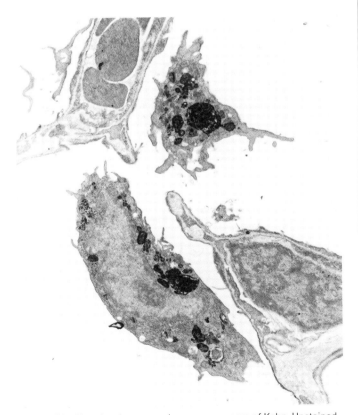

Figure 1.31 Two alveolar macrophages near a pore of Kohn. Unstained electron micrograph to show the electron-dense reaction product of lysosomal acid phosphatase, thus confirming the lysosomal nature of the cytoplasmic dense bodies. (Reproduced with permission from Corrin *et al.* Ultrastructural localisation of acid phosphatase in the rat lung. Journal of Anatomy 1969; 104:65–70.[132] With permission from Blackwell Publishing Ltd.)

the phagocytosis of a variety of inhaled pollutants.[187] Another powerful antibacterial agent formed in macrophages and other phagocytic cells, is nitric oxide.[188–190] The antibacterial activity of alveolar macrophages is depressed by hypoxia, hyperoxia, cold, alcohol, cigarette smoke, metabolic acidosis and viral infections[191–196] and is defective in chronic granulomatous disease (see p. 485). Bacteria killed within macrophages are digested by the action of lysosomal acid hydrolases.

Although primarily concerned with intracellular digestion, lysosomal enzymes are known to be released during phagocytosis. This was initially thought to represent inadvertent leakage due to premature membrane fusion, but it is now appreciated that macrophages actively secrete certain substances and the release of acid hydrolases during phagocytosis may not be fortuitous.[197,198] Indeed, the bulk of the lysozyme within macrophages appears to be destined for secretion outside the cell rather than intracellular digestion; its secretion is independent of phagocytic activity. Other antimicrobial factors secreted by macrophages include interferon. The excessive release of reactive oxygen metabolites, nitric oxide and lysosomal enzymes from macrophages may have deleterious results, possibly contributing to lung injury in processes such as septic shock (see p. 139). Macrophages can also be an abundant source of matrix metalloproteinases such as collagenase, gelatinase and elastase, the release of which is implicated in the development of emphysema.[199,200]

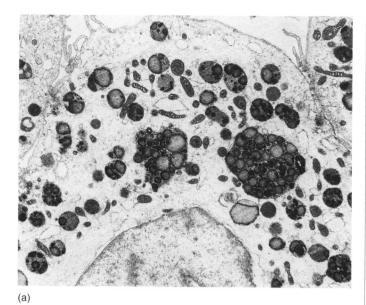

(a)

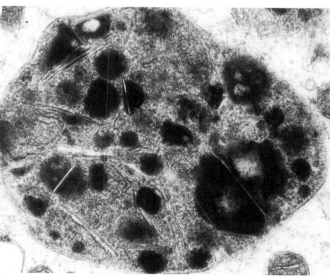

(b)

Figure 1.33 Macrophages from a cigarette smoker. The lysosomal dense bodies are increased in number and contain (a) lipidic 'tar bodies' or (b) the needle-shaped crystals of kaolinite. (Transmission electron micrographs provided by Miss A Dewar, Brompton, UK.)

Other macrophage factors of interest are those influencing the activity of other host cells and the identification of a fibroblast-stimulating substance is clearly relevant to fibrotic lung disease.[201–204] Transformation of macrophages into epithelioid and multinucleated giant cells is particularly associated with the development of organelles more associated with secretory than phagocytic cells, e.g. Golgi apparatus and vesicles (see Fig. 6.1.32, p. 289). This is associated with the secretion of an array of cytokines (see p. 288).

BLOOD SUPPLY OF THE LUNGS

The pulmonary vasculature is unique in that it receives the whole of the cardiac output, but it perfuses rather than nourishes the lungs, this latter function being undertaken by the bronchial vasculature. The pulmonary circulation is a low-pressure system. At rest a mean pressure of only 10 mmHg is sufficient to distribute the cardiac output through the lungs. This barely counteracts gravity and in the upright position, blood flow through the apices of the lungs is minimal at rest. Cardiac output may double without any increase in pulmonary artery pressure because closed capillaries in the underperfused upper zones of the lungs are first recruited. Thus there is considerable reserve in the pulmonary vascular bed and many vessels may be lost in disease or surgically without incurring a significant rise in pulmonary vascular resistance. The full extent of the pulmonary arterial system is shown in Figure 1.34.

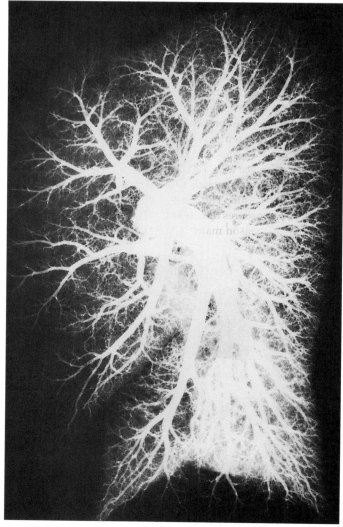

Figure 1.34 A pulmonary arteriogram produced by injecting the arteries of an excised lung with a molten barium-gelatine mixture.

Pulmonary arteries

The anatomy of the main pulmonary arteries and the relationship of their branches to the airways have been described above (see p. 1). The major pulmonary arteries are elastic vessels and at birth the pattern of their elastic laminae closely resembles that of the aorta. Within the first few months of life there is fragmentation of the elastic fibres and an irreversible 'adult pattern' is reached by about the age of 6 months (see Fig. 8.2.9, p. 423).

There is a sharp transition from elastic to muscular pulmonary arteries at a level of the bronchovascular tree where bronchi give way to bronchioles (such airways having a diameter close to 1 mm and the accompanying arteries being of similar or slightly smaller size). Muscular pulmonary arteries have well defined internal and external elastic laminae enclosing their muscular media. The whole wall is very thin compared with systemic arteries of comparable diameter, reflecting the different pressures in the two circulations. In normal uninjected lungs, the medial thickness of muscular pulmonary arteries is about 5% of the external diameter compared with 15–20% in systemic arteries.[205] Injection of the pulmonary arteries with fixative or contrast medium yields lower values. Despite blood flow being greater in the base of the lung than the apex, there is normally no quantitative difference in pulmonary artery structure between these zones (although such differences develop when venous pressure is raised).

The muscle of the media thins progressively as the arteries narrow with repeated branching and in vessels between 100 and 30 μm diameter, is represented only by a spiral, so that in cross section arteries of this size are only muscularised for part of their circumference (Fig. 1.35). Below 30 μm diameter, precapillary vessels have no muscle in their walls, which consist only of fibroelastic tissue. The existence of partially muscularised blood vessels obscures the distinction between arteries and arterioles. For this reason many workers prefer to call all precapillary vessels arteries.

The pulmonary artery endothelium has many fine cytoplasmic projections which increase the surface area considerably.[206] Myofilaments are found in the endothelium of pulmonary arteries and precapillaries, but not capillaries.[207] Distinctive inclusions first found in the endothelium of pulmonary arteries have subsequently been identified in systemic arteries and are occasionally also observed in alveolar capillaries. They consist of parallel microtubules forming rod-shaped membrane-bound granules up to 3 μm in length and are frequently termed Weibel-Palade bodies after those who first described them.[208] Their function is uncertain but it has been shown that they contain von Willebrand protein.[209]

Ventilation perfusion matching

The muscular pulmonary arteries are unique in contracting in response to hypoxia and an important consequence of defective ventilation of the lung is that it induces a corresponding fall in pulmonary perfusion. This mechanism operates at the local level. There is a remarkably fine local matching of pulmonary perfusion to ventilation, brought about by vasoconstriction in poorly ventilated areas.[210,211] It is important that such a mechanism should operate, for blood leaving the lungs is normally fully saturated with oxygen and if poorly ventilated lung tissue were perfused, hypoxaemia would inevitably result (Fig. 1.36).

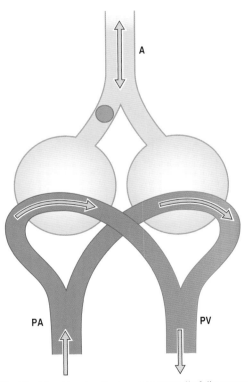

Figure 1.36   The blood leaving the lungs is normally fully oxygenated and perfusion of any poorly ventilated areas (as on the left) would inevitably result in hypoxaemia. This is prevented by matching perfusion to ventilation through arteriolar constriction at the local level, which is probably mediated by reduced nitric oxide release from the endothelium in response to low oxygen tension. A, airway; PA, pulmonary artery; PV, pulmonary vein.

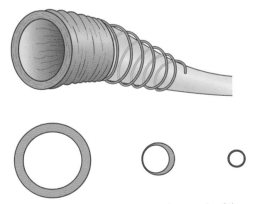

Figure 1.35   As pulmonary arteries narrow, the muscle of the media thins progressively and in vessels between 100 and 30 μm diameter it is represented only by a spiral, so that in cross section, arteries of this size are only muscularised for part of their circumference. Below 30 μm diameter, precapillary vessels have no muscle at all in their walls, which consist only of fibroelastic tissue.

Local perfusion/ventilation matching minimises the danger of hypoxaemia. This is an important adaptive mechanism and beneficial when there is focal ventilatory impairment, as with an inhaled foreign body, but if airflow limitation is generalised, as in chronic bronchitis and emphysema, there is widespread pulmonary vasoconstriction, which causes right-heart strain and eventual failure. The immediate cause of the pulmonary vasoconstriction is low oxygen tension in the inspired air but how this operates has been the subject of much debate. The rise in pulmonary vascular resistance is virtually unaffected by vagotomy, indicating that it is a local response. Mechanisms that have been suggested include a local axon reflex, paracrine activity by neuroendocrine cells in the airway mucosa (see p. 12) and a direct vascular response to the low oxygen tension.[212] The last of these mechanisms has most support; arterial endothelia synthesise and secrete various vasoactive substances, notably the vasoconstrictor, endothelin,[213] and the relaxing factor, nitric oxide. In the lungs hypoxia has the effect of increasing the release of endothelin and inhibiting the release of nitric oxide.[214] The resultant vasoconstriction is most profound in small muscular pulmonary arteries of about 30–50 μm diameter.[210,211] Generalised pulmonary vasoconstriction imposes a considerable burden on the right side of the heart, which counters by releasing atrial natriuretic factor. This decreases pulmonary vasoconstriction, as well as opposing the action of renin and aldosterone on the kidney and promoting diuresis.[215]

Alveolar capillaries

The alveolar capillaries form a tightly matted network of short intersecting tubules (Fig. 1.37),[216] rather than sheet-like vascular spaces intersected by pillars of connective tissue, as previously supposed.[217] There are about 1000 such capillary segments per alveolus[218] and a blood cell passing through the lungs would have to traverse about 60.[219] The capillary wall consists merely of endothelium of the usual continuous type and a basement membrane (see Figs 1.24, 1.25).

Pinocytotic vesicles are numerous in the endothelial cells. They open as caveolae onto both the luminal and interstitial aspects, but are more noticeable on the former where many of them have a special structure, being 'sealed' by a thin single membrane or diaphragm (Fig. 1.38). Where the caveolar membrane, diaphragm and cell membrane fuse, dense knobs are found, possibly representing a ring structure that may maintain the patency of the stoma and the integrity of the diaphragm. Nucleotide-splitting enzymes thought to minimise the risk of thrombosis have been localised within these caveolae.[220]

The capillary diameter is about 5 μm, less than that of the blood cells, but erythrocytes at least are fairly deformable. White blood cells are less deformable and transit of these cells through the alveolar capillaries is slower than that of erythrocytes.[221] This delay is increased in pulmonary inflammation. The alveolar capillaries are the vessels involved in neutrophil sequestration and migration,[222] in contrast to the systemic circulation where these processes take place in venules.

The endothelial cell is similar to the type I epithelial cell in thickness (Fig. 1.23) but covers only one-third of the area, and the alveolar wall contains many more endothelial than type I epithelial cells.[120] In contrast to the alveolar epithelium, the endothelial cell junctions readily permit the passage of small molecular weight proteins.[223] The basement membrane offers no barrier to fluid transport. Larger molecules such as albumin are retained by the intercellular junctions but small amounts of albumin cross the endothelium to reach the interstitium by pinocytotic transport.[224] Alveolar capillaries are attended by pericytes, elongated contractile cells rich in cytoplasmic filaments and which are ensheathed by the endothelial basement membrane.[155] The role of pericytes and myofibroblasts in controlling perfusion is discussed above (see p. 17, 'alveolar interstitium').

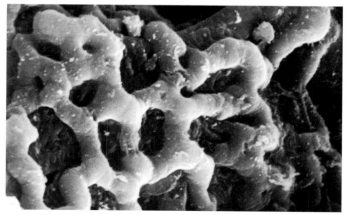

Figure 1.37 The alveolar capillaries (which are unduly prominent in this congested lung) form many short, interconnecting segments. (Scanning electron micrograph provided by Professor PK Jeffery, Brompton, UK.)

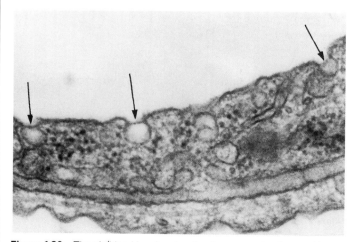

Figure 1.38 The air/blood barrier showing three caveolae (arrows) in the surface of the capillary endothelium, each sealed by a thin single membrane. (Transmission electron micrograph provided by Mrs D Bowes, Midhurst, UK.)

Pulmonary veins

The walls of pulmonary veins consist largely of multiple irregular elastic laminae and collagen with little intervening muscle. However, with increased venous pressure, veins may acquire a muscular media and become 'arterialised' (see Fig. 8.2.13, p. 429). In disease states therefore, the structure of the vessel wall is not a wholly reliable criterion in distinguishing veins from arteries. More valuable is an assessment of the location of the vessel, remembering that pulmonary veins are found at the periphery of the lung lobule and in the interlobular septa (Figs 1.4, 1.5 and 1.9). Intralobular veins less than 30 μm in diameter are identical in structure to arteries of comparable size and are distinguishable from them only by their connections to larger veins. Pulmonary veins are not valved, but sphincters have been described in the pulmonary veins of rats.[225]

Sometimes small cellular collections are observed adjacent to the pulmonary veins. They have been likened to chemoreceptor tissue but ultrastructural studies show that they have a remarkable resemblance to meningeal arachnoid cells. Some authors refer to them as arachnoid nodules and suggest that like those in the meninges that transfer interstitial fluid to the dural veins, those in the lungs may transfer interstitial lung fluid to the pulmonary veins and so minimise the danger of pulmonary oedema.[226] These structures are described more fully in the section dealing with lung tumours (see p. 688).

At the hila, the intrapulmonary veins have joined to form four main veins that drain into the left atria, two from the upper and middle lobes and two from the lower lobes.

Metabolic functions of the pulmonary endothelium

It is now recognised that many serum factors, including certain drugs and hormones, are modified as they pass through the lung and that the pulmonary endothelium is not just a smooth inert vascular lining. Some substances are merely bound to the endothelium and may be dislodged by others. For example, imipramine is a drug for which the lung has a high affinity, but no metabolic capability, and further infusions of imipramine or chlorpromazine will displace imipramine previously accumulated in the lung.[227] Other substances are taken up by the endothelium and actively metabolised, either on the surface or within the cytoplasm of the endothelial cell, resulting in the serum factor being either activated or inactivated. For example, angiotensin is activated and bradykinin inactivated by an enzyme, dipeptidyl carboxypeptidase, also known as angiotensin converting enzyme (ACE), that is distributed uniformly along the endothelial cell surface.[220] Substances taken up and metabolised within the endothelial cells include 5-hydroxytryptamine (by monoamine oxidase), noradrenaline (by catechol-o-methyl transferase) and prostaglandins of the E and F series (by 14-hydroxyprostaglandin dehydrogenase). 5-hydroxytryptamine is taken up by endothelial cells throughout the pulmonary circulation, whereas noradrenaline is preferentially taken up by small pre- and post-capillary vessels and by veins.[228,229] Some substances that the endothelium is capable of metabolising pass through the pulmonary circulation unchanged because there is no uptake mechanism. For example, despite the presence within the pulmonary endothelial cells of peptidases capable of splitting oxytocin, vasopressin and substance P, these substances are unchanged on passage through the pulmonary circulation because there is no uptake. Similarly histamine and prostaglandin A pass through the lung unchanged despite the presence of intracellular imidazole-N-methyl transferase and 14-hydroxyprostaglandin dehydrogenase, again because of the low affinity the lung has for these substances.[230]

Prostacyclin synthetase is found particularly in relation to the arterial intima.[231] Prostacyclin is spontaneously released from the lungs and it has been proposed that this represents active secretion by the endothelium.[232] Prostacyclin is vasodilatory and, in regard to platelets, anti-aggregatory: in particular, prostacyclin is antagonistic to thromboxane, the platelet-aggregating factor released from platelets themselves. Prostacyclin therefore plays an important role in minimising pulmonary thrombosis. Nucleotidases found in the endothelial caveolae described above are also thought to minimise the risk of thrombosis. However, thrombogenic factors are also found in the endothelium: for example, von Willebrand protein has been localised to Weibel–Palade bodies, which are widely distributed in vascular endothelium,[209] and factor VIII-related antigen is strongly represented in pulmonary endothelium.

The endothelium lining pulmonary arteries and to a lesser extent pulmonary veins, also secretes potent vasoactive substances outwards, that is, away from the lumen towards the smooth muscle in the medial coat of the vessel. Two substances are of note here, endothelin,[213,233] which is a particularly powerful vasoconstrictor and nitric oxide,[188,189,234] which was known as endothelium-derived relaxing factor before its simple chemical structure was appreciated. Enhanced nitric oxide activity is thought to contribute to the normal decline in pulmonary vascular resistance at birth. Neither of these vasoactive factors is unique to the pulmonary circulation, being formed in endothelia throughout the body. Indeed, neither is confined to blood vessels and both function quite differently in other tissues. In the lung, endothelin is also formed in airway epithelium[107,213] and when administered via the airways has a strong bronchoconstrictor effect. Nitric oxide, which is cytotoxic and has only a very short tissue half-life, is an important neurotransmitter and, in phagocytes, an effective bactericidal agent. In blood vessels, endothelin and nitric oxide have opposing actions and normal vascular tone depends upon them balancing one another. This equilibrium is disturbed in diseases such as pulmonary hypertension, where there is evidence of excess endothelin activity,[235] and in septic shock, where excess nitric oxide is released from activated neutrophils and macrophages.[190]

The alveolar capillary endothelium also shares antigens with a macrophage subset capable of presenting antigens to lymphocytes, suggesting that it may play a role in the immunological response of the lung.[236]

Megakaryocytes in the pulmonary circulation: the lung as a source of platelets

Megakaryocytes are produced in the bone marrow and some at least are evidently released intact for they are relatively abundant in mixed venous blood. The dimensions of megakaryocytes and pulmonary capillaries are such that any megakaryocytes arriving in the lungs would be held there. Occasional megakaryocytes are indeed seen in normal lung, trapped in alveolar capillaries.[237–239] They generally appear as irregular haematoxyphil clumps representing only the condensed nuclei of these platelet precursor cells.[239,240] They are devoid of cytoplasm and have evidently discharged their platelets. The fact that platelets are more numerous in arterial than mixed venous blood whereas the converse applies for megakaryocytes suggests that many platelets are first released from megakaryocytes trapped in the lungs,[241–247] but this does not mean that the lungs are the principal site of platelet production.[239] Megakaryocytes are particularly easy to find in pulmonary capillaries when there is an increased demand for platelets, as in conditions such as shock and carcinomatosis which lead to increased platelet consumption (see Fig. 4.21b, p. 141).[239,248,249]

Bronchial vasculature

Bronchial arteries

The bronchial arteries supply oxygenated blood to the walls of the airways, the interlobular septa and the visceral pleura. There is usually one bronchial artery on the right, which arises from the third posterior intercostal artery or from the upper left bronchial artery. The left bronchial arteries usually number two and arise from the descending thoracic aorta inferior to the origin of the third posterior intercostal artery. However, bronchial arteries may arise from the thyrocervical trunk, an internal mammary artery, the costocervical trunk, a subclavian artery, a lower intercostal artery, an inferior phrenic artery or even the abdominal aorta. They anastomose with tracheal arteries derived from the inferior thyroid artery. Bronchopulmonary anastomoses are considered below.

Within the lung, bronchial arteries are best seen at the level of the larger bronchi where the pulmonary arteries are still of the elastic type, which contrasts sharply with the muscular structure of the bronchial arteries. Bronchial arteries have a thicker medial coat than pulmonary arteries, commensurate with the higher pressure they have to withstand. They also lack an outer elastic membrane, having only a single internal elastic lamina (Fig. 1.39). Bronchial arteries also lie within the wall of the bronchi whereas pulmonary blood vessels lie alongside.

Small peripheral bronchial arteries sometimes exhibit longitudinal bundles of smooth muscle. These develop both within and outwith the elastic lamina and on occasion are so well developed that they seriously compromise or even completely obliterate the lumen (Fig. 1.40). Such 'Sperrarterien' (the German word Sperr meaning dam or valve) are generally thought to represent sphincters controlling the flow through

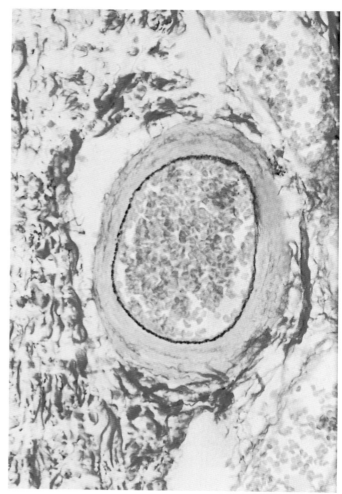

Figure 1.39   A bronchial artery, which lacks an external elastic lamina and, in comparison to pulmonary arteries, has a thick medial coat. (Elastin van Gieson stain).

arteriovenous or bronchopulmonary anastomoses (see below).[250] It is postulated that the longitudinal muscle hypertrophy is a response to intermittent stretching,[250] but this is disputed.[251]

Normally the bronchial arteries are inconspicuous but the bronchial circulation is greatly expanded in many pathological conditions: lesions as diverse as bronchiectasis and carcinoma are largely supplied by bronchial arteries.[252–255] The bronchial circulation can also make an important contribution to gas exchange in conditions where the pulmonary blood supply is reduced, as in certain forms of congenital heart disease and thromboembolic lung disease.

Bronchial capillaries

Bronchial capillaries form a profuse subepithelial network, the extent of which reflects the high metabolic rate of an epithelium involved in warming the inspired air, ion exchange and ciliary activity. The subepithelial capillaries are connected to a deeper system of muscularised sinusoidal vessels which are distensible and so influence bronchial wall thickness, thus narrowing

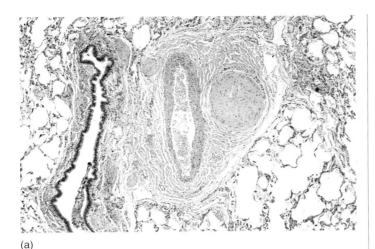

(a)

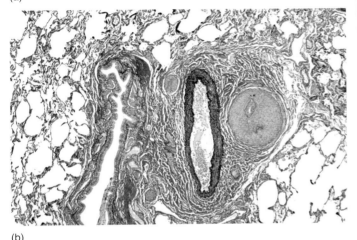

(b)

Figure 1.40 A 'Sperrarterie'. These vascular structures, believed to represent valvular arteriovenous or bronchopulmonary anastomoses, are often markedly narrowed by bundles of hyperplastic longitudinal muscle. This one lies next to a pulmonary artery (to its right) but they may be found as far out as the pleura. (a) Haematoxlin and eosin (b) Elastin van Gieson stain.

the lumen and promoting heat and water exchange,[256-258] albeit at the expense of ventilation. Bronchial capillaries generally have the usual continuous type of endothelium but a fenestrated type is found in the vicinity of neuroepithelial bodies and submucosal glands, raising the possibility that circulating or endothelial factors may regulate the function of these structures.[259-261] A fenestrated capillary endothelium is also found in many fibrotic disorders of the lung.[259,262]

Bronchial veins

The bronchial veins, usually two on each side, open into the azygos vein on the right and the superior intercostal vein, the superior hemiazygos vein or the innominate vein on the left. They drain only blood supplied to the proximal bronchi, the blood supplied to the distal airways being drained into pulmonary veins via bronchopulmonary anastomoses described below. Thus, part of this systemic blood is destined for the right side of the heart and part for the left.

Glomera (non-chromaffin paraganglia)

Glomera were identified widely distributed throughout an infant's lung in a search of 5250 serial sections, being found particularly at the branching point of pulmonary arteries in close relation to nerves.[263] In fine structure they resembled chemoreceptors and a regulatory role in respiration and pulmonary blood flow was proposed.

Pulmonary arteriovenous shunts

Shunts that bypass the capillary bed have been demonstrated in experimental animals by perfusing glass spheres 20–40 times the diameter of the capillaries.[264] In man, these shunts have been shown to be at the entry to the bronchopulmonary segments, the entry to the acini and within the visceral pleura.[265] They normally conduct little of the pulmonary blood flow but widen when small pulmonary vessels are narrowed.

Bronchopulmonary anastomoses

The bronchial and pulmonary circulations mix through precapillary, capillary and venous bronchopulmonary anastomoses, flow normally being from systemic to pulmonary vessels. At the arterial level mixing is normally very limited but up to two-thirds of the bronchial venous flow escapes the right side of the heart by entering anastomotic channels which connect with the pulmonary veins. By this means, up to 4% of the output of the left ventricle consists of blood from the bronchial circulation.[266] When the bronchial circulation expands, as in a variety of lung diseases (see above), new bronchopulmonary anastomoses are established. Large bronchopulmonary anastomoses bypass stenosed pulmonary valves or arteries in congenital heart disease. Similarly, bronchopulmonary anastomoses develop in diseases characterised by thrombotic occlusion of pulmonary arteries.[267]

At the venous level, pulmonobronchial anastomoses direct oxygenated blood back to the right ventricle in conditions such as mitral stenosis and pulmonary veno-occlusive disease, while there may be increased flow in the reverse direction when precapillary causes of pulmonary hypertension lead to right-sided heart failure and vena caval hypertension: blood from the azygos veins may then flow through the bronchial veins into the pulmonary veins and cause cyanosis.[268]

LYMPHOID TISSUE OF THE LUNGS

This section first describes the lymphatic drainage of the lungs and the three principal locations within the lung in which lymphoid cells are found and then outlines the important features of the lymphoid cells themselves.

Lymphatic drainage of the lungs

Lymphatics are not found in the alveolar walls but commence in the centriacinar region and in the interlobular septa. They accompany the blood vessels to the hilum of the lung, which they also reach by joining a pleural plexus on the outer surface of the lung. Lymph from both lower lobes drains into the infratracheal group of lymph nodes, while the tracheobronchial lymph nodes on each side of the trachea receive lymph from the remaining lobes on the respective sides. The lymph from the left tracheobronchial group of nodes drains into the thoracic duct, while that from the nodes on the right side passes into the right bronchomediastinal trunk. Each of these main channels empties into the subclavian vein on its own side but the lymphatics of the two lungs communicate freely.

Pulmonary lymphatics are wide in relation to their wall thickness and are attached to adjacent connective tissue fibres by special anchoring filaments which hold the lymphatics open when interstitial fluid accumulates, interstitial pressure rises and compression might otherwise be expected.[269] There is considerable reserve in the clearance capability of the pulmonary lymphatics which may increase their load 10-fold when pulmonary oedema threatens.[270] Pulmonary lymphatics are valved structures and, in addition to the above features, their capillaries differ from blood capillaries in that their endothelium has poorly developed junctions. Adjacent endothelial cells often merely overlap and the endothelial basal lamina is discontinuous. Although they are not found at the alveolar level their commencement near the smallest bronchioles means that no part of the lung is removed from a lymphatic vessel by much more than 2 mm.

Intrapulmonary lymph nodes

Encapsulated lymph nodes of classic structure are found within the lungs, mainly related to the bifurcations of large bronchi. They are situated in the peribronchial tissues and do not come into direct contact with respiratory epithelium. Although mainly related to bronchi of the first three or four orders, they may rarely be found in the peripheral lung, even as far out as the pleura (see Fig. 12.4.1, p. 642). Although they are not of direct clinical relevance, they are becoming more important in relation to the differential diagnosis of peripheral nodules, especially in relation to computed tomography (CT) screening for carcinomas.[271,272]

Bronchus-associated lymphoid tissue

Certain lymphoid collections are closely related to the bronchial epithelium and because of their resemblance to Peyer's patches (gut-associated lymphoid tissue or GALT) are termed bronchial mucosa-associated lymphoid tissue (MALT).[273,274] Bronchial MALT is not thought to be a normal constituent of the human bronchial tree but acquired in response to various antigenic stimuli.[275–277] It is better represented in children[278] and in smokers,[277,279] and is prominent in certain inflammatory diseases, such as follicular bronchiectasis (Fig. 1.41). It is also better developed in species such as the rabbit and rat, where again it may undergo hypertrophy when subjected to antigenic stimulation.[275,280–282] Bronchial MALT is found especially at the airway

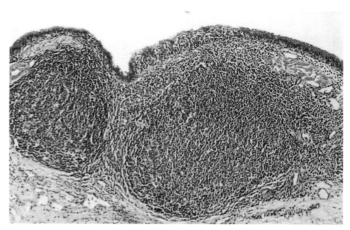

Figure 1.41 A focus of bronchial mucosa-associated lymphoid tissue shows follicular hyperplasia in a case of follicular bronchiectasis. Note how the lymphoid cells infiltrate the overlying epithelium, which at this point is not ciliated.

bifurcations, which is where inhaled antigens are particularly likely to impinge.

In many species, bronchial MALT is formed of follicular lymphoid tissue, which is closely applied to a distinctive overlying 'lymphoepithelium' consisting of flattened non-ciliated epithelial cells known as microfold or 'M cells', intimately involved with which are lymphocytes that form part of the outer mantle or dome region of the underlying lymphoid follicle (Figs 1.41, 1.42). Antigen is taken up by the M cells[282] and passed to follicular dendritic cells (see below) within the bronchial MALT.[283] The germinal centres consist of a mesh of follicular dendritic cells that sustain rapidly dividing B lymphocytes and present them with antigenic information. More than half the lymphocytes of the bronchial MALT are B cells, with IgA being the predominant isotope.[59,284] T-cells comprise about 18% of lymphocytes in bronchial MALT.

In man bronchial MALT is not so well organised or so closely applied to the surface epithelium, being better seen in the outer coat of the bronchus[279] and around the bronchial glands.[277] IgA-secreting plasma cells are concentrated about the serous acini of the bronchial glands[277,284] where the secretory component of IgA is synthesised and incorporated into the IgA dimer as this passes across the epithelium to reach the lumen (Fig. 1.17).[57–59]

After an immune response is induced in the bronchial MALT, lymphocytes enter the blood and travel to mucosal effector sites such as the lamina propria throughout the body where large amounts of IgA are produced.[285] This migratory pathway forms part of a common mucosal immune system in which responses induced in one location can be replicated elsewhere. Similarly, lymphomas arising in one part of this system tend to recur in the mucosae of other organs.

Lymphoreticular aggregates

Lymphoreticular aggregates were described before bronchial MALT and today many would probably be classified as such. However, they are more widely distributed, being found

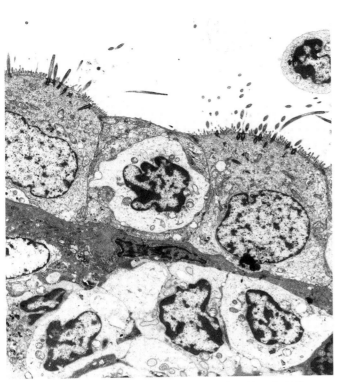

Figure 1.42 The dome region of bronchus-associated lymphoid tissue consisting of a collection of lymphocytes, one of which is located within surface epithelium that at this point is non-ciliated. (Transmission electron micrograph provided by Miss A Dewar, Brompton, UK.)

throughout the lungs, about bronchi and in alveolar tissue, interlobular septa and the pleura. They are particularly noticeable at the centres of the acini, interposed between the terminal or a respiratory bronchiole and its accompanying artery (Fig. 1.21).[286] This is the point at which lymphatics commence and the aggregates are well placed to monitor fluid and cells draining from the alveolar tissue in the interstitial plane. They consist of small collections of lymphocytes with a few plasma cells and eosinophils. Reticulin stains show a delicate connective tissue network but the sinusoidal and nodal architecture of a lymph node is lacking. Dust-laden macrophages accumulate in the lymphoreticular aggregates, leading Macklin to refer to the aggregates as 'dust sumps'.[6] On the cut surface of a city-dweller's or smoker's lung they provide a useful marker of the centres of the lung acini (Fig. 1.6).

Lymphocytes

Lymphocytes of all classes are present in the lung: B and T, T-helper and T-suppressor and T-helper-1 and -2. The functions of B and T cells in humoral and cellular immunity and hypersensitivity are well known, as are the promoter and suppressor/cytotoxic functions of T-helper (CD4) and T-suppressor (CD8) cells. T-helper cells are cytokine secretors whereas T-suppressor cells are mainly cytotoxic killer cells. Their respective roles are dealt with in some detail under various granulomatous diseases, notable tuberculosis (see p. 204) and sarcoidosis (see p. 286). The subsets of T-helper cells (T-helper-1 and -2) determine whether an immune response is directed towards phagocytosis and bacterial elimination or hypersensitivity reactions characterised by eosinophilia. The former is effected by activated T-helper-1 lymphocytes through the elaboration of cytokines such as interleukin-2 and interferon-γ and the latter by elective activation of the T-helper-2 lymphocytes resulting in interleukin 4, 5, 6 and 10 secretion. Interleukin 4 is responsible for plasma cells forming IgE rather than IgG while interleukin 5 is responsible for tissue eosinophilia (see Fig. 3.31, p. 113). Both cell types produce granulocyte-macrophage-colony stimulating factor. Further T-cell subsets identified in the lungs include alpha beta and gamma delta cells, the former thought to be important to immunological memory while the latter contribute to the early immune response.[287]

Dendritic cells

There are two types of dendritic cells, both of which are described in the lungs: follicular dendritic cells, mentioned above as a component of the bronchial MALT and S100-positive interdigitating dendritic cells.[288–294] They are both derived from bone marrow stem cells and reach the lung by the blood stream. Interdigitating dendritic cells are found in T-cell-dependent areas of lymph nodes and are widely distributed in the connective tissue of the lung, being found around and within the walls of bronchi and bronchioles and in alveolar walls, interlobular septa and the pleura. They have long cytoplasmic processes and irregular, convoluted nuclei. In the airways, they form a network at the base of the epithelium that is ideally positioned to sample inhaled antigens. They are not present at birth but develop in the respiratory mucosa after about 1 year of life, probably in response to infection.[295] Both types of dendritic cell function as antigen presenters to T-lymphocytes. They do this by processing the antigen intracellularly into short peptides before presenting it to T-lymphocytes on their surface in association with the HLA-DR histocompatibility complex. Dendritic cells are also activated by endogenous signals such as interferon-α released from virally infected cells and heat-shock proteins released by dying cells.

Langerhans cells[290]

These cells constitute a subpopulation of dendritic cells, from which they are derived by a process of differentiation. They differ from dendritic cells by expressing CD1a and by the presence of certain pentilaminar structures known as Birbeck granules[296] (see Fig. 6.1.36, p. 291), which develop in the cytoplasm during the internalisation of surface-bound antigens. They are essentially cells of the epidermis, but small numbers are found in the bronchial epithelium. Proliferation and differentiation of pulmonary dendritic cells into Langerhans cells is influenced by factors affecting the epithelium: both cell types are increased in smokers, especially where there is epithelial hyperplasia and metaplasia.[297–299] Like dendritic cells, Langerhans cells do not normally enter the air space but up to 5% Langerhans cells can be recovered by lavage from smokers and patients with epithelial hyperplasia. They are referred to again under the disease Langerhans cell histiocytosis (see p. 290).

Mast cells

Mast cells are mainly situated in the subepithelial tissues of the airways,[300–303] but some are found in the surface epithelium[304] and may be recovered by bronchoalveolar lavage. They progressively increase in number distally so that in the small bronchioles, total mast cell numbers are 100- to 150-fold greater than in the trachea. Mast cells make up about 2% of the cross-sectional area of the alveolar walls, with higher values in disease states.[305] Proliferation of mucosal mast cells is thymus dependent. In both normal and fibrotic lung, mast cells show remarkably close apposition to fibroblasts,[306] and there is evidence that they promote fibrosis.[307,308] However, they are best known for their role in type I allergic reactions and are referred to again under asthma (see p. 112).

There are at least two subtypes of mast cell. Those in the surface epithelium are more difficult to stain than mast cells in the underlying connective tissue. They are also smaller and contain heparin and tryptase rather than chymase.[309,310] Various mediators are released when the mast cell degranulates. Preformed mediators include histamine, exoglycosidases, tryptase and eosinophil and neutrophil chemotactic factors. Degranulation also stimulates the generation and release of newly formed mediators, including prostaglandin D2, platelet-activating factor and leukotrienes C4 and D4. Mast cells also produce a variety of cytokines, notably interleukins 1, 2, 3, 4 and 5, granulocyte-macrophage colony-stimulating factor, interferon-γ and tumour necrosis factor-α.[311]

INNERVATION OF THE LUNGS

Several nerve bundles enter the lung at the hilum along with the bronchus. They contain parasympathetic and sympathetic fibres derived respectively from the vagus nerve and cervical ganglia and peptidergic (non-cholinergic, non-adrenergic) fibres.[312–316]

On entering the lung, the nerves divide into peribronchial and perivascular plexuses, the former further ramifying about the cartilage plates and beneath the surface epithelium. Sensory endings include rapidly adapting receptors within the surface epithelium responding to irritants and promoting the cough reflex, those supplying the neuroepithelial chemoreceptors, slowly adapting stretch receptors associated with muscle and thought to be responsible for the Hering-Breuer reflex and juxta-capillary (J-type) receptors in the alveolar walls sensitive to rises in pulmonary venous pressure and possibly interstitial oedema.[65,68,70,71,101,317–319]

Terminals identified by vital staining in the walls of pulmonary veins and bronchial arteries, but not pulmonary arteries, are probably further pressor receptors.[320] Histochemical and ultrastructural studies have shown that the whole pulmonary vasculature is innervated by noradrenergic and cholinergic nerves and that rapid changes take place in these nerves during the postnatal adaptation of the pulmonary circulation.[321]

Motor terminals are also found in bronchial glands, muscle and surface epithelium, while ganglia containing Kultschitsky-like cells in addition to nerve cells and fibres have been identified in the bronchial submucosa.[62] Neurotransmitters include acetylcholine, catecholamines and peptides such as vasoactive intestinal peptide[322] and substance P.[323] Cholinergic innervation appears to be the most important effector drive to bronchial contraction and secretion but may be augmented by the peptide substance P. Inhibition of contraction may be by catecholamines or by peptidergic nerves, particularly those releasing vasoactive intestinal peptide.[324] Cholinergic stimulation also appears to extend to alveolar secretory cells, for bilateral vagotomy in the rat results in atelectasis,[325] while cholinergic drugs increase the production of type II cell lamellar bodies[326] and the secretion of surfactant.[327]

REFERENCES

Anatomy of the lungs and airways

1. Coppoletta JM, Wolbach SB. Body length and normal weights of more important vital organs between birth and twelve years of age. Am J Pathol 1933; 9:55.
2. Thoracic Society. The nomenclature of broncho-pulmonary anatomy. Thorax 1950; 5:222–227.
3. Weibel ER. Morphometry of the human lung. Berlin: Springer, 1963.
4. Haefeli-Bleuer B, Weibel ER. Morphometry of the human pulmonary acinus. Anat Rec 1988; 220:401–414.
5. Dunnill MS. Postnatal growth of the lung. Thorax 1962; 17:329–333.
6. Macklin CS. Pulmonary sumps, dust accumulations, alveolar fluid and lymph vessels. Acta Anat 1955; 23:1–33.
7. Horsfield K. The relation between structure and function in the airways of the lung. Br J Dis Chest 1974; 68:145–160.
8. Hasleton PS. The internal surface of the adult human lung. J Anat 1972; 112:391–399.
9. Lambert MW. Accessory bronchiole-alveolar communications. J Pathol Bacteriol 1955; 70:311–314.
10. Martin HB. Respiratory bronchioles as the pathway for collateral ventilation. J Appl Physiol 1966; 21:1443–1447.
11. Raskin SP, Harman PG. Interacinar pathways in the human lung. Am Rev Respir Dis 1975; 111:489–495.
12. Andersen JB, Jespersen W. Demonstration of intersegmental respiratory bronchioles in normal human lungs. Eur J Respir Dis 1980; 61:337–341.
13. Elliott FM, Reid L. Some new facts about the pulmonary artery and its branching pattern. Clin Radiol 1965; 16:193–198.

Microscopy of the airways

14. Monkhouse WS, Whimster WF. An account of the longitudinal mucosal corrugations of the human tracheo-bronchial tree, with observations on those of some animals. J Anat 1976; 122:681–695.
15. Whimster WF. The microanatomy of the alveolar duct system. Thorax 1970; 25:141–149.

16. Carroll NG, Perry S, Karkhanis A, et al. The airway longitudinal elastic fiber network and mucosal folding in patients with asthma. Am J Respir Crit Care Med 2000; 161:244–248.

17. Breeze RJ, Wheeldon EB. The cells of the pulmonary airways. Am Rev Respir Dis 1977; 116:705–777.

18. Jeffery PK. Morphologic features of airway surface epithelial cells and glands. Am Rev Respir Dis 1983; 128:S14–S20.

19. Jeffery PK. Airway mucosa: secretory cells, mucus and mucin genes. Eur Resp J 1997; 10:1655–1662.

20. Clara M. Zur Histobiologie des Bronchalepithels. Z Forschung 1937; 41:321–347.

21. Rogers AV, Dewar A, Corrin B, Jeffery PK. Identification of serous-like cells in the surface epithelium of human bronchioles. Eur Respir J 1993; 6:498–504.

22. Mercer RR, Russell ML, Roggli VL, Crapo JD. Cell number and distribution in human and rat airways. Am J Respir Cell Mol Biol 1994; 10:613–624.

23. Glanville AR, Tazelaar HD, Theodore J, et al. The distribution of MHC class-I and class-II antigens on bronchial epithelium. Am Rev Respir Dis 1989; 139:330–334.

24. Nakajima M, Kawanami O, Jin E, et al. Immunohistochemical and ultrastructural studies of basal cells, Clara cells and bronchiolar cuboidal cells in normal human airways. Pathol Int 1998; 48:944–953.

25. Clover J, Oates J, Edwards C. Anti-cytokeratin 5/6: A positive marker for epithelioid mesothelioma. Histopathology 1997; 31:140–143.

26. Hulbert WC. Fixation of the respiratory epithelial surface mucus. Lab Invest 1983; 48:650–652.

27. Gil J, Weibel ER. Extracellular lining of bronchioles after perfusion-fixation of rat lungs for electron microscopy. Anat Rec 1971; 169:185–199.

28. Iravani J, van As A. Mucus transport in the tracheobronchial tree of normal and bronchitic rats. J Pathol 1972; 106:81–93.

29. Inoue S, Hogg JC. Intercellular junctions of the tracheal epithelium in guinea pigs. Lab Invest 1974; 31:68–74.

30. Richardson JB, Bouchard T, Ferguson CC. Uptake and transport of exogenous proteins by respiratory epithelium. Lab Invest 1976; 35:307–314.

31. Vai F, Fournier MF, Lafuma JC, Touaty JC, Pariente R. SO$_2$ induced bronchopathy in the rat: abnormal permeability of the bronchial epithelium in vivo after anatomic recovery. Am Rev Respir Dis 1980; 121:851–858.

32. Hulbert WC, Walker DC, Jackson A, Hogg JC. Airway permeability to horseradish peroxidase in guinea pigs: the repair phase after injury by cigarette smoke. Am Rev Respir Dis 1981; 123:320–321.

33. Ayers MM, Jeffery PK. Proliferation and differentiation in mammalian airway epithelium. Eur Respir J 1988; 1:58–80.

34. Otto WR. Lung epithelial stem cells. J Pathol 2002; 197:527–535.

35. Thompson AB, Robbins RA, Romberger DJ, et al. Immunological functions of the pulmonary epithelium. Eur Respir J 1995; 8:127–149.

36. Iravani J, Melville GN. Mucociliary function in the respiratory tract influenced by physicochemical factors. Pharmac Ther 1976; 2:471–492.

37. Sleigh MA. The nature and action of respiratory tract cilia. In: Brain JD, Proctor DF, Reid LM, eds. Respiratory Defense Mechanisms Lung Biology in Health and Disease, Vol. 5 (Part 1). New York: Marcel Dekker; 1977:247–282.

38. Jeffery PK, Reid LM. New observations of rat airway epithelium: a quantitative electron microscopic study. J Anat 1975; 120:295–320.

39. Schlegel R, Banks-Schlegel S, Pinkus GS. Immunohistochemical localization of keratin in normal human tissues. Lab Invest 1980; 42:91–96.

40. Evans MJ, Cabral-Anderson LJ, Freeman G. Role of the Clara cell in renewal of the bronchiolar epithelium. Lab Invest 1978; 38:648–655.

41. Bolduc P, Jones R, Reid L. Mitotic activity of airway epithelium after short exposure to tobacco smoke and the effect of the anti-inflammatory agent phenylmethyloxadiazole. Br J Exp Pathol 1981; 62:461–468.

42. Hong KU, Reynolds SD, Watkins S, Fuchs E, Stripp BR. Basal cells are a multipotent progenitor capable of renewing the bronchial epithelium. Am J Pathol 2004; 164:577–588.

43. Evans MJ, Plopper CG. The role of basal cells in adhesion of columnar epithelium to airway basement membrane. Am Rev Respir Dis 1988; 138:481–483.

44. Evans MJ, Moller PC. Biology of airway basal cells. Exp Lung Res 1991; 17:513–531.

45. Gendler SJ, Spicer AP. Epithelial mucin genes. Annu Rev Physiol 1995; 57:607–634.

46. Sharma P, Dudus L, Nielsen PA, et al. MUC5B and MUC7 are differentially expressed in mucous and serous cells of submucosal glands in human bronchial airways. Am J Respir Cell Mol Biol 1998; 19:30–37.

47. Wickstrom C, Davies JR, Eriksen GV, Veerman EC, Carlstedt I. MUC5B is a major gel-forming, oligomeric mucin from human salivary gland, respiratory tract and endocervix: identification of glycoforms and C-terminal cleavage. Biochem J 1998; 334:685–693.

48. Hovenberg HW, Davies JR, Carlstedt I. Different mucins are produced by the surface epithelium and the submucosa in human trachea: identification of MUC5AC as a major mucin from the goblet cells. Biochem J 1996; 318:319–324.

49. Davies JR, Herrmann A, Russell W, Svitacheva N, Wickstrom C, Carlstedt I. Respiratory tract mucins: structure and expression patterns. Novartis Found Symp 2002; 248:76–88.

50. Groneberg DA, Eynott PR, Oates T, et al. Expression of MUC5AC and MUC5B mucins in normal and cystic fibrosis lung. Respir Med 2002; 96:81–86.

51. Boggaram V. Regulation of lung surfactant protein gene expression. Front Biosci 2003; 8:d751–d764.

52. Spicer SS, Schulte BA, Thomopoulos GN. Histochemical properties of the respiratory tract epithelium in different species. Am Rev Respir Dis 1983; 128:S20–S26.

53. Meyrick B, Sturgess J, Reid L. Reconstruction of the duct system and secretory tubules of the human bronchial submucosal gland. Thorax 1969; 24:729–736.

54. Bowes D, Clark AE, Corrin B. Ultrastructural localisation of lactoferrin and glycoprotein in human bronchial glands. Thorax 1981; 36:108–115.

55. Bowes D, Corrin B. Ultrastructural immunocytochemical localization of lysozyme in human bronchial glands. Thorax 1977; 32:163–170.

56. Kramps JA, Franken C, Meijer CJLM, Dijkman JH. Localization of low molecular weight protease inhibitor in serous secretory cells of the respiratory tract. J Histochem 1981; 29:712–719.

57. Brandtzaeg P. Mucosal and glandular distribution of immunoglobulin components: immunohistochemistry with a cold ethanol-fixation technique. Immunology 1974; 26:1101–1113.

58. Goodman JR, Link DW, Brown WR, Nakane PK. Ultrastructural evidence of transport of secretory IgA across bronchial epithelium. Am Rev Respir Dis 1981; 123:115–119.

59. Pilette C, Ouadrhiri Y, Godding V, Vaerman JP, Sibille Y. Lung mucosal immunity: immunoglobulin-A revisited. Eur Resp J 2001; 18:571–588.

60. Christensen TG, Janeczek AH, Gaensler EA, Hayes JA. Localisation of endogenous peroxidase in human bronchial submucosal glands. Am Rev Respir Dis 1981; 123(supplement):222.

61. Matsuba K, Takizawa T, Thurlbeck W. Oncocytes in human bronchial mucous glands. Thorax 1972; 27:181–184.

62. Bensch KG, Gordon GB, Miller LR. Studies on the bronchial counterpart of the Kultschitsky (argentaffin) cell and the innervation of bronchial glands. J Ultrastruct Res 1965; 12:668–686.

63. Bensch KG, Corrin B, Pariente R, Spencer H. Oat cell carcinoma of the lung: its origin and relationship to bronchial carcinoid. Cancer 1968; 22:1163–1172.

64. Capella C, Hage E, Solcia E, Usellini L. Ultrastructural similarity of endocrine-like cells of the human lung and some related cells of the gut. Cell Tissue Res 1978; 186:25–37.

65. Lauweryns JM, Van Lommel A. The intrapulmonary neuroepithelial bodies after vagotomy: demonstration of their sensory neuroreceptor-like innervation. Experientia 1983; 39:1123–1124.

66. Tateishi R. Distribution of argyrophil cells in adult human lungs. Arch Pathol 1973; 96:198–202.

67. Boers JE, Denbrok JLM, Koudstaal J, Arends JW, Thunnissen FBJM. Number and proliferation of neuroendocrine cells in normal human airway epithelium. Am J Respir Crit Care Med 1996; 154:758–763.

68. Lauweryns JM, Van Lommel A. Ultrastructure of nerve endings and synaptic junctions in rabbit intrapulmonary neuroepithelial bodies: a single and serial section analysis. J Anat 1987; 151:65–83.

69. Van Lommel A, Lauweryns JM, Deleyn P, Wouters P, Schreinemakers H, Lerut T. Pulmonary neuroepithelial bodies in neonatal and adult dogs: histochemistry, ultrastructure and effects of unilateral hilar lung denervation. Lung 1995; 173:13–23.

70. Brouns I, VanGenechten J, Hayashi H, et al. Dual sensory innervation of pulmonary neuroepithelial bodies. Am J Respir Cell Molec Biol 2003; 28:275–285.

71. Larson SD, Schelegle ES, Hyde DM, Plopper CG. The three-dimensional distribution of nerves along the entire intrapulmonary airway tree of the adult rat and the anatomical relationship between nerves and neuroepithelial bodies. Am J Respir Cell Mol Biol 2003; 28:592–599.

72. Cutz E, Chan W, Wong V, Conen PE. Endocrine cells in rat fetal lungs. Ultrastructural and histochemical study. Lab Invest 1974; 30:458–464.

73. Lauweryns JM, Van Ranst L. Immunocytochemical localization of aromatic L-aminoacid decarboxylase in human, rat and mouse bronchopulmonary and gastrointestinal endocrine cells. J Histochem Cytochem 1988; 36:1181–1186.

74. Lauweryns JM, de Bock V, Verhofstad AAJ, Steinbusch HWM. Immunohistochemical localization of serotonin in intrapulmonary neuro-epithelial bodies. Cell Tissue Res 1982; 226:215–223.

75. Wharton J, Polak JM, Cole GA, Marangos PJ, Pearse AGE. Neuro-specific enolase as an immunocytochemical marker for the diffuse neuroendocrine system in human fetal lung. J Histochem Cytochem 1981; 29:1359–1364.

76. Lauweryns JM, Van Ranst L, Lloyd RV, O'Connor DT. Chromogranin in bronchopulmonary neuroendocrine cells. Immunocytochemical detection in human, monkey and pig respiratory mucosa. J Histochem Cytochem 1987; 35:113–118.

77. Lee I, Gould VE, Moll R, Wiedenmann B, Franke WW. Synaptophysin expressed in the bronchopulmonary tract: neuroendocrine cells, neuroepithelial bodies and neuroendocrine neoplasms. Differentiation 1987; 34:115–125.

78. Lantuejoul S, Moro D, Michalides RJAM, Brambilla C, Brambilla E. Neural cell adhesion molecules (NCAM) and NCAM-PSA expression in neuroendocrine lung tumors. Am J Surg Pathol 1998; 22:1267–1276.

79. Wharton J, Polak JM, Bloom SR, et al. Bombesin-like immunoreactivity in the lung. Nature 1978; 273:769–770.

80. Cutz E, Chan W, Track NS. Bombesin, calcitonin and leuenkephalin immunoreactivity in endocrine cells of the human lung. Experientia 1981; 37:765–766.

81. Tsutsumi Y, Osamura Y, Watanabe K, Yanaihara N. Immunohistochemical studies on gastrin-releasing peptide and adrenocorticotropic hormone-containing cells in the human lung. Lab Invest 1983; 48:623–632.

82. Willey JC, Lechner JR, Harris CC. Bombesin and the C-terminal tetradecapeptide of gastrin-releasing peptide are growth factors for normal human bronchial epithelial cells. Exp Cell Res 1984; 153:245–248.

83. Becker KL, Monaghan KG, Silva OL. Immunocytochemical localization of calcitonin in Kulchitsky cells of human lung. Arch Pathol Lab Med 1980; 104:196–198.

84. Tsutsumi Y, Osamura Y, Watanabe K, Yanaihara N. Simultaneous immunohistochemical localization of gastrin-releasing peptide (GPR) and calcitonin (CT) in human bronchial endocrine-type cells. Virchows Arch Pathol Anat Histopathol 1983; 400:163–171.

85. Gallego R, Garciacaballero T, Roson E, Beiras A. Neuroendocrine cells of the human lung express substance-P-like immunoreactivity. Acta Anat 1990; 139:278–282.

86. Kato K, Asano T, Kamiya N, et al. Production of the alpha subunit of guanine nucleotide binding protein Go by neuroendocrine tumors. Cancer Res 1987; 47:5800–5805.

87. Brambilla E, Veale D, Moro D, Morel F, Dubois F, Brambilla C. Neuroendocrine phenotype in lung cancers – comparison of immunohistochemistry with biochemical determination of enolase isoenzymes. Am J Clin Pathol 1992; 98:88–97.

88. Gosney JR, Gosney MA, Lye M, Butt SA. Reliability of commercially available immunocytochemical markers for identification of neuroendocrine differentiation in bronchoscopic biopsies of bronchial carcinoma. Thorax 1995; 50:116–120.

89. Reznik-Schuller H. Sequential morphologic alterations in the bronchial epithelium of Syrian golden hamsters during N-nitrosomorpholine-induced pulmonary tumorigenesis. Am J Pathol 1977; 89:59–66.

90. Reynolds SD, Giangreco A, Power JHT, Stripp BR. Neuroepithelial bodies of pulmonary airways serve as a reservoir of progenitor cells capable of epithelial regeneration. Am J Pathol 2000; 156:269–278.

91. Peake JL, Reynolds SD, Stripp BR, Stephens KE, Pinkerton KE. Alteration of pulmonary neuroendocrine cells during epithelial repair of naphthalene-induced airway injury. Am J Pathol 2000; 156:279–286.

92. Johnson NF, Wagner JC, Wills HA. Endocrine cell proliferation in the rat lung following asbestos exposure. Lung 1980; 158:221–228.

93. Wilson NJE, Gosney JR, Mayall F. Endocrine cells in diffuse pulmonary fibrosis. Thorax 1993; 48:1252–1256.

94. Johnson DE, Lock JE, Elde RP, Thompson TR. Pulmonary neuroendocrine cells in hyaline membrane disease and bronchopulmonary dysplasia. Pediatr Res 1982; 16:446–454.

95. Gosney J, Heath D, Smith P, Harris P, Yacoub M. Pulmonary endocrine cells in pulmonary arterial disease. Arch Pathol Lab Med 1989; 113:337–341.

96. Gould VE, Linnoila RI, Memoli VA, Warren WH. Neuroendocrine cells and neuroendocrine neoplasms of the lung. Pathol Annu 1983; 18:287–330.

97. Lauweryns JM, Cokelaere M. Intrapulmonary neuroepithelial bodies: hypoxia-sensitive neuro (chemo-) receptors. Experientia 1973; 29:1384–1386.

98. Moosavi H, Smith P, Heath D. The Feyrter cell in hypoxia. Thorax 1973; 28:729–741.

99. Taylor W. Pulmonary argyrophil cells at high altitude. J Pathol 1977; 122:137–144.

100. Anand IS. Hypoxia and the pulmonary circulation. Thorax 1994; 49:S19–S24.

101. Lauweryns JM, Van Lommel A. Effect of various vagotomy procedures on the reaction to hypoxia of rabbit neuroepithelial bodies: modulation by intrapulmonary axon reflexes? Exp Lung Res 1986; 11:319–339.

102. Johnston CJ, Mango GW, Finkelstein JN, Stripp BR. Altered pulmonary response to hyperoxia in Clara cell secretory protein deficient mice. Am J Respir Cell Mol Biol 1997; 17:147–155.

103. Boyd MR. Evidence for the Clara cell as a site of cytochrome P450–dependent mixed-function oxidase activity in lung. Nature 1977; 269:713–715.

104. Villaschi S, Giovanetti A, Lombardi CC, Nicolai G, Garbati M, Andreozzi U. Damage and repair of mouse bronchial epithelium following acute inhalation of trichloroethylene. Exp Lung Res 1991; 17:601–614.

105. Woods LW, Wilson DW, Schiedt MJ, Giri N. Structural and biochemical changes in lungs of 3– methylindole- treated rats. Am J Pathol 1993; 142:129–138.

106. Plopper CG, VanWinkle LS, Fanucchi MV, et al. Early events in naphthalene-induced acute Clara cell toxicity - II. Comparison of glutathione depletion and histopathology by airway location. Am J Respir Cell Mol Biol 2001; 24:272–281.

107. Laporte J, Dorleansjuste P, Sirois P. Guinea pig Clara cells secrete endothelin 1 through a phosphoramidon-sensitive pathway. Am J Respir Cell Mol Biol 1996; 14:356–362.

108. Hayashi T, Ishii A, Nakai S, Hasegawa K. Ultrastructure of goblet-cell metaplasia from Clara cell in the allergic asthmatic airway inflammation in a mouse model of asthma in vivo. Virchows Arch 2004; 444; 66–73.

109. Meyrick B, Reid L. The alveolar brush cell in rat lung - a third pneumocyte. J Ultrastruct Res 1968; 23:71–80.

110. Hijiya K, Okada Y, Tankawa H. Ultrastructural study of the alveolar brush cell. J Electron Microsc 1977; 26:321–329.

Microscopy of the alveolar tissue

111. Heard BE, Izukawa T. Pulmonary emphysema in fifty consecutive male necropsies in London. J Pathol Bacteriol 1964; 88:423–431.

112. Oderr C. Architecture of the lung parenchyma. Studies with a specially designed X-ray microscope. Am Rev Respir Dis 1964; 90:401–410.

113. Ochs M, Nyengaard LR, Lung A, et al. The number of alveoli in the human lung. Am J Respir Crit Care Med 2004; 169:120–124.

114. Glazier JB, Hughes JMB, Maloney JE, West JB. Vertical gradient of alveolar size in lungs of dogs frozen intact. J Appl Physiol 1967; 23:694–705.

115. Haber PS, Colebatch HJH, Ng CKY, Greaves IA. Alveolar size as a determinant of pulmonary distensibility in mammalian lungs. J Appl Physiol 1983; 54:837–845.

116. Parra SC, Gaddy LR, Takaro T. Ultrastructural studies of canine interalveolar pores (of Kohn). Lab Invest 1978; 38:8–13.

117. Low FN. The pulmonary alveolar epithelium of laboratory mammals and man. Anat Rec 1953; 117:241–263.

118. Weibel ER, Knight BW. A morphometric study on the thickness of the pulmonary air-blood barrier. J Cell Biol 1964; 21:367–384.

119. Weibel ER. The mystery of 'non-nucleated plates' in the alveolar epithelium of the lung explained. Acta Anat 1971; 78:425–443.

120. Crapo JD, Barry BE, Gehr P, Bachofen M, Weibel ER. Cell characteristics of the normal human lung. Am Rev Respir Dis 1982; 125:740–745.

121. Crandall ED, Matthay MA. Alveolar epithelial transport - Basic science to clinical medicine. Am J Respir Crit Care Med 2001; 163:1021–1029.

122. Chesnutt MS, Nuckton TJ, Golden J, Folkesson HG, Matthay MA. Rapid alveolar epithelial fluid clearance following lung lavage in pulmonary alveolar proteinosis. Chest 2001; 120:271–274.

123. Gonzales-Crussi F, Boston RW. The absorptive function of the neonatal lung: ultrastructural study of horseradish peroxidase uptake at the onset of ventilation. Lab Invest 1972; 26:114–121.

124. Corrin B. Phagocytic potential of pulmonary alveolar epithelium with particular reference to surfactant metabolism. Thorax 1970; 25:110–115.

125. Brody AR, Hill LH, Adkins B, O'Connor RW. Chrysotile asbestos inhalation in rats: deposition pattern and reaction of alveolar epithelium and pulmonary macrophages. Am Rev Respir Dis 1981; 123:670–678.

126. Faulkner CS. The role of the granular pneumonocyte in surfactant metabolism. An autoradiographic study. Arch Pathol 1969; 87:521–525.

127. Askin FB, Kuhn C. The cellular origin of pulmonary surfactant. Lab Invest 1971; 25:260–268.

128. Massaro GD, Massaro D. Granular pneumocytes. Electron microscopic radioautographic evidence of intracellular protein transport. Am Rev Respir Dis 1972; 105:927–931.

129. Chevalier G, Collet AJ. In vivo incorporation of choline-3H , leucine-3H and galactose-3H in alveolar type II pneumocytes in relation to surfactant synthesis. A quantitative radiographic study in mouse by electron microscopy. Anat Rec 1972; 174:289–310.

130. Kikkawa Y, Yoneda K, Smith F, Packard B, Suzuki K. The type II epithelial cells of the lung. II Chemical composition and phospholipid synthesis. Lab Invest 1975; 32:295–302.

131. Corrin B, Clark AE. Lysosomal aryl sulphatase in pulmonary alveolar cells. Histochemie 1968; 15:95–98.

132. Corrin B, Clark AE, Spencer H. Ultrastructural localisation of acid phosphatase in the rat lung. J Anat 1969; 104:65–70.

133. Meban C. Localization of phosphatidic acid phosphatase activity in granular pneumocytes. J Cell Biol 1972; 53:249–252.

134. Ochs M, Johnen G, Muller KM, et al. Intracellular and intraalveolar localization of surfactant protein a (SP-A) in the parenchymal region of the human lung. Am J Respir Cell Mol Biol 2002; 26:91–98.

135. Evans MJ, Cabral LJ, Stephens RJ, Freeman G. Renewal of alveolar epithelium in the rat following exposure to NO2. Am J Pathol 1973; 70:175–198.

136. Evans MJ, Cabral LJ, Stephens RJ, Freeman G. Transformation of alveolar type 2 cells to type 1 cells following exposure to NO2. Exp Mol Pathol 1975; 22:142–150.

137. Adamson IYR, Bowden DH. Derivation of type 1 epithelium from type 2 cells in the developing rat lung. Lab Invest 1975; 32:736–745.

138. Hamm H, Kroegel C, Hohlfeld J. Surfactant: a review of its functions and relevance in adult respiratory disorders. Respir Med 1996; 90:251–270.

139. Creuwels LAJM, Vangolde LMG, Haagsman HP. The pulmonary surfactant system: biochemical and clinical aspects. Lung 1997; 175:1–39.

140. Clements JA, Avery ME. Lung surfactant and neonatal respiratory distress syndrome. Am J Respir Crit Care Med 1998; 157:S59–S66.

141. Pattle RE. Properties, function and origin of the alveolar lining layer. Proc R Soc London B Biol Sci 1958; 148:217–240.

142. Gil J, Weibel ER. Improvements in demonstration of lining layer of lung alveoli by electron microscopy. Respir Physiol 1969; 8:13–36.

143. Johansson J, Curstedt T, Robertson B. The proteins of the surfactant system. Eur Respir J 1994; 7:372–391.

144. LaForce FM, Kelly WJ, Huber GL. Inactivation of staphylococci by alveolar macrophages with preliminary observations on the importance of alveolar lining material. Am Rev Respir Dis 1973; 108:784–790.

145. Restrepo CI, Dong Q, Savov J, Mariencheck WI, Wright JR. Surfactant protein D stimulates phagocytosis of Pseudomonas aeruginosa by alveolar macrophages. Am J Respir Cell Mol Biol 1999; 21:576–585.

146. Slade R, Crissman K, Norwood J, Hatch G. Comparison of antioxidant substances in bronchoalveolar lavage cells and fluid from humans, guinea pigs and rats. Exp Lung Res 1993; 19:469–484.

147. Rao RH, Waite M, Myrvik QN. Deacylation of dipalmitoyllecithin by phospholipases A in alveolar macrophages. Exp Lung Res 1981; 2:9–15.

148. Jobe A, Ikegami M, Sarton-Miller I. The in vivo labelling with acetate and palmitate of lung phospholipids from developing and adult rabbits. Biochim Biophys Acta 1980; 617:65–75.

149. Jacobs H, Jobe A, Ikegami M, Conaway D. The significance of reutilization of surfactant phosphatidylcholine. J Biol Chem 1983; 258:4156–4165.

150. Stevens PA, Wright JR, Clements JA. Changes in quantity, composition and surface activity of alveolar surfactant at birth. J Appl Physiol 1987; 63:1049–1057.

151. Baritussio A, Bellina L, Carraro R, et al. Heterogeneity of alveolar surfactant in the rabbit: composition, morphology and labelling of subfractions isolated by centrifugation of lung lavage. Eur J Clin Invest 1984; 14:24–29.

152. Sirianni FE, Chu FSF, Walker DC. Human alveolar wall fibroblasts directly link epithelial type 2 cells to capillary endothelium. Am J Respir Crit Care Med 2003; 168:1532–1537.

153. Kapanci Y, Assimacopoulos A, Irle C, Zwahlen A, Gabbiani G. Contractile interstitial cells in pulmonary alveolar septa: a possible regulator of ventilation/perfusion ratio? J Cell Biol 1974; 60:375–392.

154. Adler KB, Low RB, Leslie KO, Mitchell J, Evans JN. Biology of disease. Contractile cells in normal and fibrotic lung. Lab Invest 1989; 60:473–485.

155. Weibel ER. On pericytes, particularly their existence in lung capillaries. Microvasc Res 1974; 8:218–235.

156. Adamson IYR, Bowden DH. Role of monocytes and interstitial cells in the generation of alveolar macrophages. II. Kinetic studies after carbon loading. Lab Invest 1980; 42:518–524.

157. Crowell RE, Heaphy E, Valdez YE, Mold C, Lehnert BE. Alveolar and interstitial macrophage populations in the murine lung. Exp Lung Res 1992; 18:435–446.

158. Sebring RJ, Lehnert BE. Morphometric comparisons of rat alveolar macrophages, pulmonary interstitial macrophages and blood monocytes. Exp Lung Res 1992; 18:479–496.

159. Johansson A, Lundborg M, Skold CM, et al. Functional, morphological and phenotypical differences between rat alveolar and interstitial macrophages. Am J Respir Cell Mol Biol 1997; 16:582–588.

160. Wallace WAH, Gillooly M, Lamb D. Intra-alveolar macrophage numbers in current smokers and non- smokers - a morphometric study of tissue sections. Thorax 1992; 47:437–440.

161. Bowden DH, Adamson IYR. Role of monocytes and interstitial cells in the generation of alveolar macrophages. I. Kinetic studies of normal mice. Lab Invest 1980; 42:511–513.

162. Takahashi K, Naito M, Takeya M. Development and heterogeneity of macrophages and their related cells through their differentiation pathways. Pathol Int 1996; 46:473–485.

163. Vijeyaratnam GS, Corrin B. Origin of the pulmonary alveolar macrophage studied in the iprindole-treated rat. J Pathol 1972; 108:115–118.

164. Bowden DH, Adamson IYR. Alveolar macrophage response to carbon in monocyte-depleted mice. Am Rev Respir Dis 1982; 126:708–711.

165. Polosukhin VV, Manouilova LS, Romberger DJ, et al. Ultrastructural heterogeneity of the alveolar macrophages from tobacco smokers with chronic bronchitis. Ultrastruct Pathol 2004; 25:5–11.

166. Evans MJ, Cabral LJ, Stephens RJ, Freeman G. Cell division of alveolar macrophages in rat lung following exposure to NO_2. Am J Pathol 1973; 70:199–206.

167. Shellito J, Esparza C, Armstrong C. Maintenance of the normal rat alveolar macrophage cell population. The roles of monocyte influx and alveolar macrophage proliferation in situ. Am Rev Respir Dis 1987; 135:78–81.

168. Cordingley JL, Nicol T. The lung: an excretory route for macromolecules and particles. J Physiol (London) 1967; 190:7.

169. Nakstad B, Lyberg T, Skjorten F, Boye NP. Subpopulations of human lung alveolar macrophages: ultrastructural features. Ultrastruct Pathol 1989; 13:1–14.

170. Spiteri MA, Poulter LW. Characteristics of immune inducer and suppressor macrophages from the normal human lung. Clin Exp Immunol 1991; 83:157–162.

171. Schaberg T, Klein U, Rau M, Eller J, Lode H. Subpopulations of alveolar macrophages in smokers and nonsmokers: relation to the expression of CD11/CD18 molecules and superoxide anion production. Am J Respir Crit Care Med 1995; 151:1551–1558.

172. Brain JD. Free cells in the lungs. Arch Intern Med 1970; 126:477–487.

173. Policard A, Collet A, Pregermain S, Reuet C. Etude au microscope electronique du granulome pulmonaire silicotique experimental. Presse Med 1957; 65:121–124.

174. Harmsen AG, Muggenburg BA, Snipes MB, Bice DE. The role of macrophages in particle translocation from lungs to lymph nodes. Science 1985; 230:1277–1280.

175. Corry D, Kulkarni P, Lipscomb MF. The migration of bronchoalveolar macrophages into hilar lymph nodes. Am J Pathol 1984; 115:321–328.

176. Oren R, Farnham AE, Saito K, Milofsky E, Karnovsky ML. Metabolic patterns in three types of phagocytosing cells. J Cell Biol 1963; 17:487–501.

177. Reynolds HY, Atkinson JP, Newball HH, Frank MM. Receptors for immunoglobulin and complement on human alveolar macrophages. J Immunol 1975; 114:1813–1819.

178. Sone S, Bucana C, Hoyer LC, Fidler IJ. Kinetics and ultrastructural studies of the induction of rat alveolar macrophage fusion by mediators released from mitogen-stimulated lymphocytes. Am J Pathol 1981; 103:234–246.

179. Hocking WG, Golde DW. The pulmonary-alveolar macrophage. N Engl J Med 1979; 301:639–645.

180. Kaltreider HB. Alveolar macrophages. Enhancers or suppressors of pulmonary immune reactivity? Chest 1982; 82:261–262.

181. Adamson IYR, Bowden DH. Adaptive responses of the pulmonary macrophagic system to carbon. II. Morphological studies. Lab Invest 1978; 38:430–438.

182. Brody AR, Craighead JE. Cytoplasmic inclusions in pulmonary macrophages of cigarette smokers. Lab Invest 1975; 32:125–132.

183. Schwartz LW, Christman CA. Lung lining material as a chemotactant for alveolar macrophages. Chest 1979; 75:284S–288S.

184. Crouch EC. Collectins and pulmonary host defense. Am J Respir Cell Mol Biol 1998; 19:177–201.

185. Gee JBL, Vassallo CL, Vogt MT, Thomas C, Basford RE. Peroxidative metabolism in alveolar macrophages. Arch Intern Med 1971; 127:1046–1049.

186. Davies P, Drath DB, Engel EE, Huber GL. The localization of catalase in the pulmonary alveolar macrophage. Lab Invest 1979; 40:221–226.

187. Hatch GE, Gardner GE, Menzel DB. Stimulation of oxidant production in alveolar macrophages by pollutant and latex particles. Environ Res 1980; 23:121–136.

188. Moncada S, Palmer RMJ, Higgs EA. Biosynthesis of nitric oxide from L-arginine: a pathway for the regulation of cell function and communication. Biochem Pharmacol 1989; 38:1709–1715.

189. Kobzik L, Bredt DS, Lowenstein CJ, et al. Nitric oxide synthase in human and rat lung - immunocytochemical and histochemical localization. Am J Respir Cell Mol Biol 1993; 9:371–377.

190. Barnes PJ, Belvisi MG. Nitric oxide and lung disease. Thorax 1993; 48:1034–1043.

191. Green GM, Kass EH. The influence of bacterial species on pulmonary resistance to infection in mice subjected to hypoxia, cold, stress and ethanolic intoxication. Br J Exp Pathol 1965; 46:360–366.

192. Green GH, Carolin D. The depressant effect of cigarette smoke on the in vitro antibacterial activity of alveolar macrophages. N Engl J Med 1967; 276:421–427.

193. Goldstein E, Green GM, Seamans C. The effect of acidosis on pulmonary bactericidal function. J Lab Clin Med 1970; 75:912–913.

194. Jakab GJ, Green GM. Defect in intracellular killing of staphylococcus aureus within alveolar macrophages in sendai virus-infected murine lungs. J Clin Invest 1976; 57:1533–1539.

195. Raffin TA, Simon LM, Braun D, Theodore J, Robin ED. Impairment of phagocytosis by moderate hyperoxia (40 to 60 per cent oxygen) in lung macrophages. Lab Invest 1980; 42:622–626.

196. Wallaert B, Aerts C, Colombel JF, Voisin C. Human alveolar macrophage antibacterial activity in the alcoholic lung. Am Rev Respir Dis 1991; 144:278–283.

197. Unanue ER, Beller DI, Calderon J, Kiely JM, Stadecker MJ. Regulation of immunity and inflammation by mediators from macrophages. Am J Pathol 1976; 85:465–478.

198. Nathan CF. Secretory products of macrophages. J Clin Invest 1987; 79:319–326.

199. Gibbs DF, Warner RL, Weiss SJ, Johnson KJ, Varani J. Characterization of matrix metalloproteinases produced by rat alveolar macrophages. Am J Respir Cell Mol Biol 1999; 20:1136–1144.

200. Gibbs DF, Shanley TP, Warner RL, Murphy HS, Varani J, Johnson KJ. Role of matrix metalloproteinases in models of macrophage-dependent acute lung injury - Evidence for alveolar macrophage as source of proteinases. Am J Respir Cell Mol Biol 1999; 20:1145–1154.

201. Leibovich SJ, Ross R. A macrophage-dependent factor that stimulates the proliferation of fibroblasts in vitro. Am J Pathol 1976; 84:501–514.

202. Lemaire I, Beaudoin H, Masse S, Grondin C. Alveolar macrophage stimulation of lung fibroblast growth in asbestos-induced pulmonary fibrosis. Am J Pathol 1986; 122:205–211.

203. Osorniovargas AR, Bonner JC, Badgett A, Brody AR. Rat alveolar macrophage derived platelet-derived growth factor is chemotactic for rat lung fibroblasts. Am J Respir Cell Mol Biol 1990; 3:595–602.

204. Denholm EM. Continuous secretion of monocyte chemotactic factors and fibroblast growth factors by alveolar macrophages following a single exposure to bleomycin in vitro. Am J Pathol 1992; 141:965–971.

Blood supply of the lung

205. Hattano S, Strasser T. Primary pulmonary hypertension. Geneva: World Health Organization, 1975.

206. Smith U, Ryan JW, Michie DD, Smith DS. Endothelial projections as revealed by scanning electron microscopy. Science 1971; 173:925–927.

207. Bensch KG, Gordon GB, Miller LR. Fibrillar structures resembling leiomyofibrils in endothelial cells of mammalian pulmonary blood vessels. Zeitschrift fur Zellforschung 1964; 63:759–766.

208. Weibel ER, Palade GE. New cytoplasmic components in arterial endothelia. J Cell Biol 1964; 23:101–112.

209. Wagner DD, Olmsted JB, Marder VJ. Immunolocalization of von Willebrand protein in Weibel-Palade bodies of human endothelial cells. J Cell Biol 1982; 95:355–360.

210. Kato M, Staub NC. Response of small pulmonary arteries to unilobar hypoxia and hypercapnia. Circ Res 1966; 19:426–439.

211. Nagasaka Y, Bhattacharya F, Nanjo S, Gropper MA, Staub NC. Micropuncture measurement of lung microvascular pressure profile during hypoxia in cats. Circ Res 1984; 54:90–95.

212. Brij SO, Peacock AJ. Cellular responses to hypoxia in the pulmonary circulation. Thorax 1998; 53:1075–1079.

213. Michael JR, Markewitz BA. Endothelins and the lung. Am J Respir Crit Care Med 1996; 154:555–581.

214. Kourembanas S, Bernfield M. Hypoxia and endothelial smooth muscle cell interactions in the lung. Am J Respir Cell Mol Biol 1994; 11:373–374.

215. Perreault T, Gutkowska J. Role of atrial natriuretic factor in lung physiology and pathology. Am J Respir Crit Care Med 1995; 151:226–242.

216. Guntheroth WG, Luchtel DL, Kawabori I. Pulmonary microcirculation: tubules rather than sheet and post. J Appl Physiol 1982; 53:510–515.

217. Sobin SS, Tremer HM, Fung YC. Morphometric basis of sheet-flow concept of the pulmonary alveolar microcirculation in the cat. Circ Res 1970; 26:397–414.

218. Weibel ER. Lung cell biology. In American physiological society ed. Handbook of physiology The respiratory system. Bethesda. 1984; 47–91.

219. Hogg JC. Neutrophil kinetics and lung injury. Physiol Rev 1987; 67:1249–1295.

220. Ryan US, Ryan JW, Whitaker C, Chiu A. Localization of angiotensin converting enzyme (kininase II). II. Immunocytochemistry and immunofluorescence. Tissue Cell 1976; 8:125–146.

221. Macnee W, Selby C. Neutrophil kinetics in the lungs. Clin Sci 1990; 79:97–107.

222. Downey GP, Worthen GS, Henson PM, Hyde DM. Neutrophil sequestration and migration in localized pulmonary inflammation – capillary localization and migration across the interalveolar septum. Am Rev Respir Dis 1993; 147:168–176.

223. Schneeberger-Keeley EE, Karnovsky MJ. The ultrastructural basis of alveolar-capillary membrane permeability to peroxidase used as a tracer. J Cell Biol 1968; 37:781–793.

224. Feldmann G, Chahinian P, Leturcq E, Bignon J. Localisation ultrastructurale par anticorps couples a la peroxydase de l'albumine extra-vasculaire dans le poumon de rat. Comptes rendus de l'Academie des Sciences 1973; 277:251.

225. Schraufnagel DE, Patel KR. Sphincters in pulmonary veins. An anatomic study in rats. Am Rev Respir Dis 1990; 141:721–726.

226. Heath D, Williams D. Arachnoid nodules in the lungs of high altitude Indians. Thorax 1993; 48:743–745.

227. Junod AE. Accumulation of 14 C-imipramine in isolated perfused rat lungs. J Pharmacol Exp Ther 1972; 183:182–187.

228. Strum JM, Junod AF. Radioautographic demonstration of 5–hydroxytryptamine-3H uptake by pulmonary endothelial cells. J Cell Biol 1972; 54:456–467.

229. Nicholas TE, Strum JM, Angelo LS, Junod AF. Site and mechanism of uptake of HL-norepinephrine by isolated perfused rat lungs. Circ Res 1974; 35:670–680.

230. Ferreira SH, Greene LJ, Salgado MCO, Krieger EM. The fate of circulating biologically active peptides in the lungs. In: Ciba foundation, ed. Symposium 78: Metabolic Activities of the Lung. Amsterdam: Excerpta Medica; 1980:129–145.

231. Moncada S, Vane JR. Pharmacology and endogenous roles of prostaglandin endoperoxides, thromboxane A2 and prostacyclin. Pharmacol Rev 1978; 30:293–331.

232. Gryglewski RJ, Korbut R, Ocetkiewicz A. Generation of prostacyclin by lungs in vivo and its release into the arterial circulation. Nature 1978; 273:765–767.

233. Yanagisawa M, Kurihara H, Kimura S, et al. A novel potent vasoconstrictor peptide produced by vascular endothelial cell. Nature 1988; 332:411–415.

234. Moncada S, Palmer RMJ, Higgs EA. Nitric oxide: physiology, pathophysiology and pharmacology. Pharmacol Rev 1991; 43:109–142.

235. Cernacek P, Stewart DJ. Immunoreactive endothelin in human plasma: marked elevations in patients in cardiogenic shock. Biochem Biophys Res Commun 1989; 161:562–567.

236. Yamamoto M, Shimokata K, Nagura H. An immunohistochemical study on phenotypic heterogeneity of human pulmonary vascular endothelial cells. Virchows Arch Pathol Anat Histopathol 1988; 412:479–486.

237. Brill R, Halpern MM. The frequency of megakaryocytes in autopsy sections. Blood 1948; 3:286–291.

238. Aabo K, Hansen KB. Megakarocytes in pulmonary blood vessels. 1. Incidences at autopsy, clinicopathological relations especially to disseminated intravascular coagulation. Acta Path Microbiol Scand 1978; 86:285–291.

239. Sharma GK, Talbot IC. Pulmonary megakaryocytes: 'missing link' between cardiovascular and respiratory disease? J Clin Pathol 1986; 39:969–976.

240. Crow J. Pulmonary haematoxyphil bodies. J Clin Pathol 1982; 35:690–691.

241. Scheinin TM, Koivuniemi AP. Megakaryocytes in the pulmonary circulation. Blood 1963; 22:82–87.

242. Melamed MR, Cliffton EE, Mercer C, Koss LG. The megakaryocyte blood count. Am J Med Sci 1966; 252:301–309.

243. Kallinikos-Maniatis A. Megakaryocytes and platelets in central venous and arterial blood. Acta Haematol 1969; 42:330–335.

244. Tinggaard Pedersen N. The pulmonary vessels as a filter for circulating megakaryocytes in rats. Scand J Haematol 1974; 13:225–231.

245. Tinggaard Pedersen N. Occurrence of megakaryocytes in various vessels and their retention in the pulmonary capillaries of man. Scand J Haematol 1978; 21:379–375.

246. Trowbridge EA, Martin JF, Slater DN. Evidence for a theory of physical fragmentation of megakaryocytes, implying that all platelets are produced in the pulmonary circulation. Thromb Res 1982; 28:461–475.

247. Slater DN, Trowbridge EA, Martin JF. The megakaryocyte in thrombocytopenia: a microscopic study which supports the theory that platelets are produced in the lungs. Thromb Res 1983; 31:163–176.

248. Hardaway RM, Johnson D. Clotting mechanism in endotoxin shock. Arch Intern Med 1963; 112:775–782.

249. Soares FA. Increased numbers of pulmonary megakaryocytes in patients with arterial pulmonary tumour embolism and with lung metastases seen at necropsy. J Clin Pathol 1992; 45:140–142.

250. Weibel E. Die Entstehung der Langsmuskulatur in den Asten der A.bronchialis. Zeitschrift fur Zellforschung 1958; 47:440–468.

251. Wagenaar SJ, Wagenvoort CA. Experimental production of longitudinal smooth muscle cells in the intima of muscular arteries. Lab Invest 1978; 39:370–374.

252. Hales MR, Liebow AA. Collateral circulation to the lungs in congenital pulmonic stenosis. Bull Assoc Med Mus 1948; 28:1–22.

253. Liebow AA, Hales MR, Lindskog GE. Enlargement of the bronchial arteries and their anastomoses with the pulmonary arteries in bronchiectasis. Am J Pathol 1949; 25:211–231.

254. Turner-Warwick M. Pre-capillary systemic-pulmonary anastomoses. Thorax 1963; 18:225–237.

255. Charan NB, Baile EM, Pare PD. Bronchial vascular congestion and angiogenesis. Eur Respir J 1997; 10:1173–1180.

256. Hill P, Goulding D, Webber SE, Widdicombe JG. Blood sinuses in the submucosa of the large airways of the sheep. J Anat 1989; 162:235–247.

257. Laitinen A, Laitinen LA, Moss R, Widdicombe JG. The organisation and structure of tracheal and bronchial blood vessels in the dog. J Anat 1989; 165:133–140.

258. Widdicombe JG. Tracheobronchial vasculature. Br Med Bull 1992; 48:108–119.

259. Suzuki Y. Fenestration of alveolar capillary endothelium in experimental pulmonary fibrosis. Lab Invest 1969; 21:304–308.

260. Wanner A. Airway circulation. Am Rev Respir Dis 1992; 146:S1–S2.

261. Renkin EM. Cellular and intercellular transport pathways in exchange vessels. Am Rev Respir Dis 1992; 146:S28–S31.

262. Kawanami O, Matsuda K, Yoneyama H, Ferrans VJ, Crystal RG. Endothelial fenestration of the alveolar capillaries in interstitial fibrotic lung diseases. Acta Pathol Jpn 1992; 42:177–184.

263. Blessing MH, Hora BI. Glomera in der lunge des menschen. Zeitschrift fur Zellforschung 1968; 87:562–570.

264. Printzmetal M, Ornitze EM, Simkin B, Bergman HC. Arterio-venous anastomoses in liver, spleen and lungs. Am J Physiol 1948; 152:48–52.

265. Tobin CE, Zariquiey MD. Arterio-venous shunts in the human lung. Proc Soc Exp Biol Med 1950; 75:827–829.

266. Fritts HW Jr, Harris P, Chidsey CAI, Clauss RH, Cournand A. Estimation of flow through bronchial-pulmonary vascular anastomoses with use of T-1824 dye. Circulation 1961; 23:390–398.

267. Heath D, Thompson IM. Bronchopulmonary anastomoses in sickle cell anaemia. Thorax 1969; 24:232–238.

268. Vanderhoeft PJ. Broncho-pulmonary circuits: a synoptic appraisal. Thorax 1963; 19:537–540.

Lymphoid tissue of the lungs
269. Lauweryns JM. The blood and lymphatic microcirculation of the lung. Pathol Annu 1971; 6:365–415.

270. Staub NC. The pathophysiology of pulmonary edema. Hum Pathol 1970; 1:419–432.

271. Trapnell DH. Recognition and incidence of intrapulmonary lymph nodes. Thorax 1964; 19:44–50.

272. Kradin RI, Spirn PW, Mark EJ. Intrapulmonary lymph nodes. Clinical, radiologic and pathologic features. Chest 1985; 87:662–667.

273. Bienenstock J, Johnston N, Perey DYE. Bronchial lymphoid tissue I morphologic characteristics. Lab Invest 1973; 28:686–692.

274. Bienenstock J, Johnston N, Perey DYE. Bronchial lymphoid tissue II functional characteristics. Lab Invest 1973; 28:693–698.

275. Pabst R, Gehrke I. Is the bronchus-associated lymphoid tissue (BALT) an integral structure of the lung in normal mammals, including humans? Am J Respir Cell Mol Biol 1990; 3:131–136.

276. Gould SJ, Isaacson PG. Bronchus-associated lymphoid tissue (BALT) in human fetal and infant lung. J Pathol 1993; 169:229–234.

277. Richmond I, Pritchard GE, Ashcroft T, Avery A, Corris PA, Walters EH. Bronchus associated lymphoid tissue (BALT) in human lung – its distribution in smokers and non-smokers. Thorax 1993; 48:1130–1134.

278. Tschernig T, Kleemann WJ, Pabst R. Bronchus-associated lymphoid tissue (BALT) in the lungs of children who had died from sudden infant death syndrome and other causes. Thorax 1995; 50:658–660.

279. Bosken CH, Hards J, Gatter K, Hogg JC. Characterization of the inflammatory reaction in the peripheral airways of cigarette smokers using immunocytochemistry. Am Rev Respir Dis 1992; 145:911–917.

280. McDermott MR, Befus AD, Bienenstock J. The structural basis for immunity in the respiratory tract. Int Rev Exp Pathol 1982; 23:47–112.

281. Rudzik R, Clancy RL, Perey DYE, Day RP, Bienenstock J. Repopulation with IgA-containing cells of bronchial and intestinal lamina propria after transfer of homologous Peyer's patch and bronchial lymphocytes. J Immunol 1975; 114:1599–1604.

282. Fournier M, Vai F, Derenne JP, Pariente R. Bronchial lymphoepithelial nodules in the rat. Morphologic features and uptake and transport of exogenous proteins. Am Rev Respir Dis 1977; 116:685–694.

283. Matsuura Y, Matsuoka T, Fuse Y. Ultrastructural and immunohistochemical studies on the ontogenic development of bronchus-associated lymphoid tissue (BALT) in the rat - special reference to follicular dendritic cells. Eur Respir J 1992; 5:824–828.

284. Soutar CA. Distribution of plasma cells and other cells containing immunoglobulin in the respiratory tract of normal man and class of immunoglobulin contained therein. Thorax 1976; 31:158–166.

285. Sato J, Chida K, Suda T, Sato A, Nakamura H. Migratory patterns of thoracic duct lymphocytes into bronchus- associated lymphoid tissue of immunized rats. Lung 2000; 178:295–308.

286. Emery JL, Dinsdale F. The postnatal development of lymphoreticular aggregates and lymph nodes in infants' lungs. J Clin Pathol 1973; 26:539–545.

287. Hayday AC, Roberts S, Ramsburg E. Gamma delta cells and the regulation of mucosal immune responses. Am J Respir Crit Care Med 2000; 162:S161+.

288. Holt PG, Schon-Hegrad MA, Oliver J, Holt BJ, McMenamin PG. A contiguous network of dendritic antigen-presenting cells within the respiratory epithelium. Int Arch Allergy Appl Immunol 1990; 91:155–159.

289. Holt PG. Regulation of antigen-presenting cell function(s) in lung and airway tissues. Eur Respir J 1993; 6:120–129.

290. Hance AJ. Pulmonary immune cells in health and disease – dendritic cells and Langerhans cells. Eur Respir J 1993; 6:1213–1220.

291. Vanhaarst JMW, Dewit HJ, Drexhage HA, Hoogsteden HC. Distribution and immunophenotype of mononuclear phagocytes and dendritic cells in the human lung. Am J Respir Cell Mol Biol 1994; 10:487–492.

292. Austyn JM. Antigen-presenting cells – Experimental and clinical studies of dendritic cells. Am J Respir Crit Care Med 2000; 162:S146.

293. Holt PG. Antigen presentation in the lung. Am J Respir Crit Care Med 2000; 162:S151–S156.

294. Lambrecht BN, Prins JB, Hoogsteden HC. Lung dendritic cells and host immunity to infection. Eur Resp J 2001; 18:692–704.

295. Tschernig T, Debertin AS, Paulsen F, Kleemann WJ, Pabst R. Dendritic cells in the mucosa of the human trachea are not regularly found in the first year of life. Thorax 2001; 56; 427–431.

296. Birbeck MS, Breathnach AS, Everall JD. An electron microscopic study of basal melanocytes and high level clear cells (Langerhans' cell) in vitiligo. J Invest Dermatol 1961; 37:51.

297. Soler P, Valeyre D, Georges R, Battesti JP, Basset F, Hance A. The role of epithelial abnormality in recruiting Langerhans cells to the lower respiratory tract. Am Rev Respir Dis 1986; 133:A-243.

298. Hosokawa S, Shinzato M, Kaneko C, Shamoto M. Migration and maturation of Langerhans cells in squamous metaplasia of the rat trachea induced by vitamin-A deficiency. Virchows Arch B Cell Pathol 1993; 63:159–166.

299. Casoloro MA, Bernaudin J-F, Saltini C, Ferrans VJ, Crystal RG. Accumulation of Langerhans' cells on the epithelial surface of the lower respiratory tract in normal subjects in association with cigarette smoking. Am Rev Respir Dis 1988; 137:406–411.

300. Guerzon GM, Pare PD, Michoud M-C, Hogg JC. The number and distribution of mast cells in monkey lungs. Am Rev Respir Dis 1979; 119:59–66.

301. Djukanovic R, Wilson JW, Britten KM, et al. Quantitation of mast cells and eosinophils in the bronchial mucosa of symptomatic asthmatics and healthy control subjects using immunohistochemistry. Am Rev Respir Dis 1990; 142:863–871.

302. Bradley BL, Azzawi M, Jacobson M, et al. Eosinophils, T-lymphocytes, mast cells, neutrophils and macrophages in bronchial biopsy specimens from atopic subjects with asthma: comparison with biopsy specimens from atopic subjects without asthma and normal controls subjects and relationship to bronchial hyperresponsiveness. J Allergy Clin Immunol 1991; 88:661–674.

303. Heard BE, Nunn AJ, Kay AB. Mast cells in human lungs. J Pathol 1989; 157:59–63.

304. Lamb D, Lumsden A. Intra-epithelial mast cells in human airway epithelium: evidence for smoking-induced changes in their frequency. Thorax 1982; 37:334–342.

305. Fox B, Bull TB, Guz A. Mast cells in the human alveolar wall: an electronmicroscopic study. J Clin Pathol 1981; 34:1333–1342.

306. Heard BE, Dewar A, Corrin B. Apposition of fibroblasts to mast cells and lymphocytes in normal human lung and in cryptogenic fibrosing alveolitis – ultrastructure and cell perimeter measurements. J Pathol 1992; 166:303–310.

307. Chanez P, Lacoste JY, Guillot B, et al. Mast cells' contribution to the fibrosing alveolitis of the scleroderma lung. Am Rev Respir Dis 1993; 147:1497–1502.

308. Qu ZH, Liebler JM, Powers MR, et al. Mast cells are a major source of basic fibroblast growth factor in chronic inflammation and cutaneous hemangioma. Am J Pathol 1995; 147:564–573.

309. Heard BE. Histochemical aspects of the staining of mast cells with particular reference to heterogeneity and quantification. In: Kay AB, ed. Asthma Clinical Pharmacology and Therapeutic Progress. Oxford: Blackwell, 1986; 286–294.

310. Heard BE, Dewar A, Nunn AJ, Kay AB. Heterogeneous ultrastructure of human bronchial mast cells: morphometric subdivision of cell types and evidence for a degranulation gradient. Am J Respir Cell Mol Biol 1990; 3:71–78.

311. Lane SJ, Lee TH. Mast cell effector mechanisms. J Allergy Clin Immunol 1996; 98:S67–S71.

Innervation of the lungs

312. Barnes PJ. Neural control of human airways in health and disease. Am Rev Respir Dis 1986; 134:1289–1314.

313. Barnes PJ. Modulation of neurotransmission in airways. Physiol Rev 1992; 72:699–729.

314. Barnes PJ, Baraniuk JN, Belvisi MG. Neuropeptides in the respiratory tract 1. Am Rev Respir Dis 1991; 144:1187–1198.

315. Barnes PJ, Baraniuk JN, Belvisi MG. Neuropeptides in the respiratory tract 2. Am Rev Respir Dis 1991; 144:1391–1399.

316. Jeffery PK. Innervation of the airway mucosa: structure, function and changes in airway disease. In: Goldie R, ed. Handbook of Immunopharmacology of Epithelial Barriers. London: Academic Press; 1994:85–118.

317. Fox B, Bull TB, Guz A. Innervation of alveolar walls in the human lung: an electron microscopical study. J Anat 1980; 131:683–692.

318. Laitinen A. Ultrastructural organisation of intraepithelial nerves in the human airway tract. Thorax 1985; 40:488–492.

319. Lauweryns JM, Van Lommel AT, Dom RJ. Innervation of rabbit intrapulmonary neuroepithelial bodies. Quantitative and qualitative ultrastructural study after vagotomy. J Neurol Sci 1985; 67:81–92.

320. Spencer H, Leof D. The innervation of the human lung. J Anat 1964; 98:599–609.

321. Wharton J, Haworth SG, Polak JM. Postnatal development of the innervation and paraganglia in the porcine pulmonary arterial bed. J Pathol 1988; 154:19–27.

322. Uddman R, Alumeta J, Densert O, Hakanson R, Sundler F. Occurrence and distribution of VIP nerves in the nasal mucosa and tracheobronchial wall. Acta Otolaryngol (Stockh) 1978; 86:443–448.

323. Wharton J, Polak JM, Bloom SR, Will JA, Brown MR, Pearse AGE. Substance P-like immunoreactive nerves in mammalian lung. Invest Cell Pathol 1979; 2:3–10.

324. Barnes PJ. The third nervous system in the lung: physiology and clinical perspectives. Thorax 1984; 39:561–567.

325. Goldenberg VE, Buckingham S, Sommers SC. Pulmonary alveolar lesions in vagotomized rats. Lab Invest 1967; 16:693–705.

326. Goldenberg VE, Buckingham S, Somers SC. Pilocarpine stimulation of granular pneumocyte secretion. Lab Invest 1969; 20:147–158.

327. Delahunty TJ, Johnston JM. Neurohumoral control of pulmonary surfactant secretion. Lung 1979; 157:45–51.

2

Development of the lungs; perinatal and developmental lung disease

The traditional division of disease into congenital and acquired is less useful in the case of the lungs than one that considers developmental as opposed to non-developmental disorders. This is because lung development continues long after birth. Developmental disease may therefore be acquired well into the postnatal period. Conversely some congenital lung disease is non-developmental but acquired *in utero*, a good example of which is congenital pneumonia. A knowledge of embryology is often helpful in understanding developmental diseases but with the exception of tracheo-oesophageal fistula and anomalous pulmonary veins this is hardly true of the lungs for the embryological basis of most developmental lung disease is poorly understood. Nor is the pathogenesis of most pulmonary malformations at all clear.

DEVELOPMENT OF THE LUNGS

Human lung development is first marked by a longitudinal groove that appears on the ventral side of the primitive foregut 26 days after fertilisation. This separates from the foregut, first at its caudal end and then progressively forward until a connection is retained only at the cranial end. This bud then bifurcates and grows on either side of the foregut as the embryonic lungs, with successive branching giving rise to the lobes and segments of the lungs and the further divisions of the airways (Fig. 2.1).[1] The developing lungs protrude into the coelomic cavity, the mesothelial lining of which forms from the mesoderm about the 14th day of gestation. With the development of the diaphragm and a pleuropericardial membrane the lungs become confined to the pleural cavities.

The phases of lung development and the major events therein are summarised in Table 2.1. The embryonic stage of lung development lasts until 6 weeks gestation, by which time the lungs have acquired a pseudoglandular appearance (Fig. 2.2). At this time, the primitive potential air spaces are widely separated by abundant mesenchyme and lined by a vacuolated columnar or cuboidal epithelium rich in glycogen. The glycogen is particularly plentiful in the budding terminal epithelium where mitoses are most frequent. The pseudoglandular stage of development lasts until 16 weeks by which time

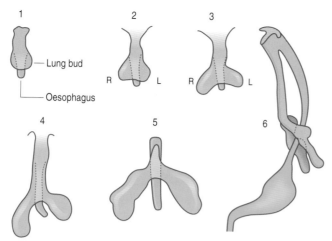

Figure 2.1 Development of the lungs from the 26th to the 33rd day of gestation. (l) A bud appears at the lower end of the laryngopharyngeal sulcus. (2–4) The bud elongates to form a primitive trachea and lungs. (5) Early lobation of the lungs. (6) The primitive lungs extend dorsally on either side of the oesophagus. R, right; L, left.

Table 2.1	Major events during lung development	
Phase	*Gestation*	*Major events*
Embryonic	→6 weeks	Lung buds form (3 weeks)
		Segmental airways appear (6 weeks)
Pseudoglandular	6–16 weeks	Bronchial smooth muscle appears (7 weeks)
		Neuroendocrine cells and submucosal glands appear (8 weeks)
		Bronchial cartilages appear (10 weeks)
		Airway branching complete (16 weeks)
Canalicula	16–28 weeks	Basal cells appear (17 weeks)
		Type II alveolar cells appear (22 weeks)
		Clara cells appear (25 weeks)
Saccular	28–36 weeks	Subdivision of saccules
Alveolar[a]	36 weeks to term	Double layer of alveolar capillaries fuses to give a single layer
	Birth	Lung liquid rapidly cleared
[a]Alveolar multiplication continues from 36 weeks well into childhood.		

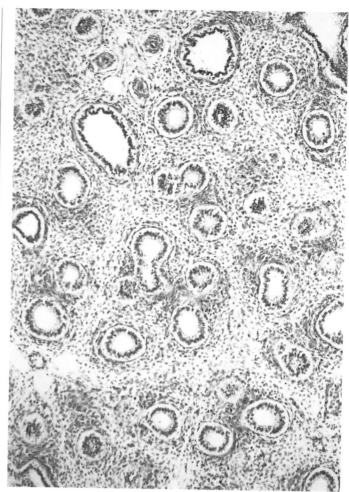

Figure 2.2 The pseudoglandular s1tage of lung development at 12 weeks gestation showing air spaces widely separated by abundant mesenchyme and lined by columnar epithelium showing marked subnuclear vacuolation.

division of the conductive airways down to the terminal bronchiole is complete.[2] This is followed by a canalicular stage marked by the appearance of further air spaces which have an attenuated lining epithelium (Fig. 2.3). During this period the epithelium loses its glycogen and differentiates into the type I and II cells seen in adult alveoli (see p. 15). Although no proper alveoli are yet present, respiration is possible towards the end of the canalicular period around 28 weeks. Substantial amounts of connective tissue still separate the air spaces at this time but in the saccular stage of intrauterine lung development the

connective tissue progressively diminishes by an apoptotic mechanism[3] as new air spaces called terminal sacs develop. These resemble adult alveoli but are shallower and their walls still have enough connective tissue to separate the capillaries abutting air spaces into two layers. The development of true alveoli, first apparent at 36 weeks gestation, is characterised by the in-folding of one of the two capillary layers, further thinning of the connective tissue and the eventual fusion of the double capillary layer into one.[4]

Alveoli develop mainly in the first year of extrauterine life and lung disease in infancy seriously impairs this. At birth, there are about 24 million terminal sacs and alveoli, compared with the adult figure of about 300 million alveoli. In the first year of life, there is a 5-fold increase in alveolar number with continued but slower increase thereafter, up to about 8 years of age and perhaps well into adolescence.[5] There is also remodelling of airways in the first year of life. This entails an increase in length of all airway generations, further branching of alveolar ducts to give more generations, transformation of distal

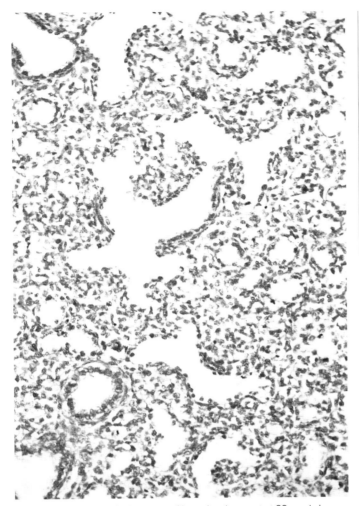

Figure 2.3 The canalicular stage of lung development at 20 weeks' gestation. Further air spaces have developed and the lining epithelium is more attenuated.

respiratory bronchioles into alveolar ducts by increasing alveolisation of their walls and transformation of terminal into respiratory bronchiole by centripetal alveolisation.[6–8] An important facet of postnatal lung development is that events in infancy and childhood may predispose to pulmonary disease in adult life. Thus, an increased frequency of respiratory infections in childhood has been identified in adults with chronic airflow obstruction.[9–11]

All the epithelial tissues of the lung, down to and including the alveoli, are of endodermal origin and all the interstitial elements are mesodermal in origin. This is contrary to older views on the development of the lung which envisaged the peripheral parts being purely mesodermal, but is demonstrated quite conclusively by electron microscopic studies of the developing mammalian lung. These show that the epithelial cells of the primitive endodermal bud extend continuously down to the smallest air spaces and that the epithelial lining of these spaces is not contributed to by any mesodermal elements.[12–14]

The endodermal and mesodermal elements of the lung are each important to the proper development of the other. The basement membrane, cell adhesion factors such as fibronectin and integrin and a variety of growth factors all play a role in this interaction.[15–21] The growth factors include epithelial signalling molecules such as bone morphogenetic factor, transforming growth factor and sonic hedgehog that influence the underlying mesenchyme while the mesenchyme expresses signalling molecules such as fibroblast growth factor that are important in pulmonary epithelial development. Contacts between interstitial and type II epithelial cells have been identified in the newborn and shown to diminish during a postnatal proliferative phase.[22] Experiments demonstrate that respiratory epithelium has an inhibitory effect on the growth of the underlying mesenchyme,[23,24] while in fetal organ culture, intestinal mesoderm will induce bronchial budding but not branching, bronchial mesoderm will induce the tracheal endoderm to branch and tracheal mesoderm will inhibit bronchial branching.[25] Furthermore, while the bronchial mesoderm of one species will induce the endoderm of another to branch, the pattern of endodermal branching is that of the species contributing the mesoderm. These experiments clearly demonstrate the interdependence of mesoderm and endoderm in pulmonary development. They are reinforced by the arrested development of endodermal lung buds within ectopic neuroglia (see p. 56).

The fetal airspaces are filled by a chloride-rich fluid secreted by their lining epithelium, which makes a substantial contribution to the production of amniotic fluid.[26] Its presence in the airways appears to be important to fetal lung growth for this is retarded if the fluid is drained.[27] Conversely, ligation of the trachea results in large lungs.[28]

Neuroendocrine cells are particularly numerous in the respiratory epithelium of the developing airways[29–33] and at least one of their products, gastrin-releasing peptide (human bombesin), is known to stimulate lung growth and maturation during the later stages of development.[34] The expression of gastrin-releasing peptide receptor gene peaks at a time and at sites of most rapid airway growth and development.[35]

Respiratory movements take place *in utero* and these too are thought to be important for fetal lung growth and maturation.[36] Section of the cervical cord above, but not below, the phrenic nucleus leads to severe pulmonary hypoplasia.[37]

Hormones are also important in lung development. The lungs bear steroid receptors and maturation, but not growth, is promoted by glucocorticosteroids and probably other hormones. Glucocorticoid treatment of the fetus accelerates epithelial glycogen depletion, differentiation into type I and II cells, the appearance of lamellar bodies in type II cells and their release into the air spaces.[38] This is utilised in clinical practice to minimise the risk of respiratory distress in premature infants (see below): a decreased incidence of the respiratory distress syndrome and increased survival is reported in premature infants exposed to maternal steroid therapy.[39] The steroids appear to act, at least in part, by stimulating lung fibroblasts to produce an oligopeptide known as fibroblast-pneumonocyte-

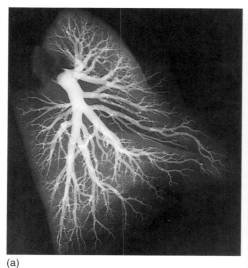

(a)

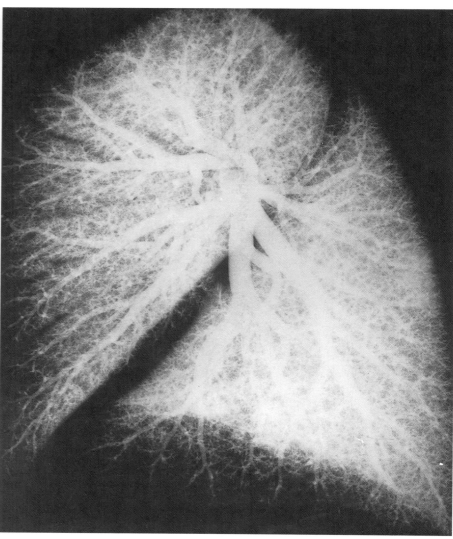

(b)

Figure 2.4 Pulmonary arteriograms showing the development of the pulmonary circulation after birth. (a) Life size pulmonary arteriogram of the left lung of a baby at term. The arterial branching pattern is complete but there is little background haze as there are as yet few peripheral arteries. (b) Life size pulmonary arteriogram of the left lung of an infant aged 18 months. The branching pattern is similar to that seen at birth but there is now a dense background haze made up of numerous peripheral arteries that have grown in the alveolar region of the lung after birth and are too small to be identified individually. (Reproduced with permission from Jeffrey PK, Hislop AA. Embryology and growth. In: Gibson GJ, et al (eds). Respiratory Medicine. Saunders 2003; 51–63.[44] With permission from Elsevier Ltd.)

factor which in turn stimulates surfactant synthesis by the type II cells, an example of paracrine activity.[40]

The blood supply to the developing lung buds is derived from the 6th pair of aortic arches. On the right, the ventral part of this arch persists as the right pulmonary artery while the dorsal part disappears. On the left, the ventral part persists as the ductus arteriosus. Within the lung buds, blood vessels are formed by two processes. Angiogenesis, or the sprouting of new vessels from pre-existing ones, underlies the formation of proximal lung vessels while vasculogenesis or the formation of vascular lakes by precursor angioblasts within the mesenchyme contributes the peripheral vascular component, the two ultimately fusing by a lytic process.[41,42] The pulmonary arteries develop alongside newly formed airways, the latter seemingly acting as templates for the arteries.[43] A well-defined branching pattern is apparent by 14 weeks gestation and all preacinar arteries are present by 16 weeks. At 20 weeks the branching pattern resembles that of adults. However, many peripheral arteries develop after birth (Fig. 2.4).[44]

The processes of vasculogenesis and angiogenesis are also involved in the development of the pulmonary veins.[45] Vessels draining the lung buds initially enter a plexus around the foregut, but later switch to a primary pulmonary vein that grows from the developing left atrium towards the lung buds. Incorporation of the primary pulmonary vein and its first two orders of branches into the wall of the left atrium results in two pulmonary veins from each lung entering the left atrium separately. Failure of the intrapulmonary veins to switch from the enteric venous plexus to the primary pulmonary vein underlies the congenital condition of anomalous pulmonary venous drainage (see p. 72).

Lymphatic development is first seen in the lung from about the 8th gestational week and by 14 weeks, the pulmonary lymphatics are well established. Neural tissue derived from the vagus nerve extends into the growing tips of the fetal airways and bronchial smooth muscle, which develops from 7 weeks gestation, contracts from early gestation in response to nervous stimulation.[46]

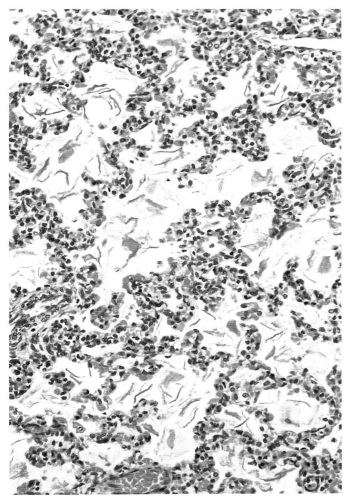

Figure 2.5 Fetal hypoxia has led to excessive respiratory movements *in utero*, resulting in the alveoli being filled with amniotic squamous cells.

PERINATAL DISORDERS

Meconium aspiration

The expulsion of meconium into the amniotic fluid occurs as a response to fetal stress from a wide range of causes and its aspiration may cause a chemical or infective fetal pneumonia,[47] which are described below. Fetal stress also increases the normal respiratory excursions that take place before birth and may so result in the airways being obstructed by numerous fetal squames and mucus (Fig. 2.5). Pathologists are likely to encounter only fatal cases, but the lungs are inherently normal and the obstruction is potentially reversible. The natural clearance mechanisms can be augmented with suction but such treatment may need to be prolonged, in which case oxygenation of the blood has to be maintained with an extracorporeal device; mechanical ventilation would only impair clearance. The mortality remains high, although corticosteroid and surfactant treatment are of some benefit.[48–50]

Massive pulmonary haemorrhage

This is a fairly common finding in perinatal necropsies and has several causes. In some cases of apparent pulmonary haemorrhage, the findings are due to heavy blood-staining of oedema fluid rather than true haemorrhage and in these patients shock and left ventricular failure are important contributory factors. A coagulopathy, usually acquired, may cause true haemorrhage but the most common cause is asphyxia. Cerebral oedema and haemorrhage are often also present and probably represent further manifestations of asphyxial damage. The condition is disproportionately frequent among pre-term babies with very low birth weights[51] and it is postulated that abnormal alveolar surface forces may contribute to the bleeding.[52]

Neonatal pneumonia

Pulmonary infection in the neonate may be due to transplacental transmission from the mother, aspiration of either infected amniotic fluid before birth or infected material during birth, or environmental contacts after birth.

With transplacental transmission, the pneumonia is only part of a generalised infection. Causative agents include cytomegalovirus, rubella virus, herpes simplex virus, mycoplasmas, *Listeria monocytogenes*, *Treponema pallidum*, *Mycobacterium tuberculosis* and *Toxoplasma gondii*. Many of these microbes elicit specific reactions that are dealt with in later chapters. However, it may be mentioned here that eosinophilic nuclear inclusions that have been shown to represent parvovirus by *in situ* DNA hybridisation, may be found in the lungs and other organs of premature stillbirths and neonates with non-immune hydrops.[53]

Pneumonia acquired by aspiration of infected amniotic fluid is known as congenital or intrauterine pneumonia. It is particularly likely if there is prolonged rupture of the membranes. Chorioamnionitis suggests this mechanism and examination of the placenta and its membranes is therefore helpful. Vaginal group B haemolytic streptococci or *Candida albicans* may be responsible, as may bowel bacteria such as *Escherichia coli*, klebsiella and *Pseudomonas aeruginosa*. The airspaces contain polymorphonuclear leukocytes and fibrin but neither of these is as prominent as in an adult with pneumonia (Fig. 2.6). The distribution of the process is that of a bronchopneumonia. In some cases, there is a combination of hyaline membrane disease and pneumonia. Bacteria may then be seen in the hyaline membranes, rendering them haematoxyphilic. It is possible that in such cases the bacteria promote the formation of the membranes by damaging the alveolar epithelium. Acute pneumonia and hyaline membranes may also result from the chemical toxicity of the bilirubin in aspirated meconium.[47] The fact that atelectasis is minimal helps to distinguish pneumonia with hyaline membranes from the infantile respiratory distress syndrome, which is dealt with next.[54]

The combination of pneumonia and hyaline membranes is also seen in immature babies requiring ventilator support.[55,56]

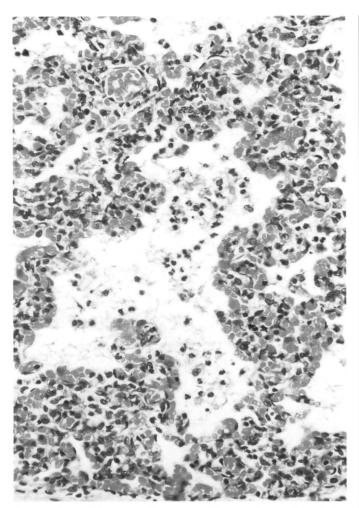

Figure 2.6 Fetal (intrauterine) pneumonia. Neutrophils are evident in the alveoli but they are not as numerous as in fatal bacterial pneumonia in an adult.

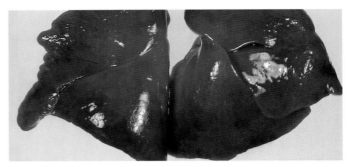

Figure 2.7 The lungs of a premature infant dying of the infantile respiratory distress syndrome (hyaline membrane disease) are dark, airless and resemble hepatic tissue.

Infantile respiratory distress syndrome (hyaline membrane disease)[57]

By 28 weeks gestation, the alveolar epithelium has differentiated into type I and type II pneumocytes, surfactant can be detected and an extrauterine existence is possible. With modern intensive care, an increasing number of babies born before 28 weeks are surviving, but without it the chances of successful respiration at this age are slim. By 34 to 36 weeks, premature birth is generally followed by successful respiration but the capacity of type II pneumocytes to replenish spent stocks of surfactant is frequently inadequate, in which case respiratory distress becomes evident within a few hours of birth. This is apparent as grunting, indrawing of the intercostal tissues on inspiration and hypoxia. Radiographically, there is opacification of the whole lung fields except for an 'air bronchogram'. Without respiratory support the death rate in the first few days is high.

Pathological findings

At necropsy, the lungs are heavy, dark and airless (Fig. 2.7). Microscopy confirms the atelectasis, with air limited to the bronchioles (Fig. 2.8). There is also lymphatic distension and interstitial oedema, which is best seen in the perivascular connective tissue sheaths (Fig. 2.8). Alveolar collapse and interstitial oedema are the expected consequences of high surface tensive forces acting on the alveolar walls. Hyaline membranes are found at the boundary of the air-filled bronchioles and the collapsed alveoli (Fig. 2.9). They are not found when death occurs in the first few hours of life and they are no longer thought to play a causal role in the alveolar collapse. The hyaline membranes represent compacted plasma exudates and cellular debris. They do not stain for fibrin with conventional histological stains but fibrin can be demonstrated in them by immunocytochemistry and epithelial necrosis by electron microscopy.[58] The hyaline membranes are yellow if there has also been unconjugated hyperbilirubinaemia (Fig. 2.10).[59,60]

Hyaline membranes are not specific to premature babies and may be found in term infants who die of birth asphyxia some hours later. Virtually identical pathological changes are seen in the adult respiratory distress syndrome (see p. 131). Hyaline membrane disease is evidently a consequence of non-specific injury to the bronchiolar and alveolar lining. In premature infants the injury is likely to be physical; ventilatory efforts in the surfactant-deficient lung put undue shear forces on the epithelium at the air-liquid interface, which at end-expiration is at the bronchiolar level, the alveoli having collapsed completely. Such mechanical stress operates during each ventilatory cycle so that it is repeated several thousand times in the first few hours of extrauterine life.[58]

Therapy and its complications

If premature birth is expected, or induction of premature labour planned, the risks of respiratory distress can be reduced by administration of steroids to the mother.[39] This promotes maturation of the fetal lung, including surfactant secretion.[38] It is a preventive measure that is only feasible when premature birth can be anticipated.

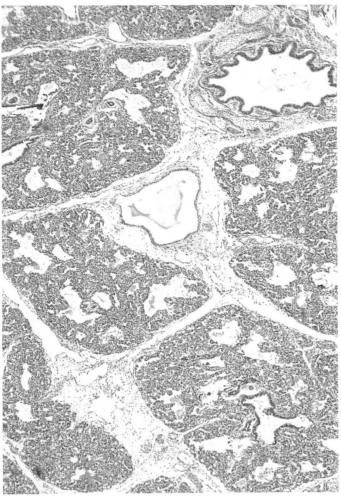

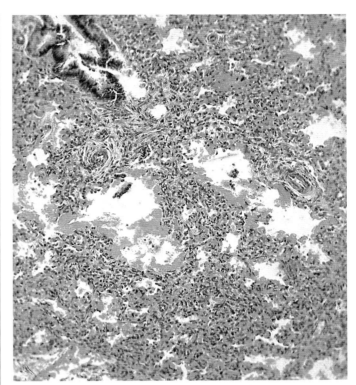

Figure 2.9 Infantile respiratory distress syndrome (hyaline membrane disease). Hyaline membranes separate collapsed alveoli from aerated bronchioles.

Figure 2.8 Infantile respiratory distress syndrome (hyaline membrane disease). The interlobular septa are broadened by oedema and lymphatics within them are dilated. Alveoli have collapsed and air is confined to the bronchioles.

After birth, mechanical respiratory support with oxygen enrichment is the main means of maintaining oxygenation. This is being increasingly supplemented by the insufflation of natural or synthetic surfactant into the infant's airways.[61] Such surfactant therapy is proving very successful but, if the infant does come to autopsy, the exogenous surfactant is seen in the air spaces as a yellow birefringent material. Another useful measure is the administration of nitric oxide gas in low concentrations (less than 80 parts per million) to induce pulmonary arterial dilatation and improve ventilation/perfusion matching. Extracorporeal oxygenation of the infant's blood may also be undertaken but results are best in babies greater than 37 weeks gestation: pre-term babies weighing less than 2 kg have blood vessels that are too fragile to withstand the damage from cannulae and are at risk of ventricular haemorrhage from the heparinised circuits.

With these measures, the survival rate of pre-term infants who develop respiratory distress has been greatly increased and hyaline membrane disease is now seen far less frequently.

However, there are cardiopulmonary complications of such treatment. Immediate complications of positive pressure ventilation include interstitial emphysema and pneumothorax (see below), while patency of the ductus arteriosus and cardiac failure (persistent fetal circulation, see below) may dominate the clinical picture after a few days. Some infants who survive the first weeks of life on ventilator support develop diffuse lung disease and die in the succeeding months from extensive bronchopulmonary dysplasia (see below). Long-term survivors tend to have impaired lung function for some months[62,63] and a high incidence of bronchiolitis and pneumonia in infancy.[64] Babies who recover spontaneously from the respiratory distress syndrome do so completely and suffer none of these pulmonary complications.

Bronchopulmonary dysplasia and chronic lung disease of early infancy

Bronchopulmonary dysplasia is the condition found in infants dying in the first months of life after having survived initial respiratory distress with the help of artificial ventilation.[65,66] As infants who recover spontaneously do not develop this condition it must be attributed to the respirator support, but it is controversial whether oxygen toxicity or barotrauma is mainly responsible.[67,68] Other factors that have been incriminated include prematurity, infection, tracheal intubation, patency of the ductus arteriosus and fluid overload.

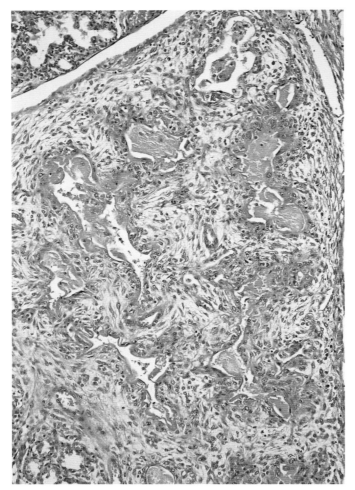

Figure 2.10 Yellow hyaline membranes in a premature infant with hyperbilirubinaemia.

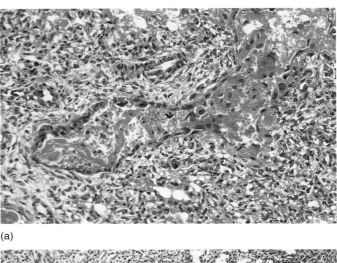

(a)

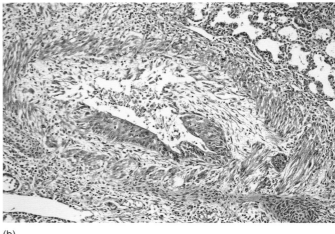

(b)

Figure 2.11 Bronchopulmonary dysplasia. (a) A bronchiole is lined by atypical regenerative epithelium. Hyaline membranes are seen in the bronchiolar lumen. Adjacent alveolar tissue shows interstitial fibroblast proliferation. (b) A bronchiole shows mucosal thickening by cellular fibrosis and there is squamous metaplasia.

It represents disordered prolongation of the healing phase of hyaline membrane disease in which the original damage is augmented by the supportive therapy. Interstitial oedema persists and granulation tissue develops in the walls of the airways and alveoli, progressing to interstitial fibrosis. The air/blood barrier is thickened and the alveolar capillaries are reduced in number. There is also organisation of the hyaline membranes and intraluminal fibrosis leads to the obliteration of many bronchioles. Regenerative hyperplasia is evident in the epithelium of alveoli, bronchioles and bronchi, often with metaplastic changes (Fig. 2.11). Distal air spaces are lined by cuboidal type II pneumocytes or atypical elongated cells which represent type II cells differentiating into type I. Severe squamous metaplasia is often evident in the larger airways. The epithelial changes resolve with time and in babies who survive longer than 3 months, the changes are more marked in the lung parenchyma. The changes are often patchy and consist of fibrotic airless areas of lung tissue alternating with distended or even emphysematous areas (Fig. 2.12). Fibrosis predominates in babies who die in the first 2 months and emphysema in those who survive 1 year or more.[69] Long-term survivors generally have impaired lung function.[70] They also show hypertrophy of the right ventricle.[71]

These may be considered the classic features of bronchopulmonary dysplasia, as described in infants born at about 32 weeks gestation. However, with improved therapy, most such babies now survive and autopsy is today largely limited to extremely immature infants, those born at about 24–26 weeks gestation. The pathological findings in these children differ sufficiently from the classic picture described above to warrant the introduction of a new term, chronic lung disease of early infancy. That the features differ from the classic ones described above should occasion no surprise given the dramatic changes that take place in the normal lung between 22 and 32 weeks gestation. This period encompasses the change from the canalicular to the saccular phase of lung development.

Chronic lung disease of early infancy is characterised by large simple airspaces lined by undifferentiated cuboidal cells and separated by cellular fibroelastic septa of even thickness. Mean linear intercept counts are low indicating reduced

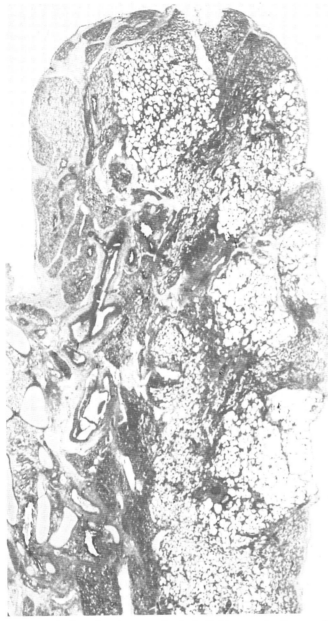

Figure 2.12 Bronchopulmonary dysplasia. Solid areas of collapse and fibrosis alternate with lighter distended areas. (Reproduced by permission of Dr W Geddie, Toronto, Canada.)

numbers of airspaces and arrested alveolar development. The squamous metaplasia and alternating areas of collapse and overinflation seen in bronchopulmonary dysplasia are not well represented in chronic lung disease of infancy.[72,73]

Surfactant protein deficiency and related disorders

The surfactant deficiency underlying the great majority of cases of hyaline membrane disease is attributable to immaturity of the lung but the infantile respiratory distress syndrome is also seen in a few mature babies who have an inherited defect in surfactant production.[74,75] The best known of these involves faults in surfactant protein B synthesis.[76–79] Various mutations of the surfactant protein B gene have been identified, resulting in considerable molecular and phenotypic variability.[80,81] These babies may die with hyaline membrane disease or bronchopulmonary dysplasia or survive the neonatal period only to develop changes that resemble pulmonary alveolar proteinosis or cholesterol pneumonitis (see pp. 316, 317).[76,82] It seems likely that in protein B deficiency the alveolar proteinosis is due to excessive amounts of surfactant being secreted in order to compensate for its defective protein content. As in idiopathic alveolar proteinosis there is an initial stage of endogenous lipid pneumonia, representing macrophage ingestion of the excess surfactant. Electron microscopy shows abnormal type II cell inclusions: these lack their normal whorled lamellae and resemble those described in mice in which the surfactant protein B gene has been disrupted.[83,84] The diagnosis of surfactant protein B deficiency may be established by immunostaining bronchoalveolar lavage material or lung tissue for the various surfactant proteins.

Abnormalities involving surfactant protein C have also been reported,[85] again with considerable phenotypic variation. Some cases have exhibited the changes described in chronic pneumonitis of infancy (see below),[86] while others have been adults displaying various patterns of interstitial pneumonitis.[87]

An absence of surfactant lamellar bodies from type II alveolar cells in a term infant who developed respiratory distress soon after birth and died at 23 days of age despite respirator support may represent a further error in surfactant production.[88] In this child all surfactant proteins were demonstrated and a defect in surfactant phospholipid synthesis or lamellar body assembly was postulated. This condition has subsequently been reported in siblings, suggesting that it has a genetic basis.[89]

Other conditions that lead to respiratory distress in term infants include congenital alveolar capillary dysplasia (misalignment of pulmonary vessels, see p. 72) and acinar dysplasia (type 0 congenital pulmonary airway malformation, see p. 59).

Interstitial emphysema

This condition is a form of barotrauma and in infancy is often a complication of mechanical ventilation. High ventilatory pressures rupture the alveolar walls and permit air to enter the interstitial tissue. The air is seen particularly in the abundant connective tissue that surrounds the pulmonary artery and bronchiole in the centre of the acinus and forms the interlobular septa. Lines of bubbles are seen through the pleura, outlining the lung lobules. Blebs may project from the pleura and cyst-like spaces up to 3 cm in diameter are found on the cut surface of the lung (Figs 2.13, 2.14).[90–92] Pneumothorax and surgical emphysema of the mediastinum and neck frequently accompany interstitial emphysema. The air may track into the other serosal cavities causing pneumopericardium or pneumoperitoneum. Rarely, large subpleural cysts develop.[93] In some cases, the changes resolve spontaneously whereas in others, they persist and may require excision of affected tissue.[94]

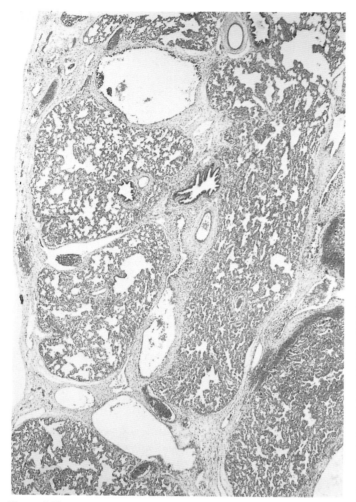

Figure 2.13 Interstitial emphysema. Air-filled spaces are seen in the interlobular septa.

Microscopically the differential diagnosis is from congenital lymphangiectasia (see p. 75). This can be extremely difficult, not least because the air tracks within lymphatics as well as the surrounding connective tissue.[95] It is therefore helpful if the nature of the content of the cysts, gaseous or fluid, is ascertained at necropsy. If the emphysema has been present for a few days before death, the diagnosis is simplified by the development of a foreign body giant cell reaction to the air (Fig. 2.15). The presence of interstitial emphysema has been used forensically as evidence of live birth.[96]

Tracheobronchomalacia acquired in infancy

Tracheobronchomalacia (softening of the major airways) may be congenital or acquired but the two are often confused because the condition is most commonly acquired as a complication of congenital lung disease or its treatment – notably intubation.[96a] This section is concerned with acquired disease. Congenital tracheobronchomalacia is dealt with below. The acquired disease is seen most commonly in premature babies who are intubated because of respiratory distress. Airway infection may

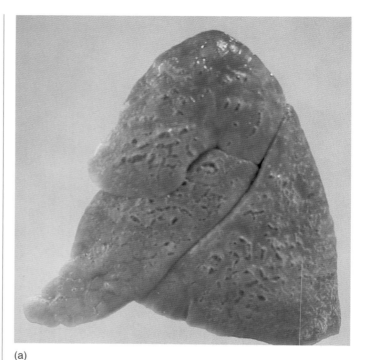

(a)

(b)

Figure 2.14 Interstitial emphysema. (a) Lines of air bubbles are seen through the pleura, outlining the lung lobules. (b) Cyst-like spaces are seen on the cut surface of the lung.

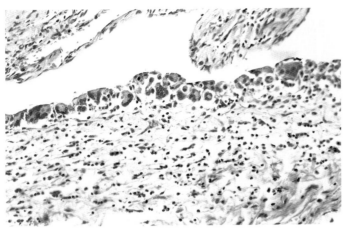

Figure 2.15 Interstitial emphysema. Within a few days the cysts are lined by a foreign body giant cell reaction to the air.

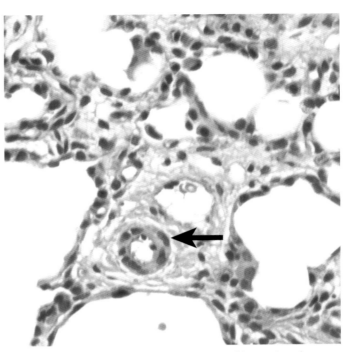

Figure 2.16 Persistent pulmonary hypertension of the newborn in a case of alveolar capillary dysplasia (see p. 72). A pulmonary artery showing marked medial hypertrophy is present within underdeveloped alveolar walls (arrow).

also contribute to tracheobronchomalacia being acquired in infancy. Other causes include pressure from congenital abnormalities such as pectus excavatum (see p. 77), bronchogenic cyst or an aberrant artery. Whatever its cause, tracheobronchomalacia causes undue collapsibility of the airways and, hence, respiratory obstruction. Histopathological examination shows fibrous replacement of the tracheobronchial cartilages.

Persistent fetal circulation (persistent pulmonary hypertension of the newborn)

In this condition, the high pulmonary blood pressure of the fetus fails to fall at birth and right to left shunting through the foramen ovale and ductus arteriosus continues in neonatal life.[97] The incidence of the condition is about 1 in 1000 live births and prior to the introduction of nitric oxide therapy the mortality was about 50%. Autopsy studies show that the muscular pulmonary arteries have a thickened media and that muscle extends into small peripheral arteries that are not normally muscular (Fig. 2.16).[98] The condition may be idiopathic or secondary to a wide variety of neonatal cardiopulmonary disorders, including hyaline membrane disease, asphyxia, meconium aspiration and diaphragmatic hernia. The idiopathic cases are poorly understood but autopsy has shown that some are secondary to alveolar capillary dysplasia (see p. 72) that was undetected until autopsy.[99,100] All these underlying causes reduce the stimuli that normally initiate pulmonary vascular dilatation at birth, namely pulmonary expansion, raised pulmonary oxygen tension and lowered pulmonary carbon dioxide tension. Notable among the agents that mediate the vasodilatation is nitric oxide (endothelium-derived relaxation factor) and the inhalation of low levels of this gas appears to reverse the hypoxaemia of persistent pulmonary hypertension of the newborn.[101,102]

Chronic pneumonitis of infancy

Chronic pneumonitis of infancy is a disease of full-term infants of either sex whose mothers experienced uncomplicated preg-

nancies and deliveries.[103] The infants are normal at birth but cough, respiratory distress and a failure to thrive develop at ages varying from 2 weeks to 11 months (average 3.6 months). Radiographs show a predominantly interstitial pattern of opacification. The prognosis is variable, some of the children recovering spontaneously and others dying of respiratory failure within 3 months of the onset of symptoms.

Biopsy shows alveolar wall thickening with a variety of airspace abnormalities. There is little inflammation. The alveolar wall thickening is due to interstitial spindle cell proliferation and type II epithelial cell hyperplasia. Collagen is not a feature in the early stages but the disease may progress to interstitial fibrosis. Within the alveolar lumen, macrophages are increased and there is often an accumulation of granular eosinophilic material in which acicular cholesterol crystal clefts may be seen. The macrophages may contain haemosiderin or have a foamy cytoplasm (Fig. 2.17).

The aetiology is unknown and may be multifactorial. It has been suggested that the condition represents recurrent or poorly cleared infection,[103] but there is no firm evidence of this. The changes within the airspaces often resemble those of alveolar proteinosis (see p. 317), suggesting that causes of this disease in infancy such as surfactant protein B or C deficiency[76–79,85] (see above) and lysinuric protein intolerance[104–106] may be responsible. Gastro-oesophageal reflux with aspiration is another possibility and has been identified in children reported as showing a combination of endogenous lipid pneumonia, cholesterol granulomas and alveolar proteinosis.[107,108] These children were older than those reported as having chronic pneumonitis of

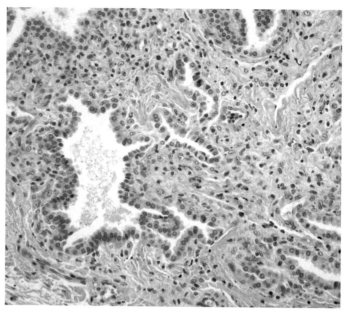

Figure 2.17 Chronic pneumonitis of infancy. The alveolar walls are thickened by immature connective tissue cells; there is little interstitial inflammation. Type II pneumocytes are hyperplastic and there is proteinaceous debris in the airspaces.

infancy but had similar pathological features. Similar cases have been reported by others in the past.[109–112]

Cellular interstitial pneumonitis[113,114] and pulmonary interstitial glycogenosis[115]

Cellular interstitial pneumonitis shows less marked interstitial thickening than chronic pneumonitis of infancy (see above) and lacks the type II cell hyperplasia and alveolar changes seen in the latter. It also appears to have a better prognosis. However, whether this means that the two represent separate conditions[86] or are variations of one[113,114] is debatable. However, those that distinguish the two equate cellular interstitial pneumonitis with what has been described as pulmonary interstitial glycogenosis,[86] a term that was coined when vacuoles in the interstitial cells were shown to represent glycogen.[115]

Idiopathic interstitial pneumonia in childhood

Interstitial lung disease is less well characterised in children than in adults and no classification is entirely satisfactory. However, it is useful to divide these diseases into those unique to infancy (e.g. persistent tachypnoea of the newborn and chronic pneumonitis of infancy), those of known aetiology (e.g. aspiration syndromes, infections, bronchopulmonary dysplasia and hypersensitivity pneumonia) and those of unknown aetiology (Fig. 2.18).[116] The first two groups are discussed elsewhere, leaving only the idiopathic interstitial pneumonias to be dealt with here.

Several groups report series of children with cryptogenic fibrosing alveolitis but most of these ante-date the recognition of non-specific interstitial pneumonia (NSIP) and the introduction of the ATS/ERS consensus classification of diffuse parenchymal lung disease in adults described in Chapter 6 (see p. 263). When the criteria recommended in this classification are applied to the paediatric cases it is found that usual interstitial pneumonia (UIP) is exceptionally rare in children.[116,117] This may explain why cryptogenic fibrosing alveolitis is reputed to have a much better prognosis in children than in adults. Most childhood cases have the pattern of NSIP rather than UIP. In adults, NSIP is suspected of being multifactorial and its recognition in children may add hitherto undiscovered gene mutations to the list of possible causes.

Lymphoid interstitial pneumonia is also more common in childhood, where it is nearly always associated with either connective tissue disease or immunodeficiency, both congenital and acquired.[116,117] It is a well described complication of paediatric AIDS, occurring in over 30% of children infected perinatally by HIV. Desquamative interstitial pneumonia is rare and its outcome worse in children, especially in infancy[118] and those with familial disease.[119] The aetiology is different in children and is probably multifactorial. Some cases represent inborn errors of metabolism such as surfactant B deficiency and lipid storage diseases.[120] Cryptogenic organising pneumonia is exceptionally rare in children and respiratory bronchiolitis has not been reported in infants.

Wilson–Mikity syndrome

This syndrome consists of late neonatal respiratory distress of obscure aetiology, typically coming on in the first month of life of premature babies. A lack of respiratory symptoms in the early postnatal period distinguishes the Wilson–Mikity syndrome from bronchopulmonary dysplasia. The onset of symptoms was 5, 10, 18, 25 and 35 days after birth in the five patients originally described by Wilson and Mikity.[121] Three of the babies died (27, 62 and 232 days after the onset of symptoms) and necropsy showed interstitial mononuclear cell infiltration and fibrosis, cuboidal hyperplasia of the alveolar epithelium, breakdown of alveolar walls, distortion of the alveolar architecture and overdistension. All five babies were premature (average birth weight 1370 g) and oxygen enrichment is recorded in four of the case histories. The suspicion exists that this syndrome is related to bronchopulmonary dysplasia (see above). An alternative view relates it to perinatal infection.[122,123]

DEVELOPMENTAL DISORDERS[124]

Laryngeal atresia

This condition is usually due to cartilaginous overgrowth just below the vocal cords leaving only a narrow channel between the pharynx and trachea that is insufficient to permit respiration. Viewed from above, the larynx appears normal but

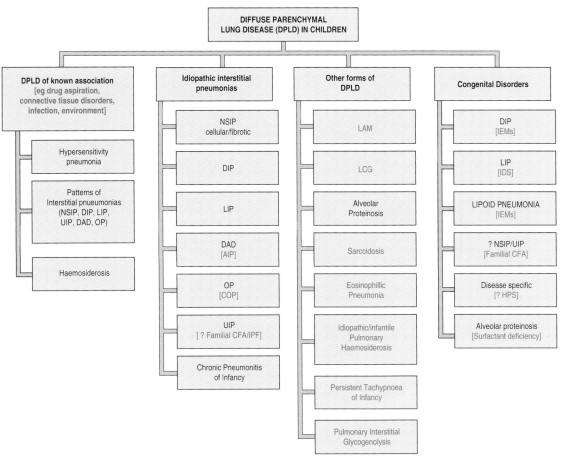

Figure 2.18 Histopathological classification of diffuse parenchymal lung disease (DPLD) in children. Histopathological patterns are in black and clinical correlates in red. DIP, desquamative interstitial pneumonia; LIP, lymphoid interstitial pneumonia; NSIP, non-specific interstitial pneumonia; DAD, diffuse alveolar damage; AIP, acute interstitial pneumonia; OP, organising pneumonia; COP, cryptogenic organising pneumonia; CFA, cryptogenic fibrosing alveolitis; IPF, idiopathic pulmonary fibrosis; LAM, lymphangioleiomyomatosis; LCG, Langerhans cell granulomatosis; UIP, usual interstitial pneumonia; IEM, inborn errors of metabolism; HPS, Hermansky–Pudlak syndrome; IDS, immunodeficiency syndrome. (Redrawn from Clement A et al. Chronic interstitial lung disease in immunocompetent children. Eur Resp J 2004; 24:686–697.)

attempts at intubation are unsuccessful and the baby quickly asphyxiates. *In utero* diagnosis may be possible because the lungs are often hyperplastic[125] and therefore hyperechogenic, in which case an immediate tracheostomy undertaken before the cord is clamped may prove life-saving. However, the condition is often associated with other congenital abnormalities, notably those comprising Fraser's syndrome.

Laryngeal webs may also be congenital, the majority involving the anterior glottis. They show a strong association with the velocardiofacial syndrome (chromosome 22q11.2 deletion). Subglottic stenosis is usually the result of prolonged intubation but may be due to a congenital abnormality of the cricoid cartilage.

Tracheal aplasia

With total or partial absence of the trachea, the main bronchi either communicate only with each other or with the oesophagus.[126] A minor degree of tracheal hypoplasia, with both the sagittal and coronal diameters being reduced, may be seen in Down's syndrome.[127] (The normal diameters of the adult trachea are given on p. 63, under 'Mounier–Kuhn's syndrome of tracheobronchomegaly', a genetic disorder which generally becomes evident in adult life.)

Tracheal stenosis

Tracheal stenosis may result from intrinsic or extrinsic lesions, which may be congenital or acquired. Congenital intrinsic stenosis may take the form of a gradual tapering, an isolated segmental narrowing or a membranous web, or be due to a nodule of ectopic oesophageal tissue. Congenital extrinsic compression may be due to various anomalies of the great vessels forming (vascular) rings or a sling around the trachea (see p. 482). The left pulmonary artery sling syndrome may form part of a (tracheal) ring-sling complex in which the tracheal cartilages form complete rings, the left bronchus is short and the right is long (bronchial pseudoisomerism).[128] The complete cartilage rings represent an absence of the posterior membranous part of the trachea (Fig. 2.19) and the abnormally long trachea is consequently narrowed, the stenosis generally being funnel-shaped. This abnormality is difficult to correct surgically and

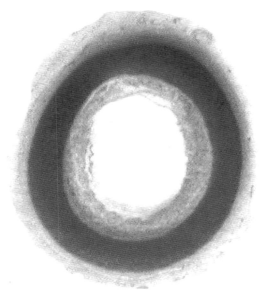

Figure 2.19 Tracheal stenosis due to segmental absence of the posterior membranous portion so that the cartilaginous plates form complete rings. In this patient the tracheal stenosis was associated with an aberrant left pulmonary artery forming a sling round the trachea, the two abnormalities making a 'ring–sling' complex. (Specimen provided by Dr M Kearney, Tromso, Norway.)

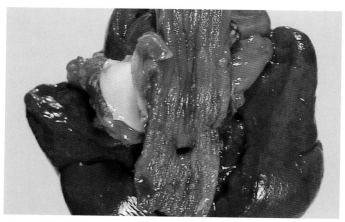

Figure 2.20 The oesophagus opened from the rear to show the orifice of a tracheo-oesophageal fistula towards its lower end. (Reproduced by permission of the late Dr AH Cameron and of Dr F Raafat, Birmingham, UK.)

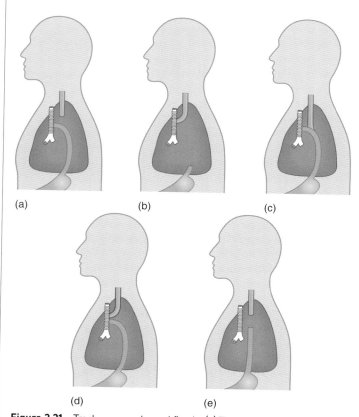

Figure 2.21 Tracheo-oesophageal fistula. (a) The arrangement found in 87% of cases where the upper oesophagus ends blindly and the lower oesophagus joins the trachea. (b–d) Rare variants of tracheo-oesophageal fistula. (e) Oesophageal atresia without fistula.

the prognosis is poor. The trachea normally has 22 cartilages. More are generally seen in the ring-sling complex and fewer in infants with a congenitally short neck. A congenitally short trachea may not be recognised until the seventh decade.[129]

Tracheo-oesophageal fistula

The mesodermal separation of those parts of the primitive foregut destined to become oesophagus and trachea may be incomplete resulting in a tracheo-oesophageal fistula (Fig. 2.20). Separation of trachea and oesophagus normally proceeds in a cephalad direction and if this is incomplete, the two may communicate. Usually the proximal part of the oesophagus ends in a blind sac and the distal part takes origin from the lower part of the trachea, but the anatomy varies (Fig. 2.21). Histological examination shows that abnormalities in the wall of the trachea extend beyond the fistula; there is often widespread loss of cartilage and squamous metaplasia.[130,131] Tracheal communication with remnants of the branchial clefts (branchial cysts) is also recorded.[132] Occasionally it is a bronchus that communicates with the oesophagus.[133]

Congenital tracheobronchomalacia[134]

Tracheobronchomalacia (softening of the major airways) may be congenital or acquired but the two are often confused because the condition is most commonly acquired as a complication of congenital disease (e.g. cardiovascular abnormalities compressing the airways) or its treatment – notably intubation.[96a] Acquired tracheobronchomalacia has been dealt with above

(see p. 46) and this section is confined to congenital tracheobronchomalacia, a condition in which there is softening of the airway cartilages, often as part of a generalised chondrodystrophy seen in several skeletal dysplasia syndromes, e.g. Kniest dysplasia.[135] The trachea and bronchi may be affected alone or

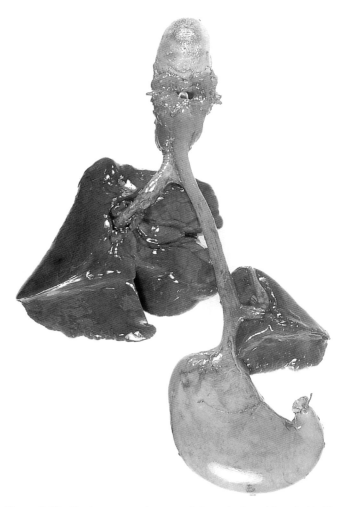

Figure 2.22 The lungs, oesophagus and stomach viewed from behind to show the right main bronchus arising from the lower oesophagus. (Reproduced by permission of the late Dr AH Cameron and of Dr F Raafat, Birmingham, UK.)

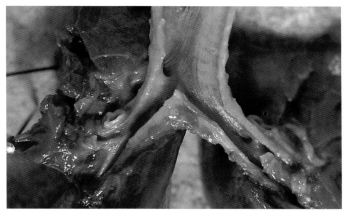

Figure 2.23 Origin of the right upper lobe bronchus from the trachea, which has been opened anteriorly. (Reproduced by permission of the late Dr AH Cameron and of Dr F Raafat, Birmingham, UK.)

in combination. Other causes of congenital tracheobronchomalacia include the presence of oesophageal remnants in the wall of the trachea, which is generally seen in association with oesophageal atresia and tracheo-oesophageal fistula.[131]

Tracheobronchomalacia causes undue collapsibility of the airways and, hence, respiratory obstruction. However, as a cause of respiratory obstruction, congenital tracheobronchomalacia is less common than focal absence of airway cartilages, the supposed basis of both congenital bronchiectasis (Williams–Campbell syndrome, see p. 62) and infantile lobar emphysema (see p. 70).

Abnormal bronchial branching and pulmonary lobation

Main bronchi may be displaced so that one or both whole lungs arise from the alimentary tract rather than the trachea (Fig. 2.22).[126] This often accompanies tracheal agenesis and probably represents a variety of tracheo-oesophageal fistula (see above),

but a bronchobiliary fistula (connecting the biliary and tracheobronchial trees, usually near the carina) may be part of a duplication of the upper alimentary tract from the level of the fistula to the ampulla of Vater.[136,137] Bile causes intense inflammation of the bronchial tree and in infancy the combination of cough with bile-stained sputum forms a distinctive clinical picture indicative of this type of fistula. An unusual case of bronchial diverticulosis possibly represents abnormal bronchial branching.[138]

Abnormalities of the lobar bronchi include a tracheal right upper lobe bronchus, either displaced or supernumerary (Fig. 2.23), a double upper lobe bronchus and an accessory cardiac lobe bronchus arising from the intermediate bronchus. There is a high incidence of tracheal upper lobe bronchus in association with the tetralogy of Fallot.[139] A 'bridging bronchus' crossing the mediastinum from left to right represents origin of the right lower lobe bronchus from the left bronchial tree.[140]

Abnormalities of segmental bronchi include double bronchi to the apical segment of either upper lobe, origin of the apical segmental bronchus of the right upper lobe from the trachea, either displaced or supernumerary, an absent right upper lobe apical segmental bronchus and separate origin of the apical segmental bronchus of the left lower lobe from the main bronchus. A crossover lung segment is one with bronchial and arterial connections from the other side.[141–143] Usually the crossover is from right to left, the right lung is hypoplastic and the venous drainage anomalous, a variant of the 'scimitar' syndrome (see p. 74). These are features that crossover lung segment shares with the equally rare condition 'horseshoe' lung, where there is fusion of the lungs behind the heart and in front of the oesophagus.[143–146] However, unlike 'horseshoe' kidney, there is no fusion of the lungs; there are separate pleural cavities and the crossover segment lies in a pleural recess behind the heart that communicates with the pleural cavity on the side from which the segment derives.[142,143]

Abnormal lobation of the lungs does not imply an abnormal pattern of bronchial branching: lack or incomplete development

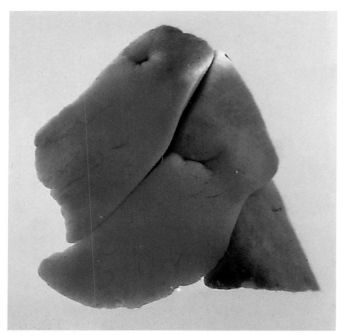

Figure 2.24 Abnormal lobation of the left lung. Extra fissures partly separate the apical segments of both lobes and the complete posterior basal segment of the lower lobe. (Reproduced by permission of the late Dr AH Cameron and of Dr F Raafat, Birmingham, UK.)

Box 2.1 Relative frequency of abnormalities of pulmonary lobation[147]

Right	Left
Deficient transverse fissure 25%	Lingular fissure 25%
Superior accessory fissure 18%	Superior accessory fissure 2%
Medial basal fissure 10%	Medial basal fissure 18%
Other 2%	

The abnormalities may be complete or partial and in 20% of cases they are multiple.

---

of one or more interlobar fissures is common despite the presence of five lobar bronchi. Extra fissures separating segments off as extra lobes are also common, particularly the lingula and the medial basal and apical segments of the lower lobes (Box 2.1, Fig. 2.24).[147] Fissures accommodating blood vessels may also be found, so that an azygos lobe may be formed by the parasagittal separation of the medial part of the right or left upper lobes by the azygos and hemiazygos veins respectively. Absence of a lobe (and its bronchus) is rare.

Bronchopulmonary isomerism represents symmetry of the lungs and bronchi, with both sides having the pattern of either the normal right lung or the normal left lung. As emphasised above, lobation is an unreliable indicator of whether a lung is 'right' or 'left'. This can however be assessed by examining the extrapulmonary bronchi and pulmonary arteries. It will be remembered that the right main bronchus is shorter than the left and enters the lung behind the pulmonary artery whereas the

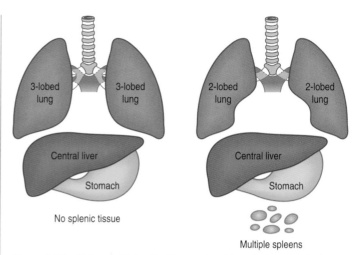

Figure 2.25 Right- and left-sided isomerism. Note the symmetrical extrapulmonary bronchoarterial anatomy (compared with the normal asymmetrical arrangement; see Figs 1.1b, p. 2 and 10.11, p. 482).

longer left main bronchus is 'hyparterial', crossing behind the main left pulmonary artery to enter the lung below the artery. Bronchopulmonary isomerism is often associated with atrial isomerism, anomalous pulmonary veins and abnormalities of the spleen and liver (Fig. 2.25).[139,148] The Ivemark asplenia syndrome consists of bilateral right-sidedness with two morphologically right lungs, absence of the spleen, a symmetrical liver, malrotation of the gut and a variety of cardiac abnormalities including a common ventricle, totally anomalous pulmonary veins and bilateral superior venae cavae and right atria. Bilateral morphologically left lungs are found in association with multiple minute spleens (polysplenia), a symmetrical liver, malrotation of the gut, partially anomalous pulmonary venous drainage and cardiac septal defects. Either right- or left-sided bronchopulmonary isomerism may be associated with multiple spleens of varying size (anisopolysplenia). Although non-familial, Ivemark's syndrome is confined to males whereas the other isomerism syndromes may affect either sex.

Bronchogenic and other foregut cysts

Bronchogenic cysts, recognisable by cartilage and glands in their wall and a lining of respiratory epithelium (Fig. 2.26), are a variety of foregut duplication cysts. They are usually situated in the mediastinum close to the carina (51%) but may be found in the right paratracheal region (19%), alongside the oesophagus (14%), the hilum of the lung (9%) or a variety of other locations (7%) including the substance of the lungs and even beneath the diaphragm.[149–154] Occasionally, air-fluid levels are demonstrated radiographically suggesting a connection with the airways. Cysts lined by respiratory epithelium but lacking cartilage in their walls should be regarded as undifferentiated foregut cysts (also termed simple congenital cysts). These differ from type I congenital cystic adenomatoid malformations as the

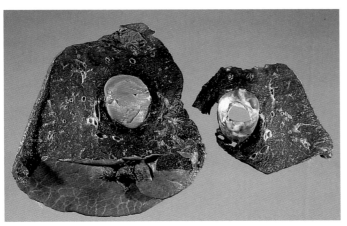

Figure 2.26   An intrapulmonary bronchogenic cyst. On the left the cyst is filled by mucus. On the right the mucus has been removed to show the cyst wall. (Reproduced by permission of Dr M Jagusch, Auckland, New Zealand.)

Box 2.2 Pulmonary 'cysts' in infancy and childhood[161]	
Developmental	**Non-developmental**
Bronchogenic and other foregut cysts[a]	Pneumatocoele
	Bronchiectasis
Sequestration	Interstitial emphysema
Congenital cystic adenomatoid malformation	
Lobar 'emphysema'	
Bronchial atresia	
Lymphangiectasia	

[a]Generally mediastinal rather than pulmonary. Other mediastinal cysts include thymic, pericardial, lymphatic (cystic hygroma) and teratomatous ('dermoid') cysts.

---

latter show polypoid infoldings, mucus cell hyperplasia and disordered parenchymal growth with smaller cysts resembling bronchioles (see p. 59).[155] Congenital lung cysts are often not discovered until adult life, either as an incidental radiographic finding or because of complications, which include infection, haemorrhage and, in rare instances, neoplastic transformation.[156–158] Occasionally, they may be mimicked by low-grade neoplasms exhibiting secondary cystic change.[159]

Enterogenous cysts are another variety of foregut cyst. Oesophageal and gastroenteric (duplication) varieties are recognised, the former being the more common. Oesophageal cysts are wholly intramural and are lined by a squamous or respiratory-type epithelium. Thoracic gastroenteric cysts may be associated with others situated in the abdomen. They are recognisable by a gastric, intestinal or squamous (oesophageal) epithelial lining, a muscle coat and an absence of cartilage. They are usually situated in the posterior mediastinum or, as they may be associated with vertebral malformations, even within the spine, when they are termed neurenteric cysts.[160] Other varieties of lung cyst encountered in childhood are listed in Box 2.2.[161]

Bronchial atresia

This anomaly is generally detected radiographically in an asymptomatic individual: the age range is therefore wide, the average age being 17 years.[162–165] The radiological appearances are virtually diagnostic, consisting of an ovoid hilar opacity, most commonly in the left upper lobe, with branches radiating out into a distal area of hyperinflation.

The opacity represents a distended, mucus-filled bronchus that is continuous with the distal airways but has no connection with the more proximal airways, the corresponding one of which ends blindly. Infection may result in inflammation and fibrosis. The interruption to the airway may take the form of a

membrane, a fibrous cord or a gap. The distal hyperinflation is due to collateral ventilation and air-trapping. Failure to identify the atresia may lead to the changes being wrongfully identified as mucous plugging. Bronchial atresia differs from infantile lobar emphysema (see p. 70) in that it is focal and does not affect a whole lobe. The continuity of the cyst with the distal airways and the hyperinflation of the distal lung distinguish bronchial atresia from bronchogenic cyst, but the two conditions are occasionally associated.[166]

Pulmonary aplasia

Absence of one lung (Fig. 2.27) is not uncommon, but absence of a lobe (as distinct from left-sided isomerism, see above) or of both lungs is distinctly rare. The bronchi may also be absent or there may be a rudimentary stump, an important point in unilateral aplasia as secretions tend to pool in the stump, become infected and spill over to infect the sole lung.[167] In bilateral pulmonary aplasia, the trachea ends blindly and the pulmonary artery joins the aorta. Aplasia is often associated with other malformations and if the aplasia is unilateral, these are often on the same side of the body.[168–170] In unilateral aplasia the single lung is enlarged and contains twice the normal number of alveoli, but the bronchi are normal.[171] Nevertheless there is a significant reduction in vital capacity and exercise tolerance.[168]

Pulmonary hypoplasia

Hypoplastic lungs are small but normal in form and it is possible that some cases are misdiagnosed as atelectasis. Hypoplasia of the lungs signifies that the alveoli are reduced in number or size. This may be assessed by counting the intercepts made by alveolar walls on a line from the terminal bronchiole to the interlobular septum.[172,173] Alternatively, the lungs may be weighed. Normal right and left lung weights at term are 21 and 18 g, respectively (see Table 1.1, p. 3), but hypoplasia is best considered to be present in term babies when the combined lung/body weight ratio is less than 0.012.[174] The reduction in alveoli may be associated with fewer airway generations, the

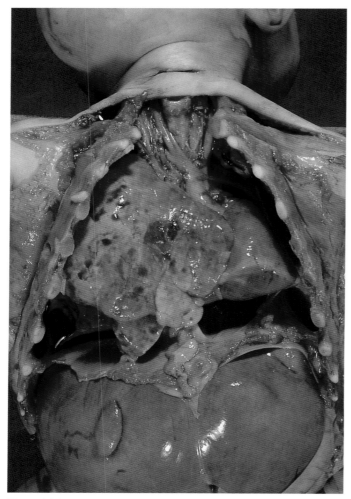

Figure 2.27 Left-sided pulmonary aplasia. The left chest cavity contains only the heart, which is partly overlapped by the anterior border of the right lung. (Reproduced by permission of the late Dr AH Cameron and of Dr F Raafat, Birmingham, UK.)

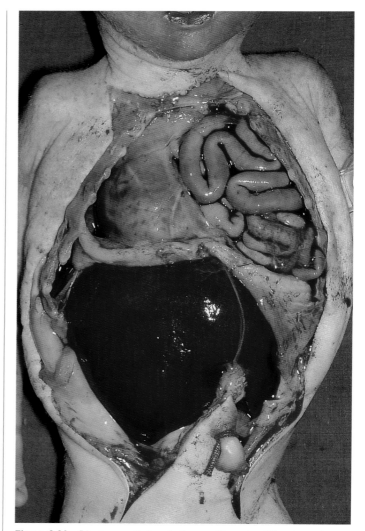

Figure 2.28 Diaphragmatic hernia. Loops of bowel and the stomach filling much of the left side of the chest. (Reproduced by permission of Dr GA Russell, Tunbridge Wells, UK.)

degree of loss depending upon how early lung development was impaired. Development of airways down to the terminal bronchioles is complete by 16 weeks and the whole gas conductive system is complete by birth, unlike the alveoli and alveolar ducts, which continue to grow throughout infancy and into childhood. It follows that correction after birth of such causes of hypoplasia as diaphragmatic hernia may permit growth of alveoli but not airways.[175]

Hypoplasia of the lungs is seldom an isolated finding. It is usually associated with a variety of other malformations.[176] These include diaphragmatic defects, renal anomalies, extralobar pulmonary sequestration and severe musculoskeletal disorders. Most of these associations have a causal relationship (see below) but some, such as that with Down's syndrome[177] and the low set ears of Potter's syndrome (see below), are not readily explained. Lung growth before birth is dependent upon blood supply, availability of space, respiratory movements taking

place *in utero* and fluid filling the airways. The causes of pulmonary hypoplasia therefore include the following:

- congenital abnormalities of blood vessels supplying the lungs, as in pulmonary valve stenosis
- compression of the lungs by intrathoracic masses, as with herniation of abdominal viscera through a congenital diaphragmatic defect (Figs 2.28, 2.29)
- compression of the lungs due to deformities of the thorax such as Jeune's asphyxiating thoracic dystrophy (see p. 77). Because the lungs continue to grow after birth, infantile scoliosis may also cause postnatal hypoplasia[178,179]
- lack of respiratory movements due to the antenatal onset of neuromuscular diseases such as myotonic dystrophy
- oligohydramnios, caused by either chronic leakage or deficient production of amniotic fluid. The mechanism whereby oligohydramnios causes pulmonary hypoplasia

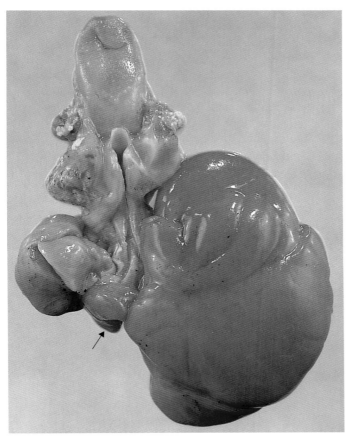

Figure 2.29 Diaphragmatic hernia. The left lung, seen as a small nodule (arrow) between the right lung and the heart, is hypoplastic.

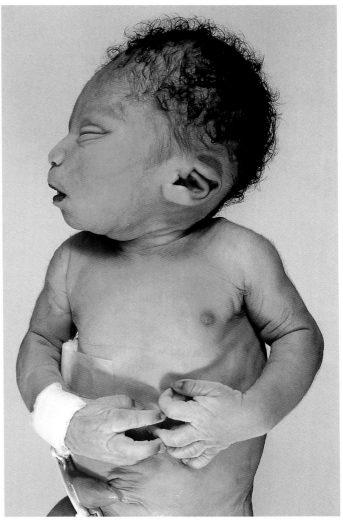

Figure 2.30 Potter facies consisting of low set ears and a small hooked nose is seen in association with renal agenesis and pulmonary hypoplasia. (Reproduced by permission of the late Dr AH Cameron and of Dr F Raafat, Birmingham, UK.)

could again be compression of the lungs, but manometry shows that amniotic pressure is reduced rather than raised in oligohydramnios.[180] Loss of lung liquid is probably more important, being implicated by the demonstration that experimental tracheal ligation prevents the adverse pulmonary effects of oligohydramnios,[181] and by the observation that human fetuses with renal agenesis do not develop pulmonary hypoplasia if there is also laryngeal atresia.[182] Indeed, laryngeal atresia is recorded in association with pulmonary hyperplasia rather than hypoplasia.[125] Lung liquid therefore appears to act as a stent and thereby provide internal support essential to proper lung development. Fetal urine contributes greatly to amniotic fluid and renal agenesis and urethral stricture are important causes of oligohydramnios-associated pulmonary hypoplasia. The Potter syndrome consists of abnormal facies (Fig. 2.30), pulmonary hypoplasia and renal agenesis: oligohydramnios due to the renal agenesis is generally thought to be the cause of the pulmonary abnormality,[183] although a lack of renal metabolites has also been proposed.[28]

Hypoplasia is evident on antenatal scans and some of these causes are amenable to various surgical interventions before birth. Thus, diaphragmatic herniae have been repaired *in utero*, the fetal trachea has been occluded by the insertion of a balloon catheter (to retain lung liquid) and lung cysts have been drained into the amniotic cavity by the insertion of a catheter.

Ectopia

Two categories of ectopia need to be considered – ectopia of non-pulmonary tissues in the thorax and ectopia of lung tissue outside the thoracic cavity. Pleural endometriosis (see p. 494) and splenosis (see p. 720), teratomas of the lung (see p. 666) and traumatic embolism of bone marrow, liver or brain tissue to the lung (see p. 411) are dealt with separately.

Ectopia of adrenocortical tissue,[184] thyroid (lacking C-cells)[185] and liver[186] has been described in the lung and pancreatic tissue has been noted within intralobar sequestrations with gastrointestinal connections.[187,188] Ectopic striated muscle is recorded in sequestered and hypoplastic lungs[189–191] and occasionally as an isolated pulmonary abnormality,[192] sometimes tumour-like.[193] Rarely, a whole kidney may be found above the diaphragm but outside the lung.[194]

Ectopia of glial tissue within the lung is well recognised.[195–201] Nodules of glial tissue may be implanted in the embryonic lung by aspiration of amniotic fluid in some cases of anencephaly[195,197,198] and in the absence of anencephaly by embolisation due to intrauterine trauma[200] or, with small macerated fetuses, merely normal uterine contractions.[201] The ectopic glial tissue lacks neurones but may contain cysts lined by ciliated epithelium: devoid of their normal mesenchyme these primitive lung buds fail to develop bronchial cartilage and muscle or differentiate into alveoli. Two patients with unexplained glial ectopia survived surgery for neonatal respiratory distress to reach adult life, one with mental retardation[196] and one without.[199]

Ectopia of lung tissue in the neck, the abdomen or the chest wall is often termed herniation, but is probably due neither to raised intrathoracic pressure nor deficiencies in the thoracic boundaries, as often proposed, for the one causes pulmonary hypoplasia and the other leads to herniation of structures into, rather than from, the thorax. Although it is often associated with skeletal or diaphragmatic abnormalities (Fig. 2.31) it appears to represent genuine ectopia. Some examples of abdominal pulmonary ectopia represent extralobar sequestration as well as ectopia.[202]

Pulmonary sequestration

The term sequestration indicates that a portion of lung exists without appropriate bronchial and vascular connections. Classically, no airway connects the lesion to the tracheobronchial tree and the blood supply is systemic, but the separation may be purely vascular.[203] Alternatively, an 'airway' may connect the sequestration to the oesophagus or stomach in a complex 'bronchopulmonary-foregut malformation',[204] or ectopic pancreatic tissue may be present within the sequestration.[187,188] Sequestrations may be associated with a variety of other malformations such as foregut duplications and venous anomalies such as the scimitar syndrome,[154,188,205] as well as sometimes showing the histologic features of congenital pulmonary airway malformations.[206,207] There is therefore a spectrum of abnormalities associated with pulmonary sequestration.[208–210] Pathologists dealing with these malformations should report on all their connections (bronchial, arterial and venous) and on the presence of any associated abnormalities.

Two forms of sequestration are recognised, extralobar, which has its own covering of visceral pleura and intralobar, which is embedded in an otherwise normal lung (Fig. 2.32). The first was called an accessory lobe until Pryce[211] described the intralobar variety, related it embryologically to accessory lobe and coined the term 'sequestration'. Intralobar sequestrations are much the more common. The major differences between the two types are summarised in Table 2.2.

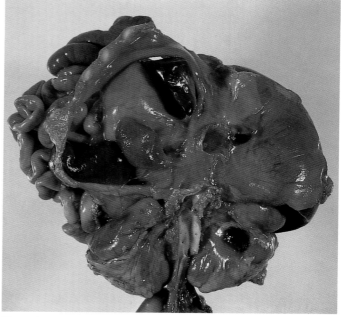

Figure 2.31 Ectopia of the lungs. The diaphragm and abdominal contents are viewed from above. The left hemidiaphragm is largely absent and through this deficiency dark unaerated lung tissue and abdominal viscera can be seen. (Reproduced by permission of the late Dr AH Cameron and of Dr F Raafat, Birmingham, UK.)

Table 2.2 Pulmonary sequestration		
	Intralobar sequestration	*Extralobar sequestration*
Age at diagnosis	50% over 20 years (15% asymptomatic)	60% less than 6 months (10% asymptomatic)
Sex ratio (M : F)	1.5 : 1	4 : 1
Typical site	Posterior basal segment of the left lower lobe	Between the left lower lobe and the diaphragm
Arterial supply	Systemic	Systemic
Venous drainage	Pulmonary	Systemic
Associated anomalies	Uncommon (6–12%)	Common (50–70%)
Aetiology	Uncertain whether developmental or acquired	Developmental anomaly

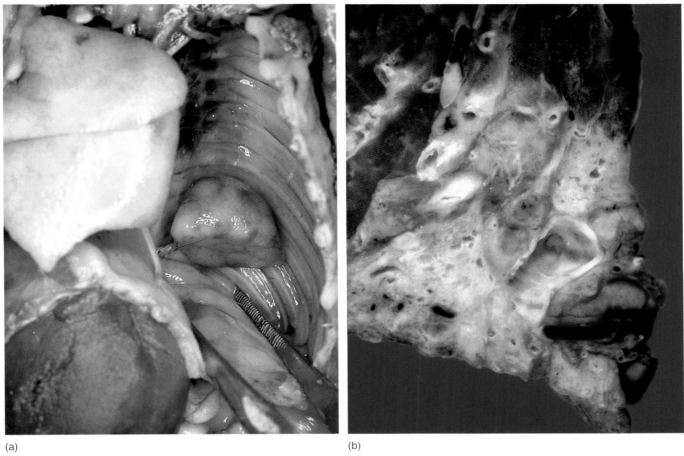

(a)　　　　　　　　　　　　　　　　　　　　　　(b)

Figure 2.32 (a) Extralobar sequestration. The left lung has been reflected to the right to reveal a separate nodule of lung tissue lying against the ribs. The sequestration is completely detached from the rest of the lung but has a thin pedicle containing systemic blood vessels through which it is supplied from the aorta. (Reproduced by permission of Dr GA Russell, Tunbridge Wells, UK). (b) An intralobar sequestration shows a systemic vessel entering the lateral aspect of the lobe and feeding a well demarcated partly solid and partly cystic area of abnormal lung parenchyma. A cystically dilated airway is seen centrally, consistent with lack of communication with the bronchial tree.

Extralobar sequestration is generally detected in infancy because of associated malformations and affects males four times more frequently than females. In contrast, intralobar sequestration is often an isolated anomaly and therefore escapes recognition until adult life and has a male to female ratio of only 1:5.[212]

Intralobar sequestrations are typically located in the posterior basal segment of the left lower lobe and extralobar sequestrations beneath the left lower lobe. There is often a defect in the diaphragm and about 15% of extralobar sequestrations are abdominal. The veins leaving an extralobar sequestration generally join the azygos or other systemic veins whereas an intralobar sequestration usually has normal pulmonary venous connections.

The embryological basis of pulmonary sequestration is poorly understood. Indeed some workers believe that the intralobar variety is an acquired condition in which the aberrant artery is a dilated systemic collateral to a focus of infection, basing this on the relative sparsity of malformations associated with this type of sequestration and its rarity in perinatal autopsies.[213,214] However, although the incidence of associated anomalies is lower than with extralobar sequestrations (50–70%), it is still appreciable (6–12%),[215] and the rarity of the condition in neonates may be because it is easily overlooked until there is cystic degeneration or infection. Advocates of a congenital aetiology generally propose that accessory lung buds are fundamental to both forms of pulmonary sequestration and liken them to intestinal duplications,[210] but are undecided whether the aberrant systemic arteries play a causative role by pulling on the developing lung[211] or are merely compensatory to a primary failure of the pulmonary arteries.[216] The absence of a bronchial connection has led some to link sequestration to bronchial atresia (see p. 53), bronchogenic and simple congenital lung cysts (see p. 52), infantile lobar emphysema (see p. 70) and congenital cystic adenomatoid malformation (which is dealt with next),[208–210] while on the basis of cases in which there is communication with the oesophagus or stomach it has been proposed that the lesions are congenital foregut malformations,[204,217] attributable to a fault within embryonic organiser centres.[218]

Although there is no bronchial connection, small bronchi may be found within the sequestration. The lung tissue in the lesion is often poorly developed and cystically dilated (Figs 2.33, 2.34). The cysts are lined by columnar or cuboidal epithelium, or the sequestered lung may be entirely composed of structures resembling bronchioles surrounded by alveolar ducts and alveoli, histologically resembling a type 2 congenital cystic adenomatoid malformation (see below). Mucous distends the multiple intercommunicating spaces and the lesion appears solid radiographically, unless air enters through an aberrant bronchial connection or, in the case of intralobar sequestration, by collateral ventilation, when fluid levels are often seen. In the absence of associated anomalies, detection is unlikely unless a radiograph is undertaken for some other reason or infection ensues, this being most likely when there is air entry. When operation is contemplated for any cystic or suppurative lesion of the lungs it is important that sequestration be considered and the possibility of unusual blood vessels investigated angiographically. Inadvertent severance of anomalous systemic arteries has led to fatal haemorrhage, while ligation of anomalous veins from adjacent non-sequestered lung has led to infarction of potentially salvable tissue.

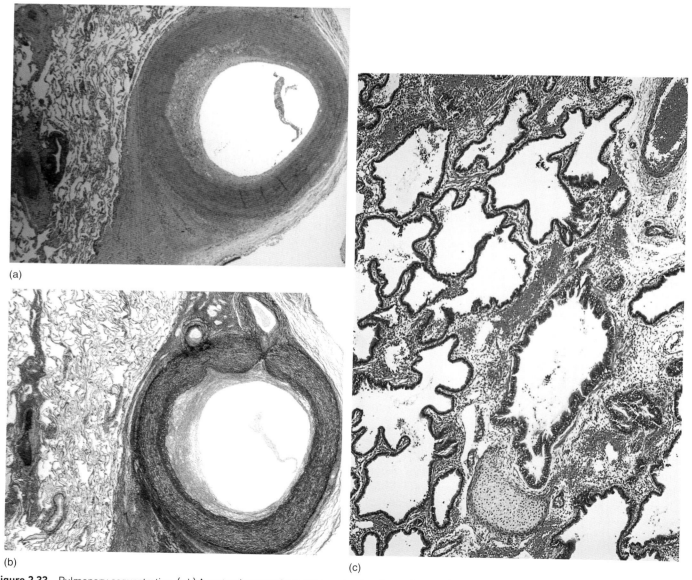

(a)

(b)

(c)

Figure 2.33   Pulmonary sequestration. (a,b) A systemic artery forms the predominant vascular supply, a pulmonary artery (left) showing fibrous obliteration. (c) In a separate case, the sequestered lung tissue is poorly developed and resembles a type 2 cystic congenital adenomatoid malformation. (b, elastin van Giesen stain).

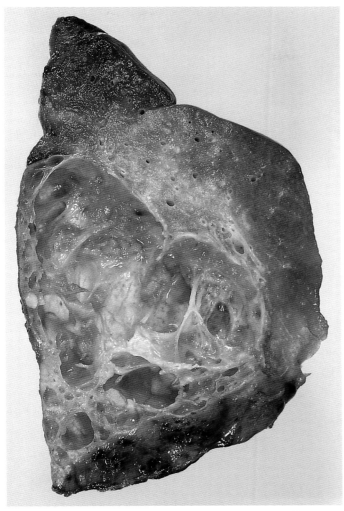

Figure 2.34 Intralobar sequestration in which the sequestered lung tissue is cystically dilated. (Reproduced by permission of the late Dr AH Cameron and of Dr F Raafat, Birmingham, UK.)

Congenital cystic adenomatoid malformation (congenital pulmonary airway malformation)

The term congenital cystic adenomatoid malformation encompasses a spectrum of conditions, the inter-relationship of which is contentious. The aetiology of the condition is obscure but a maturation defect is envisaged.[219–221]

Early reports date from 1897[222] but it was not until 1949 that the term congenital adenomatoid malformation was introduced.[223] It was applied to a newborn infant's greatly enlarged and apparently airless left lower lobe, which microscopically consisted solely of bronchiole-like structures so that it had an adenomatoid appearance. Subsequently, cystic and intermediate (microcystic) varieties were described.[219] These were initially numbered I–III but with the addition of two further lesions the numbering switched to 0–4, it now being envisaged that the spectrum represented malformations of five successive groups of airways, type 0 being tracheobronchial and type 4 alveolar.[155,159,224,225] This is not wholly convincing because except for type 4, which tends to be peripheral, the lesions are not obviously distributed along the bronchial pathway. Types 0 and 3 tend to affect a whole lobe or lung. Furthermore, although cartilaginous airways are a prominent feature of the type 0 ('tracheobronchial') lesion, the complete absence of bronchioles and alveoli cannot be overlooked. For type 0 lesions, previous workers concentrated upon the undifferentiated stroma that separates the cartilaginous airways and preferred the term acinar dysplasia, implying a developmental error affecting the periphery of the lung rather than the central airways.[226–228] A further development is the introduction of the term congenital pulmonary airway malformation in place of congenital cystic adenomatoid malformation. This is advocated because only the originally described type 3 lesion is adenomatoid and only types 1, 2 and 4 are cystic.[155] Many cases of the commoner types have now been reported.[159,219,224,229–233]

Some workers envisage an even wider 'sequestration spectrum' encompassing both sequestration and congenital cystic adenomatoid malformation[210] and others extend this by adding bronchial atresia, bronchogenic cysts, simple foregut cysts and infantile lobar emphysema.[209] Congenital cystic adenomatoid malformation is also associated with abnormalities of the bronchial tree on occasion.[234] Rare examples of extralobar sequestrations containing tissue with the distinctive features of congenital cystic adenomatoid malformation strengthen the proposed link between these two conditions.[206,207,235] The two differ in that congenital cystic adenomatoid malformation has a pulmonary rather than systemic blood supply.

The five types are compared in Table 2.3 and will now be described individually. Despite the above contentions regarding their inter-relationships and appropriate classification their distinction is important because certain varieties carry a risk of malignant transformation.

Type 0 Congenital pulmonary airway malformation (acinar dysplasia)

This rare form of the anomaly is incompatible with life, being seen in term or premature babies who are cyanosed at birth and survive only a few hours. It is usually associated with cardiovascular anomalies and dermal hypoplasia. The lungs are small and firm throughout. Microscopically, bronchial-type airways that have cartilage, smooth muscle and glands are separated by abundant mesenchymal tissue.

Type 1 Congenital pulmonary airway malformation (cystic type of congenital cystic adenomatoid malformation)

This is the most common type and the one with the best prognosis, as it is a localised lesion that typically affects only part of a lobe and lends itself to surgical resection. The boundary between the lesion and the adjacent normal lobe is sharply delineated but there is no capsule. Presentation usually takes

Table 2.3 Congenital cystic adenomatoid malformation (congenital pulmonary airway malformation)

Type	Proportional incidence	Gross appearance	Microscopy	Other features
0	1–3%	Solid	Pseudostratified ciliated cells Mucous cells Cartilage, glands	Neonates Other malformations Poor prognosis
1	60–70%	Large cysts (up to 10 cm)	Pseudostratified ciliated cells, often with rows of mucous cells	Presentation may be late Resectable Good prognosis except for rare carcinomatous change
2	10–15%	Small cysts (up to 2 cm)	Simple columnar epithelium Striated muscle in 5%	Neonates Other malformations Poor prognosis
3	5%	Solid	Simple cuboidal epithelium	Male neonates Poor prognosis
4	15%	Large cysts (up to 10 cm)	Flattened epithelium	Neonates, infants Good prognosis Uncertain relation to pleuropulmonary blastoma and mesenchymal cystic hamartoma

It is envisaged that the five types differ in the level of airway affected.
Type 0 is described as bronchial, type 1 as bronchial/bronchiolar, type 2 as bronchiolar, type 3 as bronchiolar/alveolar duct and type 4 as peripheral.[155]

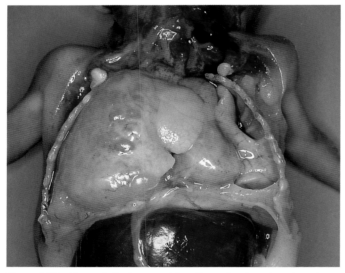

Figure 2.35 Congenital adenomatoid malformation: type 1 cystic variety, *in situ*. (Reproduced by permission of Dr GA Russell, Tunbridge Wells, UK.)

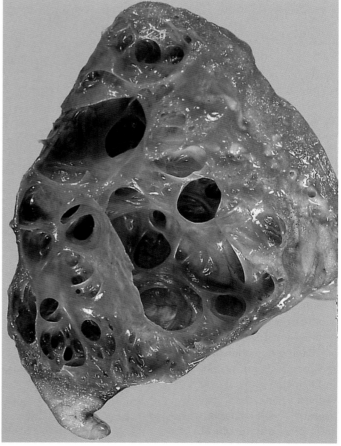

Figure 2.36 Congenital adenomatoid malformation: type 1 cystic variety. (Reproduced by permission of Professor LJ Holloway, Wellington, New Zealand.)

the form of neonatal respiratory distress but the condition may be detected *in utero* by ultrasonography[236] and surgery undertaken soon after birth. Alternatively, recurrent infections in older children or even young adults may prompt initial investigation.[237] Radiographically, air-filled cysts that are usually limited to one lobe compress the rest of the lung, depress the diaphragm and cause mediastinal shift. The cysts range in size from 1 to 10 cm (Figs 2.35, 2.36). The relevant bronchus is often atretic,[209,229,231,234,238,239] yet the cysts are usually radiolucent, presumably due to collateral ventilation. They are lined by pseudostratified ciliated columnar epithelium interspersed with

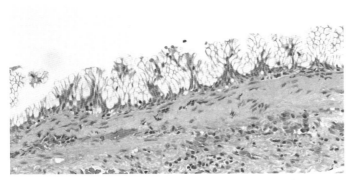

Figure 2.37 Congenital adenomatoid malformation: cystic variety, showing replacement of the respiratory epithelium by rows of mucous cells.

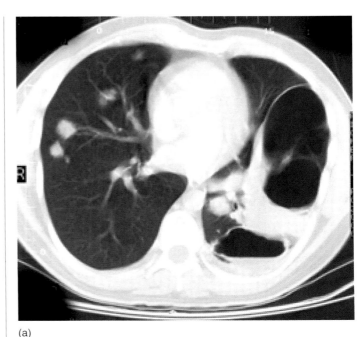

(a)

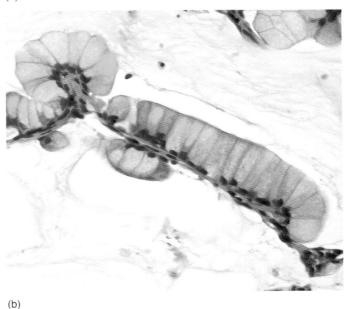

(b)

Figure 2.38 Type 1 congenital adenomatoid malformation. (a) An HRCT of a long-standing type 1 congenital adenomatoid malformation shows foci of consolidation in the ipsilateral lung adjacent to the cyst, with additional nodules of consolidation on the opposite (right) side. (b) Biopsy of the right side shows mucinous bronchioloalveolar carcinoma.

rows of mucous cells (Fig. 2.37),[155] which are probably the site of malignant transformation that occasionally complicates this lesion, usually to mucinous bronchioloalveolar cell adenocarcinoma.[157,240–242] Mucus cell proliferation within the cyst is regarded as hyperplasia whereas extensions of this process into the adjacent alveoli, where it assumes a lepidic growth pattern, is taken to represent bronchioloalveolar cell carcinoma (Fig. 2.38).[159] Genetic studies have shown chromosomal aberrations in the mucous cells similar to those seen in adenocarcinomas encountered in non-smokers.[243] As would be expected of a localised adenocarcinoma of bronchioloalveolar cell pattern, survival following excision is good and metastasis is exceptional.[244]

The sparsity of bronchial cartilage distinguishes this lesion from bronchogenic cyst and the distinctive rows of mucous cells help distinguish it from simple foregut cyst (see p. 52). The distinction from intralobar sequestration (see p. 56) may be difficult but a systemic blood supply would favour sequestration.

Type 2 Congenital pulmonary airway malformation (intermediate type of congenital cystic adenomatoid malformation)

This is the second most frequent type. It generally causes respiratory distress in the first month of life. Associated anomalies such as renal agenesis, cardiovascular defects, diaphragmatic hernia and syrenomelia often have a further adverse effect on the prognosis but occasional cases present later in childhood with infection.[237] It may be identified within extralobar sequestrations.[206,235,245] The lesion is sponge-like, consisting of multiple small cysts as well as solid pale tumour-like tissue (Fig. 2.39). Microscopically, the cysts are seen to comprise an excess of dilated structures resembling bronchioles separated by poorly developed alveoli or alveolar ducts that may be quite sparse (Fig. 2.40).[155] Occasional examples contain striated muscle.[191]

Type 3 Congenital pulmonary airway malformation (solid type of congenital cystic adenomatoid malformation)

This uncommon type occurs almost exclusively in male babies. Some view it as a form of pulmonary hyperplasia, histologically similar to that seen in laryngeal atresia.[225] It is a large, bulky lesion that typically involves and expands a whole lobe, the

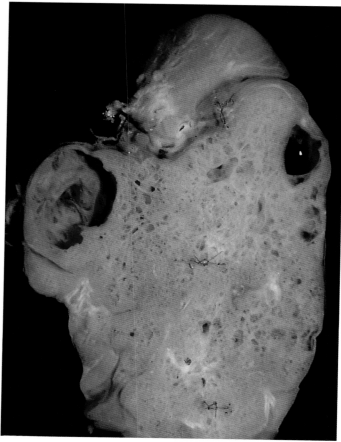

Figure 2.39 Congenital adenomatoid malformation: type 2. (Reproduced by permission of the late Dr AH Cameron and of Dr F Raafat, Birmingham, UK.)

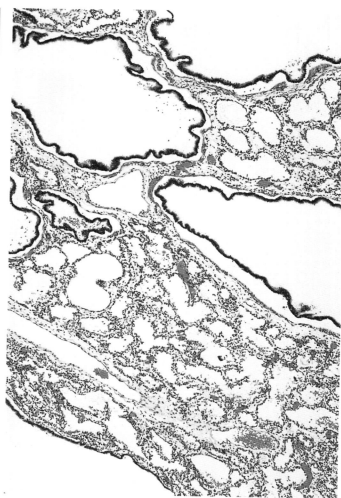

Figure 2.40 Congenital adenomatoid malformation: type 2. There is an excess of bronchioles, which are separated by underdeveloped alveolar tissue. This pattern is also sometimes seen in sequestrations (see Fig. 2.33c).

others being compressed and the mediastinum displaced. The resultant venous compression usually causes the mother to suffer from hydramnios and the baby from generalised anasarca.[236] It also results in hypoplasia of the remaining pulmonary tissue. The prognosis is dependent upon the amount of unaffected lung and hence on the size of the lesion. Microscopically, an excess of bronchiolar structures separated by air spaces that are small, have a cuboidal lining and resemble late fetal lung. There are virtually no arteries within the lesion.[155] Unlike the preceding types there is little or no cystic change.

Type 4 Congenital pulmonary airway malformation

This relatively uncommon type typically presents as infantile respiratory distress or repeated pneumonia in childhood. Radiographically, large air-filled cysts are seen with compression of the other thoracic structures and occasionally pneumothorax. The cysts are peripheral and thin-walled. They are lined by flattened alveolar or bronchiolar epithelial cells resting upon loose mesenchymal tissue (Fig. 2.41). Occasionally the stroma is focally hypercellular and one lesion underwent malignant change to recur as a high grade pleuropulmonary blas-

toma.[246] At present the inter-relationship of these two conditions is uncertain and some now advocate classifying lesions of type 4 CCAM morphology with *any* degree of hypercellularity as type 1 pleuropulmonary blastomas (see p. 612).[247]

Congenital bronchiectasis

Several congenital defects lead to the development of bronchiectasis after birth. These are dealt with in the next section. Conditions characterised by bronchiectasis at birth are less numerous but the Williams–Campbell syndrome falls into this category.

Williams–Campbell syndrome

This syndrome is characterised by bilateral diffuse cylindrical bronchiectasis associated with deficiency of bronchial cartilage.[248–250] There is also panlobular alveolar distension. The

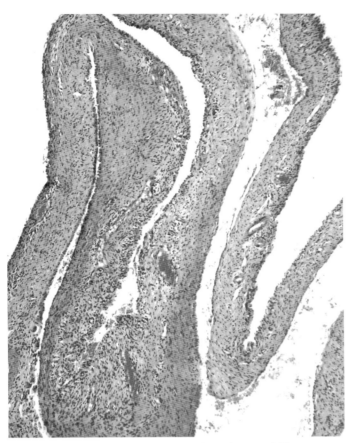

Figure 2.41 Congenital adenomatoid malformation: type 4. The cysts are thin-walled and multiloculated. They are lined by alveolar or bronchiolar cells resting upon loose mesenchymal tissue.

deficiency is similar to that found in infantile lobar emphysema (see p. 70) but more widespread. Secondary infection leads to chronic inflammation and bronchiolitis obliterans and hence confusion with the Swyer–James or Macleod syndrome of hyperlucent lung which, as explained on p. 71, is probably post-infective. The occasional association of other congenital abnormalities,[251] its early onset and rare instances of the disease in siblings all favour a congenital deficiency.[252,253] The most convincing cases are those in which there is only minimal inflammation.

Anomalies promoting bronchiectasis in later life

Certain familial diseases predispose to recurrent respiratory infections and hence bronchiectasis. The bronchiectasis develops after birth but the basic defect is congenital. These conditions are tracheobronchomegaly (Mounier–Kuhn's syndrome), Kartagener's and other primary ciliary dyskinesia syndromes, Young's syndrome and cystic fibrosis. Bronchiectasis is also recorded in a young adult with homozygous α_1-antitrypsin deficiency,[254] which is more often associated with emphysema (see p. 101).

Mounier–Kuhn's syndrome (tracheobronchomegaly or trachiectasis)

In this rare disease, the major airways are dilated by saccular bulges between the cartilages and bronchial clearance is impaired, resulting in recurrent respiratory infection.[255–260] It generally becomes manifest between the ages of 30 and 50 years and occurs predominantly in males.[261] A congenital connective tissue defect with autosomal recessive inheritance is suggested.[262] This is supported by the occasional association of Mounier–Kuhn's syndrome with Ehler–Danlos syndrome,[263] cutis laxa[264] or Kenny–Caffey syndrome.[265] When considering the diagnosis, it is useful to know that in the normal adult, the maximum transverse diameters of the trachea and main bronchi are 20 and 14.5 mm, respectively.[266]

Kartagener's syndrome and primary ciliary dyskinesia

The triad of 'situs inversus, bronchiectasis and sinusitis' was first described in 1904[267] but its usual eponym, Kartagener's syndrome, derives from the Swiss paediatrician who described four cases with these features in 1933.[268] The syndrome was given a firm pathogenetic basis when it was recognised that the respiratory infections were the consequence of a developmental anomaly consisting of a reduced number of ciliary dynein arms (Fig. 2.42).[269] Roughly half of the patients with dynein arm defects do not have situs inversus and it would appear that this ciliary abnormality is associated with random lateralisation of the viscera. The term immotile cilia syndrome was therefore introduced to encompass all patients with a developmental ciliary defect, regardless of their visceral anatomy.[270,271] Later, the term primary ciliary dyskinesia was substituted because the cilia show some movement although they do not beat effectively.[272] The condition is inherited as an autosomal recessive with variable penetrance.

Sperm tails have a similar structure to cilia and dynein arm defects often result in affected males being infertile due to immotility of their spermatozoa.[273,274] Female fertility also appears to be impaired, but the incidence of ectopic pregnancy does not appear to be increased.[275] Some patients are more concerned with their infertility than their respiratory problems, which may be relatively minor.

As well as dynein arm defects, primary ciliary dyskinesia may be caused by absence of ciliary spokes, transposition of one of the outer microtubular doublets of the cilium to replace the central pair, random ciliary orientation or abnormally long cilia (Fig. 2.42b–d).[276–280] These primary ciliary defects must not be confused with acquired ciliary abnormalities, such as compound cilia, which commonly result from infection or chemical injury (Fig. 2.42e). More recently described primary ciliary defects[281,282] require further evaluation. The various primary abnormalities do not affect every cilium and their recognition requires rather tedious electron microscopic quantitation.[283–285] This is only justified if functional studies are abnormal. These include the saccharine test, in which a saccharine particle is placed on the anterior end of the inferior turbinate and the time

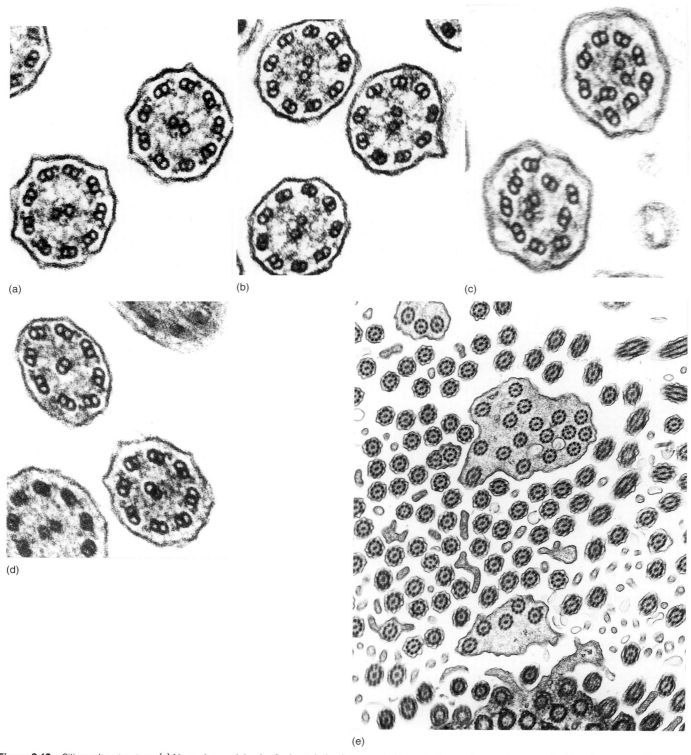

(a)

(b)

(c)

(d)

(e)

Figure 2.42 Ciliary ultrastructure. (a) Normal: an axial pair of microtubules is connected by radiating spokes to nine outer double microtubules (9 + 2 arrangement). Small dynein arms extend from one outer microtubule to one in the adjacent pair. The dynein arms are involved in the outer double microtubules sliding on each other and thereby causing the cilium to beat. (b,c,d) Ciliary dyskinesia syndromes: (b) absent dynein arms, (c) absent spokes, (d) transposition of one of the nine outer doublets to replace the central pair of microtubules, which is absent, so that there are only eight doublets in the outer ring. (e) Compound cilia, a secondary focal abnormality that is to be distinguished from the diffuse congenital abnormalities of the ciliary dyskinesia syndromes. (Reproduced by permission of Professor P Cole and Miss A Dewar, Brompton, UK.)

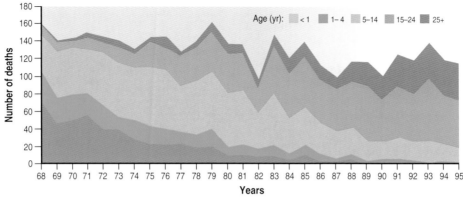

Figure 2.43 Deaths from cystic fibrosis in England and Wales from 1968 to 1995, showing that there has been a gradual increase in longevity. (Reproduced by courtesy of the Lung and Asthma Agency.)

taken for the subject to notice the taste is recorded, and in vitro assessment of ciliary beat frequency, suitable cells for which may be obtained by brushing the back of the nose.[286-289] Where possible, ultrastructural studies should be conducted on more than one occasion or on ciliated cells from different organs,[290] while in adult men, sperm tail ultrastructure may demonstrate a primary abnormality.[273,274] Nasal nitric oxide is greatly reduced in primary ciliary dyskinesia and measurement of this gas in the exhaled breath shows promise as a further screening test. The low levels probably reflect involvement of the nasal sinuses, which are the major source of the gas.[271,288]

Cystic fibrosis

Incidence and inheritance

Fifty years ago, four out of five patients with cystic fibrosis died in the first year of life, whereas today most can expect to survive until the fourth decade (Fig. 2.43).[291] This improvement in survival is attributable to a combination of earlier diagnosis, better management of meconium ileus, dietary control, pancreatic enzyme supplementation, physiotherapy, the introduction of potent antibiotics and the development of specialist centres.

Cystic fibrosis has been reported in all racial groups but is most common in white people (Table 2.4). In Great Britain, it is the most common lethal genetic disorder, affecting 1 in 2500 live births with the gene responsible for the condition being carried by 1 in 25 of the Caucasian population. About 1 in 400 marriages involves two carriers and because transmission is by an autosomal recessive gene, the children of such marriages have a 1 in 4 chance of having the disease. The carriers are entirely normal and apart from the siblings of an affected child, a family history of cystic fibrosis is unusual. Because the homozygotes have only recently survived to sexual maturity and the males are generally infertile due to agenesis of the vasa deferentia, persistence of the condition is puzzling. It suggests that there is either a high mutation rate or the heterozygotes carry some advantage, either in reproductive fitness or resistance to other diseases. One possibility is that the defect minimises dehydration when severe diarrhoeal diseases are contracted.[292]

Table 2.4   Frequency of cystic fibrosis and the carrier state in different populations

Race	Homozygotes	Heterozygotes
UK white	1:2500	1:25
US white	1:3500	1:30
Sweden	1:7700	1:45
US black	1:14000	1:60
US Asian	1:25500	1:80

The gene responsible for cystic fibrosis is located on the long arm of chromosome 7,[293-295] and DNA probes now provide a test by which, in families having an affected infant, it is possible to identify the abnormality in further pregnancies as early as the first trimester.[296] This test has also enabled the identification of carrier status in the healthy siblings of an affected person or in couples contemplating parenthood.[297-299] Although more than 800 cystic fibrosis mutations have been identified, one (δF508) accounts for about 70% of alleles[300] and another (G551D) for a further 5%.[301] The identification of specific genetic defects has led to trials of gene therapy involving the insufflation of the airways with preparations of the normal gene carried within liposomes or on a viral vector.[302-304]

Pathogenesis

Cystic fibrosis is thought to depend upon abnormal secretions,[305] as indicated by its alternative name 'mucoviscidosis' although this term has no direct relevance to the abnormally salty sweat that characterises the condition. Furthermore, the hyperviscous mucous is not the primary abnormality. Ciliary beat frequency and ultrastructure are normal,[306,307] and claims that there is a serum factor that inhibits ciliary function *in vivo* offer no explanation for the intestinal and pancreatic lesions of the disease. It is now known that an abnormality of chloride ion transport underlies both the sweat hypersalinity and the mucus hyperviscosity.[308,309] The genetic abnormalities referred to above affect a protein named the cystic fibrosis transmembrane conductance regulator (CFTR) that acts as a cyclic adenosine monophosphate-regulated chloride channel and thereby controls ion and hence water movement across the cell membrane.[310,311] This protein is made up of 1480 amino acids of which the 508th from the N terminus (phenylalanine) is deleted when there is δF508 gene homozygosity. The abnormal protein is trapped in the endoplasmic reticulum leading to defective ion transport at the apical cell membrane.[312,313] Another variant, G551D, is properly transported to the plasma membrane but is unresponsive to cyclic adenosine monophosphate.[313] Such defects result in excessive re-absorption of water and hence hyperviscosity of mucus and hypersalinity of sweat and mucosal secretions. Embryological development of the vas deferens is also dependent upon proper regulation of chloride channels and about 96% of male patients are infertile due to congenital absence or focal atresia of the vas deferens.[314,315] Female fertility is slightly impaired, probably because the cervical mucus is unduly viscid.

In the airways, hypersalinity impairs the antibacterial action of constituents such as lactoferrin and lysozyme,[316,317] and this, coupled with the difficulty in clearing hyperviscous mucus, inevitably leads to permanent infection and inflammation of the respiratory tract. A deficiency of surfactant apoproteins A and D is a further factor promoting continued bacterial infection.[318] Deoxyribonucleic acid released in large amounts from effete neutrophils[319] polymerises with glycoprotein to exacerbate the hyperviscosity of the mucus. Further neutrophil and bacterial products damage the bronchial wall, resulting in bronchiectasis.

Cystic fibrosis patients benefit from lung transplantation[320] and it is relevant to the pathogenesis that the donor lungs maintain normal membrane ion transport[321] and do not develop the changes found in the explanted lungs.

The phenotypic spectrum associated with mutations of the CFTR gene is now known to extend beyond the classic features of cystic fibrosis and now includes several monosymptomatic diseases such as isolated forms of pancreatitis, agenesis of the vasa deferentia,[322] nasal polyposis[323] or lung disease.[324]

Clinical features

Despite improvements in patient care, repeated pulmonary infection remains the major clinical problem in cystic fibrosis. Bronchopulmonary infection, respiratory failure and cor pulmonale are the usual causes of death in adults,[325] but there are also many extrapulmonary features (Boxes 2.3 and 2.4).[315] Advanced age is no bar to a new diagnosis of cystic fibrosis[326–328] but in 70% of cases the diagnosis is made in the first year of life and the mean age at diagnosis is 3 years. The diagnosis is generally confirmed by a skin test that detects high sodium levels in the sweat, but some mutations are associated with normal sweat salinity.[324] Alternative diagnostic procedures include examination of nail parings for high chloride concentrations using a scanning electron microscope fitted for elemental analysis,[329,330] recognition of an unduly negative potential difference across a mucosal surface, such as that lining the nose,[331] and genetic testing.

Box 2.3 Effects of cystic fibrosis in chronological order

Primary effects	Secondary effects
Meconium ileus	Peritonitis
	Rectal prolapse
Salty sweat	Hyponatraemia
Pancreatic duct obstruction	Failure to thrive
	Steatorrhoea
	Diabetes mellitus
Respiratory	Bronchiectasis
	Recurrent infections
	Hyperactive airways
	Atelectasis
	Subpleural cysts and pneumothorax
	Allergic bronchopulmonary aspergillosis
Hepatic duct obstruction	Biliary cirrhosis
Vas deferens atresia	Male infertility[a]

[a]Atresia of the vasa deferentia is responsible for 6% of obstructive aspermia[314] and 1–2% of male infertility.[315]

Box 2.4 Extrapulmonary manifestations of cystic fibrosis

Cardiac		Cor pulmonale
		Fibrosis of left ventricle
		Enlarged carotid bodies
Gastrointestinal	Upper	Barrett's oesophagus
		Varices (due to cirrhosis)
	Lower	Meconium ileus (leading to perforation, obstruction, prolapse)
		Appendicitis
		Fibrosing colonopathy (due to treatment)
	Liver	Sclerosing cholangitis
		Biliary cirrhosis
	Gall bladder	Cholecystitis and micro-gallbladder
	Pancreas	Pancreatic insufficiency (Steatorrhoea)
		Chronic pancreatitis
		Diabetes mellitus
Kidney		Nephrolithiasis
		Diabetic glomerulopathy
		Immune complex-mediated glomerulonephritis
Genital tract	Male	Atresia of vas deferens
	Female	Multiple follicular cysts
		Cervicitis, mucous gland hyperplasia, vaginitis
		Reduced fertility
Musculoskeletal		Osteoporosis
		Muscle wasting
		Hypertrophic pulmonary osteoarthropathy
		Clubbing
Skin		Acrodermatitis
		Dilation of eccrine and apocrine glands
General		Malnutrition
		Vitamin deficiencies (E, K[a], B12)
		Amyloidosis

[a]Vitamin K deficiency at birth may lead to bleeding.

Bacteriology

The episodic attacks of airway infection represent acute exacerbations of a permanent colonisation of the lower respiratory tract by *Staphylococcus aureus, Haemophilus influenzae* or *Pseudomonas aeruginosa*, which defies eradication with long term antibiotics. This is associated with the emergence of mucoid alginate-producing *P. aeruginosa* mutants that develop into bacterial microcolonies embedded in exopolysaccharide biofilms on the bronchial mucosa, leading to an exaggerated tissue-damaging immune response.[331a,b]

More recently, *Burkholderia* (formerly *Pseudomonas*) *cepacia* infection has also proved troublesome in cystic fibrosis.[332] This plant pathogen was previously regarded as a harmless commensal in man but is now recognised to attack the lungs of patients with cystic fibrosis and hasten their deterioration. *B. cepacia* is resistant to most antibiotics. Acquisition is by person to person transmission and advice based on this that the infected should not mix with other cystic fibrosis patients is very distressing to individuals who derive much comfort from mutual support groups.[333] *Chlamydia pneumoniae* and opportunistic mycobacteria have also been identified as troublesome pathogens in cystic fibrosis.

Immunological abnormalities

Atopy and immunological abnormalities are common in cystic fibrosis but it is uncertain whether these are primary or secondary. They include circulating immune complexes, which are deposited in the respiratory and intestinal tracts and could conceivably contribute to the tissue damage there.[334] These complexes presumably also underlie the cutaneous vasculitis and arthritis that are occasionally encountered in cystic fibrosis.[335] Bronchial hyperactivity is common, possibly due to easier penetrance of the damaged epithelium by common environmental allergens. Serum immunoglobulins are generally raised and there is a high prevalence of positive skin reactions (type I and III) to common allergens such as *Aspergillus fumigatus*.[325,336] The incidence of allergic bronchopulmonary aspergillosis is markedly increased in cystic fibrosis.[337,338] Aspergillomas are rare but the increasing use of immunosuppressive and antipseudomonal drugs in cystic fibrosis has led to an increase in invasive aspergillosis.

Structural changes in the respiratory tract

The earliest histological change in the respiratory tract in cystic fibrosis is mucus plugging of the tracheobronchial glands (Fig. 2.44).[339] This is found in infants who succumb to meconium ileus or its complications and who show no bronchopulmonary inflammation,[340] indicating that it is a primary change. The plugging develops to obstruct bronchi and infection invariably follows (Fig. 2.45), resulting in recurrent attacks of bronchitis, bronchiolitis and ultimately pneumonia. The bronchitis is characterised by secondary hyperplasia of the bronchial glands indistinguishable from that seen in the chronic bronchitis of cigarette smokers.[341,342] There may also be papillary hyperplasia of the bronchial mucosa. The bronchiolitis is accompanied by

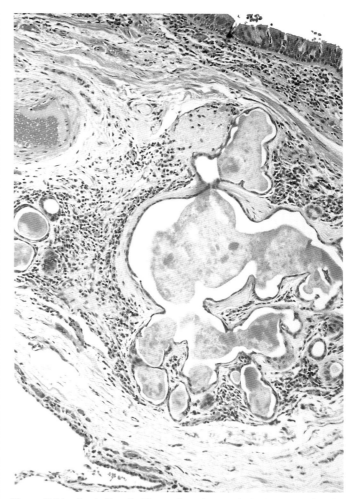

Figure 2.44 Cystic fibrosis. The earliest changes in the lungs consist of plugs of viscid mucus distending bronchial gland ducts.

peribronchiolar fibrosis, which constricts these airways.[343] An obstructive pneumonitis consisting of interstitial inflammation and fibrosis develops.[344] There may also be evidence of organising pneumonia, air-trapping and collapse. The chronic sepsis leads to bronchial ulceration, destruction of the bronchial cartilage and bronchiectasis.[345] At necropsy, pus-filled bronchiectatic cavities, abscesses and areas of pneumonic consolidation are found throughout the lungs (Figs 2.46 and 3.32a, p. 116). The upper lobes are generally more severely affected than the lower.[346] Lymphoid follicles often develop in relation to the bronchiectatic cavities.[341] Air cysts are another frequent finding in older patients.[347] Some of these are bronchiectatic cysts, some have multiple communications with bronchi showing that they are pneumatoceles derived from former abscesses, some represent interstitial emphysema and others are emphysematous bullae. Their rupture largely accounts for the high incidence of pneumothorax that is seen in adults with cystic fibrosis.[347,347a] Attenuated and shortened interalveolar septa may be evident microscopically, resulting in appearances resembling

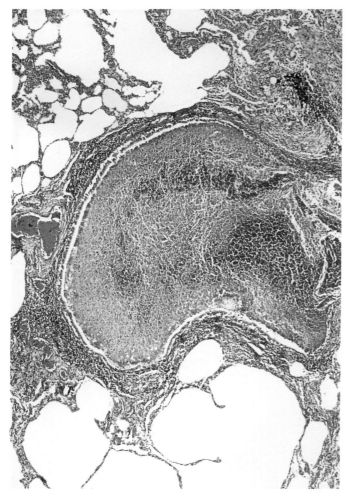

Figure 2.45 Cystic fibrosis. In advanced cases the bronchi are dilated and filled with pus.

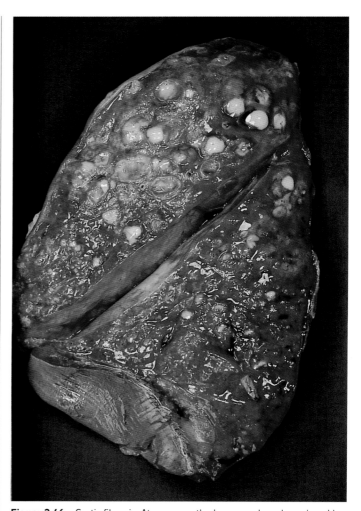

Figure 2.46 Cystic fibrosis. At necropsy the lungs are largely replaced by pus-filled bronchiectatic cavities and abscesses, more marked in the upper lobe.

panacinar emphysema but probably representing retarded postnatal lung growth.[343] In older patients pulmonary hypertension and cor pulmonale may develop.[348,349] Large haemoptyses may occur,[325] probably from the highly vascularised granulation tissue that lines the bronchiectatic cavities and which is supplied by systemic arteries. Nasal polyps are common in cystic fibrosis, but they differ from those of atopic subjects in that they lack eosinophils.[350]

Extrapulmonary disease (Box 2.4)

The many extrapulmonary effects of cystic fibrosis include serious consequences before birth, notably meconium ileus obstructing the fetal bowel to such a degree that the intestine ruptures *in utero* leading to a sterile chemical peritonitis and severe ascites, which may prolong labour. If the child dies during delivery, the deficiency in the bowel wall may have healed but extensive peritoneal calcification is often present and this gives a clue to the nature of the peritonitis. More often meconium ileus causes constipation or intestinal obstruction after birth. If bowel is resected or autopsy undertaken, the intes-

tine is found to be obstructed by hard rubbery meconium and the appropriateness of the term mucoviscidosis can be readily appreciated. Older children and even adults may be similarly affected by a 'meconium ileus-equivalent'. Microscopy shows the bowel to be filled and the crypts of Lieberkuhn distended by mucus (Fig. 2.47). Mucus may also plug the ducts of salivary and labial glands.

Pancreatic disease is a further manifestation of cystic fibrosis. Indeed the term cystic fibrosis was coined specifically for the late changes in the pancreas. The first change is mucus plugging of the pancreatic ducts, which leads to atrophy and fatty replacement of the exocrine portion of the gland. Low-grade inflammation is common and this leads to fibrosis (Fig. 2.48) while the obstructed ducts become cystically dilated. The administration of pancreatic enzymes is possibly responsible for an increasing incidence of colonic strictures. The endocrine portion of the gland is initially spared but eventually even the islets of Langerhans atrophy; diabetes mellitus is a common late result, generally preceded by years of malabsorption.

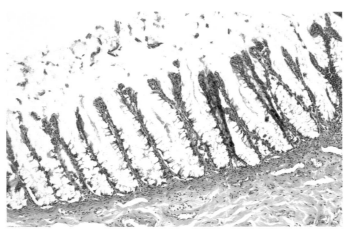

Figure 2.47 Cystic fibrosis. Meconium ileus-equivalent in an adult patient. The crypts of Lieberkuhn are distended by mucus, which also forms a thick coat on the surface.

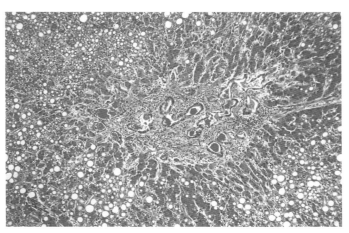

Figure 2.49 Cystic fibrosis. Liver. Small bile ducts are plugged by eosinophilic secretions.

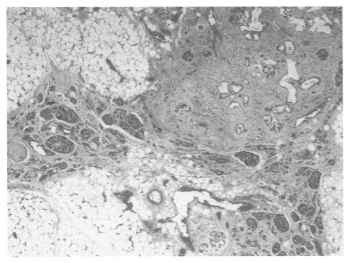

Figure 2.48 Cystic fibrosis. Pancreas. The exocrine portion is reduced to dilated ducts in a fibrous stroma or shows fatty replacement. Islets of Langerhans survive, but these too may eventually atrophy.

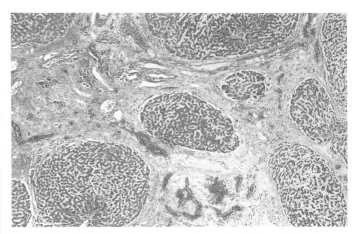

Figure 2.50 Cystic fibrosis. Liver, showing well established cirrhosis.

Hepatic disease has a similar basis to that in the pancreas. Initially small bile ducts are plugged by mucus (Fig. 2.49), leading to biliary cirrhosis (Figs 2.50, 2.51).

Renal disease includes diabetic glomerulopathy, amyloidosis and immune complex-mediated glomerulonephritis. There is also an increase in urinary oxalate excretion, which is linked to the malabsorption and results in microscopic nephrocalcinosis[351] and urolithiasis.[352,353]

Together with salty sweat, atresia of the vas deferens is one of the features of cystic fibrosis that is not based on undue viscidity of mucus. The vasa deferentia are frequently atretic and the patient is consequently sterile.[314,315] At autopsy, the epididymis and testes show obstructive features (Figs 2.52, 2.53) and the vasa cannot be identified or are represented by thin

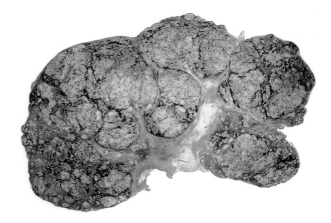

Figure 2.51 Cystic fibrosis. Liver, showing the gross appearances of macronodular biliary cirrhosis.

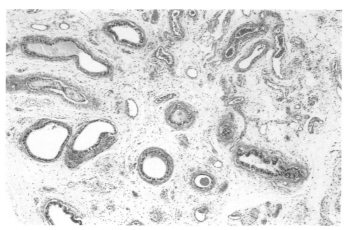

Figure 2.52 Cystic fibrosis. Epididymis, showing glandular dilatation and stromal fibrosis.

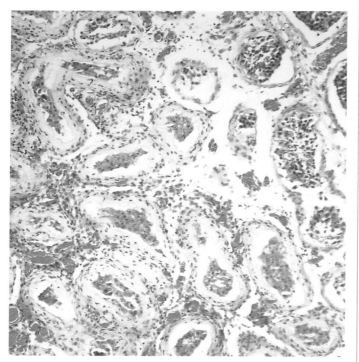

Figure 2.53 Cystic fibrosis. Testis, showing basement membrane thickening but normal spermatogenesis.

fibrous bands. The female genital tract is anatomically normal and patients reach the menarche, although this may be delayed by chronic pulmonary sepsis. However, cervical mucus is abnormal and cervicitis, cervical erosions and cervical mucous gland hyperplasia are commonly found. Nevertheless, pregnancy is possible and with improved support is now becoming more frequent.

Generalised changes include all those classically associated with the secondary effects of cystic fibrosis, including malnutrition, systemic amyloidosis and the immunological

abnormalities referred to above. Thus there may be generalised muscle wasting and osteoporosis. Other changes include hypertrophic pulmonary osteoarthropathy and clubbing and the craniofacial alterations seen in children with nasal obstruction.[354]

Young's syndrome

Young's syndrome consists of sinusitis, bronchiectasis and obstructive oligospermia caused by mucociliary dysfunction in the respiratory tract and epididymis. Spermatozoa accumulate in the head of the epididymis, which is markedly dilated. Ciliary ultrastructure and beat frequency *in vitro* are both normal[355,356] yet *in vivo* tracer studies show impaired mucociliary clearance.[357] The basic defect in Young's syndrome is obscure but it may be hyperviscosity of the respiratory and epididymal secretions.

Congenital 'emphysema'

Emphysema is defined in a later chapter as enlargement of airspaces distal to the terminal bronchiole due to breakdown of their walls. This is not found at birth: so-called congenital emphysema is a miscellany of other conditions in which the lungs are light and airy. A single segment, a lobe, a whole lung or all the lung tissue may be so affected in the neonatal period. Most of these conditions represent alveolar distension rather than destruction. Polyalveolar lobe is another condition in which the organ is large and airy. It too fails to conform to the above definition of emphysema but has been regarded as a type of congenital emphysema and is therefore considered in this section. Familial α_1-antitrypsin deficiency causes true emphysema and is congenital but the onset of the emphysema is not until adult life and this condition is therefore considered later in Chapter 3.

Alveolar distension may be compensatory to collapse or hypoplasia of the adjacent lung,[358] or it may be obstructive.[359] If the obstructed airway supplies a segment of a lobe or less, inflation of the distal lung may be by collateral ventilation, but if a lobar or main bronchus is affected collateral ventilation is not possible and a check valve mechanism is generally invoked to explain the distension. Bronchial atresia (see p. 53) typically affects a segmental bronchus and any distension is focal and due to collateral ventilation, in contrast to infantile lobar emphysema.

Infantile lobar emphysema (congenital lobar emphysema)

Infantile lobar emphysema is due to partial obstruction of the lobar bronchus leading to air-trapping. The other lobes are thereby compressed and mediastinal structures displaced causing severe respiratory distress, which generally necessitates early surgical resection. The condition generally affects neonates but cases occasionally come to light in adult life.[360,361] Males are affected more than females but the condition is not

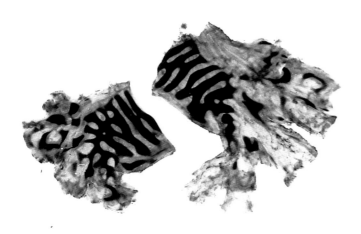

Figure 2.54 Infantile lobar emphysema. A fatal case, in which the bronchi have been dissected out, their cartilages stained with toluidine blue and the tissues cleared. Bronchi to the right are devoid of cartilage. (Reproduced by permission of the late Professor BE Heard, Brompton, UK.)

familial. The condition affects the left upper lobe in about half the cases, with the right middle and right upper lobes being involved in most of the remainder and the lower lobes in less than 10%.

The obstruction may be caused by intrinsic abnormalities of the bronchus, such as mucosal flaps, mucus plugs or twisting of the lobe on its pedicle, or by external compression from causes such as a bronchogenic cyst or abnormal blood vessels.[359] In the absence of such causes, a deficiency of bronchial cartilage is generally postulated. This may be demonstrated in the resected lobe by dissecting out the bronchi, staining the cartilage with toluidine blue and clearing the specimen with potassium hydroxide or an organic solvent such as cedarwood oil or xylol (Fig. 2.54).[362–364]

In practice, the cause is frequently not identified. Explanations based on simple air trapping are possibly too facile as the lobe is not only distended to its normal maximum but hyperinflated. This implies a connective tissue defect at the alveolar level,[365] although none has been convincingly demonstrated so far. About 20% of patients also have congenital cardiac anomalies and it is possible that the relationship is causal.[366] The bronchi supplying the lobes that are predominantly affected (the left upper and right middle lobes) are in particularly close proximity to pulmonary arteries and if these are distended, as in acyanotic congenital heart disease, they are liable to be compressed, the narrow, pliable bronchi of neonates being particularly susceptible (see Fig. 10.10, p. 481).

The causes of external compression cannot be identified by examining the excised lobe and it is therefore essential that as well as paying particular attention to the lobar bronchus the pathologist is aware of the clinical, radiological and surgical findings.

Polyalveolar lobe

A polyalveolar lobe has a normal number of conductive airways but an increased number of alveoli in each acinus.[367] The affected lobe is enlarged, light and airy but individual alveoli are not increased in size. The number of alveoli in an acinus is best assessed by counting the intercepts made by alveolar walls on a line from the terminal bronchiole to the interlobular septum.[172] The number of alveoli depends on the age of the child, but in general, fetuses have a radial count of 2 to 5, infants have a count of 5 to 10 and children a few years old have a count of 10 to 12. These figures are increased by as much as three to five times in a polyalveolar lobe.

Clinically, polyalveolar lobe resembles infantile lobar emphysema and often the true diagnosis only becomes apparent on examination of the excised specimen.[368] Affected babies are dyspnoeic and chest radiographs show lobar enlargement with displacement of the other thoracic viscera. The prognosis following surgery is good and it may be preferable to operate early rather than late to maximise compensatory lung growth.

Hyperlucent lung (hypertransradiant lung; Swyer–James or Macleod syndrome)

This is a condition in which the normal radiographic markings of the lungs, which represent the pulmonary blood vessels, are diminished. The syndrome was originally thought to be due to unilateral hypoplasia of the pulmonary artery but vascular shutdown in response to hypoventilation caused by post-infective bronchiolitis obliterans is now the favoured explanation.[369,370] The airway obstruction may add an element of distension but in contrast to the forms of overinflation discussed above the affected lung is not enlarged. This is compatible with an infective aetiology as this could well impair the normal postnatal growth of the lung at the alveolar level.

Hamartomas

Hamartomas represent abnormal mixtures of tissue elements, or an abnormal proportion of a single element normally present in an organ resulting in changes that are tumour-like but not neoplastic. Pleuropulmonary examples include vascular malformations (see below), neurofibromatosis (see pp. 488, 629) and mesenchymal malformation of the chest wall (see p. 721). However, the so-called 'chondroid hamartoma' shows an increasing incidence with age and is probably a true neoplasm. It is therefore dealt with in the tumour section (see p. 615). It is also debatable whether the so-called *mesenchymal cystic hamartoma* is a valid entity. It was first described in 1986,[371] since then only a few more cases have been reported.[372–377] Some appear to have represented metastases of endometrial stromal sarcoma[378,379] while others have resembled the type 4 congenital pulmonary airway malformation (see p. 62) or a low-grade type 1 pleuropulmonary blastoma (see p. 612). The term *muscular hamartoma* is often applied to small focal proliferations of smooth muscle that are occasionally observed incidentally in the lung. They are generally stellate in outline and almost always the muscle is intermingled with fibrous tissue. Such lesions more likely represent old scars in which there is prominent reactive smooth muscle hyperplasia. Diffuse changes of this nature are often seen in end-stage diffuse pulmonary fibrosis and the term 'muscular cirrhosis of the lung' has been used for this (see p. 272). Genuine examples of smooth muscle hamartomas are reported in the lung, sometimes associated with similar lesions in the bowel and liver,[380] but they are much rarer than focal scars.

Congenital peribronchial myofibroblastic tumour

This rare lesion is found in the newborn, sometimes causing heart failure or hydrops fetalis.[381,382] It forms a localised mass that shows a characteristic peribronchial infiltrate of spindle cells of mixed smooth muscle and fibroblast phenotype. The proliferation spreads from the bronchoarterial bundles to involve the pleura and interlobular septa. It is suggested that it develops from the condensed mesenchyme that surrounds the proximal bronchi at about the 12th week of intrauterine development. The condition is probably akin to other organ-specific lesions that are collectively termed fibromatoses of early infancy, rather than representing a neoplasm or hamartoma, as implied by some of the other terms that have been applied – congenital leiomyosarcoma, bronchopulmonary fibrosarcoma, massive congenital mesenchymal malformation.

Anomalies of the pulmonary blood vessels

Unilateral absence of a pulmonary artery

Absence of one of the main pulmonary arteries leads to the lung on that side receiving only systemic blood, either through anomalous arteries or enlarged bronchial arteries.[383,384] Either lung may be affected and the defect may be isolated or associated with other cardiovascular anomalies, typically tetralogy of Fallot with an absent left pulmonary artery and patent ductus arteriosus with an absent right pulmonary artery.[383] Patients with an isolated anomaly of this type may lead a normal life or symptoms may not arise until adult life, when they are generally attributable to pulmonary infection or to bleeding from bronchopulmonary anastomoses.[385–389] Clinically, the condition may be difficult to distinguish from embolic occlusion but an association with other congenital vascular defects would support the diagnosis.[385] Only a short segment of the artery may be lacking and surgical correction may be possible.[390] In other cases, pulmonary arteries may be difficult to identify in lung sections, where they tend to be overshadowed by hypertrophied bronchial arteries, sometimes showing plexiform lesions.[388] Pulmonary hypertension develops in 18% of patients with an isolated defect and more often when there are other vascular anomalies. Relevant to this is the observation that ligation of one main pulmonary artery, for example during pneumonectomy, has little effect on the contralateral vasculature in adults but when the ligation is conducted in the perinatal period the high fetal pulmonary pressure is maintained.[383]

Pulmonary artery stenosis

Stenosis of the main pulmonary artery belongs to the subject of systemic vascular disease but it should be noted that lobar and segmental pulmonary arteries may also be affected and that there may be multiple constrictions.

Dieulafoy's disease

This vascular malformation is best known in the gastrointestinal tract but a few cases affecting bronchial arteries have been described.[391,392,392a] The patients generally present with massive haemoptysis and are found to have an isolated aneurysmally-dilated bronchial artery that has bled into a bronchus (Fig. 2.55).

Anomalous systemic arteries

Anomalous systemic arteries to the lung are an essential feature of pulmonary sequestration. They are also found with pulmonary artery aplasia and arteriovenous malformations, or they may be an isolated abnormality. They are usually small but sometimes the right pulmonary artery arises from the aorta.[393] As well as these congenital anomalies, conditions such as bronchiectasis often acquire a systemic blood supply, usually via enlarged bronchial arteries but also from intercostal or mediastinal arteries if there are pleural adhesions.[394]

Alveolar capillary dysplasia (misalignment of lung vessels)[99,395–399]

This malformation represents a failure of capillaries to extend into the alveolar tissue of the lung and is an unusual cause of persistent pulmonary hypertension and respiratory distress of the newborn. Cases reported to date have all been fatal, survival generally not exceeding a few hours. However, there are anecdotal reports of symptomatic improvement. Many cases show associated gastrointestinal or genitourinary malformations. Occasionally, siblings are affected and an autosomal recessive genetic abnormality has been demonstrated in some cases.

The pulmonary lobules are small and radial alveolar counts are decreased. The alveolar septal connective tissue is increased and alveolar capillaries are greatly reduced (Figs 2.16, p. 47 and 2.56). Those present are in poor contact with the alveolar epithelium, which shows type II cell hyperplasia. The pulmonary veins accompany small pulmonary arteries in the centres of the acini rather than occupying their normal position in the interlobular septa (misalignment of lung vessels. The pulmonary arteries are decreased in number and show increased muscularisation.

Anomalous pulmonary veins

Anomalous pulmonary veins result in blood from the lungs returning to the right side of the heart rather than entering the left atrium. The embryological basis is a failure of the veins within the primitive lungs to switch from draining into chan-

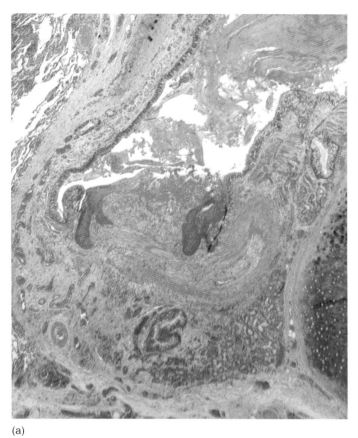

(a)

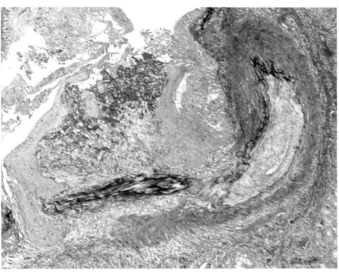

(b)

Figure 2.55 Dieulafoy's disease. (a) Rupture of an aneurysmally-dilated mucosal artery proved to be the cause of intractable haemoptysis that necessitated lobectomy. (b) An elastin stain highlights the eroded bronchial artery. (Case provided by Dr MM Burke, Harefield, UK.)

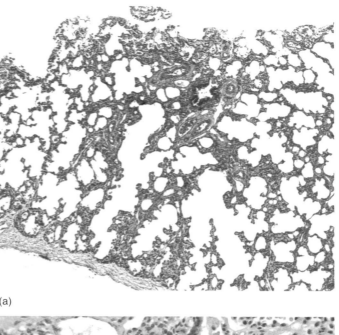

(a)

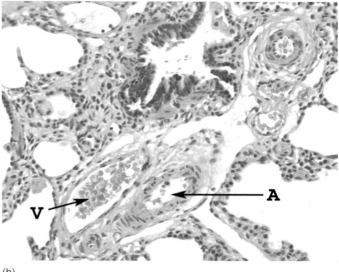

(b)

Figure 2.56 Alveolar capillary dysplasia. (a) There is a low density of alveoli. (b) High power shows misalignment of pulmonary vessels with both arteries and veins in a bronchovascular bundle (A, artery; V, vein).

nels around the foregut to a new primary pulmonary vein which grows from the developing left atrium toward the lung buds. The anomalous veins may join the inferior vena cava or hepatic, portal or splenic veins below the diaphragm, or above the diaphragm they may drain into the superior vena cava or its tributaries, the coronary sinus or the right atrium (Box 2.5). The anomaly may be total or partial, unilateral or bilateral and isolated or associated with other cardiopulmonary developmental defects. These include bronchopulmonary isomerism, dextrocardia, asplenia, pulmonary stenosis, patent ductus arteriosus and a small interatrial communication.[400] The type of isomerism gives a good indication as to whether the anomaly is

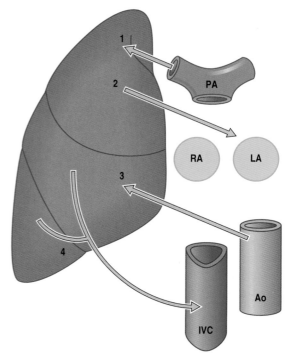

Figure 2.57 Scimitar syndrome. (1) The right upper lobe is often supplied by a hypoplastic pulmonary artery (PA). (2) The blood from the upper part of the lung drains normally into the left atrium (LA). (3) The remainder of the right lung is supplied by vessels arising from the aorta (Ao). (4) The blood from a variable part of the right lung drains by a prominent vein (evident radiologically as a curved, scimitar-shaped linear opacity) which joins the inferior vena cava (IVC) below the diaphragm. Less frequently, the drainage of the lower part of the right lung is by veins that pass directly to the right atrium (RA). (Redrawn from Brewis RAL, Corrin B, Geddes DM, Gibson GJ, eds. Respiratory Medicine, 2nd edn. London: Saunders; 1995. With permission from Elsevier.)

total or partial, right-sided isomerism suggesting totally anomalous veins and left-sided isomerism suggesting a partial anomaly.[139] Occasionally the anomalous vein runs much of its course buried within the lung substance.[401] Anomalous pulmonary venous connections are often narrow and this may cause pulmonary hypertension of the relatively mild, reversible venous variety.[402] Occasional reports of plexogenic pulmonary hypertension probably reflect the association with a patent ductus arteriosus.[400]

Atresia of the pulmonary veins[403,404] or narrowing of their ostia entering the left atrium (collectively termed pulmonary vein stenosis[403]) does not in itself constitute anomalous drainage but similarly results in pulmonary venous obstruction and may be associated with partial anomalous pulmonary venous drainage. The atresia may be unilateral or bilateral but in either case, severe hypertensive changes develop in both lungs. Small capillary-sized vessels may be found within all coats of the thickened arteries, or congeries of them may be seen alongside the larger blood vessels. They represent abortive anastomotic attempts at bypassing the obstruction, which are doomed to failure because the obstruction is extrapulmonary. They bear some resemblance to plexiform lesions but the necrotising arteritis that leads to plexogenic arteriopathy is not a feature. There is a closer resemblance to pulmonary capillary haemangiomatosis, supporting the view that this supposedly neoplastic condition merely represents a reaction to pulmonary venous occlusion (see pp. 429, 430). Congenital pulmonary vein atresia carries a very poor prognosis, few children with the condition surviving longer than 1 year.

Partial anomalous pulmonary venous drainage is an essential feature of the *scimitar syndrome*, in which an anomalous right pulmonary vein descending to join the inferior vena cava just below the diaphragm gives a characteristic, supposedly scimitar-like, vertical radiographic opacity parallel to the right side of the heart (Fig. 2.57). The arterial supply of the right lung is often largely from the aorta, so that there is some overlap with pulmonary sequestration and hypoplasia due to deficient pulmonary artery supply. Indeed, there is often hypoplasia or abnormal lobation of the right lung and mediastinal shift to the right. The vascular connections of the left lung are normal. Cardiovascular, diaphragmatic, gastrointestinal and other pulmonary anomalies are often found. The syndrome may be familial with an autosomal dominant pattern of inheritance. Some patients are asymptomatic and the lesion is detected only on routine radiographs. However, the anomaly represents a left to right shunt and surgical correction may be required if this is large.[405]

Arteriovenous fistula

Arteriovenous fistulas may be developmental or acquired. The latter result from injuries such as penetrating chest wounds or they may complicate liver disease (see p. 487). This account will be confined to the developmental variety, which was first reported in 1897,[406] since when many further cases have been reported.[407–412] The lesion is a vascular hamartoma resulting from persistence of anastomotic fetal capillaries. This results in abnormal communication between pulmonary arteries and veins, bypassing the normal pulmonary capillary bed. More rarely the lesion connects systemic and pulmonary vessels.[413–416] The lesions may be single or multiple and often increase in size with age so that the alternative term arteriovenous aneurysm is sometimes applied.[417] About 70% of patients have *hereditary haemorrhagic telangiectasia (Rendu–Osler–Weber disease)*, which is an autosomal dominant condition (see p. 483).[409,418,419] Conversely, about 15% of patients with hereditary haemorrhagic telangiectasia have pulmonary arteriovenous fistulae.[420] This association portends an increased risk of multiple fistulae and progressive symptoms, which is important as surgical correction is only possible with limited disease. Patients with multiple fistulae are more suitable for treatment by balloon occlusion or embolization. The role of lung transplantation is controversial.[421,422]

Clinical features

Although the lesion is a developmental anomaly, it may remain asymptomatic until late in life. The average age at presentation is about 40 years but the condition has been first identified in both the newborn and the very old.[408,409,414] Fistulae with an appreciable arterio-venous shunt cause cyanosis, clubbing of the fingers, breathlessness, polycythaemia and an extracardiac murmur. Haemorrhage from the lungs, as opposed to nasal telangiectasia, is an uncommon but potentially fatal complica-

tion.[423] The proximity of most malformations to the pleura explains the occasional complication of haemothorax. Systemic complications may be caused by hypoxaemia, thrombosis secondary to the polycythaemia, haemorrhage due to associated hereditary telangiectasia and paradoxical embolism or metastatic abscesses due to loss of the filtering effect of the pulmonary capillaries or, rarely, infective endarteritis within the fistula. Cerebral abscess is reported in 20% of patients, stroke in 18% and transient ischaemic attacks in 37%.[418] Sarcomatous change has been reported[424] but is very rare.

Pathology

The lower lobes are most commonly affected but any lobe may be involved. The lesions are multiple in one-third of cases and in one-sixth the condition is bilateral. Resected lesions will almost certainly have been demonstrated angiographically before operation (Fig. 2.58a,b). If not, the pathologist may do this with a barium gelatin mixture before fixing the specimen but the results are rarely better than the images produced 'in

(a)

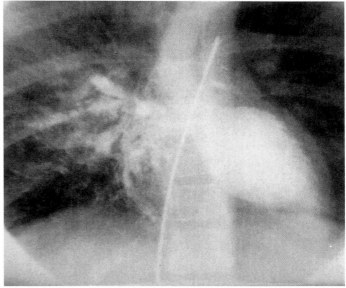

(b)

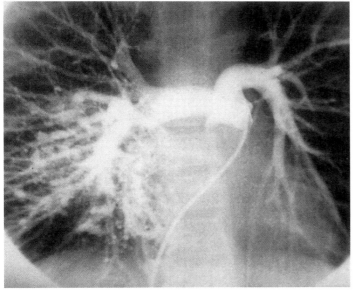

(c)

Figure 2.58 Arteriovenous malformation of the right lung demonstrated angiographically (a,b, the latter showing delayed emptying) and after lobectomy when unusually large thin-walled blood vessels are evident on the cut surface of the lung (c). (Illustrations provided by Dr M Jagusch, formerly of Auckland, New Zealand.)

vivo'. The lesion is usually peripheral and visible as a bluish swelling beneath the visceral pleura. It consists of vascular channels of various size and wall thickness, with little supportive tissue, separated by normal lung tissue (Fig. 2.58c). Individual vessels may be narrowed by intimal fibrosis or there may be dilatation associated with medial atrophy. Without prior angiography, arteriovenous communication can only be demonstrated by semi-serial sections.

Anomalies of the pulmonary lymphatics

Lymphatic hypoplasia of varied distribution underlies the *yellow nail syndrome* in which lymphoedema is accompanied by discolouration of the nails and chylous pleural effusions (see Fig. 13.3, p. 694).[425–427] Although inherited it is not usually manifest until adult life. The *Klippel-Trenaunay syndrome*, usually characterised by varicosities of systemic veins, cutaneous haemangiomas and soft tissue hypertrophy, is another congenital disorder in which pleuropulmonary abnormalities are described, including pulmonary lymphatic hyperplasia, pleural effusions, pulmonary thromboembolism and pulmonary vein varicosities.[428,429]

Congenital pulmonary lymphangiectasia

Congenital pulmonary lymphangiectasia may be caused by obstruction to pulmonary lymphatic or venous drainage or be 'primary', the latter either limited to the lung or part of generalised lymphangiectasia.[430] There is a high association of primary pulmonary lymphangiectasia with other congenital abnormalities, particularly asplenia[431] and cardiac anomalies. When the other abnormalities entail impaired pulmonary venous drainage there is obviously a causal relationship, but this is not always the case.[431]

Primary pulmonary lymphangiectasia is presumed to result from developmental failure of the pulmonary lymphatics to link with the main drainage channels. It causes severe respiratory distress and is generally fatal in the neonatal period, but some children survive, albeit with respiratory impairment,[432] and presentation may be delayed until adult life.[433,434]

The macroscopic findings can be very instructive diagnostically. The microscopic distinction of lymphangiectasia from interstitial emphysema can be extremely difficult and it is regrettable that sure macroscopic distinctions are often omitted from the autopsy report. In lymphangiectasia the lungs are heavy but this is often also the case in interstitial emphysema because of some underlying disease which necessitated artificial respiration. In both conditions the interlobular septa are widened and on the visceral pleural surface there is a pronounced reticular pattern of small cysts, which accentuates the lobular architecture of the lungs. Pricking the cysts gives invaluable evidence of their content, clear serous fluid running out in lymphangiectasia. On slicing the lungs, further fluid runs from the cut surfaces, which show a microcystic pattern (Fig. 2.59). The cysts measure up to 5 mm in diameter and are situated in

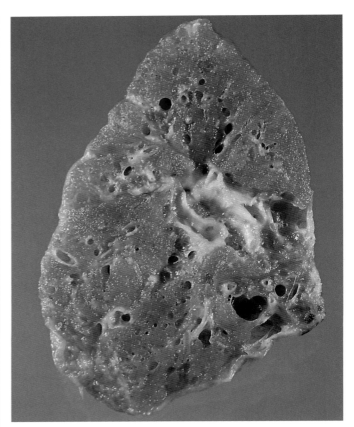

Figure 2.59 Congenital pulmonary lymphangiectasia. Cystically dilated lymphatics are evident on the cut surface of the lung. (Reproduced by permission of Dr M Jagusch, Auckland, New Zealand.)

the interlobular septa and about the bronchovascular bundles. Near the hila of the lungs the cysts are elongated.[435]

Microscopy confirms that the cysts are located in connective tissue under the pleura, in the interlobular septa and about the bronchioles and arteries (Fig. 2.60). Serial sections show that they are part of an intricate network of intercommunicating channels, which vary greatly in width and are devoid of valves.[435] The cysts are lined by an attenuated simple endothelium, an appearance which may be mimicked by compressed connective tissue cells in interstitial emphysema. Never seen in lymphangiectasia is the foreign body giant cell reaction to air, which develops after a few days in interstitial emphysema. Apart from this, the two conditions can be virtually indistinguishable microscopically, which is understandable as in interstitial emphysema the air is contained within lymphatics as well as dissecting the interstitial tissues.[95] Interstitial emphysema rather than lymphangiectasia may also be suspected if there is some other underlying disease that necessitated ventilator support.

It is important not to confuse lymphangiectasia with artefactual expansion of the interlobular septa by overzealous injection of formalin.

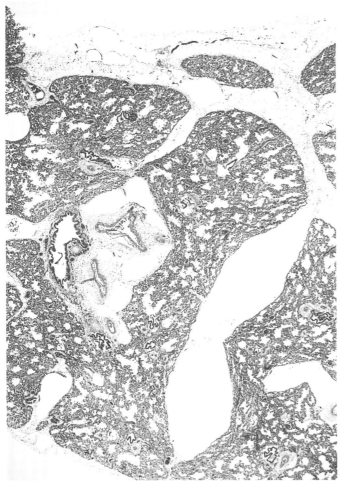

Figure 2.60   Congenital pulmonary lymphangiectasia. Lymphatics in the interlobular septa are markedly dilated.

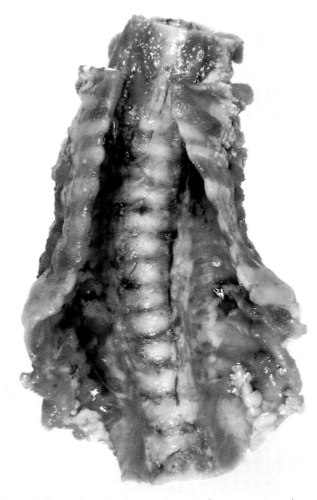

Figure 2.61   Asphyxiating thoracic dystrophy (Jeune's syndrome). Deformity of the chest wall reduces the thoracic cavity to a narrow funnel and thereby causes pulmonary hypoplasia. (Reproduced by permission of the late Dr AH Cameron and of Dr F Raafat, Birmingham, UK.)

Anomalies of the thoracic cage

Diaphragmatic anomalies

The diaphragm forms from the fetal septum transversum, which grows across the common coelomic cavity to divide the peritoneal from the pleural and pericardial cavities. The posterolateral portions containing the foramina of Bochdalek are the last to form and arrested development here results in widened foramina through which herniation of abdominal viscera is prone to occur, particularly on the left resulting in mediastinal shift to the right. Hernias of this type are among the commonest congenital defects. They occur in about 1 in 2000 fetuses but many of these have other major anomalies, in particular cardiac abnormalities, and are stillborn. If the infant is suitable for surgical correction, respiratory insufficiency and persistent fetal circulation (see p. 47) are frequent postoperative problems. The foramina are normally sealed at about 8 weeks gestation by the pleural and peritoneal membranes so that hernias forming after this time tend to be enclosed in a serosal sac.

The diaphragmatic muscle is formed between the pleural and peritoneal membranes and if it is deficient, the diaphragm is reduced to a thin membrane, which rises into the thorax, a process known as eventration. The whole diaphragm may be affected but more often the defect is unilateral (Fig. 2.31, p. 56). Posterolateral herniation and eventration are both most common on the left and affect boys twice as often as girls. Anterior and paraoesophageal hernias each account for only 5% of the total, while total absence of half or the whole diaphragm is very unusual.[436]

All these diaphragmatic defects result in abdominal viscera moving into a pleural space and compromising lung development (see pulmonary hypoplasia, p. 53 and Figs 2.28, 2.29).

Duplication of the diaphragm results in a fibromuscular septum dividing one pleural cavity in two, usually between the right upper and middle lobes. Associated anomalies of the heart and lungs are frequent.

Pectus carinatum (pigeon breast)

In this condition, the sternum protrudes anteriorly and may lie obliquely if the excessive growth of the ribs is asymmetrical. It may be present at birth but usually becomes prominent during adolescence. Respiratory function is normal, as there is no loss of lung volume and little interference with rib movement.

Pectus excavatum (funnel chest)

This condition appears soon after birth and is occasionally associated with kyphosis, scoliosis or mitral valve prolapse. It may be familial or associated with Marfan's syndrome, the Ehlers–Danlos syndrome or hyperflexibility of the joints. It may also be acquired in infancy by upper airway obstruction from enlargement of the tonsils and adenoids necessitating an increase in the force of the respiratory movements. Initially the condition is reversible but it may become permanent. The respiratory effects are minor but the heart may be compressed between the depressed sternum and the spine so that cardiac filling is impaired.[437]

Asphyxiating thoracic dystrophy (Jeune's syndrome)

This is a rare disorder of the ribs, which are shortened and the ribcage narrowed so that lung development is retarded and there is pulmonary hypoplasia (Fig. 2.61). Less severe degrees are compatible with life but respiratory movements are entirely abdominal and respiratory failure often develops in infancy or childhood. Although rare, Jeune's syndrome is the commonest of several generalised skeletal disorders that result in a small chest. In many of them the thoracic deformity is associated with short limbs, syndactyly or polydactyly.[438]

Scoliosis

Scoliosis (lateral curvature of the spine) is generally accompanied by rotation of the spine. If the condition is present at birth there is often a recognisable congenital abnormality of the spine, such as hemivertebra and other congenital skeletal abnormalities such as absent or fused ribs may also be present. However, most cases are idiopathic. Some idiopathic cases present in infancy. These tend to progress to respiratory failure in later life.[178,179] However, it is commoner for idiopathic scoliosis to appear during adolescence and not progress in this way. Scoliosis may also be secondary to neuromuscular disorders, both hereditary and acquired.

REFERENCES

Development of the lungs

1. Jeffery PK. The development of large and small airways. Am J Respir Crit Care Med 1998; 157:S174–S180.
2. Bucher U, Reid L. Development of the intrasegmental bronchial tree: The pattern of branching and development of cartilage at various stages of intra-uterine life. Thorax 1961; 16:207–218.
3. Scavo LM, Ertsey R, Chapin CJ, Allen L, Kitterman JA. Apoptosis in the development of rat and human fetal lungs. Am J Respir Cell Mol Biol 1998; 18:21–31.
4. Zeltner TB, Burri PH. The postnatal development and growth of the human lung. II. Morphology. Respir Physiol 1987; 67:269–282.
5. Thurlbeck WM, Angus GE. Growth and aging of the normal human lung. Chest 1975; 67:3S–7S.
6. Hislop A, Reid L. Development of the acinus in the human lung. Thorax 1974; 29:90–94.
7. Thurlbeck WM. Postnatal growth and development of the lung. Am Rev Respir Dis 1975; 111:803–844.
8. Thurlbeck WM. Postnatal human lung growth. Thorax 1982; 37:564–571.
9. Burrows B, Knudson RJ, Lebowitz MD. The relationship of childhood respiratory illness to adult obstructive airway disease. Am Rev Respir Dis 1977; 115:751–760.
10. Shaheen S, Barker DJP. Early lung growth and chronic airflow obstruction. Thorax 1994; 49:533–536.
11. Johnston IDA, Strachan DP, Anderson HR. Effect of pneumonia and whooping cough in childhood on adult lung function. N Engl J Med 1998; 338:581–587.
12. Campiche Ma, Gautier A, Hernandez EI, Reymond A. An electron microscope study of the fetal development of human lung. Pediatrics 1963; 32:976–994.
13. Leeson TS, Leeson CR. A light and electron microscope study of developing respiratory tissue in the rat. J Anat 1964; 98:183–193.
14. O'Hare KH, Sheridan MN. Electron microscopic observations on the morphogenesis of the albino rat lung, with special reference to pulmonary epithelial cells. Am J Anat 1970; 127:181–205.
15. Adamson IYR, Young L, King GM. Reciprocal epithelial – fibroblast interactions in the control of fetal and adult rat lung cells in culture. Exp Lung Res 1991; 17:821–835.
16. Virtanen I, Laitinen A, Tani T, et al. Differential expression of laminins and their integrin receptors in developing and adult human lung. Am J Respir Cell Mol Biol 1996; 15:184–196.
17. Arai H, Hirano H, Mushiake S, Nakayama M, Takada G, Sekiguchi K. Loss of EDB+ fibronectin isoform is associated with differentiation of alveolar epithelial cells in human fetal lung. Am J Pathol 1997; 151:403–412.
18. Shannon JM, Deterding RR. Epithelial-mesenchymal interactions in lung development. In: McDonald JA, ed. Lung Growth and Development. New York: Marcel Dekker; 1997: 81–118.
19. Warburton D, Schwarz M, Tefft D, Flores-Delgado G, Anderson KD, Cardoso WV. The molecular basis of lung morphogenesis. Mech Dev 2000; 92:55–81.
20. Cardoso WV. Molecular regulation of lung development. Annu Rev Physiol 2001; 63:471–494.
21. Bartram U, Speer CP. The role of transforming growth factor beta in lung development and disease. Chest 2004; 125(2):754–765.
22. Adamson IYR, King GM. Epithelial-mesenchymal interactions in postnatal rat lung growth. Exp Lung Res 1985; 8:261–274.
23. Terzaghi M, Nettesheim P, Williams ML. Repopulation of denuded tracheal grafts with normal, preneoplastic and neoplastic epithelial cell populations. Cancer Res 1978; 38:4546–4553.
24. Caniggia I, Tseu I, Rolland G, Edelson J, Tanswell AK, Post M. Inhibition of fibroblast growth by epithelial cells in fetal rat lung. Am J Respir Cell Mol Biol 1995; 13:91–98.
25. Taderera JV. Control of lung differentiation in vitro. Dev Biol 1967; 16:489–512.
26. Olver RE, Strang LB. Ion fluxes across the pulmonary epithelium and the secretion of lung liquid in the foetal lamb. J Physiol (London) 1974; 241:327–357.
27. Symchuch PS, Winchester P. Animal model: amniotic fluid deficiency and fetal lung growth in the rat. Am J Pathol 1978; 90:779–782.
28. Hislop A, Hey E, Reid L. The lungs in congenital bilateral renal agenesis and dysplasia. Arch Dis Child 1979; 54:32–38.
29. Cutz E, Chan W, Wong V, Conen PE. Endocrine cells in rat fetal lungs. Ultrastructural and histochemical study. Lab Invest 1974; 30:458–464.

30. Wharton J, Polak JM, Cole GA, Marangos PJ, Pearse AGE. Neuro-specific enolase as an immunocytochemical marker for the diffuse neuroendocrine system in human fetal lung. J Histochem Cytochem 1981; 29:1359–1364.

31. Stahlman MT, Gray ME. Ontogeny of neuroendocrine cells in human fetal lung. I. An electron microscopic study. Lab Invest 1984; 51:449–463.

32. Stahlman MT, Kasselberg AG, Orth DN, Gray ME. Ontogeny of neuroendocrine cells in human fetal lung. II. An immunohistochemical study. Lab Invest 1985; 52:52–60.

33. Van Lommel A, Lauweryns JM, Deleyn P, Wouters P, Schreinemakers H, Lerut T. Pulmonary neuroepithelial bodies in neonatal and adult dogs: histochemistry, ultrastructure and effects of unilateral hilar lung denervation. Lung 1995; 173:13–23.

34. Aguayo SM, Schuyler WE, Murtagh JJ, Roman J. Regulation of lung branching morphogenesis by bombesin- like peptides and neutral endopeptidase. Am J Respir Cell Mol Biol 1994; 10:635–642.

35. Wang DS, Yeger H, Cutz E. Expression of gastrin-releasing peptide receptor gene in developing lung. Am J Respir Cell Mol Biol 1996; 14:409–416.

36. Gutierrez JA, Ertsey R, Scavo LM, Collins E, Dobbs LG. Mechanical distension modulates alveolar epithelial cell phenotypic expression by transcriptional regulation. Am J Respir Cell Mol Biol 1999; 21:223–229.

37. Wigglesworth JS, Desai R. Effects on lung growth of cervical cord section in the rabbit fetus. Early Hum Dev 1979; 3:51–65.

38. Ballard PL, Benson BJ, Brehier A. Glucocorticoid effects in fetal lung. Am Rev Respir Dis 1977; 115:Supplement 36.

39. Liggins GC, Howie RN. A controlled trial of antepartum glucocorticoid treatment for prevention of the respiratory distress syndrome in premature infants. Pediatrics 1972; 50:515–525.

40. Monkhouse WS. Characterization of proteoglycans synthesized by fetal rat lung type II pneumocytes in vitro and the effects of cortisol. Exp Lung Res 1987; 12:253–264.

41. Demello DE, Sawyer D, Galvin N, Reid LM. Early fetal development of lung vasculature. Am J Respir Cell Mol Biol 1997; 16:568–581.

42. Demello DE, Reid LM. Embryonic and early fetal development of human lung vasculature and its functional implications. Pediatr Dev Pathol 2000; 3:439–449.

43. Hall SM, Hislop AA, Pierce CM, Haworth SG. Prenatal origins of human intrapulmonary arteries formation and smooth muscle maturation. Am J Respir Cell Mol Biol 2000; 23:194–203.

44. Jeffery PK, Hislop AA. Embryology and Growth. In: Gibson GJ, Geddes DM, Costabel U, Sterk PJ, Corrin B, eds. Respiratory Medicine. London: Saunders; 2003:51–63.

45. Hall SM, Hislop AA, Haworth SG. Origin, differentiation and maturation of human pulmonary veins. Am J Respir Cell Mol Biol 2002; 26:333–340.

46. Weichselbaum M, Sparrow MP. A confocal microscopic study of the formation of ganglia in the airways of fetal pig lung. Am J Respir Cell Mol Biol 1999; 21:607–620.

Perinatal disorders

47. Burgess AM, Hutchins GM. Inflammation of the lungs, umbilical cord and placenta associated with meconium passage in utero – review of 123 autopsied cases. Pathol Res Pract 1996; 192:1121–1128.

48. Finer NN. Surfactant use for neonatal lung injury: beyond respiratory distress syndrome. Paediatr Respir Rev 2004; 5(Suppl A):S289–S297.

49. Salvia-Roiges MD, Carbonell-Estrany X, Figueras-Aloy J, Rodriguez-Miguelez JM. Efficacy of three treatment schedules in severe meconium aspiration syndrome. Acta Paediatr 2004; 93:60–65.

50. Keenan WJ. Recommendations for management of the child born through meconium-stained amniotic fluid. Pediatrics 2004; 113:133–134.

51. Lin TW, Su BH, Lin HC, et al. Risk factors of pulmonary hemorrhage in very-low-birth-weight infants: a two-year retrospective study. Acta Paediatr Taiwan 2000; 41:255–258.

52. Esterly JR, Oppenheimer WH, Rowe S, Avery ME. Massive pulmonary haemorrhage in the newborn. J Pediatr 1966; 69:3–20.

53. Franciosi RA, Tattersall P. Fetal infection with human parvovirus B19. Hum Pathol 1988; 19:489–491.

54. Ablow RC, Driscoll SG, Effman EL, et al. A comparison of early onset Group B streptococcal neonatal infection and the respiratory distress syndrome of the newborn. N Engl J Med 1976; 294:65–70.

55. Cordero L, Ayers LW, Miller RR, Seguin JH, Coley BD. Surveillance of ventilator-associated pneumonia in very-low-birth-weight infants. Am J Infect Control 2002; 30:32–39.

56. Apisarnthanarak A, Holzmann-Pazgal G, Hamvas A, Olsen MA, Fraser VJ. Ventilator-associated pneumonia in extremely pre-term neonates in a neonatal intensive care unit: characteristics, risk factors and outcomes. Pediatrics 2003; 112:1283–1289.

57. Clements JA, Avery ME. Lung surfactant and neonatal respiratory distress syndrome. Am J Respir Crit Care Med 1998; 157:S59–S66.

58. Robertson B. Pathology of neonatal surfactant deficiency. In: Rosenberg HS, Bernstein J, eds. Respiratory and Alimentary Tract Diseases, Vol. 11 Perspectives in Pediatric Pathology. Basel: Karger; 1987:6–46.

59. Doshi N, Klionsky B, Fujikura T, MacDonald H. Pulmonary yellow hyaline membranes in neonates. Hum Pathol 1980; 11:520–527.

60. Morgenstern B, Klionsky B, Doshi N. Yellow hyaline membrane disease. Identification of the pigment and bilirubin binding. Lab Invest 1981; 44:514–518.

61. Kresch MJ, Lin WH, Thrall RS. Surfactant replacement therapy. Thorax 1996; 51:1137–1154.

62. Bryan MH, Hardie MJ, Reilly BJ, Swyer PR. Pulmonary function studies during the first year of life in infants recovering from the respiratory distress syndrome. Pediatrics 1973; 52:169–178.

63. Baraldi E, Filippone M, Trevisanuto D, Zanardo V, Zacchello F. Pulmonary function until two years of life in infants with bronchopulmonary dysplasia. Am J Respir Crit Care Med 1997; 155:149–155.

64. Kamper J. Long term prognosis of infants with severe idiopathic respiratory distress syndrome. Acta Paediatr Scand 1978; 67:71–76.

65. Northway WH, Rosan RC, Porter DY. Pulmonary disease following respirator therapy of hyaline membrane disease. Bronchopulmonary dysplasia. N Engl J Med 1967; 276:357–368.

66. Edwards DK, Dyer WM, Northway WH. Twelve years experience with bronchopulmonary dysplasia. Pediatrics 1977; 59:839–846.

67. Taghizadeh A, Reynolds EOR. Pathogenesis of bronchopulmonary dysplasia following hyaline membrane disease. Am J Pathol 1976; 82:241–264.

68. Chang LYL, Subramaniam M, Yoder BA, et al. A catalytic antioxidant attenuates alveolar structural remodeling in bronchopulmonary dysplasia. Am J Respir Crit Care Med 2003; 167:57–64.

69. Erickson AM, de la Monte SM, Moore GW, Hutchins GM. The progression of morphologic changes in bronchopulmonary dysplasia. Am J Pathol 1987; 127:474–484.

70. Jacob SV, Lands LC, Coates AL, et al. Exercise ability in survivors of severe bronchopulmonary dysplasia. Am J Respir Crit Care Med 1997; 155:1925–1929.

71. Anderson WR, Engel RR. Cardiopulmonary sequelae of reparative stages of bronchopulmonary dysplasia. Arch Pathol Lab Med 1983; 107:603–608.

72. Chambers HM, van Velzen D. Ventilator-related pathology in the extremely immature lung. Pathology 1989; 21:79–83.

73. Coalson JJ. Pathology of chronic lung disease in early infancy. In: Bland RD, Coalson JJ, eds. Chronic Lung Disease in Early Infancy. New York: Marcel Dekker; 2000:85–124.

74. Boggaram V. Regulation of lung surfactant protein gene expression. Front Biosci 2003; 8:d751–d764.

75. Shulenin S, Nogee LM, Annilo T, Wert SE, Whitsett JA, Dean M. ABCA3 Gene Mutations in newborns with fatal surfactant deficiency. N Engl J Med 2004; 350:1296–1303.

76. Nogee LM, Demello DE, Dehner LP, Colten HR. Brief report – deficiency of pulmonary surfactant protein-B in congenital alveolar proteinosis. N Engl J Med 1993; 328:406–410.

77. Nogee L, Garnier G, Dietz H, Singer L, Murphy A, DeMello D. A mutation in the surfactant protein B gene responsible for fatal neonatal respiratory disease in multiple kindreds. J Clin Invest 1994; 93:1860–1863.

78. Demello DE, Heyman S, Phelps DS, et al. Ultrastructure of lung in surfactant protein B deficiency. Am J Respir Cell Mol Biol 1994; 11:230–239.

79. Ball R, Chetcuti PAJ, Beverley D. Fatal familial surfactant protein B deficiency. Arch Dis Child 1995; 73:F53.

80. Demello DE, Nogee LM, Heyman S, et al. Molecular and phenotypic variability in the congenital alveolar proteinosis syndrome associated with inherited surfactant protein B deficiency. J Pediatr 1994; 125:43–50.

81. Nogee LM, Wert SE, Proffit SA, Hull WM, Whitsett JA. Allelic heterogeneity in hereditary surfactant protein B (SP-B) deficiency. Amer J Respir Crit Care Med 2000; 161:973–981.

82. Mildenberger E, Demello DE, Lin ZW, Kossel H, Hoehn T, Versmold HT. Focal congenital alveolar proteinosis associated with abnormal surfactant protein B messenger RNA. Chest 2001; 119:645–647.

83. Clark JC, Wert SE, Bachurski CJ, et al. Targeted disruption of the surfactant protein B gene disrupts surfactant homeostasis, causing respiratory failure in newborn mice. Proc Natl Acad Sci USA 1995; 92:7794–7798.

84. Stahlman MT, Gray MP, Falconieri MW, Whitsett JA, Weaver TE. Lamellar body formation in normal and surfactant protein B- deficient fetal mice. Lab Invest 2000; 80(3):395–403.

85. Nogee LM, Dunbar AE, III, Wert SE, Askin F, Hamvas A, Whitsett JA. A mutation in the surfactant protein C gene associated with familial interstitial lung disease. N Engl J Med 2001; 344:573–579.

86. Fan LL, Langston C. Pediatric interstitial lung disease – Children are not small adults. Am J Respir Crit Care Med 2002; 165:1466–1467.

87. Thomas AQ, Lane K, Phillips J, et al. Heterozygosity for a surfactant protein C gene mutation associated with usual interstitial pneumonitis and cellular nonspecific interstitial pneumonitis in one kindred. Am J Respir Crit Care Med 2002; 165:1322–1328.

88. Cutz E, Wert SE, Nogee LM, Moore AM. Deficiency of lamellar bodies in alveolar type II cells associated with fatal respiratory disease in a full-term infant. Am J Respir Crit Care Med 2000; 161:608–614.

89. Tryka AF, Wert SE, Mazursky JE, Arrington RW, Nogee LM. Absence of lamellar bodies with accumulation of dense bodies characterizes a novel form of congenital surfactant defect. Pediatr Dev Pathol 2000; 3:335–345.

90. Stocker JT, Madewell JE. Persistent interstitial pulmonary emphysema: another complication of the respiratory distress syndrome. Pediatrics 1977; 59:847–857.

91. Brewer LL, Moskowitz PS, Carrington CB, Bensch KG. Pneumatosis pulmonalis. A complication of the idiopathic respiratory distress syndrome. Am J Pathol 1979; 95:171–190.

92. Wilson JM, Mark EJ, Connolly SA, Shannon DC, Ryan DP. A pre-term newborn female triplet with diffuse cystic changes in the left lung – Pulmonary interstitial emphysema, localized, persistent. N Engl J Med 1997; 337:916–924.

93. Deroux SJ, Prendergast NC. Large sub-pleural air cysts: an extreme form of pulmonary interstitial emphysema. Pediatr Radiol 1998; 28:981–983.

94. Donnelly LF, Lucaya J, Ozelame V, et al. CT findings and temporal course of persistent pulmonary interstitial emphysema in neonates: a multiinstitutional study. Am J Roentgenol 2003; 180:1129–1133.

95. Wood BP, Anderson VM, Mauk JE, Merritt TA. Pulmonary lymphatic air: locating 'pulmonary interstitial emphysema' of the premature infant. Am J Roentgenol 1982; 138:809–814.

96. Lavezzi WA, Keough KM, Der'Ohannesian P, Person TL, Wolf BC. The use of pulmonary interstitial emphysema as an indicator of live birth. Am J Forensic Med Pathol 2003; 24:87–91.

96a. Carden KA, Boiselle PM, Waltz DA, Ernst A. Tracheomalacia and tracheobronchomalacia in children and adults: an in-depth review. Chest 2005;127:984–1005.

97. Morin FC, Stenmark KR. Persistent pulmonary hypertension of the newborn. Am J Respir Crit Care Med 1995; 151:2010–2032.

98. Haworth SG, Reid L. Persistent fetal circulation: newly recognized structural features. J Pediatr 1976; 88:614–620.

99. Boggs S, Harris MC, Hoffman DJ, et al. Misalignment of pulmonary veins with alveolar capillary dysplasia: affected siblings and variable phenotypic expression. J Pediatr 1994; 124:125–128.

100. Gutierrez C, Rodriguez A, Palenzuela S, Forteza C, Rossello JL. Congenital misalignment of pulmonary veins with alveolar capillary dysplasia causing persistent neonatal pulmonary hypertension: report of two affected siblings. Pediatr Dev Pathol 2000; 3:271–276.

101. Roberts JD, Polaner DM, Lang P, Zapol WM. Inhaled nitric oxide in persistent pulmonary hypertension of the newborn. Lancet 1992; 340:818–819.

102. Kinsella JP, Neish SR, Shaffer E, Abman SH. Low-dose inhalational nitric oxide in persistent pulmonary hypertension of the newborn. Lancet 1992; 340:819–820.

103. Katzenstein ALA, Gordon LP, Oliphant M, Swender PT. Chronic pneumonitis of infancy: a unique form of interstitial lung disease occurring in early childhood. Am J Surg Pathol 1995; 19:439–447.

104. Parto K, Maki L, Pelliniemi LJ, Simell O. Abnormal pulmonary macrophages in lysinuric protein intolerance: ultrastructural, morphometric and X-ray microanalytic study. Arch Pathol Lab Med 1994; 118:536–541.

105. Parto K, Kallajoki M, Aho H, Simell O. Pulmonary alveolar proteinosis and glomerulonephritis in lysinuric protein intolerance: case reports and autopsy findings of four pediatric patients. Hum Pathol 1994; 25:400–407.

106. McManus DT, Moore R, Hill CM, Rodgers C, Carson DJ, Love AHG. Necropsy findings in lysinuric protein intolerance. J Clin Pathol 1996; 49:345–347.

107. Fisher M, Roggli V, Merten D, Mulvihill D, Spock A. Coexisting endogenous lipoid pneumonia, cholesterol granulomas and pulmonary alveolar proteinosis in a pediatric population: a clinical, radiographic and pathologic correlation. Pediatr Pathol 1992; 12:365–383.

108. McDonald JW, Roggli VL, Bradford WD. Coexisting endogenous and exogenous lipoid pneumonia and alveolar proteinosis in a patient with neurodevelopmental disease. Pediatr Pathol 1993; 14:505–511.

109. Buchta RM, Park S, Giammona ST. Desquamative interstitial pneumonia in a 7-week-old infant. Am J Dis Child 1970; 120:341–343.

110. Bhagwat AG, Wentworth P, Conen RE. Observation on the relationship of desquamative interstitial pneumonia and pulmonary alveolar proteinosis in childhood: A pathologic and experimental study. Chest 1970; 58:326–332.

111. Wigger HJ, Berdon WE, Ores CN. Fatal desquamative interstitial pneumonia in an infant. Arch Pathol Lab Med 1977; 101:129–132.

112. Sato K, Takahashi H, Amano H, Uekusa T, Dambara T, Kira S. Diffuse progressive pulmonary interstitial and intra- alveolar cholesterol granulomas in childhood. Eur Respir J 1996; 9:2419–2422.

113. Schroeder SA, Shannon DC, Mark EJ. Cellular interstitial pneumonitis in infants. A clinicopathologic study. Chest 1992; 101:1065–1069.

114. Boyce JA, Mark EJ, Bramson RT, Shannon DC, Youth B. A four-month-old girl with chronic cyanosis and diffuse pulmonary infiltrates. Cellular interstitial pneumonitis. N Engl J Med 1999; 341:2075–2083.

115. Canakis AM, Cutz E, Manson D, Obrodovich H. Pulmonary interstitial glycogenosis - A new variant of neonatal interstitial lung disease. Am J Respir Crit Care Med 2002; 165:1557–1565.

116. Fan LL, Kozinetz CA, Wojtczak HA, Chatfield BA, Cohen AH, Rothenberg SS. Diagnostic value of transbronchial, thoracoscopic and open lung biopsy in immunocompetent children with chronic interstitial lung disease. J Pediatr 1997; 131:565–569.

117. Nicholson AG, Kim H, Corrin B, et al. The value of classifying interstitial pneumonitis in childhood according to defined histological patterns. Histopathology 1998; 33:203–211.

118. Stillwell PC, Norris DG, O'Connell EJ, Rosenow EC, III, Weiland LH, Harrison EG, Jr. Desquamative interstitial pneumonitis in children. Chest 1980; 77:165–171.

119. Tal A, Maor E, Bar-Ziv J, Gorodischer R. Fatal desquamative interstitial pneumonia in three infants siblings. J Pediatr 1984; 104:873–876.

120. Amir G, Ron N. Pulmonary pathology in Gaucher's disease. Hum Pathol 1999; 30:666–670.

121. Wilson MG, Mikity VG. A new form of respiratory disease in premature infants. J Dis Child 1960; 99:119–129.

122. Fujimura M, Takeuchi T, Kitajima H, Nakayama M. Chorioamnionitis and serum IgM in Wilson–Mikity syndrome. Arch Dis Child 1989; 64:1379–1383.

123. Reiterer F, Dornbusch HJ, Urlesberger B, et al. Cytomegalovirus associated neonatal pneumonia and Wilson–Mikity syndrome: a causal relationship? Eur Resp J 1999; 13:460–462.

Developmental disorders

124. Landing BH, Dixon LG. Congenital malformations and genetic disorders of respiratory tract. Am Rev Respir Dis 1979; 120:151–185.

125. Silver MM, Thurston WA, Patrick JE. Perinatal pulmonary hyperplasia due to laryngeal atresia. Hum Pathol 1988; 19:110–113.

126. Hopkinson JM. Congenital absence of the trachea. J Pathol 1972; 107:63–67.

127. Aboussouan LS, Odonovan PB, Moodie DS, Gragg LA, Stoller JK. Hypoplastic trachea in Down's syndrome. Am Rev Respir Dis 1993; 147:72–75.

128. Berdon WE, Baker DH, Wung J-T, et al. Complete cartilage-ring tracheal stenosis associated with anomalous left pulmonary artery: the ring-sling complex. J Radiol 1984; 152:57–64.

129. Ravenna F, Caramori G, Panella GL, et al. An unusual case of congenital short trachea with very long bronchi mimicking bronchial asthma. Thorax 2002; 57:372–373.

130. Emery JL, Haddadin AJ. Squamous epithelium in the respiratory tract of children with tracheo-oesophageal fistula. Arch Dis Child 1971; 46:236–242.

131. Wailoo MP, Emery JL. The trachea in children with tracheo-oesophageal fistula. Histopathology 1979; 3:329–338.

132. Tanaka H, Igarashi T, Teramoto S, Yoshida Y, Abe S. Lymphoepithelial cysts in the mediastinum with an opening to the trachea. Respiration 1995; 62:110–113.

133. Deb S, Ali MB, Fonseca P. Congenital bronchoesophageal fistula in an adult. Chest 1998; 114:1784–1786.

134. Jacobs IN, Wetmore RF, Tom LW, Handler SO, Potsic WP. Tracheobronchomalacia in children. Arch Otolaryngol Head Neck Surg 1994; 120:154–158.

135. Hicks J, De Jong A, Barrish J, Zhu SH, Popek E. Tracheomalacia in a neonate with Kniest dysplasia: histopathologic and ultrastructural features. Ultrastruct Pathol 2001; 25:79–83.

136. Stigol LC, Traversaro J, Trigo ER. Carinal trifurcation with congenital tracheobiliary fistula. Pediatrics 1966; 37:89–91.

137. de Carvalho CRR, Barbas CSV, Guarnieri RDdG, et al. Congenital bronchobiliary fistula: first case in an adult. Thorax 1988; 43:792–793.

138. Barbato A, Novello A, Zanolin D, Corner P, Talenti E. Diverticulosis of the main bronchi - a rare cause of recurrent bronchopneumonia in a child. Thorax 1993; 48:187–188.

139. Bloor CM, Liebow AA. In: Sonnenblick E, Parmley WW, eds. The Pulmonary and Bronchial Circulations in Congenital Heart Disease. New York and London: Plenum; 1980:96.

140. Gonzalez-Crussi F, Padilla L-M, Miller JK, Grosfeld JL. 'Bridging bronchus', a previously undescribed airway anomaly. Am J Dis Child 1976; 130:1015–1018.

141. Clements BS, Warner JO. The crossover lung segment: congenital malformation associated with a variant of scimitar syndrome. Thorax 1987; 42:417–419.

142. Warner JO, Clements BS. The crossover lung segment: congenital malformation associated with a variant of scimitar syndrome. Thorax 1987; 42:992.

143. Kelly DR, Mroczek EC, Galliani CA, Guion JC, Wells TR, Landing BH. Horseshoe lung and crossover lung segment: a unifying concept of fusion events in the lungs and other paired organs. In: Askin FB, Langston C, Rosenberg HS, Bernstein J, eds. Pulmonary Disease. Basel: Karger; 1995:183–213.

144. Frank JL, Poole CA, Rosas G. Horseshoe lung: clinical, pathologic and radiologic features and a new plain film finding. Am J Roentgenol 1986; 146:217–226.

145. Kramer MS. 'Horseshoe' lung: report of five new cases. Am J Roentgenol 1986; 146:211–215.

146. Ersoz A, Soncul H, Gokgoz L, et al. Horseshoe lung with left lung hypoplasia. Thorax 1992; 47:205–206.

147. Langlois SLP, Henderson DW. Variant pulmonary lobation. Australas Radiol 1980; 24:255–261.

148. Landing BH, Lawrence T-YK, Payne VC, Wells TR. Bronchial anatomy syndromes with abnormal visceral situs, abnormal spleen and congenital heart disease. Am J Cardiol 1971; 28:456–462.

149. Maier HC. Bronchogenic cysts of mediastinum. Ann Surg 1948; 127:476–502.

150. Aktogu S, Yuncu G, Halilcolar H, Ermete S, Buduneli T. Bronchogenic cysts: clinicopathological presentation and treatment. Eur Respir J 1996; 9:2017–2021.

151. Haddadin WJ, Reid R, Jindal RM. A retroperitoneal bronchogenic cyst: a rare cause of a mass in the adrenal region. J Clin Pathol 2001; 54:801–802.

152. Kim NR, Kim HH, Suh YL. Cutaneous bronchogenic cyst of the abdominal wall. Pathol Int 2001; 51:970–973.

153. Ingu A, Watanabe A, Ichimiya Y, Saito T, Abe T. Retroperitoneal bronchogenic cyst – A case report. Chest 2002; 121:1357–1359.

154. Matsubayashi J, Ishida T, Ozawa T, Aoki T, Koyanagi Y, Mukai K. Subphrenic bronchopulmonary foregut malformation with pulmonary-sequestration-like features. Pathol Int 2003; 53:313–316.

155. Stocker JT. Congenital pulmonary airway malformation-a new name for an expanded classification of congenital cystic adenomatoid malformation of the lung. Histopathology 2002; 41:424–458.

156. Pritchard MG, Brown PJE, Sterrett GF. Bronchioloalveolar carcinoma arising in longstanding lung cysts. Thorax 1984; 39:545–549.

157. Sheffield EA, Addis BJ, Corrin B, McCabe MM. Epithelial hyperplasia and malignant change in congenital lung cysts. J Clin Pathol 1987; 40:612–614.

158. Okada Y, Mori H, Maeda T, Obashi A, Itoh Y, Doi KJ. Congenital mediastinal bronchogenic cyst with malignant transformation: an autopsy. Pathol Int 1996; 46:594–600.

159. MacSweeney F, Papagiannopoulos K, Goldstraw P, Sheppard MN, Corrin B, Nicholson AG. An assessment of the expanded classification of congenital cystic adenomatoid malformations and their relationship to malignant transformation. Am J Surg Pathol 2003; 27:1139–1146.

160. Fallon M, Gordon ARG, Lendrum AC. Mediastinal cysts of foregut origin associated with vertebral anomalies. Br J Surg 1954; 41:520–533.

161. Soosay GN, Baudouin SV, Hanson PJV, et al. Symptomatic cysts in otherwise normal lungs of children and adults. Histopathology 1992; 20:517–522.

162. Simon G, Reid L. Atresia of an apical bronchus of the left upper lobe – report of three cases. Br J Dis Chest 1963; 57:126–132.

163. Meng RL, Jensik RJ, Faber LP, Matthews GR, Kittle LF. Bronchial atresia. Ann Thorac Surg 1978; 25:184–192.

164. Jederlinic PJ, Sicilian LS, Baigelman W, Gaensler EA. Congenital bronchial atresia. A report of 4 cases and a review of the literature. Medicine (Baltimore) 1986; 65:73–83.

165. Rossoff LJ, Steinberg H. Bronchial atresia and mucocele: a report of two cases. Respir Med 1994; 88:789–791.

166. Williams AJ, Schuster SR. Bronchial atresia associated with a bronchogenic cyst. Evidence of early appearance of atretic segments. Chest 1985; 87:396–398.

167. Borja AR, Ransdell HT, Villa S. Congenital developmental arrest of the lung. Ann Thorac Surg 1970; 10:317–326.

168. Booth JB, Berry CL. Unilateral pulmonary agenesis. Am J Dis Child 1967; 42:361–374.

169. Maltz DL, Nadas AS. Agenesis of the lung. Pediatrics 1968; 42:175–188.

170. Cunningham ML, Mann N. Pulmonary agenesis: A predictor of ipsilateral malformations. Am J Med Genet 1997; 70:391–398.

171. Ryland D, Reid L. Pulmonary aplasia – a quantitative analysis of the development of the single lung. Thorax 1971; 26:602–609.

172. Emery JL, Mithal A. The number of alveoli in the terminal respiratory unit of man during late intrauterine life and childhood. Arch Dis Child 1960; 35:544–547.

173. Nakamura Y, Yamamoto I, Fukuda S, Hashimoto T. Pulmonary acinar development in diaphragmatic hernia. Arch Pathol Lab Med 1991; 115:372–376.

174. Reale FR, Esterly JR. Pulmonary hypoplasia: a morphometric study of the lungs of infants with diaphragmatic hernia, anencephaly and renal malformations. Pediatrics 1972; 51:91–96.

175. Hislop A, Reid L. Persistent hypoplasia of the lung after repair of congenital diaphragmatic hernia. Thorax 1976; 31:450–455.

176. Page DV, Stocker JT. Anomalies associated with pulmonary hypoplasia. Am Rev Respir Dis 1982; 125:216–221.

177. Cooney TP, Thurlbeck WM. Pulmonary hypoplasia in Down's syndrome. N Engl J Med 1982; 307:1170–1173.

178. Davies G, Reid L. Effect of scoliosis on growth of alveoli and pulmonary arteries and on right ventricle. Arch Dis Child 1971; 46:623–632.

179. Boffa P, Stovin P, Shneerson J. Lung developmental abnormalities in severe scoliosis. Thorax 1984; 39:681–682.

180. Nicolini U, Fisk NM, Rodeck CH, Talbert DG, Wigglesworth JS. Low amniotic pressure in oligohydramnios - Is this the cause of pulmonary hypoplasia? Am J Obstet Gynecol 1989; 161:1098–1101.

181. Adzick NS, Harrison MR, Glick PL, Villa RL, Finkbeiner W. Experimental pulmonary hypoplasia and oligohydramnios: Relative contributions of lung fluid and fetal breathing movements. J Pediatr Surg 1984; 19:658–665.

182. Wigglesworth JS, Hislop A, Desai R. Fetal lung growth in congenital laryngeal atresia. Pediatr Pathol 1987; 7:515–525.

183. Thomas IT, Smith DW. Oligohydramnios, cause of the non-renal features of Potter's syndrome, including pulmonary hypoplasia. J Pediatr 1974; 84:811–814.

184. Armin A, Castelli M. Congenital adrenal tissue in the lung with adrenal cytomegaly. Case report and review of the literature. Am J Clin Pathol 1984; 82:225–228.

185. Bando T, Genka K, Ishikawa K, Kuniyoshi M, Kuda T. Ectopic intrapulmonary thyroid. Chest 1993; 103:1278–1279.

186. Mendoza A, Voland J, Wolf P, Benirschke K. Supradiaphragmatic liver in the lung. Arch Pathol Lab Med 1986; 110:1085–1086.

187. Beskin CA. Intralobar enteric sequestration of the lung containing aberrant pancreas. J Thorac Cardiovasc Surg 1961; 41:314–317.

188. Corrin B, Danel C, Allaway A, Warner JO, Lenney W. Intralobar pulmonary sequestration of ectopic pancreatic tissue with gastro-pancreatic duplication. Thorax 1985; 40:637–638.

189. Aterman K, Patel S. Striated muscle in the lung. Am J Anat 1970; 128:341–358.

190. Remberger K, Hubner G. Rhabdomyomatous dysplasia of the lung. Virchows Arch Pathol Anat Histopathol 1974; 363:363–369.

191. Fraggetta F, Davenport M, Magro G, Cacciaguerra S, Nash R. Striated muscle cells in non-neoplastic lung tissue: a clinicopathologic study. Hum Pathol 2000; 31:1477–1481.

192. Hardisson D, Garcia Jimenez JA, Jimenez Heffernan JA, Nistal M. Rhabdomyomatosis of the newborn lung unassociated with other malformations. Histopathology 1997; 31:474–479.

193. Ramaswamy A, Weyers I, Duda V, Bock K, Barth PJ. A tumorous type of pulmonary rhabdomyomatous dysplasia. Pathol Res Pract 1998; 194:639–642.

194. Burke EC, Wenzl JE, Utz DC. The intrathoracic kidney. Report of a case. Am J Dis Child 1967; 113:487–490.

195. Kanbour AJ, Barmada MA, Klionsky B, Moossy J. Anencephaly and heterotopic central nervous tissue in lungs. Arch Pathol Lab Med 1979; 103:116–118.

196. Gonzalez-Crussi F, Boggs JD, Raffensperger JG. Brain heterotopia in the lungs. Am J Clin Pathol 1980; 73:281–285.

197. Chen WJ, Kelly MM, Shaw CM, et al. Pathogenic mechanisms of heterotopic neural tissue associated with anencephaly. Hum Pathol 1982; 13:179–182.

198. Rakestraw MR, Masood S, Ballinger WE. Brain heterotopia and anencephaly. Arch Pathol Lab Med 1987; 111:858–860.

199. Fuller C, Gibbs AR. Heterotopic brain tissue in the lung causing acute respiratory distress in an infant. Thorax 1989; 44:1045–1046.

200. Kershisnik MM, Kaplan C, Craven CM, Carey JC, Townsend JJ, Knisely AS. Intrapulmonary neuroglial heterotopia. Arch Pathol Lab Med 1992; 116:1043–1046.

201. Langlois NEI, Gray ES. Scatterbrain fetus. J Pathol 1992; 168:347–348.

202. Lager DJ, Kuper KA, Haake GK. Subdiaphragmatic extralumbar pulmonary sequestration. Arch Pathol Lab Med 1991; 115:536–538.

203. Gustafson RA, Murray GF, Wardon HE, Hill RC, Rozar GE. Intralobar sequestration. A missed diagnosis. Ann Thorac Surg 1989; 47:841–847.

204. Gerle RD, Jaretzkia A, Ashley CA, Berne AS. Congenital bronchopulmonry-foregut malformation: pulmonary sequestration communicating with the gastrointestinal tract. N Engl J Med 1968; 278:1413–1419.

205. Flye MW, Izant RJ. Extralobar pulmonary sequestration with esophageal communication and complete duplication of the colon. Surgery 1972; 71:744–752.

206. Aulicino MR, Reis ED, Dolgin SE, Unger PD, Shah KD. Intra-abdominal pulmonary sequestration exhibiting congenital cystic adenomatoid malformation – report of a case and review of the literature. Arch Pathol Lab Med 1994; 118:1034–1037.

207. Fraggetta F, Cacciaguerra S, Nash R, Davenport M. Intra-abdominal pulmonary sequestration associated with congenital cystic adenomatoid malformation of the lung: Just an unusual combination of rare pathologies? Pathol Res Pract 1998; 194:209–211.

208. Sade RM, Clouse M, Ellis Jr FH. The spectrum of pulmonary sequestration. Ann Thorac Surg 1974; 18:644–655.

209. Demos NJ, Teresi A. Congenital lung malformations. A unified concept and a case report. J Thorac Cardiovasc Surg 1975; 70:260–264.

210. Heithoff KB, Sane SM, Williams HJ, et al. Bronchopulmonary foregut malformations. A unifying etiological concept. Am J Roentgenol 1976; 126:46–55.

211. Pryce DM. Lower accessory pulmonary artery with intralobar sequestration of lung: a report of seven cases. J Pathol Bacteriol 1946; 58:457–467.

212. Carter R. Pulmonary sequestration. Ann Thorac Surg 1969; 7:68–85.

213. Gebauer PW, Mason CB. Intralobar pulmonary sequestration associated with anomalous pulmonary vessels. Dis Chest 1959; 35:282–288.

214. Stocker JT, Malczak HT. A study of pulmonary ligament arteries. Relationship to intralobar sequestration. Chest 1984; 86:611–615.

215. Stocker JT. Sequestration of the lung. Semin Diagn Pathol 1986; 3:106–121.

216. Smith RA. A theory of the origin of intralobar sequestration of lung. Thorax 1956; 11:10–24.

217. Hruban RH, Shumway SJ, Orel SB, Dumler JS, Baker RR, Hutchins GM. Congenital bronchopulmonary foregut malformations: intralobar and extralobar pulmonary sequestrations communicating with the foregut. Am J Clin Pathol 1989; 91:403–409.

218. Baar HS, d'Abreu AL. Duplications of the foregut. Superior accessory lung (2 cases); epiphrenic oesophageal diverticulum; intrapericardial teratoid tumour; and oesophageal cyst. Br J Surg 1949; 37:220–230.

219. Van Dijk C, Wagenvoort CA. The various types of congenital adenomatoid malformation of the lung. J Pathol 1973; 110:131–134.

220. Cangiarella J, Greco MA, Askin F, Perlman E, Goswami S, Jagirdar J. Congenital cystic adenomatoid malformation of the lung: insights into the pathogenesis utilizing quantitative analysis of vascular marker CD34 (QBEND-10) and cell proliferation marker MIB-1. Mod Pathol 1995; 8:913–918.

221. Morotti RA, Cangiarella J, Gutierrez MC, et al. Congenital cystic adenomatoid malformation of the lung (CCAM): Evaluation of the cellular components. Hum Pathol 1999; 30:618–625.

222. Stoerk O. Ueber angeborene blasige mis-bildung der lung. Wien Klin Wschr 1897; 10:25–31.

223. Ch'in KY, Tang MY. Congenital adenomatoid malformation of one lobe of a lung with general anasarca. Arch Pathol 1949; 48:221–229.

224. Stocker JT, Madewell JE, Drake RM. Congenital cystic adenomatoid malformation of the lung. Hum Pathol 1977; 8:155–171.

225. Langston C. New concepts in the pathology of congenital lung malformations. Semin Pediatr Surg 2003; 12:17–37.

226. Rutledge JC, Jensen P. Acinar dysplasia: a new form of pulmonary maldevelopment. Hum Pathol 1986; 17:1290–1293.

227. Chambers HM. Congenital acinar aplasia - an extreme form of pulmonary maldevelopment. Pathology 1991; 23:69–71.

228. Davidson LA, Batman P, Fagan DG. Congenital acinar dysplasia: a rare cause of pulmonary hypoplasia. Histopathology 1998; 32:57–59.

229. Dempster AG. Adenomatoid hamartoma of the lung in a neonate. J Clin Pathol 1969; 22:401–406.

230. Ostor AG, Fortune DW. Congenital cystic adenomatoid malformation of the lung. Am J Clin Pathol 1978; 70:595–604.

231. Miller RK, Sieber WK, Yunis EJ. Congenital adenomatoid malformation of the lung. A report of 17 cases and review of the literature. In: Sommers

SC, Rosen PP, eds. Pathol Ann, Vol. 15, Part 1. New York: Appleton-Century-Crofts; 1980:387–406.

232. Avitabile AM, Hulnick DH, Greco MA, Feiner HD. Congenital cystic adenomatoid malformation of the lung in adults. Am J Surg Pathol 1984; 8:193–202.

233. Kinane TB, Mark EJ, Connolly SA, Shannon DC. A newborn triplet with episodes of respiratory distress and a pulmonary mass – congenital cystic adenomatoid malformation of the lung. N Engl J Med 1996; 334: 1726–1732.

234. Imai Y, Mark EJ. Cystic adenomatoid change is common to various forms of cystic lung diseases of children: a clinicopathologic analysis of 10 cases with emphasis on tracing the bronchial tree. Arch Pathol Lab Med 2002; 126:934–940.

235. Ajitsaria R, Awad WI, Jaffe A, et al. Congenital lung abnormality in a 1-yr old. Congenital intradiaphragmatic cystic lung abnormality, Stocker's classification type 2. Eur Resp J 2004; 23(2):348–351.

236. Mendoza A, Wolf P, Edwards DK, Leopold GR, Voland JR, Benirschke K. Prenatal ultrasonographic diagnosis of congenital adenomatoid malformation of the lung. Arch Pathol Lab Med 1986; 110:402–404.

237. Lujan M, Bosque M, Mirapeix RM, Marco MT, Asensio O, Domingo C. Late-onset congenital cystic adenomatoid malformation of the lung – embryology, clinical symptomatology, diagnostic procedures, therapeutic approach and clinical follow-up. Respiration 2002; 69:148–154.

238. Cachia R, Sobonya RE. Congenital cystic adenomatoid malformation of the lung with bronchial atresia. Hum Pathol 1981; 12:947–950.

239. Moerman P, Fryns JP, Vandenberghe K, Devlieger H, Lauweryns JM. Pathogenesis of congenital cystic adenomatoid malformation of the lung. Histopathology 1992; 21:315–321.

240. Ribet ME, Copin MC, Soots JG, Gosselin BH. Bronchioloalveolar carcinoma and congenital cystic adenomatoid malformation. Ann Thorac Surg 1995; 60:1126–1128.

241. Kaslovsky RA, Purdy S, Dangman BC, McKenna BJ, Brien T, Ilves R. Bronchioloalveolar carcinoma in a child with congenital cystic adenomatoid malformation. Chest 1997; 112:548–551.

242. Ota H, Langston C, Honda T, Katsuyama T, Genta RM. Histochemical analysis of mucous cells of congenital adenomatoid malformation of the lung: Insights into the carcinogenesis of pulmonary adenocarcinoma expressing gastric mucins. Am J Clin Pathol 1998; 110:450–455.

243. Stacher E, Ullmann R, Halbwedl I, et al. Atypical goblet cell hyperplasia in congenital cystic adenomatoid malformation as a possible preneoplasia for pulmonary adenocarcinoma in childhood: a genetic analysis. Hum Pathol 2004; 35:565–570.

244. Prichard MG, Brown PJ, Sterrett GF. Bronchioloalveolar carcinoma arising in longstanding lung cysts. Thorax 1984; 39:545–549.

245. Samuel M, Burge DM. Management of antenatally diagnosed pulmonary sequestration associated with congenital cystic adenomatoid malformation. Thorax 1999; 54:701–706.

246. Papagiannopoulos KA, Sheppard M, Bush A, Goldstraw P. Pleuropulmonary blastoma: is prophylactic resection of congenital lung cysts effective? Ann Thorac Surg 2001; 72:604–605.

247. Hill DA, Dehner LP. A cautionary note about congenital cystic adenomatoid malformation (CCAM) type 4. Am J Surg Pathol 2004; 28:554–555.

248. Williams H, Campbell P. Generalized bronchiectasis associated with deficiency of cartilage in the bronchial tree. Arch Dis Child 1960; 35:182–191.

249. Williams HE, Landau LI, Phelan PD. Generalized bronchiectasis due to extensive deficiency of bronchial cartilage. Arch Dis Child 1972; 47:423–428.

250. Mitchell RE, Bury RG. Congenital bronchiectasis due to deficiency of bronchial cartilage (Williams-Campbell syndrome). J Pediatr 1975; 87:230–234.

251. Lee P, Bush A, Warner JO. Left bronchial isomerism associated with bronchomalacia, presenting with intractable wheeze. Thorax 1991; 46:459–461.

252. Wayne KS, Taussig LM. Probable familial congenital bronchiectasis due to cartilage deficiency (Williams–Campbell syndrome). Am Rev Respir Dis 1976; 114:15–22.

253. Jones VF, Eid NS, Franco SM, Badgett JT, Buchino JJ. Familial congenital bronchiectasis: Williams-Campbell syndrome. Pediatr Pulmonol 1993; 16:263–267.

254. Rodriguez-Cintron W, Guntupalli K, Fraire AE. Bronchiectasis and homozygous (P1ZZ) α1-antitrypsin deficiency in a young man. Thorax 1995; 50:424–425.

255. Mounier-Kuhn P. Dilatation de la trachee; constatations radiographiques et bronchoscopiques. Lyon Med 1932; 150:106–109.

256. Al-Mallah Z, Quantock OP. Tracheobronchomegaly. Thorax 1968; 23:320–324.

257. Himalstein MR, Gallagher JC. Tracheobronchomegaly. Ann Otol Rhinol Laryngol 1973; 82:223–227.

258. Van Schoor J, Joos G, Pauwels R. Tracheobronchomegaly – the Mounier-Kuhn syndrome: report of two cases and a review of the literature. Eur Respir J 1991; 4:1303–1306.

259. Schwartz M, Rossoff L. Tracheobronchomegaly. Chest 1994; 106:1589–1590.

260. Schwarz MI. A 60-year-old man with recurrent pneumonias. Chest 2001; 119:1590–1592.

261. Vidal C, Pena F, Mosquera MR, Quintela AG. Tracheobronchomegaly associated with interstitial pulmonary fibrosis. Respiration 1991; 58:207–210.

262. Johnston RF, Green RA. Tracheobronchiomegaly: Report of five cases and demonstration of familial occurrence. Am Rev Respir Dis 1965; 91:35–50.

263. Aaby GV, Blake HA. Tracheobronchiomegaly. Ann Thorac Surg 1966; 2:64–70.

264. Wanderer AA, Ellis EF, Goltz RW, Cotton EK. Tracheobronchiomegaly and acquired cutis laxa in a child. Pediatrics 1969; 44:709–715.

265. Sane AC, Effmann EL, Brown SD. Tracheobronchiomegaly – the Mounier-Kuhn syndrome in a patient with the Kenny-Caffey syndrome. Chest 1992; 102:618–619.

266. Katz I, Levine M, Herman P. Tracheobronchiomegaly: the Mounier–Kuhn syndrome. Am J Roentgenol 1962; 88:1084–1093.

267. Siewert A. Uber einem fall von Bronchiektasien bei einem patienten mit situs inversus viscerum. Klin Wochenschr 1904; 41:139–141.

268. Kartagener M. Zur Pathogenese der Bronchiektasien. I Mitteilung Bronchiektasien bei situs viscerum inversus. Beitr Klin Tuberk 1933; 83:489–501.

269. Camner P, Mossberg B, Afzelius BA. Evidence for congenitally non-functioning cilia in the tracheobronchial tract in two subjects. Am Rev Respir Dis 1975; 112:807–809.

270. Eliasson R, Mossberg B, Camner P, Afzelius BA. The immotile-cilia syndrome. A congenital ciliary abnormality as an etiologic factor in chronic airway infections and male sterility. N Engl J Med 1977; 297:1–6.

271. Afzelius BA. Immotile cilia syndrome: past, present and prospects for the future. Thorax 1998; 53:894–897.

272. Rossman CM, Forrest JB, Lee RMKW, Newhouse MT. The dyskinetic cilia syndrome. Ciliary motility in immotile cilia syndrome. Chest 1980; 78:580–582.

273. Afzelius BA, Eliasson R, Johnsen O, Lindholmer C. Lack of dynein arms in immotile human spermatozoa. J Cell Biol 1975; 66:225–232.

274. Munro NC, Currie DC, Lindsay KS, et al. Fertility in men with primary ciliary dyskinesia presenting with respiratory infection. Thorax 1994; 49:684–687.

275. Afzelius BA, Eliasson R. Male and female infertility problems in the immotile-cilia syndrome. Eur J Respir Dis 1983; 64(suppl 127):144–147.

276. Sturgess JM, Chao J, Wong J, Aspin N, Turner JAP. Cilia with defective radial spokes. A cause of human respiratory disease. N Engl J Med 1979; 300:53–56.

277. Sturgess JM, Chao J, Turner JAP. Transposition of ciliary microtubules: another cause of impaired ciliary motility. N Engl J Med 1980; 303:318–322.

278. Rutland J, Deiongh RU. Random ciliary orientation – a cause of respiratory tract disease. N Engl J Med 1990; 323:1681–1684.

279. Niggemann B, Muller A, Nolte A, Schnoy N, Wahn U. Abnormal length of cilia - a cause of primary ciliary dyskinesia - a case report. Eur J Pediatr 1992; 151:73–75.

280. Rayner CFJ, Rutman A, Dewar A, Greenstone MA, Cole PJ, Wilson R. Ciliary disorientation alone as a cause of primary ciliary dyskinesia syndrome. Am J Respir Crit Care Med 1996; 153:1123–1129.

281. Tsang KWT, Tipoe G, Sun J, et al. Severe bronchiectasis in patients with 'cystlike' structures within the ciliary shafts. Am J Respir Crit Care Med 2000; 161:1300–1305.

282. Kovesi T, Sinclair B, MacCormick J, Matzinger MA, Carpenier B. Primary ciliary dyskinesia associated with a novel microtubule defect in a child with Down's syndrome. Chest 2000; 117:1207–1209.

283. Fox B, Bull TB. Letter to editor. Am Rev Respir Dis 1981; 123:142–143.

284. Mierau GW, Agostini R, Beals TF, et al. The role of electron microscopy in evaluating ciliary dysfunction – report of a workshop. Ultrastruct Pathol 1992; 16:245–254.

285. Deiongh RU, Rutland J. Ciliary defects in healthy subjects, bronchiectasis and primary ciliary dyskinesia. Am J Respir Crit Care Med 1995; 151:1559–1567.

286. Rutland J, Cole PJ. Non-invasive sampling of nasal cilia for measurement of beat frequency and study of ultrastructure. Lancet 1980; 2:564–565.

287. Rutland J, Dewar A, Cox T, Cole P. Nasal brushing for the study of ciliary ultrastructure. J Clin Pathol 1982; 35:357–359.

288. Bush A, Cole P, Hariri M, et al. Primary ciliary dyskinesia: diagnosis and standards of care. Eur Resp J 1998; 12:982–988.

289. Bush A, Cole P, Hariri M, et al. Primary ciliary dyskinesia: diagnosis and standards of care. Eur Respir J 1998; 12:982–988.

290. Rutland J, Cox T, Dewar A, Cole P, Warner JO. Transitory ultrastructural abnormalities of cilia. Br J Dis Chest 1982; 76:185–188.

291. Elborn JS, Shale DJ, Britton JR. Cystic fibrosis – current survival and population estimates to the year 2000. Thorax 1991; 46:881–885.

292. Clausiusz J. Hidden benefits. Online. Available: http://www people virginia edu/~rjh9u/cysfib html 1997.

293. Wainwright BJ, Scambler PJ, Schmidtke J, et al. Localization of cystic fibrosis locus to chromosome 7cen-q22. Nature 1985; 318:384–385.

294. Tsui LC, Buchwald M, Barker D, et al. Cystic fibrosis locus defined by a genetically linked polymorphic DNA marker. Science 1985; 230:1054–1057.

295. Davidson DJ, Porteous DJ. The genetics of cystic fibrosis lung disease. Thorax 1998; 53:389–397.

296. Farral M, Law HY, Rodek CH, et al. First-trimester prenatal diagnosis of cystic fibrosis using linked DNA probes. Lancet 1986; i:1402–1404.

297. Wald NJ. Couple screening for cystic fibrosis. Lancet 1991; 338:1318–1320.

298. Grody WW. Cystic fibrosis – Molecular diagnosis, population screening and public policy. Arch Pathol Lab Med 1999; 123:1041–1046.

299. Lyon E, Miller C. Current challenges in cystic fibrosis screening. Arch Pathol Lab Med 2003; 127(9):1133–1139.

300. Kerem B-S, Rommens JM, Buchanan JA, et al. Identification of the cystic fibrosis gene: genetic analysis. Science 1989; 245:1073–1080.

301. Cutting GR, Kasch LM, Rosenstein BJ, et al. A cluster of cystic fibrosis mutations in the first nucleotide-binding fold of the cystic fibrosis conductant regulator protein. Nature 1990; 346:366–369.

302. Alton EWFW, Geddes DM. Gene therapy for respiratory diseases: potential applications and difficulties. Thorax 1995; 50:484–486.

303. Johnson LG. Gene therapy for cystic fibrosis. Chest 1995; 107:S77–S83.

304. Korst RJ, McElvaney NG, Chu CS, et al. Gene therapy for the respiratory manifestations of cystic fibrosis. Am J Respir Crit Care Med 1995; 151:S75–S87.

305. Koch C, Hoiby N. Pathogenesis of cystic fibrosis. Lancet 1993; 341:1065–1069.

306. Rutland J, Cole PJ. Nasal mucociliary clearance and ciliary beat frequency in cystic fibrosis compared with sinusitis and bronchiectasis. Thorax 1981; 36:654–658.

307. Katz SM, Holsclaw DS. Ultrastructural features of respiratory cilia in cystic fibrosis. Am J Clin Pathol 1980; 73:682–685.

308. Quinton PM. Chloride impermeability in cystic fibrosis. Nature 1983; 301:421–422.

309. Welsh MJ, Liedtke CM. Chloride and potassium channels in cystic fibrosis airway epithelia. Nature 1986; 322:467–470.

310. Tsui LC. The cystic fibrosis transmembrane conductance regulator gene. Am J Respir Crit Care Med 1995; 151:S47–S53.

311. Frizzell RA. Function of the cystic fibrosis transmembrane conductance regulator protein. Am J Respir Crit Care Med 1995; 151:S54–S58.

312. Puchelle E, Gaillard D, Ploton D, et al. Differential localization of the cystic fibrosis transmembrane conductance regulator in normal and cystic fibrosis airway epithelium. Am J Respir Cell Mol Biol 1992; 7:485–491.

313. Yang Y, Engelhardt JF, Wilson JM. Ultrastructural localization of variant forms of cystic fibrosis transmembrane conductance regulator in human bronchial epithelia of xenografts. Am J Respir Cell Mol Biol 1994; 11:7–15.

314. Valman HB, France NE. The vas deferens in CF. Lancet 1969; ii:566–567.

315. Chillon M, Casals T, Mercier B, et al. Mutations in the cystic fibrosis gene in patients with congenital absence of the vas deferens. N Engl J Med 1995; 332:1475–1480.

316. Smith JJ, Travis SM, Greenberg EP, Welsh MJ. Cystic fibrosis airway epithelia fail to kill bacteria because of abnormal airway surface fluid [published erratum appears in Cell 1996; 87:355]. Cell 1996; 85:229–236.

317. Goldman MJ, Anderson GM, Stolzenberg ED, Kari UP, Zasloff M, Wilson JM. Human beta-defensin-1 is a salt-sensitive antibiotic in lung that is inactivated in cystic fibrosis. Cell 1997; 88:553–560.

318. Postle AD, Mander A, Reid KBM, et al. Deficient hydrophilic lung surfactant proteins A and D with normal surfactant phospholipid molecular species in cystic fibrosis. Am J Respir Cell Mol Biol 1999; 20:90–98.

319. Lethem MI, James SL, Marriott C, Burke JF. The origin of DNA associated with mucous glycoproteins in cystic fibrosis sputum. Eur Respir J 1990; 3:19–23.

320. Yacoub MH, Banner NR, Khaghani A, et al. Heart-lung transplantation for cystic fibrosis and subsequent domino heart transplantation. J Heart Transplant 1990; 9:459–467.

321. Tsang VT, Alton EWFW, Hodson ME, Yacoub M. In vitro bioelectric properties of bronchial epithelium from transplanted lungs in recipients with cystic fibrosis. Thorax 1993; 48:1006–1011.

322. Anguiano A, Oates RD, Amos J. Congenital absence of the vas deferens- a primary genital form of cystic fibrosis. JAMA 1992; 267:1794.

323. Drake-Lee AB, Pitcher-Wilmott RW. The clinical and laboratory correlates of nasal polyps in cystic fibrosis. Int J Pediatr Otorhinolaryngol 1982; 4:209.

324. Bronsveld I, Bijman J, Mekus F, Ballmann M, Veeze HJ, Tummler B. Clinical presentation of exclusive cystic fibrosis lung disease. Thorax 1999; 54:278–281.

325. Penketh ARL, Wise A, Mearns MB, Hodson ME, Batten JC. Cystic fibrosis in adolescents and adults. Thorax 1987; 42:526–532.

326. van Biezen P, Overbeek SE, Hilvering C. Cystic fibrosis in a 70 year old woman. Thorax 1992; 47:202–203.

327. Rosenbluth D, Goodenberger D. Cystic fibrosis in an elderly woman. Chest 1997; 112:1124–1126.

328. Gilljam M, Bjorck E. Cystic fibrosis diagnosed in an elderly man. Respiration 2004; 71:98–100.

329. Chapman AL, Fagley B, Cho CT. X-ray microanalysis of chloride in nails from cystic fibrosis and control patients. Eur J Respir Dis 1985; 66:218–223.

330. Roomans GM, Afzelius BA, Kollberg H, Forslind B. Electrolytes in nails analysed by X-ray microanalysis in electron microscopy. Considerations of a new method for the diagnosis of cystic fibrosis. Acta Paediatr Scand 1978; 67:89–94.

331. Alton E, Currie D, Logan-Sinclair R, Warner JO, Hodson ME, Geddes DM. Nasal potential difference: a clinical diagnostic test for cystic fibrosis. Eur Respir J 1990; 3:922–926.

331a. Donlan RM, Costerton JW. Biofilms: survival mechanisms of clinically relevant microorganisms. Clin Microbiol Rev 2002; 15:167–193.

331b. Donlan RM. Biofilms: microbial life on surfaces. Emerg Infect Dis 2002; 8:881–890.

332. Stableforth DE, Smith DL. Pseudomonas cepacia in cystic fibrosis. Thorax 1994; 49:629–630.

333. Govan JRW, Brown PH, Maddison J, et al. Evidence for transmission of pseudomonas-cepacia by social contact in cystic fibrosis. Lancet 1993; 342:15–19.

334. McFarlane H, Holzel A, Brenchley P, et al. Immune complexes in cystic fibrosis. BMJ 1975; 1:423–428.

335. Finnegan MJ, Hinchcliffe J, Russell-Jones D, et al. Vasculitis complicating cystic fibrosis. Q J Med 1989; 72:609–622.

336. Hodson M. Immunological abnormalities in cystic fibrosis: chicken or egg? Thorax 1980; 35:801–806.

337. Geller DE, Kaplowitz H, Light MJ, Colin AA. Allergic bronchopulmonary aspergillosis in cystic fibrosis – Reported prevalence, regional distribution and patient characteristics. Chest 1999; 116:639–646.

338. Mastella G, Rainisio M, Harms HK, et al. Allergic bronchopulmonary aspergillosis in cystic fibrosis. A European epidemiological study. Eur Resp J 2000; 16:464–471.

339. Bedrossian CWM, Greenberg SD, Singer DB, Hansen JJ, Rosenberg HS. The lung in cystic fibrosis. A quantitative study of pathologic findings amongst different age groups. Hum Pathol 1976; 7:195–204.

340. Oppenheimer EH, Esterly JR. Pathology of cystic fibrosis. Review of the literature and comparison with 146 autopsied cases. Perspect pediatr Pathol 1975; 2:241–278.

341. Esterly JR, Oppenheimer EH. Observations in cystic fibrosis of the pancreas. II. Pulmonary lesions. Johns Hopkins Med J 1968; 122:94–101.

342. Lamb D, Reid L. The tracheobronchial submucosal glands in cystic fibrosis: a qualitative and quantitative histochemical study. Br J Dis Chest 1972; 66:239–247.

343. Esterly JR, Oppenheimer EH. Cystic fibrosis of the pancreas: structural changes in peripheral airways. Thorax 1968; 23:670–675.

344. Tomashefski JFJr, Konstan MW, Bruce MC, Abramowsky CR. The pathologic characteristics of interstitial pneumonia in cystic fibrosis. A retrospective autopsy study. Am J Clin Pathol 1989; 91:522–530.

345. Ogrinc G, Kampalath B, Tomashefski JF. Destruction and loss of bronchial cartilage in cystic fibrosis. Hum Pathol 1998; 29:65–73.

346. Tomashefski JF, Bruce M, Goldberg HI, Dearborn DG. Regional distribution of macroscopic lung disease in cystic fibrosis. Am Rev Respir Dis 1986; 133:535–540.

347. Tomashefski JF, Bruce M, Stern RC, Dearborn DG, Dahms B. Pulmonary air cysts in cystic fibrosis: relation of pathologic features to radiologic findings and history of pneumothorax. Hum Pathol 1985; 16:253–261.

347a. Flume PA, Strange C, Ye X, et al. Pneumothorax in cystic fibrosis. Chest 2005; 128:720–728.

348. Wentworth P, Gough J, Wentworth JE. Pulmonary changes and cor pulmonale in mucoviscidosis. Thorax 1968; 23:582–589.

349. Ryland D, Reid L. The pulmonary circulation in cystic fibrosis. Thorax 1975; 30:285–292.

350. Oppenheimer EH, Rosenstein BJ. Differential pathology of nasal polyps in cystic fibrosis and atopy. Lab Invest 1979; 40:445–449.

351. Couper R, Bentur L, Kilbourn JP, Wolf P. Immunoreactive calmodulin in cystic fibrosis kidneys. Aust N Z J Med 1993; 23:484–488.

352. Turner MA, Goldwater D, David TJ. Oxalate and calcium excretion in cystic fibrosis. Arch Dis Child 2000; 83:244–247.

353. Perez-Brayfield MR, Caplan D, Gatti JM, Smith EA, Kirsch AJ. Metabolic risk factors for stone formation in patients with cystic fibrosis. J Urol 2002; 167:480–484.

354. Hellsing E, Brattstrom V, Strandvik B. Craniofacial morphology in children with cystic fibrosis. Eur J Orthod 1992; 14:147–151.

355. Hendry WF, Knight RK, Whitfield HN, et al. Obstructive azoospermia: respiratory function tests, electron microscopy and the results of surgery. Br J Urol 1978; 50:598–604.

356. Deiongh R, Ing A, Rutland J. Mucociliary function, ciliary ultrastructure and ciliary orientation in Young's syndrome. Thorax 1992; 47:184–187.

357. Pavia D, Agnew JE, Bateman JRM, et al. Lung mucociliary clearance in patients with Young's syndrome. Chest 1981; 80(suppl):892–895.

358. Henderson R, Hislop A, Reid L. New pathological findings in emphysema of childhood: 3. Unilateral congenital emphysema with hypoplasia and compensatory emphysema of the contralateral lung. Thorax 1971; 26:195–205.

359. Hislop A, Reid L. New pathological findings in emphysema in childhood: 2. Overinflation of a normal lobe. Thorax 1971; 26:190–194.

360. Critchley PS, Forrester-Wood CP, Ridley PD. Adult congenital lobar emphysema in pregnancy. Thorax 1995; 50:909–910.

361. Sedivy R, Bankl HC, Stimpfl T, Kurkciyan I. Sudden, unexpected death of a young marathon runner as a result of bronchial malformation. Mod Pathol 1997; 10:247–251.

362. Stovin PGI. Congenital lobar emphysema. Thorax 1959; 14:254–262.

363. Warner JO, Rubin S, Heard BE. Congenital lobar emphysema: a case with bronchial atresia and abnormal bronchial cartilages. Br J Dis Chest 1982; 76:177–184.

364. MonforteMunoz H, Walls RL. Intrapulmonary airways visualized by staining and clearing of whole-lung sections: the transparent human lung. Modern Pathol 2004; 17(1):22–27.

365. Leape LL, Longino LA. Infantile lobar emphysema. Pediatrics 1964; 34:246–255.

366. Stanger P, Lucas RV, Jr., Edwards JE. Anatomic factors causing respiratory distress in acyanotic congenital cardiac disease. Special reference to bronchial obstruction. Pediatrics 1969; 43:760–769.

367. Hislop A, Reid L. New pathological findings in emphysema in childhood: 1. Polyalveolar lobe with emphysema. Thorax 1970; 25:682–690.

368. Mani H, Suarez E, Stocker JT. The morphologic spectrum of infantile lobar emphysema: a study of 33 cases. Paediatr Respir Rev 2004; 5(Suppl A):S313–S320.

369. Reid L, Simon G. Unilateral lung transradiancy. Thorax 1962; 17:230–239.

370. Stokes D, Sigler A, Khouri NF, Talmo RC. Unilateral hyperlucent lung (Swyer-James syndrome) after severe Mycoplasma pneumoniae infection. Am Rev Respir Dis 1978; 117:145–152.

371. Mark EJ. Mesenchymal cystic hamartoma of the lung. N Engl J Med 1986; 315:1255–1259.

372. Hedlund GL, Bisset GSI, Bove KE. Malignant neoplasms arising in cystic hamartomas of the lung in childhood. Radiology 1989; 173:77–79.

373. Mushtaq M, Ward SP, Hutchison JT, Mann JS. Multiple cystic pulmonary hamartomas. Thorax 1992; 47:1076–1077.

374. Leroyer C, Quiot JJ, Dewitte JD, Briere J, Clavier J. Mesenchymal cystic hamartoma of the lung. Respiration 1993; 60:305–306.

375. van Klaveren RJ, Hassing HHM, Wiersma-van Tilburg JM, Lacquet LK, Cox AL. Mesenchymal cystic hamartoma of the lung: a rare cause of relapsing pneumothorax. Thorax 1994; 49:1175–1176.

376. Chadwick SL, Corrin B, Hansell DM, Geddes DM. Fatal haemorrhage from mesenchymal cystic hamartoma of the lung. Eur Respir J 1995; 8:2182–2184.

377. Cottin V, Thomas L, Loire R, Chalabreysse L, Gindre D, Cordier JF. Mesenchymal cystic hamartoma of the lung in Cowden's disease. Resp Med 2003; 97:188–191.

378. Abrams J, Talcott J, Corson JM. Pulmonary metastases in patients with low-grade endometrial stromal sarcoma. Clinicopathologic findings with immunohistochemical characterization. Am J Surg Pathol 1989; 13:133–140.

379. Chang KL, Crabtree GS, Lim-Tan SK, Kempson RL, Hendrickson MR. Primary uterine endometrial stromal neoplasms. A clinicopathologic study of 117 cases. Am J Surg Pathol 1990; 14:415–438.

380. Rosenmann E, Maayan C, Lernau O. Leiomyomatous hamartosis with congenital jejunoileal atresia. Isr J Med Sci 1980; 16:775–779.

381. McGinnis M, Jacobs G, Elnaggar A, Redline RW. Congenital peribronchial myofibroblastic tumor (so-called congenital leiomyosarcoma) – a distinct neonatal lung lesion associated with nonimmune hydrops-fetalis. Mod Pathol 1993; 6:487–492.

382. Alobeid B, Beneck D, Sreekantaiah C, Abbi RK, Slim MS. Congenital pulmonary myofibroblastic tumor: A case report with cytogenetic analysis and review of the literature. Am J Surg Pathol 1997; 21:610–614.

383. Pool PE, Vogel JHK, Blount SG. Congenital unilateral absence of a pulmonary artery. Am J Cardiol 1962; 10:706–732.

384. Brassard JM, Johnson JE. Unilateral absence of a pulmonary artery – data from cardiopulmonary exercise testing. Chest 1993; 103:293–295.

385. Arriero JM, Gil J, Martin C, Mainar V, Romero S. Unilateral absence of a pulmonary artery – congenital disease or embolic occlusion. Eur Respir J 1991; 4:1299–1300.

386. Morales P, Miravet L, Marco V. Agenesis of the right pulmonary artery in a young asymptomatic girl. Eur Respir J 1991; 4:1301–1302.

387. Ko T, Gatz MG, Reisz GR. Congenital unilateral absence of a pulmonary artery: Report of two adult cases. Am Rev Respir Dis 1990; 141:795–798.

388. Maeda S, Suzuki S, Moriya T, et al. Isolated unilateral absence of a pulmonary artery: Influence of systemic circulation on alveolar capillary vessels. Pathol Int 2001; 51:649–653.

389. TenHarkel ADJ, Blom NA, Ottenkamp J. Isolated unilateral absence of a pulmonary artery - A case report and review of the literature. Chest 2002; 122:1471–1477.

390. Presbitero P, Bull C, Haworth SG, de Laval MR. Absent or occult pulmonary artery. Br Heart J 1984; 52:178–185.

391. Sweerts M, Nicholson AG, Goldstraw P, Corrin B. Dieulafoy's disease of the bronchus. Thorax 1995; 50:697–698.

392. Stoopen E, BaqueraHeredia J, Cortes D, Green L. Dieulafoy's disease of the bronchus in association with a paravertebral neurilemoma. Chest 2001; 119:292–294.

392a. Pomplun S, Sheaff MT. Dieulafoy's disease of the bronchus: an uncommon entity. Histopathology 2005; 46:598–599.

393. Nashef SAM, Jamieson MPG, Pollock JCS, Houston AB. Aortic origin of right pulmonary artery: successful surgical correction in three consecutive patients. Ann Thorac Surg 1987; 44:536–538.

394. Liebow AA, Hales MR, Lindskog GE. Enlargement of the bronchial arteries and their anastomoses with the pulmonary arteries in bronchiectasis. Am J Pathol 1949; 25:211–231.

395. Janney CG, Askin FB, Kuhn C. Congenital alveolar capillary dysplasia – an unusual cause of respiratory distress in the newborn. Am J Clin Pathol 1981; 76:722–727.

396. Wagenvoort CA. Misalignment of lung vessels: a syndrome causing persistent neonatal pulmonary hypertension. Hum Pathol 1986; 17:727–730.

397. Cater G, Thibeault DW, Beatty EC, Kilbride HW, Huntrakoon M. Misalignment of lung vessels and alveolar capillary dysplasia: a cause of persistent pulmonary hypertension. J Pediatr 1989; 114:293–300.

398. Oldenburg J, Vanderpal HJH, Schrevel LS, Blok APR, Wagenvoort CA. Misalignment of lung vessels and alveolar capillary dysplasia. Histopathology 1995; 27:192–194.

399. Vassal HB, Malone M, Petros AJ, Winter RM. Familial persistent pulmonary hypertension of the newborn resulting from misalignment of the pulmonary vessels (congenital alveolar capillary dysplasia). J Med Genet 1998; 35:58–60.

400. Petersen RC, Edwards WD. Pulmonary vascular disease in 57 necropsy cases of total anomalous pulmonary venous connection. Histopathology 1983; 7:487–496.

401. Wang JK, Chiu IS, How SW, et al. Anomalous pulmonary venous pathway traversing pulmonary parenchyma: diagnosis and implication. Chest 1996; 110:1363–1366.

402. Haworth SG, Reid L. Structural study of pulmonary circulation and of heart in total anomalous pulmonary venous return in early infancy. Br Heart J 1977; 39:80–92.

403. Sun CC, Doyle T, Ringel RE. Pulmonary vein stenosis. Hum Pathol 1995; 26:880–886.

404. Omasa M, Hasegawa S, Bando T, et al. A case of congenital pulmonary vein stenosis in an adult. Respiration 2004; 71(1):92–94.

405. Honey M. Anomalous pulmonary venous drainage of right lung to inferior vena cava ('Scimitar Syndrome'): clinical spectrum in older patients and role of surgery. Q J Med 1977; 184:463–483.

406. Churton T. Multiple aneurysms of pulmonary artery. BMJ 1897; i:1223.

407. Le Roux BT. Pulmonary arteriovenous fistulae. Q J Med 1959; 28:1–19.

408. Utzon F, Brandup F. Pulmonary arteriovenous fistulas in children. Acta Paediatr Scand 1973; 62:422–432.

409. Dines DE, Arms RA, Bernatz PE, Gomes MR. Pulmonary arteriovenous fistulas. Mayo Clin Proc 1974; 49:460–465.

410. Przybojewski JZ, Maritz F. Pulmonary arteriovenous fistulas. A case presentation and review of the literature. S Afr Med J 1980; 57:366–373.

411. Prager RL, Laws KH, Bender Jr HW. Arteriovenous fistula of the lung. Ann Thorac Surg 1983; 36:231–239.

412. Gossage JR, Kanj G. Pulmonary arteriovenous malformations – A state of the art review. Am J Respir Crit Care Med 1998; 158:643–661.

413. Grishman A, Poppel MH, Simpson RS, Sussman ML. The roentgenographic and angiocardiographic aspects of (1) aberrant insertion of pulmonary veins associated with interatrial septal defect and (2) congenital arteriovenous aneurysm of the lung. Am J Roentgenol 1949; 62:500–508.

414. Gomes MR, Bernatz PE, Dines DE. Pulmonary arteriovenous fistulas. Ann Thorac Surg 1969; 7:582–593.

415. Pouwels HMM, Janevski BK, Penn OCKM, Sie HT, Tenvelde GPM. Systemic to pulmonary vascular malformation. Eur Respir J 1992; 5:1288–1291.

416. Akahane T, Yaegashi H, Kurokawa Y, Satomi S, Takahashi T. Systemic-to-pulmonary vascular malformation of lung visualized by computer-assisted 3-D reconstruction. Histopathology 1997; 31:252–257.

417. Hoffman R, Rabens R. Evolving pulmonary nodules: multiple pulmonary arteriovenous fistulas. Am J Roentgenol 1974; 120:861–864.

418. Hughes JMB. Intrapulmonary shunts: coils to transplantation. J R Coll Physicians Lond 1994; 28:247–253.

419. Shovlin CL, Letarte M. Hereditary haemorrhagic telangiectasia and pulmonary arteriovenous malformations: issues in clinical management and review of pathogenic mechanisms. Thorax 1999; 54:714–729.

420. Hodgson CH, Burchell HB, Good CA, Clagett OT. Hereditary hemorrhagic telangiectasia and pulmonary arteriovenous fistula. Survey of a large family. N Engl J Med 1959; 261:625–636.

421. Reynaud-Gaubert M, Thomas P, Gaubert JY, et al. Pulmonary arteriovenous malformations: lung transplantation as a therapeutic option. Eur Resp J 1999; 14:1425–1428.

422. Faughnan ME, Lui YW, Wirth JA, et al. Diffuse pulmonary arterio-venous malformations – Characteristics and prognosis. Chest 2000; 117:31–38.

423. Ference BA, Shannon TM, White RI, Zawin M, Burdge CM. Life-threatening pulmonary hemorrhage with pulmonary arteriovenous malformations and hereditary hemorrhagic telangiectasia. Chest 1994; 106:1387–1390.

424. Wang N-S, Seemayer TA, Ahmed MN, Morin J. Pulmonary leiomyosarcoma associated with an arteriovenous fistula. Arch Pathol 1974; 98:100–105.

425. Emerson PA. Yellow nails, lymphoedema and pleural effusions. Thorax 1966; 21:247–253.

426. Solal-Celigny P, Cormier Y, Fournier M. The yellow nail syndrome. Arch Pathol Lab Med 1983; 107:183–185.

427. Beer DJ, Pereira W, Snider GL. Pleural effusion associated with primary lymphedema: a perspective on the yellow nail syndrome. Am Rev Respir Dis 1978; 117:595–599.

428. Joshi M, Cole S, Knibbs D, Diana D. Pulmonary abnormalities in Klippel-Trenaunay syndrome – a histologic, ultrastructural and immunocytochemical study. Chest 1992; 102:1274–1277.

429. Gianlupi A, Harper RW, Dwyre DM, Marelich GP. Recurrent pulmonary embolism associated with Klippel–Trenaunay–Weber syndrome. Chest 1999; 115:1199–1201.

430. Faul JL, Berry GJ, Colby TV, et al. Thoracic lymphangiomas, lymphangiectasis, lymphangiomatosis and lymphatic dysplasia syndrome. Am J Respir Crit Care Med 2000; 161:1037–1046.

431. Esterly JR, Oppenheimer EH. Lymphangiectasis and other pulmonary lesions in the asplenia syndrome. Arch Pathol 1970; 90:553–560.

432. Barker PM, Esther CR Jr., Fordham LA, Maygarden SJ, Funkhouser WK. Primary pulmonary lymphangiectasia in infancy and childhood. Eur Respir J 2004; 24:413–419.

433. Wagenaar SS, Swierenga J, Wagenvoort CA. Late presentation of primary pulmonary lymphangiectasis. Thorax 1978; 33:791–795.

434. White JES, Veale D, Fishwick D, Mitchell L, Corris PA. Generalised lymphangiectasia: pulmonary presentation in an adult. Thorax 1996; 51:767–768.

435. Laurence KM. Congenital pulmonary lymphangiectasis. J Clin Pathol 1959; 12:62–69.

436. Sheehan JJ, Kearns SR, McNamara DA, Brennan RP, Deasy JM. Adult presentation of agenesis of the hemidiaphragm. Chest 2000; 117:901–902.

437. Theerthakarat R, ElHalees W, Javadpoor S, Khan MA. Severe pectus excavatum associated with cor pulmonale and chronic respiratory acidosis in a young woman. Chest 2001; 119:1957–1961.

438. Greenough A. Abnormalities of the skeleton. In: Greenough A, Milner AD, eds. Neonatal Respiratory Disorders. London: Arnold; 2003:505–518.

3

Diseases of the airways

The function of the airways is to conduct gas in and out of the lungs and all airway diseases are liable to impede this, resulting in 'obstructive lung disease', as opposed to the 'restrictive lung disease' caused by many diseases of the lung parenchyma. Airway obstruction has important effects on the lung parenchyma and this chapter first considers one of these: pulmonary collapse. Another important consequence of airway obstruction is obstructive pneumonia, which is dealt with in Chapter 5.2.

ATELECTASIS AND PULMONARY COLLAPSE

The term atelectasis literally means imperfect expansion and is applied specifically to failure of the lungs to expand fully at birth. This may be due to congenital airway obstruction or pulmonary compression and is of course found in stillbirths. Once the lungs have expanded, return to the airless state is sometimes referred to as secondary atelectasis, but is more widely known as pulmonary collapse. Two types of pulmonary collapse are recognised, one due to pressure changes and the other to absorbed alveolar gas not being replenished.

Pressure collapse may result from external forces exerted by air or fluid in the pleural cavity, enlargement of the heart or mediastinum, or a thoracic tumour. Alternatively, pressure collapse may be due to a rise in alveolar surface tension from depletion of pulmonary surfactant, as in the infantile and adult respiratory distress syndromes (see pp. 42, 131).

Absorption collapse is likely when bronchial obstruction prevents free entry of air into the lungs. The causes are listed in Box 3.1. Mucus frequently collects during anaesthesia, when respiratory movements are reduced and the cough reflex suppressed, while the inhalation of a foreign body is especially common in children. The narrow, pliable bronchi of infants are particularly liable to be compressed by distended pulmonary arteries at points where they are in close anatomical proximity (see Fig. 10.10, p. 481) or by abnormally located systemic arteries. In time, the alveolar air – first the oxygen and later the nitrogen – is removed by the blood that passes through the affected area and the alveoli then progressively collapse.

Box 3.1 Causes of absorption collapse

Intralumenal lesions
    Mucus
    Foreign body
    Broncholith
    Endobronchial tumour[a]
Mural lesions
    Bronchogenic carcinoma
    Sarcoid
Extrinsic lesions
    Lymph nodes enlarged by metastatic tumour or tuberculosis
    Distended or aneurysmally dilated arteries

[a]Tumours particularly prone to grow preferentially into the lumen of an airway include carcinosarcoma, carcinoid, bronchial gland neoplasms, metastases, lymphoma, chondroid hamartoma, papillary neoplasms, granular cell tumour and amyloid tumour.

Pulmonary collapse has been seen quite commonly in the crew of high performance aircraft. An important cause is breathing pure oxygen, which washes nitrogen from the alveoli and is more rapidly absorbed into the blood. Parts of the lung filled with oxygen but temporarily closed off by increased gravitational forces distorting airways are liable to absorption collapse. These forces operate whenever the pilot makes a tight turn at high speed or pulls out of a steep dive. Clothing designed to protect the aviator from a burst lung (see p. 370) increases the adverse effect on the basal parts of the lungs by raising the diaphragm and reducing lung volume.

Pathological findings

Whatever the cause, collapsed lungs are small and firm and have a deeply wrinkled pleural surface. Portions of collapsed lungs tend to sink when dropped into water but this is not an infallible test of airlessness. Where part of a lung has recently collapsed, the immediately adjacent, pale pink, aerated lobules are sharply separated from the dark red depressed areas of collapse by zigzag lines that correspond to the interlobular septa (see Fig. 4.3, p. 133). The collapse involves alveoli and bronchioles but bronchial cartilage maintains the patency of these larger airways. Subsequent changes differ according to whether the collapse is due to absorption or compression. With absorption collapse the affected lung resembles splenic tissue, both grossly and microscopically.[1] Alveolar walls are in apposition and their capillaries are greatly dilated so that the bulk of the collapsed lung no longer consists of air space but of sinusoidal vessels engorged with blood, although the circulation may be reduced. The interlobular septa are thickened but there is little fibrosis of the alveolar tissue. The changes are irreversible, suggesting that there is fusion of the apposed alveolar walls. With pressure collapse congestion is less marked and fibrosis of both the alveolar tissue and overlying pleura is more marked (Fig. 3.1). In either case, re-inflation is prevented.

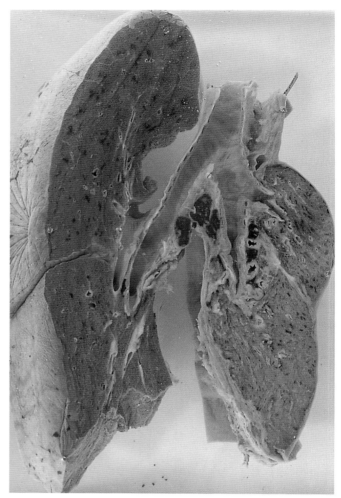

Figure 3.1 Chronic pulmonary collapse due to long-standing pleural effusion. On the right of the picture pleuropulmonary fibrosis has developed, preventing the lung from ever expanding.

Collateral ventilation

When obstruction to an airway is only partial, permitting inspiration but hindering expiration, air is retained in the affected area and there is full inflation rather than collapse (see 'infantile lobar emphysema', p. 70). Absorption collapse may also be prevented by collateral ventilation, a process by which one portion of lung is ventilated through another via the pores of Kohn, Lambert's canals and other peripheral communications (see pp. 5, 13). Collateral ventilation is best developed at the acinar level, being hindered by the interlobular septa and prevented by interlobar fissures, but because interlobular septa are incomplete, it may prevent whole segments undergoing absorption collapse. However, airflow through the tortuous bypass channels afforded by many pores of Kohn is poor and collateral ventilation plays little part in gas exchange.[2] Its function is to maintain inflation of alveoli when their supplying airways are obstructed by secretions or a foreign body. This is essential to the cough mechanism, dependent upon which are the expulsion of the obstructive material and the restoration of bronchial patency.

Middle lobe syndrome

The term 'middle lobe syndrome' was introduced in 1937 to describe a condition of chronic or recurrent absorption collapse of the right middle lobe.[3] The collapse was most frequently caused by tuberculous involvement of lymph nodes compressing the right middle lobe bronchus. Although tuberculosis is less common today, any disease enlarging these lymph nodes may have the same effect. Predilection for involvement of the middle lobe was considered to be the result of a combination of factors: the prominent collar of nodes about its bronchus, the lymphatic drainage of these nodes being from much of the right lung and parts of the left and the relatively narrow calibre and possibly undue compressibility of the middle lobe bronchus. A further possible factor is the limited capacity for collateral ventilation (see above) within the middle lobe. This stems from the fact that its two segments have relatively large proportions of their surfaces covered by pleura and, together with the inferior segment of the lingula, are the only ones that abut no more than one other segment.[4]

Patients with the middle lobe syndrome complain of chronic cough, haemoptysis, chest pain and dyspnoea, to relieve which, the diseased lobe may be removed. Pathological changes in the resected lobe include bronchiectasis, chronic bronchitis and bronchiolitis, lymphoid hyperplasia, organising pneumonia and abscess formation, in addition to collapse (Fig. 3.2).[5] A similar syndrome may affect the lingula.

OBSTRUCTION OF THE UPPER AIRWAYS

Obstruction of the upper airways may be complete and cause rapid asphyxial death, or incomplete, when there is stridor or wheezing, or distal complications such as obstructive pneumonia may ensue. Foreign bodies are an important cause, especially in children and edentulous adults. Another important cause, tumours, is dealt with in Chapter 13. Rare causes include amyloid tumours (see p. 684) and tracheobronchomalacia (see pp. 46, 50). In infancy, the airways are unduly pliable and may be compressed by distended arteries, particularly where the two are in close contact (see Fig. 10.10). Anomalous arteries may also compress airways in infancy, as in the vascular sling and ring syndromes (see Figs 10.11, 10.12, p. 482).

Obstructive sleep apnoea

Obstructive sleep apnoea is characterised by repeated periods during which the patient stops breathing for 10 s or more while asleep. The patient may not waken, but is repeatedly aroused so that the quality of the sleep is poor and daytime sleepiness is consequently excessive.[6] Snoring is a common accompaniment. The patient is generally obese and it is postulated that cervical fat pads obstruct the upper airway. Often the patient is male and excessively fond of alcohol. Other family members are often similarly affected, possibly because of similarities in cervicofacial structure. Obstructive sleep apnoea is to be

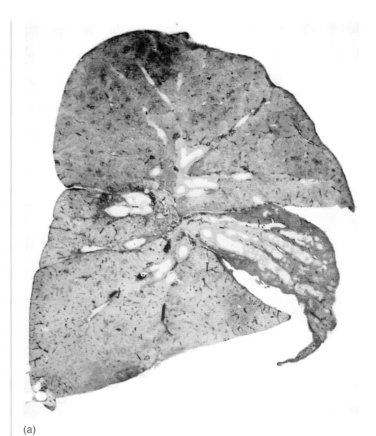

(a)

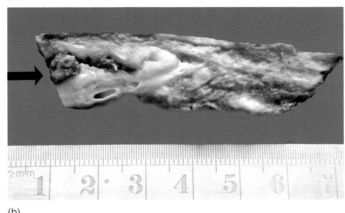

(b)

Figure 3.2 Middle lobe syndrome. (a) The middle lobe is collapsed and its bronchi are dilated. (b) In this patient, the syndrome was caused by a broncholith (arrow) blocking the lobar bronchus.

distinguished from a central variety of apnoea known as Ondine's curse. (In German legend, the water nymph Ondine, having been jilted by her mortal lover, took from him all automatic functions, requiring him to remember to breathe. When he finally fell asleep, he died.) Central apnoea has been encountered with bulbar poliomyelitis. It is likely that the central syndrome results from damage to the medullary CO_2 receptor in which airway patency is maintained but respiratory drive is weak, especially during sleep.

The principal problem in obstructive sleep apnoea is the daytime tiredness, which leads to poor performance at work and a tendency to fall sleep at inappropriate moments. The consequences of this can be very serious if, for example, the patient drives. Charles Dickens was evidently familiar with such individuals, portraying one in his novel 'The Pickwick Papers'. Such patients have therefore been termed 'Pickwickian', although the Dickensian character was the 'fat boy' rather than Mr Pickwick himself. Defects in the secretion of testosterone and growth hormone may also be identified. These are reversible and are probably due to the central effects of sleep fragmentation and hypoxaemia.

The periods of apnoea result in hypoxaemia, which in turn causes pulmonary hypertension. The apnoeic episodes are also accompanied by systemic hypertension and death may be caused by biventricular cardiac failure. The pulmonary blood vessels show the usual changes found with hypoxia, principally hypertrophy of the arterial media (see p. 425). Pulmonary haemorrhage and haemosiderosis are further features, possibly attributable to the left ventricular failure. Pronounced capillary proliferation resembling capillary haemangiomatosis (see p. 429) is also described.[7]

Tracheobronchopathia osteochondroplastica

The first descriptions of this condition date back to the middle of the nineteenth century[8,9] and it has continued to arouse interest because of its apparent rarity and disputed aetiology. It is confined to the trachea and bronchi and does not infiltrate surrounding tissues or metastasise but it endangers life through airway obstruction.[10] It affects men more often than women and is seldom recognised before the age of 50. Symptomatic cases are rare but it is possible that mild cases are overlooked[11]: four cases were reported in one series of 500 bronchoscopies.[12]

Tracheobronchoscopy reveals multiple mucosal nodules and relevant to both the diagnosis and aetiology of the condition, is the observation that the membranous portion of the trachea is spared (Fig. 3.3).[13] This suggests that the condition is related to the airway cartilage and that the lesions represent exostoses (as suggested by Virchow) rather than submucosal metaplasia (as suggested by Aschoff).[9,14] A superficial resemblance to tracheobronchial amyloidosis (which is prone to ossify) has led to erroneous suggestions that these two conditions are related.[15–17] Growth factors that induce new bone formation, have been

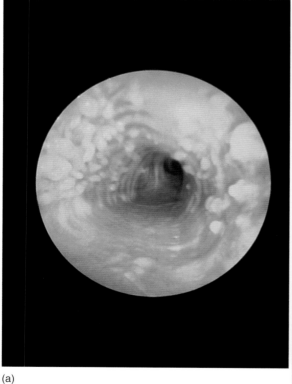

(a)

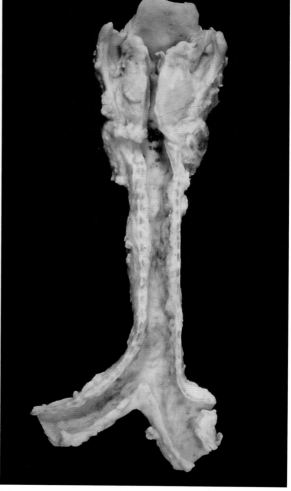

(b)

Figure 3.3 Tracheobronchopathia osteochondroplastica. (a) Bronchoscopic view. The nodules affect all but the posterior membranous portion of the trachea, compatible with them arising from the tracheal cartilages. (b) Extensive roughening of the tracheal mucosa is seen at necropsy. (Illustration provided by Dr Sj Sc Wagenaar, Utrecht, Netherlands.)

demonstrated about the ossifying nodules but not about those composed of mature lamellar bone.[18]

Pathology

At necropsy the tracheobronchial mucosa is roughened by numerous nodular excrescences (Fig. 3.3). Microscopy shows that the nodules consist of cartilage, which like the normal cartilage of the airways may calcify and ossify.[10,13,19–21] These osseo-cartilaginous nodules are situated between the normal cartilage and the surface epithelium of the airway, causing the mucosa to protrude into and compromise the lumen. The new cartilage differs from that normally found in the airways only in its abnormal position. Cytologically it is quite normal and in a small fibreoptic biopsy is likely to be mistaken for the normal cartilage of the large airways. It generally appears to have no connection with the normal cartilage but step sections show that there is indeed continuity through narrow pedicles,[13,21] supporting the view that the condition represents multiple ec-chondroses of the tracheobronchial cartilages,[19] as originally proposed by Virchow.[9] Treatment consists of nibbling the nodules away endoscopically as often as proves necessary.

Relapsing polychondritis

This condition is characterised by recurrent inflammation of cartilaginous structures and other tissues rich in glycosamino-gycans.[22–26] Immunoglobulins and complement have been identified at the chondrofibrous junction,[27] and the presence of circulating anticartilage immunoglobulin and the ability of car-tilage antigens to transform lymphocytes from these patients provide evidence that the disease has a tissue-specific auto-immune basis.[28]

Clinical features

The disease affects patients of both sexes and any age but the maximum frequency is in the fourth decade. It typically causes distortion of the pinnae and collapse of the nose. Other tissues involved include the larynx, trachea, bronchi, joints, eyes, inner ears and blood vessels. The trachea and bronchi may be spared and only very rarely are they affected in isolation.[29–32] Tracheo-bronchial involvement is characterised by airflow obstruction due to airway collapse[29–31] or, less commonly, bronchorrhoea.[33] The arthritis has a predilection for thoracic joints and may further contribute to respiratory difficulties. Blood vessel involvement is characterised by vasculitis involving vessels of all sizes and leading to aneurysms of major arteries. Occasion-ally, medium-sized arteries develop aneurysms and the changes are then those of polyarteritis nodosa.[34] Glomerulonephritis may also develop.[35]

Pathology

The affected bronchi may feel soft. Microscopically, the appear-ances vary according to the degree of inflammatory activity. In the active stage of the disease, the tracheobronchial cartilage is less basophilic than normal (Fig. 3.4a), reflecting loss of acidic proteoglycans, which may appear in the urine.[24] The tracheal and bronchial cartilages are cuffed by a chronic inflammatory

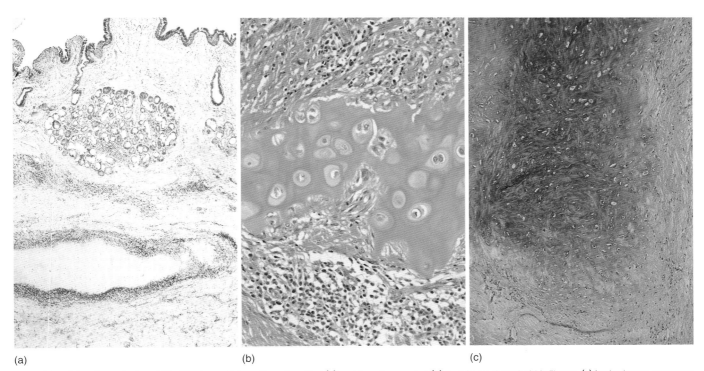

(a) (b) (c)

Figure 3.4 Relapsing polychondritis. The bronchial cartilage is cuffed (a) and its edge eroded (b) by a heavy lymphoid infiltrate. (c) In the burnt-out stage the inflammation has resolved but the bronchial cartilage is disrupted by fibrosis.

infiltrate of lymphocytes, plasma cells and occasional multinucleate histiocytes that is limited to the edge of the cartilage, which is ragged and evidently under attack (Fig. 3.4b).[23] In the late stages of the disease, the inflammation may have resolved leaving collagen surrounding and intersecting the cartilage matrix, which at this stage is fibrillary rather than amorphous and shows increased basophilia (Fig. 3.4c).[24,29,31] Other components of the airway appear normal and there is generally no evidence of vasculitis in the airways. These features are characteristic but not specific, being seen for example in a post-intubation tracheal stricture.

ACUTE TRACHEOBRONCHITIS AND BRONCHIOLITIS

Acute inflammation of the conductive airways is common, especially among young children and the elderly and a number of factors, environmental and microbial, may contribute to its causation. There is a marked seasonal incidence. In the summer months the mortality is low, but from early winter, the death rate rises steadily to reach a peak in the late winter or early spring. The time of greatest mortality varies considerably from year to year and depends partly on the severity of the weather and partly on the prevalence of two epidemic diseases, influenza and measles.

In the normal person, the defensive mechanisms of the respiratory tract usually destroy or remove any inhaled microbes that may be caught on its mucus-covered surface. But should the combined defences of mucus, ciliated epithelium and the cough reflex be weakened from any cause, such as exposure to cold, irritant dust or vapours, or certain specific infections, the potentially pathogenic bacteria that are ordinarily resident in the nose and pharynx may succeed in temporarily colonising the mucosa of the trachea and bronchi. In the pathogenesis of acute tracheobronchitis, therefore, these potentiating factors are of particular significance, for without them, the responsible organisms might be unable to establish themselves in these portions of the respiratory tract, which normally are sterile.

Environmental causes

Atmospheric pollution by hydrocarbon combustion products is common in many cities and from time to time, often in particular meteorological conditions, the level of pollution may rise to values that cause an attack of acute tracheobronchitis. Los Angeles, Liège and London have been notorious for their smogs but in recent years they have been overtaken in this respect by such rapidly growing conurbations as Athens and Sao Paulo. In some cities, smoke control has reduced the levels of visible particulates and sulphur dioxide but not pollution by ozone and oxides of nitrogen, which are chiefly derived from internal combustion engines.

In men engaged in industries in which irritant gases or dusts may be inhaled, the mucous membrane of the trachea and bronchi may become acutely inflamed and occasionally noxious gases such as ammonia and sulphur dioxide may be breathed in such concentrations that widespread injury to the respiratory mucosa may follow. Silo-fillers' disease is a consequence of acute bronchiolitis caused by oxides of nitrogen formed from fermenting grain. The use of thermal lances on steel is ordinarily safe but if special alloys of steel are attacked with these tools the inhalation of beryllium, cadmium and other hot metal fumes may cause acute bronchiolitis and diffuse alveolar damage. In the First World War, the military use of chlorine and phosgene as poisonous gases was often followed by destructive lesions throughout the respiratory tracts of the exposed troops.

The damage inflicted by soluble noxious gases and fumes is liable to be concentrated on the main airways, whereas less soluble gases are prone to damage more distal airspaces, including alveoli as well as the finer conductive airways (see Table 7.2.1, p. 373).[36] Examples of the former include chlorine and ozone, while the latter include beryllium, mercury and cadmium fume, oxides of nitrogen and high concentrations of oxygen.

Microbial causes

In recent decades, great changes have taken place in the relative importance of bacteria and viruses in the aetiology of acute tracheobronchitis. Prophylactic immunisation against diphtheria and pertussis and the availability of antibiotics effective against the bacterial causes of secondary pneumonia, particularly pneumococci, have together greatly lessened the frequency of both the primary diseases and the respiratory complications. Similarly, the bacterial complications of measles and influenza can now be effectively treated and effective immunisation against measles is available, although uptake of this vaccine is low in some countries. Most of these microbial diseases are dealt with in the chapters devoted to viral and bacterial infections but diphtheria and whooping cough will now be described.

Diphtheria

Diphtheria is caused by infection with the bacterium *Corynebacterium diphtheriae*. It formerly cost many lives each year but immunisation programmes have been highly successful and the disease is now very rare. It is characteristic of diphtheria that the bacteria responsible inhabit a surface membrane of fibrin and necrotic epithelium and that much of the ill-effects are due to powerful bacterial exotoxins that are distributed throughout the body by the bloodstream, typically causing myocardial degeneration and peripheral neuropathy. Infection is generally limited to the pharynx and only occasionally does it spread down to cause acute laryngitis, tracheitis and bronchitis. The typical membrane may obstruct the larynx and cause death from asphyxia. More often the primary injury to the respiratory mucosa by the locally released toxin lays the lungs open to invasion by various other organisms, among them *Haemophilus influenzae* and the pyogenic cocci.

Whooping cough (pertussis)

Whooping cough is a highly infectious bacterial disease of childhood caused by the bacterium *Bordetella pertussis*. It is spread by droplet infection. The incubation period is 7–10 days and a case is infectious from 7 days after exposure to 3 weeks after the onset of typical paroxysms. An initial catarrhal stage is the most infectious period. An irritating cough develops and gradually becomes paroxysmal, which is responsible for the typical 'whoop'. Whooping cough may be complicated by bronchopneumonia, post-tussive vomiting and cerebral hypoxia, most commonly in infants under 6 months of age.

At one time, whooping cough was one of the most common causes of death in children and its decline in the developed countries of the world since the Second World War represents one of the notable contributions of prophylaxis to public health. In Britain, for example, widespread immunisation resulted in a 30-fold reduction in the number of notifications, and deaths became rare. Understandably, complacency followed and when publicity was given to cerebral complications of the vaccine in 1974, its acceptance rate dropped dramatically, followed in 1977 by the biggest epidemic for 20 years (Fig. 3.5). Subsequent studies showed that the risk of permanent brain damage was very small, 1 in 310 000 injections. Increased vaccine uptake resulting from a return of public confidence cut short an expected epidemic in 1986 and in 1991, when uptake had risen to 88%, an anticipated epidemic failed to materialise. By 1994 uptake had reached a record 94% (Fig. 3.5).

B. pertussis, has a marked tendency to attach itself to respiratory epithelium.[37] In fatal cases, *B. pertussis* can be recovered from the lungs and the organisms can be seen microscopically in large numbers in the thick mucopurulent film that covers the mucosa of the trachea and the bronchi. The mucus may be so viscous that it obstructs the passage of air and so leads to segmental lung collapse.

Although *B. pertussis* itself seems to be capable of establishing an acute inflammatory reaction in the lower respiratory passages, it would appear from bacteriological studies at necropsy that the terminal, fatal bronchopneumonia is more often caused by *Haemophilus influenzae* or by one of the pyogenic cocci; these are enabled to enter the lungs by the damage caused by the bordetella, which impairs the tracheobronchial defence mechanisms. In infants, this complication is the chief cause of death in whooping cough, which in many countries is still one of the most fatal infectious diseases in the first 2 years of life. Bronchiectasis and obliterative brochiolitis are notable complications amongst survivors.

Necrotising sialometaplasia

Throughout the lower respiratory tract, regenerative processes may be so atypical that carcinomatous transformation has to be considered in the differential diagnosis. This impression is often augmented by excessive mitotic activity and metaplasia. Thus, at the alveolar level, necrotising lesions such as infarcts and the granulomatoses may be bordered by foci of atypical squamous hyperplasia that are easily mistaken for squamous cell carcinoma. Similarly, damage to the bronchial epithelium is often followed by atypical regeneration that is easily mistaken for carcinoma, particularly when exfoliated cells are being examined. Bronchoscopy inevitably involves bronchial injury and cytopathologists have to be aware of the atypicalities that follow this procedure. Necrotising lesions of the larynx are sometimes accompanied by atypical regeneration that involves both the surface epithelium and the submucosal glands: the term necrotising sialometaplasia[38] has been applied to this and to a similar process involving the trachea in patients with herpetic tracheitis undergoing repeated intubation.[39,40]

CHRONIC BRONCHITIS AND EMPHYSEMA, CHRONIC OBSTRUCTIVE LUNG DISEASE

The collective term chronic bronchitis and emphysema (chronic obstructive pulmonary disease, COPD) encompasses three quite distinct conditions that have much in common.[41] The third condition, which is not specified in the title, is one formerly thought to be a subtype of chronic bronchitis but is now being increasingly recognised as a separate disease. No specific name exists for this condition but it is generally known as small airway disease or chronic obstructive bronchiolitis. It is important to understand how these three diseases differ and what features they share. One obvious difference is that chronic bronchitis and small airway disease involve conducting airways of differing size, whereas emphysema involves the alveoli. Another is that while chronic bronchitis is hypersecretory in nature, small airway disease is essentially obstructive and emphysema is a purely destructive process. However, they are related in their causation. The most important aetiological factor in all is cigarette smoking and for this reason, they frequently co-exist. They all show airflow limitation to some degree and therefore can be difficult to distinguish clinically although the ventilatory defect is based on very different structural abnormalities. In chronic bronchitis, the airflow limitation is due to inflammatory thickening of the wall and intermittent luminal plugging, in small airway disease, to inflammatory thickening

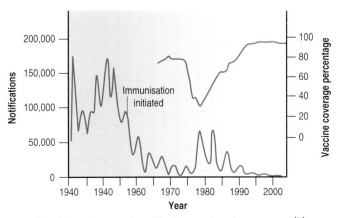

Figure 3.5 Whooping cough notifications and vaccine coverage (%), England and Wales 1940–2003.

of the wall and peribronchiolar fibrosis and in emphysema to premature closure of inherently normal or atrophic airways because of diminished pulmonary elastic recoil.

The majority of patients with generalised chronic airflow limitation suffer from both obstructive airway disease and emphysema but a minority of patients have one condition or another. Two clinical syndromes, types A ('pink puffer') and B ('blue bloater'), have been described and it is widely believed that the former indicates emphysema and the latter chronic bronchitis.[42,43] The association of the type A syndrome with emphysema is fairly well established but the association of type B with chronic bronchitis is not well substantiated morphologically. Type A patients show rapid shallow breathing and this maintains near normal blood gases at the cost of subjective breathlessness. They are usually thin and because their blood gases are not severely deranged they tend not to develop polycythaemia or cor pulmonale. Type B patients on the other hand are hypoxic and therefore suffer from polycythaemia and repeated bouts of congestive cardiac failure. They are usually obese and oedematous and have a productive cough but they are seldom severely breathless. It is important to realise that most patients with chronic airflow limitation do not fit neatly into one or other of these types. Nor do these two types reflect pure bronchitis or pure emphysema.[44] The fundamental difference between type A and type B patients may be in the brain rather than the lungs: type B patients seem to have a respiratory centre that is relatively unresponsive to the usual stimuli, an abnormality that may be genetically determined.

Chronic bronchitis

Definition

Chronic bronchitis is defined in clinical terms as a persistent or recurrent excess of secretion in the bronchial tree on most days for at least 3 months in the year, over at least 2 years.[45] The secretions of the normal human respiratory tract are believed to total less than 100 ml in 24 h, all of which is swallowed without conscious need to clear the throat or cough so that the normal person produces no sputum. The diagnosis of chronic bronchitis may be made only when other conditions that cause expectoration, such as tuberculosis and bronchiectasis, have been excluded.

Chronic bronchitis was formerly subdivided into simple mucoid bronchitis, mucopurulent bronchitis and obstructive bronchitis.[46] It was widely thought that these subdivisions represented successive phases of the disease but a strong counterargument to this was advanced by British epidemiologists.[47] These workers showed that while simple mucoid bronchitis progresses to the mucopurulent variety, this does not progress in turn to the obstructive form. In line with this, neither bronchial gland size nor sputum production are significantly related to airflow limitation.[48] The view that the development of obstructive bronchitis is independent of the repeated respiratory infections that characterise mucopurulent bronchitis has been challenged,[49] but the obstructive form of the disease is now

nevertheless widely recognised as a separate condition: small airway disease, which is dealt with below.

Aetiology

Chronic bronchitis affects mainly the middle-aged and elderly and is more common in men; cigarette smoking is by far the most important cause.[50–52] The influence of cigarette smoke often begins in infancy when the child is exposed passively to parental cigarette smoke. This is generally augmented by active cigarette smoking when the child emulates parents or schoolmates and acquires the habit, often becoming addicted for life. However, as with lung cancer, many indulge in smoking with impunity, indicating that susceptibility to disease varies considerably,[41] probably reflecting genetic differences in the control of such factors as the balance of helper and cytotoxic T-lymphocytes.[53] Marijuana smoke is likely to be recognised as a further aetiological agent as it has similar morphological effects on the airways as tobacco smoke.[54]

Other factors contributing to chronic bronchitis include general air pollution, which accounts for the higher prevalence of the disease in urban communities, occupational dust exposure,[55] fog and a damp and cold climate. The morbidity from the disease rises every winter and remains high throughout the colder, damper months. The occurrence of fog, especially the form known as smog in which the water vapour becomes heavily contaminated with smoke and sulphurous gases, causes a prompt increase in both morbidity and mortality among older people. The heavy 4-day smog in London in 1952 is believed to have precipitated 4000 deaths.

Infections by respiratory viruses and bacteria are also of importance in both initiating and promoting chronic bronchitis.[56] Some patients may recall a liability in their earlier years for head colds to go to their chest.[57] Relatives are often similarly affected. An increased frequency of respiratory infection in childhood has been identified in adults with chronic bronchitis.[58]

These various irritants initiate mucus secretion by a combination of direct action on the mucous cells and nervous reflexes involving sensory nerve endings in the airway epithelium and both local peptidergic and spinal cholinergic pathways. Upregulation of the mucin (MUC) genes is involved and epidermal growth factor is a key mediator in the mucous cell hyperplasia.

Clinical features

The excessive bronchial secretion inherent in the definition of chronic bronchitis is manifest as sputum. This is typically mucoid and white but the disease is marked by episodes of acute bronchitis when the sputum becomes purulent and yellow. Later the sputum may become purulent continuously; it accumulates in the bronchi during sleep and causes severe obstruction of the airways until it is coughed up in the morning. While a change from white to yellow sputum usually signifies infection it should be noted that large numbers of eosinophils also render the sputum yellow, a potential pitfall in the clinical distinction of bronchitis and asthma.

Microbiological examination of the sputum in chronic bronchitis has shown that the most frequent and important pathogens are *Haemophilus influenzae*, *Streptococcus pneumoniae*, *Branhamella catarrhalis* and *Chlamydia pneumoniae*.[59–63] Purulent sputum usually contains one or more of these organisms in abundance; they tend to disappear after antimicrobial therapy when the sputum becomes mucoid again.

The productive cough appears at first only in the winter months. Later, it is present all through the year, characteristically with acute exacerbations in winter that are usually precipitated by a viral infection.[64,65]

Morbidity and mortality

Chronic obstructive lung disease is a major cause of death worldwide.[52] However, death comes many years after the onset of the disease and it is therefore also a major cause of sickness and incapacity for work. The social gradient of the disease is steep, for the death rate in the poorest section of the population is some five times that in the most prosperous. Death in chronic bronchitis is often due to bronchopneumonia. There is also a 4- to 5-fold increased risk of lung cancer in patients with obstructive lung disease, as compared with controls matched for cigarette smoking.[66,67]

Morbid anatomy

When the lungs of a patient with chronic bronchitis are dissected at necropsy, the exposed bronchi, especially those in the lower lobes, are typically filled with a mixture of mucus and pus. When the purulent material is washed away from bronchi that have been opened longitudinally, the underlying mucous membrane is seen to be a dusky red. The calibre of the main bronchi may remain unchanged but distal bronchi characteristically are slightly dilated; when they are opened with fine scissors, the dilation is found to reach almost to the pleura (Fig. 3.6).[68] Some consider the dilation to be due to atrophy of the bronchial wall and describe it in association with emphysema rather than as a feature of chronic bronchitis.[69,70] Others have described degenerative changes in the bronchial cartilage in chronic bronchitis and emphysema and have correlated this with the degree of inflammation.[71] The lung substance is often emphysematous in patients with chronic bronchitis and there may be bronchopneumonia.

Histological appearances

The main features of chronic bronchitis become apparent only when the lungs are examined histologically. The submucosal glands are much enlarged and there is a shift in gland type from mixed seromucous to pure mucous (Figs 3.7, 3.8).[72] The enlargement is primarily a hyperplastic change.[73] Furthermore the usual mixture of neutral and acidic glycoprotein in bronchial mucus changes to one that is largely acidic and within the acidic mucins sulphomucin increases at the expense of sialomucin, alterations that possibly increase sputum viscosity. The mucous acini and their ducts become distended with retained mucus.[72,74]

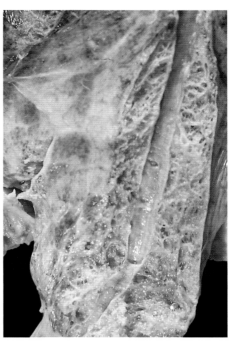

Figure 3.6 Chronic bronchitis. The bronchi do not show the normal peripheral narrowing, their calibre being maintained until they approach the pleura. (Illustration provided by the late Professor BE Heard, Brompton, UK.)

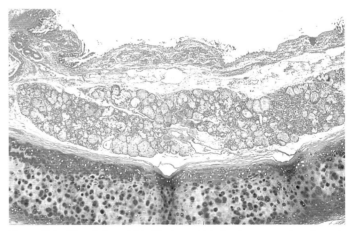

Figure 3.7 Chronic bronchitis. The bronchial glands are greatly enlarged, the Reid Index measuring 0.6, double the normal value. The bronchial glands are also almost entirely mucous in type.

It is possible to correlate the clinical history of chronic bronchitis with the size of the bronchial glands. This may be done by measuring the ratio of the thickness of the gland layer to the thickness of the wall between the base of the surface epithelium and the internal limit of the cartilage plates. The fraction occupied by the glands is known as the Reid Index.[72] In chronic bronchitis this may double from the normal value of 0.3 (Figs 3.7, 3.8). The Reid Index takes no account of the glands situated between the cartilaginous plates and a more accurate method

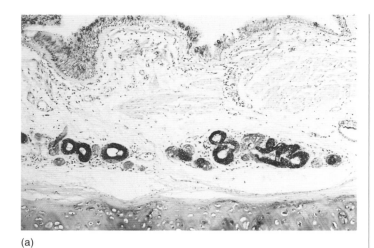

(a)

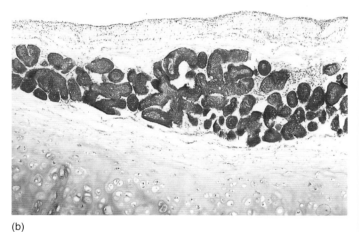

(b)

Figure 3.8 (a) Normal bronchus. (b) Chronic bronchitis. As well as enlargement of the submucosal glands, chronic bronchitis is characterised by a shift in the nature of the glands from the normal mixed seromucous pattern to one that is almost entirely mucous, while within the mucous acini there is a shift from mixed neutral and acidic (red/blue) mucus to purely acidic (blue) mucus. A further shift within the acidic mucus, one from sialomucin to sulphomucin, is not apparent with this Alcian blue-periodic acid Schiff stain.

of assessing the size of the glands is to estimate their cross-sectional area as a percentage of that of all the bronchial wall components.[75,76] This is now greatly facilitated by the use of a computerised digitising tablet rather than relying on the accurate but tedious method of point counting.

As well as the glands, the epithelium that lines the bronchi shows signs of increased mucus production, the proportion of goblet cells being increased at the expense of the ciliated cells (Fig. 3.9).[77] Also, the surface epithelium may undergo patchy squamous metaplasia. The accompanying loss of cilia, which ordinarily clear bacteria and dust particles from the lower respiratory tract, predisposes to infection.

The fall in the proportion of serous to mucous acini in the bronchial glands may also be expected to promote infection as the serous cells are a major source of the antibacterial agents lysozyme and lactoferrin[78,79]; however, these antibacterial agents continue to be detectable in patients' sputum.[80] The serous cells

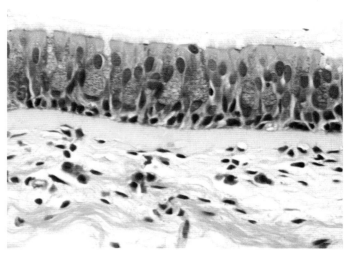

Figure 3.9 Chronic bronchitis. In the surface epithelium, goblet cells are increased at the expense of the ciliated cells.

also contribute the secretory piece to immunoglobulin A, so protecting it from proteolytic degradation. Reduced expression of this secretory piece has been demonstrated in severe COPD.[81] The serous cells are also a major source of secretory leukocyte protease inhibitor.[82] This factor can be identified in the sputum of patients with chronic bronchitis but normal values have not been established. A diminution could help explain why chronic bronchitis and emphysema are so commonly associated.

Mucus accumulates in the airways and may completely fill their lumen. With infection, neutrophil leukocytes are added to the mucus and the airway wall is swollen by oedema and an acute inflammatory infiltrate. Between acute attacks, the wall of the airways is infiltrated by lymphocytes and macrophages and its blood vessels are congested. The lymphocytes are largely CD8-positive (cytotoxic/suppressor) T cells, in contrast to the CD4-positive Th2-cells found in asthma.[83–85] Thus, although essentially hypersecretory, chronic bronchitis is also a truly inflammatory disease (Fig. 3.10).[86] Furthermore, it appears that the inflammation in turn promotes hypersecretion,[87,88] a process envisaged by an older generation of pathologists when they spoke of catarrhal inflammation. A vicious cycle is thus set in motion in chronic bronchitis, as in bronchiectasis (see p. 115).

'Wheezy' bronchitis

Hyperplasia of bronchial muscle in chronic bronchitis is reported by some observers[89] but not by others.[90] The explanation for this discrepancy may be that some patients have features of both asthma and bronchitis. The amount of muscle in the airways of these 'wheezy bronchitics' is intermediate between the normal amounts found in purely bronchitic subjects and the increased amount found in atopic asthmatics.[91]

Constitutional factors, in particular bronchial hyperactivity, may contribute to airflow limitation in certain cigarette smokers who develop 'chronic asthmatic bronchitis'.[92] This concept is embodied in what has become known as the 'Dutch hypothe-

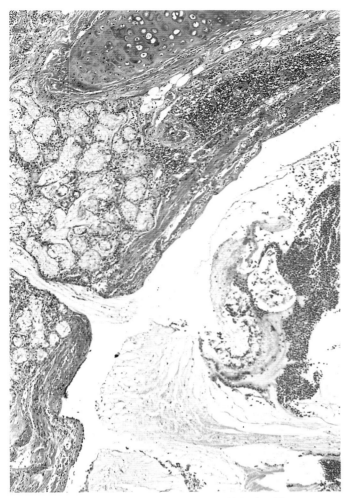

Figure 3.10 Chronic bronchitis with superadded infection. The submucosal glands are enlarged, a gland duct is plugged by mucus, mucus has accumulated in the bronchial lumen and as a consequence of secondary infection there is also pus in the lumen and chronic inflammation of the bronchial wall.

sis' – that smokers with progressive airflow limitation have increased bronchial reactivity and atopic features similar to, but less marked than, those observed in asthma.[93,94] The observation that cigarette smokers have elevated serum immunoglobulin E levels raises the possibility that some of the adverse effects of smoking might be immunologically mediated.[95] However the elevated serum immunoglobulin E in smokers does not appear to be specific for the common seasonal aeroallergens. Chronic bronchitis and asthma are compared in Table 3.1.[96]

Small airway disease (chronic obstructive bronchiolitis)

The aetiological differences between chronic bronchitis and small airway disease are as yet unclear but cigarette smoking is undoubtedly important in both. The latter condition is met more often in those patients whose breathlessness steadily increases with the years and in whom there is progressive deterioration in exercise tolerance leading to inability to continue working.

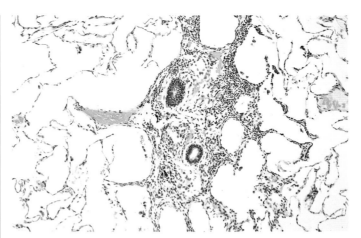

Figure 3.11 Peribronchiolitis and fibrosis in small airway disease.

Post-mortem studies have shown that in COPD, the major site of airflow obstruction is in airways of about 2 mm diameter or less.[97] Airways of this calibre, which correspond to those of approximately the ninth generation, have subsequently become generally known as 'small airways'. They include both small bronchi and proximal bronchioles.

Such small calibre airways are numerous and in health they have a large collective cross-sectional area so that they normally contribute little to total airflow resistance (see Fig. 1.7, p. 5). Many may be lost before there is any appreciable impairment of airflow. It is likely therefore that many cigarette smokers are progressively developing obstructive airway disease long before they notice any significant reduction in their respiratory capabilities. For this reason the periphery of the lung has become known as its 'silent zone'.

Histopathology

Small airway disease is characterised by bronchiolar goblet cell hyperplasia.[98] This takes place at the expense of Clara cells,[99] which, together with the serous cells of the bronchial glands, secrete an airway-specific low molecular weight protease inhibitor (anti-leukoprotease), which is a potent protective factor against the development of emphysema.[82,100–103] There is also inflammation in the smaller bronchi and bronchioles. Similar chronic inflammatory changes to those affecting the larger airways in chronic bronchitis are observed in the walls and adjacent tissues of bronchioles and small bronchi; the predominant cell again being the CD8-positive T-lymphocyte.[104] Wall thickening[105] and fibrosing peribronchiolitis[106] (Fig. 3.11) lead to the lumen becoming severely reduced. This causes irreversible obstruction and severe airflow limitation. The narrowing takes the form of focal stenoses.[107] Proximal to the stenoses the bronchioles are often dilated. Bronchographic medium pools in the dilated segments, giving what has been described as a 'mimosa flower' effect,[108] and an absence of peripheral filling.[109] The focal stenoses are difficult to identify in random sections but are well demonstrated in plastic casts of the airways (Fig. 3.12).[110,111] Alternatively, quantitative methods may

Table 3.1 Comparison of chronic bronchitis and asthma[96]

	Chronic bronchitis	Asthma
Airflow obstruction	Fixed and irreversible	Variable and reversible
Sputum	Macrophages Neutrophils	Eosinophils Charcot–Leyden crystals Creola bodies Curschmann's spirals
Postmortem appearances	Excess mucus Bronchial dilatation Associated emphysema	Mucus plugs Hyperinflation but no emphysema
Airway inflammation	CD8+ T cells Neutrophils periodically	CD4+ T cells Eosinophils Mast cells
Airway congestion and oedema	Present	Present
Airway epithelium	Intact Goblet cell hyperplasia Squamous metaplasia	Fragile with stripping Goblet cell hyperplasia Squamous metaplasia
Basement membrane reticular layer thickening	Mild-to-moderate	Marked
Bronchial glands	Marked enlargement of the mucous acini	Moderate enlargement of both mucous and serous acini
Mucin histochemistry	Shift from neutral to acid and within the acid mucins from sialo- to sulpho-	Unchanged
Airway muscle	May show hypertrophy	Marked hypertrophy
Major complications	Cor pulmonale	Allergic bronchopulmonary aspergillosis

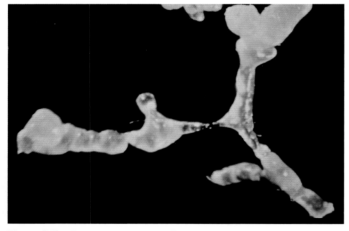

Figure 3.12 Small airway disease. Plastic cast of some small airways of a patient dying of chronic obstructive bronchiolitis, showing a focal stenosis. (Illustration provided by Professor J Bignon, Creteil, France.)

be employed; these show both organic narrowing and mucous plugging of small airways.[112] It is likely that cases of small airway disease were included among the patients with chronic lung diseases studied by McLean.[113–115] In many smokers, peribronchiolar inflammation and fibrosis involves the more distal respiratory bronchioles and thickens the walls of adjacent alveoli so that there is restrictive as well as obstructive lung disease. This so-called respiratory bronchiolitis-associated interstitial lung disease overlaps with yet another effect of cigarette smoking, namely desquamative interstitial pneumonia and is dealt with on p. 313.

Complications

Patients with small airway disease are prone to develop cor pulmonale (see p. 432), mainly as a result of widespread hypoxic pulmonary vasoconstriction and the consequent rise in pulmonary vascular resistance. Hypoxic pulmonary hypertension is dealt with on p. 425. A further consequence of the hypoxia is compensatory polycythaemia, the resultant haemoconcentration adding to the increased cardiac burden. While death from small airway disease is usually due to right-sided heart failure, obstructive respiratory failure and bronchopneumonia also contribute. These conditions are often present in combination.

Emphysema

Emphysema denotes pathological inflation of the affected tissue. Two fundamentally different forms are recognised, vesicular and interstitial (or surgical). The first affects spaces that normally contain air, while the second represents the ingress of air into the normally airless interstitial planes of the lung and contiguous connective tissues outside the lung. The distinction between vesicular and interstitial emphysema was first made by Laennec in 1819 but pathological descriptions of the condition have been traced back to as early as 1679.[116] The adjective vesicular has fallen into disuse and may be inferred when the term emphysema is used without qualification. Although interstitial emphysema does not fall within current definitions of emphysema the term interstitial (or surgical) emphysema persists and the condition is described as such on p. 105.

Vesicular emphysema is a common condition. A consecutive series of 50 male necropsies in London identified emphysema in more than trace amounts in 37, although few of the patients had respiratory symptoms.[117] Similar findings have been reported in other English cities.[118]

Airways may be normal in emphysema. Alternatively, they may be atrophic and dilated but prone to collapse prematurely,[69,70] unless there is also chronic bronchitis with its characteristic thickening of the airway wall by glandular hyperplasia and inflammatory oedema.

Definition

Emphysema was defined in 1959 as 'a condition of the lung characterised by increase beyond the normal in the size of air spaces distal to the terminal bronchiole either from dilatation or from destruction of their walls'.[45] Subsequently, this was modified by excluding purely distensive forms of pulmonary enlargement so that the definition became: 'an abnormal increase in the size of air spaces beyond the terminal bronchioles with destruction of air space walls'.[119] However, in some patients, the destruction is secondary to scarring and it has been suggested that this type of airspace enlargement should also be excluded from the definition. The American Thoracic Society accepted this recommendation and adopted the following definition: 'abnormal, permanent enlargement of the airspaces distal to the terminal bronchioles, accompanied by destruction of their walls and without obvious fibrosis'.[120,121] The exclusion of fibrosis is unfortunate for two reasons. First, the term scar emphysema is a useful one and second, those forms of emphysema that are not secondary to scarring do entail some degree of fibrosis, albeit slight.[122–124]

Pathology

Early emphysematous changes can only be detected microscopically. These include an increase in the size and number of fenestrae (pores of Kohn) in the alveolar walls.[125] When the destruction is moderate in degree, there is loss of alveolar walls, resulting in fewer alveolar attachments to bronchioles and consequent premature closure of these airways on expiration.[44,126–128] Quantitation of the microscopic changes in the lung substance can best be achieved by the application of an image analyser set to calculate factors such as mean linear intercept[129,130] or the airspace wall surface area per unit volume.[131,132] More severe changes are characterised by complete loss of most of the wall of the airspaces, bronchiolar as well as alveolar, leaving only a network of blood vessels and some interlobular septa.

These gross changes are better appreciated by the macroscopic study of whole lung slices rather than microscopy. If the lungs are fixed by distension with aqueous formalin at a pressure of 25–30 cm of water before slicing, the emphysema can be appreciated much better than in the collapsed fresh lung. Fixation overnight is adequate and if time presses a few hours is beneficial. If the fixed slices are impregnated with barium sulphate, deficiencies in the lung substance are highlighted and

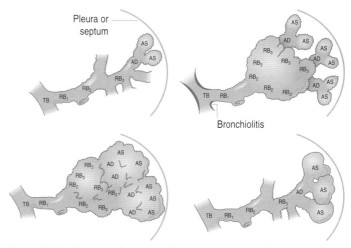

Figure 3.13 Morphological types of emphysema in relation to the acinar architecture of the lung. Upper left: The normal acinus. Upper right: Centriacinar emphysema, in which third order respiratory bronchioles are predominantly involved. Lower left: Panacinar emphysema in which there is destructive enlargement of all airspaces distal to the terminal bronchiole and the acinus is affected uniformly. Lower right: Paraseptal emphysema. TB, terminal bronchiole; RB, three orders of respiratory bronchioles; AD, alveolar duct; AS, alveolar sac. (For simplicity, only one order of alveolar duct and one of alveolar sac are drawn and they are not to scale.)

the amount of destruction and the type of emphysema can be better appreciated.[133] Barium sulphate impregnation is simply achieved by gently squeezing a slice of lung in a saturated solution of sodium sulphate and then immersing it in one of barium nitrate. Paper-mounted whole lung sections can be prepared if a permanent record is desired.[134] Various ways of quantitating the gross changes have been recommended[135] but none is as accurate or as easy as computerised image analysis.[136]

Several morphological types of emphysema are distinguished according to the part of the acinus that is affected, as observed in whole lung slices or paper-mounted whole lung sections. Three of these types, centriacinar, paraseptal and panacinar are illustrated diagrammatically in Figure 3.13. The fourth type, scar or irregular emphysema, bears no relation to the acinar architecture of the lung.

Centriacinar emphysema

This form of emphysema is characterised by focal lesions confined to the centres of the acini (Fig. 3.14). They are often pigmented with dust. The changes are more marked in the upper lobes, a feature that has been attributed to the greater gravitational forces there, consequent upon our upright posture and also upon the support afforded to the lower lobes by the diaphragm. Spaces that exceed 1 cm in size are known as bullae and may be seen in severe cases. The alveolar walls are lost, only some pulmonary vessels survive to cross the spaces as seemingly bare strands radiating outward from their parent arteries to supply the alveoli of the periphery of the acini (Fig. 3.14). Although centriacinar emphysema affects the upper lobes of the lungs more severely than the lower, any part may be involved and centriacinar emphysema is quite often accompanied by panacinar emphysema. Severe centriacinar emphysema may be difficult to distinguish from the panacinar form but an upper lobe predominance suggests that the lesions were originally confined to the centres of the acini, as does the presence of an obviously centriacinar form of emphysema in the less severely affected portions of the lung.

Panacinar emphysema

Panacinar emphysema involves all the air spaces beyond the terminal bronchiole more or less equally (Fig. 3.15). Most classic descriptions of emphysema refer to this variety. It affects all zones or is worse in the lower lobes. There may be a remarkable degree of parenchymal destruction. The lungs have a doughy feel, pit on pressure, do not collapse when the chest is opened and overlap the heart because of their great size. They appear very pale because of loss of substance; air-filled bullae, several centimetres across, may be seen.

Paraseptal emphysema

This form of emphysema affects air spaces adjacent to septa or to the pleura, thus involving only the periphery of the lung lobules (Fig. 3.16). It may result from forces pulling on the septa and perhaps also from inflammation. It may occur alone or in association with other forms of emphysema.

Particularly large solitary bullae are apt to form in paraseptal emphysema (Fig. 3.16). On inspiration, emphysematous portions of the lung in general and large bullae in particular are preferentially inflated, in accordance with Laplace's law, which states that a distending force is proportional to surface tension and inversely proportional to diameter. Inflation of these large useless air sacs prevents the expansion of adjacent normal lung and their excision may be beneficial. Subpleural bullae that are liable to rupture and cause pneumothorax are also particularly common in paraseptal emphysema. Giant bullae may be multilocular or crossed by fibrous bands containing the remnants of blood vessels. Some have oedematous papillary infoldings which bear a superficial histological

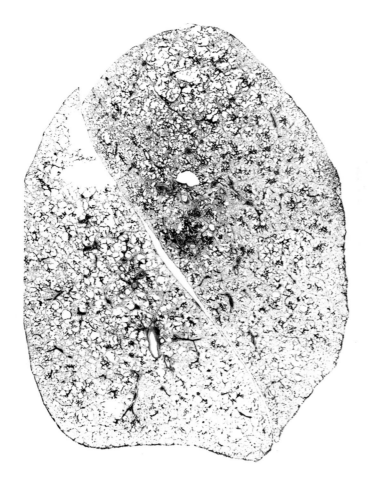

(a)

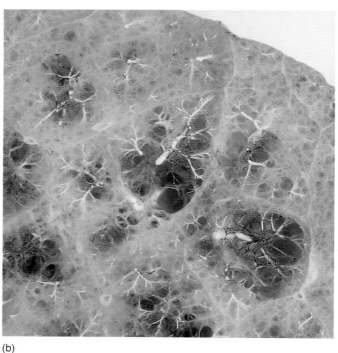

(b)

Figure 3.14 Centriacinar emphysema. (a) Paper-mounted whole lung section. (b) Inflation fixation and barium sulphate precipitation. Dust-pigmented deficiencies in the lung substance are confined to the centres of the acini. As well as using barium sulphate to emphasise the emphysema, the pulmonary arteries have been injected with a barium gelatine preparation for angiography. (Illustration (b) provided by the late Professor BE Heard, Brompton, UK.)

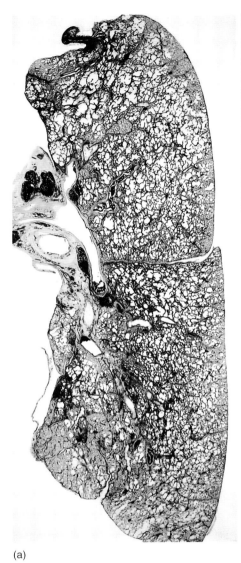

(a)

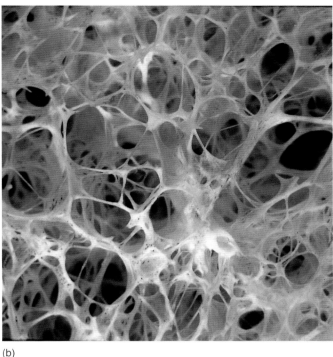

(b)

Figure 3.15 Panacinar emphysema. The whole of lung acinus is affected uniformly. (a) Paper-mounted whole lung section. (b) Barium sulphate precipitation. (Illustration (b) provided by the late Professor BE Heard, Brompton, UK.)

resemblance to chorionic villi and this has given rise to the somewhat bizarre terms placentoid bullous lesion and placental transmogrification of the lung,[137,138] or, if fat is also present, pulmonary lipomatosis.[139] Such terms have also been applied to other conditions and the papillary features are evidently non-specific.[140,141]

Irregular, scar or cicatricial 'emphysema'

This term has been used to describe permanent enlargement of air spaces distal to terminal bronchioles caused by fibrosis, a category of enlargement that is specifically excluded from the latest definition of emphysema (see above). This type of air-space enlargement does not affect the lungs in any regular pattern in relation to the acini or lobules, but occurs in focal areas near scars. It is a consequence of the scars and is therefore often known as scar or cicatricial 'emphysema'. Diffuse pulmonary fibrosis is often accompanied by widespread irregular cystic destruction of parenchyma, which together with bronchiolectasis gives a characteristic gross appearance known as 'honeycombing' that reflects end-stage fibrosis, typically in cryptogenic fibrosing alveolitis (see Figs 6.1.4–6, p. 270).

Aetiology and pathogenesis of emphysema

Better knowledge of the anatomical types of emphysema has improved our understanding of its aetiology. So too have discoveries concerning the control of tissue proteolysis.

Centriacinar emphysema is related to cigarette smoking[142] and has long been thought to be the result of airway inflammation.[106,143] Particular blame is attached to elastases released by neutrophil leukocytes during episodes of acute inflammation. That proteases can have this effect is shown by the experimental induction of a non-inflammatory panacinar form of emphysema by the intratracheal injection of the proteolytic enzyme papain.[144]

Panacinar emphysema, in contrast, is recognised as being that form associated with an inherited deficiency of α1-antitrypsin, which is normally the chief component of plasma

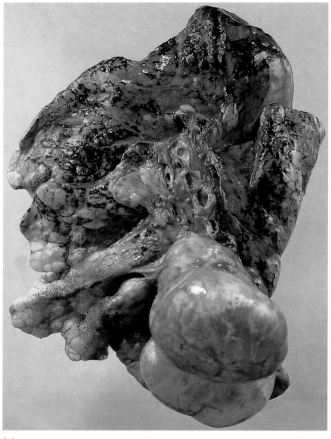

(a)

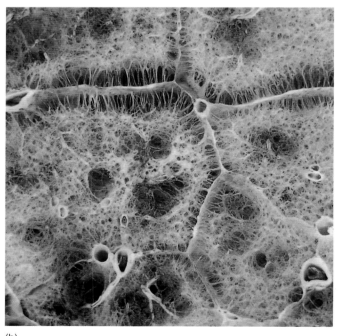

(b)

Figure 3.16 Paraseptal emphysema. (a) Giant bulla formation. (b) Barium sulphate precipitation (Illustration (b) provided by the late Professor BE Heard, Brompton, UK.)

Table 3.2 Serum α1-antitrypsin concentrations (expressed as percentage of normal level) and frequencies of the commoner phenotypes in the UK[147,148]

Phenotype	Serum concentration (%)	Frequency
MM	100	86
MS	75	9
MZ	57	3
SS	52	0.25
SZ	37	0.2
ZZ	16	0.03

α1-globulin.[145,146] Deficiency of this protein results in leukocyte elastases acting unopposed on the connective tissues of the lungs.

α1-antitrypsin deficiency is inherited through an autosomal recessive gene, which exhibits polymorphism, the variants being classified alphabetically in a Pi (protease inhibitor) nomenclature according to their electrophoretic mobility. For example, PiBB is the homozygote for an anodal variant and PiZZ for a cathodal variant, with PiMM representing the homozygote for the normal M allele. There are over 70 different variants. Those of particular medical relevance are the Z and S mutants.[147–149] The frequency of Pi types in England and Wales and the corresponding serum levels of α1-antitrypsin are shown in Table 3.2. Although α1-antitrypsin deficiency was first identified in Sweden, subsequent studies have shown that it affects all races.[150]

PiZZ homozygotes are prone to suffer hepatitis, cirrhosis or emphysema, the liver being the site of synthesis of the enzyme and the lung an important site of its action. α1-antitrypsin deficiency accounts for about 6% of all clinically significant emphysema (PiZZ 5%; PiSS and PiSZ 1%). It is debatable whether PiM heterozygotes (PiMS and PiMZ) have an increased risk of emphysema but it appears unlikely, particularly if they do not smoke.[151,152]

The emphysema associated with α1-antitrypsin deficiency develops unusually early in life, typically in the third or fourth decade. The condition is familial and patients may have seen an older relative die of the same disease. The bases of the lungs are particularly affected because their greater blood flow, which is attributable to gravity, brings more leukocytes to these regions.

α2-macroglobulin is another antiprotease that is synthesised in the liver, but it is of too large a molecular size to leave the circulation. However, as well as antiproteases that reach the lungs from the blood, antiproteases specific to the lung have been identified, notably in the serous acini of the bronchial glands and in the Clara cells of the bronchioles.[82,100–102] A reported increase in Clara cells in small airway disease[103] possibly represents a compensatory response to inactivation of antiproteases by irritants such as cigarette smoke[153,154] and to the increased release of proteases that cigarette smoke elicits from phagocytic cells.[155] Others report that the bronchiolar goblet cell proliferation seen in smokers takes place at the expense of Clara cells.[99]

Cigarette smokers have a constant increase in alveolar macrophages,[156,157] particularly in the central part of the lung

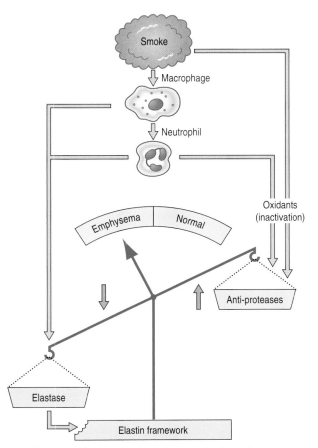

Figure 3.17 The pathogenesis of emphysema, envisaged as a consequence of imbalance between proteases and antiproteases in the lung.

acini.[158] During phagocytosis these cells release proteolytic enzymes[159] and a neutrophil-chemotactic factor,[160] and this process is enhanced by cigarette smoking.[161] The role of cigarette smoking in the development of emphysema was demonstrated in a radiological study of persistent smokers during which foci of ground-glass attenuation probably representing bronchiolocentric aggregates of alveolar macrophages progressed to emphysema over a 5-year period in about 25% of cases.[162] Neutrophils are an even richer source of proteases than macrophages and large numbers of these cells enter the lungs in the acute exacerbations that characterise chronic bronchitis. An imbalance between proteases and antiproteases is therefore considered to underlie the aetiology of emphysema.[163] The various factors contributing to this imbalance are represented in Figure 3.17. This protease-antiprotease theory may be invoked to explain both centriacinar and panacinar emphysema, which frequently co-exist.

The inflammatory component of emphysema is often maintained long after the patient gives up smoking,[164] possibly because peptides derived from degraded connective tissue are chemotactic for inflammatory cells.[165] This suggests that the disease is sometimes self-perpetuating, which may explain the progressive clinical deterioration that is seen in some ex-smokers with obstructive airway disease.

A check-valve mechanism is often envisaged to explain the formation of bullae, but pressure measurements at thoracotomy show that the air in bullae is at the same negative pressure as that in the rest of the lungs, except when they are subjected to positive pressure ventilation.[166] It would appear that bullae originate in the same way as smaller emphysematous foci, namely by a process of unchecked proteolysis rather than through undue distensive forces.

Cadmium is a further factor involved in the pathogenesis of emphysema. It has been found that occupational exposure to cadmium fumes over long periods can cause emphysema,[167] and this clinical observation has experimental support from the production of emphysema through the introduction of cadmium into the trachea of animals or its inhalation in the form of an aerosol.[168] In man, the emphysema that is attributable to inhalation of cadmium affects the upper lobes severely and is mainly of the centriacinar type.[169] Cigarette smoke is an important source of inhaled cadmium and there is a significant correlation between the degree of emphysema and the concentration of cadmium in the lungs at necropsy, even in the case of patients who have not been exposed to cadmium fumes at work.[170] A combination of occupational cadmium exposure and cigarette smoking appears to be particularly dangerous.[171]

Functional effects of emphysema

Although much emphasis is placed on elastin digestion in the pathogenesis of emphysema, it is debatable whether the actual amounts of elastin are reduced in this disease.[123,124,172] Nevertheless, if a piece of elastic material such as a rubber band is cut at merely one point, its functional integrity is completely destroyed: focal digestion of alveolar elastin may be expected to have a similar effect without there necessarily being much overall loss of this protein. Experiments inducing emphysema with elastase show that losses in elastin can be made good but that the structural derangement is irreversible.[173]

Although elastic recoil is often attributed to the connective tissue framework of the lung it is markedly reduced when alveolar air is replaced by water, showing that it is surface-tensive forces at the tissue/air interface that underlies recoil. These forces are, of course, also weakened when there is loss of alveolar tissue.

Diminished elastic recoil and severance of alveolar attachments to bronchioles results in premature closure of these airways on expiration (Fig. 3.18).[44,126–128] The resultant air trapping is responsible for the overinflation of the lungs and 'barrel chest' that are characteristic of emphysema. Respiration is conducted near maximal lung volume, which severely compromises inspiratory muscle function. Some adaptation to this is achieved by an increase in the proportion of slow ('endurance') fibres in the inspiratory muscles.[174]

Emphysema also results in there being less alveolar surface available for gas exchange but the extent of this is seldom appreciated when lung slices are examined. The relationship of diameter to surface area is logarithmic so that for a given increase in airspace diameter there is a much greater loss in surface area.

Normal alveoli are about 0.25 mm in diameter, which corresponds to an alveolar surface area of about $24\,mm^2\,mm^{-3}$ whereas by the time emphysema is just visible to the naked eye at an alveolar diameter of 1 mm, three-quarters of the surface area of the lung has been lost, the alveolar surface area being reduced to $6\,mm^2\,mm^{-3}$. Emphysema that is easily recognisable in the post-mortem room has air spaces that measure about 4 mm diameter, when the alveolar surface is less than 10% of normal (Fig. 3.19).

Emphysema is often accompanied by the small airway disease dealt with in the preceding section. In their different ways, emphysema and small airway disease both contribute to the airflow limitation that these patients suffer, one permitting premature bronchiolar closure and the other narrowing the bronchioles, but there has been much debate as to which of these mechanisms is the more important.

Treatment of emphysema

The cessation of smoking is essential to minimising progression of the disease but apart from bullectomy there has, until recently, been no effective treatment for emphysema. However, in recent years, the intravenous infusion of α1-antitrypsin,[175] lung transplantation and lung volume reduction surgery (reduction pneumoplasty)[176–179] have been introduced. In addition, there is potential in techniques that promote atelectasis by the insertion of bronchial valves or the injection of polymers, the induction of bronchopulmonary fenestrations to enhance expiratory flow and the thoracoscopic plication or compression of emphysematous lung.[180] In the future, there is also the possibility of genetic manipulation to correct α1-antitrypsin deficiency.

Bullectomy is practised to reduce the risk of pneumothorax and to eliminate tissue which, in accordance with Laplace's law, is preferentially aerated and compresses comparatively normal adjacent tissue. In contrast to bullectomy, lung volume reduction surgery often involves the resection of much comparatively normal lung tissue as well as the most severely diseased portions, a seemingly paradoxical way to treat someone who has already lost considerable lung tissue. The undoubted success of

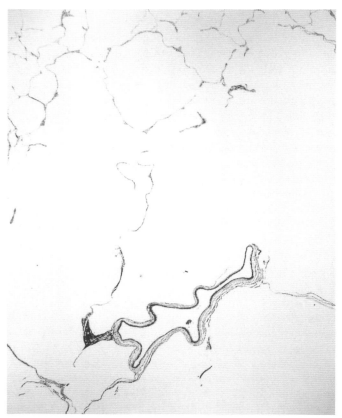

Figure 3.18 Emphysema showing bronchiolar collapse due to loss of alveolar attachments.

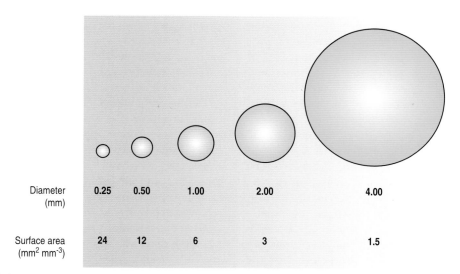

Diameter (mm)	0.25	0.50	1.00	2.00	4.00
Surface area (mm² mm⁻³)	24	12	6	3	1.5

Figure 3.19 Relationship between alveolar diameter and surface area. The normal alveolar diameter is about 0.25 mm. Emphysema is just detectable when the diameter is increased 4-fold (to 1 mm), at which time there is a 75% loss of alveolar surface area. At autopsy the emphysematous airspaces commonly have a diameter of 4 mm, representing a loss of alveolar surface of approximately 90%.

this operation probably stems from the improved efficiency of the inspiratory muscles when they are no longer operating at maximal stretch.[181,182] Pathological examination of the resected tissue is worthwhile as it occasionally reveals unexpected diseases such as fibrosis, inflammation, lymphangioleiomyomatosis and even carcinoma that adversely affect the postoperative course.[183,184]

Early attempts at treating emphysema by unilateral lung transplantation were unsuccessful and at the time this was attributed to a poor understanding of Laplace's principles, which dictate that the inspired air will enter the large volume diseased lung rather the unilateral implant. In retrospect, rejection was the probable cause of the failure. Today, transplantation of one or both lungs is firmly established in the treatment of emphysema, the success of the unilateral procedure probably depending partly upon the improved efficiency of the inspiratory muscles, as in lung volume reduction surgery.

Intervention at the molecular level has great potential in the prevention of emphysema in groups particularly at risk, such as those with α1-antitrypsin deficiency and replacement or supplemental therapy using either natural or recombinant antiproteases is being attempted. Unfortunately, the half-life of natural α1-antitrypsin is only 4 days, so weekly infusions are needed. Recombinant α1-antitrypsin has an even shorter half-life but aerosol trials are in progress. Bronchial antileukoprotease has also been produced by recombinant methods and trials of this are under way. Work is also in progress on the production of synthetic antiproteases.

Emphysema-like conditions

The term emphysema has been applied to several other conditions, none of which falls strictly within the limits of the current definition (p. 99), which requires destruction of respiratory tissue as well as the abnormal enlargement of air spaces.

Senile 'emphysema'

The condition that has been known as senile 'emphysema' is not a true form of the disease because the alterations are neither destructive nor beyond the limits of normal age change. After a developmental period of alveolar multiplication that terminates in adolescence there is a gradual alteration in the shape of the lungs coupled with progressive diminution in elastic recoil and alveolar surface area, the latter reducing by about 4% in each decade after the age of 30 years.[185] Total lung capacity remains constant throughout adult life but with increasing age, the lungs change shape, increasing in height and particularly in anteroposterior distance. There is also a gradual shift in the distribution of air from the alveoli to the alveolar ducts and bronchioles. The alveolar ducts gradually enlarge and the mouths of alveoli opening from them dilate so that the alveoli become shallower. All these changes may be regarded as part of the normal ageing process and therefore outwith the definition of emphysema. Although the ageing lungs lose some elastic recoil, this is not so great as in true emphysema and they generally

collapse when the chest is opened. This gave rise to the term atrophic emphysema as an alternative to senile emphysema and in contrast to hypertrophic emphysema, which was formerly used for true emphysema. The definition of emphysema given on p. 99 renders the terms atrophic, senile and hypertrophic emphysema redundant.

Infantile lobar 'emphysema'

Infantile lobar 'emphysema' is described on p. 70. It is the result of valvular obstruction to a lobar bronchus and is characterised by extreme distension without destruction.

Compensatory 'emphysema'

This is another condition characterised by distension without destruction. It occurs when parts of the lung collapse or are removed. Pneumonectomy leads to distension of the remaining lung rather than true (destructive) emphysema. Lung cancer is a common reason for pneumonectomy and with cigarette smoking underlying both lung cancer and emphysema, the remaining lung may well show true emphysema. The relationship between the pneumonectomy and the emphysema is not then a causal one.

Focal 'emphysema'

Focal 'emphysema' and simple pneumoconiosis of coalworkers are terms applied to a distensive bronchiolectasis that closely simulates the milder degrees of centriacinar emphysema.[186] It may represent an early form of centriacinar emphysema but is said to affect more proximal respiratory bronchioles and to be non-destructive. Until recently, the pneumoconiosis medical panels in Britain have restricted their attention to fibrosis, not attempting to distinguish focal and centriacinar emphysema and attributing both to social factors rather than occupation. Others did not accept this and believed that mine-dust causes chronic bronchitis, obstructive bronchiolitis and true emphysema, in addition to this focal dilatation of respiratory bronchioles.[187–189] This view has now prevailed so that British miners are now compensated financially if they have these diseases (see also p. 342).

Interstitial emphysema

The fundamental difference between interstitial emphysema and the forms of emphysema described above is outlined on p. 98 and may be summarised as follows: whereas all other forms of emphysema affect spaces that normally contain air, interstitial emphysema represents the ingress of air into tissues that are normally airless.

Air reaches the interstitial tissues of the lung when abnormal pressure ruptures the alveolar walls. Interstitial emphysema is therefore a form of barotrauma. The rupture may be due to excessively high pressure caused by violent artificial respiration, exposure to the blast of explosions, sudden decompression, or tearing of alveolar walls by fractured ribs or by instruments.

At operation or necropsy, interstitial emphysema is seen as small bubbles of air in the connective tissue immediately beneath the visceral pleura (see Fig. 2.14, p. 46). Large interstitial air bubbles are termed blebs, as distinct from bullae, which represent enlargement of pre-existent air spaces.[119] Air in the interstitial tissues may track along the connective tissue sheaths about the pulmonary vessels to the hila of the lungs, producing mediastinal emphysema; it may then reach the neck and present subcutaneously, as surgical emphysema. Systemic air embolism may complicate interstitial emphysema (see p. 412).

Microscopically, minute air bubbles appear as seemingly empty interstitial spaces, particularly in the abundant connective tissue that surrounds the pulmonary artery and airway and forms the interlobular septa. The differential diagnosis on microscopy is from congenital lymphangiectasia and this can be extremely difficult, not least because the air tracks within lymphatics as well as through the surrounding connective tissues. It is therefore helpful if the nature of the contents of the spaces, gaseous or fluid, is ascertained at necropsy. If the emphysema has been present for a few days before death, the diagnosis is simplified by the development of a foreign body giant cell reaction to the air (see Fig. 2.15, p. 47)[190–192] similar to that found in pneumatosis coli and following the experimental injection of gases into the subcutaneous tissues.[190]

PLASTIC BRONCHITIS

Patients with plastic bronchitis are generally well but complain of fits of coughing that often result in them involuntarily expectorating long stringy pieces of sputum, which causes them much social embarrassment.[193–197] The expectorate represents a bronchial cast of up to eight airway generations (Fig. 3.20). Microscopically the cast is seen to consist of alternating bands of fibrin and mucus, with the fibrin containing variable numbers of lymphocytes.[194,195] The appearances suggest that the cast represents an inspissated fibrinous exudate and the term fibrinous bronchitis is sometimes applied to the condition. Several associated conditions have been described[194,197,198] and it is possible that some of these have a causal relationship, notably heart failure and lymphatic abnormalities. Plastic bronchitis is often confused with the mucoid impaction of allergic bronchopulmonary aspergillosis,[199] which is characterised by the expectoration of short stubby gobbets of mucus. The two conditions are quite different. They are compared in Table 3.3.[194,200,201]

BRONCHIAL ASTHMA

Bronchial asthma is to be distinguished from the aetiologically distinct condition of cardiac asthma. The latter represents pulmonary oedema consequent upon a failing left heart. Bronchial asthma, hereafter called simply asthma, is a condition in which breathing is periodically rendered difficult by widespread narrowing of the bronchi that changes in severity over short periods of time, either spontaneously or under treatment.[45] The difficulty becomes particularly apparent during expiration because the airways normally collapse during that phase of respiration and because the expiratory muscles are less powerful than those that act during inspiration.

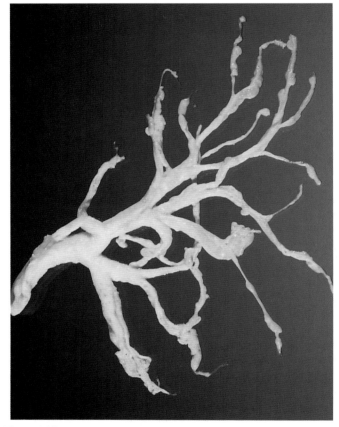

Figure 3.20 A 15 cm long bronchial cast from a patient with plastic bronchitis.

Table 3.3 A comparison of mucoid impaction and plastic bronchitis		
	Mucoid impaction	*Plastic bronchitis*
Clinical features	Aggravation of underlying asthma. Progression to hilar bronchiectasis	Expectoration of stringy sputum.
Cause	Atopy: allergic broncho-pulmonary aspergillosis complicating asthma	Unknown. Associations of questionable causal relationship include heart disease and lymphatic abnormalities
Gross appearance of expectorate	A short stubby mucoid plug	A long stringy bronchial cast of up to eight airway generations
Microscopic appearance of plug/cast	Alternating layers of mucus and inspissated eosinophils with numerous Charcot–Leyden crystals and scanty aspergillus hyphae.	Alternating layers of mucus and fibrin with variable numbers of lymphocytes. No eosinophils. No fungi.

Extrinsic and intrinsic forms of asthma

Asthma is said to be 'extrinsic' if allergy to exogenous substances is recognised and 'intrinsic' if no such exogenous factors can be identified. Extrinsic asthma is the more common. It usually begins in childhood and is generally paroxysmal, the attack starting suddenly and lasting a few hours or days. Boys are affected about twice as much as girls. Extrinsic asthma tends to become less severe as the child grows older and often ceases during adolescence. However, about 30% of asthmatic children continue to have symptoms in adult life. Extrinsic asthma is often familial and some of the genes responsible have been identified.[202–205] This form of asthma is frequently preceded by flexural infantile eczema and succeeded in adult life by perennial vasomotor rhinitis, although in such families, any one of these three diseases may affect some members much more than others. In contrast, intrinsic asthma more often has its onset in adult life, is chronic, with exacerbations and remissions less evident and tends to worsen with age. The symptoms are also apt to become more severe in winter, when the asthmatic disabilities are likely to be complicated by infection of the respiratory tract. In both types of the disease, the dyspnoea is characteristically accompanied by cough, wheezy breathing, some cyanosis and expectoration. Blood eosinophilia is more prominent in extrinsic asthma but eosinophils are found in the airways in both. Serum immunoglobulin E is often raised in extrinsic asthma and normal or low in intrinsic asthma. There is an increased incidence of nasal polyps in both forms of asthma, but especially in the intrinsic variety and in certain asthmatic patients in whom bronchospasm is triggered by aspirin. Despite these differences, the pathological features are similar and an immunological basis may be envisaged in both.[206,207]

Epidemiology

Over the past few decades the prevalence of asthma has increased considerably in most developed countries where it now stands at about 5%. The reason for this is unclear. General atmospheric pollution has been widely incriminated but there is little to support this: the increase has been experienced in countries such as New Zealand which have little atmospheric pollution and in Philadelphia at a time when atmospheric pollution declined.[208] Atmospheric pollution is more likely to aggravate asthma than cause it. Changes in the home that encourage the growth of the principal allergen, the house dust mite (higher temperature and humidity and extensive carpeting), are more likely environmental factors.[209,210]

Another possibility is the decline in childhood infections in the developed countries. Infection induces a Th1 response rather than the Th2 reactions responsible for atopy (see 'aetiology', below).[211] Indirect support for this possibility comes from studies of family size and birth order. Atopy is less common in children belonging to large families and, within such families, in the younger children – the ones that are most likely to be exposed in infancy to infections brought home by their sib-

lings.[212,213] More direct evidence comes from studies showing less atopy in those who had previously had measles,[214] were seropositive for hepatitis A[215,216] or gave a strong tuberculin reaction.[217] This raises the attractive possibility of preventive immunisation using harmless bacteria.[218]

Mortality figures have fluctuated over the past few decades, apparently being influenced adversely on occasion by the introduction of new drugs, particularly β-agonists (Fig. 3.21).[219,220] The mechanism underlying these fluctuations is not fully understood but overdosage, cardiac dysrhythmia, refractoriness to the bronchodilatory effect of the drug and a false sense of security afforded by carrying an inhaler are all thought to have contributed.[219] The prognosis is worse in late-onset intrinsic asthma. Most asthma deaths occur in the elderly, although asthma accounts for a greater proportion of deaths in the young (0.9% of those under 25 *vs* 0.3% overall). Changes in the mortality rate from 1979 to 1999 are shown in Table 3.4.

The sputum in asthma

The sputum is viscous[221] and yellow in asthma. The colour should not be taken as evidence that the sputum is infected. It is due to myeloperoxidase, which is found in both eosinophils and neutrophils. In asthma, the sputum is rich in eosinophils, but not neutrophils unless there is also infection. As well as eosinophils, microscopy shows the presence of certain formed

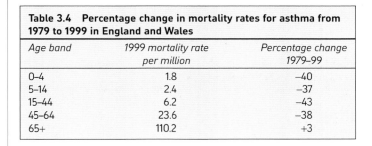

Table 3.4 Percentage change in mortality rates for asthma from 1979 to 1999 in England and Wales

Age band	1999 mortality rate per million	Percentage change 1979–99
0–4	1.8	−40
5–14	2.4	−37
15–44	6.2	−43
45–64	23.6	−38
65+	110.2	+3

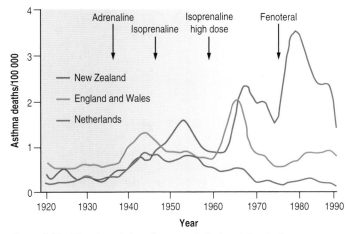

Figure 3.21 Time trends in asthma mortality in relation to the introduction of various inhaled drugs. (Reproduced from Blauw GJ, Westendorp RGJ. Asthma deaths in New Zealand: whodunnit? The Lancet 1995; 345:2–3, with permission from Elsevier.)

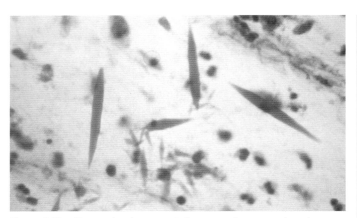

Figure 3.22 Charcot–Leyden crystals in sputum from an asthmatic patient.

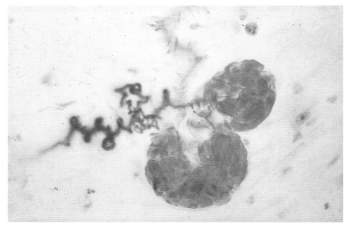

Figure 3.23 A Curschmann spiral and two Creola bodies in sputum from an asthmatic patient. (Methylene blue stain.)

elements: Charcot–Leyden crystals, Curschmann's spirals and Creola bodies.

Charcot–Leyden crystals are found when there are large numbers of eosinophils. They have the shape of a pair of long, narrow, six-sided pyramids placed base to base (Fig. 3.22). Their hexagonal shape can often be seen when they are cut across in histological preparations. Chromatographic studies suggested that they consisted of lysophospholipase derived from the cell membranes of eosinophils[222] but molecular analyses indicate that they represent a β-galactose binding lectin, galectin-10.[223]

A Curschmann spiral (Fig. 3.23) is a spiral twist of condensed mucus several millimetres long that is usually surrounded by an elongated mass of clear or opalescent material. Curschmann spirals are widely believed to represent bronchial casts, but their calibre is more commensurate with that of a bronchial gland duct or of a peripheral bronchiole. Furthermore, they have also been observed in uterine cervical smears and in peritoneal and pleural effusions.[224]

Creola bodies (Fig. 3.23) are compact clumps or strips of columnar epithelial cells shed from the bronchus. They are sometimes found in the sputum of asthmatics and care must be

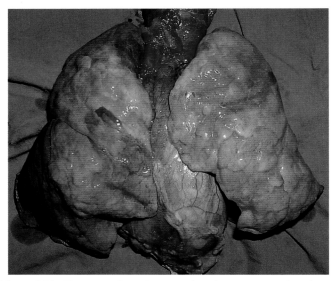

Figure 3.24 The lungs of a patient who died of status asthmaticus. After their removal from the chest and exposure to atmospheric pressure the lungs fail to collapse owing to mucus obstructing the airways. (Reproduced by permission of Dr GA Russell, Tunbridge Wells, UK.)

taken not to mistake them for exfoliated adenocarcinoma cells.[225]

Morbid anatomy

No differences are recognised between the structural changes in extrinsic and intrinsic asthma, but most of our knowledge has come from necropsies in cases of status asthmaticus. This has tended to over-emphasise the terminal features and the complications of the condition, but from the few biopsy specimens obtained from asthmatics or autopsies performed on asthmatics dying of other diseases it seems that qualitatively similar but less severe lesions are present between attacks. During non-fatal attacks, it is assumed that similar lesions of intermediate severity are present. Bronchography has shown that airway plugging is widespread between asthmatic attacks as well as being prominent in patients dying of asthma.[226]

The gross appearances are characteristic. When the chest is opened in cases of death in status asthmaticus, the lungs are found to be greatly distended: they fail to retract as normal lungs do when the negative intrapleural pressure is replaced by atmospheric pressure on opening the pleural cavities (Fig. 3.24). Contrasting with the general distension, small foci of collapse may sometimes be seen as dark, airless, firm areas, depressed below the level of the surrounding lung. The airways are occluded by plugs of thick, tenacious mucus (Fig. 3.25). These are found in airways of all sizes beyond the second order bronchi[226] but the most striking changes are seen in airways of about 5 mm diameter. When the cut surface of the lung is exposed, the bronchi of this size are seen to be filled with grey plugs of viscous mucus that can be made to protrude from the lumen by compressing the lungs. Bronchography shows that air can pass the plugs only on inspiration.[226]

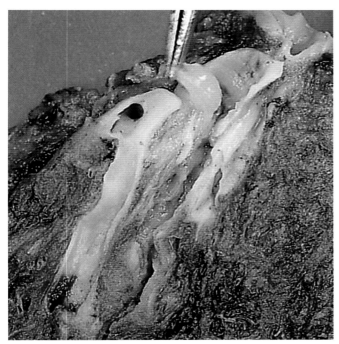

Figure 3.25 Status asthmaticus. Tenacious plugs of mucus occlude the airways. (Reproduced by permission of Dr GA Russell, Tunbridge Wells, UK.)

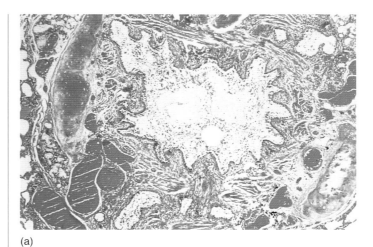

(a)

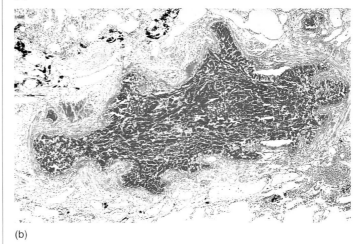

(b)

Figure 3.26 Asthma showing bronchial plugging by mucus. (a) Haematoxylin and eosin, (b) Alcian blue–periodic acid Schiff.

Patches of subpleural fibrosis and honeycombing are common, particularly in the upper lobes; these are possibly the sequel of eosinophilic pneumonia which is often most marked in the periphery of the upper lobes. It is notable in asthma that although the lungs may be fully distended with air at necropsy, very little emphysema is found. Some patients have right ventricular hypertrophy but this is uncommon in the absence of associated bronchiectasis or chronic bronchitis.

The above changes are typically found in patients dying hours after the onset of an asthmatic attack but they have also been found after death in asthmatic patients who have been well seconds earlier.[227,228] Rarely, a patient with asthma dies suddenly and the airways are found to be empty of mucus.[229] Myocardial contraction bands that have been described in such patients[230] are possibly connected with the overuse of β-adrenergic drugs, which may have contributed to these deaths.[231,232] Other such patients have been found to have inflammation of their cardiac conduction system.[233]

Mucus plugging of airways and hyperinflation of the lungs are not confined to patients with a history of asthma. They are also found in patients dying of anaphylaxis initiated by factors such as wasp or bee venom, foodstuffs and drugs.[234]

Histopathology

Microscopically, three major processes are seen to contribute to the airway narrowing: increased amounts of mucus, inflammatory oedema and muscular hypertrophy. These are found principally in bronchi but may also be found in smaller airways, including bronchioles.[235–239] The inflammation may even involve alveoli.[240]

The airway lumen is compromised by the accumulation of mucus and an exudate of eosinophils and desquamated epithelial cells mixed with components derived from the plasma but not including fibrin (Fig. 3.26).[241,242] The mucus commonly has a concentric or spiral pattern in cross section and includes cells that are often aggregated in a corresponding distribution. These cells are mostly eosinophils and desquamated epithelium. There is goblet cell hyperplasia in the surface epithelium and the bronchial glands are enlarged, but not as much as in chronic bronchitis[90,91,235]; in contrast to chronic bronchitis, the serous elements in the submucosal glands are as numerous as the mucous acini.[243] The mucus is consequently less acidic than that in chronic bronchitis.[244] Changes in the bronchioles are less obvious than those in the larger airways but there may be muscle hypertrophy and an increase in goblet cells.[235,238] The bronchioles may also contain mucous plugs and mucus may even be seen in alveolar ducts. How much of this mucus is derived from bronchiolar goblet cells and how much is aspirated from the more proximal airways is unknown.

A characteristic feature of the airways in status asthmaticus is infiltration of the walls of bronchi and proximal bronchioles

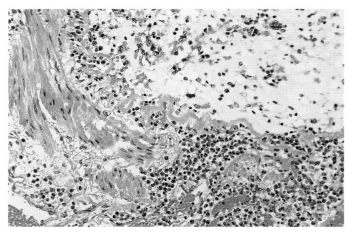

Figure 3.27 Asthma showing epithelial desquamation, hypersecretion of mucus, thickening of the epithelial basement membrane and infiltration of the bronchial wall by lymphocytes and eosinophils.

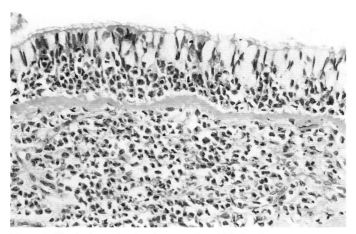

Figure 3.28 Asthma showing heavy eosinophil infiltration and marked basement membrane thickening.

by eosinophils (Figs 3.27, 3.28).[235] It has been shown immunocytochemically that the eosinophils are activated to secrete major basic protein.[245–247] Neutrophils are generally uncommon and when numerous suggest secondary bacterial infection. However, more attention is now being paid to the pathogenetic role of these cells in asthma.[248,249] It is reported that in fatal asthma of sudden onset neutrophils outnumber eosinophils,[250] or even that they are the only polymorphonuclear leukocyte present.[251] Lymphocytes (mainly T-helper cells) are generally numerous in asthma, making up half the inflammatory cells.[245,246,252] Mast cells are not usually identified in appreciable numbers, but this is only because of degranulation, which can sometimes be recognised in appropriately stained sections by the presence of clusters of free metachromatic granules.[244] Staining for mast cell tryptase shows that these cells are increased in number.[253] Eosinophil degranulation is also evident and degranulation of both eosinophils and mast cells is confirmed by electron microscopy.[254]

The eosinophil inflammation of the airways is accompanied by marked congestion and oedema and separation and detachment of the more superficial columnar epithelial cells from the underlying basal cells.[255,256] Where such exfoliation has occurred, regeneration may be evident in the form of mitotic division of the basal cells of the epithelium. The loss of ciliated cells contributes to the impaired bronchial clearance. Between attacks, patchy exfoliation of the epithelium may still be recognised,[257] and electron microscopy shows blebbing of the apical cell membrane and bizarre cilia.[258] During the regenerative process, the epithelium may show evidence of cell proliferation and squamous metaplasia.[256,259]

Loss of the surface epithelial cells also exposes intraepithelial nerves to inflammatory mediators released in the bronchial lumen: stimulation of these nerves is thought to lead to an axon reflex that is responsible for much of the vasodilatation, oedema, mucus secretion and smooth muscle contraction that characterises an asthmatic attack.[260]

The epithelial basement membrane is often thickened in asthma (Fig. 3.28). This may be a reflection of the repeated shedding of epithelial cells, for basement membrane thickening is well known in other situations where the cells it supports are rapidly replaced. However, electron microscopy shows that the thickening is confined to the deepest layer of the basement membrane, the collagen and fibronectin-rich lamina reticularis (Fig. 3.29), which is probably produced by myofibroblasts rather than the epithelium.[261–263] Tenascin, a glycoprotein concerned in repair, has been identified in the bronchial basement membrane in asthma but not in controls[264] whereas although plasma proteins, including immunoglobulins, can be demonstrated in the thickened basement membrane they are also present in the bronchial basement membrane of many non-asthmatic patients.[261] Although basement membrane thickening is frequently emphasised as being characteristic of asthma, it is by no means specific for this disease,[244,257,265] lesser degrees often being seen in biopsy specimens from non-asthmatic patients, taken for example because of suspected cancer.

A prominent increase in the amount of airway muscle is a further feature of bronchial asthma and presumably reflects sustained muscular contraction (Fig. 3.30).[89–91,237,266–268] The increase involves airways of all sizes but is most apparent in small bronchi of about 0.5 cm diameter.[89,237,238,266,269] It is attributable to hyperplasia as well as hypertrophy.[89,268] The bronchial smooth muscle is hyperactive in asthma and the peptidergic (non-adrenergic, non-cholinergic) bronchial innervation is probably important here for fatal asthma is characterised by depletion of vasoactive intestinal peptide from bronchial nerve terminals.[270]

The major changes in the airways act together and enhance the effect of each other on airway calibre. Mathematical modelling suggests that a moderate degree of inflammatory thickening of the mucosa, which by itself would have little effect on baseline resistance to gas flow, can profoundly affect the airway narrowing caused by normal smooth muscle shortening: the various processes narrowing the airways are more than additive in their effect on airway responsiveness.[236,271–273]

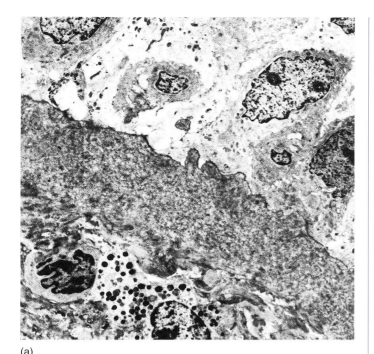

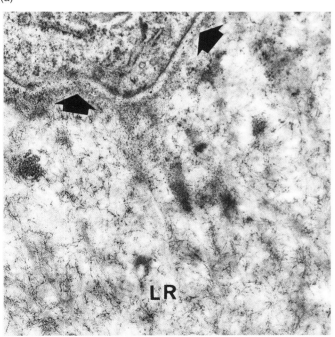

(a)

(b)

Figure 3.29 Bronchial asthma. (a) Transmission electron micrograph showing that the epithelial basement membrane dividing epithelium (above) from connective tissue (below) is greatly thickened. Immediately beneath the basement membrane there is a lymphocyte and a mast cell. (b) Higher magnification shows that the lamina rara and lamina densa (arrows) are normal and that the thickening involves the deepest layer of the basement membrane, the lamina reticularis (LR). (a) ×2500; (b) ×30 000.

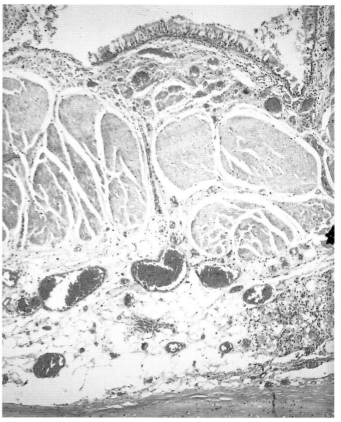

Figure 3.30 Asthma. The bronchial muscle is greatly hypertrophied due to sustained contraction.

It will be evident from the above that asthma and chronic bronchitis have features in common but that there are notable differences. The two diseases are compared in Table 3.1 (p. 98). A possible overlap condition known as 'wheezy bronchitis' is described on p. 96.

Pathogenesis and aetiology of asthma

Two major mechanisms operate in both extrinsic and intrinsic asthma, one neurological and the other inflammatory.[260,274,275] The two mechanisms may interact. Thus, inflammatory mediators are prone to trigger nerve reflexes while nerve stimuli, or loss of inhibitory activity, may, in addition to causing secretion and contraction, affect vascular permeability and promote oedema.

In both extrinsic and intrinsic asthma, there are many non-specific trigger factors. For example, many asthmatics are over-responsive to irritant dusts and to respiratory infection, reacting to either with marked bronchial narrowing. Emotional stress is another non-specific triggering factor in asthma. Exercise has a similar effect in many asthmatic patients, the large amount of cold dry air inhaled during outdoor exercise probably being the non-specific bronchial irritant. Exercise-induced asthma is rare in the warm, humid atmosphere of an indoor swimming bath. Eosinophilia is not a feature of exercise-induced asthma.[276]

Up to 10% of asthmatic patients are unduly sensitive to aspirin and other non-steroidal anti-inflammatory drugs.[277,278] Non-atopic patients with nasal polyps whose asthma is difficult to control are particularly sensitive to aspirin.[279] Aspirin-induced bronchial narrowing is attributed to inhibition of arachidonic acid metabolism by the cyclo-oxygenase pathway and its diversion to the lipoxygenase pathway with the production of bronchoconstrictor leukotrienes C4 and D4 (formerly known collectively as slow releasing factor of anaphylaxis).

Extrinsic asthma is usually associated with atopy, this being a liability to develop excessive amounts of immunoglobulin E (so-called reaginic antibodies) in response to commonplace antigens that the individual repeatedly meets in everyday life. Cutaneous prick tests usually result in an immediate wheal and flare response to a range of allergens. Specific allergens are found in many pollens, feathers, horse dander, fur and especially house dust. The most important asthma-causing allergen is probably the house dust mite, *Dermatophagoides pteronyssinus*, which is found worldwide. It feeds on shed human epidermal squames and for this reason is particularly numerous in dust from bedding, especially mattresses. Warm damp houses favour the growth of the mites more than cold dry ones, but very few samples of house dust are completely free of them. A reported increase in asthmatic attacks during thunderstorms may be due to pollen counts rising at such times.[280,281] Many environmental allergens causing asthma probably go undetected but one such agent was identified when periodic outbreaks of asthma in the vicinity of Barcelona's docks were found to coincide with the unloading of soybean.[282] Occupational factors can be identified as contributing to asthma in about 2% of adult cases (see p. 359). Such asthma occurs in many industries and over two hundred aetiological agents have been identified (see Table 7.1.8, p. 359).

Intrinsic asthma usually affects people older than those afflicted with extrinsic asthma. IgE levels are lower than in extrinsic asthma and skin tests are often negative or only weakly positive. It is therefore widely presumed that in intrinsic asthma, airway inflammation is triggered by non-immunological mechanisms. However, IgE levels and the prevalence of positive skin tests to common allergens decline throughout adult life and some workers find that a high age-corrected IgE level is as good a marker of asthma in the elderly as in the young.[283,284] When these age-related changes are taken into account the traditional separation of intrinsic and extrinsic asthma is less clear.

The reaginic antibodies are largely fixed to cells, particularly to the Fc receptors on the surface of mast cells.[285] Inhalation of the appropriate allergen then leads to an antigen-antibody reaction on the surface of the mast cells, the consequent degranulation releasing various chemical mediators from these cells.

The mast cell and the eosinophil leukocyte are central to the pathogenesis of asthma, the former cell being responsible for many of the acute manifestations of the disease and the latter for more of its chronic features. In response to both immunological and non-specific stimuli, the mast cell secretes a range of bioactive substances, while the eosinophil secretes substances antagonistic to mast cell mediators but also releases others that are detrimental to the integrity of the respiratory epithelium.

Mast cells are most numerous in relation to airway muscle and glands,[286] but they are also present within the surface epithelium[258,287] and can be recovered in bronchial washes.[288] Inhaled antigens first react with immunoglobulin E bound to mast cells free in the bronchial lumen and this causes release of mediators from these mast cells and consequent weakening of the tight junctions binding together surface epithelial cells, so facilitating access of the antigen to mast cells in the epithelium. The degranulation of these mast cells further augments epithelial permeability. Penetration of antigen into the rest of the bronchial wall is thus facilitated as successive mast cells are rapidly triggered. Differences between mucosal and connective tissue mast cells are described: the former are smaller and contain heparin and tryptase rather than chymase.[289,290] Both types have been identified in human airways.[289]

Various mediators are released when the mast cell degranulates. Some of these cause immediate effects while others are responsible for reactions that come on hours later. Preformed mediators include histamine, exoglycosidases, tryptase and eosinophil and neutrophil chemotactic factors. Histamine causes dilatation and increased permeability of blood vessels, triggers irritant nerve receptors causing coughing and stimulates smooth muscle contraction and mucus secretion, while exoglycosidases such as glucuronidase, hexosaminidase and galactosidase together with neutral proteases disrupt the integrity of the bronchial submucosa through their actions on connective tissue ground substance. Histamine release also stimulates the generation and release of newly formed mediators, including prostaglandin D2, platelet-activating factor and leukotrienes C4 and D4, that are responsible for the later effects. Prostaglandin D2 and leukotriene C4, respectively enhance vasodilation and vascular permeability, while platelet-activating factor and the leukotrienes C4 and D4 cause smooth muscle to contract. Collectively these contribute greatly to the inflammatory oedema, muscular contraction and hypersecretion of mucus that characterise an asthmatic attack. Mast cells also produce a variety of cytokines, notably interleukins 1, 2, 3, 10 and 13, granulocyte-macrophage colony-stimulating factor, interferon-γ and tumour necrosis factor-α.[291]

The eosinophil counters the action of many of these mast cell mediators by secreting degradative enzymes: these include histaminase and aryl sulphatase, which destroy histamine and leukotrienes respectively. However, further substances secreted by the eosinophil aggravate the disease. In helminthic infestation, major basic protein and eosinophil cationic protein derived from the eosinophil are probably beneficial in promoting elimination of the parasites but in asthma they appear to be responsible for the epithelial disintegration that characterises the disease.[292] *In vitro*, low concentrations of major basic protein impair ciliary motility and cause epithelial disruption, cell shedding and lysis.[292,293] *In vivo*, there is vacuolation of epithelial cells and the degree to which this occurs correlates with the number of eosinophils.[252] Major basic protein is normally confined to the core of eosinophil granules[294] but in patients dying of status asthmaticus, it is present within mucous plugs and on damaged epithelial surfaces.[295] Epithelial fragility is likely to enhance the access of allergens and non-specific irritants to mast cells, lymphocytes and nerves in the bronchial wall, thereby aggravating the condition. Nevertheless, a clear disassociation between eosinophil infiltration of the airways and bronchial hyper-responsiveness is seen in the separate condition of eosinophilic bronchitis, which is considered below.

There is increasing evidence, largely based on the demonstration of activated T-helper lymphocytes in the airways,[246,247,296–300] that cellular hypersensitivity is important in asthma. Indeed the T-lymphocyte appears to play an important role in initiating an asthmatic attack (Fig. 3.31). Selective activation of the Th2 subgroup has been identified, resulting in interleukin 4, 5, 9, 10 and 13 secretion.[217,245,301–308] Interleukins 4 and 13 cause plasma cells to form IgE rather than IgG while interleukin 5 is responsible for the tissue eosinophilia and bronchial hyper-reactivity that characterise asthma and interleukin 10 inhibits the development of Th1 cells. Conversely, Th1

cells produce interferon-α, which is a potent inhibitor of IgE production.

Both genetic and environmental factors appear to influence the relative activity of Th1 and Th2 cells. Certain infections are characterised by the production of large amounts on interferon-γ but the children of atopic parents have fewer interferon-γ producing cells in their peripheral blood. It is plausible therefore to envisage repeated viral infections, particularly in early life, selectively enhancing the development of Th1 cells and inhibiting the proliferation of Th2 clones and allergic sensitisation – the so-called hygiene hypothesis that is also touched upon above, under epidemiology. This hypothesis has led to suggestions that vaccines designed to stimulate Th1 cell development could be beneficial in preventing asthma and allied allergic diseases.[217]

Asthma is also characterised by infiltration of the bronchial surface epithelium by Langerhans cells.[301] These non-phagocytic histiocytes are rich in surface receptors and are responsible for the presentation of antigenic information to T-lymphocytes. Very few Langerhans cells are found in the normal lung although there is a rich network of the dendritic cells that are their probable precursors.[301,309–311]

The bronchial epithelium also contributes actively to the development of asthma.[274] For example, epithelial expression of the bronchoconstrictor substance endothelin is increased in asthma.[312] Other bronchoconstrictor agents, such as prostacyclins are also released when bronchial epithelium is damaged.

The association of asthma with nasal polyps and paranasal sinusitis has been ascribed to aspiration of upper respiratory tract secretions but radionuclide tracer studies do not support this.[313] Furthermore asthmatic patients' minor salivary glands show inflammatory changes similar to those in their airways,[314] suggesting that there is generalised mucosal disease affecting both upper and lower airways. The polyps themselves have an oedematous stroma infiltrated by eosinophils. Nasal polyps are common in certain other airway diseases, notably cystic fibrosis and primary ciliary dyskinesia, but in these non-allergic conditions the polyps lack the tissue eosinophilia seen in asthma.

Asthma is also associated with gastro-oesophageal reflux but it is uncertain whether the relationship is causal.[315,316] Contact of the oesophagus or the trachea with hydrochloric acid induces reflex bronchial constriction[317] but it is unclear whether the reflux is the primary event as hyperinflation of the lungs increases abdominal pressure and thus promotes reflux. Reflux may be asymptomatic[318] and some asthmatics report symptomatic improvement on medical antireflux therapy, but their lung function is generally unchanged.[316] Surgical intervention is currently considered inappropriate.

Some intriguing observations concerning asthma have emanated from transplantation centres. It is reported that the lungs of an asthmatic donor confer asthma on a non-atopic recipient and conversely that an asthmatic recipient receiving lungs from a non-asthmatic donor experiences no further attacks of asthma.[319]

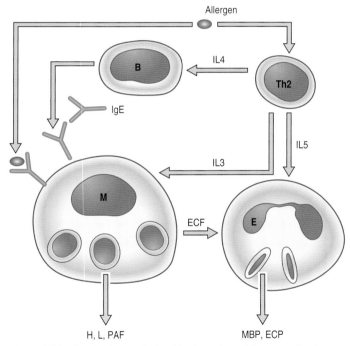

Figure 3.31 Cellular inter-relationships in asthma. Allergens stimulate Th2-lymphocytes to release interleukins which activate B-lymphocytes, mast cells and eosinophils. Interleukin-5 promotes eosinophil activation while interleukin-4 is responsible for B-lymphocyte maturation, which results in immunoglobulin E production, the adherence of which to mast cells primes the latter to degranulate on contact with the same allergen. The eosinophil modulates some of the effects of the mast cell by releasing histaminase and aryl sulphatase, which inactivate histamine and leukotrienes respectively, but also damages adjacent tissue by secreting major basic protein and eosinophil cationic protein. Th2, T-helper2-lymphocyte; B, B-lymphocyte; M, mast cell; E, eosinophil; IL, interleukin; IgE, immunoglobulin E; H, histamine; L, leukotrienes; PAF, platelet activating factor; MBP, major basic protein; ECP, eosinophil cationic protein; ECF, eosinophil chemotactic factor.

Treatment of asthma

Asthma is largely treated quite successfully by the avoidance of recognised trigger agents coupled with bronchodilator drugs and corticosteroids as required, supplemented on occasion by desensitisation to specific allergens and breathing exercises. Other treatments that have been developed more recently include leukotriene and leukotriene-receptor antagonists and antibodies directed against IgE, while several asthma genes have recently been identified suggesting that gene therapy may be introduced at some future date.

Complications of asthma

Asthma is sometimes complicated by allergic bronchopulmonary aspergillosis: it is also a frequent manifestation of the latter (see p. 225). *Aspergillus fumigatus* is the species most commonly concerned in Britain, but other species appear to be relatively more frequent causes in other parts of the world, hence the alternative term allergic bronchopulmonary fungal disease. It is important to note that in this condition the fungus does not invade the tissues. Inhalation of fungal spores sets up a reaction in the sensitised bronchial tree that is characterised by bronchospasm, accumulation of eosinophils and outpouring of abundant, very viscid mucus. The mucus forms a cast that distends the affected segment of the bronchial tree. The cast is colonised by the fungus and the preparation of histological sections of these mucous plugs, expectorated at the end of the acute episode of the illness, permits demonstration of the characteristic hyphae within their substance – silver impregnation methods are very satisfactory for this purpose. It should be noted that the hyphae are usually scanty. Immunological tests have largely superseded histological investigation in the diagnosis of this condition, although the latter is a valuable confirmatory measure and in cases with equivocal immunological results, may be the only means of recognising the disease. Immunological tests include the demonstration of precipitating antibodies to aspergillus in the blood and skin testing with aspergillus antigen which causes both immediate and delayed reactions. Some atopic individuals develop allergic aspergillosis of the paranasal sinuses similar to that in the bronchi.[320]

Bronchocentric granulomatosis (see p. 463) is a further manifestation of allergic bronchopulmonary aspergillosis. So too is eosinophilic pneumonia (see p. 459). In this latter condition, radiological examination of the chest during an attack of asthma reveals scattered opacities which biopsy shows to be foci of eosinophil exudation in the alveoli, with similar infiltration of the bronchiolar and alveolar walls. Such foci appear to be transient but healing of them by fibrosis may contribute to the subpleural honeycombing and bronchiectasis mentioned above.

Eosinophilic bronchitis

Eosinophilic bronchitis is characterised by corticosteroid-responsive cough and eosinophilia but not the variable airflow obstruction, airway hyperresponsiveness or bronchial muscle hypertrophy seen in asthma.[321,322] The inflammatory changes are similar except that mast cells are reportedly better represented in the bronchial muscle in asthma whereas they are best seen in the epithelium in eosinophilic bronchitis.[323,324] Both conditions show thickening of the reticular basement membrane.[322] Exposure to certain occupational allergens has been reported to cause eosinophilic bronchitis.[325]

BRONCHIECTASIS

In literal terms, bronchiectasis means no more than dilatation of the bronchi and it is legitimately used in this restricted sense to describe, for instance, the distensive changes that are commonly encountered distal to a bronchial tumour. More often, however, it is understood to indicate a characteristic clinical condition that has bronchial dilatation and suppuration as its pathological basis. Although such dilatation is traditionally considered to be permanent, radiologists are familiar with early cases reverting to normal with treatment.

Clinical features

Prior to the advent of antibiotics and immunisation against the common exanthems of childhood, bronchiectasis usually followed a severe respiratory infection. It was characterised by a chronic cough productive of abundant foul sputum that originated in localised saccular lesions, which were typically located in the lung bases. This form of the disease is now uncommon and has been replaced by, or its reduction has uncovered, an insidious progressive type of bronchiectasis, which is usually more extensive and cylindrical. This is also characterised by persistent purulent sputum production but patients with this form of the disease often give a history of wheezy bronchitis in childhood and have chronic rhinosinusitis.[326] The cause of this form of bronchiectasis is not easily identified and it is often termed idiopathic.

Aetiology

The historic role of childhood infections and the more recent prominence of idiopathic cases of bronchiectasis have been touched upon above. A recent investigation failed to identify a cause in 53% of adult cases and while childhood pneumonia, pertussis and measles accounted for most of the remainder several other causes were identified.[327] Another study was confined to children and excluded cystic fibrosis: multiple causes were again identified, the commonest being previous pneumonia (30%) and immunodeficiency (21%) with 18% of cases being idiopathic.[328] Recognised causes of bronchiectasis are shown in Box 3.2.[329–334]

An unexplained association of bronchiectasis is that with lymphatic obstruction and pleural effusions in the yellow nail syndrome.[335–337] It is also uncertain whether an observed association between bronchiectasis and antitrypsin deficiency is attributable to impaired defence against infection or protease-antiprotease imbalance.[338]

Box 3.2 Recognised causes of bronchiectasis

Infection	Measles, pertussis, adenovirus
Obstruction	Tumour, foreign body,[329] enlarged hilar nodes, deficiency of bronchial cartilage[330]
Impaired local defence	Cystic fibrosis (p. 65), ciliary dyskinesia (p. 63)
Impaired systemic immunity	Hypogammaglobulinaemia
Autoimmunity	Ulcerative colitis,[331,332] rheumatoid disease,[333] Sjögren's syndrome, ankylosing spondylitis, relapsing polychondritis, systemic lupus erythematosus, Marfan's syndrome.
Allergy	Aspergillosis (p. 224)
Congenital	Mounier–Kuhn's syndrome (p. 63), Williams–Campbell syndrome (p. 62).

Bacteriology

In the earlier stages of bronchiectasis, *Haemophilus influenzae* is much the commonest bacterium to be recovered from the sputum. Later, a wide variety of different organisms becomes established in the infected air passages. As well as *H. influenzae*, *Pseudomonas aeruginosa* and *Streptococcus pneumoniae* are typically present. Sometimes, various spirochaetes and anaerobes are found and it is through the activities of these organisms that the smell of the sputum is so often offensive. Probably all these bacteria are secondary colonisers rather than the primary causative agent. *P. aeruginosa* is a particularly difficult bacterium to eradicate as it secretes an alginate coating that enables it to live on the mucosal surface ensconced within a biofilm where it is protected against phagocytosis and humoral or chemical attack.[339]

Structural changes[326,340]

The terms cylindrical and saccular (Fig. 3.32) alluded to above, are self-explanatory. Follicular is another descriptive term, one that refers to an abundance of lymphoid follicles in the walls of the affected bronchi (Fig. 3.33), which are usually dilated in a cylindrical fashion. The terms follicular and cylindrical are therefore often used interchangeably. Apart from the association of saccular disease with preceding infection and cylindrical/follicular with idiopathic cases, the distribution of the disease within the lungs also gives a clue to the aetiology. Thus, post-infective bronchiectasis tends to be basal, while in cystic fibrosis and ciliary dyskinesia the bronchiectasis is generalised but with upper lobe preponderance and in allergic bronchopulmonary aspergillosis hilar bronchi are particularly affected. Bronchiectasis confined to the right middle lobe is a major feature of the middle lobe syndrome (see p. 89).

The affected bronchi are most frequently those of the third or fourth order, the first orders being spared because their more substantial cartilage prevents dilatation. By counting the number of generations of the bronchial tree from the hilum it has been shown that subpleural bronchiectatic cavities of the cystic type usually represent dilated proximal airways.[341]

The dilated airways are usually filled with a purulent exudate and their mucosal surfaces are deeply congested. Many of the normal components of the bronchial wall are partly destroyed, particularly the fibromuscular and elastic framework. The bronchial walls may be thin, but more often they are thickened by fibrosis, inflammatory oedema and a heavy infiltrate of lymphocytes and plasma cells. Lymphoid follicles may be prominent (Fig. 3.33). The mucosa may show polypoid hyperplasia and there may be squamous metaplasia. Thin-walled pus-filled bronchiectatic cavities may be mistaken for abscesses. The essential difference is that the latter entail destruction of lung tissue and consequently several airways may communicate with one abscess cavity (Fig. 3.34).

The dilated airways often end blindly, the more distal airways being obliterated by fibrosis (Fig. 3.35). Unless inflation is maintained by collateral ventilation (see p. 88), the distal lung then shows absorption collapse. The adjacent lung may be substantially normal or, particularly in follicular bronchiectasis, there may be extensive chronic interstitial pneumonia. Organising pneumonia may be found in relation to the bronchiectasis but this is not an invariable association and when present it is generally difficult to tell whether it has preceded or followed the bronchiectasis.

As with many diseases of the lung, bronchiectasis derives its blood supply chiefly from the bronchial arteries, leading to the development of large bronchopulmonary anastomoses.[342]

The airway neuroendocrine cells are often increased in bronchiectasis, sometimes leading to the formation of multiple tumourlets (see p. 588).

Pathogenesis

The pathogenesis of bronchiectasis is complex and several mechanisms have been proposed. It is likely that some of these act in conjunction establishing a 'vicious cycle' of events.[343,344] This involves initial damage to the bronchial epithelium permitting heavy secondary bacterial colonisation which in turn inhibits ciliary clearance and so promotes continued infection and inflammation. Evidence for this comes from the isolation of a heat-labile bacterial product that attacks ciliated cells and slows ciliary motility. Other bacterial products capable of perpetuating obstructive lung disease include proteinases that stimulate the secretion of mucus into the airways.[87,345] *Pseudomonas aeruginosa* is a particularly troublesome coloniser because it survives within a biofilm on the mucosal surface where it is protected against cellular and humoral attack but is nevertheless responsible for strong antigen-antibody reactions that attract neutrophils.

An undoubtedly important pathogenetic mechanism is inflammatory weakening of the walls of the bronchi, this largely stemming from proteolytic enzymes and toxic oxygen radicals released by neutrophils. The normal tractive forces that operate on the airways in inspiration may then be enough to stretch their walls unduly. Distal to an obstruction, dammed up secretions exert distensive forces, while outside the inflamed airways, increased tractive forces are brought to bear on their

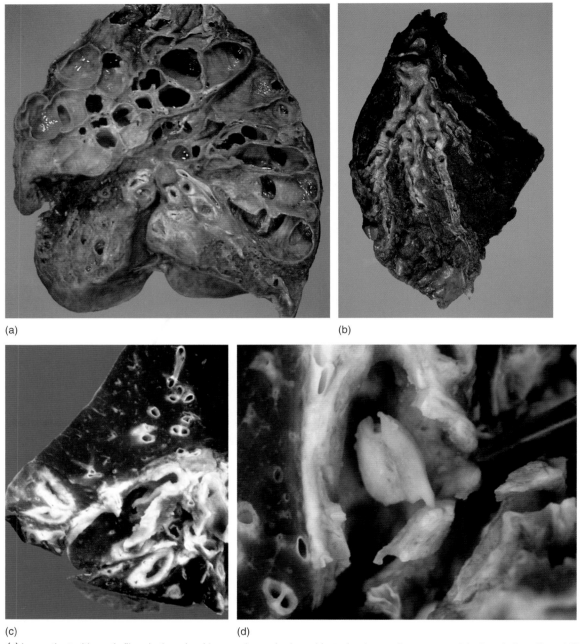

(a)

(b)

(c)

(d)

Figure 3.32 (a) In a patient with cystic fibrosis there is widespread saccular bronchiectasis, almost all segments of the lung being affected. The lung is largely replaced by saccules with thick fibrous walls, sometimes showing the remains of the mucosal folds of the bronchi from which they were derived. (b) In a patient with idiopathic bronchiectasis, the changes are cylindrical. (c) In a further patient with lower lobe bronchiectasis involving the basal segments, a peanut was identified obstructing the airway lumen (d).

weakened walls by processes such as absorption collapse and post-pneumonic fibrosis (Fig. 3.36). Coughing may be dismissed as a possible pathogenetic factor because it entails the sudden closure of airways rather than their distension.

Complications

Notable local complications of bronchiectasis include the development of lung abscess and empyema, the latter being the less common because adhesions often form early and obliterate the pleural cavity. Bronchiectasis is seldom widespread enough to cause severe pulmonary hypertension but cor pulmonale is common in the generalised form of the disease that develops in cystic fibrosis (see p. 65). Old bronchiectatic cavities may be colonised saprophytically by fungi (see p. 227). Distant complications of bronchiectasis include metastatic abscesses, particularly in the brain, generalised amyloidosis and immune-complex vasculitis.[346,347]

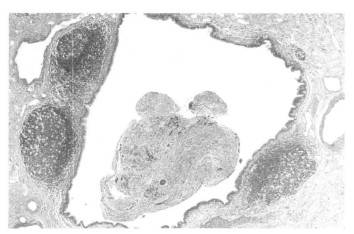

Figure 3.33 Follicular bronchiectasis. Lymphoid follicles are evident in the wall of this dilated airway, which also contains mucopus.

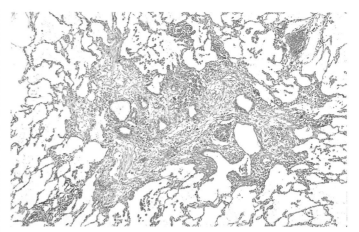

Figure 3.35 Bronchiectasis. Distal airways are obliterated by fibrosis.

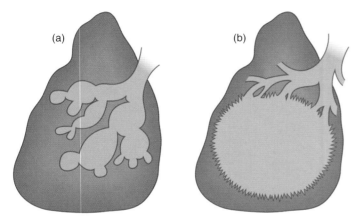

Figure 3.34 Diagrammatic representation of bronchiectasis (a) and lung abscess (b). In bronchiectasis each space represents a dilated airway that communicates only with its parent and daughter airways, in contrast to an abscess cavity brought about by 'cross-country' necrosis forming a newly formed cavity that communicates with several separate airways.

BRONCHOLITHIASIS

Occasionally the laboratory is presented with a stony hard object that a patient has coughed up. Such sputum 'liths' (or broncholiths) may derive from many conditions characterised by bronchopulmonary calcification. Analytical electron microscopy and X-ray diffraction may give information on their elemental composition and crystalline structure that can be helpful in identifying the underlying disease.[348] Generally the cause is a heavily calcified bronchial lymph node, representing healed tuberculosis, sarcoidosis or histoplasmosis, that presses upon and gradually ulcerates the wall of a bronchus until it is free in the lumen (Fig. 3.2b, p. 89). Bronchial obstruction or bleeding may necessitate intervention before the broncholith works itself free.[349] Broncholiths may also cause obstructive pneumonia, mediastinal abscess and broncho-oesophageal fistula.[350]

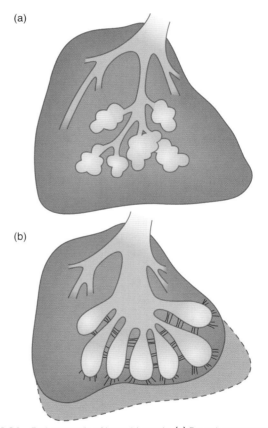

Figure 3.36 Pathogenesis of bronchiectasis. (a) Bronchopneumonia. (b) The peribronchiolar consolidation has healed by fibrosis, contracture of which exerts a tractive force on airway walls weakened by inflammation.

There is also a variety of conditions characterised by small free bodies, calcified or otherwise, that may be detected in sputum or lung tissue. These are mainly found free in the airspaces and are dealt with under 'alveolar filling defects', on pp. 321–323.

CHRONIC BRONCHIOLITIS

It is useful to separate those disorders in which bronchiolar disease is the predominant feature from those in which it represents a distal extension of what is primarily a bronchial disorder and those in which it represents a proximal extension of an essentially parenchymal condition (Box 3.3).[351] Attention here is confined to the disorders in which bronchiolar disease is the predominant feature. Bronchiolitis may be acute, chronic or acute on chronic. The more acute forms have been dealt with earlier in this chapter and this section is concerned with the chronic forms, particularly that associated with significant obstructive features. This important cause of obstructive airway disease is known as obliterative bronchiolitis (or bronchiolitis obliterans).

Chronic bronchiolitis has many causes (Box 3.4) and the appearances are often non-specific. However, some forms of chronic bronchiolitis have distinctive histological patterns and therefore their own special terms, such as follicular bronchioli-

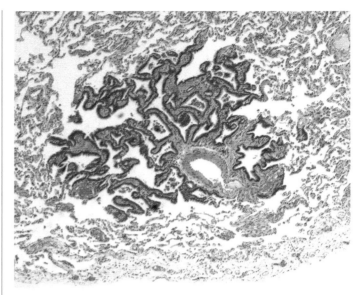

(a)

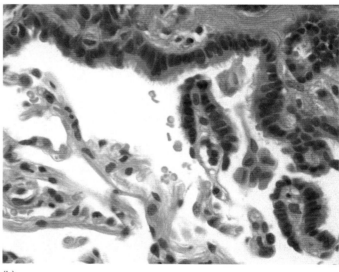

(b)

Figure 3.37 Lambertosis. (a) Centriacinar scarring with bronchiolar epithelial hyperplasia. (b) The hyperplastic cells are mainly of ciliated type. There is no atypia.

tis (see p. 642), respiratory bronchiolitis (see p. 313) and diffuse panbronchiolitis (see below). Not infrequently the inflammation is accompanied by fibrosis, which almost invariably narrows and in extreme cases obliterates the bronchiolar lumen.

Sometimes the inflammation and fibrosis extend out to affect the adjacent alveoli, resulting in a bronchiolocentric interstitial pneumonia and fibrosis, which on occasion is idiopathic.[352] There may also be a centrifugal extension of the bronchiolar epithelium through the canals of Lambert (see p. 5) so that alveolar septa thickened by fibrosis are lined by columnar epithelial cells, a process termed bronchiolisation of alveoli, peribronchiolar scarring with metaplasia, or Lambertosis (Fig. 3.37).

Obliterative bronchiolitis

Obliterative bronchiolitis represents repair of bronchiolar damage that may have been caused by a variety of harmful agents; it is not an aetiological entity. Furthermore, it may affect widely differing orders of bronchioles, sometimes extending proximally into small bronchi and in other patients extending distally to involve alveoli. For this reason, the functional effects are not uniform; whereas obliteration of proximal bronchioles causes a classic obstructive pattern of impairment, scarring in the region of respiratory bronchioles may cause restrictive functional impairment.

Pathological features

Not surprisingly for a disease of varied aetiology, the morphological changes also vary and to some extent the pathology can be correlated with the aetiology and the timing of the biopsy (Box 3.5). Two major pathological types of bronchiolar obstruction are recognised, one characterised by polypoid intraluminal buds of granulation tissue, which is sometimes termed chronic proliferative or intrusive, and a constrictive type. The polypoid type probably represents healing of damage inflicted at one point in time and the constrictive, type the result of chronic attrition from continuing damage. Thus, the polypoid form is typically seen after viral and chemical attack on the bronchioles and the constrictive type with auto-immune disease, lung transplant rejection and graft-versus-host disease. However, with time intraluminal buds of granulation tissue may be incorporated into the airway wall resulting in appearances indistinguishable from those of the constrictive type. Thus, the aetiological division is not rigid. Indeed, both patterns are the result of epithelial injury but whereas with intraluminal organisation the injury is brief, the constrictive form is the result of continuing remorseless attrition that prevents regeneration of the bronchiolar epithelium.

Organisation of luminal inflammatory exudates entails the development of granulation tissue polyps that protrude into and obstruct much of the bronchiolar lumen (Fig. 3.38). These are akin to the Masson bodies (bourgeons conjonctifs) of organising pneumonia, which may also be present. Alveoli beyond the bronchiolar obstruction may contain abundant foamy macrophages, the hallmark of endogenous lipid pneumonia, which should prompt the pathologist to examine the bronchioles.

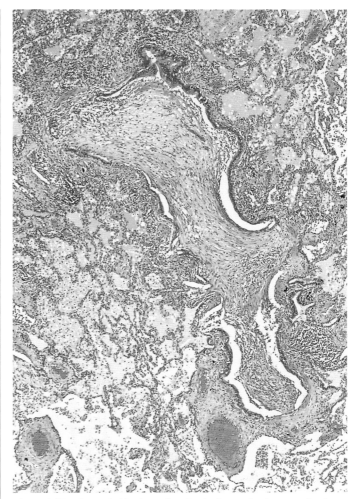

Figure 3.38 Bronchiolitis due to intraluminal organisation complicating viral infection. A granulation tissue polyp protrudes into and occupies most of the bronchiolar lumen.

In constrictive obliterative bronchiolitis[353,354] the mucosa is concentrically thickened by chronic inflammatory granulation tissue and in active cases the surface epithelium is destroyed (Figs 3.39 and 3.40). Sometimes the bronchiole is totally replaced by scar tissue. If this is the case, the presence of small fibrous scars next to pulmonary arteries that lack their usual accompanying airway should suggest that there has been bronchiolar destruction. Elastin stains may support this by showing a remnant of the bronchiolar wall in the scar, a feature that is often difficult to determine on haematoxylin and eosin staining (Fig. 3.41). The disease is often patchy and may affect only short segments of the bronchioles. More distal airways may therefore appear structurally normal although they are in fact non-functioning continuations of completely obliterated bronchioles, something that may only be appreciated by studying serial sections. As with the intraluminal pattern, peripheral accumulations of foamy alveolar macrophages may be found, suggesting that there is airway obstruction and that the bronchioles may therefore be worthy of more detailed examination (Fig. 3.42).

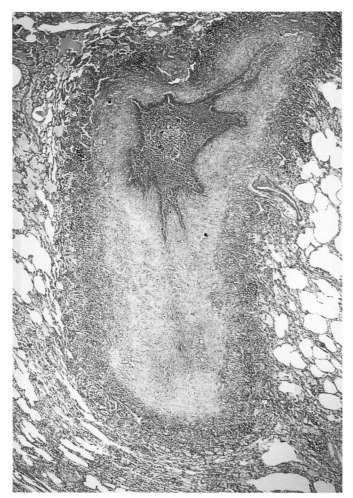

Figure 3.39 Active constrictive obliterative bronchiolitis in a rheumatoid patient. The epithelium is under constant attack and is consequently unable to regenerate, leading to the build-up of granulation tissue.

Bronchiolitis of specific aetiology

Post-infective bronchiolitis

Bronchiolar infection is a major cause of the intraluminal organising pattern of bronchiolitis. The organisation of an acute inflammatory exudate caused by viral infection complicated by bacterial superinfection results in the polypoid intraluminal buds of granulation tissue (Fig. 3.38).[113–115,355] The viruses responsible include adenoviruses, respiratory syncytial virus and influenza virus. Cases may also rarely progress to a constrictive pattern, particularly in children after an adenovirus infection.[355a,355b] These patterns of bronchiolar obstruction may also be found beyond chronic suppurative bronchial diseases, such as bronchiectasis or cystic fibrosis and in immunocompromised patients.[356,357]

Chemical causes of bronchiolitis

Intraluminal organisation is again seen in silo-fillers' disease (see also p. 358).[358–361] The pathogenesis is identical to that which follows infective bronchiolitis but here, the early damage is due

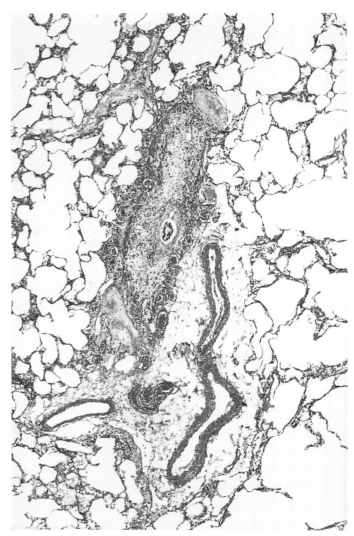

Figure 3.40 Constrictive obliterative bronchiolitis in a rheumatoid patient. Internal to the muscle coat there is a thick layer of pale staining granulation tissue which severely compromises the airway lumen. Surviving bronchiolar epithelium is reduced to a small central nidus. (Reproduced from Geddes DM et al, Progressive airway obliteration in adults and its association with rheumatoid disease. Quarterly Journal of Medicine 1977; 46:427–444,[353] by permission of Oxford University Press.)

to nitrogen dioxide fumes that the farmer entering a container of fermenting silage is liable to encounter. Further chemicals that cause intraluminal organisation include diacetyl, which is encountered by popcorn workers (see p. 357), thionyl chloride used in the manufacture of lithium batteries (see p. 359) and nylon flock (see p. 356). War gases such as phosgene and sulphur mustard and indeed many irritant gases or fumes that are inadvertently inhaled, are liable to cause a chemical bronchiolitis that may be complicated by intraluminal organisation.[362] When due to inhaled chemicals this is generally indistinguishable from that caused by infections but nylon flock workers' lung has a distinctive lymphoid pattern (see p. 356). Ingested chemicals may also cause constrictive obliterative bronchiolitis. *Sauropus androgynus* described on p. 377 is a notable example; here the damage is perpetuated by repeated

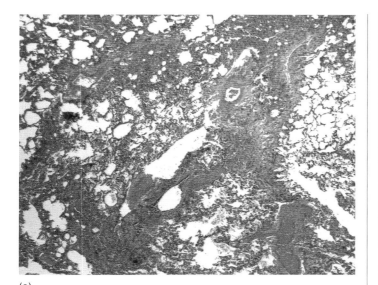

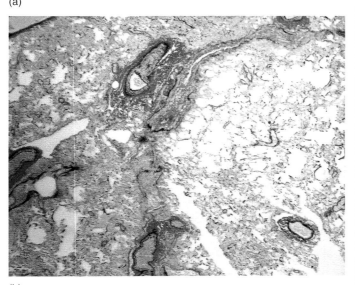

Figure 3.41 Constrictive obliterative bronchiolitis. At low power (a), there are no obvious abnormalities but an elastin stain (b) highlights the fact that what might have been interpreted as an interlobular septum is a bronchiole wholly obliterated by fibrosis. (Case provided by Dr G Taylor, Auckland, New Zealand.)

ingestion and the obliterative bronchiolitis is of the constrictive variety.

Bronchiolar involvement in the pneumoconioses

The clearance mechanisms of the alveolus result in inhaled dust being concentrated in and around the terminal bronchiole and its accompanying lymphoreticular aggregates (see Macklin's dust sumps, pp. 27, 331 and Figs 1.6, p. 5 and 7.1.12, p. 341). This is therefore a site where pneumoconiotic nodules are particularly likely to develop, with inevitable distortion of the bronchiole.[363–365] Peribronchiolar fibrosis is also an early feature of asbestosis,[364,366] probably because much inhaled fibrous dust initially penetrates no further than the bronchioles.

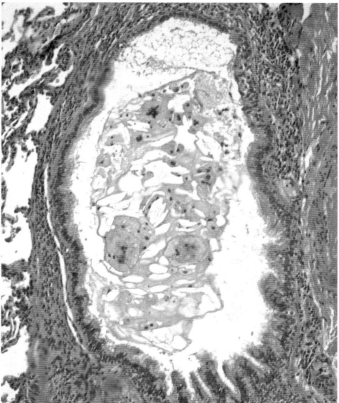

Figure 3.42 Chronic bronchiolitis. A small airway shows chronic inflammation and intralumenal accumulation of macrophages suggesting proximal obstruction.

Bronchiolar damage in cigarette smokers

Cigarette smokers are at risk of two forms of bronchiolitis. Respiratory bronchiolitis and chronic obstructive bronchiolitis (small airway disease). The former predominantly affects the peribronchiolar alveoli and is therefore dealt with in Chapter 6, while the latter is considered above under chronic obstructive lung disease (see p. 97).

Bronchiolitis and autoimmune disease

Obliterative bronchiolitis of constrictive pattern has been described in such autoimmune disorders as rheumatoid disease,[354] ankylosing spondylitis, systemic sclerosis[367] and paraneoplastic pemphigus[368] while milder but otherwise clinically similar 'cryptogenic' cases have subsequently been reported in patients free of connective tissue disease.[369] In some cases, the changes have been attributed to drugs used to treat the underlying disease but the bronchiolar narrowing is recorded in patients who have not been so treated and it is therefore more likely to be a manifestation of the connective tissue disease than an effect of the drug. Similarly, some cases of obliterative bronchiolitis attributed to chemical fumes have involved rheumatoid patients and may represent rheumatoid airway disease rather than chemical damage.[370]

The disease affects small bronchi as well as bronchioles and is rapidly progressive: affected patients may die of obstructive respiratory impairment within a year of the onset of dyspnoea. The association of lung and connective tissue disease is dealt with further in Chapter 10 (see p. 471).

Bronchiolitis and ulcerative colitis

Obstructive pulmonary disease has been recorded in several patients with ulcerative colitis.[371,372] Airways of any size from the trachea to small bronchioles may be affected and there is a spectrum of disease ranging from sclerosing tracheobronchitis to obliterative bronchiolitis of constrictive type, similar to that seen in autoimmune connective tissue disease (see above). As in rheumatoid disease, the airway narrowing is progressive and may prove fatal. The temporal relationship of disease activity in the bowel and airways is a weak one. Indeed, the pulmonary disease may appear years after the patient has undergone colectomy. The changes in the airways are comparable to those that develop in the biliary tree in sclerosing cholangitis, another extra-intestinal complication of ulcerative colitis. The association of lung and bowel disease is dealt with further in Chapter 10 (see p. 485).

Swyer–James or Macleod syndrome of unilateral hypertransradiancy of the lungs[373–376]

Vascular shutdown in response to hypoventilation underlies this syndrome. The term hypertransradiancy (or hyperlucency) denotes loss of the normal radiographic markings of the lungs. These largely represent the pulmonary blood vessels, which close down in response to poor ventilation. A whole lung, a lobe or a segment may be affected and the changes are occasionally bilateral. The condition is an acquired one with obliterative bronchiolitis as its pathological basis. The hypertransradiancy appears soon after an attack of bronchiolitis and is initially due to arterial constriction: later, structural obliteration of the vessels supervenes. Absorption collapse, which would render the lung radiopaque rather than radiolucent, is prevented by collateral ventilation (see p. 88).

DIFFUSE PANBRONCHIOLITIS

This disease is prevalent in Japan and to a lesser extent, Korea and China.[377–381] Only a few cases have been described in the West,[382–385] possibly because of genetic differences. The affected Asians show an increase in certain HLA antigens that do not occur in other races, notably B54 in Japan and A11 in Korea.[386,387] However, one Hispanic man with diffuse panbronchiolitis had visited Japan, raising the possibility that a transmissible agent was involved.[388] As diffuse panbronchiolitis mimics several other obstructive airway diseases,[379] it is possibly masquerading as one or other of these elsewhere and chest physicians and pathologists outside Japan need to be more conversant with the features of this disease.

Longstanding sinusitis generally precedes the onset of lower respiratory tract disease, which in its early stages is characterised by a productive cough and obstructive respiratory impairment. The term sinobronchial syndrome is often applied. Wheezing

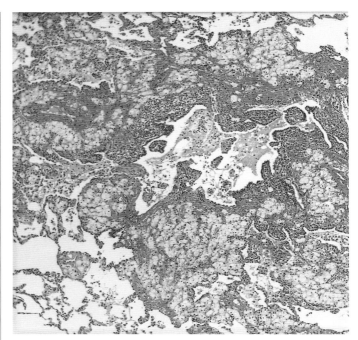

Figure 3.43 Diffuse panbronchiolitis. The bronchiolar wall is thickened by a chronic inflammatory infiltrate and the surrounding alveoli contain many foam cells, which also infiltrate the alveolar walls. (Reproduced by permission of Dr M Kitaichi, Kyoto, Japan.)

may lead to a resemblance to chronic bronchitis or asthma. In the advanced stages, large amounts of purulent sputum infected by *Haemophilus influenzae* and *Pseudomonas aeruginosa* are produced and dilatation of proximal bronchioles develops, so that the disease resembles bronchiectasis. Chest radiographs show bilateral small nodules and hyperinflation. Death from respiratory failure and cor pulmonale was formerly common but erythromycin treatment has improved the prognosis.[389,390]

The aetiology is unknown. The disease has a wide age distribution and does not appear to be related to smoking. Rheumatoid factor is often present but few patients with diffuse panbronchiolitis have overt rheumatoid disease. Cold haemagglutinins frequently develop after the disease is established but mycoplasma antibodies are generally lacking.

Pathological features

As its name suggests, diffuse panbronchiolitis is an inflammatory disease of small airways that is widely disseminated throughout both lungs, but it especially affects the bases. Radiologically, numerous small nodular opacities are scattered throughout both lung fields and, in late cases, bronchiolectasis may be demonstrated. At necropsy, numerous yellow nodules measuring up to 4 mm in diameter are seen on the cut surfaces of the lungs. Microscopically, the disease is characterised by thickening of the walls of membranous and respiratory bronchioles by granulation tissue and a lympho-plasmacytic infiltrate, prominence of the bronchus-associated lymphoid tissue, extension of the inflammatory changes into the peribronchiolar tissues and an obstructive lipid pneumonia (Fig. 3.43).[378,391]

The interstitial as well as airspace accumulation of foamy macrophages is a striking histological feature which corresponds to the fine yellow nodules observed grossly. However, the pathological changes are not specific. In a review of American archival material the changes of diffuse panbronchiolitis were identified in 20 (1.5%) of 1336 patients with a variety of other lung diseases, notably cystic fibrosis (6 of 19 patients), bronchiectasis and bronchiolitis.[392]

REFERENCES

Atelectasis and pulmonary collapse

1. MacPherson AMC, Zorab PA, Reid L. Collapse of the lung associated with primary tuberculosis: a review of 51 cases. Thorax 1960; 15:346–354.
2. Morrell NW, Roberts CM, Biggs T, Seed WA. Collateral ventilation and gas exchange during airway occlusion in the normal human lung. Am Rev Respir Dis 1993; 147:535–539.
3. Brock RC, Cann RJ, Dickinson JR. Tuberculous mediastinal lymphadenitis in childhood; secondary effects on the lungs. Guy Hosp Rep 1937; 87:295–317.
4. Inners CR, Terry PB, Traystman RJ, Menkes HA. Collateral ventilation and the middle lobe syndrome. Am Rev Respir Dis 1978; 118:305–310.
5. Kwon KY, Myers JL, Swensen SJ, Colby TV. Middle lobe syndrome: a clinicopathological study of 21 patients. Hum Pathol 1995; 26:302–307.

Obstruction of the upper airways

6. McNamara SG, Grunstein RR, Sullivan CE. Obstructive sleep apnoea. Thorax 1993; 48:754–764.
7. Ahmed Q, Chung-Park M, Tomashefski JF. Cardiopulmonary pathology in patients with sleep apnea/obesity hypoventilation syndrome. Hum Pathol 1997; 28:264–269.
8. Wilks W. Ossific deposits on the larynx, trachea and bronchi. Pathol Soc Lond 1857; 8:88.
9. Virchow R. Die Krankhaften geschwulste. Berlin: Hirschwald, 1863; 443.
10. Vilkman S, Keistinen T. Tracheobronchopathia osteochondroplastica – report of a young man with severe disease and retrospective review of 18 cases. Respiration 1995; 62:151–154.
11. Coetmeur D, Bovyn G, Leroux P, NielDuriez M. Tracheobronchopathia osteochondroplastica presenting at the time of a difficult intubation. Resp Med 1997; 91:496–498.
12. Primer G. Osteochondroplastica, tracheobronchopathy. Prax Klin Pneumol 1979; 33:1060–1063.
13. Pounder DJ, Pieterse AS. Tracheopathia osteoplastica: report of four cases. Pathology 1982; 14:429–433.
14. Aschoff L. Uber Tracheopathia osteoplastica. Verh Dtsch Pathol Ges 1910; 14:125–127.
15. Sakula A. Tracheobronchopathia osteoplastica. Its relationship to primary tracheobronchial amyloidosis. Thorax 1968; 23:105–110.
16. Alroy GG, Lichtig C, Kaftori JK. Tracheobronchopathia osteoplastica: end stage of primary lung amyloidosis? Chest 1972; 61:465–468.
17. Jones AW, Chatterji AN. Primary tracheobronchial amyloidosis with tracheobronchopathia osteoplastica. Br J Dis Chest 1977; 71:268–272.
18. Tajima K, Yamakawa M, Katagiri T, Sasaki H. Immunohistochemical detection of bone morphogenetic protein-2 and transforming growth factor beta-1 in tracheopathia osteochondroplastica. Virchows Archiv 1997; 431:359–363.
19. Baird RB, Macartney JN. Tracheopathia osteoplastica. Thorax 1966; 21:321–324.
20. Ashley DJB. Bony metaplasia in trachea and bronchi. J Pathol 1970; 102:186–188.
21. Pounder DJ, Pieterse AS. Tracheopathia osteoplastica: a study of the minimal lesion. J Pathol 1982; 138:235–239.
22. Pearson CM, Cline HM, Newcomer VD. Relapsing polychondritis. N Engl J Med 1960; 263:51–58.
23. Verity MA, Larson WM, Madden SC. Relapsing polychondritis. Report of two necropsied cases with histochemical investigation of the cartilage lesion. Am J Pathol 1963; 42:251–269.
24. Kaye RL, Sones DA. Relapsing polychondritis. Clinical and pathological features in 14 cases. Ann Intern Med 1964; 60:653–664.
25. Hughes RAC, Berry CL, Seifert M, Lessof MH. Relapsing polychondritis. Three cases in a clinico-pathological study and literature review. Q J Med 1972; 41:363–380.
26. McAdam LP, O'Hanlan MA, Bluestone R, Pearson CM. Relapsing polychondritis: prospective study of 23 patients and a review of the literature. Medicine (Baltimore) 1976; 55:193–215.
27. Valenzuela R, Cooperrider PA, Gogate P, Deodhar SD, Bergfeld WF. Relapsing polychondritis. Immunomicroscopic findings in cartilage of ear biopsy specimens. Hum Pathol 1980; 11:19–22.
28. Ebringer R, Rook G, Swana GT, Botazzo GF, Doniach D. Autoantibodies to cartilage and type II collagen in relapsing polychondritis and other rheumatic diseases. Ann Rheum Dis 1979; 40:473–479.
29. Higgenbottam T, Dixon J. Chondritis associated with fatal intramural bronchial fibrosis. Thorax 1979; 34:563–564.
30. Rogerson ME, Higgins EM, Godfrey RC. Tracheal stenosis due to relapsing polychondritis in rheumatoid arthritis. Thorax 1987; 42:905–906.
31. Sheffield E, Corrin B. Fatal bronchial stenosis due to isolated relapsing chondritis. Histopathology 1992; 20:442–443.
32. Ozbay B, Dilek FH, Yalcinkaya I, Gencer M. Relapsing polychondritis. Respiration 1998; 65:206–207.
33. Chan HS, Pang J. Relapsing polychondritis presenting with bronchorrhoea. Respir Med 1990; 84:341–343.
34. Somers G, Potvliege P. Relapsing polychondritis: relation to periarteritis nodosa. BMJ 1978; 2:603–604.
35. Neild GH, Cameron JS, Lessof MH, Ogg CS, Turner DR. Relapsing polychondritis with crescentic glomerulonephritis. BMJ 1978; 1:743–745.

Acute tracheobronchitis and bronchiolitis

36. Haggard HW. Action of irritant gases upon the respiratory tract. J Indust Hyg 1924; 5:390.
37. Holt LB. The pathology and immunology of *Bordetella pertussis* infection. J Med Microbiol 1972; 5:407–424.
38. Wenig BM. Necrotizing sialometaplasia of the larynx: a report of two cases and a review of the literature. Am J Clin Pathol 1995; 103:609–613.
39. Benizhak O, Benarieh Y. Necrotizing squamous metaplasia in herpetic tracheitis following prolonged intubation - a lesion similar to necrotizing sialometaplasia. Histopathology 1993; 22:265–269.
40. Littman CD. Necrotizing sialometaplasia (adenometaplasia) of the trachea. Histopathology 1993; 22:298–299.

Chronic bronchitis and emphysema (COPD, COLD)

41. Barnes PJ. Medical progress: Chronic obstructive pulmonary disease. N Engl J Med 2000; 343:269–280.
42. Dornhorst AC. Respiratory insufficiency. Lancet 1955; 1:1185–1187.
43. Fletcher CM, Hugh-Jones P, McNicol MW, Pride NB. The diagnosis of pulmonary emphysema in the presence of chronic bronchitis. Q J Med 1963; 32:33–49.
44. Mitchell RS, Stanford RE, Johnson JM, Silvers GW, Dart G, George MS. The morphologic features of the bronchi, bronchioles and alveoli in chronic airway obstruction: a clinicopathologic study. Am Rev Respir Dis 1976; 114:137–145.
45. Terminology, definitions and classification of chronic pulmonary emphysema and related conditions. A report of the conclusions of a CIBA guest symposium Thorax 1959; 14:286–299.
46. Medical Research Council. Definition and classification of chronic bronchitis for clinical and epidemiological purposes. Lancet 1965; 1:775–779.
47. Fletcher C, Peto R. The natural history of chronic airflow obstruction. BMJ 1977; 1:1645–1648.
48. Jamal K, Cooney TP, Fleetham JA, Thurlbeck WM. Chronic bronchitis. Correlation of morphologic findings to sputum production and flow rates. Am Rev Respir Dis 1984; 129:719–722.

49. Vestbo J, Prescott E, Lange P. Association of chronic mucus hypersecretion with FEV1 decline and chronic obstructive pulmonary disease morbidity. Copenhagen City Heart Study Group. Am J Respir Crit Care Med 1996; 153:1530–1535.

50. Doll R, Hill AB. Mortality in relation to smoking: ten years' observations of British doctors. BMJ 1964; 1:1399–1410.

51. Doll R, Hill AB. Mortality in relation to smoking: ten years' observations of British doctors. BMJ 1964; 1:1460–1467.

52. Anto JM, Vermeire P, Vestbo J, Sunyer J. Epidemiology of chronic obstructive pulmonary disease. Eur Resp J 2001; 17:982–994.

53. Amadori A, Zamarchi R, De Silvestro G, et al. Genetic control of the CD4/CD8 T-cell ratio in humans. Nat Med 1995; 1:1279–1283.

54. Hyashi M, Sornberger GC, Huber GL. A morphometric analysis of the male and female tracheal epithelium after experimental exposure to marijuana smoke. Lab Invest 1980; 42:65–69.

55. Oxman AD, Muir DCF, Shannon HS, Stock SR, Hnizdo E, Lange HJ. Occupational dust exposure and chronic obstructive pulmonary disease – a systematic overview of the evidence. Am Rev Respir Dis 1993; 148:38–48.

56. Rohde G, Wiethege A, Borg I, et al. Respiratory viruses in exacerbations of chronic obstructive pulmonary disease requiring hospitalisation: a case-control study. Thorax 2003; 58:37–42.

57. Oswald NC, Harold JT, Martin WJ. Clinical pattern of chronic bronchitis. Lancet 1953; 2:639–643.

58. Burrows B, Knudson RJ, Lebowitz MD. The relationship of childhood respiratory illness to adult obstructive airway disease. Am Rev Respir Dis 1977; 115:751–760.

59. Mannion PT. Sputum microbiology in a district general hospital. The role of *Branhamella catarrhalis*. Br J Dis Chest 1987; 81:391–396.

60. Murphy TF, Sethi S. Bacterial infection in chronic obstructive pulmonary disease. Am Rev Respir Dis 1992; 146:1067–1083.

61. Sethi S, Muscarella K, Evans N, Klingman KL, Grant BJB, Murphy TF. Airway inflammation and etiology of acute exacerbations of chronic bronchitis. Chest 2000; 118:1557–1565.

62. Sethi S, Evans N, Grant BJB, Murphy TF. New strains of bacteria and exacerbations of chronic obstructive pulmonary disease. N Engl J Med 2002; 347:465–471.

63. Blasi F, Damato S, Cosentini R, et al. *Chlamydia pneumoniae* and chronic bronchitis: association with severity and bacterial clearance following treatment. Thorax 2002; 57:672–676.

64. Stuart-Harris CH, Pownall M, Scothorne CM, Franks Z. The factor of infection in chronic bronchitis. Q J Med 1953; 22:121–132.

65. Seemungal T, HarperOwen R, Bhowmik A, et al. Respiratory viruses, symptoms and inflammatory markers in acute exacerbations and stable chronic obstructive pulmonary disease. Am J Respir Crit Care Med 2001; 164:1618–1623.

66. Davis AL. Bronchogenic carcinoma in chronic obstructive pulmonary disease. JAMA 1976; 235:621–622.

67. Skillrud DM, Offord KP, Miller RD. Higher risk of lung cancer in chronic obstructive pulmonary disease. A prospective, matched, controlled study. Ann Intern Med 1986; 105:503–507.

68. Restrepo GL, Heard BE. Air trapping in chronic bronchitis and emphysema. Am Rev Respir Dis 1964; 90:395–400.

69. Wright RR. Bronchial atrophy and collapse in chronic obstructive pulmonary emphysema. Am J Pathol 1960; 37:63–77.

70. Thurlbeck WM, Pun R, Toth J, Frazer RG. Bronchial cartilage in chronic obstructive lung disease. Am Rev Respir Dis 1974; 109:73–80.

71. Haraguchi M, Shimura S, Shirato K. Morphometric analysis of bronchial cartilage in chronic obstructive pulmonary disease and bronchial asthma. Am J Respir Crit Care Med 1999; 159:1005–1013.

72. Reid L. Measurement of the bronchial mucous gland layer: a diagnostic yardstick in chronic bronchitis. Thorax 1960; 15:132–141.

73. Douglas AN. Quantitative study of bronchial mucous gland enlargement. Thorax 1980; 35:198–201.

74. Restrepo G, Heard BE. The size of the bronchial glands in chronic bronchitis. J Pathol Bacteriol 1963; 85:305–310.

75. Matsuba K, Thurlbeck WM. A morphometric study of bronchial and bronchiolar walls in children. Am Rev Respir Dis 1972; 105:908.

76. Takizawa T, Thurlbeck WM. A comparative study of four methods of assessing the morphologic changes in chronic bronchitis. Am Rev Respir Dis 1971; 103:774–783.

77. Saetta M, Turato G, Baraldo S, et al. Goblet cell hyperplasia and epithelial inflammation in peripheral airways of smokers with both symptoms of chronic bronchitis and chronic airflow limitation. Am J Respir Crit Care Med 2000; 161:1016–1021.

78. Bowes D, Corrin B. Ultrastructural immunocytochemical localization of lysozyme in human bronchial glands. Thorax 1977; 32:163–170.

79. Bowes D, Clark AE, Corrin B. Ultrastructural localisation of lactoferrin and glycoprotein in human bronchial glands. Thorax 1981; 36:108–115.

80. Harbitz O, Jenssen AO, Smidsrod O. Lysozyme and lactoferrin in sputum from patients with chronic obstructive lung disease. Eur J Respir Dis 1984; 65:512–520.

81. Pilette C, Godding V, Kiss R, et al. Reduced epithelial expression of secretory component in small airways correlates with airflow obstruction in chronic obstructive pulmonary disease. Am J Respir Crit Care Med 2001; 163:185–194.

82. Kramps JA, Franken C, Meijer CJLM, Dijkman JH. Localization of low molecular weight protease inhibitor in serous secretory cells of the respiratory tract. J Histochem 1981; 29:712–719.

83. O'Shaughnessy TC, Ansari TW, Barnes NC, Jeffery PK. Inflammation in bronchial biopsies of subjects with chronic bronchitis: inverse relationship of CD8+ T lymphocytes with FEV1. Am J Respir Crit Care Med 1997; 155:852–7.

84. Saetta M, Turato G, Facchini FM, et al. Inflammatory cells in the bronchial glands of smokers with chronic bronchitis. Am J Respir Crit Care Med 1997; 156:1633–9.

85. Saetta M, Turato G, Baraldo S, et al. Goblet cell hyperplasia and epithelial inflammation in peripheral airways of smokers with both symptoms of chronic bronchitis and chronic airflow limitation. Am J Respir Crit Care Med 2000; 161:1016–2183.

86. Mullen JBM, Wright JL, Wiggs BR, Pare PD, Hogg JC. Reassessment of inflammation of airways in chronic bronchitis. BMJ 1985; 291:1235–1239.

87. Boat TF, Cheng PW, Klinger JD, Liedtke CM, Tandler B. Proteinases release mucin from airways goblet cells. London: Pitman; 1984:72–87.

88. Mullen JBM, Wright JL, Wiggs BR, Pare PD, Hogg JC. Structure of central airways in current smokers and ex-smokers with and without mucus hypersecretion: relationship to lung function. Thorax 1987; 42:843–848.

89. Hossain S, Heard BE. Hyperplasia of bronchial muscle in chronic bronchitis. J Pathol 1970; 101:171–184.

90. Dunnill MS, Massarella GR, Anderson JA. A comparison of the quantitative anatomy of the bronchi in normal subjects, in status asthmaticus, in chronic bronchitis and in emphysema. Thorax 1969; 24:176–179.

91. Takizawa T, Thurlbeck WM. Muscle and mucous gland size in the major bronchi of patients with chronic bronchitis, asthma and asthmatic bronchitis. Am Rev Respir Dis 1971; 104:331–336.

92. Barter CE, Campbell AH. Relationship of constitutional factors and cigarette smoking to decrease in 1-second forced expiratory volume. Am Rev Respir Dis 1976; 113:305–314.

93. Orie NGM, Sluiter HJ, deVries K, Tammeling GJ, Witkop J. The host factor in bronchitis. In: Orie NGM and Sluiter HJ. Assen, Royal van Gorcum. Bronchitis: an international symposium, Assen, Netherlands, 1961, pp. 44–59.

94. Bleecker ER. Similarities and differences in asthma and COPD: the Dutch hypothesis. Chest 2004; 126:93S–99S.

95. Burrows B, Halonen M, Barbee RA, Lebowitz MD. The relationship of serum immunoglobulin E to cigarette smoking. Am Rev Respir Dis 1981; 124:523–525.

96. Jeffery PK. Comparison of the structural and inflammatory features of COPD and asthma. Giles F. Filley Lecture. Chest 2000; 117:251S–260S.

97. Hogg JC, Macklem PT, Thurlbeck WM. Site and nature of airway obstruction in chronic obstructive lung disease. N Engl J Med 1968; 278:1355–1360.

98. Thurlbeck WM, Malaka D, Murphy K. Goblet cells in the peripheral airways in chronic bronchitis. Am Rev Respir Dis 1975; 112:65–69.

99. Lumsden AB, McLean A, Lamb D. Goblet and Clara cells of human distal airways: evidence for smoking induced changes in their numbers. Thorax 1984; 39:844–849.

100. Mooren HWD, Kramps JA, Franken C, Meijer CJLM, Dijkman JH. Localisation of a low molecular weight bronchial protease inhibitor in the peripheral human lung. Thorax 1983; 38:180–183.

101. Water D, Willems LNA, van Muijen GNP, et al. Ultrastructural localization of bronchial antileukoprotease in central and peripheral human airways by a gold-labelling technique using monoclonal antibodies. Am Rev Respir Dis 1986; 133:882–890.

102. Willems LNA, Kramps JA, Water de R, et al. Evaluation of antileukoprotease in surgical lung specimens. Eur J Respir Dis 1986; 69:242–247.

103. Willems LNA, Kramps JA, Stijnen T, Sterk PJ, Weening JJ, Dijkman JH. Antileukoprotease-containing bronchiolar cells. Relationship with morphologic disease of small airways and parenchyma. Am Rev Respir Dis 1989; 139:1244–1250.

104. Edwards C, Cayton R, Bryan R. Chronic transmural bronchiolitis – a non-specific lesion of small airways. J Clin Pathol 1992; 45:993–998.

105. Bosken CH, Wiggs BR, Pare PD, Hogg JC. Small airway dimensions in smokers with obstruction to airflow. Am Rev Respir Dis 1990; 142:563–570.

106. Leopold JG, Gough J. The centrilobular form of hypertrophic emphysema and its relation to chronic bronchitis. Thorax 1957; 12:219–235.

107. Esterly JR, Heard BE. Multiple bronchiolar stenoses in a patient with generalized airways obstruction. Thorax 1965; 20:309–316.

108. Duinker NW, Huizinga E. The 'flowers' in bronchography. Thorax 1962; 17:175.

109. Reid LM. Correlation of certain bronchographic abnormalities seen in chronic bronchitis with the pathological changes. Thorax 1955; 10:199–204.

110. Depierre A, Bignon J, Lebeau A, Brouet G. Quantitative study of parenchyma and small conductive airways in chronic nonspecific lung disease. Use of histologic stereology and bronchial casts. Chest 1972; 62:699–708.

111. Bignon J, Depierre A. L'obstruction des petites voies aeriennes: Essai de correlations structure-fonction. Poumon et Coeur 1975; 31:233–240.

112. Matsuba K, Thurlbeck WM. Disease of the small airways in chronic bronchitis. Am Rev Respir Dis 1973; 107:552–558.

113. McLean KH. The pathology of acute bronchiolitis – a study of its evolution. Part I: The exudative phase. Aust Ann Med 1956; 5:254–267.

114. McLean KH. The pathology of acute bronchiolitis – a study of its evolution. Part II: The repair phase. Aust Ann Med 1957; 6:29–43.

115. McLean KH. Bronchiolitis and chronic lung disease. Br J Tuberc Dis Chest 1958; 52:105–113.

116. Rosenblatt MB. Emphysema: historical perspective. Bull N Y Acad Med 1972; 48; 823–841.

117. Heard BE, Izukawa T. Pulmonary emphysema in fifty consecutive male necropsies in London. J Pathol Bacteriol 1964; 88:423–431.

118. Hasleton PS. Incidence of emphysema at necropsy as assessed by point-counting. Thorax 1972; 27:552–556.

119. Heard BE, Khatchatourov V, Otto H, Putov NV, Sobin L. The morphology of emphysema, chronic bronchitis and bronchiectasis: definition, nomenclature and classification. J Clin Pathol 1979; 32:882–892.

120. Snider GL, Kleinerman J, Thurlbeck WM, Bengali ZH. The definition of emphysema. Report of a National Heart, Lung and Blood Institute, Division of Lung Diseases Workshop. Am Rev Respir Dis 1985; 132:182–185.

121. American Thoracic Society. Standards for the diagnosis and care of patients with chronic obstructive pulmonary disease (COPD) and asthma. Am Rev Respir Dis 1987; 136:225–244.

122. Thurlbeck WM. Morphology of emphysema and emphysema-like conditions. In: Thurlbeck WM, ed. Chronic Airflow Obstruction in Lung Disease. Philadelphia: Saunders; 1976:98–99.

123. Cardoso WV, Sekhon HS, Hyde DM, Thurlbeck WM. Collagen and elastin in human pulmonary emphysema. Am Rev Respir Dis 1993; 147:975–981.

124. Lang MR, Fiaux GW, Gillooly M, Stewart JA, Hulmes DJS, Lamb D. Collagen content of alveolar wall tissue in emphysematous and non-emphysematous lungs. Thorax 1994; 49:319–326.

125. Wright JL. The importance of ultramicroscopic emphysema in cigarette smoke-induced lung disease. Lung 2001; 179:71–81.

126. Linhartova A anderson AE, Foraker AG. Affixment arrangements of peribronchiolar alveoli in normal and emphysematous lungs. Arch Pathol Lab Med 1982; 106:499–502.

127. Wright JL, Hobson JE, Wiggs B, Pare PD, Hogg JC. Airway inflammation and peribronchiolar attachments in the lungs of nonsmokers, current and ex-smokers. Lung 1988; 166:277–286.

128. Lamb D, McLean A, Gillooly M, Warren PM, Gould GA, Macnee W. Relation between distal airspace size, bronchiolar attachments and lung function. Thorax 1993; 48:1012–1017.

129. Dunnill MS. Quantitative methods in the study of pulmonary pathology. Thorax 1962; 17:320–328.

130. Dunnill MS. Evaluation of a simple method of sampling the lung for quantitative histological analysis. Thorax 1964; 19:443–448.

131. Gillooly M, Lamb D, Farrow ASJ. New automated technique for assessing emphysema on histological sections. J Clin Pathol 1991; 44:1007–1011.

132. McLean A, Warren PM, Gillooly M, Macnee W, Lamb D. Microscopic and macroscopic measurements of emphysema – relation to carbon monoxide gas transfer. Thorax 1992; 47:144–149.

133. Heard BE. A pathological study of emphysema of the lungs with chronic bronchitis. Thorax 1958; 13:136–149.

134. Gough J, Wentworth JE. Thin sections of entire organs mounted on paper. In: Harrison CV, ed. Recent Advances in Pathology. London: Churchill, 1960; 80–86.

135. Thurlbeck WM, Dunnill MS, Hartung W, Heard BE, Heppleston AG, Ryder RC. A comparison of three methods of measuring emphysema. Hum Pathol 1970; 1:215–226.

136. Gevenois PA, Zanen J, Demaertelaer V, Devuyst P, Dumortier P, Yernault JC. Macroscopic assessment of pulmonary emphysema by image analysis. J Clin Pathol 1995; 48:318–322.

137. Mark EJ, Muller KM, McChesney T, Donghwan S, Honig C, Mark MA. Placentoid bullous lesion of the lung. Hum Pathol 1995; 26:74–79.

138. Fidler ME, Koomen M, Sebek B, Greco MA, Rizk CC, Askin FB. Placental transmogrification of the lung, a histologic variant of giant bullous emphysema: clinicopathological study of three further cases. Am J Surg Pathol 1995; 19:563–570.

139. Hochholzer L, Moran CA, Koss MN. Pulmonary lipomatosis: A variant of placental transmogrification. Modern Pathol 1997; 10:846–849.

140. Cavazza A, Lantejoul S, Sartori G, et al. Placental transmogrification of the lung: clinicopathologic, immunohistochemical and molecular study of two cases, with particular emphasis on the interstitial clear cells. Hum Pathol, 2004; 35:517–521.

141. Xu RL, Murray M, Jagirdar J, Delgado Y, Melamed J. Placental transmogrification of the lung is a histologic pattern frequently associated with pulmonary fibrochondromatous hamartoma. Arch Pathol Lab Med 2004; 126:562–566.

142. Auerbach O, Hammond EC, Garfinkel L, Benante C. Relation of smoking and age to emphysema: whole-lung section study. N Engl J Med 1972; 286:853–857.

143. Heard BE. Further observations on the pathology of pulmonary emphysema in chronic bronchitics. Thorax 1959; 14:58–70.

144. Gross P, Pfitzer EA, Tolker E, Babyak MA, Kashak M. Experimental emphysema. Its production with papain in normal and silicotic rats. Arch Env Health 1965; 11:50–58.

145. Laurell CB, Eriksson S. The electrophoretic alpha 1-globulin pattern of serum in alpha 1-antitrypsin deficiency. Scand J Clin Lab Invest 1963; 15:132–140.

146. Mahadeva R, Lomas DA. Alpha1antitrypsin deficiency, cirrhosis and emphysema. Thorax 1998; 53:501–505.

147. Lieberman J, Gaidulis L, Garoutte B, Mittman C. Identification and characteristics of the common alpha1-antitrypsin phenotypes. Chest 1972; 62:557–564.

148. Cook PJL. Genetic aspects of the Pi system. Postgrad. Med J 1974; 50:362–364.

149. Demeo DL, Silverman EK. α1-Antitrypsin deficiency. 2: Genetic aspects of α1-antitrypsin deficiency: phenotypes and genetic modifiers of emphysema risk. Thorax 2004; 59:259–264.

150. deSerres FTJ. Worldwide racial and ethnic distribution of alpha1 antitrypsin deficiency. Summary of an analysis of published genetic epidemiologic surveys. Chest 2002; 122:1818–1829.

151. Larsson C, Eriksson S. Smoking and intermediate alpha 1-antitrypsin deficiency and lung function in middle-aged men. BMJ 1977; 2:922–925.

152. Silva GE, Sherrill DL, Guerra S, Barbee RA. A longitudinal study of alpha1antitrypsin phenotypes and decline in FEV1 in a community population. Chest 2003; 123:1435–1440.

153. Janoff A, Carp H, Lee DK, Drew RT. Cigarette smoke inhalation decreases alpha 1-antitrypsin activity in rat lung. Science 1979; 206:1313–1314.

154. Carp H, Janoff A. Inactivation of bronchial mucous proteinase inhibitor by cigarette smoke and phagocyte-derived oxidants. Exp Lung Res 1980; 1:225–237.

155. Blue M-L, Janoff A. Possible mechanisms of emphysema in cigarette smokers. Release of elastase from human polymorphonuclear leukocytes by cigarette smoke condensate in vitro. Am Rev Respir Dis 1978; 117:317–325.

156. Harris JO, Swenson EW, Johnson JE. Human alveolar macrophages: comparison of phagocytic ability, glucose utilization and ultrastructure in smokers and non-smokers. J Clin Invest 1970; 49:2086.

157. Cosio MG, Hale KA, Niewoehner DE. Morphologic and morphometric effects of prolonged cigarette smoking on the small airways. Am Rev Respir Dis 1980; 122:265–271.

158. Niewoehner DE, Kleinerman J, Rice DB. Pathologic changes in the peripheral airways of young cigarette smokers. N Engl J Med 1974; 291:755.

159. de Cremoux H, Hornebeck W, Jaurand MC, Bignon J, Robert L. Partial characterization of an elastase-like enzyme secreted by human and monkey alveolar macrophages. J Pathol 1978; 125:171–177.

160. Rodriguez RJ, White RR, Senior RM, Levine EA. Elastase release from human alveolar macrophages: comparison between smokers and non-smokers. Science 1977; 198:313.

161. Russell REK, Culpitt SV, DeMatos C, et al. Release and activity of matrix metalloproteinase-9 and tissue inhibitor of metalloproteinase-1 by alveolar macrophages from patients with chronic obstructive pulmonary disease. Am J Respir Cell Molec Biol 2002; 26:602–609.

162. Remy-Jardin M, Edme JL, Boulenguez C, Remy J, Mastora I, Sobaszek A. Longitudinal follow-up study of smoker's lung with thin-section CT in correlation with pulmonary function tests. Radiology 2002; 222:261–270.

163. Gadek JE, Hunninghake GW, Fells GA, Zimmerman RL, Keogh BA, Crystal RG. Evaluation of the protease-antiprotease theory of human destructive lung disease. Bull Eur Physiopath Resp 1980; 16:27S.

164. Retamales I, Elliott WM, Meshi B, et al. Amplification of inflammation in emphysema and its association with latent adenoviral infection. Am J Respir Crit Care Med 2001; 164:469–473.

165. Senior RM, Griffin GL, Mecham RP, Wrenn DS, Prasad KU, Urry DW. Val-Gly-Val-Ala-Pro-Gly, a repeating peptide in elastin, is chemotactic for fibroblasts and monocytes. J Cell Biol 1984; 99:870–874.

166. Morgan MD, Edwards CW, Morris J, Matthews HR. Origin and behaviour of emphysematous bullae. Thorax 1989; 44:533–538.

167. Davison AG, Newman Taylor AJ, Darbyshire J, et al. Cadmium fume inhalation and emphysema. Lancet 1988; 1:663–667.

168. Snider GL, Hayes JA, Kerthy AL, Lewis GP. Centrilobular emphysema experimentally induced by cadmium chloride aerosol. Am Rev Respir Dis 1973; 108:40–48.

169. Smith JP, Smith JC, McCall AJ. Chronic poisoning from cadmium fume. J Pathol Bacteriol 1960; 80:287–296.

170. Hirst RN, Perry HM, Cruz MG, Pierce JA. Elevated cadmium concentration in emphysematous lungs. Am Rev Respir Dis 1973; 108:30–39.

171. Leduc D, Defrancquen P, Jacobovitz D, Vandeweyer R, Lauwerys R, Devuyst P. Association of cadmium exposure with rapidly progressive emphysema in a smoker. Thorax 1993; 48:570–571.

172. Pierce JA, Hocott JB, Ebert RV. The collagen and elastin content of the lung in emphysema. Ann Intern Med 1961; 55:210–222.

173. Kuhn C, Yu S-Y, Chraplyvy M, Linder HE, Senior RM. The induction of emphysema with elastase. II. Changes in connective tissue. Lab Invest 1976; 34:372–380.

174. Levine S, Kaiser L, Leferovich J, Tikunov B. Cellular adaptations in the diaphragm in chronic obstructive pulmonary disease. N Engl J Med 1997; 337:1799–1806.

175. Stoller JK, Fallat R, Schluchter MD, et al. Augmentation therapy with alpha1antitrypsin – Patterns of use and adverse events. Chest 2003; 123:1425–1434.

176. Mannes GPM, Deboer WJ, Vanderbij W, Meuzelaar JJ. Lung transplantation and chronic obstructive pulmonary disease. Respir Med 1993; 87:61–65.

177. Davies L, Calverley PMA. Lung volume reduction surgery in chronic obstructive pulmonary disease. J Thorac Cardiovasc Surg 1995; 109:106–119.

178. Roue C, Mal H, Sleiman C, et al. Lung volume reduction in patients with severe diffuse emphysema: a retrospective study. Chest 1996; 110:28–34.

179. Brenner M, Yusen R, Mckenna R, et al. Lung volume reduction surgery for emphysema. Chest 1996; 110:205–218.

180. Maxfield RA. New and emerging minimally invasive techniques for lung volume reduction. Chest 2004; 125:777–783.

181. Hoppin FG. Theoretical basis for improvement following reduction pneumoplasty in emphysema. Am J Respir Crit Care Med 1997; 155:520–525.

182. Marchand E, Gayanramirez G, Deleyn P, Decramer M. Physiological basis of improvement after lung volume reduction surgery for severe emphysema: where are we? Eur Resp J 1999; 13:686–696.

183. Keller CA, Naunheim KS, Osterloh J, Espiritu J, McDonald JW, Ramos RR. Histopathologic diagnosis made in lung tissue resected from patients with severe emphysema undergoing lung volume reduction surgery. Chest 1997; 111:941–947.

184. Duarte IG, Gal AA, Mansour KA, Lee RB, Miller JI. Pathologic findings in lung volume reduction surgery. Chest 1998; 113:660–664.

185. Gillooly M, Lamb D. Airspace size in lungs of lifelong non-smokers – effect of age and sex. Thorax 1993; 48:39–43.

186. Heppleston AG. The pathogenesis of simple pneumokoniosis in coal workers. J Path Bact 1954; 67:51–63.

187. Lyons JP, Ryder RC, Seal RME, Wagner JC. Emphysema in smoking and non-smoking coalworkers with pneumoconiosis. Bull Europ Physiopath Resp 1981; 17:75–85.

188. Leigh J, Outhred KG, McKenzie HI, Glick M, Wiles AN. Quantified pathology of emphysema, pneumoconiosis and chronic bronchitis in coal workers. Br J Ind Med 1983; 40:258–263.

189. Ruckley VA, Gauld SJ, Chapman JS, et al. Emphysema and dust exposure in a group of coal workers. Am Rev Respir Dis 1984; 129:528–532.

190. Wright AW. The local effect of the injection of gases in the subcutaneous tissues. Am J Pathol 1930; 6:87–124.

191. Brewer LL, Moskowitz PS, Carrington CB, Bensch KG. Pneumatosis pulmonalis. A complication of the idiopathic respiratory distress syndrome. Am J Pathol 1979; 95; 171–190.

192. Wood BP, Anderson VM, Mauk JE, Merritt TA. Pulmonary lymphatic air: locating 'pulmonary interstitial emphysema' of the premature infant. Am J Roentgenol 1982; 138:809–814.

Plastic bronchitis

193. Sleigh Johnson R, Sita-Lumsden EG. Plastic bronchitis. Thorax 1960; 15:325–332.

194. Wiggins J, Sheffield E, Jeffery PK, Geddes DM, Corrin B. Bronchial casts associated with hilar lymphatic and pulmonary lymphoid abnormalities. Thorax 1989; 44:226–227.

195. Jett JR, Tazelaar HD, Keim LW, Ingrassia TS. Plastic bronchitis – an old disease revisited. Mayo Clin Proc 1991; 66:305–311.

196. Park JY, Elshami AA, Kang DS, Jung TH. Plastic bronchitis. Eur Respir J 1996; 9:612–614.

197. Castet D, Lavandier M, Asquier E, Beaulieu F, de Lajartre A-Y. Moules bronchiques associes a des anomalies lymphatiques pulmonaires. Rev Mal Resp 1998; 15:89–91.

198. Nair LG, Kurtz CP. Lymphangiomatosis presenting with bronchial cast formation. Thorax 1996; 51:765–766.

199. Sanerkin NG, Seal RME, Leopold JG. Plastic bronchitis, mucoid impaction of the bronchi and allergic broncho-pulmonary aspergillosis and their relationship to bronchial asthma. Ann Allergy 1966; 24:586–594.

200. Morgan AD, Bogomoletz W. Mucoid impaction of the bronchi in relation to asthma and plastic bronchitis. Thorax 1968; 23:356–369.

201. Seear M, Hui H, Magee F, Bohn D, Cutz E. Bronchial casts in children: a proposed classification based on nine cases and a review of the literature. Am J Respir Crit Care Med 1997; 155:364–370.

Bronchial asthma

202. Cookson WOC, Sharp P, Faux J, Hopkin JM. Linkage between immunoglobulin E responsiveness underlying asthma and rhinitis and chromosome 11q. Lancet 1989; i:1292–1295.

203. Cookson WOCM, Young RP, Sandford AJ, et al. Maternal inheritance of atopic IgE responsiveness on chromosome-11q. Lancet 1992; 340:381–384.

204. Sandford AJ, Shirakawa T, Moffatt MF, et al. Localisation of atopy and the beta subunit of the high affinity IgE receptor (FcER1) on chromosome 11q. Lancet 1993; 341:332–334.

205. Noguchi E, Shibasaki M, Arinami T, et al. Evidence for linkage between asthma/atopy in childhood and chromosome 5q31–q33 in a Japanese population. Am J Respir Crit Care Med 1997; 156:1390–1393.

206. Bentley AM, Durham SR, Kay AB. Comparison of the immunopathology of extrinsic, intrinsic and occupational asthma. J Investig Allergol Clin Immunol 1994; 4:222–232.

207. Humbert M, Durham SR, Ying S, et al. IL-4 and IL-5 mRNA and protein in bronchial biopsies from patients with atopic and nonatopic asthma: evidence against 'intrinsic' asthma being a distinct immunopathologic entity. Am J Respir Crit Care Med 1996; 154:1497–1504.

208. Lang DM, Polansky M. Patterns of asthma mortality in Philadelphia from 1969 to 1991. N Engl J Med 1994; 331:1542–1546.

209. Magnussen H, Jorres R, Nowak D. Effect of air pollution on the prevalence of asthma and allergy – lessons from the German reunification. Thorax 1993; 48:879–881.

210. Williamson IJ, Martin CJ, McGill G, Monie RDH, Fennerty AG. Damp housing and asthma: a case-control study. Thorax 1997; 52:229–234.

211. Romagnani S. Induction of Th1 and Th2 responses: a key role for the 'natural' immune response? Immunol Today 1992; 13:379–381.

212. Strachan DP. Hay fever, hygiene and household size. BMJ 1989; 299:1259–1260.

213. Strachan DP. Allergy and family size: a riddle worth solving. Clin Exp Allergy 1997; 27:235–236.

214. Shaheen SO, Aaby P, Hall AJ, et al. Measles and atopy in Guinea-Bissau. Lancet 1996; 347:1792–1796.

215. Matricardi PM, Rosmini F, Ferigno L, et al. Cross sectional retrospective study of prevalence of atopy among Italian military students with antibodies against hepatitis A virus. BMJ 1997; 314:999–1003.

216. Matricardi PM, Rosmini F, Panetta V, Ferrigno L, Bonini S. Hay fever and asthma in relation to markers of infection in the United States. J Allergy Clin Immunol 2002; 110:381–387.

217. Shirakawa T, Enomoto T, Shimazu S-I, Hopkin JM. The inverse association between tuberculin responses and atopic disorder. Science 1997; 275:77–79.

218. Holt PG. Immunoregulation of the allergic reaction in the respiratory tract. Eur Respir J 1996; 9;S85–S89.

219. Blauw GJ, Westendorp RGJ. Asthma deaths in New Zealand: whodunnit? Lancet 1995; 345; 2–3.

220. Lanes SF, Rodriguez LAG, Huerta C. Respiratory medications and risk of asthma death. Thorax 2002; 57:683–686.

221. Sheehan JK, Richardson PS, Fung DCK, Howard M, Thornton DJ. Analysis of respiratory mucus glycoproteins in asthma: a detailed study from a patient who died in status asthmaticus. Am J Respir Cell Mol Biol 1995; 13:748–756.

222. Weller PF, Bach DS, Austen KF. Biochemical characterization of human eosinophil Charcot–Leyden crystal protein (lysophospholipase). J Biol Chem 1984; 259:15100–15105.

223. Ackerman SJ, Swaminathan GJ, Leonidas DD, et al. Eosinophil proteins: structural biology of Charcot–Leyden crystal protein (Galectin-10): new insights into an old protein. Resp Med 2000; 94:1014–1016.

224. Wahl RW. Curschmann's spirals in pleural and peritoneal fluids. Report of 12 cases. Acta Cytol 1985; 30:147–151.

225. Naylor B. The shedding of the mucosa of the bronchial tree in asthma. Thorax 1962; 17:69–72.

226. Rigler L, Koucky R. Roentgen studies in pathological physiology of bronchial asthma. Am J Roentgenol 1938; 39:353–362.

227. Robin ED, Lewiston NJ. Unexpected, unexplained sudden death in young asthmatic subjects. Chest 1989; 96:790–793.

228. Kolbe J, Fergusson W, Garrett J. Rapid onset asthma: a severe but uncommon manifestation. Thorax 1998; 53:241–247.

229. Reid LM. The presence or absence of bronchial mucus in fatal asthma. J Allergy Clin Immunol 1987; 80:415–416.

230. Drislane FW, Samuels MA, Kozakewich H, Schoen FJ, Strunk RC. Myocardial contraction band lesions in patients with fatal asthma: possible neurocardiologic mechanisms. Am Rev Respir Dis 1987; 135:498–501.

231. Robin ED, McCauley R. Sudden cardiac death in bronchial asthma and inhaled beta-adrenergic agonists. Chest 1992; 101:1699–1702.

232. Ziment I. Infrequent cardiac deaths occur in bronchial asthma. Chest 1992; 101:1703–1705.

233. Bharati S, Lev M. Conduction system findings in sudden death in young adults with a history of bronchial asthma. J Am Coll Cardiol 1994; 23:741–746.

234. Pumphrey RSH, Roberts ISD. Postmortem findings after fatal anaphylactic reactions. J Clin Pathol 2000; 53:273–276.

235. Dunnill MS. The pathology of asthma, with special references to the changes in the bronchial mucosa. J Clin Pathol 1960; 13:27–33.

236. Kuwano K, Bosken CH, Pare PD, Bai TR, Wiggs BR, Hogg JC. Small airways dimensions in asthma and in chronic obstructive pulmonary disease. Am Rev Respir Dis 1993; 148:1220–1225.

237. Saetta M, Di Stefano A, Rosina C, Thiene G, Fabbri LM. Quantitative structural analysis of peripheral airways and arteries in sudden fatal asthma. Am Rev Respir Dis 1991; 143:138–143.

238. Roche WR. Inflammatory and structural changes in the small airways in bronchial asthma. Am J Respir Crit Care Med 1998; 157:S191–S194.

239. Balzar S, Wenzel SE, Chu HW. Transbronchial biopsy as a tool to evaluate small airways in asthma. Eur Resp J 2002; 20:254–259.

240. Kraft M, Martin RJ, Wilson S, Djukanovic R, Holgate ST. Lymphocyte and eosinophil influx into alveolar tissue in nocturnal asthma. Am J Respir Crit Care Med 1999; 159:228–234.

241. Sanerkin NG, Evans DMD. The sputum in bronchial asthma: pathognomonic patterns. J Pathol Bacteriol 1965; 89:535.

242. Sanerkin NG. Causes and consequences of airways obstruction in bronchial asthma. Ann Allergy 1970; 28:528.

243. Glynn AA, Michaels L. Bronchial biopsy in chronic bronchitis and asthma. Thorax 1960; 15:142–153.

244. Salvato G. Some histological changes in chronic bronchitis and asthma. Thorax 1968; 23:168–172.

245. Azzawi M, Bradley B, Jeffery PK, et al. Identification of activated T lymphocytes and eosinophils in bronchial biopsies in stable atopic asthma. Am Rev Respir Dis 1990; 142:1407–1413.

246. Azzawi M, Johnston PW, Majumdar S, Kay AB, Jeffery PK. Lymphocytes-T and activated eosinophils in airway mucosa in fatal asthma and cystic fibrosis. Am Rev Respir Dis 1992; 145:1477–1482.

247. Bentley AM, Menz G, Storz C, et al. Identification of lymphocytes-T, macrophages and activated eosinophils in the bronchial mucosa in intrinsic asthma – relationship to symptoms and bronchial responsiveness. Am Rev Respir Dis 1992; 146:500–506.

248. Jatakanon A, Uasuf C, Maziak W, Lim S, Chung KF, Barnes PJ. Neutrophilic inflammation in severe persistent asthma. Am J Respir Crit Care Med 1999; 160:1532–1539.

249. Douwes J, Gibson P, Pekkanen J, Pearce N. Non-eosinophilic asthma: importance and possible mechanisms. Thorax 2002; 57:643–648.

250. Sur S, Crotty TB, Kephart GM, et al. Sudden-onset fatal asthma – a distinct entity with few eosinophils and relatively more neutrophils in the airway submucosa. Am Rev Respir Dis 1993; 148:713–719.

251. Wenzel SE, Schwartz LB, Langmack EL, et al. Evidence that severe asthma can be divided pathologically into two inflammatory subtypes with distinct physiologic and clinical characteristics. Am J Respir Crit Care Med 1999; 160:1001–1008.

252. Ohashi Y, Motojima S, Fukuda T, Makino S. Airway hyperresponsiveness, increased intracellular spaces of bronchial epithelium and increased infiltration of eosinophils and lymphocytes in bronchial mucosa in asthma. Am Rev Respir Dis 1992; 145:1469–1476.

253. Carroll NG, Mutavdzic S, James AL. Increased mast cells and neutrophils in submucosal mucous glands and mucus plugging in patients with asthma. Thorax 2002; 57:677–682.

254. Djukanovic R, Wilson JW, Britten KM, et al. Quantitation of mast cells and eosinophils in the bronchial mucosa of symptomatic asthmatics and healthy control subjects using immunohistochemistry. Am Rev Respir Dis 1990; 142:863–871.

255. Montefort S, Roberts JA, Beasley R, Holgate ST, Roche WR. The site of disruption of the bronchial epithelium in asthmatic and non-asthmatic subjects. Thorax 1992; 47:499–503.

256. Montefort S, Roche WR, Holgate ST. Bronchial epithelial shedding in asthmatics and non-asthmatics. Respir Med 1993; 87 Supplement B:9–11.

257. Crepea SB, Harman JW. The pathology of bronchial asthma. I. Significance of membrane changes in asthmatic and non-allergic pulmonary disease. J Allergy 1955; 26:453–460.

258. Cutz E, Levison H, Cooper DM. Ultrastructure of airways in children with asthma. Histopathology 1978; 2:407–421.

259. Laitinen LA, Heino M, Laitinen A, Kava T, Haahtela T. Damage of the airway epithelium and bronchial reactivity in patients with asthma. Am Rev Respir Dis 1985; 131:599–606.

260. Barnes PJ. Asthma as an axon reflex. Lancet 1986; ii:242–245.

261. McCarter JH, Vazquez JJ. The bronchial basement membrane in asthma: immunohistochemical and ultrastructural observations. Arch Pathol 1966; 82:328–335.

262. Roche WR, Beasley R, Williams JH, Holgate ST. Subepithelial fibrosis in the bronchi of asthmatics. Lancet 1989; i:520–524.

263. Brewster CEP, Howarth PH, Djukanovic R, Wilson J, Holgate ST, Roche WR. Myofibroblasts and subepithelial fibrosis in bronchial asthma. Am J Respir Cell Mol Biol 1990; 3:507–511.

264. Laitinen A, Altraja A, Kampe M, Linden M, Virtanen I, Laitinen LA. Tenascin is increased in airway basement membrane of asthmatics and decreased by an inhaled steroid. Am J Respir Crit Care Med 1997; 156:951–958.

265. Watanabe K, Senju S, Toyoshima H, Yoshida M. Thickness of the basement membrane of bronchial epithelial cells in lung diseases as determined by transbronchial biopsy. Resp Med 1997; 91:406–410.

266. Heard BE, Hossain S. Hyperplasia of bronchial muscle in asthma. J Pathol 1972; 110:319–331.

267. Ebina M, Yaegashi H, Chiba R, Takahashi T, Motomiya M, Tanemura M. Hyperreactive site in the airway tree of asthmatic patients revealed by thickening of bronchial muscles: a morphometric study. Am Rev Respir Dis 1990; 141:1327–1332.

268. Ebina M, Takahashi T, Chiba T, Motomiya M. Cellular hypertrophy and hyperplasia of airway smooth muscles underlying bronchial asthma: a 3-D morphometric study. Am Rev Respir Dis 1993; 148:720–726.

269. Hossain S. Quantitative measurements of bronchial muscle in men with asthma. Am Rev Respir Dis 1973; 107:99–109.

270. Ollerenshaw S, Jarvis D, Woolcock A, Sullivan C, Scheiber T. Absence of immunoreactive vasoactive intestinal polypeptide in tissue from the lungs of patients with asthma. N Engl J Med 1989; 320:1244–1248.

271. Moreno RH, Hogg JC, Pare PD. Mechanics of airway narrowing in asthma. Am Rev Respir Dis 1986; 133:1171–1180.

272. James AL, Pare PD, Hogg JC. The mechanisms of airway narrowing in asthma. Am Rev Respir Dis 1989; 139:242–246.

273. Wiggs BR, Bosken C, Pare PD, James A, Hogg JC. A model of airway narrowing in asthma and in chronic obstructive pulmonary disease. Am Rev Respir Dis 1992; 145; 1251–1258.

274. Djukanovic R, Roche WR, Wilson JW, et al. Mucosal inflammation in asthma. Am Rev Respir Dis 1990; 142:434–457.

275. Barnes PJ. Cytokines as mediators of chronic asthma. Am J Respir Crit Care Med 1994; 150:S42–S49.

276. Gauvreau GM, Ronnen GM, Watson RM, OByrne PM. Exercise-induced bronchoconstriction does not cause eosinophilic airway inflammation or airway hyperresponsiveness in subjects with asthma. Am J Respir Crit Care Med 2000; 162:1302–1307.

277. Van Arsdel PP. Aspirin idiosyncrasy and tolerance. J Allergy Clin Immunol 1984; 73:431–434.

278. Ameisen JC, Capron A, Joseph M, et al. Aspirin-sensitive asthma: abnormal platelet response to drugs inducing asthmatic attacks; diagnostic and physiopathological implications. Int Arch Allergy Appl Immunol 1985; 78:438–448.

279. Lee TH. Mechanism of aspirin sensitivity. Am Rev Respir Dis 1992; 145:S34–S36.

280. Marks GB, Colquhoun JR, Girgis ST, et al. Thunderstorm outflows preceding epidemics of asthma during spring and summer. Thorax 2001; 56:468–471.

281. Dales RE, Cakmak S, Judek S, et al. The role of fungal spores in thunderstorm asthma. Chest 2003; 123:745–750.

282. Picado C. Barcelona's asthma epidemics: clinical aspects and intriguing findings. Thorax 1992; 47:197–200.

283. Barbee RA, Kaltenhorn W, Lebowitz MD, Burrows B. Longitudinal changes in allergen skin test reactivity in a community population sample. J Allergy Clin Immunol 1987; 79:16–24.

284. Burrows B, Martinez FD, Halonen M, Barbee RA, Cline MG. Association of asthma with serum IgE levels and skin-test reactivity to allergens. N Engl J Med 1989; 320:271–277.

285. Wagenaar SS, Peters A, Westermann CJJ, Oosting J. IgE bound to mast cells in bronchial mucosa and skin in atopic subjects. Respiration 1981; 41:258–263.

286. Carroll NG, Mutavdzic S, James AL. Distribution and degranulation of airway mast cells in normal and asthmatic subjects. Eur Resp J 2002; 19:879–885.

287. Guerzon GM, Pare PD, Michoud M-C, Hogg JC. The number and distribution of mast cells in monkey lungs. Am Rev Respir Dis 1979; 119:59–66.

288. Flint KC, Leung KBP, Hudspith BN, Brostoff J, Pearce FL, Johnson NM. Bronchoalveolar mast cells in extrinsic asthma: a mechanism for the initiation of antigen specific bronchoconstriction. BMJ 1985; 291:923–926.

289. Heard BE. Histochemical aspects of the staining of mast cells with particular reference to heterogeneity and quantification. In: Kay AB, ed. Asthma. Clinical Pharmacology and Therapeutic Progress. Oxford: Blackwell; 1986:286–294.

290. Heard BE, Dewar A, Nunn AJ, Kay AB. Heterogeneous ultrastructure of human bronchial mast cells: morphometric subdivision of cell types and evidence for a degranulation gradient. Am J Respir Cell Mol Biol 1990; 3:71–78.

291. Lane SJ, Lee TH. Mast cell effector mechanisms. J Allergy Clin Immunol 1996; 98:S67–S71.

292. Gleich GJ, Frigas E, Loegering DA, Wassom DL, Steinmuller D. Cytotoxic properties of the eosinophil major basic protein. J Immunol 1979; 123:2925–2927.

293. Frigas SE, Loegering DA, Gleich GJ. Cytotoxic effects of the guinea pig eosinophil major basic protein on tracheal epithelium. Lab Invest 1980; 42:35–43.

294. Peters MS, Rodriguez M, Gleich GJ. Localization of human eosinophil granule major basic protein, eosinophil cationic protein and eosinophil-derived neurotoxin by immunoelectron microscopy. Lab Invest 1986; 54:656–662.

295. Filley WV, Kephart GM, Holley KE, Gleich GJ. Identification by immunofluorescence of eosinophil granule major basic protein in lung tissues of patients with bronchial asthma. Lancet 1982; 2:11–15.

296. Corrigan CJ, Hartnell A, Kay AB. T-lymphocyte activation in acute severe asthma. Lancet 1988; i:1129–1132.

297. Wilson JW, Djukanovic R, Howarth PH, Holgate ST. Lymphocyte activation in bronchoalveolar lavage and peripheral blood in atopic asthma. Am Rev Respir Dis 1992; 145:958–960.

298. Ollerenshaw SL, Woolcock AJ. Characteristics of the inflammation in biopsies from large airways of subjects with asthma and subjects with chronic airflow limitation. Am Rev Respir Dis 1992; 145:922–927.

299. Poston RN, Chanez P, Lacoste JY, Litchfield T, Lee TH, Bousquet J. Immunohistochemical characterization of the cellular infiltration in asthmatic bronchi. Am Rev Respir Dis 1992; 145:918–921.

300. Bradley BL, Azzawi M, Jacobson M, et al. Eosinophils, T-lymphocytes, mast cells, neutrophils and macrophages in bronchial biopsy specimens from atopic subjects with asthma: comparison with biopsy specimens from atopic subjects without asthma and normal controls subjects and relationship to bronchial hyperresponsiveness. J Allergy Clin Immunol 1991; 88:661–674.

301. Bellini A, Vittori E, Marini M, Ackerman V, Mattoli S. Intraepithelial dendritic cells and selective activation of Th2-like lymphocytes in patients with atopic asthma. Chest 1993; 103:997–1005.

302. Robinson DS, Hamid Q, Ying S, et al. Predominant Th2-type bronchoalveolar lavage T lymphocyte population in atopic asthma. N Engl J Med 1992; 326:298–304.

303. Robinson DS, Durham SR, Kay AB. Cytokines in asthma. Thorax 1993; 48:845–853.

304. Hamid Q, Azzawi M, Ying S, et al. Expression of mRNA for interleukin-5 in mucosal bronchial biopsies from asthma. J Clin Invest 1991; 87:1541–1546.

305. Hamid Q, Azzawi M, Ying S, et al. Interleukin 5 mRNA in mucosal biopsies from asthmatic subjects. Int Arch Allergy Appl Immunol 1991; 94:169–170.

306. Ying S, Durham SR, Corrigan CJ, Hamid Q, Kay AB. Phenotype of cells expressing mRNA for TH2-type (interleukin 4 and interleukin 5) and TH1-type (interleukin 2 and interferon gamma) cytokines in bronchoalveolar lavage and bronchial biopsies from atopic asthmatic and normal control subjects. Am J Respir Cell Mol Biol 1995; 12:477–487.

307. Renauld JC. New insights into the role of cytokines in asthma. J Clin Pathol 2001; 54:577–589.

308. Kips JC. Cytokines in asthma. Eur Resp J 2001; 18:24S–33S:24S–33S.

309. Holt PG, Schon-Hegrad MA, Phillips MJ, McMenamin PG. Ia-positive dendritic cells form a tightly meshed network within the human airway epithelium. Clin Exp Allergy 1989; 19:597–601.

310. Holt PG, Schon-Hegrad MA, Oliver J, Holt BJ, McMenamin PG. A contiguous network of dendritic antigen-presenting cells within the respiratory epithelium. Int Arch Allergy Appl Immunol 1990; 91:155–159.

311. Holt PG. Regulation of antigen-presenting cell function(s) in lung and airway tissues. Eur Respir J 1993; 6:120–129.

312. Springall DR, Howarth PH, Counihan H, Djukanovic R, Holgate ST, Polak JM. Endothelin immunoreactivity of airway epithelium in asthmatic patients. Lancet 1991; 337:697–701.

313. Bardin PG, van Heerden BB, Joubert JR. Absence of pulmonary aspiration of sinus contents in patients with asthma and sinusitis. J Allergy Clin Immunol 1990; 86:82–88.

314. Wallaert B, Janin A, Lassalle P, et al. Airway-like inflammation of minor salivary gland in bronchial asthma. Am J Respir Crit Care Med 1994; 150:802–809.

315. Ayres JG, Miles JF. Oesophageal reflux and asthma. Eur Respir J 1996; 9:1073–1078.

316. Field SK, Sutherland LR. Does medical antireflux therapy improve asthma in asthmatics with gastroesophageal reflux? A critical review of the literature. Chest 1998; 114:275–283.

317. Wu DN, Tanifuji Y, Kobayashi H, et al. Effects of esophageal acid perfusion on airway hyperresponsiveness in patients with bronchial asthma. Chest 2000; 118:1553–1556.

318. Harding SM, Guzzo MR, Richter JE. The prevalence of gastroesophageal reflux in asthma patients without reflux symptoms. Am J Respir Crit Care Med 2000; 162:34–39.

319. Corris PA, Dark JH. Aetiology of asthma – lessons from lung transplantation. Lancet 1993; 341:1369–1371.

320. Katzenstein A, Sale SR, Greenberger PA. Allergic aspergillus sinusitis: a newly recognised form of sinusitis. J Allergy Clin Immunol 1983; 72:89–93.

321. Brightling CE, Ward R, Goh KL, Wardlaw AJ, Pavord ID. Eosinophilic bronchitis is an important cause of chronic cough. Am J Respir Crit Care Med 1999; 160:406–410.

322. Brightling CE, Symon FA, Birring SS, Bradding P, Wardlaw AJ, Pavord ID. Comparison of airway immunopathology of eosinophilic bronchitis and asthma. Thorax 2003; 58:528–532.

323. Brightling CE, Bradding P, Symon FA, Holgate ST, Wardlaw AJ, Pavord ID. Mast-cell infiltration of airway smooth muscle in asthma. N Engl J Med 2002; 346:1699–1705.

324. Birring SS, Berry M, Brightling CE, Pavord ID. Eosinophilic bronchitis: clinical features, management and pathogenesis. Am J Respir Med 2003; 2:169–173.

325. Quirce S. Eosinophilic bronchitis in the workplace. Curr Opin Allergy Clin Immunol 2004; 4:87–91.

Bronchiectasis

326. Whitwell F. A study of the pathology and pathogenesis of bronchiectasis. Thorax 1952; 7:213–239.

327. Pasteur MC, Helliwell SM, Houghton S, et al. An investigation into causative factors in patients with bronchiectasis. Am J Respir Crit Care Med 2000; 162:1277–1284.

328. Eastham KM, Fall AJ, Mitchell L, Spencer DA. The need to redefine non-cystic fibrosis bronchiectasis in childhood. Thorax 2004; 59:324–327.

329. Cleveland RH, Khaw KT, Mark EJ, Casavant DW, Kinane TB. An eight-year-old boy with bronchiectasis – Aspiration of a foreign body (plastic fastener) into the right lung, with bronchiectasis and pulmonary atelectasis and fibrosis. N Engl J Med 1998; 339:1144–1151.

330. Williams H, Campbell P. Generalized bronchiectasis associated with deficiency of cartilage in the bronchial tree. Arch Dis Child 1960; 35:182–191.

331. Butland RJA, Cole P, Citron KM, Turner-Warwick M. Chronic bronchial suppuration and inflammatory bowel disease. Q J Med 1981; 50:63–75.

332. Moles KW, Varghese G, Hayes JR. Pulmonary involvement in ulcerative colitis. Br J Dis Chest 1988; 82:79–83.

333. Takanami I, Imamuma T, Yamamoto Y, Yamamoto T, Kodaira S. Bronchiectasis complicating rheumatoid arthritis. Respir Med 1995; 89:453–454.

334. Cohen M, Sahn SA. Bronchiectasis in systemic diseases. Chest 1999; 116:1063–1074.

335. Emerson PA. Yellow nails, lymphoedema and pleural effusions. Thorax 1966; 21:247–253.

336. Beer DJ, Pereira W, Snider GL. Pleural effusion associated with primary lymphedema: a perspective on the yellow nail syndrome. Am Rev Respir Dis 1978; 117:595–599.

337. Parry CM, Powell RJ, Johnston IDA. Yellow nails, bronchiectasis and low circulating B-cells. Respir Med 1994; 88:475–476.

338. Rodriguez-Cintron W, Guntupalli K, Fraire AE. Bronchiectasis and homozygous (piZZ) α1-antitrypsin deficiency in a young man. Thorax 1995; 50:424–425.

339. Tsang KWT, Rutman A, Kanthakumar K, et al. Interaction of Pseudomonas aeruginosa with human respiratory mucosa in vitro. Eur Respir J 1994; 7:1746–1753.

340. Williams H, O'Reilly RN. Bronchiectasis in children: its multiple clinical and pathological aspects. Arch Dis Child 1959; 34:192–201.

341. Reid LM. Reduction in bronchial subdivision in bronchiectasis. Thorax 1950; 5:233–247.

342. Liebow AA, Hales MR, Lindskog GE. Enlargement of the bronchial arteries and their anastomoses with the pulmonary arteries in bronchiectasis. Am J Pathol 1949; 25:211–231.

343. Cole PJ. A new look at the pathogenesis and management of persistent bronchial sepsis: a 'vicious circle' hypothesis and its logical therapeutic consequences. In: Davies RJ, ed. Strategies for the Management of Chronic Bronchial Sepsis. Oxford: Medicine Publishing Foundation; 1984:1–20.

344. Cole P, Wilson R. Host-microbial interrelationships in respiratory infection. Chest 1989; 95:217S–221S.

345. Adler KB, Hendley DD, Davis GS. Bacteria associated with obstructive pulmonary disease elaborate extracellular products that stimulate mucus secretion by explants of guinea pig airways. Am J Pathol 1986; 125:501–514.

346. Hilton AM, Hasleton PS, Bradlow A, Leahy BC, Cooper KM, Moore M. Cutaneous vasculitis and immune complexes in severe bronchiectasis. Thorax 1984; 39:185–191.

347. Tanaka E, Tada K, Amitani R, Kuze F. Systemic hypersensitivity vasculitis associated with bronchiectasis. Chest 1992; 102:647–649.

Broncholithiasis

348. Pritzker KPH, Desai SD, Patterson MC, Cheng P-T. Calcite sputum lith. Characterization by analytic scanning electron microscopy and X-ray diffraction. Am J Clin Pathol 1981; 75:253–257.

349. Nollet AS, Vansteenkiste JF, Demedts MG. Broncholithiasis: rare but still present. Resp Med 1998; 92:963–965.

350. Studer SM, Heitmiller RF, Terry PB. Mediastinal abscess due to passage of a broncholith. Chest 2002; 121:296–297.

Chronic bronchiolitis

351. Ryu JH, Myers J, Swenson SJ. Bronchiolar disorders. Am J Respir Crit Care Med 2003; 168:1277–1292.

352. Yousem SA, Dacic S. Idiopathic bronchiolocentric interstitial pneumonia. Modern Pathol 2002; 15:1148–1153.

353. Gosink BB, Friedman PJ, Liebow AA. Bronchiolitis obliterans. Roentgenologic-pathologic correlation. Am J Roentgenol 1973; 117:816–832.

354. Geddes DM, Corrin B, Brewerton DA, Davies RJ, Turner-Warwick M. Progressive airway obliteration in adults and its association with rheumatoid disease. Q J Med 1977; 46:427–444.

355. Becroft DMO. Bronchiolitis obliterans, bronchiectasis and other sequelae of adenovirus type 21 infection in young children. J Clin Pathol 1971; 24:72–82.

335a. Mauad T, Dolhnikoff M. Histology of childhood bronchiolitis obliterans. Pediatr Pulmonol 2002; 33:466–474.

335b. Schlesinger C, Meyer CA, Veeraraghavan S, Koss MN. Constrictive (obliterative) bronchiolitis: diagnosis, etiology, and a critical review of the literature. Ann Diagn Pathol 1998; 2:321–334.

356. Diaz F, Collazos J, Martinez E, Mayo J. Bronchiolitis obliterans in a patient with HIV infection. Respir Med 1997; 91:171–173.

357. Ito M, Nakagawa A, Hirabayashi N, Asai J. Bronchiolitis obliterans in ataxia-telangiectasia. Virchows Arch 1997; 430:131–137.

358. Lowry T, Schuman LM. Silo-filler's disease – a syndrome caused by nitrogen dioxide. JAMA 1956; 162:153.

359. Ramirez-R J, Dowell AR. Silo-filler's disease: nitrogen dioxide-induced lung injury. Ann Intern Med 1971; 74:569–576.

360. Douglas WW, Hepper NGG, Colby TV. Silo filler's disease. Mayo Clin Proc 1989; 64:291–304.

361. Zwemer FL, Pratt DS, May JJ. Silo-filler's disease in New York state. Am Rev Respir Dis 1992; 146:650–653.

362. Dompeling E, Jobsis Q, Vandevijver NMA, Wesseling G, Hendriks H. Chronic bronchiolitis in a 5-yr-old child after exposure to sulphur mustard gas. Eur Resp J 2004; 23:343–346.

363. Churg A, Wright JL. Small-airway lesions in patients exposed to nonasbestos mineral dusts. Hum Pathol 1983; 14:688–693.

364. Churg A, Wright JL. Small airways disease and mineral dust exposure. Pathol Annu 1983; 18(Part 2):233–251.

365. Churg A, Wright JL, Wiggs B, Pare PD, Lazar N. Small airways disease and mineral dust exposure. Prevalence, structure and function. Am Rev Respir Dis 1985; 131:139–143.

366. Wright JL, Churg A. Morphology of small-airway lesions in patients with asbestos exposure. Hum Pathol 1984; 15:68–74.

367. Hakala M, Paakko P, Sutinen S, Huhti E, Koivisto O, Tarkka M. Association of bronchiolitis with connective tissue disorders. Ann Rheum Dis 1986; 45:656–662.

368. Hasegawa Y, Shimokata K, Ichiyama S, Saito H. Constrictive bronchiolitis obliterans and paraneoplastic pemphigus. Eur Resp J 1999; 13:934–937.

369. Turton CW, Williams G, Green M. Cryptogenic obliterative bronchiolitis in adults. Thorax 1981; 36:805–810.

370. Murphy DMF, Fairman RP, Lapp NL, Morgan WKC. Severe airway disease due to inhalation of fumes from cleansing agents. Chest 1976; 69:372–376.

371. Wilcox P, Miller R, Miller G, et al. Airway involvement in ulcerative colitis. Chest 1987; 92:18–21.

372. Rickli H, Fretz C, Hoffman M, Walser A, Knoblauch A. Severe inflammatory upper airway stenosis in ulcerative colitis. Eur Respir J 1994; 7:1899–1902.

373. Reid L, Simon G. Unilateral lung transradiancy. Thorax 1962; 17:230–239.

374. Reid L, Simon G, Zorab PA, Seidelin R. The development of unilateral hypertransradiancy of the lung. Br J Dis Chest 1967; 61:190–192.

375. Stokes D, Sigler A, Khouri NF, Talmo RC. Unilateral hyperlucent lung (Swyer–James syndrome) after severe Mycoplasma pneumoniae infection. Am Rev Respir Dis 1978; 117:145–152.

376. Avital A, Shulman DL, Bar-Yishay E, et al. Differential lung function in an infant with the Swyer–James syndrome. Thorax 1989; 44:298–302.

Diffuse panbronchiolitis

377. Homma H, Yamanaka A, Tanimoto S, et al. Diffuse panbronchiolitis. A disease of the transitional zone of the lung. Chest 1983; 83:63–69.

378. Maeda M, Saiki S, Yamanaka A. Serial section analysis of the lesions in diffuse panbronchiolitis. Acta Pathol Jpn 1987; 37:693–704.

379. Izumi T. Diffuse panbronchiolitis. Chest 1991; 100:596–597.

380. Kitaichi M, Nishimura K, Izumi T. Diffuse panbronchiolitis. In: Sharma OP, ed. Lung Disease in the Tropics. New York: Marcel Dekker; 1991:479–509.

381. Yaegashi H, Takahashi T. The site, severity and distribution of bronchiolar obstruction in lungs with chronic obstructive pulmonary disease – morphometry and computer-assisted three-dimensional reconstruction of airways. Arch Pathol Lab Med 1994; 118:975–983.

382. Poletti V, Patelli M, Poletti G, Bertanti T, Spiga L. Diffuse panbronchiolitis observed in an Italian. Chest 1990; 98:515–516.

383. Randhawa P, Hoagland MH, Yousem SA. Diffuse panbronchiolitis in North-America – report of three cases and review of the literature. Am J Surg Pathol 1991; 15:43–47.

384. Fitzgerald JE, King TE, Lynch DA, Tuder RM, Schwarz MI. Diffuse panbronchiolitis in the United States. Am J Respir Crit Care Med 1996; 154:497–503.

385. Fisher MS, Rush WL, Rosado-de-Christenson ML, et al. Diffuse panbronchiolitis: Histologic diagnosis in unsuspected cases involving North American residents of Asian descent. Arch Pathol Lab Med 1998; 122:156–160.

386. Sugiyama Y, Kudoh S, Maeda H, Suzaki H, Takaku F. Analysis of HLA antigens in patients with diffuse panbronchiolitis. Am Rev Respir Dis 1990; 141:1459–1462.

387. Park MH, Kim YW, IlYoon H, et al. Association of HLA class I antigens with diffuse panbronchiolitis in Korean patients. Am J Respir Crit Care Med 1999; 159:526–529.

388. Homer RJ, Khoo L, Smith GJW. Diffuse panbronchiolitis in a Hispanic man with travel history to Japan. Chest 1995; 107:1176–1178.

389. Ichikawa Y, Hotta M, Sumita S, Fujimoto K, Oizumi K. Reversible airway lesions in diffuse panbronchiolitis: detection by high-resolution computed tomography. Chest 1995; 107:120–125.

390. Koyama H, Geddes DM. Erythromycin and diffuse panbronchiolitis. Thorax 1997; 52:915–918.

391. Sato A, Chida K, Iwata M, Hayakawa H. Study of bronchus-associated lymphoid tissue in patients with diffuse panbronchiolitis. Am Rev Respir Dis 1992; 146:473–478.

392. Iwata M, Colby TV, Kitaichi M. Diffuse panbronchiolitis: diagnosis and distinction from various pulmonary diseases with centrilobular interstitial foam cell accumulations. Hum Pathol 1994; 25:357–363.

4

Alveolar injury and repair

DIFFUSE ALVEOLAR DAMAGE

Diffuse alveolar damage represents a non-specific pattern of acute alveolar injury caused by a variety of noxious agents.[1–4] It is the pathological basis of what was formerly known as the adult respiratory distress syndrome,[5–9] a term introduced to emphasise the similarity of the condition to that seen in premature babies suffering from the effects of deficient pulmonary surfactant production, i.e. the infantile respiratory distress syndrome (see p. 42). Following the recognition that the causes of the adult respiratory distress syndrome may also operate in children the adjective 'adult' has given way to 'acute' so that the clinical term now favoured is the acute respiratory distress syndrome. The causes of the infantile and acute respiratory distress syndromes differ markedly but all initiate a common cycle of events (Fig. 4.1) so that the end-result is the same regardless of the cause.

Clinical features

Because the pathological changes in the acute and infantile respiratory distress syndromes are similar, the clinical and radiological features also resemble each other closely. Both syndromes are characterised by refractory hypoxaemia and bilateral radiographic opacification in the absence of any evidence of an elevated left atrial pressure. These features indicate widespread alveolar collapse and exudation that cannot be attributed to left heart failure or other cause of pulmonary venous hypertension. There is generalised ground-glass opacification of the lungs, which is most pronounced in the dependent parts of the lungs. The opacification rapidly becomes increasingly dense until there is frank consolidation.[10] Air is then confined to the bronchi, which therefore appear black on plain radiographs where they stand out against the alveolar 'white-out' (so-called air bronchograms) (Fig. 4.2).[11] These changes may be modified if the cause of the lung injury is pulmonary rather than extrapulmonary.[11] The extent of radiological changes correlates with the clinical lung injury score.[12] Functional studies confirm that little of the lung substance is ventilated. There is initially mild pulmonary hypertension but the pulmonary arterial constriction responsible for this is

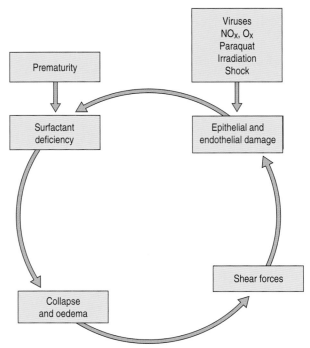

Figure 4.1 The cycle of events in the infantile and acute (formerly adult) respiratory distress syndromes. The infantile syndrome is initiated by the immature fetal lungs being unable to replenish spent surfactant whereas in the acute syndrome the cycle is initiated by a variety of causes that damage the delicate alveolar epithelium.

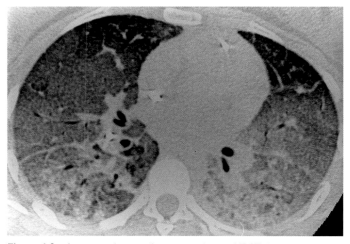

Figure 4.2 Acute respiratory distress syndrome. HRCT shows dense consolidation of both lungs, especially the dependent regions.

succeeded by vascular non-responsiveness so that the normal vasoconstrictor response to hypoxia is diminished. The consequent ventilation/perfusion mismatching aggravates the hypoxaemia. Other organs suffer both hypoxia and the effects of inflammatory mediators initiated by the pulmonary injury once these gain access to the general circulation. The end stages of the acute respiratory distress syndrome are therefore frequently associated with multiple organ failure.[13] Before this,

lung biopsy may be undertaken to exclude other causes of acute respiratory distress, notably pulmonary infection and haemorrhage,[14,15] in which case it is essential that some of the specimen goes to the microbiology department. The pathologist is also often asked to advise on the reversibility or otherwise of the process: diffuse alveolar damage is potentially reversible in its exudative phase whereas widespread fibrosis with loss of the lung architecture is not.

Pathological features

The pathological changes of diffuse alveolar damage can be divided into the overlapping phases of exudation, regeneration and repair.[16]

Exudative phase

To facilitate gas exchange, the alveolar wall is highly specialised in structure. Unfortunately this specialisation renders it susceptible to injury by a wide variety of agents. The principal cells of the air/blood barrier, the type I alveolar epithelial cell and the capillary endothelial cell, are exceptionally thin (see Figs 1.25, 1.26, p. 15) and this makes them particularly vulnerable to non-specific damage. Injury to these two cells underlies the development of diffuse alveolar damage. At an early stage of alveolar injury the type I epithelial cells show cytoplasmic blebbing, which is soon followed by necrosis resulting in denudation of the basement membrane (see Fig. 7.2.3, p. 376).[17,18] Similar blebbing is seen in the alveolar capillary endothelium but denudation of the endothelial basement membrane is seldom observed, probably because of differences in the ways epithelial and endothelial cells regenerate (see below). The consequences of this damage include the escape of fibrin-rich exudates into the interstitial and air spaces, loss of the surface-active alveolar lining film and pulmonary collapse.

The exudative phase lasts about 1 week, during which the lungs are heavy, often weighing over 1 kg each, dark and airless. The changes are often patchy, with the dorsal and basal regions being most severely affected (Fig. 4.3).[19–21] Slicing shows that they are wet, the cut surface exuding blood or heavily blood-stained watery fluid. Microscopically there is widespread collapse, intense congestion of the capillaries, interstitial oedema and distension of the lymphatics, a pattern that is sometimes known as congestive atelectasis (Fig. 4.4). Alternatively, there may be haemorrhagic oedema (Fig. 4.5). At the air/tissue interface, which in these collapsed lungs is at the respiratory bronchiole or alveolar duct level, respiratory movements compact a fibrin-rich exudate mixed with necrotic epithelial debris into a thin layer that covers an otherwise denuded epithelial basement membrane (Fig. 4.6), leading to the formation of hyaline membranes (Fig. 4.7):[1–3,22,23] these are identical to those that paediatric pathologists recognise as the hallmark of the infantile respiratory distress syndrome (compare Fig. 4.3 with Fig. 2.7, p. 42).

The congested alveolar capillaries sometimes contain increased numbers of platelets or neutrophil leukocytes. This

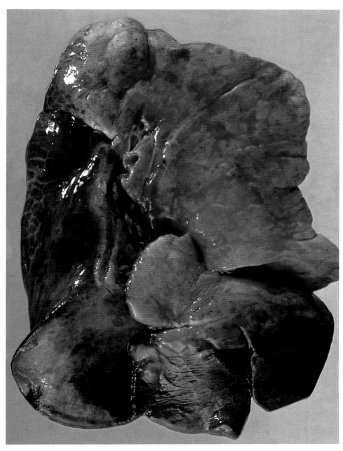

Figure 4.3 Shock lung. The lower lobe shows large irregular areas of collapse and congestion. (Reproduced with permission from Corrin B. Lung pathology in septic shock. Journal of Clinical Pathology 1980; 33:891–894.[19] With permission from BMJ Publishing Group.)

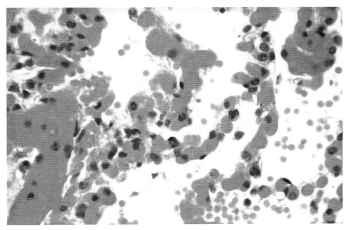

Figure 4.4 Congestive atelectasis in septic shock. There is severe capillary congestion and alveolar collapse.

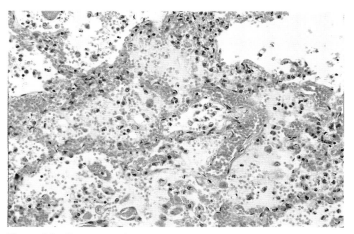

Figure 4.5 Haemorrhagic pulmonary oedema in septic shock. The alveolar capillaries are congested and the alveolar spaces are filled by oedema fluid in which there are free erythrocytes.

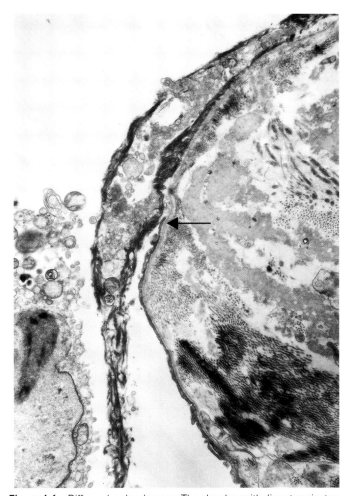

Figure 4.6 Diffuse alveolar damage. The alveolar epithelium terminates just above centre and from this point (arrow) upwards a mixture of electron-dense fibrin and cell debris (seen at the light microscopic level as a hyaline membrane) is closely applied to the denuded basement membrane. Part of a necrotic cell is seen within the alveolus. (Transmission electron micrograph provided by Miss A Dewar, Brompton, UK.)

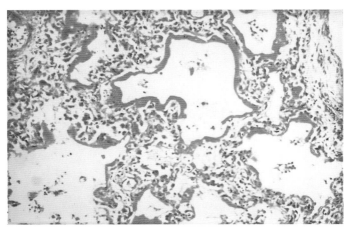

Figure 4.7 Diffuse alveolar damage, exudative phase. Hyaline membranes are a conspicuous feature. They often outline alveolar ducts. From a pregnant woman who suffered respiratory arrest due to angioneurotic oedema. She needed to be ventilated for 2 weeks before death and the oxygen concentration in the inspired air was constantly increased to prevent hypoxaemia, reaching 70% for the last 8 days of her life. (Material provided by Dr D Melcher, Brighton, UK.)

selective sequestration of formed blood elements in the microvasculature of the lungs is particularly noticeable in shock and is considered in more detail under that heading below (see p. 138).

Regenerative phase

As with any exudative process, healing may be by resolution, which involves fibrinolysis and permits the lungs to return to normal, or repair, which involves fibrosis and leaves the lungs permanently scarred. Resolution and repair are both accompanied by epithelial and endothelial regeneration.

The regenerative (or proliferative) phase becomes prominent 1–2 weeks after the initial injury. It involves proliferation of both epithelial and connective tissue cells. The stem cell concerned in epithelial regeneration is the type II alveolar epithelial cell.[24,25] These cells first proliferate and then differentiate into type I cells, thereby re-epithelialising the denuded basement membranes. The dividing type II cells. form a simple cuboidal epithelium (Fig. 4.8), or the alveoli may be lined by plump pleomorphic spindle cells that represent cell forms intermediate between types II and I epithelial cells (Figs 4.9, 4.10). Sometimes there is squamous metaplasia instead of orderly differentiation into type I cells and the unwary pathologist may mistake this for neoplasia.[26]

The regenerating epithelium usually grows beneath the exudates lining the denuded basement membrane, casting the hyaline membranes off into the airspace (Fig. 4.11), but it may grow over them so that they are incorporated into the interstitium (Figs 4.12, 4.13),[1–3] where their subsequent organisation contributes to the fibrosis.[23] The regenerating epithelial cells may also bridge the mouths of collapsed alveoli so that these air spaces never re-expand and there is permanent shrinkage of the lung, a process termed atelectatic induration (Figs 4.14, 4.15).[27–29]

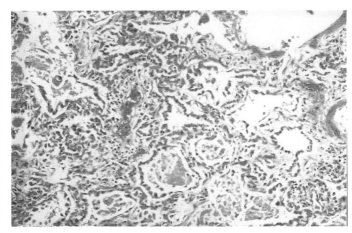

(a)

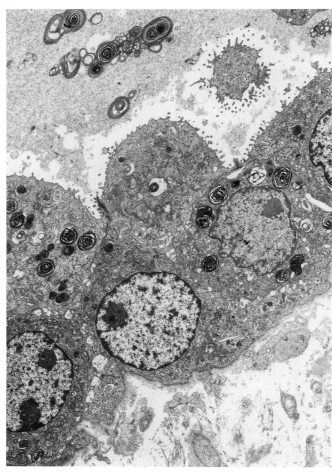

(b)

Figure 4.8 Diffuse alveolar damage, regenerative phase. (a) The alveoli have a simple cuboidal epithelial lining. (b) Electron microscopy shows that such cells represent hyperplastic type II pneumocytes, which form a continuous row rather than being scattered singly in the corners of the alveoli. They are readily recognisable by their surface microvilli and the osmiophilic lamellar secretory vacuoles of alveolar surfactant. (Material for (a) provided by Dr D Melcher, Brighton, UK; transmission electron micrograph provided by Mrs D Bowes, Midhurst, UK.)

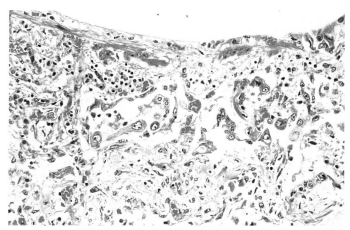

Figure 4.9 Diffuse alveolar damage, regenerative phase. Regenerating alveolar epithelial cells are atypical, consisting of plump, elongated forms that represent type II pneumocytes differentiating into type I.

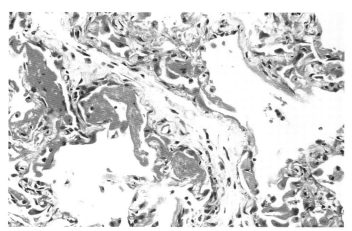

Figure 4.11 Diffuse alveolar damage, regenerative phase. The regenerating alveolar epithelium grows underneath the hyaline membranes, casting them off into the air space.

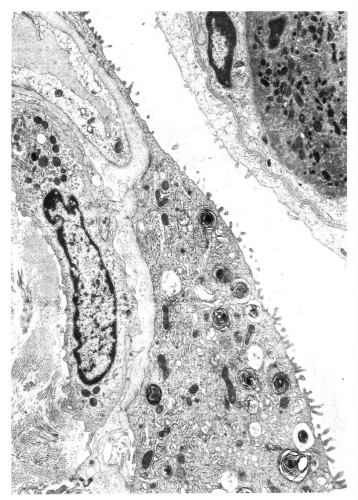

Figure 4.10 Diffuse alveolar damage, regenerative phase. An alveolar epithelial cell having the squamous form of a type I cell but the microvilli and lamellar vacuoles of a type II cell. Such intermediate cells are indicative of epithelial regeneration. (Transmission electron micrograph.)

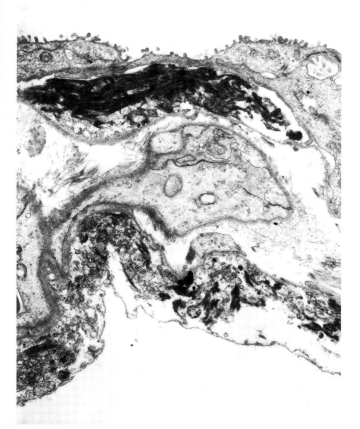

Figure 4.12 Diffuse alveolar damage, regenerative phase. The regenerating alveolar epithelium may also grow over the hyaline membranes to incorporate them into the alveolar wall. In this electron micrograph the hyaline membranes are largely represented by electron-dense fibrin, which is closely applied to previously denuded alveolar epithelial basement membrane and are in turn covered by regenerating epithelium laying down a new basement membrane. (Transmission electron micrograph provided by Miss A Dewar, Brompton, UK.)

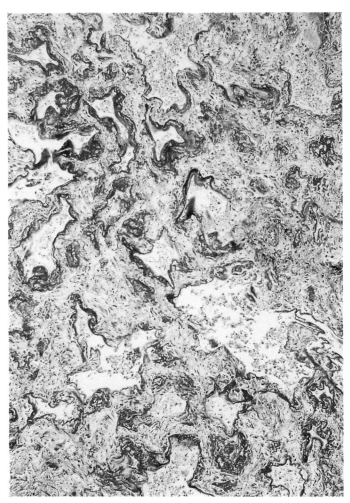

Figure 4.13 Diffuse alveolar damage, repair phase. Hyaline membranes, which are stained red, are in the process of being incorporated into the alveolar interstitium. (Martius scarlet blue stain).

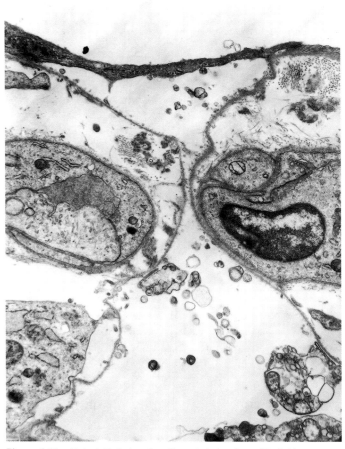

Figure 4.14 Atelectatic induration. Denuded alveolar epithelial basement membranes are closely apposed (centre). The regenerating alveolar epithelium (top) bridges the mouth of the alveolus, which consequently has little chance of ever re-expanding. (Transmission electron micrograph provided by Miss A Dewar, Brompton, UK.)

In contrast to the type I epithelial cells, which have no regenerative powers and are replaced by differentiation of proliferating type II cells, endothelial cells are replaced by lateral spread of their own kind. An effete endothelial cell is first undermined by its healthy neighbours and only cast off when these have completely covered the basement membrane.[30] Therefore, although segments of bare basement membrane have been described on the vascular side of the air/blood barrier,[31,32] they are not seen to the same extent as on the epithelial side. Nevertheless, thrombosis may complicate such endothelial damage[22,31] and subsequent organisation of such thrombi is probably responsible for some of the vascular remodelling that is seen in the repair phase of diffuse alveolar damage. This remodelling consists of fibrocellular intimal thickening that narrows the lumen of small vessels throughout the lung and can be visualised as decreased background filling on *post mortem* arteriograms.[33]

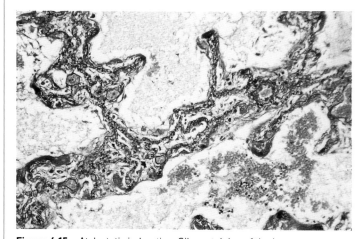

Figure 4.15 Atelectatic induration. Silver staining of the basement membranes shows that what appear to be thickened single alveolar walls represent the closely apposed walls of several collapsed alveoli.

Repair phase

If healing is by repair, interstitial connective tissue cells proliferate and as in any scarring, myofibroblasts are involved at an early stage.[34] While myofibroblast contracture is beneficial when it promotes early closure of an open wound, in the lungs it largely results in harmful distortion of the bronchioloalveolar architecture and shrinkage of the lungs.

Fibroblasts proliferate and lay down collagen, leading to the development of interstitial fibrosis.[35,36] Interactions between fibroblasts and the alveolar epithelium through gaps in the basement membrane have been described, suggesting that the regenerating epithelial cells play a role in the underlying process of fibrosis.[37–41] These cells also synthesise fibrogenic cytokines such as tumour necrosis factor-α, the secretion of which into the underlying connective tissue further promotes interstitial fibrosis.[42,43]

Fibroblasts also migrate into the alveolar exudates through defects in the epithelial basement membrane to lay down collagen within the hyaline membranes.[44,45] As epithelial cells grow over the newly formed connective tissue, a new basement membrane is formed, thereby incorporating the collagen into the interstitium,[45] a process known as fibrosis by accretion. Less frequently, the organised exudates retain a predominantly intra-alveolar position, resulting in loose buds of granulation tissue similar to those seen in organising pneumonia due to other causes (see Table 6.2.1, p. 308). However, here they are more widespread and there is more prominent type II cell hyperplasia, interstitial fibroblastic proliferation and interstitial inflammation (Fig. 4.16).

An increase in lung collagen can be detected in patients with the acute respiratory distress syndrome who survive longer than 14 days and this progressively increases with the duration of the disease.[46] The identification of pulmonary fibrosis on transbronchial biopsy is closely related to mortality,[47] while survivors may suffer from debilitating fibrotic lung disease. Fibrosis can be well established by 2 weeks, at which time the lungs may be contracted and firm with a fine sponge-like pattern on their cut surfaces, this representing bronchiolectasis and irregular microcystic distortion of the alveolar architecture (Figs 4.17, 4.18).[48–51] The changes are similar to the end-stage of any fibrotic process but are reached remarkably quickly (Fig. 4.18).[23] However, at this early stage the fibrosis differs from that seen in chronic fibrosis in being more cellular and less collagenous: extensive fibroblast proliferation is evident. With small air cysts alternating with solid areas of fibrosis and foci of squamous metaplasia there is a resemblance to the bronchopulmonary dysplasia seen in the late stages of the infantile respiratory distress syndrome.[49,50]

Causes

The causes of diffuse alveolar damage are quite diverse (Box 4.1). So too are the pathways by which the injurious agents reach the lungs. Some enter the lungs directly via the airways, e.g. oxygen in high concentrations, poisonous gases such as phosgene and metallic fumes such as those of beryllium, mercury and cadmium. Other agents responsible for diffuse

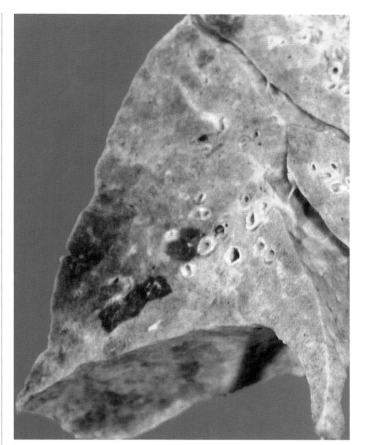

(a)

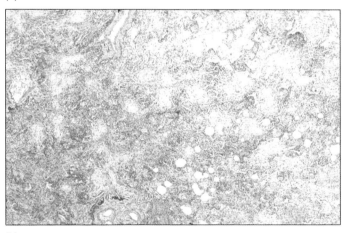

(b)

Figure 4.16 Diffuse alveolar damage, repair phase. (a) A lower lobe seen at autopsy shows diffuse fibrosis except for occasional lobules that show congestion. (b) Microscopy shows diffuse intra-alveolar organisation and marked interstitial inflammation.

alveolar damage penetrate the chest wall to damage the lungs (e.g. ionising radiation) and some reach the lungs via the bloodstream, having been ingested or injected (e.g. paraquat and cytotoxic chemotherapeutic agents). The bloodstream also conveys many of the endogenous factors that underlie the diffuse alveolar damage of shock.

Box 4.1 Causes of diffuse alveolar damage

Via the airways
   Infection – especially viral
   Inhaled smoke, fume and toxic gases, including oxygen in high
      concentrations
   Aspiration of gastric contents
Through the chest wall
   X-irradiation
Via the bloodstream
   Various mediators generated in shock (see below)
   Re-perfusion of ischaemic tissue
   Acute pancreatitis
   Cardiopulmonary bypass
   Transfusion of stored blood
   Fat embolism
   Paraquat ingestion
   Cytotoxic chemotherapeutic agents

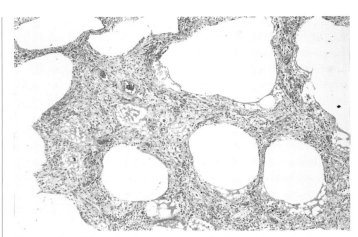

Figure 4.17 Diffuse alveolar damage, repair phase characterised by interstitial fibrosis.

Multiple causes may operate in one patient. For example, trauma may be combined with blood loss, fat embolism and sepsis, while therapeutic efforts to correct these may themselves be hazardous. The transfusion of stored blood is not without danger, while to prevent hypoxaemia, damaged lungs that require rest often have to be forcibly ventilated and subjected to injurious concentrations of oxygen, although it is known that this can only aggravate the injury to the lungs.[23] The damaged lung also appears to be unduly susceptible to infection,[52] partly because of impaired neutrophil migration into the air spaces.[53] It is therefore common in clinical practice for the lungs to be subjected to several injurious agents and since these all contribute to a non-specific pattern of disease it may be difficult for the pathologist to distinguish the initiating factor from the effects of treatment. Consideration of events in the intensive care unit is essential in these circumstances.

Many of the causes of diffuse alveolar damage listed in Box 4.1 are dealt with elsewhere, leaving only a few to be considered here. In numerical terms, septic shock is the most important.[54,54a]

Shock

Shock is a state of prolonged hypotension, generally attributable to trauma, hypovolaemia, cardiac failure, sepsis or anaphylaxis.[55,56] The hypotension leads to inadequate tissue perfusion and if this is not corrected, multiorgan failure is inevitable. At necropsy, the lungs are the organs most commonly affected.[57–59]

Severe pulmonary injury was well described in patients suffering from shock in the second world war[60] but it was not until the war in Vietnam that the importance of respiratory failure as a complication of shock was fully appreciated.[61,62] By this time, there had been major improvements in medical care. Casualties could be transported rapidly by helicopter to well-equipped field hospitals where intensive care with mechanical ventilatory support was available. Despite this, injured patients often developed fatal respiratory insufficiency, typically after an interval of between 48 and 72 hours. A number of terms graphically described this syndrome – 'shock lung', 'post-traumatic

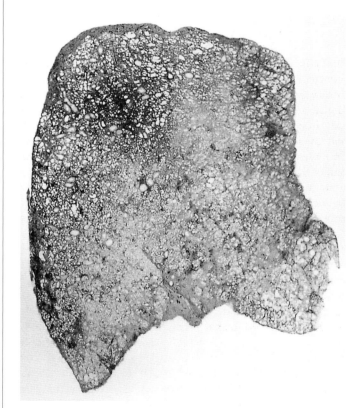

Figure 4.18 Suicidal ingestion of kerosene resulting in advanced pulmonary fibrosis and honeycombing within 2 weeks of the initial injury.

respiratory insufficiency', 'traumatic wet lung' and 'Da Nang lung'. Pathological examination showed congestive atelectasis or haemorrhagic oedema proceeding to fully developed diffuse alveolar damage, as described above.

Pathogenesis of 'shock lung'

The pathogenesis of 'shock lung' is complex and requires special consideration. In hypovolaemic and cardiogenic shock, compensatory mechanisms such as peripheral vasoconstriction initially maintain cerebral oxygenation, but if the underlying cause is untreated, there follows a state of decompensation characterised by vascular unresponsiveness: vasodilatation develops, the blood pressure plummets and there is widespread hypoxic cell death. Anaphylactic and septic shock are characterised from the outset by such vasodilatation, which is caused by a variety of mediators that are released from inflammatory and other cells. The identification of the same mediators in experimental hypovolaemia[63] suggests that the pathogenesis of shock may be similar regardless of the cause.

Lipopolysaccharide derived from the cell walls of Gram-negative bacteria is particularly important in the pathogenesis of septic shock.[64–68] Its many effects include the release of tumour necrosis factor from monocytes, macrophages and polymorphonuclear leukocytes,[65–67,69,70] the production of cytokines such as interleukin-1 and interferon-γ that act synergistically with tumour necrosis factor,[71] the widespread induction of nitric oxide synthesis[72–74] and the activation of both the coagulation and complement cascades.[75]

Tumour necrosis factor has been demonstrated on the luminal surface of pulmonary endothelium in endotoxin-induced shock.[76] It causes vascular smooth muscle to relax but this action is reduced if the endothelium is removed,[77] indicating that tumour necrosis factor-induced vasodilatation is partially dependent upon the integrity of the endothelium. A factor that causes vascular dilatation has been detected as coming from the vascular endothelium and acting on the medial muscle coat of the vessel. At first termed endothelium-derived relaxing factor, this factor is now known to be nitric oxide, a remarkably simple chemical that has long been recognised to be poisonous.[78] Fortunately, its half life in the vessel wall is very short, timed in seconds rather than minutes. The enzyme responsible for its production (from L-arginine) is nitric oxide synthase, which is found in endothelium and can be induced in the vascular medial smooth muscle. Both the constitutive and inducible forms of the enzyme are activated by bacterial lipopolysaccharide and it therefore seems likely that in septic shock bacterial products act directly on the vessel wall resulting in the production of excess amounts of nitric oxide. Even momentarily increased levels of nitric oxide might be expected to cause arterial dilatation and hence capillary congestion. It would appear that in septic shock, circulating bacterial products such as lipopolysaccharide cause vascular dilatation and possibly increased permeability by direct action on the blood vessels and indirectly through the induction of nitric oxide synthase and the release of the cytokines mentioned in the preceding paragraph.

Nitric oxide is a powerful vasodilator but it also mediates many other processes throughout the body. In host defence, nitric oxide plays a very different and more aggressive role. It enables macrophages to generate free oxygen radicals, the principal means by which these cells eliminate both bacteria and cancer cells, but which, if not inactivated, also damage healthy host cells.[79] Macrophages release much more nitric oxide than endothelial cells but as in the blood vessels, the amounts released are generally inactivated within seconds. However, overwhelming bacterial infections result in the release of very large amounts of nitric oxide and the overproduction of toxic oxygen radicals. Although the oxygen radicals are countered by the protective action of enzymes such as superoxide dismutase, their excessive release results in oxidation of lipids and protein sulphydryl groups and DNA damage.[80] Damaged cell membrane phospholipids release free arachidonic acid which in turn is degraded to produce leukotrienes, such as prostaglandins and thromboxane, that are capable of altering vessel calibre and permeability.

The direct vasodilatory action of nitric oxide and the toxic action of the free oxygen radicals that nitric oxide generates account for most of the pathological features of shock but there are other processes in the microvasculature of the lung that contribute to the pulmonary damage. The vascular engorgement characteristic of shock lung is occasionally accompanied by sequestration of neutrophil polymorphonuclear leukocytes in the pulmonary microvasculature (Figs 4.19, 4.20).[19,81–83] Acting through the complement cascade,[75,84,85] endotoxin activates these cells within the systemic circulation so that they lose their normal deformability and aggregate into microemboli, with the result that they cannot traverse the alveolar capillaries.[64,86,87] Their arrest there is promoted by activated endothelial intercellular adhesion molecules.[88–92] The unique position of the pulmonary capillaries in the circulation is probably responsible for the lungs being the organs most severely affected in shock.[57–59] Trapped in the alveolar capillaries, activated neutrophils damage the alveolar wall by producing reactive oxygen radicals and releasing enzymes such as elastase, collagenase and cathepsins that are able to degrade protein constituents of the wall.[93–99] Impairment of neutrophil migration into the air spaces has been referred to above.[53]

Patients suffering from the acute respiratory distress syndrome frequently have haematological evidence of disseminated intravascular coagulation[100] and it is then generally possible to demonstrate platelet and fibrin thrombi and increased numbers of megakaryocytes in their alveolar capillaries *post mortem* (Fig. 4.21).[19,101–105] It is uncertain whether intravascular coagulation initiates lung injury,[64,106,107] but histamine released from platelets is likely to increase vascular permeability while fibrin degradation products, which are elevated in patients with the respiratory distress syndrome,[108] are known to induce pulmonary oedema.[109] Larger pulmonary thrombi, formed *in situ* or embolic, are common in patients with the acute respiratory distress syndrome.[33] Any infarction they cause increases the risk of interstitial emphysema and pneumothorax, forms of barotrauma to which all patients on ventilators are prone.

Infection

In assessing the role of infection in causing diffuse alveolar damage, it is important to distinguish between primary infection of the lung and infection elsewhere in the body. Septic shock has been dealt with above and attention has been drawn to the increased risk of secondary lung infection when the lungs

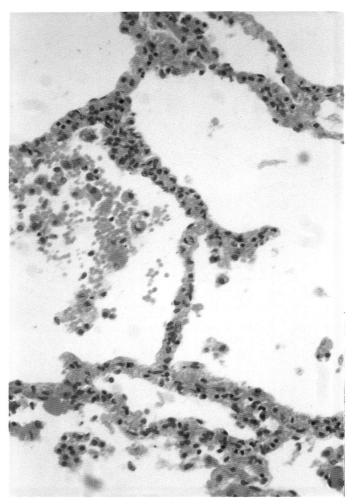

Figure 4.19 Shock lung. In shock, the alveolar walls are sometimes hypercellular due to the accumulation of neutrophil polymorphonuclear leukocytes.

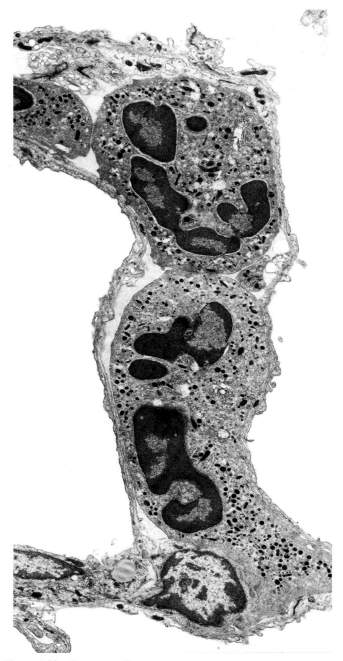

Figure 4.20 Shock lung. Electron microscopy shows that the neutrophil leukocytes are sequestered in the alveolar capillaries. (Transmission electron micrograph provided by Professor PK Jeffery, Brompton, UK.)

are damaged.[53] This section is confined to consideration of some primary pneumonias that can produce diffuse alveolar damage.

Diffuse alveolar damage is characteristic of mycoplasma and some viral infections, most recently the SARS-related coronavirus (see p. 157). Some patients with viral pneumonia succumb during the acute exudative phase and are found to have prominent hyaline membranes, while others suffer less severe damage, allowing regeneration and fibrosis. Indications that the disease is viral include the presence of specific inclusions, such as those seen in cytomegalovirus infection, or of syncytial giant cell formation, most typically seen in measles pneumonia.

The changes of diffuse alveolar damage are not typically seen in bacterial pneumonia, but may occur in fulminating infection with organisms such as *Streptococcus pyogenes* and *Haemophilus influenzae*. In pneumonic plague and anthrax pneumonia, the overwhelming alveolar damage leads to intensely haemorrhagic pulmonary oedema similar to that sometimes seen in shock (Fig. 4.5). Diffuse alveolar damage may also accompany miliary tuberculosis and pneumocystis pneumonia,

particularly the non-reactive forms seen in the severely immunocompromised.

Aspiration of gastric contents

Pulmonary aspiration of gastric contents is a frequent event in unconscious or semiconscious patients. If the aspirated material is infected it is likely to cause pneumonia and lung abscess but if sterile and highly acid the consequences are liable to be even more dire. Mendelson reported 66 instances of patients

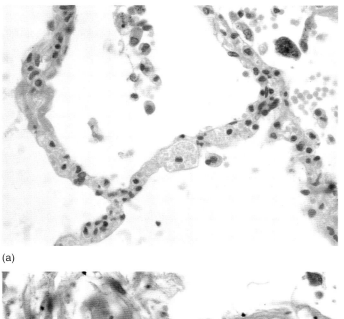

(a)

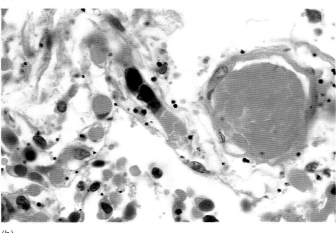

(b)

Figure 4.21   Shock lung. Shock is often accompanied by disseminated intravascular coagulation, consumptive coagulopathy and the release of megakaryocytes from the bone marrow. (a) Platelets fill the alveolar capillaries (b) Megakaryocytes released from the bone marrow are arrested in the pulmonary capillary bed, from whence they release their platelets. Occasional megakaryocytes may be observed in normal lung but they are more noticeable in shock. They are seen as clumps of basophilic nuclear material within alveolar capillaries (centre). To the right a blood vessel contains a globular hyaline microthrombus.

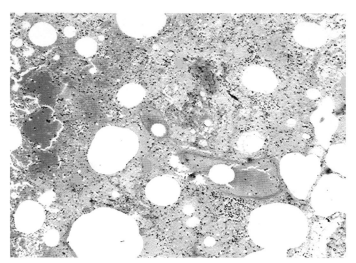

Figure 4.22   Aspiration of gastric acid (Mendelson's syndrome). There is haemorrhagic oedema and centrally the extravasated blood is discoloured due to the production of brown acid haematin.

aspirating stomach contents during obstetric anaesthesia. The aspiration of abundant solid material resulted in suffocation but Mendelson was more interested in the larger number of patients who aspirated liquids and developed pulmonary oedema. He suspected that the pH of the aspirate was important and confirmed this in experiments on rabbits.[110] The aspiration of gastric acid is now known as Mendelson's syndrome. The mortality is high,[111,112] reaching 94% in some series.[113]

Ultrastructural studies on experimental animals in which fluids of differing pH and osmolarity have been instilled into the lungs show features of alveolar injury that are most severe when the fluid is strongly acid, but even distilled water or saline is able to produce minor damage. Disturbance of the osmotic gradient across the alveolar capillary membrane may therefore be an additional factor. Damage occurs to both epithelial and endothelial cells, which separate from their basement membranes.[114] The most severe changes include necrosis and neutrophil exudation. Pulmonary haemorrhage is generally found and often shows a brown discolouration microscopically, due to the production of acid haematin (Fig. 4.22). The alveolar changes are accompanied by acute bronchitis and bronchiolitis with sloughing of the mucosa. The pathological changes after acid aspiration are best described as those of a severe chemical burn.

Preventive measures include the administration of antacids to postoperative or obstetric patients, but this often results in colonisation of the stomach by Gram-negative bacteria and a bacterial, rather than a chemical pneumonia if there is aspiration.[115]

Idiopathic acute alveolar injury

In some cases of rapidly progressive diffuse alveolar damage, no cause is evident. Such patients were described by Hamman and Rich,[116] since when these authors' names have often been applied eponymously to rapidly progressive idiopathic pulmonary fibrosis. Others favour the term acute interstitial pneumonia for such cases and emphasise the differences from chronic interstitial pneumonia,[117,118] but intermediate stages are encountered. Furthermore, some patients with idiopathic pulmonary fibrosis that for the most part has run a typically chronic course exhibit acute exacerbations. If they die of such a flare-up of their disease autopsy shows the hyaline membranes of diffuse alveolar damage superimposed upon long-established collagenous fibrosis, typically usual interstitial pneumonia (see Fig. 6.1.12, p. 275).[119]

Treatment of acute respiratory distress

The treatment of the acute respiratory distress syndrome is based upon minimising whichever of the several causes of the condition are deemed to be operating and achieving a balance between maintaining blood oxygen levels and affording the lungs the rest that all tissues recovering from injury require. Ideally, the lungs would be rested completely and the blood oxygenated in some other way. Indeed, this is attempted, with some success in the case of the infantile respiratory distress syndrome, by a process of extracorporeal oxygenation in which the systemic blood is diverted through an artificial lung in the form of a membrane oxygenator that sits alongside the patient. This is a major procedure that generally occupies a surgical operating theatre and is often attended by problems with haemostasis and if prolonged, haemolysis. The patient has therefore often been *in extremis* before such extracorporeal oxygenation has been undertaken, which possibly explains the poor initial results. The insertion of an intravenous oxygenator is less of a major procedure but this device only oxygenates a fraction of the blood leaving the heart.

More often, blood oxygenation is maintained by artificial ventilation, sacrificing the optimal conditions for lung recovery in favour of supplying other organs, particularly the brain, with oxygen. Simply allowing the mechanically expanded lung to collapse again several times a minute would establish a pattern of respiration quite unlike the normal and one that would incur further damage to the lungs. With a normal lining of surfactant, the alveoli do not collapse completely at the end of expiration. A considerable residual volume of gas is normally retained but when the alveolar lining film is lost, as in diffuse alveolar damage, the alveoli collapse completely at the end of each respiratory excursion and the inspiratory phase commences from a much lower baseline. It is now recognised that this exerts considerable mechanical stress upon the delicate alveolar epithelial lining,[120] the integrity of which is already severely compromised in the acute respiratory distress syndrome. These purely mechanical forces result in the generation and release of a variety of injurious cytokines (e.g. tumour necrosis factor-α) and reactive oxygen species without necessarily involving any inflammation.[121,122] To minimise this, positive pressure is usually maintained throughout the respiratory cycle, a form of ventilation termed positive end-expiratory pressure, frequently referred to as PEEP.[123] If, despite PEEP, hypoxaemia approaches dangerous levels the intensivist has no choice but to raise the concentration of oxygen in the inspired air although it is recognised that high concentrations of oxygen are themselves injurious to the lung. With severe lung damage, a situation is often reached where to prevent cerebral injury increasingly higher concentrations of oxygen have to be employed. The initial damage to the lung is then compounded by a combination of mechanical and chemical injury, resulting in an aggravated form of diffuse alveolar damage to which the term 'respirator lung' is often applied.

A promising technique that is now under experimental investigation follows the recent recognition that bone marrow stem cells are capable of differentiating into a variety of mature cell types, including those that constitute the alveolar epithelium. The successful application of this would hasten the healing process and minimise the likelihood of the damaged lung developing irreversible fibrosis.

Prognosis

Diffuse alveolar damage carries a high mortality rate, around 50% overall but reaching 94% when aspiration of gastric acid is the cause.[113] The diffuse alveolar damage associated with septic shock also carries a particularly high mortality rate. Survivors may appear to recover completely but tests of lung function often show that they have a mild restrictive or diffusion defect.[124,125]

PULMONARY FIBROSIS

The healing of diffuse alveolar damage by fibrosis leads to a consideration of pulmonary fibrosis in general. This is not an inevitable consequence of injury for if the damaged tissue is capable of regeneration, healing by resolution is possible and normality is regained. However, if tissue is irretrievably lost, healing can only take place by repair, this entailing the replacement of the lost tissue by fibrous tissue and resulting in scar formation. Various patterns of pulmonary fibrosis are recognised.

Focal scars are quite commonly found in the lungs at necropsy, particularly at the apices of the upper lobes where they consist of narrow bands of contracted, often blackened, lung covered by thickened pleura, the so-called apical cap.[126–128] When such apical scars are accompanied by calcification and pleural adhesions, they have probably followed tuberculosis, but this is now unusual in developed countries. Most apical scars in these countries are probably attributable to the relative ischaemia of the apices of the lungs, which due to our upright posture are barely perfused at all for much of the day. Quite minor apical scars are often associated with bullae and rupture of these underlies many spontaneous pneumothoraces (see also p. 694). Apical scarring also develops in ankylosing spondylitis (see p. 478). In other parts of the lungs, a focal subpleural scar may be the result of a primary tuberculous lesion or the corresponding primary lesions of fungal infections such as histoplasmosis. Focal scars also result from embolic infarction and pneumonia. In such scars combined stains for elastin and collagen (such as the elastin-van Gieson stain) often show that the alveolar framework of the lung is completely lost, reflecting total destruction of the affected area. Such scars are generally rich in elastin, a feature common to organs such as the lungs and the heart that are subject to repeated movement and one that is not seen to the same degree in scars of organs such as the liver and kidneys that are subjected to less movement.

With more widespread pulmonary fibrosis, elastin stains often show that the framework of the alveolar walls is maintained,[129] and one of three patterns of fibrosis may then be recognised: intra-alveolar, interstitial and obliterative.[130,131] These patterns are not mutually exclusive. For example, interstitial fibrosis may result from the incorporation of organising airspace exudates into the alveolar wall,[132,133] as described above in the proliferative phase of diffuse alveolar damage. This is particularly likely if the epithelium is lost on a broad front and its regeneration is delayed. Whether the fibrosis has an intra-alveolar, interstitial or obliterative pattern largely depends on the severity and duration of the initial injury. To some extent therefore these patterns are of prognostic significance.

Intra-alveolar fibrosis (organising pneumonia, bronchiolitis obliterans organising pneumonia)[134]

Intra-alveolar fibrosis represents organisation of an alveolar exudate. It is characterised by the presence within the alveoli of polypoid knots of myxoid granulation tissue, rich in glycosaminoglycans, fibroblasts and myofibroblasts[135] but containing little polymerised collagen. These intra-alveolar knots of granulation tissue are known as Masson bodies[136] or bourgeons conjonctifs (see Figs 4.16b, 5.2.4, p. 176 and 6.2.2c,d, p. 309). This is the classic pattern of post-pneumonic carnification, found particularly when bacterial pneumonia fails to resolve. It is familiar to all pathologists conducting autopsies and must have been well known to the great morbid anatomists of the nineteenth century. Twentieth century descriptions date back at least to 1912.[137–139]

Organising pneumonia may also represent incomplete resolution of eosinophilic pneumonia or the fibrin-rich transudate of severe left ventricular failure, or be caused by inhaled irritants,[140] viral infection, including human immunodeficiency virus,[141] drugs,[142,143] radiation[144–146] and connective tissue disease.[147,148] Organising pneumonia is also found in transplanted lungs[149] and is commonly seen around tumours or other localised lung lesions. Although organising pneumonia is readily recognisable in transbronchial biopsies such specimens may not include these underlying lesions, which may therefore remain undetected unless a surgical biopsy is obtained.

There is also an idiopathic variety of organising pneumonia, known as cryptogenic organising pneumonia or idiopathic bronchiolitis obliterans organising pneumonia. This is described in Chapter 6.2.

Obliterative alveolar fibrosis

Pulmonary fibrosis sometimes effaces the lumen of several adjacent alveoli completely, rendering them totally airless (Fig. 4.23). This obliterative pattern of fibrosis is the result of severe lung injury due to any of the causes of diffuse alveolar damage considered above. Intraalveolar and obliterative pulmonary fibrosis have many causes in common. The pattern of fibrosis depends not so much on the nature of the damage as its severity. With very severe injury the alveolar lumen is flooded with a fibrin-rich exudate, organisation of which completely obliterates the air spaces over broad tracts of lung. Within these areas, however, the framework of the alveolar walls can often still be appreciated, particularly with elastin or basement membrane stains. Parts of the lung affected by obliterative fibrosis are completely non-functioning. This pattern of fibrosis is unlikely to resolve.

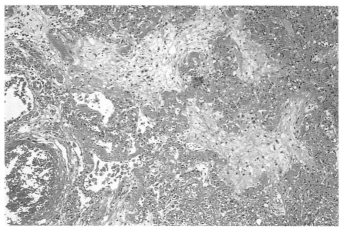

(a)

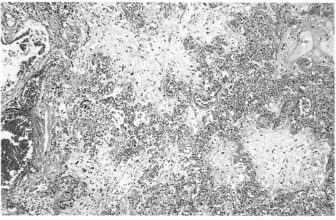

(b)

Figure 4.23 Accidental paraquat poisoning. The patient died from pulmonary fibrosis within 10 days of ingesting a relatively small amount of the chemical. The fibrosis is of the obliterative pattern, resulting from organisation of exudate that flooded many alveoli so that the air spaces are completely obliterated although the alveolar walls can still be identified. (a) Haematoxylin and eosin. (b) Masson stain.

Interstitial fibrosis

This pattern of pulmonary fibrosis involves the interstitial compartment of the alveolar walls and largely spares the airspaces (Fig. 4.24). It often entails the laying down of connective tissue within the alveolar walls but it may also be brought about by an accretive process involving incorporation into the interstitium of exudates or connective tissue first formed in airspaces.[132,133,150] The causes are varied but may be divided into two broad groups, one involving the formation of exudates and transudates and the other involving the formation of what may be loosely termed granulomas (Box 4.2). It is particularly notable that the 'exudate and transudate' group of diseases predominantly affects the basal portion of the lungs and the 'granulomatous' group more the upper parts. The reason for this is not well understood but it can be a helpful diagnostic pointer in advanced disease. It requires no great skill in interpreting chest radiographs to assign a patient with widespread

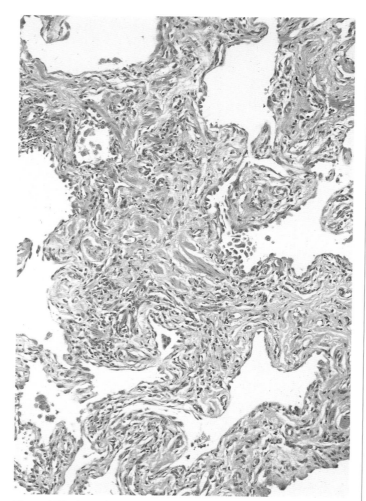

Figure 4.24 Interstitial fibrosis as seen in the fibrotic interstitial pneumonias.

reticulonodular opacities to one or other of these two broad groups on the basis of the distribution of the disease. This criterion is also useful when assessing widespread pulmonary fibrosis post mortem.

In the 'exudate and transudate' group, many cases are unexplained but some represent the outcome of diffuse alveolar damage caused by agents that range from fumes to viruses, irradiation, the aspiration of regurgitated gastric acid and the ingestion of various chemicals (Box 4.1). These causes may also lead to an obliterative pattern of pulmonary fibrosis (see above) but in the present context, instead of exudates flooding alveoli, they line the denuded alveolar walls as hyaline membranes, the organisation of which leads to their incorporation into the alveolar interstitium (Figs 4.12 and 4.13). This augments the activity of interstitial fibroblasts, the two processes combining to cause fibrosis of the alveolar walls. A similar process, albeit at a slower tempo, is envisaged in fibrosing alveolitis (usual interstitial pneumonia), which is dealt with in Chapter 6.1. Most of these conditions entail damage to the delicate lining cells of the

alveoli and capillaries with consequent exudation. It is perhaps because of this that the subsequent interstitial fibrosis is most marked in the dependent parts of the lungs. This distribution is also seen in the interstitial fibrosis that follows long standing interstitial oedema in conditions such as mitral stenosis and pulmonary veno-occlusive disease.

The other major group of causes of interstitial fibrosis may be termed 'granulomatous' because focal collections of activated macrophages are involved in the development of the fibrosis. This group includes sarcoidosis, extrinsic allergic alveolitis and Langerhans cell histiocytosis (eosinophilic granuloma), all of which are described later in Chapter 6. The fibrosis they cause is predominantly mid or upper zonal.

The pneumoconioses constitute an important group of diseases causing interstitial pulmonary fibrosis. They are dealt with separately (see Ch. 7.1) but it is possible to allocate individual pneumoconioses to one or other of the above two groups (Box 4.2). Thus, asbestosis resembles the idiopathic cases in having a predominantly basal distribution, whereas others, e.g. silicosis and chronic berylliosis, resemble the granulomatous diseases morphologically (given that early silicotic nodules resemble granulomas) and in their upper zone distribution.

'Honeycomb lung'

In advanced cases of pulmonary fibrosis, the normal alveolar architecture is lost and the three patterns just described can no longer be distinguished. At this stage, the lung is replaced by a series of cystic spaces giving an appearance that has been termed 'honeycomb lung'. The spaces represent a combination of disrupted alveoli and bronchiolectasis (see Figs 6.1.4–6, 6.1.9 and 6.1.12a, pp. 270, 272, 275). 'Honeycomb lung' is not a specific disease but represents the final result of many, being an end-stage pattern of injury comparable to the granular contracted kidney and cirrhosis of the liver. Idiopathic pulmonary fibrosis is its most common cause, particularly those cases with the pattern of usual interstitial pneumonia. Other causes include extrinsic allergic alveolitis, Langerhans cell histiocytosis, sarcoidosis and berylliosis. Lymphangioleiomyomatosis also produces widespread cystic change but generally lacks the fibrosis seen in these other conditions.

Dystrophic calcification and ossification

Dystrophic calcification is very common in pulmonary scars, particularly those resulting from tuberculosis, chickenpox and histoplasmosis. Pulmonary calcification in the absence of hypercalcaemia also occurs in the tracheobronchial cartilages of the elderly, the cartilaginous nodules of tracheobronchopathia osteochondroplastica and bronchopulmonary amyloid tumours. Pulmonary calcification also accompanies haemosiderin deposition in the lungs and is therefore found in chronic haemorrhagic conditions such as idiopathic haemosiderosis and the post-capillary pulmonary hypertension of mitral stenosis, lymphangioleiomyomatosis and veno-occlusive disease. Pulmonary calcification secondary to hypercalcaemia (metastatic calcification) is described on p. 489.

Dystrophic pulmonary ossification takes place in similar circumstances to dystrophic pulmonary calcification. It is found with scarring, ageing of the bronchial cartilages, tracheobronchopathia osteochondroplastica and amyloid tumour formation. Lamellar bone, readily recognisable as such, is laid down and marrow spaces are often evident. Sometimes branching spicules of bone extend through the lung in a racemose or dendriform manner.[151-156] Isolated foci of laminated bone may also be found within alveoli of otherwise normal appearance (see Fig. 6.2.27, p. 323).

REFERENCES

Diffuse alveolar damage

1. Liebow AA. New concepts and entities in pulmonary disease. In: International Academy of Pathology, ed. Monograph No. 8. The Lung. Baltimore: Williams and Wilkins; 1967:332–365.
2. Liebow AA. Definition and classification of interstitial pneumonias in human pathology. Prog Resp Res 1975; 8:1–33.
3. Katzenstein A-LA, Bloor CM, Liebow AA. Diffuse alveolar damage – the role of oxygen, shock and related factors. Am J Pathol 1976; 85:210–222.
4. Corrin B. Diffuse alveolar damage. In: Evans TW, Haslett C, eds. ARDS Acute Respiratory Distress in Adults. London: Chapman and Hall Medical; 1996:37–46.
5. Ashbaugh DG, Bigelow DB, Petty TL, Levine BE. Acute respiratory distress in adults. Lancet 1967; 2:319–323.
6. Ashbaugh DG, Petty TL, Bigelow DB, Harris TM. Continuous positive-pressure breathing (CPPB) in adult respiratory distress syndrome. J Thorac Cardiovasc Surg 1969; 57:31–41.
7. Petty TL, Ashbaugh DG. The adult respiratory distress syndrome. Clinical features, factors influencing prognosis and principles of management. Chest 1971; 60:233–239.
8. Petty TL. The acute respiratory distress syndrome – historic perspective. Chest 1994; 105:S44–S47.
9. Ware LB, Matthay MA. Medical progress – The acute respiratory distress syndrome. N Engl J Med 2000; 342:1334–1349.
10. Desai SR. Acute respiratory distress syndrome: imaging of the injured lung. Clin Radiol 2002; 57:8–17.
11. Desai SR, Wells AU, Suntharalingam G, Rubens MB, Evans TW, Hansell DM. Acute respiratory distress syndrome caused by pulmonary and extrapulmonary injury: a comparative CT study. Radiology 2001; 218:689–693.
12. Owens CM, Evans TW, Keogh BF, Hansell DM. Computed tomography in established adult respiratory distress syndrome. Correlation with lung injury score. Chest 1994; 106:1815–1821.
13. Bone RC, Balk R, Slotman G, et al. Adult Respiratory Distress Syndrome – sequence and importance of development of multiple organ failure. Chest 1992; 101:320–326.
14. Bulpa PA, Dive AM, Mertens L, et al. Combined bronchoalveolar lavage and transbronchial lung biopsy: safety and yield in ventilated patients. Eur Resp J 2003; 21:489–494.
15. Patel SR, Karmpaliotis D, Ayas NT, et al. The role of open-lung biopsy in ARDS. Chest 2004; 125:197–202.
16. Matsubara O. Pathogenesis of diffuse alveolar damage. Histopathology 2002; 41(Suppl.2):438–441.
17. Vijeyaratnam GS, Corrin B. Experimental paraquat poisoning. J Pathol 1971; 103:123–129.
18. Bachofen M, Weibel ER. Alterations of the gas exchange apparatus in adult respiratory insufficiency associated with septicaemia. Am Rev Respir Dis 1977; 116:589–615.
19. Corrin B. Lung pathology in septic shock. J Clin Pathol 1980; 33:891–894.
20. Yazdy AM, Tomashefski JF, Yagan R, Kleinerman J. Regional alveolar damage (RAD). A localized counterpart of diffuse alveolar damage. Am J Clin Pathol 1989; 92:10–15.
21. Barth PJ, Holtermann W, Muller B. The spatial distribution of pulmonary lesions in severe ARDS – An autopsy study of 35 cases. Pathol Res Pract 1998; 194:465–471.
22. Hill JD, Ratcliff JL, Parrott JCW, et al. Pulmonary pathology in acute respiratory insufficiency: lung biopsy as a diagnostic tool. J Thorac Cardiovasc Surg 1976; 71:64–69.
23. Pratt PC, Vollmer RT, Shelburne JD, Crapo JD. Pulmonary morphology in a multihospital collaborative extracorporeal membrane oxygenation project. Am J Pathol 1979; 95:191–214.
24. Evans MJ, Cabral LJ, Stephens RJ, Freeman G. Renewal of alveolar epithelium in the rat following exposure to NO_2. Am J Pathol 1973; 70:175–198.
25. Adamson IYR, Bowden DH. The type 2 cells as progenitor of alveolar epithelial regeneration. Lab Invest 1974; 30:25–42.
26. Ogino S, Franks TJ, Yong M, Koss MN. Extensive squamous metaplasia with cytologic atypia in diffuse alveolar damage mimicking squamous cell carcinoma: A report of 2 cases. Hum Pathol 2002; 33:1052–1054.
27. Katzenstein A-LA. Pathogenesis of 'fibrosis' in interstitial pneumonia: an electron microscopic study. Hum Pathol 1985; 16:1015–1024.
28. Burkhardt A. Pathogenesis of pulmonary fibrosis. Hum Pathol 1986; 17:971–973.
29. Burkhardt A. Alveolitis and collapse in the pathogenesis of pulmonary fibrosis. Am Rev Respir Dis 1989; 140:513–524.
30. Reidy MA, Schwartz SM. Endothelial regeneration. III. Time course of intimal changes after small defined injury to rat aortic endothelium. Lab Invest 1981; 44:301.
31. Kapanci Y, Weibel ER, Kaplan HP, Robinson FR. Pathogenesis and reversibility of the pulmonary lesions of oxygen toxicity in monkeys. II. Ultrastructural and morphometric studies. Lab Invest 1969; 20:101–118.
32. Kapanci Y, Tosco R, Eggermann J, Gould VE. Oxygen pneumonitis in man. Chest 1972; 62:162–169.
33. Tomashefski JF, Davies P, Boggis C, Greene R, Zapol WM, Reid LM. The pulmonary vascular lesions of the adult respiratory distress syndrome. Am J Pathol 1983; 112:112–116.
34. Pache JC, Christakos PG, Gannon DE, Mitchell JJ, Low RB, Leslie KO. Myofibroblasts in diffuse alveolar damage of the lung. Modern Pathol 1998; 11:1064–1070.
35. Bachofen M, Weibel ER. Basic pattern of tissue repair in human lungs following unspecific injury. Chest 1974; 65(suppl):14s–19s.
36. Meduri GU, Chinn A. Fibroproliferation in late adult respiratory distress syndrome – pathophysiology, clinical and laboratory manifestations and response to corticosteroid rescue treatment. Chest 1994; 105:S127–S129.
37. Brody AR, Craighead JE. Interstitial associations of cells lining air spaces in human pulmonary fibrosis. Virchows Arch Pathol Anat Histopathol 1976; 372:39–49.
38. Brody AR, Soler P, Basset F, Haschek WM, Witschi H. Epithelial-mesenchymal associations of cells in human pulmonary fibrosis and in BHT-oxygen-induced fibrosis in mice. Exp Lung Res 1981; 2:207–220.

39. Adamson IYR, Young L, Bowden DH. Relationship of alveolar epithelial injury and repair to the induction of pulmonary fibrosis. Am J Pathol 1988; 130:377–383.

40. Adamson IYR, Hedgecock C, Bowden DH. Epithelial cell-fibroblast interactions in lung injury and repair. Am J Pathol 1990; 137:385–392.

41. Matsubara O, Tamura A, Ohdama S, Mark EJ. Alveolar basement membrane breaks down in diffuse alveolar damage: an immunohistochemical study. Pathol Int 1995; 45:473–482.

42. Nash JRG, McLaughlin PJ, Hoyle C, Roberts D. Immunolocalization of tumour necrosis factor-alpha in lung tissue from patients dying with adult respiratory distress syndrome. Histopathology 1991; 19:395–402.

43. Pan L-H, Ohtani H, Yamauchi K, Nagura H. Co-expression of TNF alpha and IL-1 beta in human acute pulmonary fibrotic diseases: an immunohistochemical analysis. Pathol Int 1996; 46:91–99.

44. Fukuda Y, Ferrans VJ, Schoenberger CI, Rennard SI, Crystal RG. Patterns of pulmonary structural remodeling after experimental paraquat toxicity. Am J Pathol 1985; 118:452–475.

45. Fukuda Y, Ishizaki M, Masuda Y, Kimura G, Kawanami O, Masuji Y. The role of intraalveolar fibrosis in the process of pulmonary structural remodeling in patients with diffuse alveolar damage. Am J Pathol 1987; 126:171–182.

46. Zapol WM, Trelstad RL, Coffey JW, Tsai I, Salvadore RA. Pulmonary fibrosis in severe acute respiratory failure. Am Rev Respir Dis 1979; 119:547–554.

47. Martin C, Papazian L, Payan MJ, Saux P, Gouin F. Pulmonary fibrosis correlates with outcome in adult respiratory distress syndrome: a study in mechanically ventilated patients. Chest 1995; 107:196–200.

48. Slavin G, Nunn J, Crow J, Dore C. Bronchiolectasis: a complication of artificial respiration. BMJ 1982; 285:931–934.

49. Churg A, Golden J, Fligiel S, Hogg JC. Bronchopulmonary dysplasia in the adult. Am Rev Respir Dis 1983; 127:117–120.

50. Wohl MEB. Bronchopulmonary dysplasia in adulthood. N Engl J Med 1990; 323:1834–1836.

51. Hert R, Albert RK. Sequelae of the adult respiratory distress syndrome. Thorax 1994; 49:8–13.

52. Markowicz P, Wolff M, Djedaini K, et al. Multicenter prospective study of ventilator-associated pneumonia during acute respiratory distress syndrome. Incidence, prognosis and risk factors. ARDS Study Group. Am J Respir Crit Care Med 2000; 161:1942–1948.

53. Frevert CW, Warner AE, Kobzik L. Defective pulmonary recruitment of neutrophils in a rat model of endotoxemia. Am J Respir Cell Mol Biol 1994; 11:716–723.

54. Hudson LD, Milberg JA, Anardi D, Maunder RJ. Clinical risks for development of the acute respiratory distress syndrome. Am J Respir Crit Care Med 1995; 151:293–301.

54a. Stapleton RD, Wang BM, Hudson LD, et al. Causes and timing of death in patients with ARDS. Chest 2005; 128:525–532.

55. Parrillo JE. Mechanisms of disease – pathogenetic mechanisms of septic shock. N Engl J Med 1993; 328:1471–1477.

56. Evans TJ, Krausz T. Pathogenesis and pathology of shock. In: Anthony PP, MacSween RNM, eds. Recent Advances in Histopathology, Vol. 16. Edinburgh: Churchill Livingstone; 1994:21–47.

57. McGovern VJ. Shock. Pathol Annu 1971; 6:279–298.

58. McGovern VJ. The pathophysiology of gram-negative septicaemia. Pathology 1972; 4:265–271.

59. McGovern VJ. Hypovolaemic shock with particular reference to the myocardial and pulmonary lesions. Pathology 1980; 12:63–72.

60. Moon VH. The pathology of secondary shock. Am J Pathol 1948; 24:235–273.

61. Martin AM, Soloway HB, Simmons RL. Pathologic anatomy of the lungs following shock and trauma. J Trauma 1968; 8:687–699.

62. Bredenburg CE, James PM, Collins J, Anderson RW, Martin AH, Hardaway RM. Respiratory failure in shock. Ann Surg 1969; 169:392–403.

63. Thiemermann C, Szabo C, Mitchell JA, et al. Vascular hyporeactivity to vasoconstrictor agents and hemodynamic decompensation in hemorrhagic shock is mediated by nitric oxide. Proc Natl Acad Sci USA 1993; 90:267–271.

64. Clowes GHA. Pulmonary abnormalities in sepsis. Surg Clin North Am 1974; 54:993–1013.

65. Stephens KE, Ishizaka A, Larrick JW, Raffin TA. Tumor necrosis factor causes increased pulmonary permeability and edema. Am Rev Respir Dis 1988; 137:1364–1370.

66. Millar AB, Singer M, Meager A, Foley NM, Johnson NM, Rook GAW. Tumour necrosis factor in bronchopulmonary secretions of patients with adult respiratory distress syndrome. Lancet 1989; ii:712–714.

67. Johnson J, Brigham KL, Jesmok G, Meyrick B. Morphologic changes in lungs of anesthetized sheep following intravenous infusion of recombinant tumor necrosis factor-alpha. Am Rev Respir Dis 1991; 144:179–186.

68. Monick MM, Hunninghake GW. Activation of second messenger pathways in alveolar macrophages by endotoxin. Eur Resp J 2002; 20:210–222.

69. Xing Z, Kirpalani H, Torry D, Jordana M, Gauldie J. Polymorphonuclear leukocytes as a significant source of tumor necrosis factor-alpha in endotoxin-challenged lung tissue. Am J Pathol 1993; 143:1009–1015.

70. Vannhieu JT, Misset B, Lebargy F, Carlet J, Bernaudin JF. Expression of tumor necrosis factor-alpha gene in alveolar macrophages from patients with the adult respiratory distress syndrome. Am Rev Respir Dis 1993; 147:1585–1589.

71. Martin TR. Lung cytokines and ARDS. Chest 1999; 116:2S–8S.

72. Lui SF, Adcock IM, Old RW, Barnes PJ, Evans TW. Lipopolysaccharide treatment in vivo induces widespread tissue expression of inducible nitric oxide synthase mRNA. Biochem Biophys Res Comm 1993; 196:1208–1213.

73. Buttery LDK, Evans TJ, Springall DR, Carpenter A, Cohen J, Polak JM. Immunochemical localization of inducible nitric oxide synthase in endotoxin-treated rats. Lab Invest 1994; 71:755–764.

74. Ermert M, Ruppert C, Gunther A, Duncker HR, Seeger W, Ermert L. Cell-specific nitric oxide synthase-isoenzyme expression and regulation in response to endotoxin in intact rat lungs. Lab Invest 2002; 82:425–441.

75. Ward PA. Role of complement in lung inflammatory injury. Am J Pathol 1996; 149:1079.

76. Tanaka N, Kita T, Kasai K, Nagano T. The immunocytochemical localization of tumour necrosis factor and leukotriene in the rat heart and lung during endotoxin shock. Virchows Arch 1994; 424:273–277.

77. Hollenberg SM, Cunnion RE, Parrillo JE. The effect of tumour necrosis factor on vascular smooth muscle: in vitro studies using rat aorta rings. Chest 1991; 100:1133–1137.

78. Moncada S, Palmer RMJ, Higgs EA. Nitric oxide: physiology, pathophysiology and pharmacology. Pharmacol Rev 1991; 43:109–142.

79. Freeman B. Free radical chemistry of nitric oxide – looking at the dark side. Chest 1994; 105:S79–S84.

80. Rinaldo JE, Rogers RM. Adult respiratory distress syndrome: changing concepts of lung injury and repair. N Engl J Med 1982; 306:900–909.

81. Wilson JW, Ratliff NB, Hackel DB. The lung in haemorrhagic shock. 1. In vivo observations of pulmonary microcirculation in cats. Am J Pathol 1970; 58:337–345.

82. Ratliff NB, Wilson JW, Hackel DB, Martin AM. The lung in hemorrhagic shock. II.Observations on alveolar and vascular ultrastructure. Am J Pathol 1970; 58:353–373.

83. Kasajima K, Wax SD, Webb WR. Effects of methylprednisolone on pulmonary microcirculation. Surg Gynecol Obstet 1974; 139:1–5.

84. Craddock PR, Hammerschmidt DE, White JG, Dalmasso AP, Jacob HS. Complement (C5a)-induced granulocyte aggregation in vitro: a possible mechanism of complement-mediated leukostasis and leukopenia. J Clin Invest 1977; 60:260–264.

85. Tate RM, Repine JE. Neutrophils and the adult respiratory distress syndrome. Am Rev Respir Dis 1983; 128:552–559.

86. Yodice PC, Astiz ME, Kurian BM, Lin RY, Rackow EC. Neutrophil rheologic changes in septic shock. Am J Respir Crit Care Med 1997; 155:38–42.

87. Drost EM, Kassabian G, Meiselman HJ, Gelmont D, Fisher TC. Increased rigidity and priming of polymorphonuclear leukocytes in sepsis. Am J Respir Crit Care Med 1999; 159:1696–1702.

88. Wegner CD, Wolyniec WW, Laplante AM, et al. Intercellular adhesion molecule-1 contributes to pulmonary oxygen toxicity in mice – role of leukocytes revised. Lung 1992; 170:267–279.

89. Seekamp A, Mulligan MS, Till GO, et al. Role of beta-2 integrins and ICAM-1 in lung injury following ischemia-reperfusion of rat hind limbs. Am J Pathol 1993; 143:464–472.

90. Zimmerman GA, Albertine KH, Carveth HJ, et al. Endothelial activation in ARDS. Chest 1999; 116:18S–24S.

91. Doerschuk CM, Mizgerd JP, Kubo H, Qin L, Kumasaka T. Adhesion molecules and cellular biomechanical changes in acute lung injury. Chest 1999; 116:37S–43S.

92. Laudes IJ, Guo RF, Riedemann NC, et al. Disturbed homeostasis of lung intercellular adhesion molecule-1 and vascular cell adhesion molecule-1 during sepsis. Am J Pathol 2004; 164:1435–1445.

93. Sacks T, Moldow CF, Craddock PR, Bowers TK, Jacob HS. Oxygen radicals mediate endothelial cell damage by complement-stimulated granulocytes. J Clin Invest 1978; 61:1161–1167.

94. Repine JE. Scientific perspectives on adult respiratory distress syndrome. Lancet 1992; 339:466–469.

95. Donnelly SC, Haslett C. Cellular mechanisms of acute lung injury – implications for future treatment in the adult respiratory distress syndrome. Thorax 1992; 47:260–263.

96. Williams JH, Patel SK, Hatakeyama D, et al. Activated pulmonary vascular neutrophils as early mediators of endotoxin-induced lung inflammation. Am J Respir Cell Mol Biol 1993; 8:134–144.

97. Varani J, Fligiel SEG, Till GO, Kunkel RG, Ryan US, Ward PA. Pulmonary endothelial cell killing by human neutrophils: possible involvement of hydroxyl radical. Lab Invest 1985; 53:656–663.

98. Donnelly SC, Macgregor I, Zamani A, et al. Plasma elastase levels and the development of the adult respiratory distress syndrome. Am J Respir Crit Care Med 1995; 151:1428–1433.

99. Torii K, Iida KI, Miyazaki Y, et al. Higher concentrations of matrix metalloproteinases in bronchoalveolar lavage fluid of patients with adult respiratory distress syndrome. Am J Respir Crit Care Med 1997; 155:43–46.

100. Bone RC, Francis PB, Pierce AK. Intravascular coagulation associated with the adult respiratory distress syndrome. Am J Med 1976; 61:585–589.

101. Bleyl U, Rossner JA. Globular hyaline microthrombi – their nature and morphogenesis. Virchows Arch Pathol Anat Histopathol 1976; 370:113–128.

102. Hardaway RM. Disseminated intravascular coagulation as possible cause of acute respiratory failure. Surg Gynecol Obstet 1973; 137:1–5.

103. Schneider RC, Zapol WM, Carvalho AC. Platelet consumption and sequestration in severe acute respiratory failure. Am Rev Respir Dis 1980; 122:445–451.

104. Aabo K, Hansen KB. Megakarocytes in pulmonary blood vessels. 1.Incidences at autopsy, clinicopathological relations especially to disseminated intravascular coagulation. Acta Path Microbiol Scand 1978; 86:285–291.

105. Shimamura K, Oka K, Nakazawa M, Kojima M. Distribution patterns of microthrombi in disseminated intravascular coagulation. Arch Pathol Lab Med 1983; 107:543–547.

106. Blaisdell FW, Lim RC, Stallone RJ. The mechanism of pulmonary damage following traumatic shock. Surg Gynecol Obstet 1970; 130:15–22.

107. Sankey EA, Crow J, Mallett SV, et al. Pulmonary platelet aggregates – possible cause of sudden peroperative death in adults undergoing liver transplantation. J Clin Pathol 1993; 46:222–227.

108. Haynes JB, Hyers TM, Giclas PC, Franks JJ, Petty TL. Elevated fibrin(ogen) degradation products in adult respiratory distress syndrome. Am Rev Respir Dis 1980; 122:841–847.

109. Manwaring D, Thorning D, Currer PW. Mechanisms of acute pulmonary dysfunction induced by fibrinogen degradation product D. Surgery 1978; 84:45–53.

110. Mendelson CL. The aspiration of stomach contents into the lungs during obstetric anesthesia. Am J Obstet Gynecol 1946; 52:191–205.

111. Ribando CA, Grace WJ. Pulmonary aspiration. Am J Med 1971; 50:510–520.

112. Matthay MA, Rosen GD. Acid aspiration induced lung injury: new insights and therapeutic options. Am J Respir Crit Care Med 1996; 154:277–278.

113. Fowler AA, Hamman RF, Good JT, et al. Adult respiratory distress syndrome: risk with common predispositions. Ann Intern Med 1983; 98:593–597.

114. Alexander IGS. The ultrastructure of the pulmonary alveolar vessels in Mendelson's (acid pulmonary aspiration) syndrome. Br J Anaesth 1968; 40:408–414.

115. du Moulin GC, Paterson DG, Hedley-Whyte J, Lisbon A. Aspiration of gastric bacteria in antacid-treated patients: a frequent cause of postoperative colonisation of the airway. Lancet 1982; i:242–245.

116. Hamman L, Rich AR. Acute diffuse interstitial fibrosis of the lungs. Bull Johns Hopkins Hospital 1944; 74:177–212.

117. Katzenstein A-LA, Myers JL, Mazur MT. Acute interstitial pneumonia. A clinicopathologic, ultrastructural and cell kinetic study. Am J Surg Pathol 1986; 10:256–267.

118. Olson J, Colby TV, Elliott CG. Hamman-Rich syndrome revisited. Mayo Clin Proc 1990; 65:1538–1548.

119. Kondo A, Saiki S. Acute exacerbation in idiopathic interstitial pneumonia. In: Harasawa M, Fukuchi Y, Morinari H, eds. Interstitial Pneumonia of Unknown Etiology. Tokyo: University of Tokyo Press; 1989:33–42.

120. Muscedere JG, Mullen JB, Gan K, Slutsky AS. Tidal ventilation at low airway pressures can augment lung injury. Am J Respir Crit Care Med 1994; 149:1327–1334.

121. Steinberg JM, Schiller HJ, Halter JM, et al. Alveolar instability causes early ventilator-induced lung injury independent of neutrophils. Am J Respir Crit Care Med 2004; 169:57–63.

122. Bhatia M, Moochhala S. Role of inflammatory mediators in the pathophysiology of acute respiratory distress syndrome. J Pathol 2004; 202:145–156.

123. Halter JM, Steinberg JM, Schiller HJ, et al. Positive end-expiratory pressure after a recruitment maneuver prevents both alveolar collapse and recruitment/derecruitment. Am J Respir Crit Care Med 2003; 167:1620–1626.

124. Hudson LD. What happens to survivors of the adult respiratory distress syndrome. Chest 1994; 105:S123–S126.

125. Neff TA, Stocker R, Frey HR, Stein S, Russi EW. Long-term assessment of lung function in survivors of severe ARDS. Chest 2003; 123:845–853.

Pulmonary fibrosis

126. Davson J, Susman W. Apical scars and their relationship to siliceous dust accumulation in non-silicotic lungs. J Path Bact 1937; 45:597–612.

127. Butler C, Kleinerman J. The pulmonary apical cap. Am J Pathol 1970; 60:205–216.

128. Yousem SA. Pulmonary apical cap – A distinctive but poorly recognized lesion in pulmonary surgical pathology. Am J Surg Pathol 2001; 25:679–683.

129. Negri EM, Montes GS, Saldiva PHN, Capelozzi VL. Architectural remodelling in acute and chronic interstitial lung disease: fibrosis or fibroelastosis? Histopathology 2000; 37:393–401.

130. Basset F, Ferrans VJ, Soler P, Takemura T, Fukuda Y, Crystal RG. Intraluminal fibrosis in interstitial lung disorders. Am J Pathol 1986; 122:443–461.

131. Usuki J, Fukuda Y. Evolution of three patterns of intra-alveolar fibrosis produced by bleomycin in rats. Pathol Int 1995; 45:552–564.

132. Hogg JC. Chronic interstitial lung disease of unknown cause – a new classification based on pathogenesis. Am J Roentgenol 1991; 156:225–233.

133. Cohen AJ, King TE Jr, Downey GP. Rapidly progressive bronchiolitis obliterans with organizing pneumonia. Am J Respir Crit Care Med 1994; 149:1670–1675.

134. Cordier JF. Organising pneumonia. Thorax 2000; 55(4):318–328.

135. Kuhn C, McDonald JA. The roles of the myofibroblast in idiopathic pulmonary fibrosis – ultrastructural and immunohistochemical features of sites of active extracellular matrix synthesis. Am J Pathol 1991; 138:1257–1265.

136. Masson P, Riopelle JL, Martin P. Poumon rheumatismal. Ann Anat Path 1937; 14:359–382.

137. Kidd P. Some moot points in the pathology and clinical history of pneumonia. Lancet 1912; i:1665–1670.

138. Floyd R. Organization of pneumonic exudates. Am J Med Sci 1922; 163:527–548.

139. Auerbach SH, Mims OM, Goodpasture EW. Pulmonary fibrosis secondary to pneumonia. Am J Pathol 1952; 28:69–87.

140. Moya C, Anto JM, Taylor AJN, et al. Outbreak of organising pneumonia in textile printing sprayers. Lancet 1994; 344:498–502.

141. Allen JN, Wewers MD. HIV-associated bronchiolitis obliterans organising pneumonia. Chest 1989; 96:197–198.

142. Camus P, Lombard JN, Perrichon M, et al. Bronchiolitis obliterans organizing pneumonia during treatment with acebutolol and amiodarone. Thorax 1989; 44:711–715.

143. Mar KE, Sen P, Tan K, Krishnan R, Ratkalkar K. Bronchiolitis obliterans organizing pneumonia associated with massive L-tryptophan ingestion. Chest 1993; 104:1924–1926.

144. Crestani B, Kambouchner M, Soler P, et al. Migratory bronchiolitis obliterans organizing pneumonia after unilateral radiation therapy for breast carcinoma. Eur Respir J 1995; 8:318–321.

145. Bayle JY, Nesme P, Bejui-Thivolet F, Loire R, Guerin JC, Cordier JF. Migratory organizing pneumonitis 'primed' by radiation therapy. Eur Respir J 1995; 8:322–326.

146. Stover DE, Milite F, Zakowski M. A newly recognized syndrome – Radiation related bronchiolitis obliterans and organizing pneumonia. Respiration 2001; 68:540–544.

147. Yousem SA, Colby TV, Carrington CB. Lung biopsy in rheumatoid arthritis. Am Rev Respir Dis 1985; 131:770–777.

148. Rees JH, Woodhead MA, Sheppard MN, Dubois RM. Rheumatoid arthritis and cryptogenic organising pneumonitis. Respir Med 1991; 85:243–246.

149. Yousem SA, Duncan SR, Griffith BP. Interstitial and airspace granulation tissue reactions in lung transplant recipients. Am J Surg Pathol 1992; 16:877–884.

150. Spencer H. Interstitial pneumonia. Ann Rev Med 1967; 18:423–442.

151. Muller KM, Kriemann J, Stichroth E. Dendriform pulmonary ossification. Pathol Res Pract 1980; 168:163–172.

152. Pounder DJ, Pieterse AS. Dendriform pulmonary ossification. Arch Pathol Lab Med 1987; 111:1062–1064.

153. Joines RW, Roggli VL. Dendriform pulmonary ossification: report of two cases with unique findings. Am J Clin Pathol 1989; 91:398–402.

154. Chow LTC, Shum BSF, Chow WH, Tso CB. Diffuse pulmonary ossification - a rare complication of tuberculosis. Histopathology 1992; 20:435–437.

155. Ikeda Y, Yamashita H, Tamura T. Diffuse pulmonary ossification and recurrent spontaneous pneumothorax in a patient with bronchial asthma. Resp Med 1998; 92:887–889.

156. Lara JF, Catroppo JF, Kim DU, da Costa D. Dendriform pulmonary ossification, a form of diffuse pulmonary ossification: report of a 26-year autopsy experience. Arch Pathol Lab Med 2005; 129:348–353.

5

Infectious diseases

5.1

Viral, mycoplasmal and rickettsial infections

The agents considered here may strike any part or all of the respiratory tract but on the whole, each tends to affect particular parts and thereby elicit characteristic clinical effects (Fig. 5.1.1). This pattern varies however if there is some predisposing cause. Thus, the rhinoviruses, which usually cause nothing more serious than a cold, are the commonest viral trigger of acute exacerbations of chronic bronchitis, while in the immunodeficient herpes simplex virus and cytomegalovirus are serious pathogens in the lower respiratory tract. At the alveolar level, viruses cause an atypical pneumonia characterised by a chronic inflammatory interstitial infiltrate rather than the acute inflammatory exudates that fill the airspaces in the bacterial pneumonias.

VIRAL INFECTIONS

Many viruses infect the lower respiratory tract. They include the orthomyxoviruses (influenza virus), paramyxoviruses (parainfluenza viruses, measles virus and respiratory syncytial virus), adenoviruses, herpes viruses (cytomegalovirus, varicella-zoster virus and herpes simplex virus) and formerly variola virus. Many of these viruses are of course also responsible for non-respiratory disease. The role of papilloma virus in neoplasia of the respiratory tract is discussed on p. 531 and parvovirus is mentioned as a cause of hydrops fetalis on p. 41. The role of herpes-like viruses in Kaposi's sarcoma and body cavity-based lymphomas is discussed on pp. 624, 718, respectively.

Viral infection of the lower respiratory tract occurs in three general situations: infections confined to the respiratory tract, systemic infections that involve the lung and opportunistic infection of the lungs in the immunocompromised (Box 5.1.1).

The frequency of these various infections also differs in children and adults. In children, respiratory syncytial virus is the most important viral cause of lower respiratory tract disease, typically causing an obstructive bronchiolitis. Parainfluenza viruses are the most frequent cause of viral pneumonia in

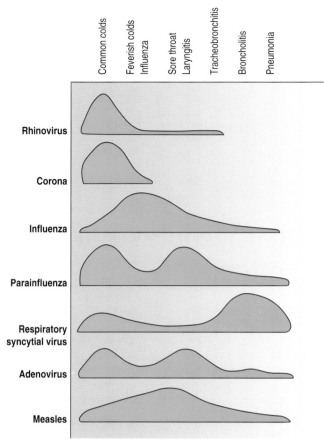

Figure 5.1.1 Clinical features of the common respiratory virus infections. RSV, respiratory syncytial virus.

Box 5.1.1 Classification of viruses that infect the lower respiratory tract

Immunocompetent host
  Primary respiratory infection
    Respiratory syncytial virus
    Parainfluenza
    Influenza
    Adenovirus
  Secondary to systemic infection
    Measles
    Varicella-zoster virus
    Adenovirus
Immunocompromised host
  Cytomegalovirus
  Herpes simplex virus
  Varicella-zoster virus
  Adenovirus

---

children and the influenza virus in adults. These are followed by the measles and adenoviruses in children and varicella virus in adults, while the immunocompromised are also susceptible to cytomegalovirus and herpes simplex virus.

The virus responsible can be cultured from sputum or nasopharyngeal washings and evidence of infection by partic-

ular viruses may be provided by the demonstration of a rising titre of specific antibodies in the patient's serum. The advent of monoclonal antibodies has provided specific, sensitive and reproducible probes that can be directly conjugated to a fluorescent tag so that the examination of exfoliated cells for viral antigen by immunofluorescent techniques is now the method of choice for the rapid identification of most respiratory viruses. In tissue, the particular virus may be identified by immunocytochemistry,[1] electron microscopy or gene probes.[2–6]

Most respiratory viral infections end in recovery. In fatal cases, the pathological changes in the lungs are often dominated by the effects of secondary bacterial infection, which is a very frequent complication. Few bacterial species have developed mechanisms for attachment to normal, intact human respiratory epithelium (notable exceptions being *Bordetella pertussis* and *Mycoplasma pneumoniae*) but viral injury to the epithelium permits bacterial attachment to take place and is associated with a greatly increased incidence of bacterial pneumonia.

From the occasional post-mortem studies that have been undertaken in uncomplicated cases of viral pneumonia it is apparent that the inflammatory reaction in the lung is mainly lymphocytic and interstitial. Neutrophils are numerous only when there is a complicating bacterial infection. The pathology is modified to some extent by the type of virus responsible but infections caused by different viruses have many features in common.[7] In the lungs, as in other organs, some viruses have a cytopathic effect and kill the infected host cells, while others stimulate proliferative activity. Thus, influenza, adenovirus, varicella and herpes simplex pneumonia are all characterised by epithelial cell necrosis (Figs 5.1.2 and 5.1.3), while respiratory syncytial virus and measles virus stimulate mitotic division and cause characteristic proliferative changes in the bronchioles and alveoli respectively. The distribution of the changes is often characteristic of a particular virus, but not specific. Thus, within the alveoli, influenza tends to affect the epithelium diffusely. The effects of adenovirus, on the other hand, are generally maximal in the region of the terminal bronchioles, while varicella pneumonia is also focal but lacks any particular relationship to the acinar architecture. Viral inclusions are evident in certain viral pneumonias, notably measles, adenovirus, cytomegalovirus, varicella and herpes simplex pneumonia, but not in others.

Alveolar epithelial necrosis is a particularly common feature of viral pneumonia. It causes the formation of hyaline membranes (Fig. 5.1.3) and the pathology of such viral pneumonia is essentially that of diffuse alveolar damage (see p. 131). Regenerative changes similar to those seen in diffuse alveolar damage are also evident and may similarly involve epithelial metaplasia.

Much of the damage caused by respiratory viruses is due to a direct cytopathic effect on the infected cells but there may also be indirect injury. The latter may be due to normal immune mechanisms such as cytotoxic T-lymphocytes attacking infected host cells, depression of immunity by the virus (facilitating secondary infections), or the development of autoimmunity initiated by the virus.

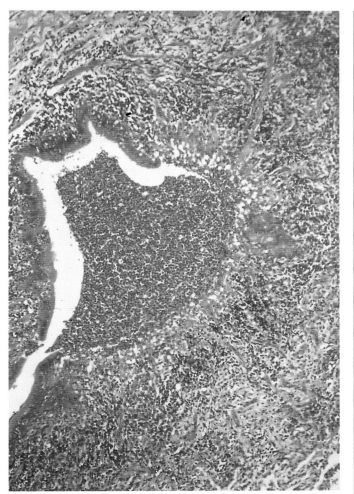

Figure 5.1.2 Necrotising viral bronchiolitis. The bronchiolar epithelium is partly destroyed and the lumen is largely filled with pus due to secondary bacterial infection.

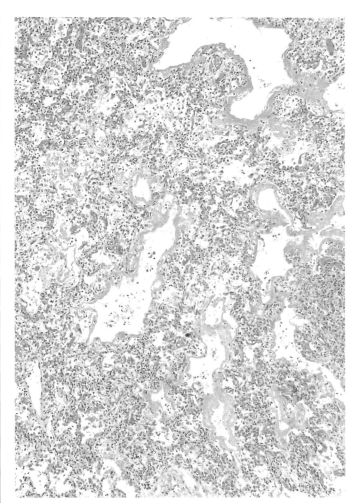

Figure 5.1.3 Viral pneumonia causing necrosis of the alveolar epithelium with the formation of hyaline membranes. The virus responsible in this patient was that of measles but many respiratory viruses have a similar effect, as do several other cytotoxic factors: (see diffuse alveolar damage, Ch. 4; material provided by Dr V Chrystal, Durban, South Africa.)

The possible threat of bioterrorism is a feature of life today and because of the ease with which they may be widely dispersed respiratory pathogens figure large in the thinking of defence forces. The United States Centers for Disease Control have classified six agents as category A threats. Several of these will be considered in this infectious disease section. The six category A agents are *Bacillus anthracis* (anthrax), *Variola major* (smallpox), *Yersinia pestis* (plague), *Francisella tularensis* (tularaemia), viral haemorrhagic agents and *Clostridium botulinum* toxin. Category B and C agents, which are seen as posing less of a threat, include the respiratory pathogens *Coxiella burnetii* (Q fever), Hantavirus and multidrug-resistant *Mycobacterium tuberculosis*.

INFLUENZA

Microbiology and epidemiology

This disease is epidemic almost annually in the winter months in many parts of the world and at long intervals the disease occurs in pandemic form, notably in 1889–1892, 1918–1919, 1957–1958 and 1968. It is estimated that in the pandemic that followed the First World War, some 20–30 million people died from the disease in little more than 1 year; more than were killed in the war itself. Until 1933, it was widely believed that the disease was caused by *Haemophilus influenzae*. The discovery in 1933 that the disease could be transmitted to ferrets by intranasal inoculation of filtered washings from the noses of patients established its viral nature.[8]

There are several types of influenza virus and constant changes in the antigenic make-up of the strain predominant at any one time defy attempts to produce a satisfactory vaccine. Those involved in the most serious infections belong to types A and B, with the former much the more virulent and including the notorious Hong Kong strain. Outbreaks of infection with influenza A occur most years, with epidemics every 5–15 years. Influenza B also causes epidemics, but less frequently. Influenza C does not appear to cause epidemics.

Antigenic lability involves changes in the principal surface antigens of the virus, haemagglutinin and neuraminidase. Minor changes ('antigenic drift') are seen progressively from season to season. Major changes ('antigenic shift') due to acquisition of a 'new' haemagglutinin occur periodically and are responsible for the emergence of new subtypes to which populations have little immunity and which therefore cause epidemics or pandemics. Influenza epidemics occur in the winter months and often start in countries south of the equator or in the east, giving northern and western countries time to prepare and distribute appropriate vaccines to those most at risk, notably the infirm. Influenza A viruses are named after their haemagglutinins (H1, H2, etc.), their neuraminidases (N1, N2, N3, etc.) and the place and year where and when the strain was first identified. Thus, the 1968 pandemic virus was H2N3 influenza A/Hong Kong/68.

The haemagglutinin molecule enables the virus to attach to host cells prior to infecting them. Although there are considerable differences between the influenza viruses that infect different species, the haemagglutinin molecule's lability occasionally permits its virus to switch from one host species to another, in which the disease is likely to spread in epidemic form. It appears that all the devastating influenza pandemics of the twentieth century, such as Spanish 'flu in 1918, Asian 'flu in 1957 and Hong Kong 'flu in 1968, were caused by viruses that made the switch from birds to man.[9] More recently, the H5N1 strain of the influenza A virus has devastated flocks of poultry in Asia and has been responsible for the deaths of some humans from what is currently termed 'Asian bird 'flu'. The switch from animals to man in the 'wet markets' of the Far East is also relevant to SARS (see p. 157).

Clinical features

The severity of influenza varies from one epidemic to another and from case to case. In its uncomplicated form it is relatively mild, with fever, coryza, headache and body aches as its main features and recovery after a few days. When the viral infection is followed by invasion of the lungs by staphylococci, pneumococci, streptococci or *Haemophilus influenzae*, the condition assumes a much graver form and the fatality rate may rise alarmingly. Infection rates are highest among school children and decrease with age but death is commonest in infants, the elderly and those with underlying lung or heart disease and is generally due to complications.

Primary influenzal pneumonia is generally rare but figured prominently in the 1918–1919 pandemic. It carries a high case fatality rate and in the 1918–1919 pandemic it was notable that mortality was highest in adults aged 25–34, possibly because older people had been exposed much earlier to a similar strain of the virus.[10,11] This form of the disease may be fulminant, leading to the death of a previously healthy person within a few hours of the onset of symptoms.[12]

Bacterial superinfection in influenza

Although pneumonia is the usual cause of death in epidemics of influenza, it is often a secondary bacterial pneumonia that is responsible. Neutrophilic exudates, organising pneumonia and bronchiolitis obliterans are then added to or replace the changes seen in uncomplicated cases.[12–14] The impact an influenza epidemic has on respiratory death rates in general is shown in Figure 5.1.4.

Before the discovery of the influenza virus in 1933, the changes that are now known to be due to the viral infection were often confused with those of complicating infections, mainly caused by bacteria. *Haemophilus influenzae* was first isolated in the 1889–90 pandemic and so named because its discoverer, Pfeiffer recovered it from a large proportion of cases and mistook it for the cause of influenza. In the 1918–1919 pandemic the predominant bacterium was again *H. influenzae* but *Streptococcus pneumoniae*, *Streptococcus pyogenes* and *Staphylococcus aureus* were also found. With the advent of antibiotics, resistant strains of *Staphylococcus aureus* emerged and in the

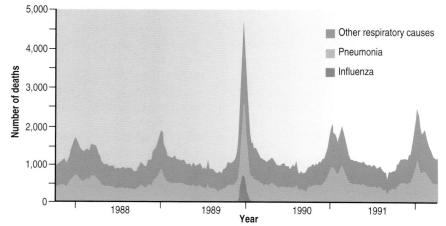

Figure 5.1.4 Weekly deaths from respiratory disease in England and Wales 1987–1992, showing the impact of an influenza epidemic in 1989/90 on deaths from other respiratory diseases. (Data supplied by the Lung and Asthma Information Centre.)

1957–1958 pandemic staphylococcal superinfection of the lungs was the major fatal complication of influenza. In the 1968 epidemic *S. pneumoniae* was the principal bacterial pathogen in the elderly and *S. aureus* in the young.[13]

The relationship of the staphylococcus and the influenza virus has been much studied and there is evidence that each promotes the growth of the other.[15] Thus, certain staphylococci have a protein in their cell wall that binds to the Fc region of immunoglobulin G. In the presence of anti-influenzal serum this protein enhances staphylococcal binding to cells infected by the influenza virus[16] and in this way the staphylococcus takes advantage of the host's immune reaction to the influenza virus. In turn, the staphylococcus aids entry of the virus into the host's cell. It does this by secreting a protease that activates a viral surface protein necessary for penetration of the host's cells[17]: normally such proteases are in short supply, so limiting the rate at which influenza virus can infect cells and reproduce. The relationship of influenza and *S. pneumoniae* infection has been studied in less detail but there is evidence of similar enhancement of bacterial adherence to tracheal epithelium following influenza infection.[18]

Pathology of uncomplicated influenzal pneumonia

In the 1918–1919 pandemic many patients died within a few days of the onset of symptoms of uncomplicated influenza viral pneumonia. In such cases the lungs are bulky, hyperaemic and often of a characteristic plum colour.[12] Blood-stained, frothy fluid oozes freely from the cut surface. Areas of haemorrhage are present and may be extensive. The mucosa of the bronchial tree is very hyperaemic.

The cytopathic effect of influenza virus is seen microscopically in characteristic degenerative changes in the epithelial cells of the bronchial and bronchiolar mucosa. These changes involve all cells of the surface epithelium and often the cells lining the bronchial glands: swelling of the cells, vacuolation of their cytoplasm and degeneration of the nucleus proceed to cell loss and frank necrosis (Fig. 5.1.5). Viral inclusions are not evident but the virus can be identified in tissue sections by immunocytochemistry and *in situ* hybridization.[19] The deeper tissues show oedema, hyperaemia and a moderate to marked accumulation of lymphocytes; neutrophils are present but account for only a small proportion of the cellular infiltrate.

Alveolar involvement is unusual but cases of fulminating influenzal viral pneumonia are occasionally encountered, especially during the course of a major epidemic of influenza. Such cases were common during the 1918–1919 pandemic. This otherwise rare condition is characterised by the exceptional rapidity of the course of the illness, death resulting within 1–2 days, or even within hours, of the clinical onset of illness. The alveoli contain a fibrin-rich oedema fluid, often frankly haemorrhagic and macrophages may be numerous in the exudate. Hyaline membranes are often found lining the alveoli. Focal necrosis of alveolar walls and thrombosis of capillaries are conspicuous features in the parts most severely affected. This form of influenzal pneumonia is often associated with changes in other parts of the body that indicate the occurrence of influenzal viraemia.

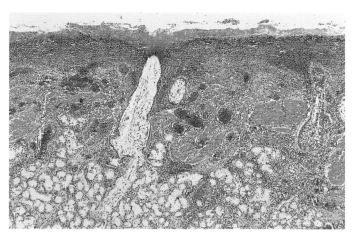

Figure 5.1.5 Influenza. This cytopathic virus has totally destroyed the bronchial epithelium, predisposing to bacterial superinfection.

Among these are haemorrhagic encephalomyelitis, which is an acute infective condition distinct from postinfluenzal encephalomyelopathy and rhabdomyolysis.[20] In the healing phase of influenzal pneumonia, there is conspicuous swelling of the alveolar lining cells, which proliferate and in places may virtually fill the lumen. The proliferation of alveolar lining cells may be so marked as to produce appearances somewhat resembling a neoplastic state. The changes reach their peak on about the 3rd–5th day of the disease and then regress, eventually subsiding completely. Also during the phase of recovery, regeneration of the bronchial epithelium may involve squamous metaplasia, but this soon gives place to normal ciliated pseudostratified respiratory tract epithelium.

Parainfluenza

Parainfluenza is caused by the parainfluenza viruses, not by *Haemophilus parainfluenzae*. It is commoner in children and particularly affects the larynx, causing croup. There may be necrosis of the mucosae, as in influenza, and quite frequently small polypoid growths of the bronchial and bronchiolar epithelium develop, similar to those associated with infection by respiratory syncytial virus (see below). In the lung there is hyperplasia of the alveolar epithelium and a serous exudate containing increased numbers of macrophages is seen. In immunosuppressed individuals, parainfluenza type III virus may result in a giant cell pneumonia that is indistinguishable from that of measles except that the inclusion bodies typical of measles pneumonia are not a feature (Fig. 5.1.6).[21–24]

RESPIRATORY SYNCYTIAL VIRUS

Epidemiology

The respiratory syncytial virus was first isolated in 1956 from an outbreak of coryza in a colony of chimpanzees and its

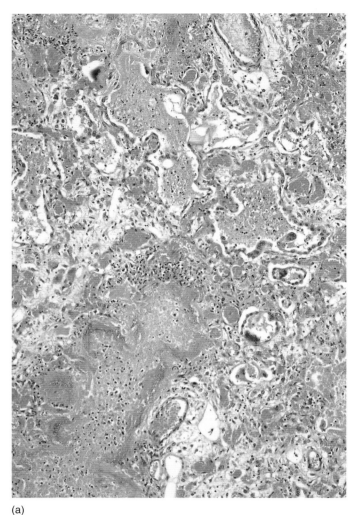

(a)

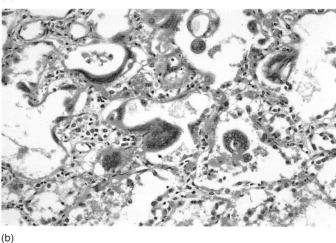

(b)

Figure 5.1.6 Parainfluenza. (a) The bronchiolar epithelium has been destroyed and giant multinucleate epithelial cells can be seen in adjacent airspaces. (b) Higher magnification of the giant cell pneumonia.

infectivity for man was shown when one of the investigators of this epizootic illness contracted the disease. It has since been shown that the virus frequently infects the lower respiratory passages of man. Specific neutralising antibodies indicative of an earlier infection are found in the serum of almost all children over the age of 5 years in Britain. However, the immunity is incomplete and reinfections may occur throughout life.

Respiratory syncytial virus shows a marked seasonal pattern, producing annual epidemics each winter in temperate climates and in the hot rainy season in tropical countries. During an incubation period of 3–6 days, the virus replicates in the upper respiratory tract causing fever, cough and coryza. Spread from the upper to the lower respiratory tract may occur, with consequent bronchiolitis and pneumonia.

Particularly important is the bronchiolitis that respiratory syncytial virus is prone to cause in infants. The conductive airways of small infants are quite narrow and easily blocked by relatively small amounts of inflammatory exudate. Because of this, fatal asphyxia is liable to follow respiratory syncytial virus infection. Several epidemics of acute bronchiolitis due to this virus have been described among infants. These outbreaks are often remarkably focal in distribution, affecting only a comparatively small area or community. As with other viral respiratory infections, secondary bacterial infection is common and babies under about 7 months, among whom fatalities are highest, frequently require intensive antibiotic treatment. Infants with bronchopulmonary dysplasia and those who have congenital heart disease or are immunocompromised are particularly at risk and units specialising in these underlying conditions have to guard against nosocomial spread of infection.[25–27] However, even previously healthy children may suffer fatal infection.[28]

It is notable that infants under 6 months of age are particularly prone to respiratory syncytial virus infection. Although this is a period when the infant benefits from the presence of maternal antibodies, placental antibody transmission is selective, being better for immunoglobulin G than A. Breast-feeding protects against respiratory syncytial virus infection,[29] presumably by virtue of breast milk being rich in immunoglobulin A. High levels of immunoglobulin G, on the other hand, may be harmful. It was noted that infants immunised against the virus and subsequently infected naturally, suffered a more severe illness than those not so immunised,[30] suggesting that the damage was mediated immunologically.[31,32] This is supported by the finding that the typical bronchiolitis is characterised by scanty virus, whereas in the rarer pneumonic form of the disease, the virus is abundant. This is compatible with the bronchiolitis representing an allergic reaction dependent on a seasonal encounter with the virus and the pneumonia being the result of direct viral damage to the lungs.[33] The cytokine profile suggests that the allergy involved in the bronchiolitis involves a predominantly type 2 response characterised by high interleukin-10/interleukin-12 and interleukin-4/γ-interferon ratios.[34] Passive immunisation, conferred by monthly injection, is free of the allergy induced by active immunisation and is recommended for high-risk babies.[35]

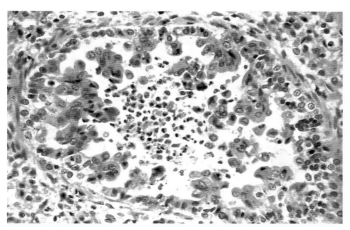

Figure 5.1.7 Respiratory syncytial virus infection in which the patency of the bronchioles is compromised by epithelial proliferation forming micropolypoid intrusions into the lumen. The bronchiolar lumen is further narrowed by a neutrophil exudate in response to secondary bacterial infection.

MEASLES

Clinical features and epidemiology

Measles is characterised by fever, coryza and a rash. In those parts of the world where it has been prevalent for centuries, the disease is almost invariably mild and, unless complicated by bacterial pneumonia, it has a very low mortality. In contrast, the mortality from measles may be appallingly high in lands to which the virus is newly introduced. When the disease was carried to Fiji from Australia in 1875, almost the whole population contracted it and one-quarter of them succumbed. Similar outbreaks have occurred in more recent times, when the infection first reached Greenland for instance.

In many parts of the world measles is still regarded as one of the inevitable infections of childhood but with an effective safe vaccine now available this is no longer necessary. In many developed countries immunisation against measles has been promoted vigourously and with uptake rates exceeding 90% the disease has nearly been eradicated.[39] However, recent unfounded claims that the vaccine is responsible for autism have led to declining vaccine uptake with consequent focal outbreaks of measles.[40]

Where measles is prevalent, the incidence is usually highest in the early spring, when droplet infections are particularly rife. The epidemics have a remarkably consistent biennial character and the explanation of this has been the subject of several interesting hypotheses. The one most favoured envisages waning immunity over the succeeding 2 years in those children who had only a subclinical illness in the last epidemic. With the influx of two further entries into infant schools, a new population of susceptible children is formed that is liable to contract overt disease when the seasonal conditions are again favourable for the spread of the virus. In this way, a fresh epidemic develops. Overt clinical disease, on the other hand, confers life-long immunity.

If the lower respiratory tract is infected, the measles virus propagates in the epithelial cells of the main respiratory passages, leading to the destruction of many of the infected cells. In time, there is recovery and multiplication of surviving cells, but at the height of the disease the natural defences of the lower respiratory tract are greatly compromised and secondary invading bacteria can successfully establish themselves in the lungs, causing bronchiolitis and pneumonia.

Pneumonia is a rare complication of measles in the western world but is common in malnourished African children, in whom it frequently proves fatal.[41] That pneumonic foci may develop in prosperous countries in the course of severe but non-fatal attacks of measles is shown by the demonstration in some such cases of patchy opacities on chest radiography; in almost all these cases the condition resolves rapidly. The cause is usually one of the common bacterial pathogens but it can be another virus taking advantage of the patient's debility and impaired cellular immunity. Measles virus infection is characterised both by the development of a strong anti-viral immune response and abnormalities of immune regulation. There is

Histopathology

The virus infects the bronchiolar epithelium and usually leads to its destruction.[36] Occasionally cytoplasmic inclusion bodies may be seen in degenerating bronchiolar epithelial cells or the virus may be demonstrated by immunocytochemistry.[1] Regeneration involves the proliferation of poorly differentiated cells which form a stratified non-ciliated epithelium. Occasionally micropolypoid epithelial protrusions are evident (Fig. 5.1.7).[7] The bronchioles are occluded by plugs of mucus, fibrin and epithelial cell debris and cuffed by an infiltrate of lymphocytes, plasma cells and histiocytes. Except in the immediate vicinity of the bronchioles, alveoli are generally not involved in the inflammatory process. If, however, infection is on a major scale there may be a pneumonia with the general features of a viral pneumonia, as described above.[28] In severe immunodeficiency, respiratory syncytial virus may cause giant cell pneumonia,[37] a condition that is more often caused by measles virus.

METAPNEUMOVIRUS

Metapneumovirus has recently been identified as a leading cause of lower respiratory tract infections in young children. The virus or its DNA was found in 20% of nasal-wash specimens previously declared virus-negative that had been collected from previously healthy infants and children suffering from a lower respiratory tract illness.[38] The virus was associated with bronchiolitis in 59% of cases, pneumonia in 8%, croup in 18% and exacerbation of asthma in 14%, a spectrum of disease similar to that found with respiratory syncytial virus.

often a poor skin response to common antigens and helper/ suppressor T-cell ratios may be low in both the blood and bronchoalveolar lavage, suggesting that cellular immunity is impaired.[42] Thus, measles has predisposed to both adenovirus and herpes virus pneumonia.[43,44] Secondary pulmonary infection is responsible for about half the mortality in measles.[45] Other causes of death include measles pneumonia and measles encephalitis.

Measles may also be very severe when it affects immuno-deficient patients, whether they are suffering from primary immunological defects, acquired diseases such as leukaemia, or conditions which require treatment with cytotoxic or immuno-suppressant drugs.[46] Such patients may have unpredictable responses to measles virus. They may have a rash but fail to produce antibodies, or they may fail to develop a rash although infected with the virus. Fatal measles pneumonia in a previously healthy adult is very rare.[47]

Pathology of measles pneumonia

Death from measles pneumonia[48,49] occurs typically about 2 weeks after the appearance of the rash. At necropsy, the lungs are heavy and of rubbery consistency and their cut surface is pale pink. Close examination may show that the small bronchi are cuffed by a greyish zone. Extensive vascular thrombosis has been a feature of some cases.

Microscopically, there are degenerative changes in the epithelium of the bronchi and bronchioles, often accompanied by hyperplasia, particularly in the small airways. As in influenzal pneumonia, squamous metaplasia may occur and mitotic figures may be numerous. Measles pneumonia may take the form of diffuse alveolar damage with hyaline membrane formation (Fig. 5.1.3), or, more characteristically, multinucleate giant cells may line the alveolar ducts and alveoli (Fig. 5.1.8). Electron microscopy shows that the giant cells are formed from type II alveolar epithelial cells.[49,50] The giant cells contain prominent cytoplasmic and nuclear viral inclusion bodies that stain with phloxine tartrazine but which are also clearly evident in eosin-stained sections. Being epithelial, the pulmonary giant cells are quite different from the Warthin–Finkeldey giant cells that are found in lymphoid tissue throughout the body in measles, particularly in the immediately pre-exanthematous stage.

As well as the epithelial changes, there is a heavy accumulation of macrophages, lymphocytes and plasma cells in the alveolar walls. This cellular infiltrate extends into the connective tissue surrounding the bronchioles and small bronchi, accounting for the pale cuff that is seen around them on naked eye examination. Neutrophils are not numerous unless there is a secondary bacterial infection. The appearances are closely comparable with those found in the lungs of dogs that have died of distemper (Carré's disease), which is also caused by a paramyxovirus.

Hecht's giant cell pneumonia is histologically indistinguishable from measles pneumonia and measles virus is now thought to be the most common cause. Although clinical evidence of measles may be lacking and there is no history of a rash, this

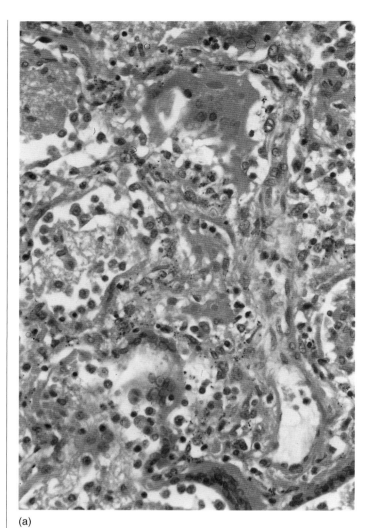

(a)

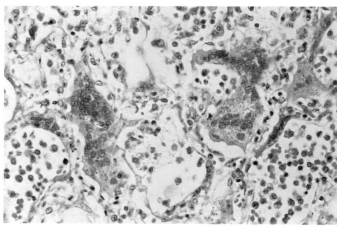

(b)

Figure 5.1.8 Measles giant cell pneumonia. There is a syncytial proliferation of type II pneumocytes containing cytoplasmic viral inclusions (a), which stain red with phloxine tartrazine (b). This response is typical of measles pneumonia but is occasionally encountered with other forms of viral pneumonia (see Fig. 5.1.6) and is also seen in hard metal workers (see p. 354). These other causes, however, lack the viral inclusions of measles pneumonia.

may be explicable on the basis of an evanescent exanthematous stage, followed by persistence of the virus as a result of deficient antibody formation. Measles virus has been isolated from the affected tissue in a number of cases. Ordinarily, measles virus can be isolated only during the first 3 days after the appearance of the skin rash. In cases of measles pneumonia it is still recoverable 1–2 weeks after the rash developed and in cases of giant cell pneumonia with no history of a rash, the infection may well have been present for a similar or longer period. In immunocompromised patients, parainfluenza, respiratory syncytial and varicella zoster viruses are further causes of giant cell pneumonia.[21,37,51]

ADENOVIRUS

Like measles, adenovirus causes a febrile rash and infects the upper respiratory tract much more commonly than the lungs. However, adenovirus may infect the lower respiratory tract at all levels and it is a relatively common cause of pneumonia in malnourished children throughout the world.

Adenovirus pneumonia occurs sporadically and in epidemics, particularly in children and young adults, and occasionally complicates measles.[43,44] Adenovirus pneumonia is usually combined with bronchiolitis and the lesions are most severe at the centres of the acini, being concentrated on the bronchioles. The virus causes necrosis of the bronchioles, many of which are totally destroyed or are recognisable only by their muscle coat: hyaline membranes replace the necrotic epithelium (Fig. 5.1.9a). Surviving epithelial cells show nuclear inclusions of varying staining reaction. Some are diffusely basophilic or amphiphilic and fill the entire nucleus apart from a rim of chromatin (Cowdry type B), while others are eosinophilic and surrounded by a clear halo (Cowdry type A). The bronchioles are cuffed by a lymphoid infiltrate and may show proliferative epithelial activity, variously interpreted as being the result of viral stimulation or of regeneration.[36,52] The alveolar tissue shows a mononuclear interstitial pneumonia. The intranuclear viral inclusions measure up to 5 μm and eventually disrupt the nucleus, leaving so-called 'smudge cells' (Fig. 5.1.9b). Healing may be by complete resolution or the pneumonia may be complicated by bronchiolitis obliterans or bronchiectasis.[53]

SEVERE ACUTE RESPIRATORY SYNDROME

Severe acute respiratory syndrome (SARS) is caused by a previously unknown coronavirus (SARS-CoV) that has probably switched from another species and adapted to human transmission.[54,55] It has now been identified in the civet cat in food markets where the disease first appeared in late 2002, namely Guangdong Province of Southern China.[56–58] From

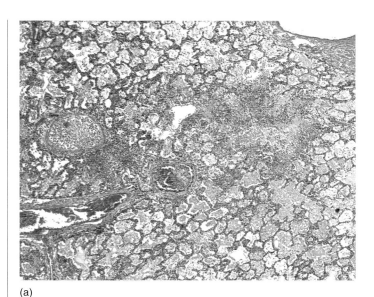

(a)

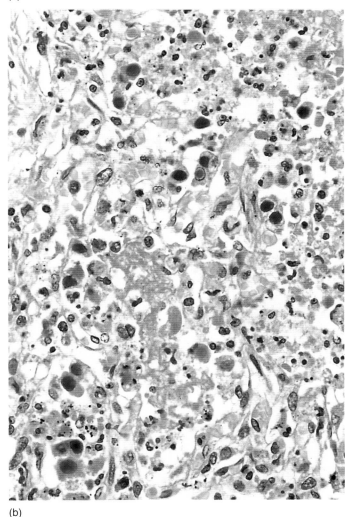

(b)

Figure 5.1.9   Adenovirus pneumonia. (a) Bronchioles bear the brunt of the damage and here show necrosis of their lining epithelium. (b) Alveolar lining cells contain basophilic nuclear inclusions. (From sections provided by the late Dr N Rossouw, Tygerberg, South Africa and Dr V Chrystal, Durban, South Africa.)

there, it quickly traversed the globe, primarily facilitated by international air travel and coming to international attention particularly after an outbreak in Hong Kong in 2003.[59–61] Since then, cases have been identified in many countries and about 10% of those affected have died.[62–65] Transmission is air-borne but requires close person-to-person contact. There is no evidence of transmission following casual contact.

Clinical features

The incubation period ranges from 1 to 10 days, following which there is a prodromal fever, cough and dyspnoea. Less common symptoms include headache, diarrhoea, dizziness, myalgia, chills, nausea, vomiting and rigor.[66] There is no sex predilection and the age distribution is wide. Common laboratory features include lymphopenia involving both CD4 and CD8 lymphocytes, thrombocytopenia, prolonged thromboplastin time, elevated alanine transaminase, lactate dehydrogenase and creatinine kinase. Positive viral recovery rates from urine, nasopharyngeal aspirate and stool specimen have been reported to be 42%, 68% and 97% respectively on day 14 of illness, whereas serological confirmation may take 28 days to reach a detection rate above 90%. However, quantitative measurement of blood SARS CoV RNA using real-time RT-PCR techniques has a detection rate of 80% as early as day 1 of hospital admission.[67]

Radiographic abnormalities include focal, multifocal or diffuse opacities. CT scanning is more sensitive, sometimes showing extensive consolidation in patients with normal chest radiographs. However, the radiological features are not specific and need to be correlated with the clinical and histological findings.[68]

Pathology

The histology varies according to the duration of illness but the predominant pattern is diffuse alveolar damage (see Chapter 4).[69–74] Cases of less than 10 days duration show airspace oedema and hyaline membranes whereas those of longer duration exhibit type II pneumocyte hyperplasia, squamous metaplasia, multinucleated giant cells and acute bronchopneumonia.[69] The alveolar pneumocytes may also show striking cytomegaly with granular amphophilic cytoplasm (Fig. 5.1.10).[70] Less common features include haemophagocytosis and thrombosis.[70,72] The virus can be identified by reverse transcriptase-polymerase chain reaction in fresh or formalin-fixed, paraffin-embedded lung tissue. Electron microscopy may reveal the viral particles in the cytoplasm of epithelial cells.[70–72]

Treatment and prognosis

Treatment with corticosteroids, broad spectrum antibiotics and antiviral agents have been beneficial.[71,75] Interferon-α may also have a role.[76] However, infection control is as important as pharmacological therapy in this disease.

In the acute phase, SARS is associated with considerable morbidity and mortality, with a global case fatality rate ranging from 7 to 27% (average about 11%). Adverse prognostic factors include advanced age, co-existent disease, high lactate dehy-

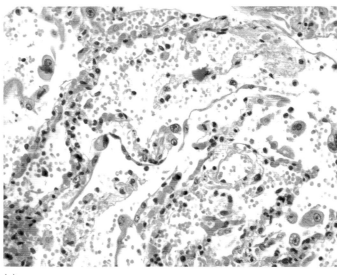

(a)

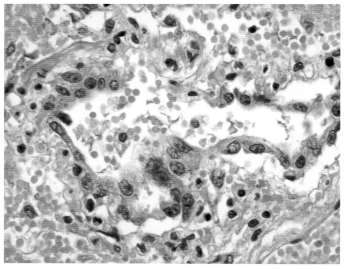

(b)

Figure 5.1.10 Severe acute respiratory syndrome. (a) Early diffuse alveolar damage represented by extravasation of red blood cells, desquamation of alveolar epithelial cells, an acute and chronic interstitial inflammatory infiltrate and a few hyaline membranes. (b) Regenerating epithelial cells show nuclear atypia.

drogenase levels and high initial neutrophil counts. CT data on the extent of the disease are also useful in assessing prognosis.[77] Clinical follow-up of patients who recover has demonstrated residual abnormalities of varying degree, including abnormal lung function and patchy fibrosis.[77a]

HERPES SIMPLEX[78,79]

Herpes simplex virus typically causes mucocutaneous vesiculation but in the immunocompromised there may be generalised disease. Generalised disease is also found in neonates,[80,81] suggesting that the infection is via the placenta rather than from the birth canal. Infection of the lower respiratory tract takes the form of tracheobronchitis or pneumonia; the latter may occur through extension of herpes tracheobronchitis or from haematogenous dissemination of oral or genital disease. Herpes simplex tracheobronchitis is predisposed to by damage to the respiratory epithelium, especially factors that lead to squamous metaplasia, such as endotracheal intubation and burns.[82–85] Risk factors for herpes simplex pneumonia include transplantation,[86] cytotoxic chemotherapy and HIV infection.[87] Herpes simplex pneumonia is rare in the immunocompetent.[88]

In herpes simplex tracheobronchitis there is extensive mucosal ulceration and pseudomembrane formation. Viral inclusions are most prominent at the periphery of the ulcers (Fig. 5.1.11). If they are not well developed an immunostain may establish the diagnosis. Longstanding airway infection leads to luminal narrowing and obstructive features. In the lungs the changes are very similar to those of adenovirus pneumonia, including the presence of Cowdry type B ground glass intra-nuclear viral inclusions, although these are more eosinophilic than those of adenovirus. Both adenovirus and herpes simplex pneumonia bear a superficial resemblance to bacterial bron-chopneumonia but the similarity is in the distribution of the lesions rather than their character: the bronchioles and cen-triacinar alveoli are mainly affected but the lesions are charac-terised by necrosis and the accumulation of nuclear debris rather than exudation of neutrophils. Occasionally herpes simplex infection takes the form of a focal necrotising pneumo-nia more typical of varicella infection (see below). Alternatively there may be arterial involvement in herpes simplex pneumo-nia with a necrotising vasculitis affecting small and medium sized pulmonary arteries.[89] Sometimes the pneumonia is diffuse. It is suggested that focal disease represents extension of oral mucocutaneous herpes virus infection down the tracheo-bronchial tree into the lung whereas diffuse pneumonia is the result of haematogenous spread.[78]

CYTOMEGALOVIRUS

Cytomegalovirus is the largest of the herpes viruses and is widespread in most communities. It is transmitted in saliva and blood and by sexual contact and organ transplantation. Seropositivity, taken to indicate carriage of the virus, steadily increases with age. The prevalence of seropositivity in adults is generally over 50% and approaches 100% in homosexual men. However, carriage of the virus does not necessarily equate with disease. The immunocompetent host is unlikely to experience any recognisable clinical effects of cytomegalovirus infection.

Symptomatic cytomegalovirus infection is seen in newborn children infected before birth by virus carried by their mother and in adults who have undergone organ transplantation or have been infected with the human immunodeficiency virus. In the newborn, the disease presents as an acute fatal infection with jaundice and leukoerythroblastic anaemia.

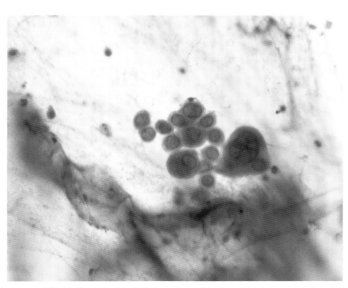

Figure 5.1.11 Herpes simplex virus. Bronchial brushings from an ulcer in the lower trachea show multinucleate epithelial cells with glassy nuclear features. From a patient with oral herpes who had started steroid therapy for asthma.

Cytomegalovirus is a serious pathogen in transplantation recipients,[90] possibly because the virus replicates best in cells that are activated, as in a transplanted organ. The risk is great-est with bone marrow transplantation, intermediate with heart, lung and liver transplantation and lowest with renal transplantation. However, donor and recipient matching for cytomegalovirus status has reduced the incidence of trans-mission from the donor. Before the introduction of this policy, fatal cytomegalovirus pneumonia or systemic infection was common. Today reactivation of latent infection is a more common problem but it is important to distinguish the mere presence of viral inclusions from pneumonitis. When a lym-phoid infiltrate accompanies the viral inclusions it is also important to distinguish an infective pneumonitis from lung allograft rejection; generally, the infiltrate of cytomegalovirus pneumonia lacks the perivascular lymphocyte distribution seen in rejection. As well as causing a pneumonitis that has to be distinguished from rejection, cytomegalovirus may also be involved in chronic lung rejection.[91] It has been speculated that cytomegalovirus could promote allograft rejection by stimulat-ing the production of proinflammatory cytokines or increasing the expression of major histocompatibility complex molecules.

The position of cytomegalovirus in regard to pulmonary disease in AIDS can also be difficult to determine. Cyto-megalovirus inclusions are frequently encountered in AIDS but it is often difficult to determine whether pathological changes are due to the virus or to accompanying bacterial or pneumo-cystis infection. Only occasionally is cytomegalovirus the only pathogen identified in severe pneumonia in AIDS patients.[92] Some investigators claim that cytomegalovirus contributes to the high mortality from pneumonia in AIDS patients,[93] while others view it merely as a bystander rather than the primary pathogen in these patients.[94] Sometimes, replication of the virus is unaccompanied by any significant degree of pulmonary inflammation or damage,[95] indicating a poor host response, which as in other viral infections largely involves T lymphocytes, cells that are particularly defective in AIDS. The differing roles of cytomegalovirus in AIDS and transplant recipients have led to the view that the pathological changes are not a direct effect of the virus but an immunopathological condition attributable to the T-cell response to the virus.[96]

Pathological features

The pneumonia may be unilateral or bilateral and generally involves the lower lobes; advanced lesions may appear as reddish purple nodular areas. Two patterns of pulmonary involvement have been described in bone marrow transplant recipients, a fulminant systemic infection characterised by a miliary pattern of disease and a more insidious disease with a more diffuse distribution in the lungs.[90]

Histologically, there is a chronic interstitial pneumonitis and some of the alveolar epithelial cells are enlarged and contain characteristic inclusions. These measure up to as much as $10\,\mu m$ diameter and are surrounded by a clear zone inside the nuclear membrane. These Cowdry type A intranuclear inclusions have been likened to an owl's eyes. The inclusions represent clumped chromatin and the clear zone the virus (Fig. 5.1.12). Cytoplasmic inclusions up to $2\,\mu m$ diameter are often also present. Severe cases may show a necrotising pneumonia or tracheobronchitis without the inclusions being well developed, in which case immunocytochemistry or *in situ* hybridisation may be used to advantage as these techniques show that many more cells are infected than those containing the characteristic inclusions (Fig. 5.1.10d).[5,6,97] Diffuse alveolar damage (see Chapter 4) is a further pattern of disease that is occasionally seen in cytomegalovirus pneumonia.

HUMAN IMMUNODEFICIENCY VIRUSES (HIV) AND AIDS

The human immunodeficiency viruses belong to the lentivirus subfamily of the retroviruses. They are the cause of the acquired immune deficiency syndrome (AIDS) and are transmitted primarily through sexual contact, by anal or vaginal intercourse with an HIV positive person. Other routes of transmission are by exposure to infected blood, generally through the use of contaminated needles and syringes by drug addicts. Infected blood products and donor tissues are other potential sources of infection. An infected woman can pass the virus to her child *in utero*, at delivery or through breast-feeding. Occupational acquisition of HIV is unusual but has occurred, chiefly through needlestick injuries. In histopathology departments, particular care is required in handling unfixed tissues, as in preparing frozen sections and conducting autopsies. Fixed tissues do not present a risk of infection. Most national bodies have produced guidelines for safe laboratory practice in the AIDS era.[98] HIV infec-

tion is not always recognisable and a practical approach is therefore to treat every cadaver and all unfixed tissue as if it were infectious.

HIV attacks the CD4-positive helper T lymphocytes and blood levels of these cells below $200/\mu l$ are associated with the development of a variety of AIDS-defining conditions. The interferon-γ-secreting Th1 cells that are central to immune defence against a variety of other infections are particularly vulnerable to attack. Once HIV infection has occurred, antibody develops, generally within a month and after a period that is usually measured in years CD4 counts drop and manifestations of AIDS develop. Concentrations of virus in the blood and body fluids are particularly high around the time of seroconversion and when AIDS develops.

Few organs escape the ravages of fully developed AIDS but the lungs are those most frequently involved in many series.[99,100] AIDS has many pulmonary manifestations, the commonest of which are listed in Table 5.1.1.[101–111] Rarer pulmonary manifestations include infection by herpes simplex[87,112] and varicellazoster[113] viruses, *Blastomyces dermatitidis*,[114] candida species,[113] cryptosporidia,[115] microsporidia[116] and *Strongyloides stercoralis*.[113] There is also an increased incidence of respiratory infection by

Table 5.1.1 The varieties of pulmonary disease described in 131 patients with AIDS[101,102]

	Patients (%)
Opportunistic infection	
Pneumocystis carinii pneumonia[a]	63
Cytomegalovirus pneumonia	19
Mycobacterial pneumonia	13
Bacterial pneumonia[a]	8
Invasive candidiasis	2
Toxoplasmosis	2
Cryptococcosis	1
Invasive aspergillosis	1
Histoplasmosis	1
Non-infectious diseases	
Diffuse alveolar damage	15
Kaposi's sarcoma	9
Non-specific pneumonitis	5
Pulmonary haemorrhage	3
Pulmonary lymphoid hyperplasia[b]	0
Lymphoid interstitial pneumonia	2
Lymphoma[a]	2

The opportunistic invaders are often present in combination and the inflammatory reaction to them is often atypical: for example, the reaction to mycobacterial infection (frequently *M. avium-intracellulare*) is often non-granulomatous, while *Pneumocystis carinii* may provoke a granulomatous response or diffuse alveolar damage, rather than the usual foamy alveolar exudate.

[a]Since the introduction of highly active antiretroviral therapy (HAART) *P. carinii* pneumonia has become less common while bacterial pneumonia and lymphoma have increased.[103–105]

[b]Pulmonary lymphoid hyperplasia is seen particularly in children suffering from AIDS[106–109] but is also recorded in occasional adults.[110] Together with lymphoid interstitial pneumonia, pulmonary lymphoma and the sicca syndrome[111] it forms a spectrum of pulmonary lymphoproliferative disease in AIDS and other conditions (see p. 642).

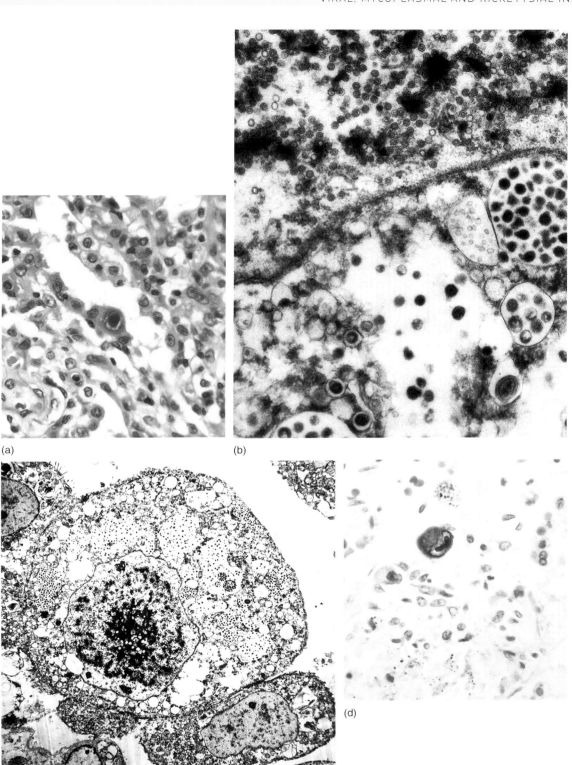

(a)

(b)

(c)

(d)

Figure 5.1.12 Cytomegalovirus pneumonia. (a) There is a prominent nuclear inclusion in the centre of the field. (b) Electron micrograph of an alveolar epithelial cell infected by cytomegalovirus. Numerous viral particles are evident in both nucleus (above) and cytoplasm (below). As the viral particles leave the nucleus and enter the cytoplasm they acquire a coating derived from the nuclear envelope and consequently enlarge. (c) Low-power electron micrograph of the cell seen in (b), showing that it is greatly enlarged compared with its neighbours. Coated viral particles are evident in the cytoplasm but uncoated particles in the nucleus are too small to be recognised at this magnification. However, characteristic central clumping of the chromatin is evident. (d) Immunocytochemistry shows abundant virus in the cytoplasm as well as the nucleus (immunoperoxidase stain). (Figs (b) and (c) were provided by Miss A Dewar, Brompton, UK.)

common pyogenic organisms,[104,117,118] especially *Streptococcus pneumoniae* and *Haemophilus influenzae*,[113] sometimes resulting in bronchiolitis obliterans[119] or unusual diseases such as bacterial tracheitis,[120] where the trachea is narrowed by pus or necrotic material containing colonies of mixed bacteria. Tuberculosis has also made an unwelcome resurgence since the advent of AIDS.[121–123] Opportunistic mycobacterial infection,[124] malakoplakia,[125,126] bacillary angiomatosis,[127] secondary alveolar lipoproteinosis,[128] follicular bronchitis and bronchiolitis[110] are also encountered in AIDS patients. However, there are marked geographical differences in the incidences of these manifestations of AIDS: tuberculosis is particularly common in poor countries whereas pneumocystis, non-tuberculous mycobacteriosis and lymphoma are more common in richer communities. In recent years, there has been a trend towards multiple infections, more mycobacterial disease and less pneumocystis infection and Kaposi's sarcoma.[99,103,129]

Since the introduction of highly active antiretroviral therapy (HAART) mortality rates have declined and life expectancy improved among those so treated, but these benefits have so far been largely confined to the industrialised countries. However, in these countries HAART drug toxicity contributes up to 2% of deaths among HIV infected patients. The toxicity is mainly hepatic but sarcoid-like nodules have been reported in the lungs,[130] possibly reflecting immune restoration. Recovery of immune status may give rise to an active, and often dramatic, inflammatory response to previously indolent infections, which has been termed the immune reconstitution inflammatory syndrome (IRIS).[130a]

In most cases the secondary pulmonary infections can be diagnosed from material obtained through the fibreoptic bronchoscope (brushings, washings, lavage or biopsy)[131] or from sputum[132] but occasionally a particular pulmonary manifestation of AIDS is not revealed until open biopsy is undertaken or examination is made post mortem.

Most of the conditions listed above are secondary to the immunodeficiency but it is possible that certain lymphocytic infiltrates reflect HIV infection of the lung. These are generally non-specific T-cell infiltrates, which are largely CD8 positive and milder than those that characterise lymphoid interstitial pneumonia[133–137]; HIV has been identified in the lung tissue by *in situ* hybridisation in a minority of cases.[136] The heavier lymphoid infiltrates of lymphoid interstitial pneumonia seen in HIV-infected children largely comprise CD8 positive HIV-specific lymphocytes. Such children have fewer opportunistic infections and survive longer than other HIV-positive children, suggesting that in this setting lymphoid interstitial pneumonia reflects an effective immune response.[138] Experiments in mice suggest that viral persistence and interferon-γ production are involved.[139,140]

Rapidly progressive plexogenic pulmonary hypertension is also reported in persons infected by HIV but generally not evincing AIDS.[141–146] The lungs are often otherwise normal. The virus has not been identified in the pulmonary vessels but tubuloreticular structures suggestive of cytokine accumulation have been identified there by electron microscopy in HIV-

positive individuals.[147] Less frequently, veno-occlusive disease or thrombotic arteriopathy is the basis of HIV-associated pulmonary hypertension. Emboli of foreign particulate material may also be found in the lungs of patients who have acquired their HIV infection through the intravenous injection of drugs formulated for oral use, while a variety of vasculitides affecting various organs including the lungs is described.[148]

As well as the neoplastic manifestations of AIDS listed in Table 5.1.1 (Kaposi's sarcoma and lymphoma) it is reported that the incidence of carcinoma of the lung is increased in AIDS and that the affected patients are younger than those in the general population.[149,150] All these tumours may present as endobronchial lesions, as may tuberculosis and aspergillosis in AIDS patients.[151] The lymphomas include diffuse large B-cell lymphomas that take the form of mass lesions within the lungs and primary effusion lymphomas affecting the pleura.

CHICKENPOX (VARICELLA) AND HERPES ZOSTER

The manifestations of chickenpox and herpes zoster are generally confined to the skin but visceral involvement occurs on rare occasions.[152,153] Since chickenpox is so common in childhood, most adults are immune. However, when chickenpox affects adults, especially pregnant women, it carries a risk of fulminating varicella pneumonia, which can be rapidly fatal. The fetus is also at risk: in the first two trimesters of pregnancy, chickenpox may result in embryopathy and in the last trimester it may cause neonatal pneumonia. The immunocompromised, including those receiving systemic steroids, are particularly prone to suffer severe infections, including pneumonia.[154] The severe forms of chickenpox sometimes encountered in otherwise healthy adults may involve the lungs but recognition of this is often retrospective, the healed lesions producing characteristic radiographic changes, namely innumerable small foci of calcification.[155,156] Such patients are generally cigarette smokers.[157]

Pathological features

The pneumonias of varicella and herpes zoster pneumonia are identical.[158] They represent a focal necrotising condition that lacks any apparent relation to the acinar architecture (Fig. 5.1.13a). It starts as a fibrinous exudate, involving several adjacent alveoli and goes on to destroy the intervening alveolar walls. Eosinophilic intranuclear viral inclusions may be evident in bronchiolar or alveolar epithelial cells. Giant cell pneumonia is a rare manifestation of varicella/zoster infection.[51]

Healing results in circumscribed fibrous nodules that measure up to 5 mm in diameter and are prone to calcify (Fig. 5.1.13b,c).[155,156] Numerous calcified opacities scattered throughout the lung fields present a radiographic appearance that, outside America and other countries where histoplasmosis is endemic, is virtually diagnostic of previous chickenpox pneumonia.

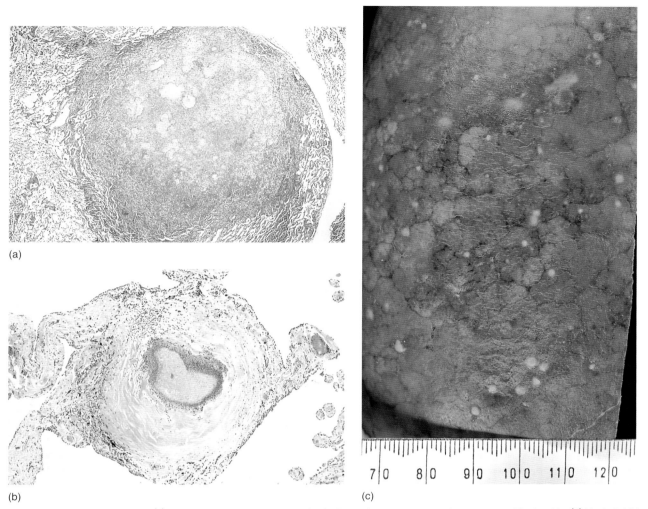

Figure 5.1.13 Chickenpox pneumonia. (a) Lung showing a focus of necrosis similar to that more commonly encountered in the skin. (b) Healed chickenpox pneumonia showing central dystrophic calcification. (c) Healed chickenpox pneumonia evident macroscopically as numerous hard, pale micronodules scattered through the lungs. (Fig. (c) was provided by Dr GA Russell, Tunbridge Wells, UK.)

SMALLPOX (VARIOLA)

In 1980 the world was declared free of smallpox and it is to be hoped that this section is only of historical interest. Severe smallpox was often accompanied by acute ulcerative tracheo-bronchitis and pneumonia. The latter was ordinarily due to secondary bacterial infection, but interstitial lesions of viral type were also found.

A condition described as 'smallpox handler's lung' was also observed. This affected nursing and medical staff attending patients with smallpox. It was characterised by high fever and prostration: radiological examination showed widespread mottling of the lungs with shadows up to several millimetres across. Typically, there were no catarrhal symptoms and recovery appeared to be the rule. These patients were well immunised by previous vaccination against smallpox and did not develop a rash. The pulmonary changes may have represented an allergic reaction to smallpox virus inhaled in the dust of scales desquamated by their patients, but it was never possible to study the pathological changes.

HANTAVIRUS

Hantaviruses are best known as the cause of haemorrhagic renal fever. Pulmonary disease was not recognised until 1993 when an unusual respiratory illness was noted in rural communities in the south-west of the USA.[159–161] It was soon identified as a previously unrecognised hantavirus infection, now known as hantavirus pulmonary syndrome. As with previously recognised hantaviruses, that responsible for the pulmonary syndrome is maintained in the wild in a single species of rodent, in this case the deer mouse, *Peromyscus maniculatus*, which is widely distributed across North America. There had been a marked increase in the number of deer mice in the south-west of America in 1993. Like other mice they are inclined to impinge on man in their hunt for food. Transmission of the virus is believed to be by inhalation of dried mouse excreta. Further cases have subsequently been identified in other parts of the USA and retrospective studies of archival material have shown that cases existed before 1993; the earliest in 1978.[162] The name Muerto Canyon virus was initially proposed for the hantavirus responsible for the pulmonary syndrome but this has given way to Sin Nombre virus. It is now known to be a member of the Bunyaviridae family of RNA viruses.

Cases of hantavirus pulmonary syndrome have subsequently been identified in several South American countries, with one outbreak in southern Argentina being unusual in that there appeared to be person-to-person transmission[163]; a feature that has so far not been observed in any other form of hantavirus infection.

Clinical features

The hantavirus pulmonary syndrome[159,160] commences with a prodromal illness characterised by fever and myalgia and perhaps nausea, vomiting, abdominal pain, headache and dizziness. After a few days, a cardiopulmonary phase is heralded by a progressive cough and shortness of breath. Common physical findings at this stage are tachypnoea, tachycardia, hypotension and fever. Radiographic findings include the rapid development of pulmonary oedema. Most of the original 17 patients with laboratory confirmed disease required intubation and mechanical ventilation and this led to the large volumes of clear proteinaceous fluid being obtained by endotracheal suction. In 13 cases (76%), intractable hypotension terminated in cardiac dysrhythmia and death within 2–16 (median 7) days of the onset of symptoms.

Pathological features

Autopsy shows heavy oedematous lungs and large, serous pleural effusions. Microscopy confirms the oedema and shows interstitial lymphocytic infiltrates.[160,161,164] Hyaline membranes have been described in some studies.[165,166] Neutrophils are scarce and viral inclusions are not found. Despite the profound circulatory failure the heart is normal. Lymphocytosis is evident in the liver, spleen and lymph nodes. Immunocytochemistry shows viral antigen in pulmonary endothelial cells and virus-like particles are evident in these cells on electron microscopy. The target of infection appears to be the capillary endothelium in all organs, with particularly heavy involvement of those in the lung, this resulting in increased pulmonary vascular permeability.

The diagnosis is now made by serological tests that detect specific IgM antibodies or a 4-fold rise in IgG antibodies. Immunocytochemistry and a polymerase chain reaction are used to detect the virus in tissue. The danger to mortuary and laboratory staff is unknown but in view of the high mortality rate full precautionary measures are advocated.[167] Treatment is supportive. Prevention is based on methods that minimise contact with the rodent vectors.

MYCOPLASMAL PNEUMONIA

Epidemiology and microbiology

During the 1930s, cases of a mild form of pneumonia were reported that clinically were unlike those attributable to bacterial infection. None of the bacteria known to cause pneumonia could be recovered from the sputum and as long as the condition was uncomplicated by secondary bacterial infection, the leukocyte count in the blood showed little tendency to rise. Cases occurred sporadically, but more often appeared in small community epidemics in schools, colleges and camps, although even under these conditions, which are usually conducive to the spread of respiratory infections, the disease was not highly contagious. It became known as primary atypical pneumonia.

The aetiology of primary atypical pneumonia attracted much interest and the first advance came in 1944 with the isolation of an organism that became widely known as the 'Eaton agent' after its discoverer. That this agent is specifically concerned with the clinical disease is indicated by the rise in specific antibodies that occurs during the course of the illness. The infection, mainly in subclinical form, has become widely prevalent, as is shown by the frequency with which specific antibodies can be detected in the serum of healthy people in the general population. The clinical disease accounts for 18% of all community-acquired pneumonia requiring admission to hospital, a frequency second only to that of pneumococcal pneumonia.[168]

Because the disease could be transmitted to both experimental animals and human volunteers by filtrates of sputum from cases of primary atypical pneumonia, the Eaton agent was at first regarded as a virus. Later studies indicated instead that it belongs to the group of 'pleuropneumonia-like' organisms (PPLO) – the mycoplasmas which can pass through a coarse bacterial filter. The organism is now known as *Mycoplasma pneumoniae*; it is one of the considerable number of mycoplasmas that have been recognised in man, animals, plants and soil. Because of their ubiquity in rats and mice, any experiments involving the lungs of these animals are soon bedevilled by the development of bronchiectasis, pneumonia, lung abscess and empyema unless specific pathogen-free strains are used.

For a time, *M. pneumoniae* was regarded as the L form of *Streptococcus MG*, a non-haemolytic streptococcus that is agglutinated by the serum of some 10% of patients with mycoplasma pneumonia and that was isolated originally from a case of the latter at necropsy. Comparative studies of the nucleic acids of the two organisms however, have shown that they are in fact unrelated. The explanation of the presence of agglutinins against *Streptococcus MG* is probably a matter of shared antigens. In about half the cases the patient's serum agglutinates Group O red blood cells at a temperature between 0° and 5°C (cold haemagglutination test), but the diagnosis is best established by demonstrating antibodies to *M. pneumoniae* in the patient's serum or more recently by PCR assay.[169,170]

Clinical features

The organism generally follows a 4-yearly epidemic cycle and predominantly affects younger patients. There is a wide spectrum of respiratory disease, including sore throat, otitis media, sinusitis, laryngitis, bronchitis, bronchiolitis and pneumonia. The chief clinical features are cough, fever, headache and malaise, sometimes associated with rashes, arthritis and haemolytic anaemia. Pneumonia develops in about 10% of cases and is characterised by a more gradual onset than acute bacterial pneumonia. Chest radiography shows irregular, ill-defined opacities, usually in the hilar region and sometimes bilateral. It is characteristic of the disease that the radiological changes are much more extensive than the comparatively mild clinical manifestations indicate. The case fatality rate is low, of the order of 1 in 1000 patients and the pulmonary opacities that are conspicuous during the 10 days or so that the illness lasts gradually resolve during the ensuing days of convalescence.

Pathogenesis

The pathogenesis of *M. pneumoniae* infection has been studied in animal models and organ cultures of human respiratory epithelium. The organisms adhere to the respiratory epithelial cells and inhibit ciliary activity. Infected cells show cytoplasmic vacuolation and nuclear swelling, with progression to complete loss of cilia.[171,172] The loss of cilia predisposes the more distal lung to secondary bacterial superinfection but the mycoplasma may also affect the distal parenchyma directly.

Immunodeficient animals show reduced severity of mycoplasmal pneumonia and it is likely that immune mechanisms are involved in the pathogenicity of the disease. Autoantibodies are produced in response to mycoplasma infection, probably as a result of mycoplasmal antigens being shared by host cells; such antibodies could account for many of the bronchopulmonary and extrapulmonary manifestations of the disease.

Histopathology

There have been few opportunities for histological study of the lesions in primary atypical pneumonia but when undertaken it generally discloses widespread bronchiolitis and chronic interstitial pneumonia similar to that caused by many respiratory viruses.[173,174] The bronchiolitis sometimes progresses to epithelial ulceration. Lymphocytic infiltration of the walls of alveolar ducts and alveoli characterises the interstitial pneumonia, while oedema fluid, red blood cells and macrophages are found in many groups of alveoli and an occasional alveolus may contain hyaline membranes. Neutrophils are generally less numerous, both in the bronchioles and the alveoli, than in the bacterial forms of pneumonia, but bacterial superinfection is a common complication.[173] The more heavily involved parts may become fibrotic and pleural adhesions may develop. There is nothing pathognomonic about any of these changes. Rarely, *M.*

pneumoniae is responsible for fatal respiratory disease, in which case the histological appearances are those of diffuse alveolar damage.[175]

RICKETTSIAL INFECTION

Rickettsia are rod-like or coccobacillary organisms that are similar to but smaller than bacteria. However, rickettsial pneumonia is dealt with in this chapter rather than with the bacterial pneumonias because its clinical and pathological features more closely resemble those of mycoplasmal pneumonia. Of the tribe rickettsiae, three genera contain organisms pathogenic to man: *Rickettsia*, *Bartonella* (formerly *Rochalimaea*) and *Coxiella*. *Rickettsia* species are responsible for typhus and certain spotted fevers and while pneumonia may occur in several of these,[176–178] the most frequent rickettsial pneumonia is that which occurs in Q fever, the causative organism of which is *Coxiella burnetii*. Respiratory disease is rarely caused by *Bartonellae*, but bacillary angiomatosis is one example.

COXIELLA BURNETII PNEUMONIA (Q FEVER)[179,180]

Q fever ('query fever') was so named because of its 'questionable' nature prior to the isolation of the causative organism, now recognised to be a rickettsia known as *Coxiella burnetii*. The disease was first recognised in a meat packing plant in Queensland, Australia, in 1937 and is now known to have a virtually global distribution. It is essentially an infection of cattle, sheep and goats that is transmitted to man, probably more frequently than is apparent from the incidence of the disease for many people who have never had Q fever possess circulating antibodies against *C. burnetii*. Among cattle, the disease is sometimes transmitted by ticks, but possibly more frequently by the inhalation of contaminated dust from the floor of milking sheds. The organisms are excreted in milk, urine and faeces and particularly during calving, when amniotic fluid and placentae are a rich source of infection. In man, the disease may be acquired by the inhalation of infected dust through close contact with cattle, as in dairy farms, abattoirs and hide factories, or through drinking milk that has been inadequately pasteurised. *C. burnetii* is resistant to drying and may survive exposure to a temperature of 60°C, an important characteristic in regard to the pasteurisation of milk.

Clinical features

Q fever is a disease of sudden onset marked by general malaise, severe frontal or retro-orbital headache, high fever and muscle pain. Men are more often symptomatic than women, despite equal seroprevalence and there is evidence that sex hormones such as 17-β-estradiol play a protective role.[181] Pneumonia develops in only a very small proportion of those infected. In these patients, chest radiographs at the height of the disease disclose numerous, relatively small, but widely distributed, opacities. The symptoms generally subside after about 1 week and most patients recover completely within a few months without treatment. Chronic Q fever, characterised by infection that persists for more than 6 months, is uncommon but more serious. This form of the disease may also represent a recrudescence of acute Q fever years after apparent recovery. It generally takes the form of endocarditis, usually developing in patients with pre-existent valvular heart disease, transplant recipients or those with cancer. Q fever responds to treatment with doxycycline, quinolones or macrolides.

The organism can generally be recovered during the height of the disease by inoculation of the patient's blood or sputum into guinea pigs but few laboratories offer this test because of the danger of laboratory infection. The detection of specific antibodies is the laboratory test of choice.

Pathology

The case fatality rate in acute Q fever is very low and few necropsies on cases uncomplicated by bacterial superinfection have been recorded. In these, the lungs show nodular or confluent areas of grey consolidation. The development of an inflammatory pseudotumour is recorded but is a very rare complication.[182]

Microscopically, the changes in the lungs resemble those seen in viral or mycoplasmal pneumonias. There is a diffuse interstitial infiltrate of lymphocytes and plasma cells and an alveolar exudate of fibrinous oedema fluid containing mainly macrophages and only a few neutrophils. Lymphocytic cuffing is seen about the bronchioles and small pulmonary arteries. The bronchioles contain an exudate similar to that in the alveoli and often lose their epithelial lining. Organisation of the exudates may lead to bronchiolitis obliterans and organising pneumonia.[183]

The causative organisms may be demonstrable in some cases: they usually measure about 0.25 by 0.45 μm but bacillary forms measuring up to 1.5 μm in length also occur. The organisms form micro-colonies in infected cells, such as alveolar epithelium and this facilitates their recognition in Giemsa-stained preparations. C. burnetii may also be identified in infected tissues by immunohistochemical staining and DNA detection. If the organisms are not demonstrable the changes are non-specific and, therefore, in suspected cases, coming to necropsy, blood should be taken for serology. It should be noted that there is a real risk of pathologists and post-mortem room staff contracting the disease if precautions to avoid splashing and drying of body fluids are not taken. This infectivity has raised its profile as a potential agent in bioterrorism.[184]

BACILLARY ANGIOMATOSIS

Bacillary angiomatosis is a reactive vascular proliferation that was originally described in the skin and regional lymph nodes

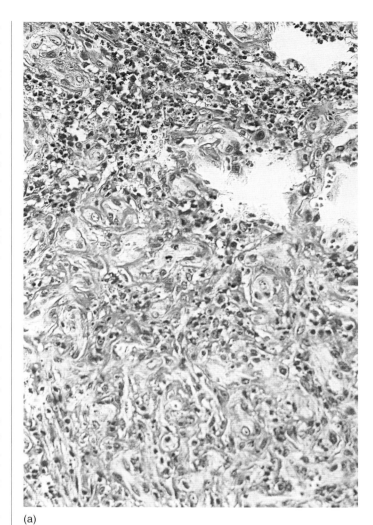

(a)

(b)

Figure 5.1.14 Bacillary angiomatosis. (a) There are many capillaries lined by plump endothelial cells, neutrophils and prominent cell debris. (b) Warthin–Starry staining reveals clumps of rickettsial coccobacilli. (Sections provided by Dr I Abdalsamad, Creteil, France.)

of patients infected by the human immunodeficiency virus.[185,186] Mucosal surfaces may also be involved, sometimes in the absence of cutaneous disease. In the respiratory tract this results in polypoid endobronchial lesions.[127,187] Chest wall involvement with intrathoracic spread is also recorded.[188] The disease has subsequently been described in other forms of immunodeficiency and even in immunocompetent patients, implying that unrecognised cases preceded the AIDS epidemic. The organisms involved have been identified as the rickettsial coccobacilli *Bartonella* (formerly *Rochalimaea*) *henselae* and *quintana*,[189,190] These microbes also cause trench foot and bacillary peliosis hepatis and are responsible for some cases of cat scratch disease (which is also caused by the related bacillus *Afipia felis*).[191]

Histologically, the lesions are likely to be mistaken for granulation tissue or Kaposi's sarcoma. Capillaries lined by plump endothelial cells are separated by neutrophils and cell debris, often surrounding clumps of bacilli (Fig. 5.1.14a). The bacilli are easily overlooked in haematoxylin and eosin stained sections and do not stain well with conventional stains for bacteria. However, aggregates of them are evident in sections stained by the Warthin–Starry or Dieterle silver techniques, predominantly in the extracellular tissue surrounding blood vessels (Fig. 5.1.14b). It should be remembered that these techniques stain many different types of micro-organisms and a positive result is only meaningful if conventional methods for bacteria fail to stain the bacilli.

The lesions lack the spindle cells of Kaposi's sarcoma and the endothelial cells are more readily recognisable as such, carrying a wide variety of endothelial markers (CD34, factor VIII-related antigen and *Ulex europaeus* lectin positivity) rather than the more restricted CD34 positivity of Kaposi's sarcoma. Similarly, Weibel–Palade bodies are readily identified on electron microscopy, which is not the case with Kaposi's sarcoma.[192] Bacillary angiomatosis responds well to treatment with erythromycin and its distinction from Kaposi's sarcoma is therefore important.

REFERENCES

1. Wright C, Oliver KC, Fenwick FI, Smith NM, Toms GL. A monoclonal antibody pool for routine immunohistochemical detection of human respiratory syncytial virus antigens in formalin-fixed, paraffin-embedded tissue. J Pathol 1997; 182:238–244.
2. Unger ER, Budgeon LR, Myerson D, Brigati DJ. Viral diagnosis by in situ hybridization. Description of a rapid simplified colorimetric method. Am J Surg Pathol 1986; 10:1–8.
3. Tomita T, Chiga M, Lenahan M, et al. Identification of herpes simplex virus infection by immunoperoxidase and in situ hybridization methods. Virchows Arch Pathol Anat Histopathol 1991; 419:99–105.
4. Hogg JC, Irving WL, Porter H, Evans M, Dunnill MS, Fleming K. In situ hybridization studies of adenoviral infections of the lung and their relationship to follicular bronchiectasis. Am Rev Respir Dis 1989; 139:1531–1535.
5. Myerson D, Lingenfelter PA, Gleaves CA, Meyers JD, Bowden RA. Diagnosis of cytomegalovirus pneumonia by the polymerase chain reaction with archived frozen lung tissue and bronchoalveolar lavage fluid. Am J Clin Pathol 1993; 100:407–413.

6. Delvenne P, Arrese JE, Thiry A, Borleehermans G, Pierard GE, Boniver J. Detection of cytomegalovirus, pneumocystis-carinii and aspergillus species in bronchoalveolar lavage fluid – a comparison of techniques. Am J Clin Pathol 1993; 100:414–418.
7. Zinserling A. Peculiarities of lesions in viral and mycoplasma infections of the respiratory tract. Virchows Arch A Pathol Anat Histopathol 1972; 356:259–273.

Influenza

8. Oxford JS, Schild GC. The orthomyxoviridae and influenza. In: Parker MT, Collier LH, eds. Topley and Wilson's Principles of Bacteriology, Virology and Immunity, Vol. 4. London: Arnold; 1990:292.
9. Gamblin SJ, Haire LF, Russell RJ, et al. The structure and receptor-binding properties of the 1918 influenza hemagglutinin. Science 2004; 303:1838–1842.
10. Reid AH, Taubenberger JK. The 1918 flu and other influenza pandemics: 'Over there' and back again. Lab Invest 1999; 79:95–101.
11. Luk J, Gross P, Thompson WW. Observations on mortality during the 1918 influenza pandemic. Clin Infect Dis 2001; 33:1375–1378.
12. Oseasohn R, Adelson L, Kaji M. Clinicopathologic study of thirty-three fatal cases of Asian influenza. N Engl J Med 1959; 260:509–518.
13. Parker MT. Necropsy studies of the bacterial complications of influenza. J Infect 1979; 1(Suppl.2):9–16.
14. Yeldandi AV, Colby TV. Pathologic features of lung biopsy specimens from influenza pneumonia cases. Hum Pathol 1994; 25:47–53.
15. Loosli CG. Influenza and the interaction of viruses and bacteria in the respiratory tract. Medicine (Baltimore) 1973; 52:369–384.
16. Austin RM, Daniels CA. The role of protein A in the attachment of staphylococci to influenza-infected cells. Lab Invest 1978; 39:128–132.
17. Tashiro M, Ciborowski P, Klenk HD, Pulverar G, Rott R. Role of Staphylococcus protease in the development of influenza pneumonia. Nature 1987; 325:536–537.
18. Plotkowski MC, Puchelle E, Beck G, Jacquot J, Hannoun C. Adherence of type I Streptococcus pneumoniae to tracheal epithelium of mice infected with influenza A/PR8 virus. Am Rev Respir Dis 1986; 134: 1040–1044.
19. Guarner J, Shieh WJ, Dawson J, et al. Immunohistochemical and in situ hybridization studies of influenza A virus infection in human lungs. Am J Clin Pathol 2000; 114:227–233.
20. Gerberding JL, Morgan JG, Shepard JA, Kradin RL. Case 9–2004 - An 18-year-old man with respiratory symptoms and shock. N Engl J Med 2004; 350:1236–1247.
21. Weintrub PS, Sullender WM, Lombard C, Link MP, Arvin A. Giant cell pneumonia caused by parainfluenza type 3 in a patient with acute myelomonocytic leukemia. Arch Pathol Lab Med 1987; 111:569–570.
22. Akizuki S, Nasu N, Setoguchi M, Yoshida S, Higuchi Y, Yamamoto S. Parainfluenza virus pneumonitis in an adult. Arch Pathol Lab Med 1991; 115:824–826.
23. Mansell AL, Bramson RT, Shannon DC, et al. An 18-month-old immunosuppressed boy with bilateral pulmonary infiltrates - parainfluenza virus type 3 pneumonia with giant cells (giant-cell pneumonia). N Engl J Med 1996; 335:1133–1140.
24. Madden JF, Burchette J, Hale LP. Pathology of parainfluenza virus infection in patients with congenital immunodeficiency syndromes. Hum Pathol 2004; 35:594–603.

Respiratory syncytial virus

25. Sinnot JT, Cullison JP, Sweery MS, Hammond M, Douglas AH. Respiratory syncytial virus pneumonia in a cardiac transplant recipient. J Infect Dis 1989; 158:650–651.
26. Harrington SW, Hooton TM, Hackman RC, et al. An outbreak of respiratory syncytial virus in a bone marrow transplant center. J Infect Dis 1989; 158:987–993.
27. Kramer MR, Marshall SE, Starnes VA, Gamberg P, Amitai Z, Theodore J. Infectious complications in heart-lung transplantation. Arch Intern Med 1993; 153:2010–2016.

28. Kurlandsky LE, French G, Webb PM, Porter DD. Fatal respiratory syncytial virus pneumonitis in a previously healthy child. Am Rev Respir Dis 1988; 138:468–472.

29. Downham MAPS, Scott R, Sims DG, Webb JKG, Gardner PS. Breast-feeding protects against respiratory syncytial virus infections. BMJ 1976; 2:274–276.

30. Zapikian AZ, Mitchell RH, Chanock RM, Shvedoff RA, Stewart CE. An epidemiologic study of altered clinical reactivity to respiratory syncytial (RS) virus infection in children previously vaccinated with an inactivated RS virus vaccine. Am J Epidemiol 1969; 89:405–421.

31. Openshaw PJM. Immunity and immunopathology to respiratory syncytial virus: the mouse model. Am J Respir Crit Care Med 1995; 152:S59–S62.

32. Graham BS. Pathogenesis of respiratory syncytial virus vaccine-augmented pathology. Am J Respir Crit Care Med 1995; 152:S63–S66.

33. Gardner PS, McQuillen J, Court SDM. Speculation on pathogenesis in death from respiratory syncytial virus infection. BMJ 1970; 1:327–330.

34. Legg JP, Hussain IR, Warner JA, Johnston SL, Warner JO. Type 1 and type 2 cytokine imbalance in acute respiratory syncytial virus bronchiolitis. Am J Respir Crit Care Med 2003; 168:633–639.

35. The IMpact-RSV study group. Palivizumab, a humanized respiratory syncytial virus monoclonal antibody, reduces hospitalization from respiratory syncytial virus infection in high-risk infants. Pediatrics 1998; 102:531–537.

36. Aherne W, Bird T, Court SDM, Gardner PS, McQuillen J. Pathological changes in virus infections of the lower respiratory tract in children. J Clin Pathol 1970; 23: 7–18.

37. Delage G, Brochu P, Robillard L, Jasmin G, Joncas JH, Lapointe N. Giant cell pneumonia due to respiratory syncytial virus. Occurrence in severe combined immunodeficiency syndrome. Arch Pathol Lab Med 1984; 108:623–625.

Metapneumovirus

38. Williams JV, Harris PA, Tollefson SJ, et al. Human metapneumovirus and lower respiratory tract disease in otherwise healthy infants and children. N Engl J Med 2004; 350:443–450.

Measles

39. Department of Health. Immunisation against infectious disease. London: HMSO; 1992.

40. Jansen VA, Stollenwerk N, Jensen HJ, Ramsay ME, Edmunds WJ, Rhodes CJ. Measles outbreaks in a population with declining vaccine uptake. Science 2003; 301:804.

41. Morley D. Severe measles in the tropics. BMJ 1969; l:297–300.

42. Myou S, Fujimura M, Yasui M, Ueno T, Matsuda T. Bronchoalveolar lavage cell analysis in measles viral pneumonia. Eur Respir J 1993; 6:1437–1442.

43. Kipps A, Kaschula ROC. Virus pneumonia following measles. A virological and histological study of autopsy material. S Afr Med J 1976; 50:1083–1088.

44. Warner JO, Marshall NC. Crippling lung disease after measles and adenovirus infection. Br J Dis Chest 1976; 70:89–94.

45. Miller DC. Frequency of complications of measles. BMJ 1964; 2:75–78.

46. Joliat G, Abetel G, Schindler A-M, Kapanci Y. Measles giant cell pneumonia without rash in a case of lymphocytic lymphosarcoma. Virchows Arch A Pathol Anat Histopathol 1973; 358:215–224.

47. Sobonya RE, Hiller FC, Pingleton W, Watanabe I. Fatal measles (rubeola) pneumonia in adults. Arch Pathol Lab Med 1978; 102:366–371.

48. Becroft DMO, Osborne DRS. The lungs in fatal measles infection in childhood: pathological, radiological and immunological correlation. Histopathology 1980; 4:401–412.

49. Rahman SM, Eto H, Morshed SA, Itakura H. Giant cell pneumonia: light microscopy, immunohistochemical and ultrastructural study of an autopsy case. Ultrastruct Pathol 1996; 20:585–591.

50. Archibald RWR, Weller RD, Meadow SR. Measles pneumonia and the nature of inclusion-bearing giant cells: a light- and electron-microscope study. J Pathol 1971; 103: 27–34.

51. Saito F, Yutani C, Imakita M, Ishibashi-Ueda H, Kanzaki T, Chiba Y. Giant cell pneumonia caused by varicella zoster virus in a neonate. Arch Pathol Lab Med 1989; 113:201–203.

Adenovirus

52. Becroft DMO. Histopathology of fatal adenovirus infection of the respiratory tract in young children. J Clin Pathol 1967; 20:561–569.

53. Becroft DMO. Bronchiolitis obliterans, bronchiectasis and other sequelae of adenovirus type 21 infection in young children. J Clin Pathol 1971; 24:72–82.

SARS

54. Ksiazek TG, Erdman D, Goldsmith CS, et al. A novel coronavirus associated with severe acute respiratory syndrome. N Engl J Med 2003; 348:1953–1966.

55. Drosten C, Gunther S, Preiser W, et al. Identification of a novel coronavirus in patients with severe acute respiratory syndrome. N Engl J Med 2003; 348:1967–1976.

56. Webster RG. Wet markets—a continuing source of severe acute respiratory syndrome and influenza? Lancet 2004; 363:234–236.

57. Guan Y, Zheng BJ, He YQ, et al. Isolation and characterization of viruses related to the SARS coronavirus from animals in southern China. Science 2003; 302:276–278.

58. Parry J. WHO confirms SARS in Chinese journalist. BMJ 2004; 328:65.

59. Chan-Yeung M, Yu WC. Outbreak of severe acute respiratory syndrome in Hong Kong Special Administrative Region: case report. BMJ 2003; 326:850–852.

60. Tsang KW, Ho PL, Ooi GC, et al. A cluster of cases of severe acute respiratory syndrome in Hong Kong. N Engl J Med 2003; 348:1977–1985.

61. Lee N, Hui D, Wu A, et al. A major outbreak of severe acute respiratory syndrome in Hong Kong. N Engl J Med 2003; 348:1986–1994.

62. Poutanen SM, Low DE, Henry B, et al. Identification of severe acute respiratory syndrome in Canada. N Engl J Med 2003; 348:1995–2005.

63. Vu HT, Leitmeyer KC, Le DH, et al. Clinical description of a completed outbreak of SARS in Vietnam, February-May 2003. Emerg Infect Dis 2004; 10:334–338.

64. Schrag SJ, Brooks JT, Van Beneden C, et al. SARS surveillance during emergency public health response, United States, March-July 2003. Emerg Infect Dis 2004; 10:185–194.

65. Desenclos JC, van der WS, Bonmarin I, et al. Introduction of SARS in France, March-April, 2003. Emerg Infect Dis 2004; 10:195–200.

66. Tiwari A, Chan S, Wong A, et al. Severe acute respiratory syndrome (SARS) in Hong Kong: patients' experiences. Nurs Outlook 2003; 51:212–219.

67. Hui DS, Wong PC, Wang C. SARS: clinical features and diagnosis. Respirology 2003; 8(Suppl.):S20–S24.

68. Paul NS, Roberts H, Butany J, et al. Radiologic pattern of disease in patients with severe acute respiratory syndrome: the Toronto experience. Radiographics 2004; 24:553–563.

69. Franks TJ, Chong PY, Chui P, et al. Lung pathology of severe acute respiratory syndrome (SARS): A study of 8 autopsy cases from Singapore. Hum Pathol 2003; 34:743–748.

70. Nicholls JM, Poon LL, Lee KC, et al. Lung pathology of fatal severe acute respiratory syndrome. Lancet 2003; 361:1773–1778.

71. Tse GMK, To KF, Chan PKS, et al. Pulmonary pathological features in coronavirus associated severe acute respiratory syndrome (SARS). J Clin Pathol 2004; 57:260–265.

72. Chong PY, Chui P, Ling AE, et al. Analysis of deaths during the severe acute respiratory syndrome (SARS) epidemic in Singapore – Challenges in determining a SARS diagnosis. Arch Pathol Lab Med 2004; 128(2):195–204.

73. Tse GMK, To KF, Chan PKS, et al. The spectrum of pathological changes in severe acute respiratory syndrome (SARS). Histopathology 2004; 45:119–124.

74. Cheung OY, Chan JWM, Ng CK, Koo CK. Pulmonary pathological features in coronavirus associated sever acute respiratory syndrome (SARS). J Clin Pathol. 2004; 57: 260–265.

75. Chu CM, Cheng VC, Hung IF, et al. Role of lopinavir/ritonavir in the treatment of SARS: initial virological and clinical findings. Thorax 2004; 59:252–256.

76. Stroher U, DiCaro A, Li Y, et al. Severe acute respiratory syndrome-related coronavirus is inhibited by interferon-alpha. J Infect Dis 2004; 189:1164–1167.

77. Paul NS, Chung T, Konen E, et al. Prognostic significance of the radiographic pattern of disease in patients with severe acute respiratory syndrome. Am J Roentgenol 2004; 182:493–498.

77a. Hui DS, Joynt GM, Wong KT, et al. Impact of severe acute respiratory syndrome (SARS) on pulmonary function, functional capacity and quality of life in a cohort of survivors. Thorax 2005; 60:401–409.

Herpes simplex

78. Ramsey PG, Fife KH, Hackman RC, Meyers JD, Corey L. Herpes simplex virus pneumonia - clinical, virologic and pathological features in 20 patients. Ann Intern Med 1982; 97:813–820.

79. Greenberg SB. Respiratory herpesvirus infections: an overview. Chest 1994; 106:S1–S2.

80. Francis DP, Herrman KL, MacMahon JR, Chavigny KH, Sanderlin KC. Nosocomial and maternally acquired herpesvirus hominis infections: a report of four fatal cases in neonates. Am J Dis Child 1975; 129:889–893.

81. Greene GR, King D, Romansky SG, Marble RD. Primary herpes simplex pneumonia in a neonate. Am J Dis Child 1983; 137:464–465.

82. Schuller D. Lower respiratory tract reactivation of herpes simplex virus - comparison of immunocompromised and immunocompetent hosts. Chest 1994; 106:S3–S7.

83. Klainer AS, Oud L, Randazzo J, Freiheiter J, Bisaccia E, Gerhard H. Herpes simplex virus involvement of the lower respiratory tract following surgery. Chest 1994; 106:S8–S14.

84. Hayden FG, Himel HN, Heggers JP. Herpesvirus infections in burn patients. Chest 1994; 106:S15–S21.

85. Byers RJ, Hasleton PS, Quigley A, et al. Pulmonary herpes simplex in burns patients. Eur Respir J 1996; 9:2313–2317.

86. Smyth RL, Higenbottam TW, Scott JP, et al. Herpes simplex virus infection in heart-lung transplant recipients. Transplantation 1990; 49:735–739.

87. Baras L, Farber CM, Vanvooren JP, Parent D. Herpes simplex virus tracheitis in a patient with the acquired immunodeficiency syndrome. Eur Respir J 1994; 7:2091–2093.

88. Martinez E, Dediego A, Paradis A, Perpina M, Hernandez M. Herpes simplex pneumonia in a young immunocompetent man. Eur Respir J 1994; 7:1185–1188.

89. Phinney PR, Fligiel S, Bryson YJ, Porter DD. Necrotizing vasculitis in a case of disseminated neonatal herpes simplex infection. Arch Pathol Lab Med 1982; 106:64–67.

Cytomegalovirus

90. Beschorner WE, Hutchins GM, Burns WH, Saral R, Tutschka PJ, Santos GW. Cytomegalovirus pneumonia in bone marrow transplant recipients: miliary and diffuse patterns. Am Rev Respir Dis 1980; 122:107–114.

91. Ettinger NA, Bailey TC, Trulock EP, et al. Cytomegalovirus infection and pneumonitis - impact after isolated lung transplantation. Am Rev Respir Dis 1993; 147:1017–1023.

92. Wallace JM, Hannah J. Cytomegalovirus pneumonitis in patients with AIDS. Findings in an autopsy series. Chest 1987; 92:198–203.

93. Waxman AB, Goldie SJ, Brettsmith H, Matthay RA. Cytomegalovirus as a primary pulmonary pathogen in AIDS. Chest 1997; 111:128–134.

94. Millar AB, Patou G, Miller RF, et al. Cytomegalovirus in the lungs of patients with AIDS. Respiratory pathogen or passenger? Am Rev Respir Dis 1990; 141:1474–1479.

95. Klatt EC, Shibata D. Cytomegalovirus infection in the acquired immunodeficiency syndrome. Clinical and autopsy findings. Arch Pathol Lab Med 1988; 112:540–544.

96. Grundy JE, Shanley JD, Griffiths PD. Is cytomegalovirus interstitial pneumonitis in transplant recipients an immunopathological condition? Lancet 1987; 2:996–999.

97. Weiss LM, Movahed LA, Berry GJ, Billingham ME. In situ hybridization studies for viral nucleic acids in heart and lung allograft biopsies. Am J Clin Pathol 1990; 93:675–679.

HIV

98. Royal College of Pathologists. HIV and the practice of pathology. 1995.

99. Hofman P, SaintPaul MC, Battaglione V, Michiels JF, Loubiere R. Autopsy findings in the acquired immunodeficiency syndrome (AIDS). A report of 395 cases from the South of France. Pathol Res Pract 1999; 195:209–217.

100. Cury PM, Pulido CF, Furtado VMG, daPalma FMC. Autopsy findings in AIDS patients from a reference hospital in Brazil: Analysis of 92 cases. Pathol Res Pract 2003; 199(12):811–814.

101. Marchevsky A, Rosen MJ, Chrystal G, Kleinerman J. Pulmonary complications of the acquired immunodeficiency syndrome: a clinicopathologic study of 70 cases. Hum Pathol 1985; 16:659–670.

102. Stover DE, White DA, Romano PA, Gellene RA, Robeson WA. Spectrum of pulmonary diseases associated with the acquired immune deficiency syndrome. Am J Med 1985; 78: 429–437.

103. Klatt EC, Nichols L, Noguchi TT. Evolving trends revealed by autopsies of patients with the acquired immunodeficiency syndrome - 565 autopsies in adults with the acquired immunodeficiency syndrome, Los Angeles, Calif, 1992– 1993. Arch Pathol Lab Med 1994; 118:884–890.

104. Afessa B, Green W, Chiao J, Frederick W. Pulmonary complications of HIV infection: Autopsy findings. Chest 1998; 113:1225–1229.

105. Wolff AJ, ODonnell AE. Pulmonary manifestations of HIV infection in the era of highly active antiretroviral therapy. Chest 2001; 120:1888–1893.

106. Joshi VV, Oleske JM, Minnefor AB, et al. Pathologic pulmonary findings in children with the acquired immunodeficiency syndrome: a study of ten cases. Hum Pathol 1985; 16:241–246.

107. Joshi VV, Oleske JM. Pulmonary lesions in children with the acquired immunodeficiency syndrome. A reappraisal based on data in additional cases and follow-up study of previously reported cases. Hum Pathol 1986; l7:641–642.

108. Joshi VV. Pathology of AIDS in children. Pathol Annu 1989; 24(Pt.1):355–381.

109. Moran CA, Suster S, Pavlova Z, Mullick FG, Koss MN. The spectrum of pathological changes in the lung in children with the acquired immunodeficiency syndrome: an autopsy study of 36 cases. Hum Pathol 1994; 25:877–882.

110. Yousem SA, Colby TV, Carrington CB. Follicular bronchitis/bronchiolitis. Hum Pathol 1985; 16:700–706.

111. Itescu S, Brancato LJ, Winchester R. A sicca syndrome in HIV infection: association with HLA-DR5 and CD8 lymphocytosis. Lancet 1989; ii:466–468.

112. Carson PJ, Goldsmith JC. Atypical pulmonary diseases associated with AIDS. Chest 1991; 100:675–677.

113. Murray JF, Mills J. Pulmonary infectious complications of human immunodeficiency virus infection. Am Rev Respir Dis 1990; 1416:1356–1372.

114. Harding CV. Blastomycosis and opportunistic infections in patients with Acquired Immunodeficiency Syndrome - an autopsy study. Arch Pathol Lab Med 1991; 115:1133–1136.

115. Moore JA, Frenkel JK. Respiratory and enteric cryptosporidiosis in humans. Arch Pathol Lab Med 1991; 115:1160–1162.

116. Scaglia M, Sacchi L, Croppo GP, et al. Pulmonary microsporidiosis due to Encephalitozoon hellem in a patient with AIDS. J Infect 1997; 34:119–126.

117. Nichols L, Balogh K, Silverman M. Bacterial infections in the acquired immune deficiency syndrome. Clinicopathologic correlations in a series of autopsy cases. Am J Clin Pathol 1989; 92:787–790.

118. Hirschtick RE, Glassroth J, Jordan MC, et al. Bacterial pneumonia in persons infected with the human immunodeficiency virus. N Engl J Med 1995; 333:845–851.

119. Diaz F, Collazos J, Martinez E, Mayo J. Bronchiolitis obliterans in a patient with HIV infection. Respir Med 1997; 91:171–173.

120. Valor RR, Polnitsky CA, Tanis DJ, Sherter CB. Bacterial tracheitis with upper airway obstruction in a patient with the acquired immunodeficiency syndrome. Am Rev Respir Dis 1992; 146:1598–1599.

121. Brudney K, Dobkin J. Resurgent tuberculosis in New York City – human immunodeficiency virus, homelessness and the decline of tuberculosis control programs. Am Rev Respir Dis 1991; 144:745–749.

122. Hill AR, Premkumar S, Brustein S, et al. Disseminated tuberculosis in the acquired immunodeficiency syndrome era. Am Rev Respir Dis 1991; 144:1164–1170.

123. Dolin PJ, Raviglione MC, Kochi A. Global tuberculosis incidence and mortality during 1990–2000. Bulletin of the World Health Organisation 1994; 72:213–220.

124. Rigsby MO, Curtis AM. Pulmonary disease from nontuberculous mycobacteria in patients with human immunodeficiency virus. Chest 1994; 106:913–919.

125. Schwartz DA, Ogden PO, Blumberg HM, Honig E. Pulmonary malakoplakia in a patient with the acquired immunodeficiency syndrome – differential diagnostic considerations. Arch Pathol Lab Med 1990; 114:1267–1272.

126. Bishopric GA, d'Agay MF, Schlemmer B, Sarfati E, Brocheriou C. Pulmonary pseudotumor due to Corynebacterium equi in a patient with the acquired immunodeficiency syndrome. Thorax 1988; 43:486–487.

127. Foltzer MA, Guiney WB, Wager GC, Alpern HD. Bronchopulmonary bacillary angiomatosis. Chest 1993; 104:973–975.

128. Ruben FL, Talamo TS. Secondary pulmonary alveolar proteinosis occurring in two patients with acquired immune deficiency syndrome. Am J Med 1986; 80:1187–1190.

129. Sehonanda A, Choi YJ, Blum S. Changing patterns of autopsy findings among persons with acquired immunodeficiency syndrome in an inner-city population: a 12-year retrospective study. Arch Pathol Lab Med 1996; 120:459–464.

130. Naccache JM, Antoine M, Wislez M, et al. Sarcoid-like pulmonary disorder in human immunodeficiency virus- infected patients receiving antiretroviral therapy. Am J Respir Crit Care Med 1999; 159:2009–2013.

130a. Shelburne SA, Hamill RJ. The immune reconstitution inflammatory syndrome. AIDS Rev 2003; 5:67–79.

131. Francis ND, Goldin RD, Forster SM, et al. Diagnosis of lung disease in acquired immune deficiency syndrome: biopsy or cytology and implications for management. J Clin Pathol 1987; 40:1269–1273.

132. del Rio C, Guarner J, Honig EG, Slade BA. Sputum examination in the diagnosis of pneumocystis carinii pneumonia in the acquired immunodeficiency syndrome. Arch Pathol Lab Med 1988; 112:1229–1232.

133. Suffredini AF, Ognibene FP, Lack EE, et al. Non-specific interstitial pneumonitis: a common cause of pulmonary disease in the acquired immunodeficiency syndrome. Ann Intern Med 1987; 107:7–13.

134. Colclough AB. Interstitial pneumonia in human immunodeficiency virus infection: a report of a fatal case in childhood. Histopathology 1988; 12:211–219.

135. Ognibene FP, Masur H, Rogers P, et al. Nonspecific interstitial pneumonitis without evidence of pneumocystis carinii in asymptomatic patients infected with human immunodeficiency virus (HIV). Ann Intern Med 1988; 109:874–879.

136. Travis WD, Fox CH, Devaney KO, et al. Lymphoid pneumonitis in 50 adult patients infected with the human immunodeficiency virus – lymphocytic interstitial pneumonitis versus nonspecific interstitial pneumonitis. Hum Pathol 1992; 23:529–541.

137. Griffiths MH, Miller RF, Semple SJG. Interstitial pneumonitis in patients infected with the human immunodeficiency virus. Thorax 1995; 50:1141–1146.

138. Mankowski JL, Carter DL, Spelman JP, et al. Pathogenesis of simian immunodeficiency virus pneumonia: An immunopathological response to virus. Am J Pathol 1998; 153:1123–1130.

139. Fitzpatrick EA, Avdiushko M, Kaplan AM, Cohen DA. Role of virus replication in a murine model of AIDS-associated interstitial pneumonitis. Exp Lung Res 1999; 25:647–661.

140. Fitzpatrick EA, Avdiushko M, Kaplan AM, Cohen DA. Role of T cell subsets in the development of AIDS-associated interstitial pneumonitis in mice. Exp Lung Res 1999; 25:671–687.

141. Coplan NL, Shimony RY, Ioachim HL, et al. Primary pulmonary hypertension associated with human immunodeficiency viral infection. Am J Med 1990; 89:96–99.

142. Speich R, Jenni R, Opravil M, Pfab M, Russi EW. Primary pulmonary hypertension in HIV infection. Chest 1991; 100:1268–1271.

143. Jacques C, Richmond G, Tierney L, Curtis JL, McKerrow J, Warnock ML. Primary pulmonary hypertension and human immunodeficiency virus infection in a non-hemophiliac man. Hum Pathol 1992; 23:191–194.

144. Mette SA, Palevsky HI, Pietra GG, et al. Primary pulmonary hypertension in association with human immunodeficiency virus infection – a possible viral etiology for some forms of hypertensive pulmonary arteriopathy. Am Rev Respir Dis 1992; 145:1196–1200.

145. Cool CD, Kennedy D, Voelkel NF, Tuder RM. Pathogenesis and evolution of plexiform lesions in pulmonary hypertension associated with scleroderma and human immunodeficiency virus infection. Hum Pathol 1997; 28:434–442.

146. Mehta NJ, Khan IA, Mehta RN, Sepkowitz DA. HIV-related pulmonary hypertension - Analytic review of 131 cases. Chest 2000; 118:1133–1141.

147. Orenstein JM, Preble OT, Kind P, Schulof R. The relationship of serum alpha-interferon and ultrastructural markers in HIV-seropositive individuals. Ultrastruct Pathol 1987; 11:673–679.

148. Chetty R. Vasculitides associated with HIV infection. J Clin Pathol 2001; 54:275–278.

149. Aaron SD, Warner E, Edelson JD. Bronchogenic carcinoma in patients seropositive for human immunodeficiency virus. Chest 1994; 106:640–642.

150. Cadranel J, Naccache JM, Wislez M, Mayaud C. Pulmonary malignancies in the immunocompromised patient. Respiration 1999; 66:289–309.

151. Judson MA, Sahn SA. Endobronchial lesions in HIV-infected individuals. Chest 1994; 105:1314–1323.

Chickenpox and herpes zoster

152. Feldman S. Varicella-zoster virus pneumonitis. Chest 1994; 106:S22–S27.

153. Mohsen AH, McKendrick M. Varicella pneumonia in adults. Eur Resp J 2003; 21:886–891.

154. Rice P, Banatvala J, Simmons K, Carr R. Near fatal chickenpox during prednisolone treatment. BMJ 1994; 309:1069–1070.

155. Raider L. Calcification in chickenpox pneumonia. Chest 1971; 60:504–507.

156. Sargent EN, Carson MJ, Reilly ED. Roentgenographic manifestations of varicella pneumonia with postmortem correlation. Am J Roentgenol 1966; 98:305–317.

157. Ellis ME, Neal KR, Webb AK. Is smoking a risk factor for pneumonia in adults with chickenpox? BMJ 1987; 294:1002.

158. Pek S, Gikas PW. Pneumonia due to herpes zoster. Report of a case and review of the literature. Ann Intern Med 1965; 62:350–358.

Hantavirus

159. Duchin JS, Koster FT, Peters CJ, et al. Hantavirus pulmonary syndrome – a clinical description of 17 patients with a newly recognized disease. N Engl J Med 1994; 330:949–955.

160. Butler JC, Peters CJ. Hantaviruses and hantavirus pulmonary syndrome. Clin Infect Dis 1994; 19:387–395.

161. Foucar K, Nolte KB, Feddersen RM, et al. Outbreak of Hantavirus pulmonary syndrome in the southwestern United States. Response of pathologists and other laboratorians. Am J Clin Pathol 1994; 101(Suppl):S1–S5.

162. Zaki SR, Khan AS, Goodman RA, et al. Retrospective diagnosis of hantavirus pulmonary syndrome, 1978–1993: implications for emerging infectious diseases. Arch Pathol Lab Med 1996; 120:134–139.

163. Wells RM, Sosa Estani S, Yadon ZE, et al. An unusual hantavirus outbreak in southern Argentina: person-to-person transmission? Hantavirus Pulmonary Syndrome Study Group for Patagonia. Emerg Infect Dis 1997; 3:171–174.

164. Nolte KB, Feddersen RM, Foucar K, et al. Hantavirus pulmonary syndrome in the United States: a pathological description of a disease caused by a new agent. Hum Pathol 1995; 26:110–120.

165. Zaki SR, Greer PW, Coffield LM, et al. Hantavirus pulmonary syndrome: pathogenesis of an emerging infectious disease. Am J Pathol 1995; 146:552–579.

166. Colby TV, Zaki SR, Feddersen RM, Nolte KB. Hantavirus pulmonary syndrome is distinguishable from acute interstitial pneumonia. Arch Pathol Lab Med 2000; 124:1463–1466.

167. Nolte KB, Foucar K, Richmond JY. Hantaviral biosafety issues in the autopsy room and laboratory: concerns and recommendation. Hum Pathol 1996; 27:1253–1254.

Mycoplasma

168. British Thoracic Society Research Committee. Community acquired pneumonia in adults in British hospitals in 1982–83: a survey of aetiology, mortality, prognostic factors and outcome. Q J Med 1987; 62:195–220.

169. Abele-Horn M, Busch U, Nitschko H, et al. Molecular approaches to diagnosis of pulmonary diseases due to Mycoplasma pneumoniae. J Clin Microbiol 1998; 36:548–551.

170. Templeton KE, Scheltinga SA, Graffelman AW, et al. Comparison and evaluation of real-time PCR, real-time nucleic acid sequence-based amplification, conventional PCR and serology for diagnosis of Mycoplasma pneumoniae. J Clin Microbiol 2003; 41:4366–4371.

171. Collier AM, Clyde WA. Relationships between Mycoplasma pneumoniae and human respiratory epithelium. Diag Radiology 1971; 3:694–701.

172. Rosendal S, Vinther O. Experimental Mycoplasmal pneumonia in dogs: electron microscopy of infected tissue. Acta Path Microbiol Scand Sect B 1977; 85:462–465.

173. Rollins S, Colby T, Clayton F. Open lung biopsy in Mycoplasma pneumoniae pneumonia. Arch Pathol Lab Med 1986; ll0:34–4l.

174. Ebnother M, Schoenenberger RA, Perruchoud AP, Soler M, Gudat F, Dalquen P. Severe bronchiolitis in acute Mycoplasma pneumoniae infection. Virchows Archiv 2001; 439: 818–822.

175. Donat WE, Shepard JAO, Mark EJ, Kalams SA, Doody DP. A 20-year-old man with diffuse pulmonary infiltrates and disseminated intravascular coagulation – Mycoplasma pneumonia, with diffuse alveolar damage and disseminated intravascular coagulation. N Engl J Med 1992; 326:324–336.

Rickettsia

176. Chayakul P, Panich V, Silpapojakul K. Scrub typhus pneumonitis: an entity which is frequently missed. Q J Med 1988; 68:595–602.

177. Walker DH, Crawford CG, Cain BG. Rickettsial infection of the pulmonary microcirculation: the basis for interstitial pneumonitis in Rocky Mountain spotted fever. Hum Pathol 1980; 11:263–272.

178. Samuels MA, Newell KL, Trotman Dickenson B. A 43-year-old woman with rapidly changing pulmonary infiltrates and markedly increased intracranial pressure – Rocky Mountain spotted fever with meningoencephalomyelitis, vasculitis and focal myocarditis. N Engl J Med 1997; 337:1149–1156.

179. Spelman DW. Q fever. A study of 111 consecutive cases. Med J Aust 1959; 1:547–553.

Coxiella

180. Marrie TJ. Coxiella burnetii pneumonia. Eur Resp J 2003; 21:713–719.

181. Leone M, Honstettre A, Lepidi H, et al. Effect of sex on Coxiella burnetii infection: protective role of 17beta-estradiol. J Infect Dis 2004; 189:339–345.

182. Janigan DJ, Marrie TJ. An inflammatory pseudotumor of the lung in Q fever pneumonia. N Engl J Med 1983; 308:86–87.

183. deLlano LAP, Racamonde AV, Bande MJR, Piquer MO, Nieves FB, Feijoo AR. Bronchiolitis obliterans with organizing pneumonia associated with acute Coxiella burnetii infection. Respiration 2001; 68:425–427.

184. Kagawa FT, Wehner JH, Mohindra V. Q fever as a biological weapon. Semin Respir Infect 2003; 18:183–195.

Bacilliary angiomatosis

185. Walford N, Van der Wouw PA, Das PK, Ten Velden JJAM, Hulsebosch HJ. Epithelioid angiomatosis in the acquired immunodeficiency syndrome: morphology and differential diagnosis. Histopathology 1990; 16:83–88.

186. Stoler M, Bonfiglio T, Steigbigel R, Pereira M. An atypical subcutaneous infection associated with acquired immune deficiency virus. Am J Clin Pathol 1993; 80:714–718.

187. Slater LN, Min KW. Polypoid endobronchial lesions – a manifestation of bacillary angiomatosis. Chest 1992; 102:972–974.

188. Finet JF, Abdalsamad I, Bakdach H, Maitre B, Laporte JL, Le Charpentier Y. Intrathoracic localization of bacillary angiomatosis. Histopathology 1996; 28:183–185.

189. Koehler JE, Quinn FD, Berger TG, Leboit PE, Tappero JW. Isolation of Rochalimaea species from cutaneous and osseous lesions of bacillary angiomatosis. N Engl J Med 1992; 327:1625–1631.

190. Leboit PE. In consultation – bacillary angiomatosis. Mod Pathol 1995; 8:218–222.

191. Adal KA, Cockerell CJ, Petri WA. Cat scratch disease, bacillary angiomatosis and other infections due to Rochalimaea. N Engl J Med 1994; 330:1509–1515.

192. Kostianovsky M, Lamy Y, Greco MA. Immunohistochemical and electron microscopic profiles of cutaneous Kaposi's sarcoma and bacillary angiomatosis. Ultrastruct Pathol 1992; 16:629–640.

5

Infectious diseases

5.2

Acute bacterial pneumonia

Acute bacterial infection of the lungs is still one of the commonest causes of death, especially in the young and in the aged, but very often it is merely a terminal event secondary to some other debilitating process. Primary pneumonia is one that develops in a previously healthy individual. While it is still possible to classify pneumonia on the classic basis of its lobar, bronchial (lobular) or interstitial distribution, an aetiological classification facilitates the choice of an appropriate antibiotic and will be followed here as far as possible. Consideration of the clinical situation provides important clues to the likely bacterium responsible (Table 5.2.1) and so aids the initial treatment. Most bacterial pneumonia is endogenous, caused by microorganisms that make up the flora of the pharynx. Cultures taken at autopsy have identified similar bacterial species in lung and pharynx.[1–3]

Of outstanding importance is the Gram-positive diplococcus *Streptococcus pneumoniae*, which is generally known as the pneumococcus. This bacterium is responsible for almost all cases of lobar pneumonia and for most cases of bronchopneumonia. Other varieties of bacteria that may produce pneumonia, almost always in its bronchopneumonic form, include *Staphylococcus aureus*, *Streptococcus pyogenes*, *Haemophilus influenzae* (Pfeiffer's bacillus), *Klebsiella pneumoniae* (Friedlander's bacillus) and *Legionella pneumophila*.

Streptococcus pneumoniae is much the commonest cause of adult cases of community-acquired pneumonia requiring admission to hospital (Table 5.2.2).[4–8] However, the situation is very different in patients who develop pneumonia after admission to hospital (nosocomial pneumonia), in whom Gram-negative enteric bacilli such as *Pseudomonas aeruginosa* and members of the Enterobacteriaceae family (*Escherichia coli*, *Proteus* and *Klebsiella* species) are most commonly responsible.[9–13] This is largely due to the administration of wide spectrum antibiotics. Soon after such antibacterial drugs are administered, the oral flora changes and the upper respiratory tract commonly becomes colonised by bowel organisms.[14,15] In intensive care units, colonisation of the upper respiratory tract is also promoted by measures designed to reduce gastric pH in an attempt to minimise the risk of gastric stress ulceration.[10] This counters an important natural defence mechanism against bacterial growth in the stomach and upper small intestine. Sometimes the lungs are infected by way of the bloodstream and on rare occasions an exogenous source such as a contaminated ventilator has been identified.[16] The mechanisms involved in nosocomial pneumonia are summarised in Figure 5.2.1.

Bacteriological diagnosis is usually made from the direct examination or culture of expectorated sputum. Sputum is prone to be contaminated by upper respiratory tract commensals and bronchoscopic or transcutaneous tracheal aspirates free of this problem have much to commend them. At autopsy, bacterial contamination is unavoidable and microbiological sampling of a consolidated area of lung should be through a surface sterilised by searing with a hot iron rod. A more elegant method entails the *in situ* culture of bacteria in the whole frozen organ using large Petri dishes.[17] By this method bacteria can be matched topographically to foci of consolidation and contaminants recognised as being on the pleural surface of the lung.

BRONCHOPNEUMONIA

Although it has been resolved to follow an aetiological classification as far as possible, many bacteria cause a common mor-

Table 5.2.1 Acute pneumonia: inference of the bacterium responsible from the clinical situation	
Clinical situation	*Likely bacterium*
1 Previously healthy individual	*Streptococcus pneumoniae*
2 Complication of viral infection	*Staphylococcus aureus*
	Streptococcus pneumoniae
3 Chronic bronchitis	*Streptococcus pneumoniae*
	Haemophilus influenzae
4 Cystic fibrosis	*Staphylococcus aureus*
	Haemophilus influenzae
	Pseudomonas aeruginosa
	Burkholderia cepacia
5 Immunosuppression	*Streptococcus pneumoniae*
	Staphylococcus aureus
	Pseudomonas aeruginosa
	Klebsiella pneumoniae
	Anaerobes
6 Hospital inpatient	*Pseudomonas aeruginosa*
	Enterobacteriaceae spp.
	Staphylococcus aureus (often methicillin-resistant)
7 Bronchial tumour	*Streptococcus pneumoniae*
	Staphylococcus aureus
	Anaerobes
8 Aspiration	Anaerobes
9 Alcoholism	*Streptococcus milleri*
	Haemophilus influenzae
	Anaerobes
	Klebsiella pneumoniae

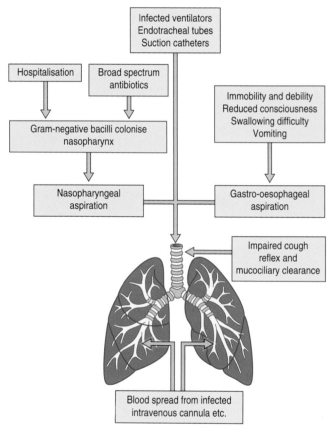

Figure 5.2.1 Mechanisms involved in the development of nosocomial pneumonia. Other risk factors include older age, underlying diseases such as cancer and diabetes mellitus, obesity and cigarette smoking.

Table 5.2.2 Microbial diagnoses (%) in adults admitted to hospital with community-acquired pneumonia					
	UK[4]	*New Zealand*[7]	*Spain*[8]	*Netherlands*[5]	*North America*[a,6]
Streptococcus pneumoniae	34	27	39	20–60	11
Mycoplasma pneumoniae	18	6	16	1–6	4
Viruses	7	8	–	2–15	14
Haemophilus influenzae	6	8	11	3–10	0.4
Chlamydia	3	3	–	4–6	9
Legionella pneumophila	2	2	11	2–8	2
Staphylococcus aureus	1	–	–	3–5	–
Microbiologically negative	33	45	27	–	57
[a]Based on 15 separate reports.					

phological pattern of disease and this will be described before proceeding to specific aetiological agents. This pattern of pneumonia results from the successive infection of conductive airways and is therefore called bronchopneumonia.

Predisposing causes

Bronchopneumonia occurs most frequently in infants, debilitated young children and elderly people and in such patients often proves fatal. The disease is particularly likely to complicate a condition that predisposes to infection by weakening either the local or general defence mechanisms. Local predisposing conditions include other acute infections of the respiratory tract, such as influenza, measles, pertussis and mycoplasma infection and chronic infective conditions such as chronic bronchitis and cystic fibrosis. Bronchopneumonia may also follow inhalation of irritant gases, aspiration of food or vomit and obstruction of a bronchus by a foreign body or tumour.

Bronchopneumonia is also common after surgical operations. The pathogenesis of postoperative bronchopneumonia is complex. Tracheal intubation bypasses the nose, which normally warms and moistens the inspired air, while ether or other irritant vapours may further impair the ciliary defence mechanism of the bronchial tree. The unconscious patient may inhale infected material from the mouth or nose and the temporary depression of the cough reflex may allow micro-organisms to establish themselves in the lungs. Once the effect of the anaesthetic has worn off, the pain associated with movement, particularly of the abdominal wall, may restrict the normal aeration of the lower parts of the lungs. The haemorrhage and shock that may accompany any major surgical operation also result in some general depression of resistance to infection.

Other factors predisposing to bronchopneumonia include generalised metabolic disorders such as diabetes mellitus. Finally, bronchopneumonia is a very common terminal event in patients debilitated by cancer.

Clinical features

The onset of bronchopneumonia is insidious but once established it may have serious effects on respiratory function. The filling of many air spaces with exudate excludes air from much of the lungs and may lead to serious peripheral hypoxia. Healing is slow and the patient's temperature, which is seldom as high as in lobar pneumonia, subsides only gradually: resolution is said to be 'by lysis' rather than 'by crisis'.

Pathological features

Bronchopneumonia is characterised by widespread patchy areas of inflammation that begin as a widely dispersed bronchitis and bronchiolitis: focal areas of pneumonia then develop in the centres of the acini. The consolidated areas are generally larger and more numerous in the lower lobes, where they may be several millimetres across. In the freshly cut lung they are commonly seen as pale, solid, centriacinar foci, often somewhat raised above the surface of the surrounding lung substance (Fig. 5.2.2). These consolidated areas can be felt as well as seen. Small

beads of yellow mucopus can often be expressed from the bronchioles on the cut surface of the lung. In severe cases, the patches of consolidation may become confluent but even when this happens the affected area seldom presents the uniformity of texture and colour that is characteristic of lobar pneumonia, in which all parts of the lobe are involved almost simultaneously.

Once the organisms are established in the small bronchioles, they spread partly by the aspiration of pus and partly by penetrating the inflamed bronchiolar walls. When the bacteria reach the alveoli they excite an acute inflammation, with copious exudation of fluid and migration of neutrophils into the alveoli (Fig. 5.2.3). The airspaces nearest to the bronchioles show the most advanced degree of inflammation; those at a greater distance may be filled merely with fluid exudate.

The point at which neutrophils interact with the pulmonary vasculature is unusual. In contrast to other tissues where neutrophil migration takes place in post-capillary venules, in the lungs neutrophils leave the circulation through the thin walls of the alveolar capillaries, a difference that may serve to localise the inflammation to the alveoli.[18]

When recovery from bronchopneumonia takes place the exudate liquefies and is expectorated or absorbed and

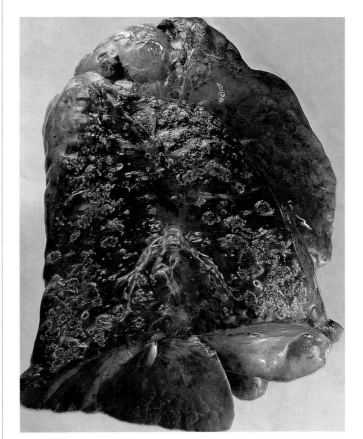

Figure 5.2.2 Bronchopneumonia. There are focal areas of pale consolidation surrounding small airways.

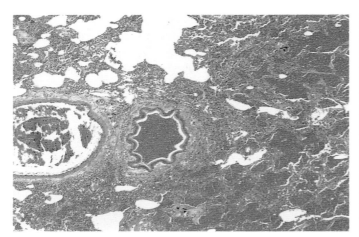

Figure 5.2.3 Bronchopneumonia. Pus fills a bronchiole (centre) and some of the adjacent alveoli.

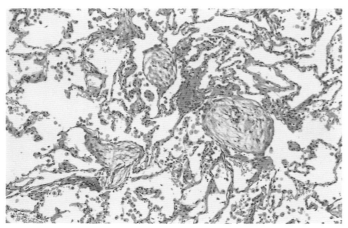

Figure 5.2.4 Organising pneumonia. Micropolypoid buds of pale, myxoid, granulation tissue (Masson bodies) are seen in three alveoli.

respiratory function is restored. However, healing by fibrosis rather than resolution is commoner in bronchopneumonia than in lobar pneumonia. Bronchopneumonia healing by fibrosis is the commonest cause of organising pneumonia. It takes the form of granulation tissue polyps, which are often known as 'Masson bodies', protruding into the alveoli and bronchioles (Fig. 5.2.4).

PNEUMOCOCCAL PNEUMONIA

In 1880, Sternberg and Pasteur independently recovered pneumococci from saliva of ill patients[19,20] and it was soon recognised that this bacterium was an important cause of lobar pneumonia. At least 90 types of pneumococcus are distinguished serologically on the basis of antigenic differences between their capsular polysaccharides.[21] Any serological type may be found

from time to time in sputum from normal people and most, if not all, are capable of causing serious disease in man. However, some types are more pathogenic than others. Type 3 is particularly pathogenic and is commonly isolated from patients with acute respiratory illness[22] and pneumococcal bacteraemia.[23] The distribution of the various serotypes differs from country to country and between different age groups but overall type 14 is the most common, particularly in young children, followed by types 4, 1, 6 and 3.[21]

Host resistance is very dependent upon the development of opsonic anticapsular antibodies because the polysaccharide capsule of the pneumococcus impairs phagocytosis. The identification of the serological type of the pneumococcus responsible for each case of pneumonia was of great importance when effective treatment depended on the prompt administration of the appropriate type-specific antiserum but the introduction of sulphonamides and then antibiotics made serum therapy obsolete. Unfortunately, penicillin-resistant strains have now emerged. Serological typing is based on the Quellung reaction, an easily recognisable swelling of the bacterial capsule when the specific antiserum is applied.

Pathogenesis

The widespread distribution of all types of pneumococcus in the throats of healthy people is relevant to the pathogenesis of pneumococcal pneumonia, the development of which must be regarded as attributable to circumstances that sharply lower resistance to a potentially pathogenic strain of pneumococcus that has been carried in the nose or throat, perhaps over a long period. Pneumococcal pneumonia is, essentially, an endogenous infection, due to failure of the natural defences of the respiratory tract to prevent the spread of a potentially pathogenic strain of pneumococcus from the nasopharynx to the lungs, where it causes acute inflammation. Pneumococci may also cause bacteraemia and meningitis.

Although most cases of pneumococcal pneumonia occur sporadically, minor epidemics sometimes occur as a result of the spread of newly introduced pathogenic strains into a community, such as a school or military camp, where personal contacts are especially close. Under these circumstances, a rise in the carrier rate for the responsible type generally precedes the outbreak.

In temperate climates, pneumococcal infections of the lungs, especially in infants and the elderly, are much more common in winter than in summer. Low external temperature probably has the greatest bearing on the seasonal occurrence of pneumonia, partly by impairing the natural defences of the respiratory tract through cold air chilling its mucosa and partly indirectly, by aggravating the overcrowding that occurs in inclement weather. Both these mechanisms also promote viral infections of the respiratory tract that predispose to subsequent pneumococcal infection. The carrier rate for pneumococci in the general population also tends to rise considerably during the winter and thus to increase dispersal of the more pathogenic strains by droplet spread.

An absent or non-functioning spleen (perhaps removed because of trauma or destroyed by sickle cell disease) also predisposes to pneumococcal infection. Other contributory conditions include chronic chest disease, respiratory depressant drugs, debilitating metabolic diseases such as diabetes mellitus, cirrhosis, the nephrotic syndrome, carcinomatosis, immunodeficiency or immunosuppression due to treatment or disease, including HIV infection, and any condition, such as coma, that depresses the cough reflex and so impairs clearance of the respiratory tract.[23] Chronically high risk individuals benefit from a polyvalent vaccine containing purified capsular polysaccharide that is now available.

Pneumococcal infection of the lungs may result in either lobar pneumonia or bronchopneumonia. These two forms of pneumonia differ greatly in their clinical and pathological features but the contributory conditions outlined above underlie both.[24] Whether the pneumonia has a lobar or bronchial distribution appears to depend more on the virulence of the particular serotype than on host defence. However, host factors involving hypersensitivity have been implicated in the development of lobar pneumonia, largely because of the rapidity with which the disease spreads to involve a whole lobe. Bronchopneumonia is dealt with above and only lobar pneumonia will be considered here.

Clinical features

The onset of lobar pneumonia is typically abrupt. The patient feels ill, complains of a sharp pain in the side of the chest that is made worse by deep breathing, coughs up 'rusty' sputum and quickly develops a fever of about 40°C. The respiration is shallow and its rate becomes fast, sometimes reaching 50 or more a minute: the ratio of pulse to respiration may fall from its usual 4:1 to 2:1. Cyanosis usually appears as the disease advances. A leucocytosis of 15–$20 \times 10^9/l$, mainly neutrophils, is frequently found. In many cases, pneumococci can be cultured from the blood during the height of the fever. The patient is delirious and before effective treatment became available the death rate was high. Before the days of chemotherapy, resolution generally began on about the eighth or ninth day of the illness, if the patient survived that long. Quite frequently, the fever fell suddenly, sweating was profuse, respiration became deeper and less rapid, the delirium abated and the temperature quickly returned to normal. The healing was said to be 'by crisis', as opposed to the gradual abatement of symptoms seen in bronchopneumonia, which was described as healing 'by lysis'. This rapid recovery followed the appearance of specific antibodies against the pneumococcus responsible.

Structural changes in the lungs

As the name lobar pneumonia implies, it is usual for the typical changes to be uniform throughout the affected lobe. Sometimes two or even three lobes may be involved simultaneously or after brief intervals, in which case, 2 or 3 days may separate the onset of involvement of the different lobes. The lower lobes are most commonly affected; there is no significant difference in the frequency of involvement of the two lungs. Before the introduction of effective treatment, the morphological alterations in the lungs generally followed a classic sequence which, following Laennec's original description, comprised four stages:

1. congestion
2. red hepatisation
3. grey hepatisation
4. resolution.

It should be realised that these terms apply to typical appearances and that each stage shades into the next. Antibiotic treatment has curtailed and modified the natural course of lobar pneumonia and reduced both its incidence and its mortality so that the classic morbid anatomical appearances are now rare.

Congestion

The stage of congestion generally lasts less than 24 h. It is exceptional for patients to die so early in the disease, but when such cases are seen at necropsy, the affected lobe is more or less uniformly involved and appears disproportionately large in comparison with the other lobes, which collapse in the usual way when the pleural sacs are opened. The pneumonic lobe is heavy and congested with blood. A blood-stained, frothy fluid oozes freely from the cut surface.

Histological examination shows that alveolar capillaries are much dilated and the air spaces are filled with pale eosinophilic fluid in which there are a few red cells and neutrophils. The uniformity of the appearances throughout the lobe is taken to indicate widespread, rapid dissemination of the bacteria through the pores of Kohn by a flood of oedema fluid. In Gram-stained sections, the paired, lanceolate pneumococci can often be seen, mainly free, in the alveolar fluid. At this stage, little fibrin has formed and the affected lobe has not yet acquired the firm consistence typical of hepatisation.

Red hepatisation

The feature that led Laennec to popularise Morgagni's term 'hepatisation' is the consistency of the affected lobe, which resembles that of the liver. The cut surface of the lung is dry and there is a serofibrinous pleurisy. Small rough tags of fibrin cover much of the visceral pleura of the affected lobe. Congestion persists and the lung remains red.

The changes in the gross features of the affected lobe are readily explained by the histological changes that have taken place during the preceding few hours. The copious fluid exudate, which at the time of its formation contained abundant fibrinogen, has clotted in the alveolar spaces and interlacing strands of fibrin now occupy each airspace and can often be seen connecting with those in neighbouring alveoli through the pores of Kohn. At the same time, more and more neutrophils have migrated from the congested capillaries into the fibrin meshwork. Usually, at this stage, the pneumococci are numerous and many of them have been ingested by neutrophils.

Grey hepatisation

After 2–3 days, the affected lobe gradually loses its red colour and assumes the grey appearance that it retains for the next few days (Fig. 5.2.5). This change in colour, which starts at the hilum and spreads towards the periphery, is brought about by a lessening of the capillary congestion and by the migration of large numbers of leukocytes, at first mainly neutrophils but later macrophages, into the fibrin in the alveoli. An almost complete shutdown of the vasculature of the affected lobe can be demonstrated in radiographs of the lungs after their injection at necropsy with radio-opaque material. The temporary virtual cessation of blood flow through the unventilated lobe lessens the liability to systemic hypoxia that might otherwise develop, a good example of ventilation/perfusion matching (see p. 21).

The cut surface of the lung is now moist as the fibrin has contracted, expelling serum. Toward the end of the stage of grey hepatisation, pneumococci are less numerous and appear in degenerate forms, varying much in size and often no longer Gram-positive.

Resolution

Resolution proceeds in a patchy yet progressive manner by liquefaction of the previously solid, fibrinous constituent of the exudate in the air spaces. Soon the affected lobe becomes more crepitant as the air spaces reopen. Liquefaction of the fibrin is thought to be due to a fibrinolytic enzyme liberated from senescent neutrophils. However, excessive neutrophil breakdown would probably damage the lung and an alternative form of cell death is also utilised, namely apoptosis: apoptotic neutrophils are ingested by macrophages and excessive lysosomal enzyme release is thereby avoided.[25]

The now fluid contents of the alveoli are removed, partly by expectoration but mainly through the lymphatics, resulting in the hilar lymph nodes being soft, moist and swollen. By the end of the stage of resolution, completion of which is shown by chest radiographs to require several weeks, the lung has recovered its normal structure.

Complications

Lobar pneumonia may be complicated by dissemination of the pneumococci throughout the lungs and to other organs. In some patients, acute pneumococcal bronchitis and foci of bronchopneumonia may be present in lobes other than that mainly involved. These accessory lesions, if severe, may exacerbate the disease by further impairing the respiratory exchange in the lungs. In many cases of lobar pneumonia there is a bacteraemia or even septicaemia at the height of the infection. Acute endocarditis may then develop and this is sometimes followed by the formation of an abscess in the brain after lodgement of an infected embolus. Pneumococcal meningitis, peritonitis and arthritis are rarer manifestations of the dissemination of the organisms by the blood.

Although, in patients who recover, the area of lobar consolidation usually resolves completely, several complications may interfere with the healing process. Resolution may be delayed through incomplete digestion of the fibrin in the exudate within the alveoli and organisation, followed by fibrosis ('carnification'), may develop. The fibrosis is essentially intraluminal, taking the form of micropolypoid buds of granulation tissue (Masson bodies) that largely fill alveoli and extend into alveolar ducts and respiratory bronchioles (organising pneumonia), as described above under bronchopneumonia (Fig. 5.2.4). The contracting fibrous tissue may exert traction on the airways, leading to bronchiectasis, which may affect the whole or part of the lobe. Alternatively, part of the affected tissue may break down, especially in cases of infection by pneumococci of serotype 3 and a lung abscess form. On the pleural surface, the serofibrinous exudate may develop into empyema (see Fig. 13.5, p. 696) or be complicated by suppurative pericarditis.

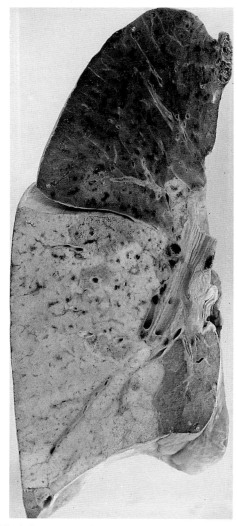

Figure 5.2.5 Lobar pneumonia in the stage of grey hepatisation. The lower lobe is uniformly consolidated.

STAPHYLOCOCCAL PNEUMONIA

Staphylococcal pneumonia is a serious but relatively uncommon disease with a high case fatality rate. It often complicates influenza. The special relationship of staphylococci and influenza virus has been dealt with on p. 153. In children, staphylococcal pneumonia may follow measles or whooping cough. In infants, a primary staphylococcal bronchopneumonia is known, with a case fatality rate as high as 80% in the pre-antibiotic era. The infection is generally endogenous, the bacteria frequently being derived from the patient's skin or nose and the infection air-borne. However, staphylococcal pneumonia or lung abscess sometimes follows bacteraemia or septicaemia,[26] particularly in drug addicts with right-sided bacterial endocarditis.

Although the mortality from most forms of pneumonia has been reduced by modern drugs, many strains of staphylococcus now widely distributed in the population are resistant to the generally used antibiotics. Even relatively new antibiotics such as methicillin are inactive against some of these staphylococci. Such strains periodically become prevalent in hospitals,[13] carried in the nose by staff and patient and fatalities from staphylococcal infection, often with pneumonia, have occurred among surgical patients who otherwise should have recovered from their operation.

At necropsy, the bronchi are acutely inflamed and the lungs contain many bright yellow centrilobular foci of suppuration (Fig. 5.2.6), which in the more advanced cases may have enlarged and coalesced to form abscesses 1 cm or more in diameter. Adjacent air spaces contain a purulent exudate. A superficial abscess may rupture into the pleura and cause empyema, this being a common complication of staphylococcal pneumonia. If the patient survives, there may be permanent damage to the lungs in the form of pulmonary fibrosis, bronchiectasis or large air-filled cysts known as pneumatoceles (Fig. 5.2.7).

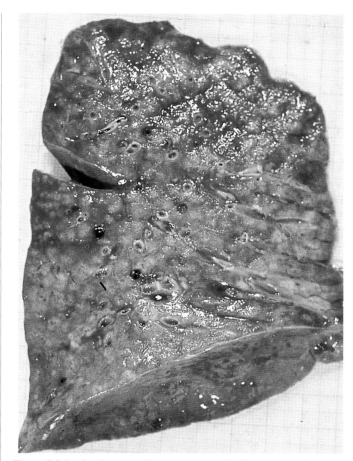

Figure 5.2.6 Staphylococcal bronchopneumonia. The pneumonic foci show early suppuration.

STREPTOCOCCAL PNEUMONIA

In the pre-antibiotic era, up to 5% of all acute pneumonias were caused by group A β-haemolytic streptococci but *Streptococcus pyogenes* is now a rare cause of serious pulmonary infection; nevertheless, occasional cases of streptococcal pneumonia are still encountered,[27] and infective pulmonary embolism is recorded in streptococcal toxic shock.[28] Streptococcal pneumonia typically follows viral infections of the respiratory tract and is thought to have been a prominent bacterial superinfection during the 1919 influenza pandemic. Patients present with abrupt fever, dyspnoea and pleuritic chest pain. They often develop haemoptysis and cynosis. Death may take place within 2–3 days of the onset, in which case the lungs show haemorrhagic oedema and pneumonic consolidation is not well developed. In subacute cases there is bronchopneumonic consolidation, which is characteristically accompanied by early pleural involvement and effusion.

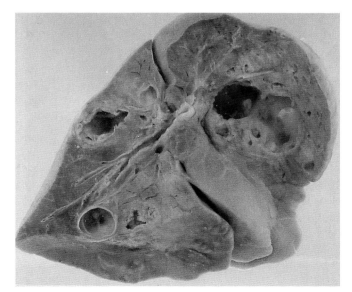

Figure 5.2.7 Pneumatoceles in a child's lung, the consequence of staphylococcal pneumonia.

The anaerobic streptococcus *S. milleri* is now recognised to be an important cause of necrotising lung disease, causing lung abscess and empyema. The patients are often elderly men with periodontal disease, excessive alcohol consumption, malignant disease or recent thoracic surgery.[29]

HAEMOPHILUS PNEUMONIA

The Gram-negative bacillus *Haemophilus influenzae* is a frequent isolate from the upper respiratory tract of healthy individuals and can often be cultured from the sputum of patients with pneumonia due to other organisms, the true pathogen being identified by lung aspiration or blood culture. Occasionally however *H. influenzae* is itself the cause of pneumonia.[30] The patient is often elderly or predisposed to pneumonia by alcoholism or chronic bronchitis. The consolidation may take the form of either lobar pneumonia or bronchopneumonia. The changes in the lung are similar to those in pneumococcal pneumonia (see above) and pleural effusion is common.

BRANHAMELLA PNEUMONIA

The Gram-positive diplococcus *Branhamella catarrhalis*, also known as *Moraxella catarrhalis* and previously as *Neisseria catarrhalis*, is usually a harmless pharyngeal commensal but in the immunodeficient it can cause many serious infections, including pneumonia.[31-33] *Br. catarrhalis* is one of the bacteria that colonise the bronchi in chronic bronchitis and are responsible for acute exacerbations of this disease.[34] Chronic bronchitis and lung cancer both predispose to *Br. catarrhalis* pneumonia.[35-37] Other conditions predisposing to *Br. catarrhalis* infection include old age, heart failure, diabetes mellitus and corticosteroid treatment. The incidence of *Br. catarrhalis* colonisation and infection is highest in winter. The pathological appearances are those of acute bronchitis and bronchopneumonia.

LEGIONELLA PNEUMONIA (LEGIONNAIRES' DISEASE)[38-40]

Aetiology and epidemiology

The legionellae were only discovered after prolonged investigations into the deaths of 34 of some 4500 members of the American Legion attending a convention in a Philadelphia hotel in 1976.[41,42] The investigations took so long because the responsible bacterium, subsequently named *Legionella pneumophila*, is resistant to conventional stains and fastidious in its culture requirements. Once identified, it was possible to recognise retrospectively from stored sera that legionella had been responsible for pneumonia in the past. Sporadic cases were subsequently recognised.[43,44] These are more common than those encountered in epidemic outbreaks but nevertheless only form a small proportion of community acquired pneumonia (Table 5.2.2). In addition to causing pneumonia (legionnaires' disease), legionella is responsible for a less severe, non-pneumonic, acute febrile illness known as Pontiac fever. The term legionellosis embraces both diseases.

Although legionella pneumonia occurs in epidemics, the bacterium is seldom transmitted from person to person. Spread is usually due to atmospheric contamination. It is ironic that a bacterium so hard to grow in the laboratory can succeed so well in air-conditioning plants. These provide the necessary warm, moist conditions that the bacterium requires, drawing it in from the outside, fostering its growth and dispersing it around a building. The contaminated buildings are therefore generally modern, but with neglected engineering plants. Colonisation of the plant by certain free-living amoebae may also promote the growth and survival of legionellae for these bacteria are resistant to amoebic digestion and may survive exposure to disinfectants when the amoeba encysts.[45]

Passers-by as well as those within the building may be infected. In 1985, the 2-year-old Stafford General Hospital in England, was the setting of one of the biggest outbreaks: some 46 people died there of legionnaires' disease, mostly patients rather than staff. It is no coincidence that outbreaks affect hospitals or conventions of ex-servicemen; for the old, the infirm, heavy smokers and those who drink to excess are at particular risk. Hospital acquired infection is particularly likely to affect immunocompromised patients, such as transplant recipients.[44] Also, mixed infections involving legionellae may be more common than previously thought.[46]

Bacteriology

Legionellae are aerobic, 1–2 μm, Gram-negative bacilli that differ from other such bacilli in the fatty acid profile of their cell wall. They fail to grow on standard media and require buffered charcoal yeast extract, which is also useful for isolating nocardia. The number of species has been continually increasing since the original isolation of *L. pneumophila* and now exceeds 50, of which about half are pathogenic to man. In the USA, *L. pneumophila* accounts for about 85% of legionella infections, *L. micadadei* for about 8% and *L. longbeachae* for 1–3%. The legionellae are facultative intracellular organisms that are able to proliferate within phagocytic cells. They are also able to invade and proliferate within alveolar epithelial cells.[47]

Host defence

Humoral mechanisms of defence appear to be limited to opsonic enhancement of phagocytosis. The role of neutrophils is unclear: neutropenic patients are not particularly susceptible to legionnaires' disease but macrophages activated by T-cell lymphokines appear to be more important.[48]

Clinical features

Legionnaires' disease is heralded by a vague prodromal illness that lasts about 5 days. Malaise and muscle pain are followed by rapidly rising fever, rigors, cough, chest pain and dyspnoea. There may also be confusion, diarrhoea and proteinuria. There is usually a moderate leukocytosis. Thus, the clinical features of legionnaires' disease are similar to those encountered in other bacterial pneumonias. The radiographic findings are similarly non-specific but detection of legionella antigen in urine provides a reliable diagnostic test.[49] Macrolides, fluoroquinolones and rifampin (rifampicin) are the most widely used drugs in treatment.

Pathology[38,39,43,50–54]

The gross appearances of the lungs are those of a confluent or multifocal lobular pneumonia with a fibrinous pleurisy and a serosanguineous pleural effusion. If confluent, the boundaries of the consolidation generally fail to match the interlobar fissures (Fig. 5.2.8). There may be abscess formation[55] but this is not typical. A miliary distribution is another atypical manifestation.[56]

Microscopically, airways do not appear to be particularly involved in the inflammatory process, so the disease is not a bronchopneumonia. An acute, leukocytoclastic, fibrinopurulent pneumonia is characteristic (Fig. 5.2.9) but sometimes macrophages are more prominent than neutrophils. The legionellae resist digestion and multiply within the phagocytes, which they eventually destroy so that intense necrosis of the inflammatory cells is often observed. At low magnifications, alveolar walls may be difficult to recognise but even when there is extensive necrosis of the exudate, close inspection, perhaps aided by reticulin stains, shows that the alveolar architecture is generally intact. Occasionally however there are breaks in the alveolar walls or more widespread destruction may be seen. This may be due to vasculitis and thrombosis, which is sometimes evident in small blood vessels.

Demonstration of the organisms is difficult, the fickle and non-specific Dieterle silver impregnation method being the best of the non-immunological techniques used to stain the small cocco-bacilli. Fortunately, the bacterial antigens withstand formalin fixation and routine processing, permitting immunostaining to be applied to paraffin sections.[57] Electron microscopy of the bacteria shows features that are indistinguishable from those of Gram-negative bacilli.[58] In practice, most cases are diagnosed without recourse to pathology.

The hilar lymph nodes are often infected and there is haematogenous dissemination to sites such as the spleen and bone marrow in 27% of cases.[43]

The process generally resolves completely but healing by organisation may be recognised in fatal cases as buds of connective tissue (Masson bodies) in the lumen of alveoli, alveolar ducts and respiratory bronchioles. Such post-pneumonic fibrosis presumably accounts for the permanent impairment of lung function that has frequently been noted in patients who recover.

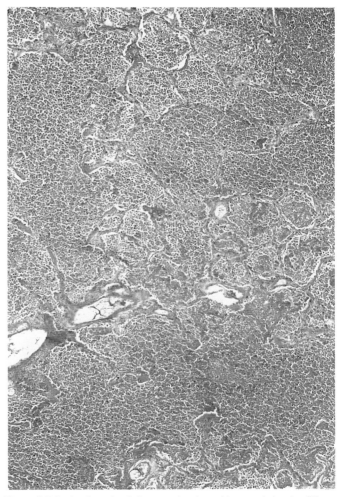

Figure 5.2.9 Legionnaires' disease, showing widespread alveolar filling by fibrin and necrotic neutrophils.

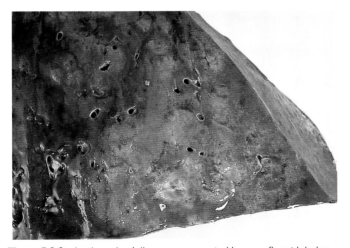

Figure 5.2.8 Legionnaires' disease represented by a confluent lobular pneumonia that does not show the uniform involvement of the affected lobe seen in lobar pneumonia.

KLEBSIELLA PNEUMONIA

Klebsiella pneumoniae (Friedlander's bacillus) is a rare cause of community acquired pneumonia but accounts for a higher proportion of pneumonia acquired in hospital, where patients are more likely to be treated with antibiotics that permit this bacterium to dominate the pharyngeal flora.[59] *K. pneumoniae* is also a particularly common inhabitant of the oral cavity in those with poor dental hygiene and such persons are accordingly at increased risk of klebsiella pneumonia. Alcoholics are also particularly susceptible to klebsiella pneumonia, constituting about half the patients dying of klebsiella infection.[60] Others at particular risk are the elderly and diabetics. The mortality of klebsiella pneumonia is much higher than that of pneumococcal pneumonia, 21% in the general population and 64% in alcoholics.[60,61] Bacteraemia is a particularly adverse prognostic factor.[60]

Klebsiella pneumonia has a predilection for the upper lobes. There is often uniform diffuse consolidation but with only part of the lobe involved, a sharply demarcated edge abutting interlobular septa rather than interlobar fissures: the part of the lobe affected by such consolidation enlarges by the progressive involvement of adjacent lobules (Fig. 5.2.10). The abundant mucoid coat of the klebsiellae gives the pneumonic lesions a distinctively slimy appearance and feel. This material is mucicarminophilic, a characteristic that is often helpful in identifying the infection in histological sections. Klebsiella pneumonia is particularly liable to suppurate and form lung abscesses (Fig. 5.2.11). These may progress to massive pulmonary gangrene.[62] Chronic klebsiella pneumonia may mimic tuberculosis by presenting with cavitating upper lobe disease.

PSEUDOMONAS PNEUMONIA

The species of pseudomonas involved in lung infections is usually *Pseudomonas aeruginosa*, which is the most common bacterium isolated in hospital-acquired pneumonia.[13] Infection may be inhalational or blood-borne. Infection via the airways generally follows colonisation of the pharynx, especially in patients on antibiotics that destroy the normal flora of the upper respiratory tract. As with many bacterial infections, prior viral injury promotes adhesion to the bronchial mucosa[63,64] for it is difficult for *P. aeruginosa* to adhere to normal epithelial cells. Adhesion of the bacteria is dependent upon the transient expression of a sialoganglioside at the apex of the regenerating epithelial cells.[65] Inhalational pseudomonas pneumonia has also developed in patients treated by tracheostomy and mechanical ventilation due to contamination and inadequate disinfection of the ventilators.[16] More recently, several outbreaks in the USA have been attributed to faulty bronchoscopes.[66,67]

Pseudomonas pneumonia is often characterised by well-demarcated pale areas of necrosis, which histologically are composed of an amorphous coagulum containing many bacteria, the nuclear debris of necrotic neutrophils and small numbers of lymphocytes and macrophages.[68,69] Pseudomonas appears to be able not only to resist, but also to destroy neutrophils.[70] It is debatable whether the tissue necrosis is due to bacterial toxins or an immunological response.

Pseudomonas septicaemia may complicate pseudomonas pneumonia or abdominal infection. It results in further changes, notably prominent colonisation of blood vessels. So pronounced is this feature that the vessels exhibit a distinctive blue haze with haematoxylin, or a red one with a Gram stain.[71] The rod-like form of the bacteria is usually readily apparent at high

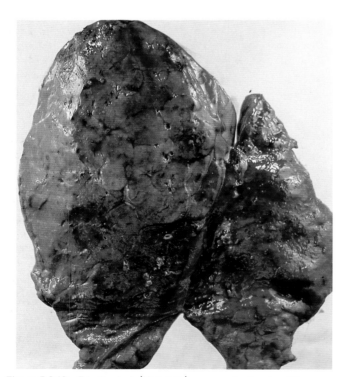

Figure 5.2.10 Friedlander's (*Klebsiella*) pneumonia showing diffuse consolidation of the upper part of the upper lobe. The unaffected lower portion is partly collapsed but the consolidated, airless upper portion has retained its shape.

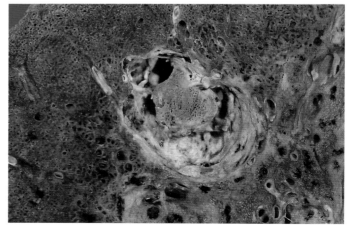

Figure 5.2.11 Abscess formation complicating Friedlander's (*Klebsiella*) pneumonia.

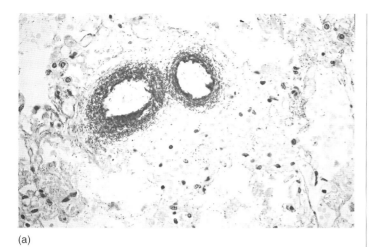

(a)

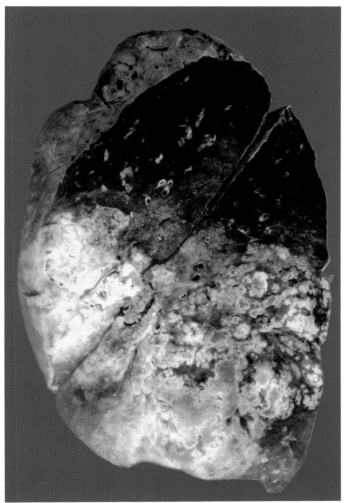

(b)

Figure 5.2.12 Blood-borne *Pseudomonas aeruginosa* pneumonia. (a) A Gram-Sandiford stain shows heavy colonisation of arterial walls by Gram-negative bacilli. (b) The consequent vasculitis has led to extensive infarction of the lower part of the lung.

magnification but the Sandiford modification of the Gram stain is especially useful for demonstrating Gram-negative bacteria in tissue sections (Fig. 5.2.12a).[72] The bacterial colonisation causes a vasculitis with resultant thrombosis and ischaemic necrosis (Fig. 5.2.12b). Such necrotising arteritis is not found in non-bacteraemic pseudomonas pneumonia.[73] Meningitis, arthritis and jaundice are further manifestations of pseudomonas septicaemia. There may also be striking skin lesions, including vesicles and sharply demarcated foci of cellulitis that enlarge rapidly and become haemorrhagic and necrotic.

ACUTE MELIOIDOSIS

Melioidosis is a generalised infection caused by *Burkholderia* (formerly *Pseudomonas*) *pseudomallei*, a Gram-negative bacillus found in watery environments in certain tropical areas, notably south-eastern Asia and northern Australia.[74] However, isolated cases have been described in many other countries.[75,76] The route of infection is most often through the skin but may be through the respiratory tract, when cystic fibrosis appears to be a predisposing factor.[77] Early studies were made during the British occupation of Burma, while French and American servicemen were infected in Vietnam.[78] The prognosis was initially thought to be very poor but improved serological testing indicated that subclinical and mild forms of the disease are common in certain tropical areas.[78] The bacterium may lie dormant in an infected person for many years before causing disease and it is estimated on the basis of high antibody titres that many thousands of American veterans of the Vietnam war are so at risk. Acute and chronic forms are recognised and in both, lesions are commonest in the lungs. Melioidosis is very similar clinically (but not epidemiologically) to the equine disease, glanders, which is caused by infection with *Malleomyces mallei*, with which *B. pseudomallei* shares certain antigenic determinants. (Chronic melioidosis is described on p. 210.)

Acute melioidosis is characterised by the sudden onset of severe diarrhoea, overwhelming pneumonia and septicaemia and if untreated is rapidly fatal. Numerous abscesses are found throughout the body. In chest radiographs these are seen as disseminated nodules.[79] The early lesions take the form of small foci of neutrophils surrounded by haemorrhagic zones. As the abscess enlarges, fibrin becomes more prominent and necrosis ensues. Cases with prominent pulmonary features are characterised by a confluent necrotizing pneumonia which has a bronchitis element that is not evident when there are only discrete abscesses. Vasculitis, a feature of *Ps. aeruginosa* pneumonia, is not seen in melioidosis. Bacilli are generally quite numerous and often form distinct collections within multinucleate macrophages that are scattered amongst the numerous neutrophils.[80] They have been shown to survive and multiply within cells, including neutrophils. The bacteria are most easily identified by the Giemsa stain, which can then be supplemented by a Gram preparation. Staining is strongest at the ends of the bacilli, which therefore have a bipolar appearance that has been likened to that of a closed safety pin.

BURKHOLDERIA CEPACIA PNEUMONIA

Burkholderia cepacia[81] (formerly *Pseudomonas cepacia*) is an important pathogen in cystic fibrosis[82] but is seldom isolated in the immunocompetent. The few reported cases of *B. cepacia* pneumonia have shown necrotizing granulomatous inflammation merging with areas of more conventional necrotising bronchopneumonia, occasionally with necrotising granulomas in the mediastinal lymph nodes.[83]

PNEUMONIC PLAGUE

In man, infection with the Gram-negative bacillus *Yersinia pestis* takes two main forms: bubonic plague, in which the bacillus is transmitted to man by the bite of infected rat fleas and pneumonic plague, in which the organism is usually spread from man to man by infected sputum droplets. Before the era of effective antibiotics both forms had a high case fatality rate; indeed, the plague bacillus has been the cause of some of the most widespread and devastating epidemics in human history.

In the pneumonic form, the lungs show many areas of bronchopneumonia. These are sometimes confluent but the course of the untreated disease is generally too short for massive consolidation to develop. The pulmonary lesions are often haemorrhagic and they are usually accompanied by serofibrinous pleurisy and great enlargement of the hilar lymph nodes. Histologically, the alveolar capillaries are engorged and the air spaces are full of fluid exudate containing few leukocytes but many bacilli. In successfully treated cases, progression to consolidation and rarely cavitation has been noted radiologically.[84]

TULARAEMIC PNEUMONIA

Tularaemia[85] is caused by *Francisella* (formerly *Pasteurella) tularensis*, a Gram-negative coccobacillus that infects many wild animals in North America and to a lesser extent Scandinavia, Japan and elsewhere, including Britain. The bacterium was named after Tulare County in California where human infection was first identified. The infected animals include rabbits, hares, muskrats and ground squirrels. Man is infected when handling these animals or when bitten by ticks that act as vectors of the disease. Direct infection takes place through skin abrasions, mucous membranes, the conjunctivae and less commonly the lungs. The bacterium is highly virulent and its handling poses an extreme hazard to microbiology staff. It is a facultative intracellular pathogen with its primary target being the macrophage.

Pulmonary involvement is usually by septicaemic spread from a lesion in the skin or eyes, via the local lymph nodes, but may be primary. Many patients show neither septicaemia nor pulmonary involvement but in fatal cases the incidence of pneumonia rises to 70%.

At necropsy, the lungs show necrotising bronchiolitis, bronchopneumonia, pleurisy and pleural effusions. The consolidation tends to become confluent and undergo necrosis.[86] The alveoli then contain abundant fibrin and necrotic macrophages, resembling the changes seen in legionella pneumonia. Vasculitis and thrombosis may lead to necrosis of the alveolar walls. The bacteria are difficult to demonstrate in sections with conventional stains but can be identified by immunocytochemistry. Culture is important and the demonstration of a rising titre of antibodies is also helpful in establishing the diagnosis.

ANTHRAX PNEUMONIA (WOOLSORTERS' DISEASE)

Anthrax occurs in many species of domestic animals, especially herbivores. Spores of the causative organism, *Bacillus anthracis*, occasionally infect man, most commonly by skin inoculation, where they cause a 'malignant pustule', least commonly by ingestion, or with devastating effect by inhalation, resulting in 'woolsorters' disease'.

Woolsorters' disease was formerly seen in the Yorkshire textile towns, where it was acquired by inhalation of dust from imported wool contaminated with anthrax spores. Other workers at risk include those exposed to infected hides, hair, bristle, bonemeal and animal carcasses. In one fatal case there was no such industrial contact but the patient had been treating his garden with bonemeal fertiliser.[87] The spores are very resistant to drying but effective measures are now directed to their destruction by exposure of imported materials to antiseptics before they are handled and, as a result, anthrax is now very rare in the UK. In 1979 there was a major epidemic of anthrax resulting in over 60 deaths in a narrow corridor of land downwind of a military establishment near Sverdlovsk, Russia, which was suspected of conducting microbiological warfare research.[88,89] Anthrax spores were also used as a bioweapon by terrorists operating in the USA in 2001; of the 11 people who were infected, five died. Screening procedures and plans to deal with the possibility of similar attacks have subsequently been put in place.[90,91]

If inhaled, the spores are rapidly transmitted to the mediastinal lymph nodes. It is here that the bacilli form and the disease starts. From the lymph nodes the bacilli reach the bloodstream and are distributed in large numbers throughout the body. The septicaemia is often so severe that the organisms are recognisable in films of the circulating blood. Although the lungs may have provided the portal of entry, they are affected secondarily as part of a systemic blood-borne disease.[92,93]

The course of inhalational anthrax is dramatic. Non-specific influenza-like symptoms rapidly progress to cardiopulmonary failure and death within a few days.[94] Necropsy shows haemorrhagic necrosis of the infected tissues. The process is most advanced in the lymph nodes draining the site of primary infection.[89] Thus, in woolsorters' disease a haemorrhagic mediastinal mass is one of the principal findings at necropsy. Other changes commonly encountered at necropsy include a large, dark, soft spleen, haemorrhagic effusions, haemorrhagic intestinal ulceration, haemorrhagic meningitis (which is often limited to the top of the cerebral hemispheres in a so-called 'cardinal's cap'), haemorrhagic bronchitis and widespread, often confluent, areas of haemorrhagic pneumonia. As in other organs, the haemorrhagic inflammatory oedema that constitutes the exudate in the alveoli contains large numbers of the characteristic, large, Gram-positive bacilli, which are readily seen in haematoxylin-eosin preparations.[87,88,93] However, immunohistochemistry is proving more reliable than Gram staining in identifying the bacteria.[90,91]

LEPTOSPIRAL PNEUMONIA

Leptospirosis is a zoonosis of worldwide distribution with many wild and domestic animal reservoirs. Human infection occurs through direct contact with infected animals or, more commonly, through contact with water or soil contaminated with the urine of infected animals. Sewage workers, farmers, animal handlers and veterinarians are at particular risk. Pulmonary disease may be seen in cases of infection by leptospires of various serogroups – they are severest in cases of infection by *Leptospira icterohaemorrhagiae*, which is acquired from rats, but have been a conspicuous feature in a small proportion of cases of canicola fever (infection by *L. canicola*, acquired from dogs) and of infection by *L. bataviae*, which occurs in parts of south-eastern Asia. The spirochaetal leptospires can be demonstrated in the lesions by Levaditi's silver impregnation method, immunocytochemistry or *in situ* hybridisation.

Pulmonary involvement is manifest as cough and haemoptysis in association with patchy consolidation of the lungs. Occasionally, severe pulmonary haemorrhage is the predominant or only manifestation of the infection,[95–97] but provided the disease is recognised and treated early and efficiently, the case fatality rate is low.

The pulmonary lesions are foci of haemorrhagic pneumonia or, in some cases, of simple haemorrhage.[96] In the pneumonic foci, there is a haemorrhagic fibrinous exudate that contains a few neutrophils and occasional macrophages. The exudate is most conspicuous within the alveoli but is seen also in the interalveolar septa, which are correspondingly thickened. Diffuse alveolar damage is occasionally observed. In cases of simple pulmonary haemorrhage, the bleeding is often associated with the profound thrombocytopenia that is an occasional accompaniment of leptospirosis but electron microscopy reveals that there is also profound capillary damage, culminating in endothelial necrosis.[98] A paucity of bacteria near the lesions supports the suggestion that they are due to toxins released elsewhere.[99]

CHLAMYDOPHILA PNEUMONIA (PSITTACOSIS, ORNITHOSIS)

The chlamydophilae, formerly known as the chlamydiae or bedsoniae and once considered to be viruses, are obligate, intracellular organisms, 0.25–0.50 μm diameter, that are now classed as bacteria. The genus includes three species pathogenic for man, *Chlamydophila psittaci*, *C. trachomatis* and *C. pneumoniae*.

C. psittaci pneumonia is contracted from infected birds, particularly parrots imported from South America, where the disease is enzootic. In contrast, *C. trachomatis* is almost exclusively confined to man, causing trachoma, lymphogranuloma venereum and other genital diseases and, in infants, pneumonia, which is usually accompanied by ocular infection.[100,101] *C. pneumoniae* was described as a separate pathogen in 1986 and in some communities is responsible for as many as 10% of pneumonia admissions to hospital,[102–105] although generally causing milder disease than *C. psittaci*.

Organisms similar to *C. psittaci* are found in many species of wild and domesticated birds in various parts of the world and at least some of these are pathogenic for man. For this reason, the more generally applicable name, ornithosis, is more appropriate to this group of diseases rather than psittacosis (parrots' disease). Budgerigars are now the most common source of ornithosis in Britain.[106] Outbreaks have also been associated with ducks, chickens and turkeys.[107,108]

Infected birds, which may show no signs of disease, excrete the organisms in droppings that eventually form a highly infected dust. It is usually through the inhalation of such dust while attending to the birds that man becomes infected, but the disease may also be contracted in poultry processing plants or pillow-filling factories.[107] The infectivity of ornithosis is high and numerous instances have been recorded of nurses and relatives contracting the disease while caring for patients. The disease has also been acquired through exposure to the organism in the laboratory and in the performance of necropsies.

Clinical features

The clinical presentation of ornithosis varies from a mild influenza-like illness to fulminating pneumonia complicated by lesions in other systems. Fulminating cases carry a high mortality. Symptoms usually start within 1–2 weeks of exposure. The organism may be cultured from the patient's blood, but more usually the diagnosis is established by demonstrating a rising titre of complement-fixing antibodies. Cross-reactions with other organisms of the psittacosis-lymphogranuloma-trachoma group occur but should not be confusing in practice. Many patients with ornithosis give a positive skin reaction to Frei (lymphogranuloma venereum) antigen.

Pathology

At necropsy, the lungs are bulky and patchily consolidated. The consolidated areas, which are usually haemorrhagic, are more numerous in the lower lobes than elsewhere. Where they abut the pleura there is local fibrinous pleurisy but pleural effusion is uncommon.

Microscopically, the changes are appropriate to a bacterial rather than to a viral pneumonia, for exudation within the alveoli is more marked than interstitial changes. However, the inflammatory cells are a mixture of those found in bacterial and viral pneumonia, macrophages predominating in the air spaces and a mixed lymphocytic and neutrophil infiltrate being seen in the interstitium. The changes are concentrated on the terminal bronchioles, from which they spread to involve adjacent alveoli and then the whole lobule, by which time there is often necrosis of the bronchiolar and bronchial epithelium.[109] There is engorgement and often thrombosis of capillaries that can result in foci of alveolar necrosis. Later, the alveoli develop a conspicuous lining of swollen epithelial cells. The chlamydiae are just visible with the light microscope as cytoplasmic inclusion bodies (known as Levinthal-Coles-Lillie bodies, LCL bodies, or Levinthal bodies) that range from about 0.25–0.50 μm in diameter. They are to be seen in the cytoplasm of a variable proportion of the alveolar lining cells. They are basophilic and may most easily be found in preparations stained by the prolonged Giemsa method. As with many bacterial pneumonias, healing may be by repair rather than resolution, resulting in organising pneumonia.[110]

C. pneumoniae pneumonia

C. pneumoniae is spread from person to person rather than from birds, infecting both upper and lower respiratory tracts and causing prolonged bronchitis and mild pneumonia of rather non-specific character, somewhat similar to that caused by *Mycoplasma pneumoniae*.[105] Retrospective studies of stored sera have shown that many patients diagnosed as having psittacosis on the basis of a positive serological test were actually infected with *C. pneumoniae*. Antibodies to *C. pneumoniae* have also been identified in many persons who give no history of respiratory disease.[111]

C. pneumoniae infection has a bimodal age distribution, affecting schoolchildren and the elderly. *C. pneumoniae* pneumonia is not fatal and there have consequently been few histopathological studies in man. Experimental studies suggest that the bacterium causes a non-specific acute pneumonia.[105] *C. pneumoniae* has been linked to chronic obstructive lung disease[105,112] and an intriguing relationship between *C. pneumoniae* and atheroma has been identified.[104,113,114]

ASPIRATION PNEUMONIA[115]

Causes of aspiration pneumonia

Aspiration lesions include infective processes such as pneumonia and lung abscess, which are dealt with here and non-infective processes such as exogenous lipid pneumonia and the chemical pneumonias or pulmonary fibrosis that result from the aspiration of gastric acid and other irritants. Aspiration is promoted by loss of consciousness and suppression of the cough reflex, particularly the latter.[116] It is therefore likely to complicate drunkenness, general anaesthesia, cerebrovascular accidents, drug overdosage or other causes of coma. Aspiration is also promoted by dysphagia, whether it be neurological or due to oesophageal diseases such as achalasia, stricture, diverticulum or involvement in systemic sclerosis.[117] Aspiration

pneumonia and lung abscess are also promoted by poor oropharyngeal hygiene: they are rare in the edentulous.

Anatomical location

Aspiration lesions affect the dependent parts of the lungs so that their anatomical location is dictated by the position of the individual when aspiration occurs. Common sites of aspiration pneumonia include the apical segment of the lower lobe (Fig. 5.2.13) and the lateral parts of the basal segments of the upper lobe because gravity carries the aspirated material into these lung segments when the patient is in the prone and lateral positions, respectively.[118] Conversely, the right middle lobe was affected when gasoline was accidentally aspirated when it was being syphoned from a motor vehicle; a procedure that necessitates the person bending forward so that the right middle lobe and the lingula become the most dependent parts of the lungs.[119]

Pathological findings

Aspiration pneumonia is a bronchopneumonia in that the conductive air passages as well as the alveoli are filled with pus

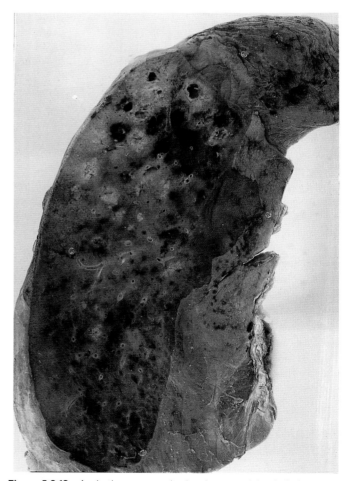

Figure 5.2.13 Aspiration pneumonia showing necrotising foci of consolidation in the apical segment of the lower lobe.

and the consolidation is peribronchiolar. The consolidation is particularly florid, individual foci often being much larger than those encountered in the more usual type of bronchopneumonia. The lesions also tend to undergo necrosis (Fig. 5.2.13). Microscopically, particles of undigested food may sometimes be observed in the pus. These are generally attended by foreign body giant cells (Fig. 5.2.14) and a florid granulomatous reaction may be provoked (Fig. 5.2.15).[120,121] In such cases, the surgeon palpitating the lung at thoracotomy may suspect metastatic carcinoma but the pathologist is more likely to mistake the microscopic changes for a specific infective granulomatous disease, such as miliary tuberculosis, if the aspirated debris goes unrecognised.

Clinical features

Fever, consolidation of the lung and leukocytosis may develop soon after the aspiration. Alternatively, the precipitating episode may not be recognised and the onset of the pneumonia

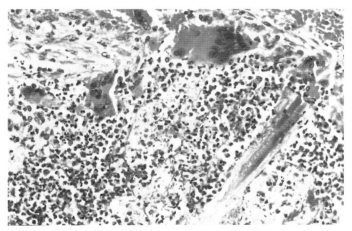

Figure 5.2.14   Aspiration pneumonia showing a bronchiole filled with pus in which there is a spicule of foreign material with attendant foreign body giant cells.

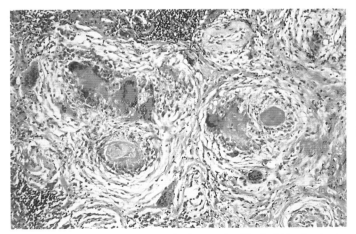

Figure 5.2.15   Aspiration pneumonia characterised by florid foreign body granulomas.

may be insidious. Cavitation and the production of foul purulent sputum are common late manifestations of aspiration pneumonia.

Bacteriology

The bacteria responsible for aspiration pneumonia are the dominant components of the indigenous flora of the upper respiratory tract and mouth. Because of this, specimen contamination bedevils the interpretation of sputum samples. Cultures of blood, pleural fluid or transcutaneous tracheal aspirates are more informative. Facilities for anaerobic culture are essential as anaerobes outnumber aerobes by 10 to 1, as they do in the mouth and pharynx. Mixed infections are the rule, comprising either a variety of different anaerobes or mixed anaerobes and aerobes. The commonest isolates are *Bacteroides melaninogenicus*, *Fusobacterium necrophorum*, anaerobic or microaerophilic cocci and *Bacteroides fragilis*.[122] It is fortunate that all except the last of these are sensitive to penicillin. *Bact. fragilis* is sensitive to the cephamycin, cefoxitin. A predilection for opportunistic mycobacteria to infect lungs containing aspirated lipids, such as those in milk, is referred to on p. 209.

LUNG ABSCESS

An abscess is a focus of suppuration consisting of a collection of pus that is walled off by chronic inflammatory granulation tissue and fibrous tissue. Although abscesses are very familiar lesions, in the lung they are often confused with other pus-filled cavities, particularly those of bronchiectasis. Similarly, when a lung abscess discharges into the air passages, as it is prone to do, the air-filled space that results is often confused with an empty bronchiectatic cavity. Lung abscess and bronchiectasis are fundamentally different diseases. The essential structural difference between them is that several airways communicate with an abscess cavity, whereas if multiple airways are ectatic, they only communicate at their normal branching points (see Fig. 3.34, p. 117). This is because the formation of an abscess entails 'cross-country' destruction of lung tissue, something that is unique to an abscess, regardless of its aetiology.

Spontaneous rupture of an abscess into a bronchus is a likely event and if the patient survives this by coughing up the pus instead of disseminating it throughout the bronchial tree, a marked improvement in his general condition can be expected. With time, the granulation tissue bordering the now empty cavity may become epithelialized. Also, the many airways cut across when the abscess formed may be sealed off by scar tissue. The cavity may then resemble a congenital cyst. A congenital bronchogenic cyst is distinguished by the presence of cartilage and glands in its wall, but a simple congenital cyst may be indistinguishable morphologically from a cavity that started as an abscess. Other congenital cysts have their own special features (see Box 2.2, p. 53).

Sometimes the airways leading into a post-infective cavity only open in inspiration so that they act as check valves. The fibrous wall is then stretched progressively, resulting in a very thin-walled air sac that is often termed a pneumatocele. This process is seen particularly after staphylococcal infection (Fig. 5.2.7). Pneumatoceles resemble emphysematous bullae but, although they are often multiple, the remainder of the lung tissue is generally free of emphysema, something that is unlikely with bullae.

Secondary lung abscess

Abscesses develop in the lungs as a complication of several conditions. Pneumococcal pneumonia was formerly a common cause but pneumonia due to staphylococci, klebsiellae (Fig. 5.2.11) and anaerobic bacteria is now more important in this respect.[123] Local predisposing conditions include bronchial cancer and the presence of a foreign body. Septic embolism and multiple pyaemic abscesses of the lung were formerly common complications of such staphylococcal infections as osteomyelitis and carbuncle but antibiotics have rendered these rare. Still seen on occasion is *necrobacillosis (Lemierre's disease)*, a severe septicaemic illness in which pharyngitis caused by the anaerobe *Fusobacterium necrophorum* is complicated by multiple metastatic abscesses, particularly in the lungs.[124–127]

Primary lung abscess: an aspiration lesion

The development of a secondary lung abscess is easily understood and clearly dependent upon some other underlying disease. On occasion, however, a lung abscess has no apparent cause and is therefore termed primary. The available evidence indicates that primary lung abscesses are nearly always a consequence of the aspiration of infected oropharyngeal secretions. First, there is usually some condition predisposing to aspiration or impairing the cough reflex, for example, alcoholic stupor, general anaesthesia, head injury or neurological disease causing loss of consciousness, dysphagia, or primary oesophageal dysfunction. Second, dental hygiene is usually poor, there often being periodontitis or gingivitis. Third, primary lung abscesses are usually found in the dependent parts of the lungs. They are more common on the right, probably because the right main bronchus is a more direct continuation of the trachea than the left and in the apical segment of the lower lobe and the lateral parts of the basal segments of the upper lobe (Fig. 5.2.16), these being the most dependent parts in the prone and lateral positions respectively (Figs 5.2.17, 5.2.18).[118] Fourth, the bacteria responsible are usually the mixed anaerobes that predominate in the oropharynx, particularly in people with bad teeth (*Fusobacterium*, *Bacteroides* and *Peptostreptococcus* species) and aerobes such as *Streptococcus milleri*.[29,128,129] Thus, primary lung abscess has much in common with aspiration pneumonia and it is for this reason that it is dealt with here, rather than in the chapter on chronic bacterial infection, which its indolent nature would justify. The bacteriology of empyema is similar to that of aspiration pneumonia and primary lung abscess but this condition is dealt with in the chapter on pleural disease.

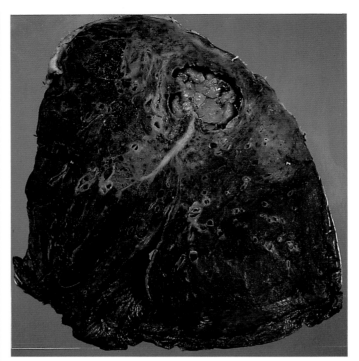

Figure 5.2.16 Primary lung abscess straddling the fissure and involving the lateral parts of the basal segments of the upper lobe and the apical segment of the lower lobe.

BOTRYOMYCOSIS

The term botryomycosis is used to describe colonies of pyogenic bacteria growing within tissues such as the skin, muscle, bone and various viscera, including the lungs. The colonies generally exist within pus-filled cavities and are often enclosed within sheaths of eosinophilic hyaline material (Splendore-Hoeppli reaction – see p. 229). They are indistinguishable from the granules of actinomycosis in sections stained by haematoxylin and eosin but Gram stains show cocci or bacilli rather than filamentous bacteria. The bacteria are viable but the growth of the colonies is slow and there is no invasion of the adjacent tissues. Something approaching a state of balance exists between the body defences and the bacteria.

The size of the bacterial colonies varies (Fig. 5.2.19). They may only be identifiable with the aid of a microscope[130] or they may form visible flecks within the pus, similar to the sulphur granules of actinomycosis. Rarely the colonies are considerably larger, sometimes a single mass of bacteria attaining a size of 5 cm diameter. One such colony simulated an aspergilloma and was called a 'botryomycoma'.[131]

The bacteria involved are often of mixed species but generally include anaerobes such as bacteroides or peptostreptococci.[131] These are normal inhabitants of the pharynx and are generally found in aspiration pneumonia and primary lung

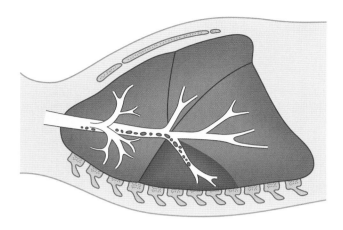

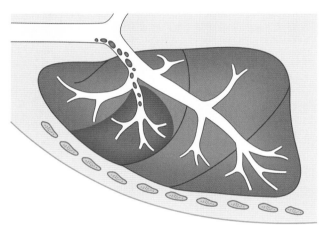

Figure 5.2.17 The effect of posture on the distribution of aspirated material. When the patient is fully supine (above) aspirated material is preferentially distributed by gravity to the apical segment of the lower lobe, whereas when tilted to one side (below) the lateral portions of the anterior and posterior basal segments of the upper lobe are affected. (Redrawn from Brock, Hodgkiss, Jones.[118])

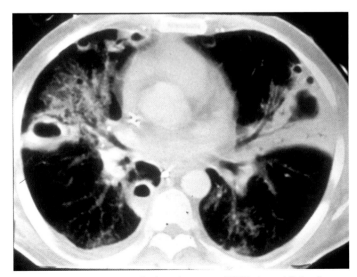

Figure 5.2.18 Bilateral aspiration abscesses. HRCT shows bilateral consolidation and cavitation. Culture grew anaerobic bacteria.

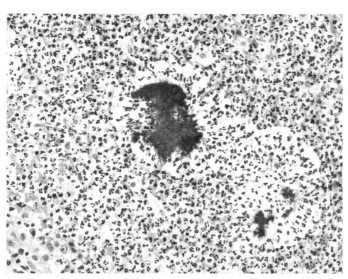

Figure 5.2.19 A case of botryomycosis shows a mixed colony of bacteria within a purulent exudate.

abscess, thus relating botryomycosis to these aspiration lesions. Botryomycosis is also a complication of cystic fibrosis,[132] AIDS[133] and tracheopathia osteochondroplastica.[134]

REFERENCES

1. Smillie WG, Duerschner DR. The epidemiology of terminal bronchopneumonia II. The selectivity of nasopharyngeal bacteria in invasion of the lungs. Am J Hyg 1947; 45:13–18.
2. Kneeland YJr, Price KM. Antibiotics and terminal pneumonia: a postmortem microbiological study. Am J Med 1960; 29:967–979.
3. Knapp BE, Kent TH. Post-mortem lung cultures. Arch Pathol Lab Med 1968; 85:200–203.
4. British Thoracic Society Research Committee. Community acquired pneumonia in adults in British hospitals in 1982–83: a survey of aetiology, mortality, prognostic factors and outcome. Q J Med 1987; 62:195–220.
5. Bohte R, Vanfurth R, Vandenbroek PJ. Aetiology of community-acquired pneumonia: a prospective study among adults requiring admission to hospital. Thorax 1995; 50:543–547.
6. Bartlett JG, Mundy LM. Current concepts: community-acquired pneumonia. N Engl J Med 1995; 333:1618–1624.
7. Neill AM, Martin IR, Weir R, et al. Community acquired pneumonia: aetiology and usefulness of severity criteria on admission. Thorax 1996; 51:1010–1016.
8. Almirall J, Bolibar I, Vidal J, et al. Epidemiology of community-acquired pneumonia in adults: a population-based study. Eur Resp J 2000; 15:757–763.
9. Heyland D, Mandell LA. Gastric colonization by Gram-negative bacilli and nosocomial pneumonia in the Intensive Care Unit patient – evidence for causation. Chest 1992; 101:187–193.
10. Acourt C, Garrard CS. Nosocomial pneumonia in the Intensive Care Unit – mechanisms and significance. 1. Thorax 1992; 47:465–473.
11. Vincent JL, Bihari DJ, Suter PM, et al. The prevalence of nosocomial infection in intensive care units in Europe. Results of the European Prevalence of Infection in Intensive Care (EPIC) Study. EPIC International Advisory Committee. JAMA 1995; 274:639–644.
12. Lynch JP. Hospital-acquired pneumonia: risk factors, microbiology and treatment. Chest 2001; 119; 373S–384S.

13. Leroy O, Giradie P, Yazdanpanah Y, et al. Hospital-acquired pneumonia: microbiological data and potential adequacy of antimicrobial regimens. Eur Resp J 2002; 20:432–439.
14. Johanson WG, Pierce AK, Sanford JP. Changing pharyngeal bacterial flora of hospitalized patients. N Engl J Med 1969; 281:1137–1140.
15. Craven DE, Steger KA. Epidemiology of nosocomial pneumonia: new perspectives on an old disease. Chest 1995; 108; S1–S16.
16. Phillips I. Pseudomonas aeruginosa respiratory tract infections in patients receiving mechanical ventilation. J Hyg 1967; 65:229–235.
17. Zanen-Lim OG, Zanen HC. Postmortem bacteriology of the lung by printculture of frozen tissue. A technique for in situ culture of microorganisms in whole frozen organs. J Clin Pathol 1980; 33:474–480.
18. Lien DC, Henson PM, Capen RL, et al. Neutrophil kinetics in the pulmonary microcirculation during acute inflammation. Lab Invest 1991; 65:145–159.

Pneumococcus

19. Sternberg GM. A fatal form of septicemia, produced by the injection of human saliva. An experimental research. Bull Nat Board Health USA 1881; 2:781–783.
20. Pasteur L. Sur une maladie nouvelle, provoquee par la salive d'une enfant mort de la rage. Comptes rendus de l'Academie des Sciences 1881; 92:159–165.
21. Kalin M. Pneumococcal serotypes and their clinical relevance. Thorax 1998; 53:159–162.
22. Gould GA, Rhind GB, Morgan AD, Williamson G, Calder MA. Pneumococcal serotypes in sputum isolates during acute respiratory illness in Edinburgh. Thorax 1987; 42:589–592.
23. Gransden WR, Eykyn SJ, Phillips I. Pneumococcal bacteraemia:325 episodes diagnosed at St Thomas's Hospital. BMJ 1985; 290:505–508.
24. Ort S, Ryan JL, Barden G, D'Esopo N. Pneumococcal pneumonia in hospitalized patients. Clinical and radiological presentations. JAMA 1983; 249:214–218.
25. Haslett C. Resolution of acute inflammation and the role of apoptosis in the tissue fate of granulocytes. Clin Sci 1992; 83:639–648.

Staphylococcus

26. Naraqi S, McDonnell G. Hematogenous staphylococcal pneumonia secondary to soft tissue infection. Chest 1981; 79:173–175.

Streptococcus pyogenes

27. McMurray JJ, Fraser DM, Brogan O. Fatal Streptococcus pyogenes pneumonia. J R Soc Med 1987; 80:525–526.
28. Cramer SF, Tomkiewicz ZM. Septic pulmonary thrombosis in streptococcal toxic shock syndrome. Hum Pathol 1995; 26:1157–1160.
29. Wong CA, Donald F, Macfarlane JT. Streptococcus milleri pulmonary disease: a review and clinical description of 25 patients. Thorax 1995; 50:1093–1096.

Haemophilus

30. Barnes DJ, Naraqi S, Igo JD. Haemophilus influenzae pneumonia in Melanesian adults: report of 15 cases. Thorax 1987; 42:889–891.

Branhamella

31. Diamond LA, Lorber B. Branhamella catarrhalis pneumonia and immunoglobulin abnormalities: A new association. Am Rev Respir Dis 1984; 129:876–878.
32. Verghese A, Berk SL. Branhamella-catarrhalis. A microbiologic and clinical update. Am J Med 1990; 88(Suppl.5A):S1–S56.
33. Murphy TF. Branhamella catarrhalis: epidemiological and clinical aspects of a human respiratory tract pathogen. Thorax 1998; 53:124–128.
34. Mannion PT. Sputum microbiology in a district general hospital. The role of Branhamella catarrhalis. Br J Dis Chest 1987; 81:391–396.
35. McLeod DT, Ahmad F, Capewell S, Croughan MJ, Calder MA, Seaton A. Increase in bronchopulmonary infection due to Branhamella catarrhalis. BMJ 1986; 292:1103–1105.

36. Black AJ, Wilson TS. Immunoglobulin G (IgG) serological response to Branhamella catarrhalis in patients with acute bronchopulmonary infections. J Clin Pathol 1988; 41:329–333.
37. Capewell S, McLeod DT, Croughan MJ, Ahmad F, Calder MA, Seaton A. Pneumonia due to Branhamella catarrhalis. Thorax 1988; 43:929–930.

Legionella

38. Winn WC, Myerowitz RL. The pathology of the legionella pneumonias. A review of 74 cases and the literature. Hum Pathol 1981; 12:401–422.
39. Roig J, Domingo C, Morera J. Legionnaires' disease. Chest 1994; 105:1817–1825.
40. Stout JE, Yu VL. Current Concepts: Legionellosis. N Engl J Med 1997; 337:682–687.
41. Fraser DW, Tsai TR, Orenstein W, et al. Legionnaires' disease. Description of an epidemic of pneumonia. N Engl J Med 1977; 297:1189–1197.
42. McDade JE, Shepard CC, Fraser DW, Tsai TR, Redus MA, Dowdle WR. Legionnaires' disease. Isolation of a bacterium and demonstration of its role in other respiratory disease. N Engl J Med 1977; 297:1197–1203.
43. Weisenberger DD, Helms CM, Renner ED. Sporadic legionnaires' disease. A pathologic study of 23 fatal cases. Arch Pathol Lab Med 1981; 105:130–137.
44. England AC, Fraser DW, Plikaytis BD, Tsai TF, Storch G, Broome CV. Sporadic legionellosis in the United States: the first thousand cases. Ann Intern Med 1981; 94:164–170.
45. Barker J, Brown MR, Collier PJ, Farrell I, Gilbert P. Relationship between Legionella pneumophila and Acanthamoeba polyphaga: physiological status and susceptibility to chemical inactivation. Appl Environ Microbiol 1992; 58:2420–2425.
46. Roig J, Sabria M, Pedro-Botet ML. Legionella spp.: community acquired and nosocomial infections. Curr Opin Infect Dis 2003; 16:145–151.
47. Maruta K, Miyamoto H, Hamada T, Ogawa M, Taniguchi H, Yoshida S. Entry and intracellular growth of Legionella dumoffii in alveolar epithelial cells. Am J Respir Crit Care Med 1998; 157:1967–1974.
48. Skerrett SJ, Martin TR. Alveolar macrophage activation in experimental legionellosis. J Immunol 1991; 147:337–345.
49. Sabria M, Campins M. Legionnaires' disease: update on epidemiology and management options. Am J Respir Med 2003; 2:235–243.
50. Blackmon JA, Chandler FW, Cherry WB, et al. Legionellosis. Am J Pathol 1981; 103:429–465.
51. Winn WC, Glavin FL, Perl DP, et al. The pathology of legionnaires' disease. Fourteen fatal cases from the 1977 outbreak in Vermont. Arch Pathol Lab Med 1978; 102:344–350.
52. Blackmon JA, Hicklin MD, Chandler FW. Legionnaires' disease. Pathological and historical aspects of a 'new' disease. Arch Pathol Lab Med 1978; 102:337–343.
53. Lattimer GL, Rachman RA, Scarlato M. Legionnaires' disease pneumonia: histopathologic features and comparison with microbial and chemical pneumonias. Ann Clin Lab Sci 1979; 9:353–361.
54. Hernandez FJ, Kirby BD, Stanley TM, Edelstein PH. Legionnaires' disease. Postmortem pathologic findings of 20 cases. Am J Clin Pathol 1980; 73:488–495.
55. Edwards D, Finlayson DM. Legionnaires' disease causing severe lung abscesses. CMA Journal 1980; 123:524–526.
56. Cluroe AD. Legionnaire's disease mimicking pulmonary miliary tuberculosis in the immunocompromised. Histopathology 1993; 22:73–75.
57. Theaker JM, Tobin OJ, Jones SEC, Kirkpatrick P, Vina MI, Fleming KA. Immunohistological detection of Legionella pneumophila in lung sections. J Clin Pathol 1987; 40:143–146.
58. Chandler FW, Cole RM, Hicklin MD, Blackmon JA, Callaway CS. Ultrastructure of the legionnaires' disease bacterium. A study using transmission electron microscopy. Ann Intern Med 1979; 90:642–647.

Klebsiella

59. Garb JL, Brown RB, Garb JR, Tuthill RW. Differences in etiology of pneumonia in nursing home and community patients. JAMA 1978; 240:2169–2172.

60. Jong GM, Hsiue TR, Chen CR, Chang HY, Chen CW. Rapidly fatal outcome of bacteremic Klebsiella pneumoniae pneumonia in alcoholics. Chest 1995; 107:214–217.

61. Dorff GJ, Rytel MW, Farmer SG, Scanlon G. Etiologies and characteristic features of pneumonias in a municipal hospital. Am J Med Sci 1973; 266:349–358.

62. Schamaun M, von Buren U, Pirozynski W. Ausgedehnte Lungennekrose bei Klebsiellen-Pneumonie (sogenannte massive Gangran der Lunge). Schweiz Med Wochenschr 1980; 110:223–225.

Pseudomonas

63. Philippon S, Streckert HJ, Morgenroth K. Invitro study of the bronchial mucosa during Pseudomonas- aeruginosa infection. Virchows Arch A Pathol Anat Histopathol 1993; 423:39–43.

64. Tsang KWT, Rutman A, Kanthakumar K, et al. Interaction of Pseudomonas aeruginosa with human respiratory mucosa in vitro. Eur Respir J 1994; 7:1746–1753.

65. Debentzmann S, Roger P, Puchelle E. Pseudomonas aeruginosa adherence to remodelling respiratory epithelium. Eur Respir J 1996; 9:2145–2150.

66. Kirschke DL, Jones TF, Craig AS, et al. Pseudomonas aeruginosa and Serratia marcescens contamination associated with a manufacturing defect in bronchoscopes. N Engl J Med 2003; 348:214–220.

67. Srinivasan A, Wolfenden LL, Song XY, et al. An outbreak of Pseudomonas aeruginosa infections associated with flexible bronchoscopes. N Engl J Med 2003; 348:221–227.

68. Fetzer AE, Werner AS, Hagstrom JWC. Pathologic features of pseudomonal pneumonia. Am Rev Respir Dis 1967; 96:1121–1130.

69. Bonifacio SL, Kitterman JA, Ursell PC. Pseudomonas pneumonia in infants: An autopsy study. Hum Pathol 2003; 34(9):929–938.

70. Teplitz C. Pathogenesis of Pseudomonas vasculitis and septic lesions. Arch Pathol 1965; 80:297–307.

71. Barson AJ. Fatal pseudomonas aeruginosa bronchopneumonia in a children's hospital. Arch Dis Child 1971; 46:55–60.

72. Leaver RE, Evans BJ, Corrin B. Identification of Gram-negative bacteria in histological sections using Sandiford's counterstain. J Clin Pathol 1977; 30:290–291.

73. Tillotson JR, Lerner AM. Characteristics of non-bacteremic Pseudomonas pneumonia. Ann Intern Med 1968; 68:295–307.

Acute melioidosis

74. Currie BJ. Melioidosis: an important cause of pneumonia in residents of and travellers returned from endemic regions. Eur Resp J 2003; 22(3):542–550.

75. Barnes PF, Appleman MD, Cosgrove MM. A case of melioidosis originating in North America. Am Rev Respir Dis 1986; 134:170–171.

76. Ip M, Osterberg LG, Chau PY, Raffin TA. Pulmonary melioidosis. Chest 1995; 108:1420–1424.

77. O'Carroll MR, Kidd TJ, Coulter C, et al. Burkholderia pseudomallei: another emerging pathogen in cystic fibrosis. Thorax 2003; 58(12):1087–1091.

78. Piggott JA, Hochholzer L. Human melioidosis. A histopathologic study of acute and chronic melioidosis. Arch Pathol 1970; 90:101–111.

79. Dhiensiri T, Puapairoj S, Susaengrat W. Pulmonary melioidosis: clinical-radiologic correlation in 183 cases in northeastern Thailand. Radiology 1988; 166:711–715.

80. Wong KT, Puthucheary SD, Vadivelu J. The histopathology of human melioidosis. Histopathology 1995; 26:51–55.

Burkholderia cepacia

81. Jones AL, Beveridge TJ, Woods DE. Intracellular survival of Burkholderia pseudomallei. Infect Immun 1996; 64:782–790.

82. Stableforth DE, Smith DL. Pseudomonas cepacia in cystic fibrosis. Thorax 1994; 49:629–630.

83. Belchis DA, Simpson E, Colby T. Histopathologic features of Burkholderia cepacia pneumonia in patients without cystic fibrosis. Modern Pathol 2000; 13(4):369–372.

Pneumonic plague

84. Florman AL, Spencer RR, Sheward S. Multiple lung cavities in a 12-year-old girl with bubonic plague, sepsis and secondary pneumonia. Am J Med 1986; 80:1191–1193.

Tularaemic pneumonia

85. Tarnvik A, Berglund L. Tularaemia. Eur Resp J 2003; 21:361–373.

86. Shapiro DS, Mark EJ, Sabloff B, Perakis C, Demeo DL. A 60-year-old farm worker with bilateral pneumonia. Tularemic pneumonia. N Engl J Med 2000; 342:1430–1438.

Anthrax

87. Severn M. A fatal case of pulmonary anthrax. BMJ 1976; 1:748.

88. Abramova FA, Grinberg LM, Yampolskaya OV, Walker DH. Pathology of inhalational anthrax in 42 cases from the Sverdlovsk outbreak of 1979. Proc Natl Acad Sci USA 1993; 90:2291–2294.

89. Grinberg LM, Abramova FA, Yampolskaya OV, Walker DH, Smith JH. Quantitative pathology of inhalational anthrax I: Quantitative microscopic findings. Modern Pathol 2001; 14(5):482–495.

90. Guarner J, Jernigan JA, Shieh WJ, et al. Pathology and pathogenesis of bioterrorism-related inhalational anthrax. Am J Pathol 2003; 163:701–709.

91. Hupert N, Bearman GM, Mushlin AI, Callahan MA. Accuracy of screening for inhalational anthrax after a bioterrorist attack. Ann Intern Med 2003; 139:337–345.

92. Ross JM. The pathogenesis of anthrax following the administration of spores by the respiratory route. J Path Bact 1957; 73:485–494.

93. Zaucha GM, Pitt MLM, Estep J, Ivins BE, Friedlander AM. The pathology of experimental anthrax in rabbits exposed by inhalation and subcutaneous inoculation. Arch Pathol Lab Med 1998; 122:982–992.

94. Shafazand S, Doyle R, Ruoss S, Weinacker A, Raffin TA. Inhalational anthrax - Epidemiology, diagnosis and management. Chest 1999; 116:1369–1376.

Leptospira

95. Teglia OF, Battagliotti C, Villavicencio RL, Cunha BA. Leptospiral pneumonia. Chest 1995; 108:874–875.

96. Zaki SR, Shieh WJ. Leptospirosis associated with outbreak of acute febrile illness and pulmonary haemorrhage, Nicaragua, 1995. The Epidemic Working Group at Ministry of Health in Nicaragua. Lancet 1996; 347:535–536.

97. Silva JJ, Dalston MO, Carvalho JE, Setubal S, Oliveira JM, Pereira MM. Clinicopathological and immunohistochemical features of the severe pulmonary form of leptospirosis. Rev Soc Bras Med Trop 2002; 35:395–399.

98. Nicodemo AC, Duarte MI, Alves VA, Takakura CF, Santos RT, Nicodemo EL. Lung lesions in human leptospirosis: microscopic, immunohistochemical and ultrastructural features related to thrombocytopenia. Am J Trop Med Hyg 1997; 56:181–187.

99. de Brito T, Bohm GM, Yasuda PH. Vascular damage in acute experimental leptospirosis of the guinea pig. J Pathol 1979; 128:177–182.

Chlamydia

100. Beem MO, Saxon EM. Respiratory tract colonization and a distinctive pneumonia syndrome in infants infected with Chlamydia trachomatis. N Engl J Med 1977; 296:306–310.

101. Harrison HR, Enlish MG, Lee CK, Alexander ER. Chlamydia trachomatis infant pneumonitis. Comparison with matched controls and other infant pneumonitis. N Engl J Med 1978; 298:702–708.

102. Grayston JT, Wang SP, Kuo CC, Campbell LA. Current knowledge on Chlamydia pneumoniae, strain TWAR: an important cause of pneumonia and other acute respiratory diseases. Eur J Clin Microbiol Infect Dis 1989; 8:191–202.

103. Grayston IT, Campbell LA, Kuo C-C, et al. A new respiratory tract pathogen: Chlamydia pneumoniae strain TWAR. J Infect Dis 1990; 161:618–625.

104. Marrie TJ. Chlamydia pneumoniae. Thorax 1993; 48:1–4.

105. Hammerschlag MR. Chlamydia pneumoniae and the lung. Eur Resp J 2000; 16:1001–1007.

106. Grist NR, McLean C. Infections by organisms of psittacosis/lymphogranuloma venereum group in the west of Scotland. BMJ 1964; 2:21–25.

107. Andrews BE, Major R, Palmer SR. Ornithosis in poultry workers. Lancet 1981; i:632–634.

108. Irons JV, Sullivan TD, Rowan J. Outbreak of psittacosis [ornithosis] from working with turkeys or chickens. Am J Public Health 1951; 41:931–937.

109. Sax PE, Trotman-Dickenson B, Klein RS, Mark EJ. Pneumonia and the acute respiratory distress syndrome in a 24–year-old man – Psittacosis, causing the acute respiratory distress syndrome. N Engl J Med 1998; 338:1527–1535.

110. Diehl JL, Gisselbrecht M, Meyer G, Israelbiet D, Sors H. Bronchiolitis obliterans organizing pneumonia associated with chlamydial infection. Eur Respir J 1996; 9:1320–1322.

111. BenYaakov M, Eshel G, Zaksonski L, Lazarovich Z, Boldur I. Prevalence of antibodies to Chlamydia pneumoniae in an Israeli population without clinical evidence of respiratory infection. J Clin Pathol 2002; 55:355–358.

112. Wu L, Skinner SJM, Lambie N, Vuletic JC, Blasi F, Black PN. Immunohistochemical staining for Chlamydia pneumoniae is increased in lung tissue from subjects with chronic obstructive pulmonary disease. Am J Respir Crit Care Med 2000; 162:1148–1151.

113. Jackson LA, Campbell LA, Schmidt RA, et al. Specificity of detection of Chlamydia pneumoniae in cardiovascular atheroma: Evaluation of the innocent bystander hypothesis. Am J Pathol 1997; 150:1785–1790.

114. Shor A, Phillips JI, Ong G, Thomas BJ, Taylor Robinson D. Chlamydia pneumoniae in atheroma: consideration of criteria for causality. J Clin Pathol 1998; 51:812–817.

Aspiration pneumonia

115. Marik PE. Primary care: Aspiration pneumonitis and aspiration pneumonia. N Engl J Med 2001; 344:665–671.

116. Huxley EJ, Viroslav J, Gray WR, Pierce AK. Pharyngeal aspiration in normal adults and patients with depressed consciousness. Am J Med 1978; 64:564–568.

117. Kennedy JH. 'Silent' gastroeosophageal reflux: an important but little known cause of pulmonary complications. Dis Chest 1962; 42:42–45.

118. Brock RC, Hodgkiss F, Jones HO. Bronchial embolism and posture in relation to lung disease. Guy Hosp Rep 1942; 91:131–139.

119. Carlson DH. Right middle lobe aspiration pneumonia following gasoline siphonage. Chest 1981; 80:246–247.

120. Crome L, Valentine JC. Lentil soup inhalation? J Clin Pathol 1962; 5x15:21–25.

121. Matsuse T, Oka T, Kida K, Fukuchi Y. Importance of diffuse aspiration bronchiolitis caused by chronic occult aspiration in the elderly. Chest 1996; 110:1289–1293.

122. Bartlett JG, Gorbach SL, Finegold SM. The bacteriology of aspiration pneumonia. Am J Med 1974; 56:202–207.

123. Penner C, Maycher B, Long R. Pulmonary gangrene. A complication of bacterial pneumonia. Chest 1994; 105:567–573.

Lung abscess

124. Lemiere A. On certain septicaemias due to anaerobic organisms. Lancet 1936; i:701–703.

125. Moore-Gillon J, Lee TH, Eykyn SJ, Phillips I. Necrobacillosis: a forgotten disease. BMJ 1984; 288:1526–1527.

126. Dykhuizen RS, Olson ES, Clive S, Douglas JG. Necrobacillosis (Lemiere's syndrome): a rare cause of necrotizing pneumonia. Eur Respir J 1994; 7:2246–2248.

127. Riordan T, Wilson M. Lemierre's syndrome: more than a historical curiosa. Postgrad Med J 2004; 80:328–334.

128. Bartlett JG, Gorbach SL, Tally FP, Fingold SM. Bacteriology and treatment of primary lung abscess. Am Rev Respir Dis 1974; 109:510–518.

129. Neild JE, Eykyn SJ, Phillips I. Lung abscess and empyema. Q J Med 1985; 57:875–882.

Botryomycosis

130. Multz AS, Cohen R, Azeuta V. Bacterial pseudomycosis: a rare cause of haemoptysis. Eur Respir J 1994; 7:1712–1713.

131. Naidech H, Ruttenberg N, Axelrod R, Fisher MS. Pulmonary botryomycoma. Chest 1976; 70:385–387.

132. Katznelsen D, Vawter GF, Foley GE, Shwachman H. Botryomycosis: a complication in cystic fibrosis. Report of 7 cases. J Pediatr 1964; 65:525–539.

133. Katapadi K, Pujol F, Vuletin JC, Katapadi M, Pachter BR. Pulmonary botryomycosis in a patient with AIDS. Chest 1996; 109:276–278.

134. Shih JY, Hsueh PR, Chang YL, et al. Tracheal botryomycosis in a patient with tracheopathia osteochondroplastica. Thorax 1998; 53:73–75.

5

Infectious diseases

5.3

Chronic bacterial infections

TUBERCULOSIS

Bacteriology

Tuberculosis is caused by certain mycobacteria. In the laboratory, these microbes are difficult to stain and in the body they are difficult to kill. Their comparative resistance to the normal body defences is due to an ability to inhibit phagosome-lysosome fusion, permitting them to survive within the host's phagocytes.[1,2] Their resistance to ordinary stains is attributed to their cell walls being rich in mycolic acid waxes. This necessitates the use of hot concentrated carbol fuchsin for their demonstration, as in the Ziehl-Neelsen stain. Once stained in this way, they are difficult to decolourise, even with strong acids and alcohol, hence references to the acid- and alcohol-fast bacilli. Mycobacteria also show some resistance to formalin: of 138 tissue specimens from autopsy lungs fixed in formalin and showing histological evidence of acid-fast bacilli, 12 grew mycobacteria, including three *Mycobacterium tuberculosis* isolates.[3]

The bacilli are normally scanty in tuberculous tissue and their identification with the Ziehl–Neelsen stain may require tedious examination of many sections.[4] They are easier to identify in rhodamine-auramine stained sections examined by fluorescence microscopy.[5–7] Tissue containing necrotising granulomas is most likely to give positive results whereas specimens showing only non-necrotising granulomas, poorly formed granulomas or acute inflammation are less likely to reveal acid-fast bacilli.[8] Culture is no more likely to identify the mycobacteria than the examination of tissue sections.[8,9] Failure to demonstrate them does not exclude a diagnosis of tuberculosis. The future lies in molecular techniques such as the polymerase chain reaction, which can be adapted for application to paraffin sections.[10,11] The detection of mycobacterial RNA indicates that the bacilli are viable and is therefore preferable to tests for mycobacterial DNA. Molecular techniques are also useful in identifying drug resistance, distinguishing mycobacterial species and identifying specific strains of *M. tuberculosis*.[12,12a,12b]

The mycobacteria that cause tuberculosis in man are sometimes listed as *M. tuberculosis, M. bovis, M. africanum* and *M. microti*, the so-called 'tuberculosis complex', although these four organisms are probably just variants of a single species. The first two correspond to the human and bovine tubercle bacilli while *M. africanum* includes a heterogeneous group of strains, with properties intermediate between the former two, isolated from man in equatorial Africa and from African immigrants in Europe. The features and management of tuberculosis in man caused by these three variants are very similar. *M. microti*, the vole tubercle bacillus, is of attenuated pathogenicity for man and has been used as a vaccine.

M. tuberculosis is largely responsible for the disease and the infection is predominantly pulmonary, acquired through inhalation of this organism into the lungs. Formerly, intestinal tuberculosis, acquired by drinking milk infected with *M. bovis*, was much commoner, but the eradication of mycobacteriosis from cattle and the widespread pasteurisation of milk brought about a virtual disappearance of this form of disease in developed countries.

In addition to the human, bovine and vole types, the term 'tubercle bacillus' includes the avian and the 'cold blooded' types. The avian tubercle bacillus is a distinct species, *M. avium*, while the 'cold blooded' group includes the fish, turtle and frog tubercle bacilli, which are known as *M. marinum, M. chelonei* and *M. fortuitum*, respectively. All these other 'tubercle bacilli' can cause opportunistic infections in man and, together with a number of other opportunistic species, are often referred to as the atypical, anonymous or opportunistic mycobacteria. *M. intracellulare* is no longer distinguished from *M. avium* and the collective *M. avium-intracellulare* is often used. Similarly, reference is sometimes made to *M. fortuitum-chelonei*. The opportunistic mycobacteria are dealt with separately later in this chapter (see p. 209).

Route of infection in pulmonary tuberculosis

In the past, there was much speculation about the possible routes of infection in tuberculosis. Today, there is little doubt that when the lesions are present in the lungs, the infection has taken place as a result of inhalation of tubercle bacilli. That the respiratory tract should be the chief portal of entry is scarcely surprising in view of the great preponderance of the pulmonary form of chronic tuberculosis in man and of the enormous numbers of tubercle bacilli that are eliminated daily in the sputum of most untreated active cases. Those in close contact with such patients are liable to inhale the bacilli and acquire the infection in their lungs. Although the smaller droplets of expectorated sputum, which may remain for many minutes suspended in the air after a cough, are probably the chief vehicle for the transmission of tubercle bacilli, it should be realised that the organisms are resistant to desiccation and that in consequence, dried 'droplet nuclei', or the dust that they ultimately contaminate, may long remain as potential carriers of the infection.

Other routes of infection which may have operated in pulmonary mycobacteriosis in the past include haematogenous dissemination from a primary focus of *M. bovis* infection in the intestine, acquired by drinking infected milk and similar spread from a primary focus in the skin acquired by traumatic inoculation (a rare occupational hazard of pathologists and butchers, hence the old term 'butcher's wart'), but these have never been as important as droplet spread.

Epidemiology

In most developed countries there has been a considerable fall in the incidence of tuberculosis and its mortality over the last 100 years (Fig. 5.3.1). This is attributable to a variety of factors that began to operate among the prosperous classes and subsequently extended to all strata of society. During almost the

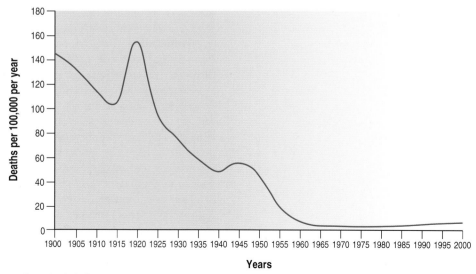

Figure 5.3.1 Deaths from tuberculosis in England and Wales in the twentieth century. The decline in mortality, temporarily checked by two world wars, was established well before specific chemotherapy became available and is largely attributable to improved living standards.

whole of this period, an amelioration in social conditions has been taking place in an almost uninterrupted, unspectacular, manner and it is to these unspecific factors that for many years the progressive fall in mortality was essentially due, although it was aided by public health measures such as the eradication of tuberculous cattle and mass radiography screening. After 1950, the decline in mortality from tuberculosis was hastened by the introduction of effective anti-tuberculosis drugs. By bringing about a great fall in the number (often even the complete disappearance) of bacilli in the sputum in cases of active respiratory tuberculosis, these drugs have much reduced the hazard of infection that was formerly incurred by those who inadvertently or by obligatory associations were brought into contact, at work or at home with an infectious case of the disease.

The reduced incidence of the disease in developed countries led to changes in the ages of the affected patients. Whereas it was formerly a disease of the young, tuberculosis came to be largely limited to the elderly in these countries, the disease representing recrudescence of quiescent infection acquired in youth. Many of these elderly patients suffered from an insidiously progressive form of the disease and this is still the case today (see p. 208).

The situation remained very different elsewhere. Much of the world has still not shared the economic and health benefits enjoyed in the West and in many countries, tuberculosis remains one of the most important specific communicable diseases. Furthermore, the considerable gains that have slowly been achieved are now in peril because of the acquired immune deficiency syndrome and other factors. There has been a resurgence of tuberculosis recently, even in groups where the acquired immune deficiency syndrome has yet to make a major impact, possibly due to new levels of urban deprivation and the influx of immigrants and refugees from countries with a high incidence of the disease.[13,14] In Britain for example, immigrants from the Indian subcontinent have rates of tuberculosis about 25 times as high as that of the white population.[15] The decline in the incidence of tuberculosis in Britain slowed towards 1987 and has subsequently reversed: since that date case numbers have risen, particularly in inner London. The situation is similar in many other developed countries. Tuberculosis can therefore be regarded once more as a worldwide problem. However, there are significant differences between countries. While in Europe (and some of its eastern neighbours) as a whole, the number of notified cases of tuberculosis rose from 242 000 to 382 000 between 1990 and 1999 the incidence is 4.3 per 100 000 in Iceland but 154 per 100 000 in Kazakhstan. Mortality rates show similar variations in relation to economic development. There are therefore major health costs, estimated at 2.1 billion annually, impacting far more on Central and Eastern Europe than the more Western European countries.[16]

In 1990 the World Health Organization undertook a special study to determine the nature and magnitude of the global tuberculosis problem, the findings of which are summarised in Table 5.3.1[17,18] It was found that one-third of the world's population (about 1700 million people) had latent tuberculosis,

caused by *M. tuberculosis* infection. The overall proportion of infected people was similar in the industrialised and developing nations, but 80% of infected individuals in the former were aged 50 years or more, while 75% of those in the latter were less than 50 years old. From this pool, roughly 8 million cases of active tuberculosis emerge annually, 95% of them in the developing countries. The prevalence of the disease is estimated at more than 20 million worldwide and tuberculosis is judged to cause 3 million deaths annually, making it the largest cause of death from a single pathogen in the world. Most of these deaths occur in developing countries, but more than 40 000 deaths are still occurring annually in the industrialised nations. In developing countries, tuberculosis frequently affects children under the age of 15 years but the greatest incidence and mortality is in the economically most productive age group of the population (15–59 years); more than 80% of the tuberculosis toll in the developing world falling on this age group. Furthermore, tuberculosis accounts for 26% of avoidable deaths, killing twice as many adults as AIDS, malaria and other parasitic diseases combined. By 1993 WHO had declared tuberculosis a global emergency.[19,20]

Despite the prevalence of tuberculosis, the human response to infection is good. In the absence of immunosuppressive disorders such as HIV infection, only about 10% of those infected develop clinically evident disease. The basis of these patients' susceptibility is not well understood but tobacco smoking is a predisposing cause[21] and genetic factors may be involved.[22]

The impact of HIV infection

Following the advent of AIDS, the downward trend in tuberculosis stabilised or was reversed.[23,24] An alarming resurgence of the disease is being witnessed, particularly in the poorer communities where drug abuse is prevalent (Table 5.3.1).[17,18,25] Furthermore, multidrug-resistant strains have emerged and now represent a global problem.[26–29] The mortality is high with such strains, even in patients who are not immunodeficient, but it is particularly high in AIDS. Extrapulmonary tuberculosis was initially one of the clinical criteria for the diagnosis of AIDS, but pulmonary tuberculosis is now recognised to be part of the syndrome. Tuberculosis may develop shortly after seroconversion or much later.

It is estimated that worldwide, more than 6 million people are dually infected with the tubercle bacillus and HIV, the majority in 10 sub-Saharan African countries. In these countries, the AIDS epidemic is having a devastating effect on tuberculosis control programmes, with up to 100% increases in reported tuberculosis cases. The annual risk of active tuberculosis in those who are doubly infected is 10%, compared with a 10% lifetime risk in those who harbour the tubercle bacillus but are HIV-negative.[30] The situation in richer countries may not be so bad because HIV infected persons tend to be young and those harbouring tuberculosis old, rendering recrudescence unlikely.[30] However, within HIV units, cross-infection is being reported.[28] Such nosocomial transmission has involved patients and hospital staff who are immunocompetent as well as other HIV positive patients.[31]

Table 5.3.1 The global toll of tuberculosis[17,18]

Region	People infected (millions)	New cases	Deaths	HIV-attributed
Western Pacific[a]	574	2 560 000	890 000	19 000
South-East Asia	426	2 480 000	940 000	66 000
Africa	171	1 400 000	660 000	194 000
Eastern Mediterranean	52	594 000	160 000	9 000
Americas[b]	117	560 000	220 000	20 000
The industrialised countries[c]	382	410 000	40 000	6 000
Total	1 722	8 004 000	2 910 000	315 000

[a]Excluding Japan, Australia and New Zealand
[b]Excluding USA and Canada
[c]Western Europe, USA, Japan, Australia and New Zealand.

The mechanism whereby HIV infection promotes tuberculosis is probably related to the pattern of cytokines produced by T-lymphocyte subsets. T-helper-1 lymphocytes produce interferon-γ and are central to antimycobacterial immune defence. However, when peripheral blood lymphocytes from HIV-infected patients with tuberculosis are exposed to tubercle bacilli *in vitro*, they produce less interferon-γ than lymphocytes from HIV-negative patients with tuberculosis, suggesting that a reduced T-helper-1 response contributes to HIV-infected patients' susceptibility to tuberculosis.[32] It is also noteworthy that there is a reciprocal relationship between tuberculosis and HIV infection: tuberculosis appears to promote the course of HIV infection, probably by inducing macrophages to secrete cytokines that increase HIV replication.[33–35]

Not surprisingly in view of the inter-relationship of HIV and the tubercle bacillus, the tuberculosis associated with HIV infection is particularly aggressive, being characterised by widespread dissemination throughout the body and a poor host response.[36] This non-reactive form of tuberculosis is similar to the insidious disease of elderly patients referred to above and described on p. 208.

Primary and post-primary types of tuberculosis

For many years it has been recognised that although the morbid anatomical changes that develop in tuberculosis assume a variety of forms, the great majority of cases fall into one or other of two distinctive types. The first type was formerly found mainly in children and became known as the 'childhood type' of tuberculosis. Further experience has shown that it is not so much the youth of these patients as the fact that they are infected for the first time that accounts for the distinctive structural features of their lesions. In consequence, this form of tuberculosis is now known as the 'primary type' and as the incidence of the disease in the general population has declined and the age of first infection has correspondingly risen, it is now met with increasing frequency in adults. The second morphological form – previously known as the 'adult type' of the disease – occurs in those patients who have been sensitised by an earlier exposure to tuberculosis; this type of disease is now generally termed 'post-primary tuberculosis'. Post-primary tuberculosis

Table 5.3.2 Summary of patterns of tuberculous infection of the lungs

Primary tuberculosis[a]
  Ghon focus + Regional lymph node = Primary complex
  Reparative
  Quiescent
  Progressive
    Pleural involvement
    Airway dissemination (tuberculous bronchopneumonia, laryngeal lesions)
    Epituberculosis (segmental tuberculosis)
    Haematogenous (miliary tuberculosis, meningitis, solitary lesions in organs with a rich systemic blood supply and therefore a high oxygen tension eg kidney. Also the lung apices because of their high ventilation/perfusion ratio)
Post-primary tuberculosis[a] (reactivation or re-infection)
  Fibrocaseous apical cavitation (high oxygen tension)
  Reparative
  Quiescent
  Progressive
    Local extension
    Pleural involvement
    Airway dissemination (tuberculous bronchopneumonia)
    Haematogenous (miliary tuberculosis)
Non-reactive tuberculosis (Immunocompromised or elderly)

[a]Primary tuberculosis usually heals but if it progresses there is a greater chance of widespread dissemination than in post-primary disease, in which progression is more often local.

is due to either fresh infection or reactivation of a dormant primary lesion. Reinfection is common in countries in which tuberculosis is prevalent but in the developed countries reactivation of infection acquired decades earlier is commoner. The various patterns of tuberculous infection are summarised in Table 5.3.2.

Primary tuberculosis

The very early stages of a tuberculous lesion in the human lung have seldom been seen and our ideas on its pathogenesis have been derived almost wholly from study of lesions in experimental animals.[37] Initially, the presence of tubercle bacilli in an alveolus excites little immediate reaction and for the first day

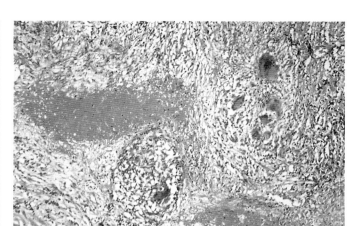

Figure 5.3.3 More advanced tuberculous granulomas showing central coagulative necrosis.

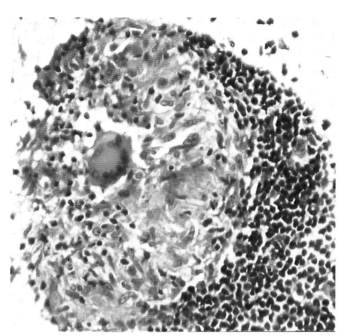

Figure 5.3.2 A tuberculous granuloma consisting of a central collection of epithelioid macrophages surrounded by lymphocytes. A Langhans giant cell is seen among the epithelioid cells.

or two, the only change may be a small amount of exudate and a few neutrophils round the organisms. Within the next few days, macrophages collect in increasing numbers and ingest most of the bacilli.

Gradually, the macrophages, with living bacilli in their cytoplasm, aggregate to form microscopical nodules that deform the alveolar architecture of the surrounding lung. The macrophages develop an abundant eosinophilic cytoplasm and are described as 'epithelioid'. This represents a switch from their basic phagocytic function to a secretory one (see sarcoidosis, p. 287 and Fig. 6.1.32, p. 289), modulated by lymphokines from T lymphocytes, notably interferon-γ.[22,38,39] This change promotes the antibacterial properties of the macrophage but also contributes to tissue necrosis, as outlined below. After about two weeks some of the more centrally placed macrophages fuse to form multinucleate cells of Langhans type. Lymphocytes, variously reported as being predominantly CD4 (helper) or CD8 (cytotoxic), are mixed with the epithelioid and giant cells and outside these there develops a mantle of B lymphocytes.[40–42] Bronchoalveolar lavage shows a raised CD4:CD8 ratio.[43] The localised collection of epithelioid macrophages, Langhans giant cells and lymphocytes constitutes a tuberculous granuloma (Fig. 5.3.2).

By the 3rd week, the granuloma has usually grown sufficiently to be visible to the naked eye as a small, grey nodule, or tubercle, which gives the disease its name. As the tubercle enlarges, its centre turns yellow. Microscopical examination at this stage shows that the granuloma has undergone necrosis (Fig. 5.3.3). By this time a ring of satellite tubercles has developed and as these undergo central necrosis they fuse together. In this way the original granuloma gradually increases in size.

The growth of a tuberculosis lesion by this progressive development and subsequent incorporation of satellite tubercles is also seen in post-primary tuberculosis (see Fig. 5.3.13, p. 207).

It is characteristic of the classic active tuberculous lesions that the tubercle bacilli are scanty, probably reflecting a state of relatively strong immunity/hypersensitivity (see below). Also characteristic of tuberculosis is prolonged survival of the tubercle bacilli within the tissues, despite a vigorous host reaction. This is attributable to the tubercle bacillus inhibiting the fusion of macrophage lysosomes and phagosomes and so avoiding the bactericidal contents of the lysosomes.[1,2]

The type of necrosis found in a classic tuberculous lesion is distinctive, being dry, crumbling and cheesy (hence the term caseous as a macroscopic description). It is of the coagulative rather than liquefactive type, probably because of the relative dearth of polymorphonuclear leukocytes. The necrosis is a hypersensitivity phenomenon; no mycobacterial toxins have been identified. It is brought about by cytotoxic T cells and macrophages activated by subsets of T-helper cells, which are described below.

The elastic tissue of the lung persists for a long time in necrotising tuberculous lesions. When stained appropriately, its distribution and pattern give information about the position of blood vessels and of alveolar walls within the necrotic centre that cannot be recognised clearly, if at all, in haematoxylin-eosin preparations. Ultimately, however, all trace of the lung's elastin framework is lost.

In the comparatively small number of cases in man in which there is an opportunity to examine the lungs while the lesion of primary tuberculosis is still active, the latter – often known as the 'Ghon focus'[44] – is generally visible as a pale yellow, caseous nodule, a few millimetres to 1–2 cm diameter. Characteristically, it is situated in the peripheral part of the lung underlying a localised area of chronic inflammation and thickening of the pleura. Usually, only one such focus is present, but if the lungs are searched carefully, preferably with the help of post-mortem radiography, it will be found that there is more than one focus

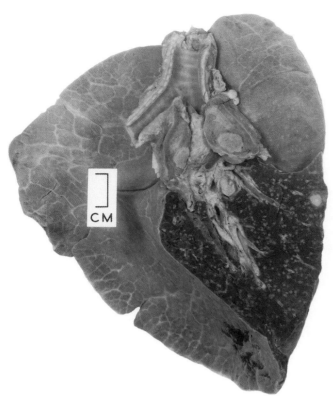

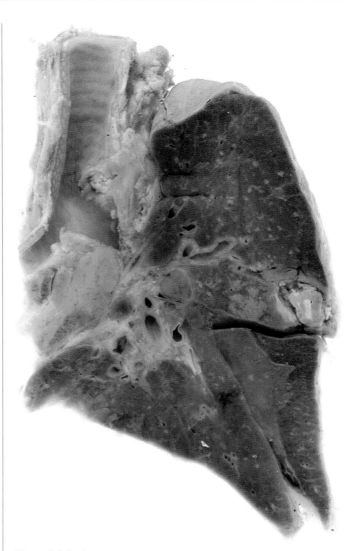

Figure 5.3.4 Primary complex of tuberculosis with miliary spread. A small Ghon focus in the lower lobe of the lung is accompanied by prominent caseating tuberculous lymphadenitis. The infection has spread from one of the lymph nodes into a branch of a pulmonary artery, resulting in miliary haematogenous tuberculosis of the lower lobe. (Reproduced with permission of the Curator of the Pathology Museum, Charing Cross and Westminster Medical School, London, UK.)

Figure 5.3.5 Primary complex of tuberculosis comprising a large caseating Ghon focus and marked enlargement of the infected mediastinal lymph nodes. Tuberculous bronchopneumonia is also seen. A caseating lymph node to the right of the lower end of the trachea has become adherent to the latter and the tuberculous process has extended through the tracheal wall to form a sinus. Aspiration of infective material from this sinus has led to the development of the bronchopneumonia. (Reproduced with permission of the Curator of the Gordon Museum, Guy's Hospital, London, UK.)

in a small proportion of cases. It is a point of importance in the distinction between primary and post-primary tuberculosis of the lungs that in the latter, the lesions are almost invariably in the apical region of an upper lobe, whereas in the former they may be found in any of the five lobes, their frequency there being closely related to the sizes of the lobes.

There is little doubt from studies on primary tuberculosis in both man and experimental animals, that within a few days of their deposition in subpleural alveoli some of the bacilli are carried centripetally in the lymphatics to establish infection in hilar lymph nodes. Thereafter, the granulomatous changes in the lung and lymph nodes and the smaller foci that may have formed along the course of the intrapulmonary lymphatics, all develop at about the same rate but the caseating lesions in the lymph nodes tend to be larger than the primary focus in the lung. This combination of a peripheral Ghon focus with the corresponding focus of caseation in the regional lymph nodes is known as the primary complex of Ranke (Figs 5.3.4, 5.3.5). The complex is the typical result of a primary tuberculous infection of the lungs.

In a small proportion of cases of primary pulmonary tuberculosis, the infection spreads to the pleura, either directly from the primary focus itself or by extension along the lymphatics. The result is often the formation of a pleural effusion. Sometimes this is the presenting manifestation, and occasionally the only clinical evidence, of the disease.

The primary complex may undergo a series of reparative changes, or it may continue to enlarge and in so doing implicate further structures and thus promote dissemination of the infection. The pathological features of healing and progressive primary complexes and the relative frequency of these processes will be considered next.

Reparative changes

The slow enlargement of the caseating primary complex is accompanied by the development of a fibrous capsule. The fibroblasts that take part in this encapsulating fibrosis come to lie more or less circumferentially round the caseous mass. As the weeks pass, they produce collagen fibres and, in time, the more or less spherical mass of caseous matter becomes enclosed by fibrous tissue that impedes further centrifugal dispersal of the bacilli should any still remain alive.

Later, further changes generally take place in these fibro-caseous masses, though the tempo of the reparative process is much diminished. One of these changes is the deposition of calcium salts. Calcium carbonate and phosphate are generally laid down diffusely through the caseous material but some-times, under the microscope, the focal deposition is seen to occur in more or less concentric rings. The rapidity with which calcification takes place varies, but many patients first show radiographic evidence of calcification 12–16 months after recovery from primary pulmonary tuberculosis. Histologically, calcification may be more rapid than this. It has been shown by serial radiography that calcified foci in the lungs and sometimes calcified hilar lymph nodes, occasionally undergo resorption, leaving no trace of their presence. This phenomenon is probably more common than has been appreciated in the past. Alternatively, after a long interval, usually several years, such calcified foci may undergo ossification. This begins at the boundary between the calcified mass and its fibrous envelope. The calcified material is slowly transformed through the complementary activities of osteoclasts and osteoblasts: lamellae of bone are formed within the capsule and eventually take the place of much or all of the originally amorphous, calcified mass. Fatty and sometimes haemopoietic marrow may form within the bone. Diffuse racemose ossification differs from this common dystrophic calcification and ossification but has also been reported in association with pulmonary tuberculosis.[45]

These old foci of caseous necrosis, walled off by fibrous tissue, may contain viable bacilli, despite an absence of inflammation. Such latent lesions, which are known as quiescent tuberculosis, are potential sites of recrudescence. Active disease is denoted by granulomatous inflammation.

Progressive changes

In a small proportion of cases of primary tuberculosis, the reparative changes fail to stem the progress of the disease. As the infected tissues undergo caseation, the bacilli tend to die in the central areas but to survive and multiply in the surviving zone of granulation tissue that borders the lesion, leading to its peripheral extension. As a result of this, a caseous mass, several centimetres in diameter, may form either in the lung itself or in the now much enlarged and generally matted regional lymph nodes. If the lesion erodes into a bronchus, loss of the necrotic material through the airway leads to the creation of a cavity, often of a size a little less than that of the parent caseous mass and surrounded by a ragged lining of partly necrotic tuberculous granulation tissue. If the necrotic focus breaks through the pleura, the result is pleural effusion, pneumothorax, tuber-

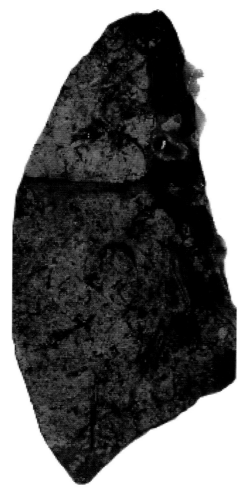

Figure 5.3.6 Tuberculous bronchopneumonia. Almost the whole of the lung shows pale, confluent areas of caseation. (Reproduced with permission of the Curator of the Gordon Museum, Guy's Hospital, London, UK.)

culous empyema or pyopneumothorax. In the last two, the matter in the pleural sac is caseous and not purulent, in spite of the traditional terminology, unless there is a secondary infection by pyogenic organisms.

Dissemination through the airways

When the infected, semifluid, caseous material enters the main respiratory passages, much of it is expectorated but some is dispersed to other parts of the lungs by the deep inspiration that usually accompanies coughing. Such dispersion of large numbers of organisms within the bronchial tree may lead to widespread tuberculous bronchopneumonia ('galloping consumption'), an often fatal condition (Figs 5.3.5 and 5.3.6). Smaller numbers of bacilli may infect the bronchial, tracheal or laryngeal mucosa, or by being swallowed, the intestine. Infection of a bronchus causes ulceration, mucosal thickening or concentric scarring which may be complicated by collapse of the distal lung.

Caseous hilar nodes may compress a bronchus and lead to absorption collapse (see 'middle lobe syndrome', p. 89).[46–48] Partial obstruction may lead to air trapping and severe distension of a lobe, proper ventilation of which may be obtainable only by surgical evacuation of the caseous contents of the nodes responsible. Massive enlargement of paratracheal nodes, particularly those of the right side, may result in compression of the trachea, causing stridor and sometimes cyanosis.

A caseating hilar lymph node may also erupt into a bronchus. Very rarely, so much matter escapes suddenly that the patient, usually a child, is quickly asphyxiated. More often there is progressive change in the affected segment. This is the condition known as epituberculosis.

Epituberculosis (segmental tuberculosis)

Epituberculosis[49] is a fairly frequent radiological finding in cases of primary pulmonary tuberculosis. The radiographic picture is that of a segmental opacity. It is associated with little clinical disturbance and usually resolves completely over a period of months. It was once commonly assumed to represent absorption collapse due to compression of the segmental bronchus by the lymph node component of the primary complex, but this explanation is now recognised to be inadequate in many cases. The great majority of these lesions represent inflammatory consolidation caused by the lymph node component of the complex perforating into the segmental bronchus so that infected caseous material is disseminated throughout the distal air passages.

The affected segment is pale grey and the lobular markings are accentuated by thickening of the interlobular septa. There is exudation of both fluid and macrophages into the alveoli and lymphocytic infiltration of the alveolar walls. That the lesion is not merely a non-specific obstructive pneumonitis is clear from the constant presence of numerous epithelioid cell granulomas. Initially the granulomas are non-necrotising but quite extensive caseation may develop. Tubercle bacilli are to be found in the caseous node but are usually very sparse in the consolidated lung.

The lesion can be reproduced experimentally by introducing either killed tubercle bacilli or the purified protein derivative of tuberculin into previously sensitised animals. The condition is therefore considered to represent a local hypersensitivity reaction to the aspiration of caseous material from the perforated hilar nodes. This is supported by the acceleration of the resolution that is achieved by adding steroids to the usual specific anti-tuberculous drugs and by the dramatic re-appearance of the disease if the steroids are withdrawn.

The outcome of epituberculosis is variable. There may be complete resolution or patchy fibrosis with contracture and perhaps bronchiectasis. The perforation of the bronchus usually heals with only minor scarring, but occasionally it causes fibrous constriction of the bronchus similar to that caused by aerogenous spread to the bronchus from a lesion in the lung, as described above. A rare sequel, comparable in pathogenesis to the traction diverticula of the oesophagus, is the formation of a bronchial diverticulum.

Haematogenous dissemination

Tuberculous bacillaemia is a common early event in primary tuberculosis. Strom provided evidence of this when he used radiolabelled tubercle bacilli to induce the disease experimentally.[50,51] The bacilli are generally destroyed by phagocytes throughout the body but occasional organisms may escape this fate and – after their lodgement in a kidney, bone or joint, the central nervous system, an adrenal gland or some other organ favourable to their growth – set up an isolated focus of tuberculosis that may either remain latent for years or progress. The apices of the lungs are among the tissues that favour the establishment of blood-borne tuberculosis (see below).

When many bacilli enter the circulation simultaneously and a massive haematogenous dissemination ensues, generalised miliary tuberculosis develops. In this condition, as in all forms of bacteraemia, the organisms are removed from the circulating blood by phagocytic cells lining sinusoids in the liver, spleen, bone marrow and elsewhere. Although, to judge from experimental tuberculous bacillaemias, the phagocytes promptly destroy most of the circulating bacilli, enough survive ingestion to set up innumerable small metastatic foci of infection.

The massive bloodstream invasion by tubercle bacilli necessary to produce miliary tuberculosis is often brought about by a caseating tuberculous focus involving the wall of a neighbouring blood vessel. This is particularly likely to complicate the hilar lymph node component of a primary complex, for these caseous masses are not only larger than those in the lungs, but they develop in proximity to the large veins in the mediastinum (Fig. 5.3.4). The wall of the affected blood vessel becomes replaced by tuberculous granulation tissue. In time, caseation develops, the lesion ulcerates through the intima and tubercle bacilli escape into the bloodstream. In exceptional cases, the aorta may be eroded, with consequent rupture and rapidly fatal bleeding. It is not always possible to demonstrate vascular erosion and it seems likely that the organisms may on occasion reach the blood by way of the lymphatics.

Generalised miliary tuberculosis is usually fatal unless treated quickly and appropriately, particularly if the infection has involved the central nervous system and given rise to tuberculous meningitis. Necropsy in cases of miliary tuberculosis shows enormous numbers of small, grey tubercles, a millimetre or less in diameter, most notably in the liver, spleen, bone marrow, lungs and meninges and more sparsely in other organs (Fig. 5.3.7). The term miliary derives from a supposed likeness of the tubercles to millet seeds. The preponderant distribution and typically uniform dispersal of tubercles in the parts affected may be ascribed partly to the particularly large number of phagocytic cells in the walls of the blood sinusoids of the tissues and partly to the situation of the vessel invaded. If it is a systemic vein in the mediastinum, or the main thoracic duct, the bacilli are first carried to the lungs, where many are filtered out in the pulmonary capillaries to give origin to a preponderance of the miliary tubercles in the lungs; if it is a tributary of the pulmonary veins, they are carried to other organs in the systemic arterial circulation.

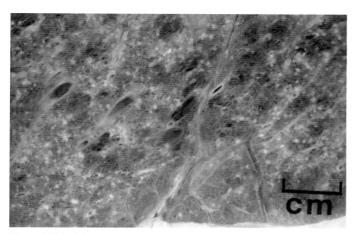

Figure 5.3.7 Miliary tuberculosis. The lung is studded with numerous tubercles, each the size of a millet seed. (Illustration provided by Dr M Kearney, Tromso, Norway.)

Histologically, miliary tubercles have a characteristic structure. A Langhans multinucleate giant cell commonly forms the centre and is enclosed by a zone of epithelioid macrophages and an outer shell of lymphocytes. If the patient survives for a month or more, the tubercles will be larger and their centres yellow because of early caseation. Microscopically, these more advanced lesions consist of small groups of satellite tubercles that have a general resemblance to the original one and surround the central caseous area that has taken its place.

Today, when many of those patients who develop generalised haematogenous dissemination of the infection are successfully treated, the progressive changes in the tubercles in the lungs can sometimes be followed in serial radiographs and the findings compared with those in histological preparations of the lungs of patients who died at the corresponding stage. Gradually, during the weeks following the institution of the treatment, when the clinical manifestations of the disease come to an end, the finely dispersed opacities can be seen to regress until their presence is no longer detectable radiologically. At this stage, microscopical examination of the tubercle shows merely a minute scar composed almost wholly of hyaline collagen with no trace of the former distinctive cellular structure. Should a cure follow at a more advanced stage of the disease, after caseation has occurred, the caseous material becomes calcified. This results in a fine mottling of the lung fields that may be seen radiologically for years after.

Subclinical primary tuberculosis

The true prevalence of tuberculous infection in the general population is very much higher than overt clinical manifestations suggest. This inference is based on two main sources of evidence: first, identification of healed tuberculous lesions in necropsy studies on long series of consecutive cases of patients dying from all causes in large general hospitals; and second, immunological surveys on large samples of the population employing the tuberculin skin test as an indicator of previous infection.

The realisation that primary tuberculosis is followed by recovery in the great majority of those infected was the most important outcome of a pioneer study by Naegeli at the end of the nineteenth century in the post-mortem room of the Zurich General Hospital. Employing acceptable anatomical criteria for the identification of healed and active tuberculous lesions, he reached two very significant conclusions. First, that practically all the adults who had died in that hospital from diseases of all kinds had, at some site in their body, recognisable tuberculous foci that, in the great majority, had healed and second, that in only a minority of these patients could death be attributed to tuberculosis. Some 40 years later, a similar study was made at the same hospital and again traces of a previous tuberculous infection were detected in the bodies of from 80 to 90% of all adult patients.

The interest and surprise aroused by Naegeli's work stimulated numerous similar studies elsewhere. His general conclusions were fully confirmed and it was recognised that signs of past tuberculous infection, notably calcified mediastinal and mesenteric lymph nodes, were common in any population studied. Although in elderly people, the frequency of evidence of such healed infections changed little over the ensuing half-century, in children and young adults it showed a decline that reflected the diminished incidence of clinical tuberculosis in western countries. A much larger fraction of the population than formerly became liable to reach adult life without a primary infection and, as a corollary, also without the valuable, if partial, immunity that results from an infection that has been overcome. Prophylactic immunisation in childhood was therefore instituted and is now widely practised.

The tuberculin skin test

As well as first identifying the tubercle bacillus in 1882, Robert Koch went on to develop a vaccine against the disease based upon the subcutaneous injection of a sterilised extract of the bacteria. It was not successful therapeutically but von Pirquet used Koch's 'Old Tuberculin' as a skin-testing agent after showing that reactivity to it indicates that a person has been infected by the tubercle bacillus. In the original test, a drop of Old Tuberculin was placed on the skin and a scratch was made through the drop, but reagents are now administered by intradermal injection (the Mantoux method) or by use of multiple-pronged devices (Heaf and tine tests). Old Tuberculin has given way to Purified Protein Derivative (PPD) but the principle of the test remains unchanged and it provides a useful indication of the extent of transmission of tuberculosis in countries where tuberculin reactivity has not been artificially induced by BCG vaccination (see below) or heavy exposure to the opportunistic environmental mycobacteria.

The tuberculin skin test becomes positive within a few weeks of tuberculous infection being acquired and remains so in the great majority. Confidence in the reliability and specificity of the test is based mainly upon evidence from two sources. The first comes from surveys made on cattle just before slaughter; the result of the test correlated very closely with the presence or

Table 5.3.3 Comparison by age of positive tuberculin reactors in a sample London population with deaths from tuberculosis for England and Wales in 1931

Age group (years)	Positive reactors (%)	Deaths from tuberculosis (%)
0–5	12	0.076
6–10	30	0.026
11–20	61	0.060

Table 5.3.4 Incidence of clinical tuberculosis among positive and negative reactors to tuberculin in London, 1934–1944[52]

Tuberculin reaction at outset	Number of people examined	Cases of tuberculosis recorded	Incidence (%)
Positive	7130	95	1.33
Negative	1745	69	3.95

absence of tuberculous lesions in the carcass. The second is derived from tests on clinically tuberculous and clinically non-tuberculous children under 5 years of age: 94% of the former and only 12% of the latter, were positive.

Tuberculin surveys have given incontestable support to the general conclusion drawn from necropsy studies that tuberculosis has been widespread in urban populations. In a tuberculin survey in London between the two World Wars, the percentage of positive reactors was found to rise progressively from well below ten in children under 2 years to 90 in adults. Yet despite the great frequency of infection and the large number of deaths from the disease, the case fatality rate – the only numerical indicator of the probable outcome of an infection – is comparatively low. This is exemplified by the figures set out in Table 5.3.3 which shows that even in 1931 only one out of several thousand children who became infected actually died from the disease. A fatal outcome is even less frequent today.

The immunity and hypersensitivity that result from tuberculous infection

The frequency with which a primary tuberculous infection is overcome, usually without the patient being aware of its presence, roused interest in the possibility that in tuberculosis, as in many other infectious diseases, recovery from an attack might leave a heightened resistance to infection in the event of subsequent exposure to the same organism. Further, as some degree of immunity generally results from a natural infection, the question was raised whether similar protection could be conferred by some controllable prophylactic procedure. An affirmative answer has been given to both these questions.

The first study that disclosed convincingly that a primary infection conferred some protection was made by Heimbeck in Oslo. His conclusions were based on studying follow-up records of positive and negative tuberculin reactors among probationer nurses entering the municipal hospital in that city. Through a comparative study of the findings on enrolment and the subsequent medical history while nursing, it became apparent that, although all were equally exposed to the same general hospital environment and its hazards, the incidence of overt tuberculosis was significantly less in those girls who were positive reactors at the time of their entry.

Heimbeck's conclusions have since been scrutinised and confirmed in many studies elsewhere. The most extensive of these – the Prophit Fund Tuberculosis Survey – was carried out on nearly 10000 young people, mainly nurses and medical students, in London over the period from 1934 to 1944.[52] The results of this investigation are summarised in Table 5.3.4, which shows that there was about three times as high an incidence of clinical tuberculosis among young adults who were negative reactors at the start of the study as among similarly exposed positive reactors in London. This is almost the same as the average ratio derived from nearly 30 comparable surveys elsewhere in Europe and in America. It establishes the conclusion that although a primary infection does not confer absolute immunity, it does give a valuable degree of protection against developing the disease in a clinical form after subsequent exposure to the same organism.

Specific prophylactic immunisation

Numerous efforts have been made to confer immunity to tuberculosis through prophylactic inoculation, many by veterinary surgeons who hoped to free cattle from the disease. The most significant conclusion from their work was that, unlike what had been found for many other infectious diseases, killed organisms were relatively impotent as immunising agents. Protection could be conferred only through an infection that had been overcome. In consequence of this, the search for an effective prophylactic agent became one for strains of the bacillus that were of such low natural virulence, or that had been so attenuated by appropriate methods of culture, that they could be inoculated safely while still alive. Such strains, it was hoped, would produce only a self-limiting infection. Of those that have been found, the organism now widely known, after those who developed it, as bacillus Calmette Guérin (BCG) has established itself as the agent of choice and is now widely employed in anti-tuberculosis schemes in many parts of the world. Yet although the effectiveness of BCG has been demonstrated on many occasions (Table 5.3.5), in other studies it appears to have conferred no protection whatsoever.[53] The reason for these marked differences is poorly understood but may be connected with the fact that since its introduction, numerous daughter strains of varying antigenicity have developed, which is not surprising as being a live bacterium it has had to be passaged in vitro over 1000 times.[54] Another possible reason is the variable prevalence of other mycobacteria in the environment as these confer some protection against tuberculosis.

In developing countries, where the prevalence of tuberculosis is high, BCG immunisation of the newborn is recommended to prevent the dangerous forms of childhood tuberculosis, but in Britain, where there is little tuberculosis, BCG is not administered until the age of 10–13 years. However, it is recommended

Table 5.3.5 The protective effect of BCG found in nine major studies[53]

Group studied	Date of commencement	Duration (years)	Age range	Protection (%)
North American Indian	1935–38	9–11	0–20 years	80
Chicago, USA	1937–48	12–23	3 months	75
Georgia, USA	1947	20	6–17 years	0
Illinois, USA	1947–48	19–20	Young adults	0
Puerto Rico	1949–51	5–7.5	1–18 years	31
Georgia/Alabama, USA	1950	14	Over 5 years	14
Great Britain	1950–52	15	14–15 years	78
South India (Bangalore)	1950–55	9–14	All ages	30
South India (Madras)	1969–71	7.5[a]	All ages	0

[a]15-year follow-up has revealed some protection amongst those administered BCG as neonates.

for the Mantoux-negative members of certain high risk groups: health workers including mortuary and laboratory staff, veterinarians, case contacts, immigrants from countries with a high prevalence of tuberculosis together with their children and infants wherever born and those intending to stay in Asia, Africa or central or south America for longer than 1 month.

Although BCG inoculation is generally harmless, disastrous dissemination of the infection has been known to occur.[55] Impaired host immunity may be presumed to account for these rare instances as the dose and batch of the vaccine used in these exceptional cases have not differed from those used successfully in other children. Cases have been reported in the context of AIDS and inherited immunodeficiency states such as severe combined immunodeficiency and chronic granulomatous disease. However, in half the cases reported no well-defined inherited immunodeficiency state has been recognised. Some of these patients have been able to mount a good granulomatous response against the infection but others have developed disease similar to lepromatous leprosy, characterised by florid proliferation of the bacilli and an apparently ineffective non-granulomatous macrophage response.[56] It follows that any form of immunosuppression is a contraindication to BCG immunisation; this includes corticosteroid treatment and HIV infection.

BCG immunisation may confer advantages other than protection against tuberculosis. It has been suggested that children so immunised suffer less leukaemia and other malignancies. However, for the present such claims must be regarded as somewhat tenuous.[57] BCG has also been injected into the pleural cavity or the bladder of patients with inoperable cancer of these regions in the hope that it would have a non-specific adjuvant effect on the immune reaction to the cancer and, as with its use in preventing tuberculosis, there are rare instances of the bacillus being disseminated widely throughout the body.[58]

The relationship of immunity to hypersensitivity in tuberculosis

The pathological characteristics of pulmonary tuberculosis in patients who have had a previous infection by *M. tuberculosis* are different in some important respects from those of a first infection with the tubercle bacillus. Notable differences include the rapid translocation of tubercle bacilli to the regional lymph nodes and perhaps beyond, on first infection, whereas post-primary tuberculosis is less likely to disseminate and the development of caseation at a time when cellular immune mechanisms may be expected to take effect. These differences depend upon both hypersensitivity and immunity acquired as a consequence of a natural primary mycobacterial infection or BCG inoculation. Long ago, Rich showed that guinea pigs made allergic by the injection of non-virulent tubercle bacilli still retained resistance after gradual desensitisation with tuberculin, suggesting that hypersensitivity and immunity were distinct,[59] a proposition for which there is now considerable support.[60,61] Hypersensitivity and specific acquired immunity are both cell-mediated, but T-cell cloning suggests that different T-cell subsets are involved.

Antigens are processed by specific cells, such as dendritic cells and are presented in association with products of the major histocompatibility complex genes to T lymphocytes. Cytotoxic (CD8-positive) T cells are activated by products of the class I major histocompatibility genes (HLA-A and -B), which are expressed on the surface of antigen presenting cells if microbial proliferation proceeds unchecked within phagocytes, the bacteria-containing phagocytes then being eliminated by the T cells. On the other hand, effective processing of the bacteria results in the antigen presenting cells expressing class II major histocompatibility genes (HLA-D), the products of which activate (CD4-positive) T-helper cells, so enhancing bacterial elimination (Fig. 5.3.8).[62]

Two types of T-helper cells are recognised: one concerned mainly in immunity and the other with hypersensitivity. Type 1 T-helper lymphocytes (Th1) secrete interleukin 2 and the macrophage activating cytokine interferon-γ, resulting in enhanced bacterial elimination. However, it also results in the secretion of tumour necrosis factor by the macrophage, which contributes to the hypersensitivity that results from the activation of type 2 helper T-cells (Th2). The Th2 pathway facilitates antibody production, particularly IgE and is effective in the elimination of parasitic worms by causing gross tissue destruction around the parasite. Th2 cells secrete interleukins 4, 5, 6 and 10, which prime tissue cells to the necrotising action of tumour necrosis factor secreted by macrophages activated by Th1 cells. Thus, type 1 reactions are essentially protective but also contribute to the type 2 cell-mediated hypersensitivity (Fig. 5.3.9).[38,39,63]

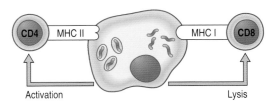

Figure 5.3.8 Antigens are processed and presented by T lymphocytes in association with products of the major histocompatibility complex genes. Cytotoxic T cells (CD8) are activated by products of the class I major histocompatibility genes (MHC I), which are expressed on the surface of antigen presenting cells if microbial proliferation proceeds unchecked within phagocytes, such cells then being eliminated by these T cells. Conversely, T-helper cells (CD4) are activated by MHC II gene products if bacterial processing is effective, resulting in enhanced elimination of the bacteria. (Redrawn after Grange JM. The immunophysiology and immunopathy of tuberculosis. In: Davies PDO (ed). Tuberculosis. London: Chapman and Hall, 1998.[62] By permission from Edward Arnold.)

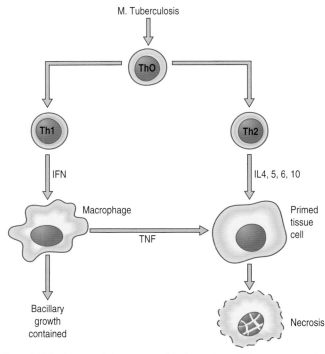

Figure 5.3.9 Types of T-helper cell (Th-) reactions. IFN, interferon-γ; IL, interleukin; TNF, tumour necrosis factor-α. (Redrawn after Grange JM. The immunophysiology and immunopathy of tuberculosis. In: Davies PDO (ed). Tuberculosis. London: Chapman and Hall, 1998.[62] By permission from Edward Arnold.)

Many chronic infections are first characterised by a Th1 response, which then shifts to a Th2 response, with detriment to the host. Animal models suggest that necrosis occurs in T-cell-dependent granulomas when Th2 involvement is superimposed on a Th1 reaction.[64]

Post-primary tuberculosis

Reinfection and reactivation

There has been a notable lack of agreement among epidemiologists in the past about the origin of post-primary tuberculosis

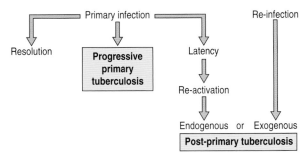

Figure 5.3.10 Possible events following infection by tubercle bacilli. (Redrawn after Grange JM. The immunophysiology and immunopathy of tuberculosis. In: Davies PDO (ed). Tuberculosis. London: Chapman and Hall, 1998.[62] By permission from Edward Arnold.)

and a difference of opinion still exists as to how often it is endogenous (that is, the result of reactivation of a primary lesion) and how often it is exogenous (that is, reinfection tuberculosis – tuberculosis due to a fresh infection from outside the patient's body). Evidence of endogenous reactivation can sometimes be demonstrated: for example, a post-primary lesion may be continuous with an old calcified primary lesion. In contrast, in exceptional instances, *M. bovis* has been isolated from the primary lesion and *M. tuberculosis* from the post-primary. Similar evidence has been provided by the recognition of typical post-primary pulmonary tuberculosis, caused by *M. tuberculosis*, in a small proportion of individuals whose primary infection was not naturally acquired but the result of inoculation with BCG.

The alternative view that post-primary tuberculous lesions develop at the site of foci of infection resulting from haematogenous dissemination of the bacilli during the primary stage was particularly favoured by some epidemiologists and pathologists of the German school. Essentially, they considered that the organisms survive in a dormant state for many years, both in the lesions of the primary complex and at sites of metastatic infection resulting from carriage in the blood. It was considered that such foci, often symmetrically situated near the apex of each lung, might long remain potential centres for recrudescence of the infection, even when clinically the disease appears to have been arrested. In this way, the development of active pulmonary tuberculosis in adults is attributable to activation of the latent infection at the vulnerable sites in the subapical region of one or both lungs, perhaps as a result of a breakdown of resistance associated with such processes as ageing. Certain factors are known to be associated with activation of latent tuberculosis, notably alcoholism, diabetes, the accumulation of silica in the lungs and immunosuppression.

Today in Britain, most pulmonary tuberculosis in the native population is seen in the elderly and probably represents recrudescence of infection first contracted many years previously when tuberculosis was much more prevalent. It seems that where there is a low incidence of disease, most post-primary cases are due to endogenous reactivation but that where the incidence of disease is high, many more cases are due to exogenous reinfection. The possible events following infection with tubercle bacilli are outlined diagrammatically in Figure 5.3.10.

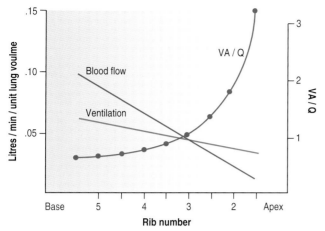

Figure 5.3.11 Regional differences in pulmonary blood flow, ventilation and ventilation/perfusion ratios (V̇A/Q̇), consequent upon gravitational forces. These result in a higher oxygen tension and poorer lymphatic drainage at the apices, thereby promoting the development of tuberculosis at this site. (Redrawn after West.[66])

The pulmonary lesions of post-primary tuberculosis

In contrast to primary tuberculosis of the lungs, where the Ghon focus may develop in any lobe, the early lesions in the post-primary disease are almost invariably found near the apex of one of the upper lobes. Post-primary pulmonary tuberculosis obviously involves considerable spread of the infection. The dissemination is believed to be blood-borne. Using radio-labelled bacilli, Strom provided experimental evidence that tuberculous bacillaemia is a common and early event in primary tuberculosis.[50,51] In the great majority of people, both the primary complex and its haematogenous dissemination are quickly overcome, but in some the distant foci progress or remain latent. If tributaries of the pulmonary veins are involved in the spread of the infection, the bacilli pass out of the thorax, but if the bloodstream is colonised via the lymphatics, the pulmonary capillaries are the first to be reached and so the infection returns to the lungs.

Oxygen tension governs the predilection for blood-borne tuberculosis to favour the apical regions of the lungs and also sites such as the kidneys, meninges and metaphyses. These extrapulmonary sites are well vascularised and therefore have a relatively high oxygen tension. The tubercle bacillus is a strict aerobe and thrives in such organs. In the lung, more complex factors govern oxygen tension. The apices of the lungs are poorly perfused, but the pulmonary arteries bring de-oxygenated blood. Ventilation on the other hand promotes oxygen tension, but the apices are also the most poorly ventilated parts of the lungs. The oxygen tension in the lungs is in fact dependent upon the ventilation/perfusion ratio. In the upright position, this declines from the apices to the bases of the lungs (Fig. 5.3.11),[65,66] and the oxygen tension is therefore highest at the top of the lungs, thus favouring the development of post-primary tuberculosis at the apices.

If the disease progresses, radiological opacities appear in the apex of one or both upper lobes. The early opacities usually disappear with adequate treatment, so that little is known of the histological structure of these transient infiltrates. Necropsy in more advanced cases indicates that such lesions are probably confluent areas of exudative inflammation, with fluid and many macrophages in the alveoli. Epithelioid cell granulomas develop and in time the central granulomas undergo caseation and merge together to produce large areas of necrosis. It is through the liquefaction of this dead tissue and its expulsion through the regional bronchi that the cavities, so typical of the advanced lesions, originate.

If the liquefying contents of a cavity escape into the bronchial tree, the bacilli become widely dispersed to other parts of both lungs, partly by gravity and partly by coughing, as in progressive primary tuberculosis. This diffuse bronchogenic infection gives rise to innumerable small areas of caseous pneumonia, mostly in the lower lobes and occasionally, a rapidly developing confluent tuberculous bronchopneumonia involves almost the whole lower lobe. Microscopical examination may show tubercle bacilli and macrophages in very large numbers in the consolidated areas. Occasionally, such regions undergo caseation. They may become so confluent as to involve a whole lobe.

At necropsy, the lungs of a patient with long-standing, progressive, post-primary tuberculosis have a characteristic appearance. Large cavities may replace much of an upper lobe and one or more smaller, but otherwise similar, cavities may be present in the apical part of the lower lobe. The cavities may be filled with caseous material (Fig. 5.3.12a) or the contents may have been evacuated through communicating bronchi (Fig. 5.3.12b, c). The cavities may be several centimetres in diameter, with walls formed by tuberculous granulation tissue in which the fibrotic remains of the larger bronchi and of branches of the pulmonary arteries form coarse, irregular bands (Fig. 5.3.12c). Usually the disease is bilateral, with similar, but often less advanced, changes in the opposite lung. As in progressive primary tuberculosis satellite nodules are evident at the advancing edge (Fig. 5.3.13). The lower lobes are typically mottled with pale yellow, caseous areas, often in small clusters and the nearby lung substance is fibrotic. In these fibrotic areas, large amounts of sooty pigment have usually collected, so that the pale caseous areas stand out prominently against a blackened background.

The hilar lymph nodes are less obviously involved in the post-primary form of tuberculosis than in the primary form of the disease but, on histological examination, tuberculous foci, often with small areas of caseation can generally be seen in them.

The loss of so much parenchyma naturally impairs the respiratory function of the lungs. That the involvement of the blood vessels is not more frequently accompanied by haemoptysis is accounted for by the fact that the destructive process usually advances slowly, so that obliterative endarteritis leads to the closure of the lumen of the pulmonary and bronchial arteries before their walls have been penetrated. Sometimes caseation advances too quickly for the artery to become completely blocked and an aneurysm may form where the muscu-

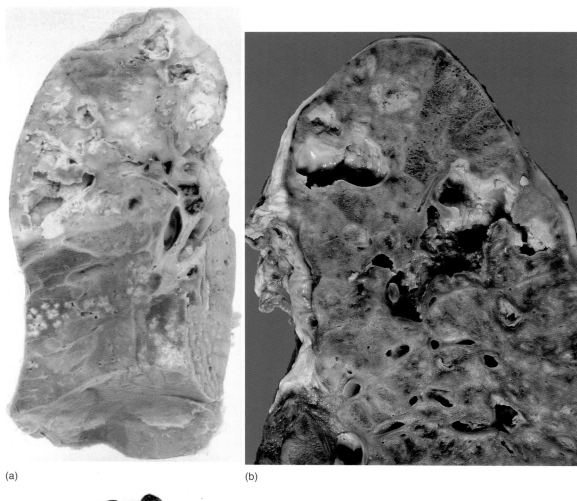

(a)

(b)

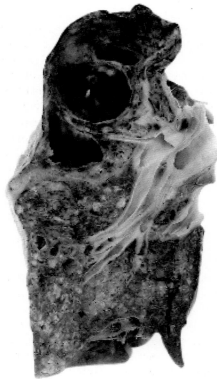

(c)

Figure 5.3.12 Post-primary tuberculosis. (a) The upper lobe is consolidated and several large foci of caseous necrosis are evident. Smaller foci are also seen in the lower lobe. (b) The caseous contents of this cavitating upper lobe lesion have been partially evacuated through communicating airways. (c) The upper lobe is almost completely replaced by a large, chronic, tuberculous cavity. The cords that cross it are the remains of blood vessels. The lower lobe shows many foci of tuberculous bronchopneumonia, the palest areas representing foci of caseation. (Figs (a) and (c) reproduced by permission of the Curator of the Gordon Museum, Guy's Hospital, London, UK; (b) provided by Dr M Kearney, Tromso, Norway.)

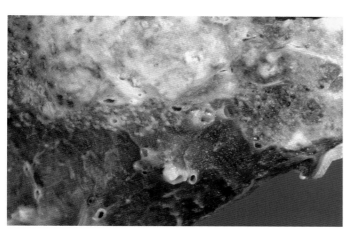

Figure 5.3.13 Post-primary pulmonary tuberculosis. Satellite tubercles are evident at the advancing edge of a chronic caseating focus of infection.

lar and elastic coats are destroyed on the side nearer the cavity. It is through the rupture of such aneurysms (Rasmussen's aneurysms) that sudden and sometimes fatal haemorrhages occur. In view of the extensive destruction of lung substance and of its blood vessels in most cases of cavitating tuberculosis, it is surprising how relatively uncommon this serious complication is.

Histological examination of the wall of a cavity usually discloses several zones, each grading into the next. The yellowish-grey lining is formed largely of granulation tissue that has undergone caseation but not yet liquefied. Acid-fast bacilli can generally be seen in this zone: their multiplication there and subsequent escape into the cavity largely accounts for the high infectivity of the sputum expectorated by patients with advanced pulmonary tuberculosis. Just deep to this is a zone of granulation tissue containing a profusion of macrophages and lymphocytes and occasional multinucleate giant cells. If the cavity has been infected secondarily by other organisms, as often happens, this zone may also contain many neutrophils. Outside this zone there is generally a mantle of satellite tubercles. Still deeper in the wall are traces of residual parenchyma, often with alveoli obliterated by compression and fibrosis. The cavities enlarge by incorporation of the satellite tubercles, more of which are constantly forming more peripherally (Fig. 5.3.13). In this way, tuberculous granulation tissue extends into the surrounding lung substance as its lining progressively caseates, liquefies and is expectorated. Eventually the process of cavitation may reach the pleura, but perforation into the sac hardly ever takes place, for the chronic pleurisy that accompanies the changes within the lungs results in the formation of firm adhesions between the visceral and parietal layers, with obliteration of the pleural sac.

Although the formation of a cavity is a serious development in the progress of a post-primary tuberculous infection of the lung, it does not represent an irreversible stage in the course of the disease. As long as it is small, a cavity may heal by scarring.

Ultimately, such a lesion may only be recognisable as an area of fibrosis that stands out from the surrounding parenchyma because of its black pigmentation and the radiating pale strands of fibrous tissue that pucker the neighbouring lung substance. Alternatively, a balance may be achieved whereby the tubercle bacilli are not destroyed but their spread is halted and the process is held in check, typically by a fibrous capsule forming. Such an encapsulated mass of caseous material is sometimes termed a tuberculoma. In such quiescent tuberculosis there is no inflammation but viable bacilli may survive in the central caseation, ready to reactivate the disease should host defence weaken. Any granulomatous inflammation in the vicinity of such a lesion indicates active tuberculosis.

Local complications of post-primary pulmonary tuberculosis

When tuberculous cavities are larger than 1–2 cm in diameter, particularly when their walls are thick and densely fibrotic, they may persist indefinitely once the tuberculous infection has been overcome. In some such cases, the cavity acquires an epithelial lining; the latter may be of modified respiratory type or squamous. A squamous lining may be simple or stratified; sometimes keratinisation develops and the lumen of the cavity may become filled by compressed desquamated cells, the appearances then being reminiscent of an epidermoid cyst. Squamous carcinoma occasionally arises from such areas of metaplasia. If the cavity is not able to drain freely into the bronchial tree, secretion may accumulate in it and predispose to secondary bacterial infection, sometimes with the formation of a lung abscess. Fungal colonisation may also take place, leading to the formation of an aspergilloma or other variety of intracavitary ball colony[67] (see p. 227).

Chronic tuberculosis of the lungs is usually accompanied by pleurisy. Although this begins in the neighbourhood of the most active lesions, in time it may extend to involve the whole surface of the lung (see Fig. 13.6, p. 697). The condition advances slowly, generally without the formation of much exudate; by the time of necropsy the pleural lesions have usually undergone fibrosis. The damaged lung becomes firmly attached to the chest wall – indeed the fibrosis may be so firm and extensive that the lung can be removed from the body only by dissection outside the parietal pleura. Occasionally, the entire lung may be enclosed by a dense white layer of hyaline connective tissue, several millimetres thick.

Extrapulmonary complications of post-primary respiratory tuberculosis

The proliferation of tubercle bacilli that takes place in the caseating lining of cavities in the lungs is often so great that it leads to heavy infection of the exudate and secretions, most of which are expelled by coughing, sometimes aided by the adoption of a posture that promotes gravitational drainage. These organisms form a potent reservoir for infection of the upper respiratory tract and of the alimentary canal.

In advanced cases of chronic respiratory tuberculosis small ulcers, each a few millimetres in diameter, often develop in the tracheobronchial mucosa,[68] as described above under the dissemination of primary pulmonary tuberculosis via the airways. Occasionally it may mimic a neoplasm but generally there is just slight destruction of tissue and the ulceration amounts to little more than loss of epithelium; occasionally, it may extend more deeply and expose one or more rings of tracheal cartilage. Such tracheobronchial disease was identified in 42% of cases in the preantibiotic era.[68] Subsequently, it was rarely encountered, until AIDS appeared, since then there have been several reports of endobronchial tuberculosis.[69–72] Similar infection may involve the larynx, particularly the glottis and the aryepiglottic folds; the subsequent injury to the vocal cords leads both to hoarseness and to frequent stimulation of the cough reflex.

The passage through the mouth of sputum teeming with tubercle bacilli may also lead to infection of the oral mucous membrane. Most commonly, the lesions appear as ulcers on the margin of the tongue; these are probably initiated by some minor damage to the mucosa such as results from abrasion by a nearby carious tooth, the resulting breach in the epithelial surface giving access to the organisms. Once these ulcers form, they may penetrate deeply into the muscle. Sometimes, the organisms gain entry to the tonsils and there produce typical changes.

Unless trained not to do so, many patients with respiratory tuberculosis swallow much of their sputum and thus maintain a constant infection of the alimentary canal. Since tubercle bacilli are relatively resistant to acid in the concentrations found in gastric juice, they escape destruction in the stomach and enter the small intestine. The most typical lesions occur in the lowest 2 m of the ileum; these are chronic, circumferentially oriented ulcers that begin in and finally destroy, Peyer's patches and then extend towards the mesentery along the mucosal lymphatics.

Amyloidosis eventually develops in many cases of slowly progressive pulmonary tuberculosis. Although many organs become infiltrated with the amyloid material, renal involvement is the commonest serious manifestation and the lungs are seldom involved. As in other forms of secondary amyloidosis, the amyloid is a polymer of the hepatic acute phase protein A.

Tuberculosis in the elderly and immunodeficient: non-reactive tuberculosis

In developed countries, miliary tuberculosis is now a commoner cause of death in the elderly than the young.[73] It is thought to result from activation of old tuberculous foci, primary or post-primary, as a consequence of waning of the immunological defences. In many cases the disease takes a 'cryptic' form,[73–75] characterised by insidious onset and progression and often lacking any evidence of miliary mottling in the chest radiograph. The diagnosis is usually not made until necropsy. Both cryptic and overt miliary tuberculosis in the elderly may be accompanied by changes in the blood, including pancytopenia and leukaemoid reactions; these may be the first manifestation of the illness and their significance in such cases is sometimes overlooked. In the elderly and especially in the immunodeficient, the disease may be non-reactive. Non-reactive tuberculosis differs from ordinary tuberculosis in lacking the usual giant cell granuloma formation.

At necropsy, disseminated miliary tuberculous lesions are found to be widespread. Microscopy shows that the lesions comprise foci of virtually structureless necrotic matter, sharply defined from the surrounding tissue, which shows little or no abnormality. There is little or no granulomatous response. Appropriate staining shows that they teem with tubercle bacilli and unlike the caseation of classic tuberculosis the necrotic material may contain much nuclear debris.[36,76,77] Neutrophil polymorphonuclear leukocytes are commonly seen.

Other forms of non-reactive tuberculosis include diffuse alveolar damage (see Chapter 4) and vasculitis. In the former tubercle bacilli are generally demonstrable in the hyaline membranes[77] while in the latter they teem within the vessel walls.

Non-reactive tuberculosis is the result of a deficiency in the body's cellular defences. In some cases it develops as a complication of lymphoid neoplasia, particularly Hodgkin's disease and leukaemia. In other cases it has followed treatment with immunosuppressant drugs. More recently it has been seen in patients suffering from the acquired immune deficiency syndrome.[36,78] Often, however, no predisposing cause is found; such patients are generally elderly.

If the diagnosis of non-reactive tuberculosis is suspected during life, tubercle bacilli should be looked for in films of bone marrow. Biopsy may be helpful, any suggestion of a tuberculous reaction being potentially an important diagnostic guide. When any biopsy section includes unexplained areas of necrosis, particularly when there is little in the way of a related cellular reaction, it is imperative to look for tubercle bacilli.

It is to be remembered that the tissues in this form of tuberculosis are highly infective. Several cases of tuberculous infection in laboratory staff, including those working in mortuaries, have been traced to this source.

Post-mortem recognition of pulmonary tuberculosis

It is estimated that many cases of active tuberculosis of the lungs go unrecognised until necropsy. This is particularly true of the elderly, whose resistance to the infection is lowered as an accompaniment of ageing: dormant lesions become active and spread of the disease follows, often with little in the way of clinical manifestations to indicate the seriousness of the danger. Similarly, at any age, patients, whose resistance is lowered by conditions such as lymphoma and poorly controlled diabetes mellitus, are prone to reactivation of dormant tuberculosis and vulnerable to exogenous reinfection: often the presence of the infection is overlooked, even when it is the immediate cause of death, until disclosed in the post-mortem room. Now that the necropsy rate is falling markedly in so many countries, many cases of active tuberculosis must go unrecognised. The danger that persists after the patient's death is that the infection may have been passed to relatives or associates without awareness of the need for treatment.

Treatment of tuberculosis

The treatment of tuberculosis is based on a combination of drugs (classically triple therapy) but is bedevilled by the emergence of drug resistant strains, an inability of many countries to provide the drugs and poor compliance on the part of the patient.[79–82]

INFECTION BY OPPORTUNISTIC MYCOBACTERIA

Bacteriology

The organisms responsible for tuberculosis and leprosy are only two of about 40 species of mycobacteria, most of which live freely in the environment, particularly where water abounds, and seldom infect man. Occasionally, however, especially when resistance is low, several of these environmental mycobacteria cause serious disease.[83,84] Their distinction from *M. tuberculosis* is important because they require special drug regimens; they do not respond to anti-tuberculosis treatment. Formerly dismissed as 'atypical' or 'anonymous', these species are better described as the opportunistic mycobacteria. They include *M. marinum* and *M. ulcerans*, the causes of swimming pool granuloma and Buruli ulcer respectively, and a group that cause disease that is very like tuberculosis. In infection by members of the latter group, as in tuberculosis itself, the lungs are the organs most often involved and there may be spread to lymph nodes, bone, meninges, kidneys and elsewhere, or massive dissemination throughout the body akin to miliary tuberculosis. The similarity to tuberculosis is also seen in that the gastrointestinal tract is another portal of entry.[85]

The most common opportunistic mycobacteria infecting the lungs are *M. avium-intracellulare*, *M. kansasii* and *M. xenopi*. Less frequent causes of tuberculosis-like disease are *M. scrofulaceum*, *M. malmoense*, *M. szulgai*, *M. simiae*, *M. chelonei*, *M. fortuitum* and *M. gordonae*. *M. avium-intracellulare* and *M. scrofulaceum* are often said to comprise the MAIS complex. They are all acid-fast but unlike *M. tuberculosis* many of them can also be demonstrated with periodic acid-Schiff and Grocott's stains. *M. kansasii* has a distinctive shape, being long, broad, beaded and bent.[86] Species-specific probes are available.

Infection with these organisms comes from the environment, in contrast to tuberculosis, which is always transmitted from an infected individual or animal. The infection rate of tuberculosis in the community bears a direct relation to the number of infectious cases but this is not the case with the opportunistic mycobacteria. The prevalence of opportunistic mycobacterial infection in a community is independent of that of tuberculosis and is not controlled by public health measures aimed at reducing the spread of tuberculosis.

Interpretation of cultured isolates

The interpretation of cultured isolates must always take account of the possibility that specimens may be contaminated with opportunistic mycobacteria from the environment. Whereas *M. tuberculosis* is an obligate parasite and its isolation indicates tuberculosis, the culture of opportunist mycobacteria does not necessarily indicate that they are the cause of the disease. Their isolation from granulomatous tissue strongly suggests that they have played a causative role, but sputum isolates need to be obtained consistently over a period of weeks and other causes of granulomatous disease, especially tuberculosis, thoroughly excluded before a clinical diagnosis of opportunistic mycobacterial infection can be advanced with confidence.[87,88]

Predisposing causes

Factors predisposing to opportunistic mycobacterial infection may be general or local. General factors include any congenital or acquired immunodeficiency, but especially AIDS,[85,89,90] therapeutic immunosuppression and auto-immune disease. Local factors include pneumoconiosis, chronic bronchitis, cystic fibrosis, bronchiectasis and old tuberculosis. The virulence of mycobacteria is enhanced by lipid[91] and the growth of opportunistic mycobacteria, especially *M. fortuitum-chelonei*, appears to be promoted by lipid pneumonia.[92–94] The aspiration of milk may explain an observed association between achalasia and *M. fortuitum-chelonei* infection.[95,96]

Although some impairment of host defence is generally necessary for these bacteria to establish themselves in man, heavy exposure may result in healthy individuals being infected. An example of this is the increasingly frequent presentation in affluent societies of diffuse lung disease by these bacteria due to the inhalation of infected aerosols from hot tubs and showers.[87,97] Only rarely is no predisposing cause recognised.[98,99]

Pathological changes

The pathological changes produced by opportunistic mycobacteria are generally very similar, if not identical, to those of tuberculosis (Fig. 5.3.14), but there is more airway involvement leading to bronchiectasis[100–102] and a higher proportion of cases that lack the classic granulomatous response.[103] In one study of cervical lymph nodes, four histological features were identified that favoured non-tuberculous mycobacterial infection: the presence of microabscesses, the granulomas being ill-defined, an absence of necrosis and a comparatively small number of giant cells,[104] but these are not absolute points of distinction.

Granulomatous disease indicates a strong immune response and the mycobacteria are then scanty, as in classic tuberculosis. However, in very severe immunodeficiency, as for example the acquired immunodeficiency syndrome, the lesions may consist of numerous swollen macrophages, all of which contain large numbers of acid-fast bacilli (Fig. 5.3.15). Necrosis is not seen and granulomas are poorly formed or absent. The changes then resemble those of lepromatous leprosy[85] or, if the macrophages are spindle-shaped, inflammatory myofibroblastic tumour (see p. 611).[105–108] A leproma-like pattern has also been described in disseminated BCG infection (see p. 203) but is unusual in non-reactive tuberculosis (see p. 208),[109] which is characterised by sheets of necrosis unattended by the usual granulomas, the

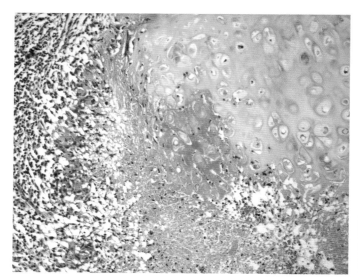

Figure 5.3.14 *M. avium-intracellulare* infection. There is necrotising granulomatous inflammation with destruction of bronchial cartilage, similar to that seen in tuberculosis.

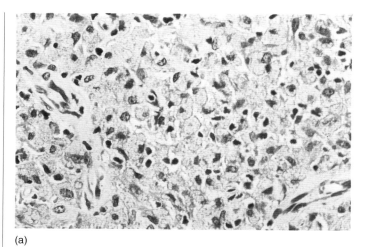

(a)

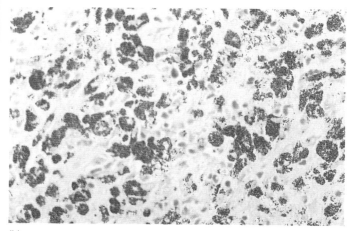

(b)

Figure 5.3.15 *M. avium-intracellulare* infection in an AIDS patient. Whereas the tissue reaction to opportunistic mycobacteria is usually identical to that seen in tuberculosis, in the immunodeficient it resembles the lepromatous form of leprosy, consisting of numerous macrophages with abundant pale cytoplasm (a), which Ziehl-Neelsen staining shows to contain innumerable acid-fast bacilli (b).

tubercle bacillus being more toxic to the macrophage than the opportunistic mycobacteria.[110]

Treatment

The treatment of opportunist mycobacteriosis is less well defined than for tuberculosis, there being few large clinical trials. However, the British Thoracic Society has published a set of guidelines.[88]

BRUCELLOSIS

Pneumonia is a rare form of brucellosis but has been reported in countries such as Kuwait and Arabia,[111,112] where this zoonosis is endemic and in farmers and meat packers in North America and Europe.[113,114] Cattle, sheep, goats and camels are common sources of infection, which is usually acquired by consuming unpasteurized milk or milk products. Close contact with infected animals or their carcasses may also be responsible for transmission of the disease to man, either orally or, in the case of pneumonia, by inhalation.

Patients with brucella pneumonia develop a cough productive of mucopurulent sputum or present with fever of unknown cause.[115] Perihilar or peribronchial infiltrates, or less frequently coin lesions, are evident radiographically. Pleural effusion with a predominance of monocytic or lymphocytic infiltrates is also described.[116]

Histology shows interstitial pneumonia with epithelioid and giant cell granulomas that occasionally undergo caseation.[111,117] As in other organs, the appearances are very similar to those of tuberculosis. Diagnosis is dependent upon excluding tuberculosis and culturing brucellae from blood or tissue. Examination of sputum and bronchial washings is generally unrewarding.

CHRONIC MELIOIDOSIS

The general features and acute form of melioidosis have been described on p. 183. Chronic melioidosis is acquired in the same way as the acute form and may represent persistence or recrudescence of acute disease or arise insidiously in someone unknown to have had acute disease. The disease progresses gradually over months or years. It takes the form of localised lesions that may affect any organ but most commonly involve the lungs, where chronic cavitatory melioidosis may closely mimic tuberculosis apart from relative sparing of the apices.[118-120] Pleural effusion and empyema are less common in chronic than acute disease. Before cavitation takes place, there are abscesses surrounded by granulomatous inflammation. The central necrotic zone is often stellate and may be suppurative or caseous. The surrounding granulomatous reaction consists of epithelioid and Langhans giant cells and is itself encompassed by a fibrous mantle. When necrosis is suppurative, the histological features mimic those of cat scratch disease or lymphogranuloma venereum and, especially in the lungs, tularaemia (see p. 184) or sporotrichosis (see p. 242). When the necrosis is caseous, the histological picture is very similar to that of tuberculosis. In contrast to the acute form of the disease, the causative bacterium (*Burkholderia pseudomallei*) can be difficult to demonstrate in tissue sections (see p. 183 for staining methods). The diagnosis is then largely dependent upon serological techniques.

ACTINOMYCOSIS

Bacteriology

Actinomycetaceae (which include the genera *Actinomyces*, *Nocardia* and *Rhodococcus*) and Mycobacteriaceae (which include the genus *Mycobacterium*) are both families of the order Actinomycetales. Although Actinomycetales are classed as bacteria and mycobacterial diseases are invariably considered among bacterial infections, some of the pathogenic Actinomycetaceae are often mistakenly referred to as fungi and the diseases they cause are commonly grouped with those caused by the true fungi under the general heading of mycoses. It will be difficult to correct this misconception, particularly in view of such entrenched nosological nomenclature as actinomycosis, which by virtue of the ending '-mycosis' – its etymology is usually misinterpreted – is unlikely to be displaced from its common association with the true mycoses, in spite of such other well-understood terminological paradoxes and pitfalls as mycosis fungoides and mycotic aneurysm. However, as well as differing from fungi in size, structure and metabolism, the Actinomycetaceae are susceptible to antibacterial agents and resistant to specifically antifungal drugs.

Actinomyces israelii is by far the most frequent cause of actinomycosis in man. *A. bovis*, the cause of actinomycosis in cattle, is an exceptionally rare cause of the disease in man. Other species that occasionally cause actinomycosis in man include *A. eriksonii*, *A. meyerii* and *A. naeslundii*. *A. propionicus* (*Arachnia propionica*), an organism closely related to *A. israelii*, also causes disease indistinguishable from actinomycosis.

A. israelii is a strictly anaerobic, Gram-positive bacterium, formed of branching filaments from 0.5 to 1.0 μm wide. The filaments readily break into bacillus-like fragments. They are not acid-fast. Like those of the nocardiae (see below), fragments of the actinomyces may be mistaken for contaminant corynebacteria.

A. israelii is a common commensal or saprophyte in the human mouth and intestine and it is probable that most infections by this organism are endogenous. About 60% of cases of actinomycosis present with lesions in the region of the mouth, face or neck, the portal of entry being dental or tonsillar. About 25% of cases of actinomycosis involve the ileocaecal region and in the remaining 15% of cases the infection is in the lungs. It is presumed that pulmonary actinomycosis is the outcome of aspiration of infected matter from the tonsillar crypts or mouth,

apart from the very small proportion of cases in which the disease has extended from known foci of infection in the abdomen. The diagnosis should therefore be particularly suspected in patients with dental caries or a history of unconsciousness with aspiration.

Most cases of actinomycosis are of mixed microbial aetiology, the pathogenicity of actinomyces being enhanced by the synergistic action of other bacteria, notably microaerophilic streptococci, other anaerobes such as *Bacteroides* and *Fusobacterium* and aerobic streptococci and staphylococci. *Actinobacillus actinomycetem comitans* is another constituent of the mouth flora, one that is seldom recovered in pure culture[121] but is often found in association with *A. israelii* in actinomycotic lesions. It secretes a powerful leukotoxin, which probably contributes to the virulence of these mixed infections.

Clinical features

Pulmonary actinomycosis is promoted by poor dental hygiene, smoking and heavy drinking[122] and is recorded in AIDS.[123] It is usually a disease of adults, though may rarely occur in children.[124,125] It is characterised by fever and expectoration of mucopurulent sputum. Contrary to a common belief, 'sulphur granules' – the yellow colonial granules of the organisms – are not often to be found in the sputum. Haemoptysis is a significant complication and may require surgical treatment.[126] The diagnosis depends on recognition of the fine, Gram-positive, sometimes branching filaments in films and isolation of the organism. It has to be remembered that the organism may be present in sputum only in short bacillary forms that are liable to be misinterpreted. The chest radiograph may show opacities of various sizes scattered through both lungs, particularly in the middle and lower zones. Alternatively, there may be a large pneumonic area, sometimes associated with an empyema. This type of the disease may be accompanied by new bone formation on the inner aspects of several contiguous ribs due to elevation of the periosteum by the inflammatory infiltrate. Occasionally, infiltration of the chest wall suggests malignancy (Fig. 5.3.16). The presence of discharging sinuses on the chest wall is characteristic of advanced thoracic actinomycosis[127] but this stage is seldom encountered today.[128,129] It is in the pus discharging from these sinuses that the 'sulphur granules' referred to above are to be found. Recent series have been characterised by less specific features that have suggested tuberculosis or cancer.[122,123,130] The diagnosis has often been made only after lung tissue has been resected, but may be possible by biopsy, particularly when the process involves major airways.[123,131] It should be confirmed by culture and because *A. israelii* is a strict anaerobe and will die on exposure to atmospheric oxygen prompt delivery to the laboratory for appropriate processing is imperative.

Pathological findings

Actinomycosis of the lungs typically affects the lower lobes but may involve any part. Characteristically, the affected tissue is riddled with chronic abscesses that range in diameter from a few millimetres to 3 cm. These lesions may communicate with

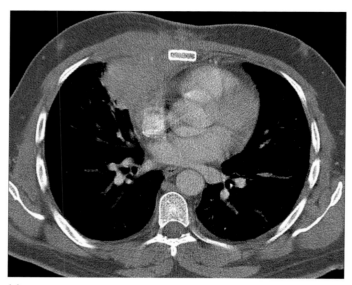

(a)

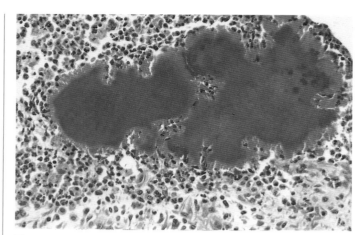

Figure 5.3.17 Actinomycosis. Pus containing a colony of actinomyces surrounded by an eosinophilic mantle of immune material (the Splendore–Hoeppli phenomenon).

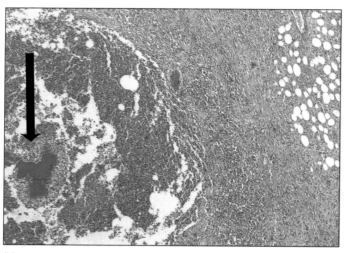

(b)

Figure 5.3.16 Actinomycosis. (a) CT shows a mass in the right middle lobe extending through the chest wall and mimicking an invasive carcinoma. (b) The lobectomy specimen shows colonies (arrow) of actinomyces within abscesses that extend into the fat of the chest wall.

such as schistosomes and helminths and even around foreign material.) Fibrosis surrounds the suppurative foci and extends more widely through the lungs, particularly involving the septa. The infection may spread to the pleura and on into the spine and ribs, whether or not there is an actinomycotic empyema: the latter may be loculated or involve the entire pleural sac. Obliteration of the sac prevents empyema formation but does not present a barrier to the infection as it spreads outwards to involve not only the thoracic skeleton but also the soft tissues and skin of the chest wall, often with the establishment of the draining sinuses that are a classic if rare feature of the disease. Actinomycotic bacteraemia is uncommon but arises more frequently from pulmonary foci than from any other form of actinomycosis; it may give rise to metastatic abscesses in other viscera, the skeleton or soft tissues. Actinomycosis is occasionally complicated by amyloidosis.

NOCARDIOSIS

Bacteriology

Nocardiosis is caused by several genera of aerobic Actinomycetaceae. Their classification is unsettled but *Nocardia* species are the usual cause, with *N. asteroides* being encountered most frequently. *N. brasiliensis* and *N. caviae* are less common human pathogens. *Nocardia* species are not part of the normal human flora. They are soil saprophytes that are often found in decaying organic matter. Human infection is thought to be exogenous. *Nocardia* were first identified in cattle suffering from farcy in 1888.[132] Human disease was described shortly afterwards.[133,134]

In contrast to *A. israelii*, *N. asteroides* is an aerobic bacterium. It is formed of filaments measuring 0.5–1.0 μm in width, which are so highly branched that they have been likened to Chinese characters. They often break into bacillus-like fragments during preparation of films of infected exudate. They are Gram-positive but often weakly so and although commonly acid-fast, they are seldom as strongly so as tubercle bacilli and they are

one another, drain into the bronchial tree or extend to the pleural surface and open into the pleural sac. 'Sulphur granules' are often to be found within the abscesses. These colonies of actinomyces consist of numerous radiating bacterial filaments that often terminate in a prominent club-like cap of eosinophilic material that represents immune material, a reaction known as the Splendore–Hoeppli phenomenon (Figs 5.3.16b, 5.3.17). (Splendore described eosinophilic material around sporotrichum in 1908 and erroneously assumed that it was a new species, while Hoeppli described the same material around schistosomes in 1932 and erroneously suggested that it was secreted by the parasite. The material is now considered to consist of immunoglobulin, complement and cellular debris. It is especially striking in actinomycosis, botryomycosis and various fungal infections, but may also be seen around parasites

not alcohol-fast; silver impregnation methods offer the best means of demonstrating this organism in tissue sections. In contrast to *A. israelii* and to *N. brasiliensis* and *N. caviae*, *N. asteroides* does not form macroscopically evident colonial granules in infected tissues.

Clinical features

Nocardiosis is typically acquired by inhalation but may extend beyond the respiratory tract. Infection may develop in a previously healthy person,[135] but in most cases there are predisposing factors, particularly those that compromise cellular immunity.[136–139] The disease is ordinarily chronic but may progress rapidly in the severely immunocompromised. Predisposing factors include diseases such as leukaemia and AIDS that interfere with resistance, therapeutic agents such as corticosteroids and cytotoxic drugs that similarly suppress immunity and underlying pulmonary diseases, including alveolar lipoproteinosis.[140,141] The overall incidence of nocardiosis appears to be rising, probably in the main because of the increasing use of the drugs that predispose to its occurrence. The disease is more common in adults than children.

Pulmonary nocardiosis causes fever and cough productive of thick, sticky, purulent sputum that may be streaked with blood. The radiological findings vary from minor infiltrates to extensive consolidation, sometimes with abscess formation or empyema.[142,143] Less commonly, nocardiosis results in bronchial obstruction.[144–146]

Pathological findings

In general, the picture of nocardiosis is that of suppuration, with the development of multiple abscesses. The lesions have a notable tendency to confluence. Pulmonary nocardiosis may affect one or both lungs very widely, with extensive consolidation round the suppurative foci. The exudate in the alveoli of these pneumonic foci initially contains much fibrinogen and a fibrin coagulum forms, often with relatively little leukocytic infiltration. The organisms are present in the exudate and may be very numerous. Their number is often only inadequately disclosed by Gram or Ziehl-Neelsen stains: the Grocott-Gomori method is generally more reliable (Fig. 5.3.18).[147] Healing may result in extensive organising pneumonia.[148] Very rarely, pulmonary nocardiosis may take the form of an intracavitary nocardioma[149] or invade contiguous vertebrae and compress the spinal cord.[150] *N. asteroides* has a particular affinity for the central nervous system, nocardial brain abscess and nocardial meningitis being frequent complications of pulmonary infection. Co-existing microbial agents are commonly identified. Treatment of nocardiosis is generally medical, typically employing sulphonamides or co-trimoxazole. Abscesses and empyema may require additional surgery.

RHODOCOCCUS PNEUMONIA

Rhodococcus equi (formerly *Corynebacterium equi*) is an aerobic, Gram-positive and acid-fast bacillus belonging to the order

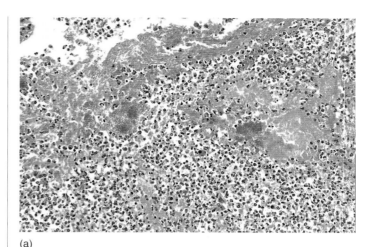

(a)

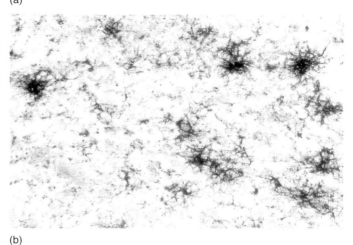

(b)

Figure 5.3.18 Nocardiosis. Pus containing three colonies of basophilic nocardia (a), which are better demonstrated by Grocott staining (b).

Actinomycetales and is therefore closely related to the mycobacteria and nocardia. Its natural habitat is the soil and its transmission is aerogenous. It is best known as a pathogen in foals, cattle, swine and sheep, where it is a lethal cause of suppurative granulomatous pneumonia, lymphadenitis, mediastinitis and pyometra. It has only recently been recognised as pathogenic to man. Infection in man often follows exposure to farm animals or to stockyards contaminated with animal excreta. Virtually all Rhodococcus-infected patients have been severely immunocompromised, typically suffering from AIDS, of which it is an infrequent complication.[151] The clinical presentation is often insidious, consisting of fatigue, fever and a non-productive cough.

R. equi infection causes pneumonic consolidation with abscesses. The disease typically affects the upper lobes and may simulate tuberculosis radiologically.[152–154] Spread to sites such as the brain and bone may occur. The inflammation is histiocytic in nature and may result in pulmonary malakoplakia.

Malakoplakia

Malakoplakia is a rare inflammatory disorder characterised by tumour-like accumulations of swollen macrophages. It usually affects the lower genitourinary or gastrointestinal tracts and until recently few cases had been described with lung involvement. However, several cases of malakoplakia confined to the lungs have now been described, chiefly in the setting of AIDS but also associated with general debilitation, organ transplantation, haematopoietic malignancy and alcoholism.[152,153,155–164]

Bacteriology

Malakoplakia is associated with infection by various bacteria and fungi. In the urinary tract the organism is usually *Escherichia coli* but in the lungs *Rhodococcus equi* (formerly *Corynebacterium equi*) is generally involved, although rare cases associated with other infections are described.[165] Rhodococci are Gram-positive coccobacilli that may be mistaken for commensal diphtheroids in sputum. They are sometimes acid-fast. *R. equi* has been recognised as an agent causing bronchopneumonia in horses and other domesticated animals since its first isolation from infected foals in 1923. Its habitat is the soil. Infection of both man and beast is thought to be acquired through the lungs. Human infection almost always involves patients who have defects in cell-mediated immunity. A history of exposure to animals is not invariably obtained. The pathogenesis of malakoplakia appears to involve defective macrophage function. Bacteria are ingested normally but are not killed within the cell, suggesting that the fault lies in the lysosomes. The condition is acquired.[166]

Pathological and clinical features

Malakoplakia of the lungs may form solitary or multiple bilateral lesions, mimicking either primary or metastatic neoplasms radiologically. The gross appearances also mimic neoplastic disease. The lesions are well demarcated, firm and either solid or cavitating. Microscopically, the lung tissue is replaced by sheets of swollen macrophages with abundant eosinophilic, granular or vacuolated cytoplasm that stains well with periodic acid-Schiff reagents and is diastase-resistant. The appearances may suggest a granular cell tumour (see p. 629). A characteristic feature is the presence of Michaelis–Gutmann bodies in the macrophage cytoplasm or free between the cells. These are faintly basophilic, round, target-like structures that measure up to 20 μm diameter (Fig. 5.3.19). They contain calcium and are therefore well shown by von Kossa's stain. The Michaelis–Gutmann bodies represent mineralised bacteria-containing phagolysosomes.[164] Aggregates of bacteria can sometimes be demonstrated within macrophages by Gram stains.

SYPHILIS

Syphilitic lesions have never been particularly frequent in the lungs and congenital pulmonary syphilis ('pneumonia alba') has probably always been the commonest manifestation.

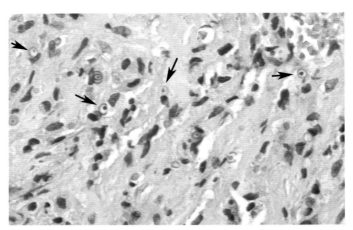

Figure 5.3.19 Pulmonary malakoplakia. A mass lesion composed of histiocytes with abundant eosinophilic cytoplasm. Several Michaelis-Gutmann bodies are evident (arrows). (Case provided by Dr B. Addis, Southampton, UK.)

However, there has recently been an increase in syphilis and its protean manifestations should not be forgotten.[167,168]

Congenital pulmonary syphilis

The pallor and firmness of the lungs, which are larger than normal, account for this condition's old name, pneumonia alba. It is usually seen in stillborn syphilitic babies or those who die within a few hours of birth: in the latter, the aerated lobules stand out above the indurated parts. Microscopically, there is widespread thickening of the alveolar walls by fibroblastic connective tissue accompanied by an accumulation of plasma cells with some lymphocytes. In places there are microscopical foci of necrosis, maybe with histiocytic proliferation round them, as well as some accumulation of neutrophils. These lesions occasionally merge to form gummatous foci that may be evident macroscopically. Usually there is a conspicuous lining of cuboidal type II alveolar epithelial cells and many alveoli may be filled with macrophages. Silver impregnation methods show the presence of great numbers of treponemes in the tissues. The bacteria may also be demonstrated immunohistochemically.[169] Imaging may show diffuse pulmonary infiltrates, which persist long after adequate antibiotic treatment.[170]

Somewhat similar macroscopical and microscopical changes may result from viral infections in the neonatal period. Also, pneumocystis pneumonia may be mistaken for syphilitic pneumonia in those cases in which interstitial accumulation of plasma cells is particularly marked (see p. 222).

Acquired pulmonary syphilis

Gummas and interstitial fibrosis are the manifestations of acquired syphilis in the lungs. The gummas may be solitary or multiple and small or large. They may occur in the trachea and bronchi as ulcerative lesions, with a tendency to destroy the cartilage of the wall. These cause cough and haemmorrhage whereas gummas in the lung substance may be clinically silent.

Bronchopulmonary gummas have the structure that is common to these lesions wherever they occur in the body. They consist of a necrotic core surrounded by granulation tissue that is heavily infiltrated by plasma cells and lymphocytes with scanty giant cells. Satellite lesions, as seen in tuberculosis, are not a feature. As elsewhere, gummas tend ultimately to produce dense scars that contract and produce deep cicatricial fissures in the surface of the lungs, an appearance comparable to that of the classic hepar lobatum of tertiary syphilis.

It is very important to consider and exclude other types of infection, particularly mycobacterioses and mycoses, before a diagnosis of gumma can be sustained, even when the patient's serological tests indicate the presence of syphilis. Moreover, primary and secondary tumours are commoner causes of discrete shadows in chest radiographs than gummas, even in patients with syphilis. The necrotic pulmonary lesions of Wegener's granulomatosis and even pulmonary infarcts are among other conditions to be considered in the differential diagnosis.

Other thoracic manifestations of acquired syphilis include diffuse pulmonary fibrosis of non-specific character, hilar lymphadenopathy and pleural fibrosis.[167,168]

REFERENCES

Tuberculosis

1. Armstrong JA, D'Arcy Hart P. Response of cultured macrophages to Mycobacterium tuberculosis with observations on fusion of lysosomes and phagosomes. J Exp Med 1971; 134:713–740.
2. Lowrie DB, Andrew PW. Macrophage antimycobacterial mechanisms. Br Med Bull 1988; 44:624–634.
3. Gerston KF, Blumberg L, Tshabalala VA, Murray J. Viability of mycobacteria in formalin-fixed lungs. Hum Pathol 2004; 35:571–575.
4. Fukunaga H, Murakami T, Gondo T, Sugi K, Ishihara T. Sensitivity of acid-fast staining for Mycobacterium tuberculosis in formalin-fixed tissue. Am J Respir Crit Care Med 2002; 166:994–997.
5. Cserni G. Auramine fluorescence for acid-fast bacilli in formalin-fixed paraffin-embedded tissues. Am J Clin Pathol 1995; 103:114.
6. Popper HH. Auramine fluorescence for acid-fast bacilli in formalin-fixed paraffin-embedded tissues – reply. Am J Clin Pathol 1995; 103:114.
7. Wockel W. Auramine fluorescence for acid-fast bacilli in formalin-fixed, paraffin-embedded tissues. Am J Clin Pathol 1995; 103:667–668.
8. Tang YW, Procop GW, Zheng XT, Myers JL, Roberts GD. Histologic parameters predictive of mycobacterial infection. Am J Clin Pathol 1998; 109:331–334.
9. Chitkara YK. Evaluation of cultures of percutaneous core needle biopsy specimens in the diagnosis of pulmonary nodules. Am J Clin Pathol 1997; 107:224–228.
10. Cheng VCC, Yam WC, Hung IFN, et al. Clinical evaluation of the polymerase chain reaction for the rapid diagnosis of tuberculosis. J Clin Pathol 2004; 57:281–285.
11. Selva E, Hofman V, Berto F, et al. The value of polymerase chain reaction detection of Mycobacterium tuberculosis in granulomas isolated by laser capture microdissection. Pathology 2004; 36(1):77–81.
12. Drobniewski FA, Watt B, Smith EG, et al. A national audit of the laboratory diagnosis of tuberculosis and other mycobacterial diseases within the United Kingdom. J Clin Pathol 1999; 52:334–337.
12a. Zink AR, Nerlich AG. Molecular strain identification of the Mycobacterium tuberculosis complex in archival tissue samples. J Clin Pathol 2004; 57:1185–1192.
12b. Schulz S, Cabras AD, Kremer M, et al. Species identification of mycobacteria in paraffin-embedded tissues: frequent detection of nontuberculous mycobacteria. Med Pathol 2005; 18:274–282.
13. Sehonanda A, Choi YJ, Blum S. Changing patterns of autopsy findings among persons with acquired immunodeficiency syndrome in an inner-city population: a 12-year retrospective study. Arch Pathol Lab Med 1996; 120:459–464.
14. Callister ME, Barringer J, Thanabalasingam ST, Gair R, Davidson RN. Pulmonary tuberculosis among political asylum seekers screened at Heathrow Airport, London, 1995–9. Thorax 2002; 57:152–156.
15. Meredith SK, Nunn AJ, Byfield SP, et al. National survey of notifications of tuberculosis in England and Wales in 1988. Thorax 1992; 47:770–775.
16. Loddenkemper R, Gibson GJ, Sibelle Y, eds. Major Respiratory Diseases – Tuberculosis. In: European Lung White Book. Lausanne: European Respiratory Society; 2004:66–73.
17. Kochi A. The global tuberculosis situation and the new control strategy of the World Health Organization. Tubercle 1991; 72:1–6.
18. Dolin PJ, Raviglione MC, Kochi A. Global tuberculosis incidence and mortality during 1990–2000. Bulletin of the World Health Organization 1994; 72:213–220.
19. World Health Organization. TB: a global emergency. Geneva: World Health Organization, 1994.
20. Raviglione MC, Snider DE, Kochi A. Global epidemiology of tuberculosis. Morbidity and mortality of a worldwide epidemic. JAMA 1995; 273:220–226.
21. Kolappan C, Gopi PG. Tobacco smoking and pulmonary tuberculosis. Thorax 2002; 57:964–966.
22. Levin M, Newport M. Unravelling the genetic basis of susceptibility to mycobacterial infection. J Pathol 1997; 181:5–7.
23. Murray JF. Cursed duet: HIV infection and tuberculosis. Respiration 1990; 57:210–220.
24. Heckbert SR, Elarth A, Nolan CM. The impact of human immunodeficiency virus infection on tuberculosis in young men in Seattle-King county, Washington. Chest 1992; 102:433–437.
25. Brudney K, Dobkin J. Resurgent tuberculosis in New York City – human immunodeficiency virus, homelessness and the decline of tuberculosis control programs. Am Rev Respir Dis 1991; 144:745–749.
26. Busillo CP, Lessnau KD, Sanjana V, et al. Multidrug resistant mycobacterium-tuberculosis in patients with human immunodeficiency virus infection. Chest 1992; 102:797–801.
27. Chawla PK, Klapper PJ, Kamholz SL, Pollack AH, Heurich AE. Drug-resistant tuberculosis in an urban population including patients at risk for human immunodeficiency virus infection. Am Rev Respir Dis 1992; 146:280–284.
28. Edlin BR, Tokars JI, Grieco MH, et al. An outbreak of multidrug-resistant tuberculosis among hospitalized patients with the acquired immunodeficiency syndrome. N Engl J Med 1992; 326:1514–1521.
29. PablosMendez A, Raviglione MC, Laszlo A, et al. Global surveillance for antituberculosis-drug resistance, 1994– 1997. N Engl J Med 1998; 338:1641–1649.
30. Selwyn PA, Hartel D, Lewis VA, et al. A prospective study of the risk of tuberculosis among intravenous drug users with human immunodeficiency virus infection. N Engl J Med 1989; 320:545–550.
31. Centre for Disease Control. Nosocomial transmission of multidrug-resistant tuberculosis to health-care workers and HIV-infected patients in an urban hospital – Florida. Mortality and Morbidity Weekly Reports 1990; 39:718–722.
32. Havlir DV, Barnes PF. Tuberculosis in patients with human immunodeficiency virus infection. N Engl J Med 1999; 340:367–373.
33. Goletti D, Weissman D, Jackson RW, et al. Effect of Mycobacterium tuberculosis on HIV replication. Role of immune activation. J Immunol 1996; 157:1271–1278.
34. Toossi Z, Nicolacakis K, Xia L, Ferrari NA, Rich EA. Activation of latent HIV-1 by Mycobacterium tuberculosis and its purified protein derivative in alveolar macrophages from HIV-infected individuals in vitro. J Acquir Immune Defic Syndr Hum Retrovirol 1997; 15:325–331.
35. Garrait V, Cadranel J, Esvant H, et al. Tuberculosis generates a microenvironment enhancing the productive infection of local lymphocytes by HIV. J Immunol 1997; 159:2824–2830.

36. Hill AR, Premkumar S, Brustein S, et al. Disseminated tuberculosis in the acquired immunodeficiency syndrome era. Am Rev Respir Dis 1991; 144:1164–1170.

37. Medlar EM. The behavior of pulmonary tuberculosis lesions: a pathological study. Am Rev Tuberc 1955; 71(suppl 1):1–244.

38. Rook GAW, Al Attiyah R. Cytokines and the Koch phenomenon. Tubercle 1991; 72:13–20.

39. Chensue SW, Warmington K, Ruth J, Lincoln P, Kuo MC, Kunkel SL. Cytokine responses during mycobacterial and schistosomal antigen-induced pulmonary granuloma formation – production of Th1 and Th2 cytokines and relative contribution of tumor necrosis factor. Am J Pathol 1994; 145:1105–1113.

40. van den Oord JJ, de Wolf-Peeters C, Fachetti F, Desmet VJ. Cellular composition of hypersensitivity-type granulomas: immunohistochemical analysis of tuberculous and sarcoidal lymphadenitis. Hum Pathol 1984; 15:559–565.

41. Brincker H, Pedersen NT. Immunological marker patterns in granulomatous lymph node lesions. Histopathology 1989; 15:495–503.

42. Randhawa PS. Lymphocyte subsets in granulomas of human tuberculosis: an in situ immunofluorescence study using monoclonal antibodies. Pathology 1990; 22:153–155.

43. Kuo HP, Yu CT. Alveolar macrophage subpopulations in patients with active pulmonary tuberculosis. Chest 1993; 104:1773–1778.

44. Ober WB. Ghon but not forgotten: Anton Ghon and his complex. Pathol Annu 1983; 18(Part 2):79–85.

45. Chow LTC, Shum BSF, Chow WH, Tso CB. Diffuse pulmonary ossification – a rare complication of tuberculosis. Histopathology 1992; 20:435–437.

46. Brock RC, Cann RJ, Dickinson JR. Tuberculous mediastinal lymphadenitis in childhood; secondary effects on the lungs. Guy Hosp Rep 1937; 87:295–317.

47. MacPherson AMC, Zorab PA, Reid L. Collapse of the lung associated with primary tuberculosis: a review of 51 cases. Thorax 1960; 15:346–354.

48. Husson RN, Bramson RT, Newton AW, Pasternak MS, Mark EJ. A 10-month-old girl with fever, upper-lobe pneumonia and a pleural effusion: Pulmonary tuberculosis, infantile. N Engl J Med 1999; 341:353–360.

49. Seal RME. The pathology of tuberculosis. Br J Hosp Med 1971; 5:783–790.

50. Strom L. Experiments with radioactive Calmette (BCG) vaccine. Acta Paed 1950; 39:453–454.

51. Strom L, Rudback L. On labelling tubercle bacteria with radioactive phosphorus. Acta tuberculosea Scandinavica 1949; 21:98–101.

52. Daniels M, Ridehalgh F, Springett VH, Hall IM. Tuberculosis in young adults. Report on the Prophit Tuberculosis Survey 1935–1944. London: Lewis, HK; 1948.

53. Grange JM. Mycobacteria and Human Disease. London: Edward Arnold, 1988; 88.

54. Behr MA, Wilson MA, Gill WP, et al. Comparative genomics of BCG vaccines by whole-genome DNA microarray. Science 1999; 284:1520–1523.

55. Abramowsky C, Gonzalez B, Sorensen RU. Disseminated bacillus Calmette-Guerin infections in patients with primary immunodeficiences. Am J Clin Pathol 1993; 100:52.

56. Emile J-F, Patey N, Altare F, et al. Correlation of granuloma structure with clinical outcome defines two types of idiopathic disseminated BCG infection. J Pathol 1997; 181:25–30.

57. Grange JM, Stanford JL. BCG vaccination and cancer. Tubercle 1990; 71:61–64.

58. Tan L, Testa G, Yung T. Diffuse alveolar damage in BCGosis: A rare complication of intravesical bacillus Calmette–Guerin therapy for transitional cell carcinoma. Pathology 1999; 31:55–56.

59. Rich AR. The pathogenesis of tuberculosis. Springfield, IL: Charles C Thomas; 1951:500–560.

60. Youmans GP. Mechanisms of immunity in tuberculosis. In: Loachim HL, ed. Pathology Annual, Vol 9. New York: Raven Press; 1979:137–157.

61. Bothamley GH, Grange JM. The Koch phenomenon and delayed hypersensitivity: 1891–1991. Tubercle 1991; 72:7–11.

62. Grange JM. The immunophysiology and immunopathology of tuberculosis. In: Davies PDO, ed. Tuberculosis. London: Chapman and Hall; 1998.

63. Myatt N, Coghill G, Morrison K, Jones D, Cree IA. Detection of tumour necrosis factor alpha in sarcoidosis and tuberculosis granulomas using in situ hybridisation. J Clin Pathol 1994; 47:423–426.

64. Grange JM, Stanford JL, Rook G, Onyebujoh P, Bretscher PA. Tuberculosis and HIV: light after darkness. Thorax 1994; 49:537–539.

65. Dock W. Apical localization of phthisis. Am Rev Tuberc 1946; 53:297–305.

66. West JB. Ventilation/blood flow and gas exchange. Oxford: Blackwell; 1977:30.

67. British Thoracic and Tuberculosis Association. Aspergilloma and residual tuberculous cavities – the results of a resurvey. Tubercle 1970; 51:227–245.

68. Auerbach O. Tuberculosis of the trachea and major bronchi. Am Rev Tuberc 1949; 60: 604–620.

69. Vandenbrande P, Lambrechts M, Tack J, Demedts M. Endobronchial tuberculosis mimicking lung cancer in elderly patients. Respir Med 1991; 85:107–109.

70. Wasser LS, Shaw GW, Talavera W. Endobronchial tuberculosis in the acquired immunodeficiency syndrome. Chest 1988; 94:1240–1244.

71. Lee JH, Park SS, Lee DH, Shin DH, Yang SC, Yoo BM. Endobronchial tuberculosis - clinical and bronchoscopic features in 121 cases. Chest 1992; 102:990–994.

72. Hoheisel G, Chan BKM, Chan CHS, Chan KS, Teschler H, Costabel U. Endobronchial tuberculosis: diagnostic features and therapeutic outcome. Respir Med 1994; 88:593–597.

73. King D, Davies PDO. Disseminated tuberculosis in the elderly: still a diagnosis overlooked. J R Soc Med 1992; 85:48–50.

74. Proudfoot AT. Cryptic disseminated tuberculosis. Br J Hosp Med 1971; 5:773–780.

75. Morris CDW. Pulmonary tuberculosis in the elderly – a different disease. Thorax 1990; 45:912–913.

76. Singh R, Joshi RC, Christie J. Generalised non-reactive tuberculosis: a clinicopathological study of four patients. Thorax 1989; 44:952–955.

77. Benatar SR, Mark EJ, McLoud TC, Kesselman H, Ko A. A 44-year-old woman with pulmonary infiltrates, respiratory failure and pancytopenia – pulmonary tuberculosis, nonreactive and miliary, with diffuse alveolar damage (adult respirator distress syndrome), with miliary tuberculosis in the liver, spleen, adrenal glands, bone marrow and kidneys. Kaposi's sarcoma of the jejunum. N Engl J Med 1995; 333: 241–248.

78. Nambuya A, Sewankambo N, Mugerwa J, Goodgame R, Lucas S. Tuberculous lymphadenitis associated with human immunodeficiency virus (HIV) in Uganda. J Clin Pathol 1988; 41:91–96.

79. Iseman MD. Tuberculosis therapy: past, present and future. Eur Respir J Suppl 2002; 36:87s–94s.

80. Loddenkemper R, Sagebiel D, Brendel A. Strategies against multidrug-resistant tuberculosis. Eur Respir J Suppl 2002; 36:66s–77s.

81. Blumberg HM, Burman WJ, Chaisson RE, et al. American Thoracic Society/Centers for Disease Control and Prevention/Infectious Diseases Society of America: treatment of tuberculosis. Am J Respir Crit Care Med 2003; 167:603–662.

82. Caminero JA, de March P. Statements of ATS, CDC and IDSA on treatment of tuberculosis. Am J Respir Crit Care Med 2004; 169:316–317.

Opportunistic mycobacteria

83. Chester AC, Winn WC. Unusual and newly recognised patterns of nontuberculous mycobacterial infection with emphasis on the immunocompromised host. Pathol Annu 1986; 21(Part 1):251–270.

84. Grange JM, Yates MD. Infections caused by opportunist mycobacteria: a review. J R Soc Med 1986; 79:226–229.

85. Wallace JM, Hannah JB. Mycobacterium avium complex infection in patients with the acquired immunodeficiency syndrome. A clinicopathologic study. Chest 1988; 93:926–932.

86. Smith MB, Molina CP, Schnadig VJ, Boyars MC, Aronson JF. Pathologic features of Mycobacterium kansasii infection in patients with acquired immunodeficiency syndrome. Arch Pathol Lab Med 2003; 127:554–560.

87. Kahana LM, Kay JM, Yakrus MA, Waserman S. Mycobacterium avium complex infection in an immunocompetent young adult related to hot tub exposure. Chest 1997; 111:242–245.

88. Management of opportunist mycobacterial infections: Joint Tuberculosis Committee Guidelines 1999. Subcommittee of the Joint Tuberculosis Committee of the British Thoracic Society Thorax 2000; 55:210–218.

89. Rigsby MO, Curtis AM. Pulmonary disease from nontuberculous mycobacteria in patients with human immunodeficiency virus. Chest 1994; 106:913–919.

90. Nash G, Said JW, Nash SV, Degirolami U. The pathology of AIDS - intestinal mycobacterium avium complex (MAC) infection in AIDS. Mod Pathol 1995; 8:209–211.

91. Laporte R. A l'etudes des bacillus paratuberculeux. I Proprietes pathogenes II Histo-cytologie des lesions paratuberculeuses. Ann Inst Pasteur 1940; 65:415–434.

92. Guest JL, Arean VM, Brenner HA. Group IV atypical mycobacterium infection occurring in association with mineral oil granuloma of lungs. Am Rev Respir Dis 1967; 95:656–662.

93. Greenberger PA, Katzenstein A-LA. Lipid pneumonia with atypical mycobacterial colonization. Association with allergic bronchopulmonary aspergillosis. Arch Intern Med 1983; 143:2003–2005.

94. Jouannic I, Desrues B, Lena H, Quinquenel ML, Donnio PY, Delaval P. Exogenous lipoid pneumonia complicated by Mycobacterium fortuitum and Aspergillus fumigatus infections. Eur Respir J 1996; 9:172–174.

95. Gibson JB. Infection of the lungs by 'saprophytic' mycobacteria in achalasia of the cardia, with report of a fatal case showing lipoid pneumonia due to milk. J Pathol Bacteriol 1953; 65:239–251.

96. Burke DS, Ullian RB. Megaesophagus and pneumonia associated with mycobacterium chelonei. A case report and a literature review. Am Rev Respir Dis 1977; 116:1101–1107.

97. Khoor A, Leslie KO, Tazelaar HD, Helmers RA, Colby TV. Diffuse pulmonary disease caused by nontuberculous mycobacteria in immunocompetent people (Hot tub lung). Am J Pathol 2001; 115:755–762.

98. Levin M, Newport M, D'Souza S, et al. Familial disseminated atypical mycobacterial infection in childhood: a human mycobacterial susceptibility gene? Lancet 1995; 345:79–83.

99. Asano T, Itoh G, Itoh M. Disseminated Mycobacterium intracellulare infection in an HIV-negative, nonimmunosuppressed patient with multiple endobronchial polyps. Respiration 2002; 69:175–177.

100. Fujita J, Ohtsuki Y, Suemitsu I, et al. Pathological and radiological changes in resected lung specimens in Mycobacterium avium intracellulare complex disease. Eur Resp J 1999; 13:535–540.

101. Fujita J, Ohtsuki Y, Shigeto E, et al. Pathological findings of bronchiectases caused by Mycobacterium avium intracellulare complex. Resp Med 2003; 97(8):933–938.

102. Fukuoka K, Nakano Y, Nakajima A, Hontsu S, Kimura H. Endobronchial lesions involved in Mycobacterium avium infection. Resp Med 2003; 97(12):1261–1264.

103. Christianson LC, Dewlett HJ. Pulmonary disease in adults associated with unclassified mycobacteria. Am J Med 1960; 29:980–991.

104. Kraus M, Benharroch D, Kaplan D, et al. Mycobacterial cervical lymphadenitis: the histological features of non-tuberculous mycobacterial infection. Histopathology 1999; 35:534–538.

105. Loo KT, Seneviratne S, Chan JKC. Mycobacterial infection mimicking inflammatory 'pseudotumour' of the lung. Histopathology 1989; 14:217–219.

106. Umlas J, Federman M, Crawford C, Ohara CJ, Fitzgibbon JS, Modeste A. Spindle cell pseudotumor due to Mycobacterium-avium-intracellulare in patients with acquired immunodeficiency syndrome (AIDS) – positive staining of mycobacteria for cytoskeleton filaments. Am J Surg Pathol 1991; 15:1181–1187.

107. Chen KTK. Mycobacterial spindle cell pseudotumor of lymph nodes. Am J Surg Pathol 1992; 16:276–281.

108. Suster S, Moran CA, Blanco M. Mycobacterial spindle-cell pseudotumor of the spleen. Am J Clin Pathol 1994; 101:539–542.

109. Sekosan M, Cleto M, Senseng C, Farolan M, Sekosan J. Spindle cell pseudotumors in the lungs due to Mycobacterium tuberculosis in a transplant patient. Am J Surg Pathol 1994; 18:1065–1068.

110. Lucas SB. Mycobacteria and the tissues of man. In: Ratledge C, Stanford JL, Grange JM, eds. Biology of Mycobacteria, Vol 3. London: Academic Press; 1989:107–176.

Brucellosis

111. Lubani MM, Lulu AR, Araj GF, Khateeb MI, Qurtom MAF, Dudin KI. Pulmonary brucellosis. Q J Med 1989; 71:319–324.

112. Al-Jam'a AH, Elbashier AM, Al-Faris SS. Brucella pneumonia: a case report. Ann Saudi Med 1993; 13:74–77.

113. Greer AE. Pulmonary brucellosis. Dis Chest 1956; 29:508–519.

114. Hunt AC, Bothwell PW. Histological findings in human brucellosis. J Clin Pathol 1967; 20:267–272.

115. Saltoglu N, Tasova Y, Midikli D, Aksu HS, Sanli A, Dundar IH. Fever of unknown origin in Turkey: evaluation of 87 cases during a nine-year-period of study. J Infect 2004; 48:81–85.

116. Pappas G, Bosilkovski M, Akritidis N, Mastora M, Krteva L, Tsianos E. Brucellosis and the respiratory system. Clin Infect Dis 2003; 37:e95-e99.

117. Weed LA, Sloss PT, Clagett OT. Chronic localised pulmonary brucellosis. JAMA 1956; 161:1044–1047.

Chronic melioidosis

118. Piggott JA, Hochholzer L. Human melioidosis. A histopathologic study of acute and chronic melioidosis. Arch Pathol 1970; 90:101–111.

119. Wong KT, Puthucheary SD, Vadivelu J. The histopathology of human melioidosis. Histopathology 1995; 26:51–55.

120. Dhiensiri T, Puapairoj S, Susaengrat W. Pulmonary melioidosis: clinical-radiologic correlation in 183 cases in northeastern Thailand. Radiology 1988; 166:711–715.

Actinomycosis

121. Bowker CM, Connellan SJ, Freeth MG. A case of thoracic actinobacillus infection. Respir Med 1992; 86:53–54.

122. Hsieh MJ, Liu HP, Chang JP, Chang CH. Thoracic actinomycosis. Chest 1993; 104:366–370.

123. Cendan I, Klapholz A, Talavera W. Pulmonary actinomycosis – a cause of endobronchial disease in a patient with AIDS. Chest 1993; 103:1886–1887.

124. Lee JP, Rudoy R. Pediatric thoracic actinomycosis. Hawaii Med J 2003; 62:30–32.

125. Mabeza GF, Macfarlane J. Pulmonary actinomycosis. Eur Respir J 2003; 21:545–551.

126. Lu MS, Liu HP, Yeh CH, et al. The role of surgery in hemoptysis caused by thoracic actinomycosis; a forgotten disease. Eur J Cardiothorac Surg 2003; 24:694–698.

127. Bates M, Cruickshank G. Thoracic actinomycosis. Thorax 1957; 12:99–124.

128. Brown JR. Human actinomycosis. A study of 181 subjects. Hum Pathol 1973; 4:319–330.

129. Slade PR, Slesser BV, Southgate J. Thoracic actinomycosis. Thorax 1973; 28:73–85.

130. Dalhoff K, Wallner S, Finck C, Gatermann S, Wiessmann KJ. Endobronchial actinomycosis. Eur Respir J 1994; 7:1189–1191.

131. Ariel I, Breuer R, Kamal NS, Ben-Dov I, Mogle P, Rosenmann E. Endobronchial actinomycosis simulating bronchogenic carcinoma. Diagnosis by bronchial biopsy. Chest 1991; 99:493–495.

Nocardia

132. Nocard ME. Note sur la maladie des boeufs de la Guadeloupe connue sous le nom de farcin. Ann Inst Pasteur 1888; 2:293–302.

133. Eppinger H. Ueber eine neue pathogene Cladothrix und eine durch sie hervorgerufene Pseudotuberculose. Wien Klin Wschr 1890; 3:321.

134. Eppinger H. Uber eine neue, pathogene Cladothrix und eine durch sie hervorgerufene Pseudotuberculosis (cladothrichica). Beitr Pathol Anat 1891; 9:287–328.

135. Brechot JM, Capron F, Prudent J, Rochemaure J. Unexpected pulmonary nocardiosis in a non-immunocompromised patient. Thorax 1987; 42:479–480.

136. Saltzman HA, Chick EW, Conant NF. Nocardiosis as a complication of other diseases. Lab Invest 1962; 11:1110–1117.

137. Uttamchandani RB, Daikos GL, Reyes RR, et al. Nocardiosis in 30 patients with advanced human immunodeficiency virus infection: clinical features and outcome. Clin Infect Dis 1994; 18:348–353.

138. Menendez R, Cordero PJ, Santos M, Gobernado M, Marco V. Pulmonary infection with Nocardia species: a report of 10 cases and review. Eur Respir J 1997; 10:1542–1546.

139. Hui CH, Au VWK, Rowland K, Slavotinek JP, Gordon DL. Pulmonary nocardiosis re-visited: experience of 35 patients at diagnosis. Resp Med 2003; 97:709–717.

140. Burbank B, Morrione TG, Cutler SS. Pulmonary alveolar proteinosis and nocardiosis. Am J Med 1960; 28:1002–1007.

141. Summers JE. Pulmonary alveolar proteinosis. Review of the literature with follow-up studies and report of two new cases. Calif Med 1966; 104:428–436.

142. Frazier AR, Rosenow ECI, Roberts GD. Nocardiosis: a review of 25 cases occurring during 24 months. Mayo Clin Proc 1975; 50:657–663.

143. Wada R, Itabashi C, Nakayama Y, Ono Y, Murakami C, Yagihashi S. Chronic granulomatous pleuritis caused by nocardia: PCR based diagnosis by nocardial 16S rDNA in pathological specimens. J Clin Pathol 2003; 56:966–969.

144. McNeil KD, Johnson DW, Oliver WA. Endobronchial nocardial infection. Thorax 1993; 48:1281–1282.

145. Fielding DI, Oliver WA. Endobronchial nocardial infection. Thorax 1994; 49:385.

146. Casty FE, Wencel M. Endobronchial nocardiosis. Eur Respir J 1994; 7:1903–1905.

147. Robboy SJ, Vickery AL Jr. Tinctorial and morphologic properties distinguishing actinomycosis and nocardiosis. N Engl J Med 1970; 282:593–596.

148. Camp M, Mehta JB, Whitson M. Bronchiolitis obliterans and Nocardia asteroides infection of the lung. Chest 1987; 92:1107–1108.

149. Murray JF, Finegold SM, Froman S, Will DW. The changing spectrum of nocardiosis. A review and presentation of nine cases. Am Rev Respir Dis 1961; 83:315–330.

150. Petersen JM, Awad I, Ahmad M, Bay JW, McHenry MC. Nocardia osteomyelitis and epidural abscess in the nonimmunosuppressed host. Cleve Clin Q 1983; 50:453–459.

Rhodococcus and malakoplakia

151. Torres Tortosa M, Arrizabalaga J, Villanueva JL, et al. Prognosis and clinical evaluation of infection caused by Rhodococcus equi in HIV-infected patients – A multicenter study of 67 cases. Chest 2003; 123:1970–1976.

152. Kwon KY, Colby TV. Rhodococcus equi pneumonia and pulmonary malakoplakia in acquired immunodeficiency syndrome – pathologic features. Arch Pathol Lab Med 1994; 118:744–748.

153. Scott MA, Graham BS, Verrall R, Dixon R, Schaffner W, Tham KT. Rhodococcus equi – an increasingly recognised opportunistic pathogen: report of 12 cases and review of 65 cases in the literature. Am J Clin Pathol 1995; 103:649–655.

154. Hamrock D, Azmi FH, ODonnell E, Gunning WT, Philips ER, Zaher A. Infection by Rhodococcus equi in a patient with AIDS: histological appearance mimicking Whipple's disease and Mycobacterium avium-intracellulare infection. J Clin Pathol 1999; 52:68–71.

155. Gupta RK, Schuster RA, Christian WD. Autopsy findings in a unique case of malacoplakia. A cytoimmunohistochemical study of Michaelis-Gutmann bodies. Arch Pathol Lab Med 1972; 93:42–48.

156. Colby TV, Hunt S, Pelzmann K, Carrington CB. Malakoplakia of the lung. A report of two cases. Respiration 1980; 39:295–299.

157. Hodder RV, St George-Hyslop P, Chalvardjian A, Bear RA, Thomas P. Pulmonary malakoplakia. Thorax 1984; 39:70–71.

158. Crouch E, Wright J, White V, Churg A. Malakoplakia mimicking carcinoma metastatic to lung. Am J Surg Pathol 1984; 8:151–156.

159. Byard RW, Thorner PS, Edwards V, Greenberg M. Pulmonary malakoplakia in a child. Pediatr Pathol 1990; 10:417–424.

160. Scannel KA, Portoni EJ, Finkel HI, Rice M. Pulmonary malakoplakia and Rhodococcus equi infection in a patient with AIDS. Chest 1990; 97:1000–1001.

161. Schwartz DA, Ogden PO, Blumberg HM, Honig E. Pulmonary malakoplakia in a patient with the acquired immunodeficiency syndrome – differential diagnostic considerations. Arch Pathol Lab Med 1990; 114:1267–1272.

162. Mollo JL, Groussard O, Baldeyrou P, Molas G, Fournier M, Pariente R. Tracheal malakoplakia. Chest 1994; 105:608–610.

163. Deperalta-Venturina MN, Clubb FJ, Kielhofner MA. Pulmonary malakoplakia associated with Rhodococcus equi infection in a patient with acquired immunodeficiency syndrome. Am J Clin Pathol 1994; 102:459–463.

164. Yuoh G, Hove MGM, Wen J, Haque AK. Pulmonary malakoplakia in acquired immunodeficiency syndrome: an ultrastructural study of morphogenesis of Michaelis-Gutmann bodies. Mod Pathol 1996; 9:476–483.

165. Bastas A, Markou N, Botsi C, et al. Malakoplakia of the lung caused by Pasteurella multocida in a patient with AIDS. Scand J Infect Dis 2002; 34:536–538.

166. Biggar WD, Keating A, Bear RA. Malakoplakia: evidence for an acquired disease secondary to immunosuppression. Transplantation 1981; 31:109–112.

Syphilis

167. Edmonds LC, Stubbs SE, Ryu JH. Syphilis – a disease to exclude in diagnosing sarcoidosis. Mayo Clin Proc 1992; 67:37–41.

168. Dooley DP, Tomski S. Syphilitic pneumonitis in an HIV-infected patient. Chest 1994; 105:629–631.

169. Guarner J, Greer PW, Bartlett T, et al. Congenital syphilis in a newborn: An immunopathologic study. Modern Pathol 1999; 12:82–87.

170. Austin R, Melhem RE. Pulmonary changes in congenital syphilis. Pediatr Radiol 1991; 21:404–405.

5

Infectious diseases

5.4

Fungal infections

In certain regions of the world, environmental soil conditions support the saprophytic phase of pathogenic fungi such as *Histoplasma capsulatum*, *Blastomyces dermatitidis*, *Coccidioides immitis* and *Paracoccidioides brasiliensis* that are able to cause disease in previously healthy people. Other fungi invade the tissues only because of lowering of the patient's resistance by some other disease or as a side effect of treatment. Some of the fungi that cause these so-called opportunistic infections are seldom, if ever, responsible for illness in healthy individuals: this is particularly so of mucormycetes. Others cause disease in healthy individuals of a type very different from the progressive, destructive, disseminated infection that they set up in those whose resistance has been reduced: asthma from sensitisation to aspergilli and saprophytic growth in previously formed cavities are examples of such disease.

Many fungi that infect man are dimorphic – that is, they grow as yeast-like organisms at certain temperatures and in mycelial form at others. Spores released by macroconidia that form on the mycelial hyphae when there is plentiful oxygen are inhaled and germinate in the lungs. Speciation generally requires culture but the size and shape of the fungus often enable the histopathologist to identify the genus (Box 5.4.1).

The ease and frequency of international travel make many hitherto 'exotic' diseases the immediate practical concern of doctors who have no personal experience in their recognition and management. The fact that fungi which are frequently the cause of disease in other parts of the world are not indigenous where the doctor is in practice is no longer an excuse for not considering the possibility that a patient may have acquired infection while visiting another country or through exposure to contaminated, imported materials. Neither histoplasmosis nor coccidioidomycosis, for instance, occurs naturally in western Europe, yet every year in countries such as Britain, patients are seen whose symptoms are due to these diseases: the cardinal importance of the patient's geographical history and of the doctor's knowledge of geographical medicine, is self-evident.

Box 5.4.1 Microscopical differentiation of common fungi in lung tissue

Yeasts
  Small
    Pneumocystis
    Histoplasma
    Torula
  Medium-sized
    Candida
    Cryptococcus
    Blastomyces
    Paracoccidioides
  Large
    Coccidioides
Hyphae
  Short
    Candida (pseudohyphae)
  Long and regular
    Aspergillus
  Long and irregular
    Mucormycetes

PNEUMOCYSTOSIS[1,2]

Microbiology

Pneumocystosis is caused by organisms discovered in the early twentieth century by Chagas and, soon after, by Carini. They both thought the organism to be a stage in the life cycle of trypanosomes as they found it in the lungs of rats experimentally infected with trypanosomiasis. The Delanoës recognised that it was a distinct species, *Pneumocystis carinii*. Pneumocystis organisms were first identified as a cause of human disease in 1942, in Belgium, in association with cases of the condition, previously of unknown causation that had been described in 1937 as interstitial plasma cell pneumonia. Outbreaks of the latter occurred during the Second World War and for some years after, in orphanages and other institutions that housed malnourished children, particularly in eastern Europe and the Middle East.[3] The causative role of the pneumocystis in this type of pneumonia in young children was generally recognised following the work of Jirovec in Czechoslovakia in the years immediately after the war.[4,5] Subsequently it has been recognised that the human pathogen is a separate species, *P. jiroveci*. Although pneumocysts were long thought to be protozoal, they are now regarded as a primitive fungus in which the mycelium is reduced to a unicellular state but is still able to sporulate.[6–8]

Electron microscopy[6,9–12] provides an insight into the structure of the organism and the pathogenesis of pneumocystis pneumonia. It shows that the organism forms cysts measuring 3–6 µm in diameter, which have a thick wall or pellicle (Fig. 5.4.1). The pellicle is particularly thick at one point, a feature that is evident by light microscopy in silver-stained preparations as a peripheral dot on the cyst wall. The pellicle is triple-layered, consisting of an outer electron-dense zone about 75 nm thick, an electron-lucent intermediate zone 250 nm thick and an inner 7 nm membrane. Numerous small tubular structures are associated with the inner layer. Up to eight nucleated

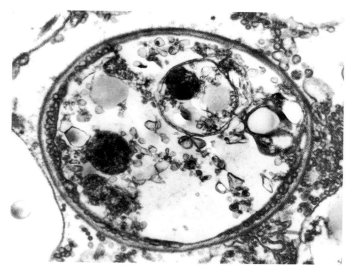

Figure 5.4.1 *Pneumocystis jiroveci.* Cyst form. The cyst wall has three layers: an outer electron-dense zone about 75 nm thick, an electron-lucent intermediate zone 250 nm thick and an inner 7 nm membrane. Numerous small tubular structures are associated with the inner layer, which also spawns up to eight intracystic bodies or sporozoites, one of which is visible here. Electron micrograph. (Reproduced with permission from Corrin B and Dewar A. Respiratory diseases. In Papadimitriou JM, et al (eds). Diagnostic Ultrastructure of Non-Neoplastic Diseases. Edinburgh: Churchill Livingstone 1992; 264–286.[12] With permission from Elsevier Ltd.)

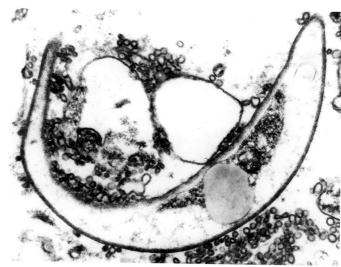

Figure 5.4.2 *Pneumocystis jiroveci.* Collapsed cyst releasing its contents. Electron micrograph. (Reproduced with permission from Corrin B and Dewar A. Respiratory diseases. In Papadimitriou JM, et al (eds). Diagnostic Ultrastructure of Non-Neoplastic Diseases. Edinburgh: Churchill Livingstone 1992; 264–286.[12] With permission from Elsevier Ltd.)

intracystic bodies are also probably derived from this membrane. These are released when the cyst ruptures (Fig. 5.4.2). Collapsed cysts are largely empty and the innermost membrane of the wall is either detached or absent. The released intracystic bodies grow from about 1.5 to 6 µm, have a thin pellicle and are highly irregular in shape (Fig. 5.4.3). They possibly undergo binary fission before entering a pre-cyst stage in which their pellicles thicken (Fig. 5.4.4). The intracystic bodies are still

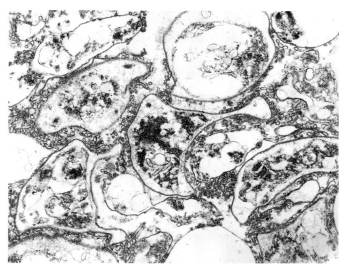

Figure 5.4.3 *Pneumocystis jiroveci.* Trophozoites. These are irregular in shape and have a thin unit membrane wall. Electron micrograph. (Reproduced with permission from Corrin B and Dewar A. Respiratory diseases. In: Papadimitriou JM, et al (eds). Diagnostic Ultrastructure of Non-Neoplastic Diseases. Edinburgh: Churchill Livingstone 1992; 264–286.[12] With permission from Elsevier Ltd.)

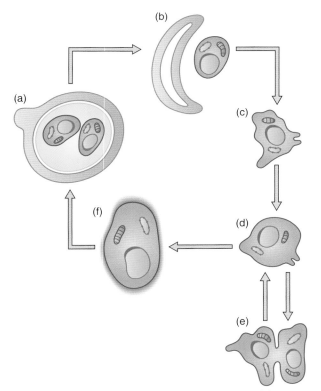

Figure 5.4.4 Proposed life cycle of *Pneumocystis jiroveci.* (a) Cystic form containing two intracystic bodies. Note the focal thickening of the pellicle. (b) Discharge of cyst contents and collapse of the cyst. (c–e) Trophozoites, which possibly undergo binary fission. (f) Trophozoite in pre-cystic stage.

generally referred to as sporozoa and in their extracystic form as trophozoites, despite the now accepted fungal nature of the organism.

Cysts tend to be sparse near the alveolar walls, which are bordered chiefly by trophozoites, suggesting that limitation of some nutritional factor promotes cyst formation. In successfully treated cases only empty cysts are found, indicating that all viable forms of the parasite, whether free-living or encysted, are vulnerable to chemotherapy. Although there is not a heavy cellular reaction within the alveolus, degenerate cysts and trophozoites may be found within alveolar macrophages.

Electron microscopy also shows that the trophozoites attach to type I alveolar epithelial cells, eventually causing these cells to slough away from the alveolar walls.[13] Tracer studies show that there is increased permeability in the lung, even before epithelial cells are lost.[14] In severe cases, trophozoites are observed within the alveolar interstitium. From here they may gain access to the bloodstream and disseminate widely.[15]

Epidemiology

The epidemic pneumocystis pneumonia mentioned above, as a feature of malnourished children, is no longer seen in Europe but is still encountered in parts of the world where poverty and malnutrition are rife. Pneumocystis pneumonia is also recognised as a complication of immunodeficiency states, both congenital and acquired. Until the appearance of the acquired immune deficiency syndrome (AIDS) such immunodeficiency was generally due to lymphoproliferative disease or immunosuppressive therapy but interest now centres on pneumocystis pneumonia as being by far the commonest opportunistic infection in AIDS (see Table 5.1.1, p. 160). *P. jiroveci* is kept in check by T lymphocytes and suppression of these cells, as in AIDS, allows the parasite to proliferate and cause pneumonia. In very severe T-lymphocyte depletion, extrapulmonary dissemination is found (see below). Patients who have undergone heart/lung transplantation are also at risk of developing pneumocystis pneumonia,[16] as are those with cancer.[17] Whatever the cause of the immunoparesis, pneumocystis pneumonia in immunodeficient individuals lacks the intense plasma cell infiltration seen in malnourished children.

Antibodies to *P. jiroveci* can be detected in most of the population by the age of 4 years[18] but the absence of the organism from normal lungs suggests that the pneumonia represents re-infection rather than re-activation.[8,19,20] Infection is presumed to be by inhalation from an as yet poorly characterised environmental source. Although *P. jiroveci* has been found in a wide range of animals it shows host specificity and is the species prevalent in man.

Clinical features

Pneumocystis pneumonia is characterised by breathlessness, cough and fever, generally of insidious onset. Untreated, the disease progresses with mounting tachypnoea, hypoxaemia and cyanosis. Radiographs typically show widespread bilateral opacification. Late features include calcification, cavitation and pneumothorax. Diagnosis requires demonstration of the organ-

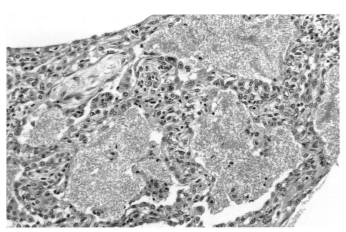

Figure 5.4.5 *Pneumocystis jiroveci* pneumonia. The alveoli are filled by a foamy exudate and the alveolar walls are thickened by a lymphoid infiltrate.

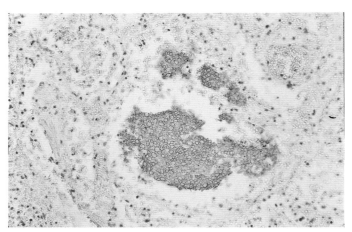

Figure 5.4.7 Immunocytochemical staining of *Pneumocystis jiroveci* demonstrates the trophozoites as well as the cysts.

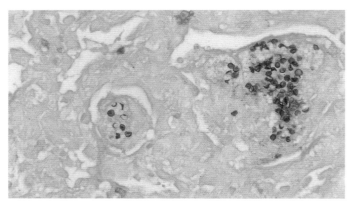

Figure 5.4.6 *Pneumocystis jiroveci* demonstrated by Grocott's methenamine silver stain. The smaller group includes crescentic forms representing collapsed cysts and other cysts that show a characteristic dot representing focal thickening of the cyst wall.

isms, for which sputum production is generally induced by the inhalation of a saline aerosol or bronchoalveolar lavage is undertaken.[21] The organisms may be demonstrated with toluidine blue, Geimsa stain, Grocott's methenamine silver stain or by immunofluorescence but detection of pneumocystis DNA by the polymerase chain reaction is much more sensitive.[22–28]

Morbid anatomy

Autopsy in cases of pneumocystis pneumonia presents no danger except in AIDS where there is a possibility of mortuary staff being infected by the HIV virus. Fatal pneumocystis pneumonia is generally characterised by widespread bilateral consolidation with relative sparing of the bases and apices of the lungs. Rarely, the disease takes the form of solid or cavitating pulmonary nodules.[29,30]

Histological appearances

Microscopically, the alveoli are filled by a foamy, pale, eosinophilic exudate (Fig. 5.4.5). The parasite is unstained in haematoxylin and eosin preparations but with Grocott's

methenamine silver stain, the alveoli are seen to contain numerous round cysts that measure about 5 μm across. Crescent-shaped forms (Fig. 5.4.6) represent collapsed cysts and their presence is helpful if there is concern that erythrocytes have not been successfully differentiated in the staining procedure, especially if bronchial washings or bronchoalveolar lavage fluids are being examined and the topographical features provided by a biopsy cannot be studied. Another helpful feature is a dot, generally seen on the edge of the cyst (Fig. 5.4.6); this represents a focal thickening of cyst wall.[31] Various quick modifications of fixation and processing and of the Grocott stain have been introduced to speed the diagnosis,[32–34] but the importance of fixation in killing any concomitant human immunodeficiency virus should not be overlooked. Other special stains that find favour include the Gram Weigert and Giemsa methods[35,36] and those using monoclonal antibodies (Fig. 5.4.7).[22] The last two methods stain the trophozoite as well as the encysted form of the parasite, but as the cysts are invariably present in pneumocystis pneumonia (and are shown by Grocott's stain), this is a dubious advantage: the Grocott stain is clearer and has the advantage of staining any other fungi that may also be present.[37] However, in sputa and other cytological specimens where the pneumocysts may be sparse the greater sensitivity of immunochemical stains and molecular techniques is advantageous.[23–27] *In situ* hybridisation has also been used to demonstrate pneumocysts in tissue sections.[38]

The alveolar exudate in which the parasites are found is virtually free of host cells except for a mild increase in the number of alveolar macrophages. The reaction to the parasite is largely an interstitial infiltrate of lymphocytes and plasma cells (Fig. 5.4.5). In most immunodeficient patients the infiltrate is generally mild but in malnourished children it is intense, warranting the original descriptive term interstitial plasma cell pneumonia.

Changes other than the classic one of foamy alveolar exudates may be found in pneumocystis pneumonia, particularly in AIDS (Table 5.4.1, Fig. 5.4.8),[29,30,39–46] demonstrating that pathological changes in infective disorders are dependent on host factors as well as the parasite. As well as the cavitating nodules mentioned above,[29,30] necrotising granulomatous inflammation,[26,39,42–44,47] diffuse alveolar damage[41], calcification,[40,45,48] lymphoid interstitial pneumonia (particularly in children – see p. 644)[49–51] and interstitial[52,53] and vascular invasion have been described, the latter sometimes resulting in a

necrotising vasculitis.[30] The invasion of the interstitium and pulmonary blood vessels probably causes the necrosis that underlies the cavitating nodules.[30,53,54] The cavities develop into air cysts, which are prone to rupture into the pleural cavities, resulting in both pneumothorax and pneumocystis infection of the pleura.[55] Alternatively, there may be interstitial spread and infection of the pleural cavities in the absence of any direct fistulous communication.[52]

In view of the vascular invasion it is not surprising that widespread blood-borne dissemination is also reported, particularly in AIDS.[15,39,56–60] The fact that this sometimes develops in the absence of obvious pneumonia has been attributed to the prophylactic use of inhaled pentamidine which reduces the risk of pneumocystis pneumonia but does not prevent the organism spreading to other organs. Restitution of the immune response following effective anti-viral therapy is sometimes accompanied by an 'immune reaction inflammation syndrome' (IRIS)[60a] and this may ultimately result in widespread interstitial pulmonary fibrosis.

Although opportunistic infections are often multiple, there appears to be a special relationship between *P. jiroveci* and

Table 5.4.1 *Pneumocystis jiroveci* pneumonia: atypical histological features[43]

		Cases (n)	(%)
Fibrosis	Interstitial	77	63
	Intraluminal	44	36
Absence of typical exudates		23	19
Numerous alveolar macrophages		11	9
Granulomatous inflammation		6	5
Hyaline membranes		5	4
Marked interstitial pneumonitis		4	3
Parenchymal cavities		3	2
Interstitial microcalcification		3	2
Minimal histological reaction		2	2
Vascular permeation		1	1

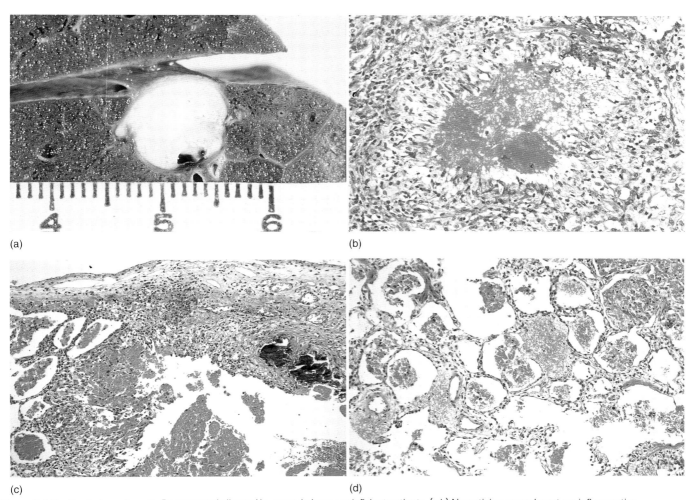

(a)

(b)

(c)

(d)

Figure 5.4.8 Atypical reactions to *Pneumocystis jiroveci* in severely immunodeficient patients. (a,b) Necrotising, granulomatous inflammation. (c) Necrosis, cavitation and dystrophic calcification. (d) Invasion of the interstitium, evident from the foamy exudate expanding alveolar walls as well as occupying alveoli. (Illustrations/sections supplied by Dr R Steele, Brisbane, Australia, Professor F Capron, Paris, France and Dr I Abdalsamad, Paris, France.)

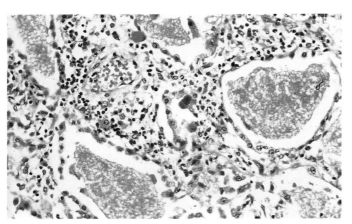

Figure 5.4.9 *Pneumocystis jiroveci* and cytomegalovirus pneumonia. As well as the foamy exudate of pneumocystis pneumonia there are prominent viral inclusions (centre).

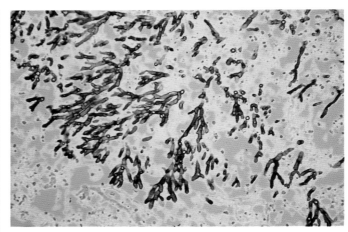

Figure 5.4.10 Aspergillus. The hyphae are septate, of fairly uniform thickness (3–6 μm diameter) and branch dichotomously at 35° to 45°. (Grocott's methenamine silver stain.)

cytomegalovirus, because these two organisms co-exist particularly frequently in the infected lung (Fig. 5.4.9). It has been suggested that *P. jiroveci* acts as an intermediate host for cytomegalovirus.[61]

Differential diagnosis

The differential diagnosis of classic pneumocystis pneumonia is from pulmonary oedema and alveolar lipoproteinosis. These three conditions are all characterised by the alveoli being filled by a largely acellular material, but whereas in oedema the material is amorphous, in lipoproteinosis it is granular and in pneumocystis pneumonia it has a foamy appearance. Alveolar lipoproteinosis is further distinguished from pneumocystis pneumonia by the presence of cholesterol crystal clefts and a few foamy fat-filled macrophages in the alveolar deposit and by the strong PAS-positivity of the deposit (compare Fig. 5.4.5 with Fig. 6.2.19).

ASPERGILLOSIS

Mycology

Aspergilli are common saprophytes found throughout the world in decaying organic matter where their spores may be so numerous that they can be seen as a dense dust cloud when piles of such material are disturbed. Several species have been identified as causes of human disease but *Aspergillus fumigatus* is by far the most frequent, particularly in European cases of pulmonary disease and septicaemia. Other species responsible for disease in man include *A. flavus* and *A. niger*, the latter more common in America.

Definitive diagnosis requires culture but this is not always successful. In histological preparations an aspergillus has a characteristic appearance and can be generically identified by the morphology of its hyphae (Fig. 5.4.10). Aspergillus hyphae are usually visible in haematoxylin-eosin preparations and sometimes are so intensely haematoxyphil that they are imme-

diately evident at low magnifications. Although the periodic-acid/Schiff stain and the Gridley stain for fungi facilitate their recognition, the Grocott-Gomori methenamine silver nitrate method is very much more reliable. The hyphae are septate and their hyphal diameter, which varies from 3 to 6 μm, is fairly regular. Typically, the hyphae branch dichotomously at relatively narrow angles (35° to 45°), the branches then tending to orient themselves parallel to each other. Rare fungi of similar morphology, such as *Chaetomium globosum*, can be distinguished by immunocytochemistry,[62–64] or culture.

The conidiophores (or fruiting heads) that are so striking a feature of aspergilli when growing as saprophytes, are seen in infected tissues only when the fungus is exposed to air: they are never found within the solid structure of colonised organs and tissues, but may occasionally be seen in the lung if the lesion communicates with a bronchus (Fig. 5.4.11). Species identification is based on colonial characteristics and on the structure of the conidiophores, which is best studied in culture (Figs 5.4.11–5.4.13).

Oxalate crystal deposition

Crystals of calcium oxalate have been identified in tissues infected by aspergilli, particularly *A. niger*, of which oxalic acid is a fermentation product. In some cases, local tissue injury and even generalised acute oxalosis and renal failure have resulted from the production of oxalic acid by the fungus.[65] Its widespread deposition as insoluble calcium oxalate may be accompanied by sudden hypocalcaemia.[66] Tissue toxicity is attributed to calcium oxalate complexing with iron, this resulting in the production of free oxidants.[67] Oxalosis is commonest with saprophytic aspergillosis but is also recorded with the allergic and invasive varieties of the infection (described below). The demonstration of oxalate crystals in biopsy and cytology specimens can be a useful aid in the diagnosis of pulmonary aspergillosis.[68–70] The crystals are birefringent (Fig. 5.4.14), stain with alizarin red[71] and can be confirmed as oxalate by crystallography and X-ray diffraction.[72]

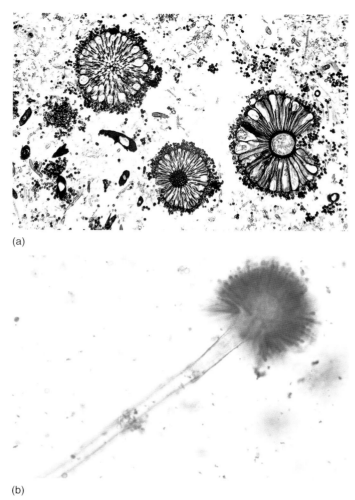

(a)

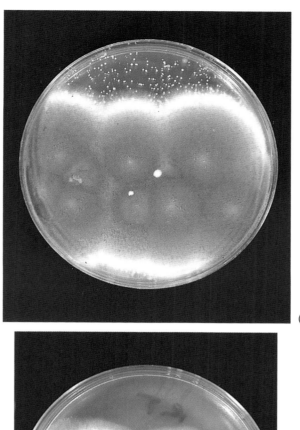

(a)

(b)

Figure 5.4.11 The fruiting heads or conidiophores of aspergillus in a pulmonary cavity that communicated with the bronchi, so affording the fungus the oxygen that stimulates this form of reproduction. (a) Grocott's methenamine silver stain, (b) lactophenol cotton blue stain on culture specimen.

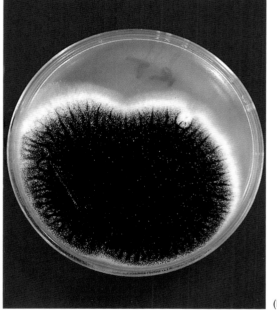

(b)

Figure 5.4.12 Aspergillus colonies in culture. The hyphal mycelium is white in all species but the conidiophores' colour is distinctive. (a) *A. fumigatus*; (b) *A. niger*.

Predisposing causes and types of pulmonary aspergillosis

Although exposure to aspergillus spores is common, the fungus is not a frequent pathogen. Only if the individual is atopic, or the lungs have been previously damaged, or general resistance is lowered by other conditions are ill-effects likely to occur. Bronchopulmonary disease caused by aspergilli may accordingly be classified respectively as allergic, saprophytic and invasive.[73,74] Rarely, different forms of pulmonary aspergillosis occur in the same patient. For example, an aspergilloma may be complicated by allergic aspergillosis,[75,76] even in a non-atopic patient, whilst an aspergilloma may develop within the bronchiectasis resulting from allergic aspergillosis.[77,78]

Allergic bronchopulmonary aspergillosis

Persons suffering from this form of aspergillosis are generally atopic and give a history of worsening asthma.[79–81a] There is also an increased incidence of allergic aspergillosis in patients with cystic fibrosis, but nearly half those so affected are also atopic.[82] It is important to reiterate that this form of aspergillosis is not characterised by invasion of the tissues by the fungus; it is an allergic response to aspergillus that remains confined to the airways. Furthermore, as the disease is a hypersensitivity phenomenon, hyphae are very sparse and have to be searched for diligently, in contrast to both the other main forms of aspergillosis (saprophytic and invasive) in which hyphae are numerous.

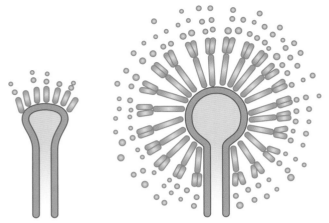

Figure 5.4.13 The structure of the conidiophores shows marked species variation. Diagrammatic appearances of *A. fumigatus* on the left and *A. flavus* on the right.

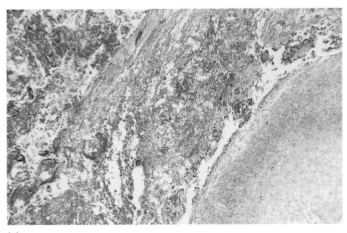

(a)

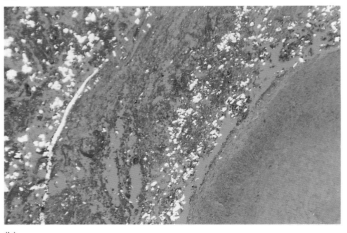

(b)

Figure 5.4.14 Calcium oxalate crystal deposition in the tissues bordering an aspergilloma viewed with (a) non-polarised and (b) polarised light. As is usually the case, much of the fungal colony is dead but here the adjacent host tissue is also necrotic, this change being attributable to oxalic acid secretion by the fungus. The oxalic acid combines with free calcium ions in the tissues to precipitate as insoluble, birefringent crystals.

The allergic reaction in the lung is frequently reflected in a raised blood eosinophil count. Eosinophilia is also seen in lung tissue and sputum. Circulating precipitating antibodies to aspergillus antigens may be demonstrable and immunoglobulin E, both total and specific, is generally raised; indeed, these immunological tests, together with the demonstration of immediate (and late) skin reactions to aspergillus antigens, are now the main means of confirming the clinical diagnosis of allergic aspergillosis. There is, however, a wide range of specific antibodies to various antigenic components of the fungus and concentration of the serum may be necessary to detect them for they are often not present in the high concentrations found in association with an aspergilloma. Poor antigens may give false negative results and steroids may depress the antibody response and thus both skin and serological reactions. Culture of the sputum is not always positive and on occasion the diagnosis of allergic bronchopulmonary aspergillosis is first made by the histopathologist after surgery has been undertaken for a suspected malignancy (Fig 5.4.15 and see Fig. 9.7, p. 465).[83]

The term allergic bronchopulmonary aspergillosis is generally limited to a syndrome that is chiefly characterised by the expectoration of mucus plugs or the impaction of such plugs and the consequent development of bronchiectasis. However, allergy to aspergillus may have further bronchopulmonary consequences, notably bronchocentric granulomatosis and eosinophilic pneumonia, both of which are dealt with elsewhere (see pp. 461, 463). Attention here will be limited to mucoid impaction.

Mucoid impaction

In some asthmatic individuals, particularly large mucus plugs develop, typically 1–2 cm thick and 2–5 cm long. They generally form in proximal bronchi (Fig. 5.4.15) and can be clearly seen in plain radiographs as finger-like opacities near the hilum of the lung. They are frequently expectorated spontaneously. The airway involved is dilated and its wall shows non-specific chronic inflammatory changes which vary from a mild infiltrate to a severe reaction that includes many eosinophils. The affected airway may be merely distended and therefore returns to normal after the plug is expectorated, or its wall may be largely destroyed by the inflammation so that there is permanent bronchiectasis (Fig. 5.4.16). The proximal distribution of this form of bronchiectasis contrasts with that of the post-infective form, which generally affects the bases.

The mucus plugs undergo inspissation and often have the consistence of hard rubber. Although they may form casts of several generations of bronchi, they tend to be shorter and stubbier than the long stringy casts expectorated in plastic bronchitis (see p. 106). The microscopic appearances also differ. Mucus plugs characteristically consist of bands of agglutinated eosinophils alternating with layers of mucus (Fig. 5.4.15b). The bands of eosinophils are arranged parallel to the airway wall and frequently diminish in length towards the centre of the lumen so that wedges of alternating cellular and mucus bands

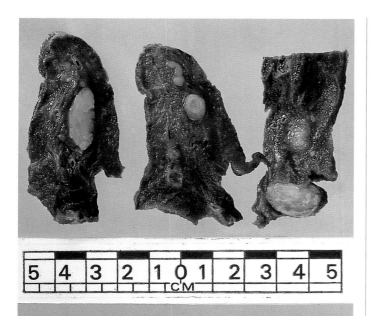

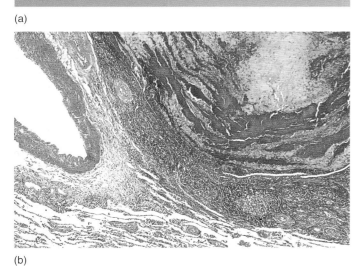

Figure 5.4.15 Allergic bronchopulmonary aspergillosis. (a) Several bronchi are distended by plugs of viscous mucus. (b) Microscopy shows alternating eosinophilic bands, the pink ones representing mucus and the red conglomerations of eosinophils. The walls of the bronchi show chronic inflammation, which weakens them and leads to proximal bronchiectasis. (Specimen submitted by Professor DH Wright, Southampton, UK.)

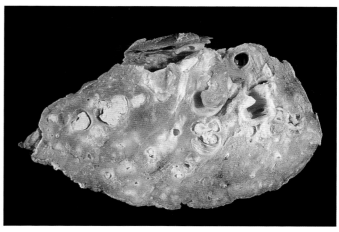

Figure 5.4.16 Allergic bronchopulmonary aspergillosis. The proximal bronchi (top) are dilated and some contain mucus plugs. More peripherally there is coagulative necrosis representing bronchocentric granulomatosis and beyond that pale foci of eosinophilic pneumonia are seen. (Illustration provided by the late Dr AA Liebow, San Diego, USA.)

Extrinsic allergic alveolitis

Extrinsic allergic alveolitis may also be a manifestation of allergy to aspergillus, but here it is heavily exposed non-atopic individuals that are affected. One example is 'malt workers' lung', which occurs in brewery staff working with mouldy barley; the species of aspergillus involved here is usually *A. clavatus*. Extrinsic allergic alveolitis may also develop in patients harbouring an aspergilloma.[76] These forms of allergy to aspergillus are similar, both clinically and pathologically, to the extrinsic allergic alveolitis that develops in response to other allergens (see p. 280).

Saprophytic aspergillosis

Aspergilli may grow saprophytically within stagnant secretions in the bronchi in cases of chronic bronchitis and, less often, bronchiectasis. In certain circumstances, this may be very marked, resulting in obstructive aspergillosis (see below). Other varieties of saprophytic aspergillosis include the colonisation of an infarct,[92] a tumour,[93] the bronchial anastomosis following transplantation[94,95] and a pre-formed cavity, resulting in the last case in the formation of an aspergilloma (intracavitary aspergillus ball colony).[96]

Aspergilloma

In an aspergilloma the fungus grows in the lumen of a cavity in the lung without invading the tissues to any appreciable extent, drawing its nutriment from such exudate as may be present. The ball usually forms in an existing cavity, particularly an old tuberculous cavity[96] but sometimes in a cavity resulting from conditions such as sarcoidosis, bronchiectasis, abscess or emphysema, or in a congenital cyst. Aspergilloma formation has been observed both in the bronchiectatic lung distal to an

point inwards, presenting an appearance that has been likened to fir trees.[84] Sparse aspergillus hyphae are generally to be found in the mucus plugs.

In exceptional cases, other fungi are responsible for similar changes, resulting in reports of allergic bronchopulmonary stemphyliosis, curvulariosis, drechsleriasis, candidosis, helminthosporiosis, penicilliosis, torulopsosis, fusariosis and pseudallescheriosis.[85–90] and the term allergic bronchopulmonary fungal disease is therefore sometimes preferred.[91]

obstructing carcinoma and within the cavity resulting from necrosis at the centre of a peripheral carcinoma.[97] Although usually single, aspergillomas may be present in cavities in both lungs and in some cases there are several such lesions.

The term mycetoma is frequently misapplied to intracavitary fungal balls, such as aspergillomas. The term is correctly limited to a type of fungal granuloma that is characterised by the formation of multiple sinuses and is usually the outcome of penetration of the soft tissues by a thorn, or the like, contaminated by the causative organism. Such lesions are most frequent on the extremities and 'Madura foot' is the type example. In this sense, a mycetoma represents a lesion caused by invasion of the tissues by the organism concerned, in contrast to an intracavitary fungal ball, which is essentially outside the tissues and does not, except in unusual circumstances, lead to extension of the infection into the wall of the cavity itself. Many varieties of fungus cause mycetomas; most of them seldom, if ever, cause other disease.

While most intracavitary fungal ball colonies are formed by *A. fumigatus*, other species of *Aspergillus* have been identified in some cases and, exceptionally, fungi such as *Pseudallescheria (Petriellidium) boydii*,[98] *Cladosporium cladosporidioides*[99] and species of *Penicillium, Candida* or *Syncephalastrum*[100] have been responsible. Also, ball colonies similar to an aspergilloma may on rare occasions consist solely of bacteria (see 'nocardioma' on p. 213 and 'botryomycoma' on p. 188).

Radiology

The radiological appearances of an aspergilloma are often characteristic, the fungal ball appearing as a sharply demarcated radio-opaque spheroid that rests on the wall of the dependent part of the cavity and is separated from it elsewhere by a crescent of air. In cases of long standing the colony may fill the cavity completely but the fungal ball is often able to move within the cavity in accordance with the patient's posture. However, although these features are characteristic of an aspergilloma, they may also be given by an indolent necrotising form of invasive aspergillosis which is considered below (see chronic necrotising aspergillus pneumonia, p. 231). A true aspergilloma is often demonstrated in radiographs over a period of several years, sometimes with little or no detectable change in its appearance, sometimes with appreciable phases of shrinkage and enlargement (Fig. 5.4.17).

Antibody production

Most patients with an aspergilloma have strong serum precipitins against aspergillus antigens but, unless allergy with asthma has developed, skin tests against extracts of the fungus are negative. Occasionally the circulating precipitins combine with fungal antigen disseminated via the airways to produce the changes of extrinsic allergic alveolitis elsewhere in the lung or there may be immune complex-mediated vasculitis elsewhere in the body.

Morbid anatomy

The fungal colony appears macroscopically as a grey or reddish brown, rarely white or green-tinged, mass, sometimes firm or

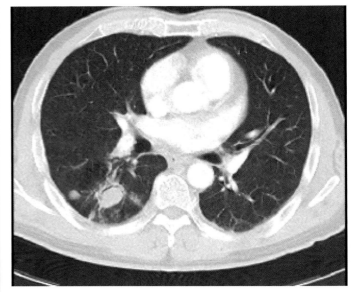

(a)

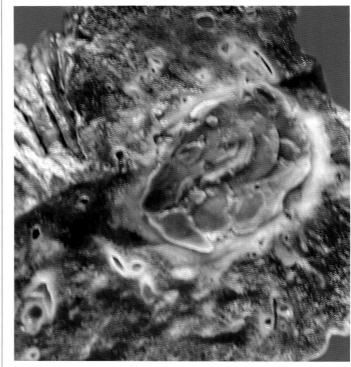

(b)

Figure 5.4.17 Aspergilloma. (a) CT shows a cavity in the apical segment of the right lower lobe, containing an intracavitary body consistent with an aspergilloma. (b) The resected lobe shows a solid, well-circumscribed brown mass lying within a bronchiectatic cavity.

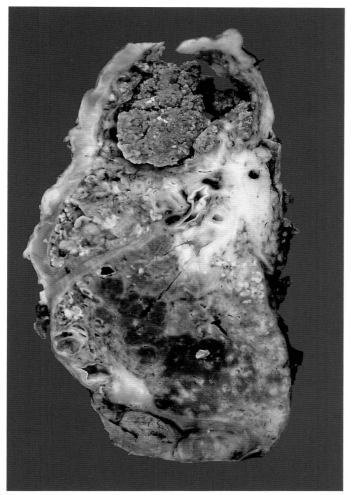

Figure 5.4.18 An aspergillus fungal ball (an aspergilloma) filling an apical cavity. In its fresh state the fungal ball forms a soft, brown, pultaceous mass but as seen here after fixation it is more friable.

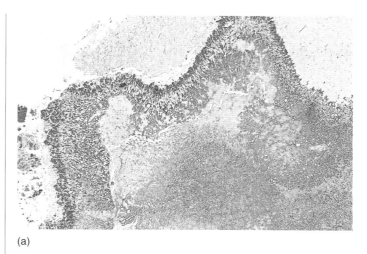

(a)

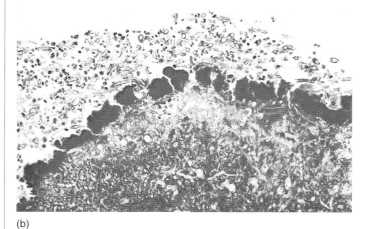

(b)

Figure 5.4.19 Aspergilloma. (a) The centre of the fungus ball consists of a dense feltwork of dead fungal hyphae. Only at the periphery is the fungus viable. (b) The edge of the fungus ball is coated by a layer of eosinophilic immune material (Splendore–Hoeppli phenomenon).

rubbery in consistency but often friable or pultaceous (Figs 5.4.17b, 5.4.18). Old colonies may have a gritty feel, from deposition of calcium salts and exceptionally, there may be so much calcification that the ball becomes stony and may be classified among the so-called 'pneumonoliths'.

Histological appearances

Microscopically, an aspergilloma consists of a dense feltwork of hyphae, most of which are dead. Only the hyphae at the surface are well preserved. The tips of these may be abundantly coated with hyaline eosinophilic material of probable immune origin (Splendore–Hoeppli phenomenon), giving the edge of the aspergilloma a distinctive appearance (Fig. 5.4.19). The lining of the cavity that contains an aspergilloma varies according to the nature of the condition that has given rise to it. The wall of an old tuberculous cavity may consist of dense, hyaline fibrous tissue, sometimes devoid of an epithelial covering; in other cases there may be a lining zone of chronic inflammatory granulation tissue, which usually is without specific features of tuberculosis or other former disease. When present, an epithelial lining may be of either respiratory or squamous type.

Chronic inflammatory changes in the lining of the cavity that are attributable to the fungal ball are variable but their presence underlies any enlargement of the cavity. It is mentioned above that numerous calcium oxalate crystals are occasionally present. These are found in the cavity lining, particularly near the surface and in relation to the sides of blood vessels that face the fungus ball (Fig. 5.4.14). The toxic nature of oxalic acid contributes to the progressive enlargement of the cavity but proteinases secreted by the fungus are probably more important in this respect.[101] Sometimes non-specific chronic inflammation is due to secondary bacterial infection.

It is exceptional for the fungus to invade the tissues, although this has been observed. Such a change from saprophytosis to invasive growth is more likely to occur when the patient's resistance is lowered, particularly by immunosuppressant and cytotoxic therapy and less often by administration of corticosteroids.

Haemorrhage

Haemoptysis is a common feature of aspergilloma. Usually it causes no more than anaemia, but in some cases it has been massive and death has resulted. It often accompanies the development of further excavation of the lung tissue round the colonised lesion. The rich capillary bed of a granulation tissue lining is generally the source of the haemorrhage,[102] but larger vessels are occasionally involved, the endarteritis obliterans usually found in chronic inflammation failing to seal them completely. The blood supply to the wall of an aspergilloma cavity ultimately derives from the bronchial circulation and the haemoptysis can sometimes be controlled by cannulation of the bronchial arteries concerned under radiographic control and the introduction of occlusive synthetic emboli (see Fig. 8.1.14, p. 412).

Obstructive aspergillosis

This form of aspergillosis was first described in the acquired immune deficiency syndrome[103] and subsequently in the recipients of organ transplants.[104] It is characterised by a progressive cough, which is sometimes productive of bronchial casts composed entirely of aspergillus hyphae, in contrast to the mucus plugs of allergic bronchopulmonary aspergillosis in which hyphae are scanty. There is no wheezing or eosinophilia but the patient rapidly develops hypoxaemia. Chest radiographs show areas of collapse and at bronchoscopy some airways are found to be completely obstructed by fungal casts. When these are removed, the bronchial mucosa appears normal. The condition therefore represents saprophytic infection. Nevertheless, it is probably a precursor of the locally invasive pseudomembranous aspergillus tracheobronchitis described below.

Invasive and septicaemic aspergillosis

Excluding saprophytic colonisation of pulmonary infarcts and superficial invasion round an aspergilloma – each a relatively rare occurrence – most instances of aspergillus pneumonia are due to the patient's resistance being undermined by factors that cause prolonged granulocytopenia, such as lymphoproliferative disease, leukaemia and corticosteroid therapy.[105–109] Less often, invasive pulmonary aspergillosis complicates influenza or other viral infection[110,111] or chronic obstructive pulmonary disease.[112] AIDS is another predisposing cause[113–116] but the incidence of invasive aspergillosis is nevertheless lower than that of many other opportunistic infections in this group of patients,[103,117,118] probably because the human immunodeficiency virus attacks lymphocytes rather than granulocytes. Rarely, the patient is apparently immuncompetent.[119] In severely immunodeficient patients the infection spreads quickly and often disseminates via the bloodstream, whereas in less debilitated patients infection results in more indolent localised lesions.

Invasive aspergillosis

Invasive aspergillosis is characterised by an outpouring of fibrinous exudate into the alveoli, often with many neutrophils,

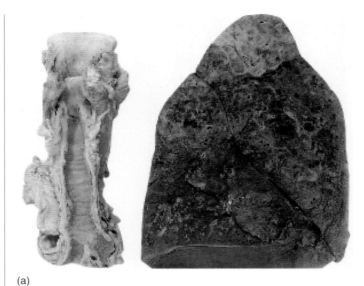

(a)

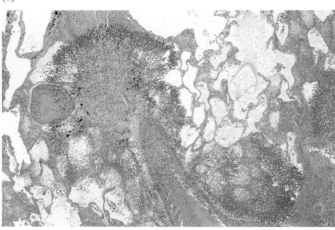

(b)

Figure 5.4.20 Invasive aspergillosis. (a) The lung and lower end of the trachea show multiple foci of necrotising inflammation. (b) The fungal hyphae grow through all constituents of the lung tissue, including blood vessels, which thrombose, resulting in infarction. (Fig (a) provided by WGJ Edwards, London, UK.)

thrombosis of the capillaries and necrosis of the tissue, which is heavily infected by the fungus (Fig. 5.4.20a). In the early lesions each alveolus may contain a small, star-like-cluster of radiating hyphae that clearly have developed from germination of one or more spores; later, the hyphae penetrate the alveolar wall and extend widely into the tissues (Fig. 5.4.20b). In the severely immunodeficient the extension is widespread and invasion of the larger blood vessels leads quickly to generalisation of the infection through the body.

Septicaemic aspergillosis

Septicaemic aspergillosis is commonly first recognised at necropsy and often not until the tissues are examined with the microscope. In many cases the portal of invasion of the bloodstream by the fungus is not apparent. In others it is a recognisable local infection such as aspergillus pneumonia. There may be a

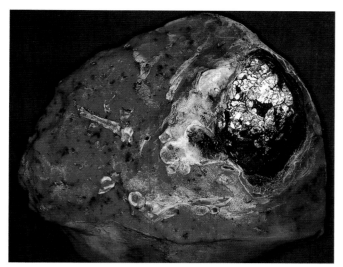

Figure 5.4.21 Chronic necrotising aspergillus pneumonia. The lung contains a cavity partly lined by a plaque of *Aspergillus nigra*. The appearances simulate those of an aspergilloma but the cavity is newly formed and its contents consist of necrotic lung tissue heavily infiltrated by the fungus. Compare the colour of this non-sporing mycelium with the cultured colony of the same species, which is exposed to oxygen and is therefore producing black conidiophores in Fig. 5.4.12, right. (Reproduced with permission from Wiggins J, et al. Chronic necrotising pneumonia caused by Aspergillus niger. Thorax 1989; 44:440–441.[125] With permission from the British Medical Association.).

rapidly overwhelming septicaemia, with little to show in the way of focal lesions, or there may be many large foci of necrosis, most frequently in the brain, heart and kidneys. The lesions are often so heavily colonised by the aspergillus that, very soon after exposure to the air at necropsy, condiophores develop and colour the necrotic tissue – green in the case of *A. fumigatus* and *flavus* and black if the fungus is *A. niger*. There may even be an obvious growth of the pigmented mould on the surface. Microscopical examination often shows that the hyphae of the invading fungus are surrounded by a spreading zone of necrosis in advance of their progress through the tissues: this is probably a result of diffusion from the infected part of toxins and degradative enzymes produced by the aspergillus.[65,101] Occasionally, the lesions are suppurative. Infection by other fungi may be present at the same time.

Chronic necrotising aspergillus pneumonia (acute cavitary pulmonary aspergillosis)

This is a localised form of invasive aspergillosis in which the necrotic lung tissue may separate away as a sequestrum and mimic an aspergilloma both radiographically and macroscopically (Fig. 5.4.21);[120–128a] microscopically, however, infected lung tissue is easily distinguishable from an intraluminal ball colony of fungus, even though both are largely necrotic.

Pseudomembranous aspergillus tracheobronchitis

Pseudomembranous aspergillus tracheobronchitis involves only a narrow zone of tissue bordering the major airways, the

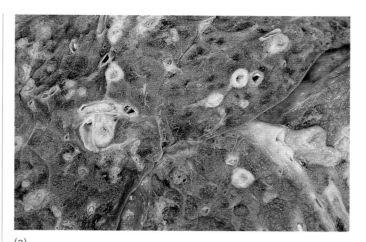

(a)

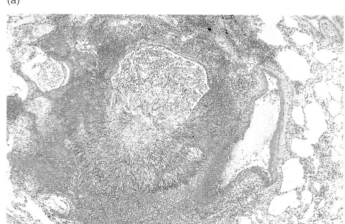

(b)

Figure 5.4.22 Pseudomembranous aspergillus bronchitis. Many airways are plugged by fungal hyphae and necrotic debris. Invasion is generally limited but in this patient the process has already affected the adjacent pulmonary artery. (a) Gross appearances, (b) Microscopy.

intervening lung parenchyma being spared.[113,129–133] In this form of invasive aspergillosis the airways are occluded by a mixture of necrotic debris and fungal hyphae (Fig. 5.4.22). It may be preceded by the obstructive form of saprophytic aspergillosis described above. A granulomatous response to the fungus may develop, mimicking bronchocentric granulomatosis (see p. 463).[134,135]

MUCORMYCOSIS

Mycology

Mucormycosis (formerly zygomycosis or phycomycosis) is the name most widely familiar for any infection caused by a fungus that is a member of the class Zygomycetes (formerly Phycomycetes). This class includes the orders Mucorales and Entomophthorales. They are found in soil, dung and dust throughout the world and are common causes of food spoilage. The classic form of mucormycosis is rhinocerebral, where the fungi grow from an infected ulcer in the nasal space to invade the cranial cavity, cerebral blood vessels and the contents of one or both orbits.[136,137] Some of the mucormycoses are primary subcutaneous or orificial mucosal infections, occurring without predisposing disease. Very rarely, dissemination of the fungus from these primary sites results in visceral infection, including pulmonary mucormycosis due to the Entomophthorales *Basidiobolus haptosporus (B. meristosporus)* and *Conidiobolus coronatus (Entomophthora coronata)*. Much more commonly, pulmonary mucormycosis is direct and attributable to lowering of resistance to invasion of the tissues by Mucorales of the species *Absidia, Mucor* and *Rhizopus* which ordinarily are saprophytes on decaying organic matter. It is quite exceptional for one of these moulds to set up progressive infection in a patient who is otherwise in good health.[138]

The Mucorales that cause pulmonary infection are recognisable as such in histological sections by their characteristic morphology (Fig. 5.4.23a) but this does not allow identification of genus or species, which requires immunohistochemistry.[64] The hyphae are characteristically of variable but generally broad diameter, ranging from 3 to 20 µm. They tend to branch perpendicularly and septation of the hyphae is absent or at most very infrequent. A false impression of septum formation may be given by folds that result from shrinkage. Because of their irregular appearance and the sometimes-striking effects of shrinkage during histological processing the hyphae have been likened to lengths of crushed ribbon. Although visible in haematoxylin-eosin preparations, the mucoraceous fungi are best shown by special methods: the methenamine silver stain is often useful, but better results may be obtained by the silver impregnation methods used in the demonstration of reticulin fibres. As in the case of aspergilli, such morphologically specific structures as sporangiophores develop only when the mould is growing in air. They are seldom, if ever, seen in pulmonary lesions in the fresh state, but they may form if a specimen has inadvertently been left exposed before being placed in fixative solution. Culture often fails and histology may then be the first means of identification.

Predisposing causes

Conditions predisposing to visceral mucormycosis include the acquired immune deficiency syndrome, leukaemia, pancytopenia, myelomatosis, diabetes mellitus and immunosuppression to prevent graft rejection.[135,139,140] Certain therapeutic measures also predispose to these infections, particularly desferrioxamine and the administration of cytotoxic and immunosuppressant drugs, including corticosteroids. Cannulation of blood vessels, when long continued, is a further occasional factor, being a potential portal of infection. Burns, too, have repeatedly become not merely a site of superficial infection but the source of haematogenous dissemination. The predisposing factors to some extent determine the site of predominant infection. For instance, the syndrome of naso-orbitomeningingocerebral mucormycosis occurs usually as a complication of diabetes mellitus or renal failure. These metabolic disorders are comparatively seldom responsible for the development of pulmonary or primarily septicaemic mucormycosis, which in most cases occur as complications of severe blood disease or of the resistance-lowering side-effects of drugs.

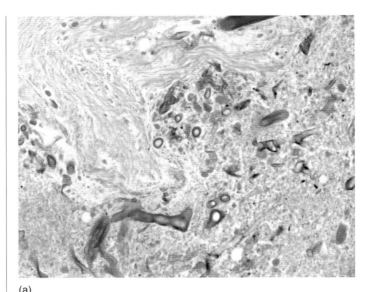

(a)

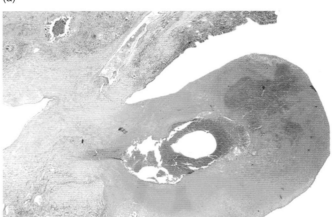

(b)

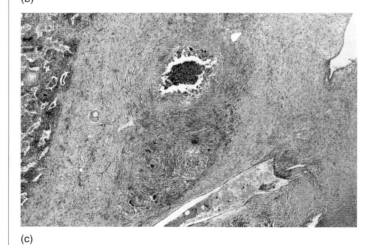

(c)

Figure 5.4.23 Mucor. (a) Mucor hyphae have few septa and are irregular in outline. The rounded structures that resemble spores are hyphae cut transversely. (b) Mucormycosis in a lung excised because of massive haemoptysis. Haemorrhage surrounds a partially thrombosed ruptured blood vessel. (c) The wall of the ruptured vessel shows necrotising granulomatous angiitis.

Similarly, severe malnutrition predisposes to mucormycosis of the stomach or intestine.

Pathological findings

Mucormycotic lesions in the lungs vary greatly in size and number. Multiple lesions are usually the result of haematogenous dissemination, as may occur in cases of naso-orbitocerebral mucormycosis, whereas lesions that are single or few may be the result of direct infection of the lungs by way of the airways. The lesions are firm, hyperaemic or haemorrhagic and often necrotic. If they extend to the pleura, a fibrinous exudate is found over them and there are often petechial or larger foci of bleeding. Central lesions tend to be spherical and peripheral ones wedge-shaped,[141] the former resembling chronic necrotising pulmonary aspergillosis (see p. 231) and the latter representing infarcts.

Microscopically, the most significant finding is fungal invasion of blood vessels of all sizes, with thrombosis and colonisation of the thrombus by the fungus and infarction (Fig. 5.4.23b,c). It is clear that many strains of these fungi are thrombogenic and staining the lesions with phosphotungstic acid haematoxylin or by other appropriate methods clearly demonstrates the formation of fine radiating threads of fibrin on the surface of the hyphae within the blood vessels. Perineural invasion is also commonly seen.[137] The hyphae may be present in great number, not only in the thrombi but throughout the resulting infarcts. The latter soon liquefy and there may be secondary bacterial infection.

As with other fungal infections occurring as a consequence of predisposing illnesses and drug-induced failure of resistance, mucormycosis is often accompanied by one or more other opportunistic infections, even of the same part. Frequent associations are of mucormycosis with aspergillosis or candidosis but bacterial, viral and protozoal infections may also be present.

CANDIDOSIS (MONILIASIS)

Candida is a yeast-like fungus that forms round or oval budding cells (blastospores), septate hyphae and intermediate structures called pseudohyphae. Candidosis generally represents infection by *Candida albicans* (formerly known as *Monilia albicans*) but other species may be involved.[142] Speciation requires culture as the species are morphologically identical. *C. (Torulopsis) glabrata* is dealt with separately (see p. 241).

The commonest form of candidosis is oral thrush, but the organism can attack any mucous or moist cutaneous surface. The fungus is often found in the sputum but its presence there generally represents no more than saprophytic growth. The diagnosis of bronchopulmonary candidosis therefore often depends on finding the organism histologically. It is found as a secondary invader of the lower respiratory tract in cases of chronic bronchitis, bronchiectasis and bronchial carcinoma and in severely ill patients with immunosuppression, including

AIDS.[114] In sections, candida may be seen within a pseudomembrane consisting of purulent exudate on the surface of a bronchus, or very rarely in lung tissue as a cause of pneumonia or even lung abscess. In agranulocytic patients there is necrosis with minimal inflammation. Candida pneumonia may represent a peripheral extension of candida bronchitis or result from haematogenous dissemination complicating diseases or therapeutic measures that lower resistance. Pulmonary vascular candidosis is reported as a complication of central venous catheters inserted for prolonged parenteral feeding.[143,144] Features that distinguish *Candida* from *P. jiroveci* and other yeast-forming fungi such as *Histoplasma* include the mixture of budding yeast cells with pseudohyphae and the pyogenic or necrotising host reaction. The invariable presence of yeasts distinguishes candidosis from aspergillosis and mucormycosis.

CRYPTOCOCCOSIS

Mycology

Cryptococcosis, a disease of worldwide distribution, is caused by the monomorphic yeast-like fungus, *Cryptococcus neoformans*. This organism was formerly known as *Torula histolytica* and the disease as torulosis. Because it was first recognised in Europe and is caused by a fungus the cells of which reproduce by budding, cryptococcosis was also sometimes known as European blastomycosis, in contrast to the so-called North and South American blastomycoses (now blastomycosis and paracoccidioidomycosis respectively).

Although perhaps most familiar as a complication of leukaemia or lymphoma, in which the infection typically presents as a progressive meningoencephalitis, cryptococcosis is also known as a primary disease of the lungs without predisposing conditions, particularly when *Cryptococcus neoformans var. gattii* is involved.[145,146] The lung is the principal portal of entry for this fungus and infection of the lungs is probably much commoner than at present recognised. The primary pulmonary lesion of cryptococcosis is comparable to the initial lesion of histoplasmosis and coccidioidomycosis and to the Ghon focus of tuberculosis. Other diseases predisposing to secondary pulmonary cryptococcosis include alveolar lipoproteinosis and AIDS.[114,147]

C. neoformans is a spheroidal or ovoid organism. A characteristic feature is variability in size, the cell body measuring from 3 to 20 μm diameter although in many instances within the range of 6 to 9 μm (Fig. 5.4.24a). Another prominent feature is single, narrow-based budding, as opposed to the single, broad-based budding of *Blastomyces dermatitidis* and the multiple narrow-based budding of *Paracoccidioides brasiliensis*. The organism has a mucoid capsule that usually stains with mucicarmine, a reaction that is not given by any other pathogenic yeast-like fungus. Cryptococci can be seen in haematoxylin eosin preparations because they are refractile and, in polarised light, birefringent. They can also be demonstrated by any of the special methods for staining fungi (Fig. 5.4.24b). The capsule is sometimes deficient, in which case the fungus is not

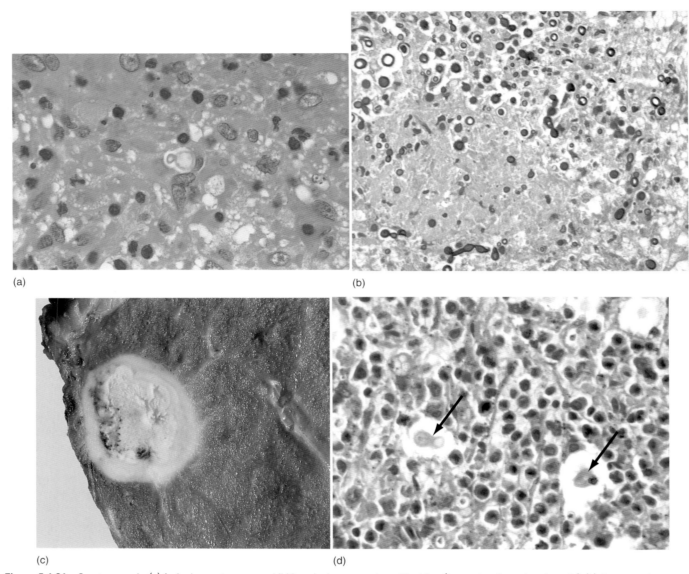

(a)

(b)

(c)

(d)

Figure 5.4.24 Cryptococcosis. (a) A single cryptococcus exhibiting single narrow-based budding (haematoxylin and eosin stain). (b) Cryptococci demonstrated by periodic acid–Schiff staining. (c) A necrotising 4 cm cryptococcoma excised after its chance radiographic discovery. (d) Fungal spores (arrows) are seen among neutrophils in an immunosuppressed patient with disseminated disease. (Illustrations (a) provided by Dr A Paiva-Correia, Oporto, Portugal and (c) Dr M Jagusch, formerly of Auckland, New Zealand. Case (b and d) provided by Dr PM Cury, Sao Jose do Rio Preto, Brazil.)

mucicarminophilic.[148] However, in most cases of capsule-deficient cryptococcosis some carminophilic capsular material can be identified around a few yeasts. A Masson–Fontana stain can also help in the recognition of capsule-deficient cryptococci because unlike other yeasts cryptococci produce a melanin-like pigment.[149]

The cryptococci may be found in the sputum in cases of pulmonary involvement. They may be seen on microscopical examination of wet films, particularly when the sputum has been mixed with India ink or nigrosin to display the capsule. In dry films, the fungal cells disintegrate or become smudged and usually cannot be recognised, although sometimes staining with mucicarmine is conclusive. Cultures are generally the preferred means of confirming the diagnosis, but some strains of the cryptococcus do not grow well and several attempts may have to be made before the organism is isolated. It is notable that the cryptococcus is only exceptionally, if ever, found in sputum in the absence of infection, in spite of its near ubiquity in our environment.

The fungus is often found in the dried droppings of birds, particularly pigeons and starlings. These provide a good culture medium and pathogenic cryptococci can often be isolated from buildings on which these birds roost. Isolation from soil is less frequent, probably because of the avidity with which cryptococci are phagocytosed by soil amoebae. As in the case of histoplasmosis, cryptococcosis has been known to develop in people who have worked in bird-infested buildings, particularly during demolition. The infection in such patients is slow to appear, in contrast to the acute pneumonic form of histoplasmosis. It is clear that exposure to cryptococci must occur very frequently: equally, the great majority of people must have a high immunity, for cryptococcosis is rare in any population.

It is important to remember that any patient with active cryptococcosis is at risk of developing infection of the central nervous system because of the peculiar affinity of the organism for the brain and meninges and the frequency of its dissemination in the blood.

Morbid anatomy

Pulmonary cryptococcosis takes several forms: primary, cryptococcoma, cavitary, pneumonic and miliary.[147,150–152] Isolated, discrete, encapsulated, subpleural granulomas are occasionally seen at necropsy: these are healed or healing lesions and the implication of their presence is that they are a manifestation of a primary and non-progressive infection. Less rarely, routine radiographs unexpectedly disclose one or more focal 'coin' lesions in the lungs, up to several centimetres in diameter, that prove to be foci of progressive cryptococcal infection. These are known as cryptococcomas (formerly torulomas) (Fig. 5.4.24c). They are firm, pale tan and rather sharply defined but are encapsulated only when healing. Their cut surface may be dry or gelatinous: the latter is the case when there is less inflammatory reaction to the organisms, which, packed closely in great numbers, account for the mucoid appearance and consistence of such lesions. Cavity formation is rare, but may occur when the focus is centred on a bronchus. Confluence and continuing enlargement of multiple foci may produce a gelatinous pneumonia involving the greater part of one or more lobes. In cases of generalised haematogenous dissemination of cryptococcosis both lungs may be studded with miliary or larger foci: close inspection of these discloses their gelatinous nature; they tend to be sharper in outline than miliary tubercles or pyaemic abscesses. The gelatinous collection of cryptococci at the centre of the lesion may be washed out during examination of the tissue, leaving a minute cavity.

Histological appearances

Microscopically, the lesions may be composed largely of the cryptococci themselves, with little cellular reaction: the alveoli and interstitial tissue contain the closely packed organisms, their cell bodies separated by the variable extent of their mucoid capsule. In other cases, particularly those involving capsule-deficient strains, there may be a tuberculoid reaction, the fungal cells being found within the cytoplasm of multinucleate giant cells and of mononuclear macrophages as well as free in the tissue spaces. In lesions of long standing, lymphocytes and plasma cells may be present in large numbers and fibrosis may be a feature, although not often conspicuous. Occasionally, neutrophils accumulate in considerable numbers (Fig. 5.4.24d), particularly in miliary haematogenous lesions, but in the absence of bacterial infection frank suppuration is not found. Caseation is a rare development and has to be distinguished from the somewhat similar appearance that may result when large numbers of cryptococci have died and disintegrated into an amorphous, finely granular, eosinophile mass.

HISTOPLASMOSIS

The first report of histoplasma infection was by Samuel Darling, a US Army pathologist stationed in Panama around the time of the building of the canal. Darling observed the organisms in histiocytes (hence the term 'histo'), likened them to plasmodia (hence 'plasma') and incorrectly assumed that an artefactual clear space around each organism was a capsule (hence 'capsulatum').

Mycology

Two species of *Histoplasma* are pathogenic in man, *H. capsulatum* and *H. duboisii*. The latter is found exclusively in tropical Africa and the disease that it causes differs significantly from that caused by *H. capsulatum*, an organism that is geographically far more widespread. In general, when the word histoplasmosis is used without elaboration it refers to disease caused by *H. capsulatum*.

The histoplasmas are dimorphic fungi, growing as ovoid, yeast-like organisms in cultures at 37°C and in infected tissues (parasitic phase) and in mycelial form, producing characteristic tuberculate macroconidia, in cultures at laboratory temperature (about 18°C) and in their free-living state in the soil (saprophytic phase). Spores released by the macroconidia are inhaled and at body temperature germinate into yeasts that grow by binary fission.

Histoplasmas can rarely be demonstrated in sputum, even by culture, but complement fixation and precipitin tests may be helpful. However, on occasion, biopsy may be necessary. When this is undertaken, the opportunity to set up cultures must not be lost. The fungi may be quite focal in their distribution and therefore difficult to find, but within these foci the spores are usually present in large numbers within the cytoplasm of macrophages or in areas of necrosis. They are readily seen in haematoxylin-eosin preparations, but only if recently viable. They measure from 1–3 μm by 3–5 μm and may contain a distinct nucleus. Histoplasmas that have been dead for some time may escape detection in such preparations, although sometimes birefringence, induced by histological processing, may make a proportion of them visible in polarised light. Fortunately, the methenamine silver stain commonly demonstrates histoplasmas very clearly even when they have long been dead. Unfortunately, they are difficult to distinguish from other budding yeasts but a granulomatous reaction, their intracellular location and an absence of pseudohyphae help separate them from *Candida* species and *P. jiroveci*.

Epidemiology

H. capsulatum is a soil-inhabiting fungus that requires organic nitrates for growth. These are generally provided by bird droppings. Histoplasmosis results from inhalation of infective spores and the geographical distribution of the disease is determined by environmental conditions. In regions where the fungus cannot survive to complete its saprophytic phase in soil or other organic debris, histoplasmosis does not occur naturally – infection does not ordinarily take place from person to person, the tissue form of the fungus being in general unable to convey the disease. In those parts of the world where the soil or the climate is unsuitable for the saprophytic phase of *H. capsulatum*, the disease is found only among those who have acquired the infection in lands where the fungus is present in the environment, or, much more rarely, as a result of exposure to imported materials contaminated by the infective spores[153] or to laboratory cultures of the saprophytic phase, which develops when the tissue form is grown at laboratory temperature.

Histoplasmosis is endemic in many parts of North, Central and South America, Asia and Africa. In North America, infection is particularly common in the basin of the Ohio and Mississippi River valleys where as many as 90% of the population give a positive reaction to the histoplasmin skin test. The histoplasmin test has the same significance in relation to histoplasmosis as the tuberculin test in relation to infection by *Mycobacterium tuberculosis*. In Africa, infection by *H. capsulatum* is endemic over an area far greater than that in which infection by the 'African histoplasma', *H. duboisii*, occurs. Histoplasmosis is also endemic in central and south America, India and south-east Asia but it has not been recognised as an indigenous infection in Australia. Its occurrence in Europe, other than as a result of travel to an endemic area or accidental exposure to the fungus, is exceptionally rare.

Most people who acquire histoplasmosis have no more than a subclinical infection. It has been estimated that clinical manifestations occur in only about 1% of cases and that few of these patients develop serious illness. Histoplasmosis is seen in rural communities exposed to bird droppings and in urban dwellers exposed to demolition and building sites. Bat guano is rich in organic phosphates and histoplasmas and the likely cause of an acute illness of cave explorers. Several forms of histoplasmosis are described, which will now be considered.

Primary pulmonary histoplasmosis

The primary focus of histoplasmosis resembles that of tuberculosis. As with mycobacteria, the main line of host defence is the macrophage. Specific T-cell immunity appears about 10–14 days after infection and macrophages so activated usually terminate the infection. If not, the organisms continue to grow within the macrophage cytoplasm. The disease is spread during its primary stage by infected macrophages migrating to the regional lymph nodes and beyond to disseminate by the bloodstream to all organs, but being filtered out particularly well by those rich in reticuloendothelial cells so that the liver and spleen are commonly involved.

The primary lesion may be solitary or there may be two or more, sometimes many, primary lesions in the lungs, the number depending on the heaviness of the exposure to the

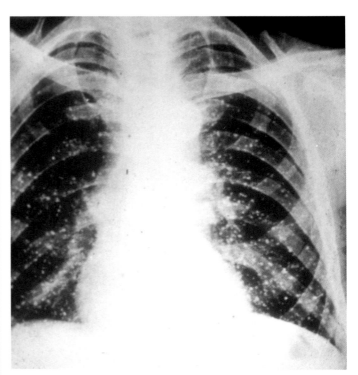

Figure 5.4.25 Histoplasmosis. A chest radiograph shows multiple bilateral calcific nodules in a patient with quiescent histoplasmosis.

infecting spores. It may occur in any part of the lungs. Generally and especially when solitary, it is larger than the corresponding lesion of primary tuberculosis but otherwise similar, showing epithelioid and giant cell granulomatous inflammation. Caseation develops within a few weeks of infection and its appearance is believed to coincide with the development of skin reactivity to histoplasmin, an observation comparable with the corresponding occurrence in tuberculosis. Early calcification and the formation of a fibrous capsule are common (Fig. 5.4.25). As in tuberculosis, there is spread of the infection to the hilar lymph nodes, which undergo comparable changes. It is a characteristic of calcified lesions of histoplasmosis that they have a massively chalky appearance and often show a peculiar stippled pattern in radiographs, particularly lesions in lymph nodes. Occasionally, the calcified foci in the lungs have a target-like radiographic shadow because of concentric zones of greater and lesser transradiancy.

Histoplasmoma

The name histoplasmoma is given to any circumscribed, persistent focus of histoplasma infection in a lung. The lesion is an outcome of a primary focus, akin to a tuberculoma rather than an aspergilloma. It occurs typically just under the pleura and is roughly spherical and from 1–4 cm, sometimes more, in diameter. Both in radiographs and when examined with the naked eye it has a characteristically concentric pattern of closely set laminae, which may contain appreciable amounts of calcium salts, although by no means invariably. This laminar structure is so characteristic of chronic caseous granulomas of fungal origin that in some centres it is regarded as proof of the non-neoplastic nature of 'coin shadows': this is not necessarily justified, for it has been known for carcinoma to arise in the fibrotic capsular zone round such a long-standing mycotic lesion. In general, histoplasmomas are altogether benign in outlook and may be left in situ with little chance that the infection will be activated and progress; they may become more heavily calcified as the years pass. If resected, they usually prove to be sterile on culture. The causative organism may then be demonstrated most reliably by the methenamine silver stain, even though it is no longer viable.

Cavitary histoplasmosis

Histoplasmosis may closely reproduce the clinical and radiological picture of cavitating pulmonary tuberculosis. Moreover, if such patients are exposed to a substantial risk of infection by *Mycobacterium tuberculosis*, as may occur if they are nursed in company with tuberculous patients, tuberculosis may be superimposed on the histoplasmic lesions, with detriment to the chances of successfully treating either infection. In general, cavitary histoplasmosis is seen most frequently in older patients, particularly men and is attributed to a local breakdown in immunity at the site of dormant subapical histoplasmic granulomas. In some cases, it is possible that the condition is due to reinfection, thus adding to the similarities between histoplasmosis tuberculosis. Like the cavities of chronic pulmonary tuberculosis, the lesion of cavitary histoplasmosis may become the site of an aspergilloma. Tuberculoid granulomatous tissue in the lining and vicinity of the cavities contains typical intracellular histoplasmas.

'Epidemic' pulmonary histoplasmosis

The condition that has been described as 'epidemic' pulmonary histoplasmosis, is a form of acute histoplasmosis characterised by a severe influenza-like illness that occurs as a result of a particularly heavy inhalational infection in an unprotected individual. The epithet 'epidemic' has been applied because such cases are commonly seen in several patients simultaneously, all of them exposed on the same occasion to a massive contamination of the air by infective spores. It is an unfortunate name, for such cases may occur singly when individuals are so unfortunate as to stir up large numbers of spores when working alone in a contaminated environment. These outbreaks have occurred when infected dust is disturbed in the course of cleaning or demolishing buildings, ranging from hen houses to city halls, that have harboured birds that over years have left the droppings that so perfectly favour the growth of the saprophytic

phase of *H. capsulatum*. Similarly, those who enter caves where bat and bird droppings have encouraged the histoplasma to proliferate may suffer comparable group outbreaks of acute histoplasmic pneumonia. The multiple foci of histoplasmosis that form in the lungs of heavily infected patients have the same structure and run the same course as the solitary primary foci described above. In some cases the infection is so heavy and the resulting changes in the lungs are so widespread, that death occurs. Those who have not previously had a histoplasmic infection tend to suffer the severest illness in these outbreaks, but even those already known to have had a primary infection may develop fatal pneumonic lesions under such conditions of massive re-infection. Fatal opportunistic histoplasma pneumonia is recorded[154] but immunosuppression is by no means necessary.

Progressive disseminated histoplasmosis

Mention has been made above of haematogenous dissemination of the infection during its primary stage. In most such cases the widespread lesions heal without ill effects. However, there is another form of disseminated histoplasmosis in which the disease progresses and eventually kills the patient. In some cases of this sort there are no obvious predisposing causes but in most the patient's resistance is lowered by the presence of serious underlying disease leading to defective T-cell function.[155] AIDS is now an important cause of such progressive disease (Fig. 5.4.26).[156,157]

Fatal disseminated histoplasmosis is characterised by heavy parasitisation of the reticuloendothelial cells resulting in hepatosplenomegaly and leukoerythroblastic anaemia. Painful ulcers develop at mucocutaneous junction zones or within the orifices of the body or in the pharynx and larynx. Organising pneumonic exudates and thin-walled cavities may be found in the lungs. Well-formed granulomas are not usually found. Fatal adrenal cortical insufficiency is another important manifestation.

Fibrosing mediastinitis

In those countries where histoplasmosis is prevalent mediastinal fibrosis with obstruction of some, or all, of the mediastinal contents is recorded as a complication of such infection.[158]

African histoplasmosis

Histoplasma duboisii, an organism larger than *H. capsulatum*, has been recognised as a cause of disease throughout much of Africa between the Sahara and the Zambesi. Its distribution overlaps that of *H. capsulatum*, which, however, is much more widespread on the continent. The source of the infection and the portal of entry of the fungus remain debatable. There is growing evidence that the organism has a saprophytic phase, probably in soil and that it may enter the body either through the lungs

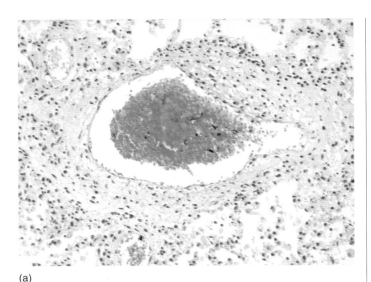

(a)

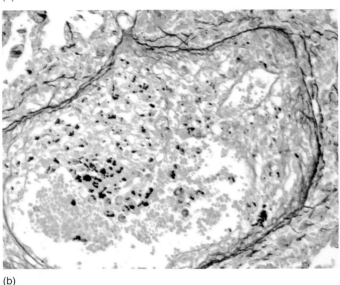

(b)

Figure 5.4.26 Progressive disseminated histoplasmosis. In a patient dying of AIDS, a pulmonary vessel shows only slight granulomatous inflammation (a) but Grocott staining shows extensive infiltration of the vessel by histoplasma (b). (Case provided by Dr PM Cury, Sao Jose do Rio Preto, Brazil.)

or, in certain cases, by inoculation into the skin. Pulmonary disease as one of its manifestations has attracted less attention than cutaneous and skeletal involvement, but it is possible that in many cases the lesions in the skin, like those in bones, are the result of dissemination in the blood from inapparent pulmonary foci.

A feature typical of African histoplasmosis is that the fungal cells provoke a foreign body giant cell reaction, not a simple histiocytosis with or without tuberculoid metamorphosis as occurs in cases of infection by *H. capsulatum*. The organism is ovoid, has a distinct cell wall and some internal structure

and measures from 5 to 12 μm in its longer dimension. It stains well with all the fungal stains, but is unlikely to be overlooked by the careful microscopist in haematoxylin-eosin preparations.

COCCIDIOIDOMYCOSIS[159–161]

Epidemiology

This disease is endemic in certain parts of North and South America, occurring especially in hot semi-arid regions such as Arizona and the San Joaquin valley of California, but also in other such areas of the Americas down to Argentina. It is caused by the fungus *Coccidioides immitis*, the saprophytic, free-living form of which requires special environmental conditions of soil and climate for its survival: these determine its geographical distribution. *C. immitis* grows best in soils free of competing microflora, losing out to competitors when the soil is irrigated. Upsurges of infection may follow dust storms that release the fungus into the air. The fungus may also be transported on inanimate objects such as crops or native artefacts and infect persons outside endemic areas and of course patients may travel to non-endemic regions while incubating the disease.[162] For example, the 2001 model airplane-flying world championship was held in an endemic region of California and several of those attending from other areas were found to have contracted coccidioidomycosis when they returned home.[163]

Mycology

C. immitis is a dimorphic fungus. Saprophytically, it grows as a mould that produces highly infective arthroconidia: these, inhaled in soil dust, establish the disease. As a parasite, the organism is found almost exclusively in the form of spherules. Hyphae develop occasionally in the wall of coccidioidal cavities when air is admitted by them communicating with an airway, but this is exceptional: only spherules and their released spores are usually present, even when air is admitted (Figs 5.4.27, 5.4.28).

Coccidioides is one of the most dangerous of all organisms in terms of risk of accidental infection of laboratory personnel. It is imperative that clinicians communicate to the laboratory any suspicion that a specimen may contain *C. immitis*. Laboratories dealing with coccidioidal cultures must operate with stringent precautions, including the exclusion of staff not known to have acquired some natural immunity through previous infection. The coccidioidin skin reaction is an invaluable screening test.

Once in the lungs, the arthroconidia develop into endosporulating spherules. These range from 30 to 60 μm or more in diameter and contain from scores to hundreds of endospores (Fig. 5.4.28). The maturing spherule is usually accompanied by a histiocytic reaction, with the formation of many multinucleate giant cells; the parasite may be enclosed by the latter or lie free in the tissues. The mature spherule attracts neutrophils,

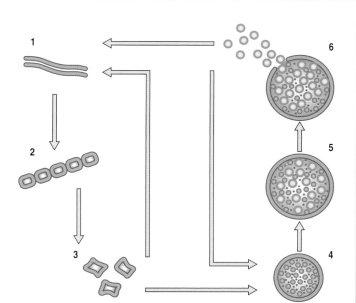

Figure 5.4.27 Life cycle of *Coccidioides immitis*. 1–3: Saprophytic phase in soil; 4–6: Parasitic phase in lungs. Mycelial strands (1) growing in soil mature into chains of barrel-shaped arthroconidia (2), which disarticulate (3), become air-borne and are returned to the soil, or are inhaled. The parasitic phase in the lungs begins with the enlargement of the inhaled arthroconidia and their development into thick-walled spherules (4), within which endospores form (5). Released spores (6) can initiate the development of a new spherule in the lungs or if infected material returns to the soil, mycelia (1), so completing the cycle.

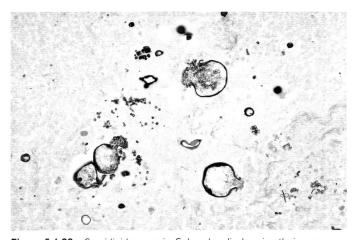

Figure 5.4.28 Coccidioidomycosis. Spherules discharging their spores within lung tissue. (Grocott methenamine-silver stain. Section provided by Dr JT Gmelich, Pasadena, USA.)

which collect to form microabscesses at the centre of the histiocytic granulomatous foci. When the spherule ruptures, the freshly released spores, which range from 5 to 10 µm in diameter, at first lie free in the purulent exudate but soon are engulfed by mononucleate or multinucleate macrophages. They grow and eventually become transformed into further

spherules, thus repeating the cycle and leading to extension of the infection.

The fungal cells are usually well seen in haematoxylin eosin preparations, except in the early stages when only a few, newly released spores are present, which may be so inconspicuous as to escape detection. The methenamine silver and other stains for fungi demonstrate all forms of the organism very clearly (Fig. 5.4.28). While the mature or even ruptured spherule is diagnostic, immature spherules or free spores are not; the former may be confused with blastomyces or paracoccidioides and the latter with cryptococci or histoplasmas.

Clinical features

The initial coccidioidal infection is symptomless in about 60% of persons.[164] When disease develops, there is usually an influenza-like fever, which characteristically may be accompanied by erythema nodosum – hence its popular name of 'the bumps' in the San Joaquin valley, where it is also called 'valley fever'. In most cases there is spontaneous recovery from the primary infection. When the disease is more severe, which is likelier to be the case in patients of African or Asian ethnic origin, it may mimic tuberculosis in any of its manifestations. In severe infections generalisation through the bloodstream is a frequent and particularly grave complication. Meningitis is another common complication. Many patients are left with quiescent pulmonary foci.

Pathological findings

At necropsy, the lungs may show focal consolidation, necrotic haemorrhagic areas or extensive necrotic excavating granulomatous nodules. Histologically, there may be a suppurative exudate in the alveoli, or necrotic haemorrhagic and fibrinous lesions, or a tuberculoid granulomatous reaction. Granulomatous inflammation is in general associated with good resistance and purulent inflammation with poor resistance. However, when a spherule ruptures to release its spores (Fig. 5.4.28), there may be a transient neutrophil response whatever the underlying pattern of inflammation. Also, the type of reaction is also partly determined by the maturity of the developing fungal cells. Patients whose resistance is lowered by other diseases may develop generalised haematogenous coccidioidomycosis as a consequence of activation of a dormant pulmonary focus. The lesion of quiescent pulmonary coccidioidomycosis is typically a fibrocaseous nodule containing a few viable organisms.

BLASTOMYCOSIS ('NORTH AMERICAN' BLASTOMYCOSIS)[165]

Epidemiology

It is now recognised that infection with *Blastomyces dermatitidis* occurs very widely throughout Africa and that the geographical designation 'North American', intended to distinguish this disease from 'European blastomycosis' (cryptococcosis) and

'South American blastomycosis' (paracoccidioidomycosis), is inappropriate.

In North America, the greatest prevalence is in the south-east of the USA, the area drained by the Mississippi, Missouri and Ohio rivers, the Great Lakes region and the eastern provinces of Canada. The natural habitat of the fungus is soil, particularly that subjected to flooding. Infection is believed to occur by inhalation. The usual site of primary infection is the lung. Most infection occurs in previously healthy persons and is subclinical but progressive pulmonary disease may result in disseminated extrapulmonary lesions such as meningoencephalitis, particularly in immunocompromised patients.

In Africa, lung disease is not so predominant. Many patients present with bone lesions or skin disease. Also, the antigenic make-up of the fungus differs from that encountered in North America, suggesting that there are at least two variants of blastomycosis, one seen in North America and in scattered foci in other countries (Mexico, Lebanon, Israel, Saudi Arabia and India), the other restricted to Africa.

Cultural characteristics and pathological findings

Like the histoplasmas, *B. dermatitidis* is a diphasic fungus. In tissues and in cultures at 37°C it grows as a yeast, whereas in cultures at laboratory temperature and presumably in nature, it grows as a mycelium from which project special slender hyphae known as conidiophores which bear conidia, the infective agents. The lungs are the usual portal of entry.

In the lung, the upper lobes are predominately involved.[166] Pathologically, the pulmonary lesions of blastomycosis may reproduce any of the features seen in histoplasmosis but the lesions are usually suppurative, with the fungal cells either lying free in the purulent exudate or engulfed by phagocytes. Most cases are first identified on cytology or histology with subsequent positive culture.[167] The organisms are rounded and usually within the range of 7–15 μm in diameter, although some cells may be as much as 30 μm across (Fig. 5.4.29). They have a thick wall, which may give them a double contoured appearance but they differ from the spores of *Cryptococcus neoformans*, which they otherwise resemble, in lacking a capsule and therefore failing to stain with mucicarmine. It is a special feature of *B. dermatitidis* that it reproduces in tissues by the formation of a single broad-necked bud that protrudes from the surface of the parent cell, enlarging even until it has reached as much as half the diameter of the latter, or more, before the two separate.

Although neutrophils are generally conspicuous in the reaction to the fungi, tuberculoid granulomas also form: a characteristic feature is the so-called 'suppurating pseudotubercle', in which a central microabscess is enclosed within a complex of epithelioid histiocytes and multinucleate giant cells (Fig. 5.4.29). Alternatively, an overwhelming infection may cause diffuse alveolar damage.[168–170] The infection is usually confined to the lungs and hilar lymph nodes but with impaired immunity dissemination may occur. However, blastomycosis is not a common manifestation of AIDS.

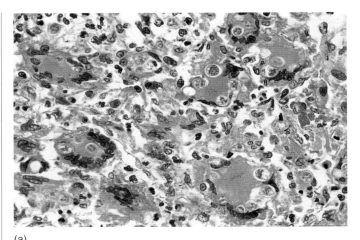

(a)

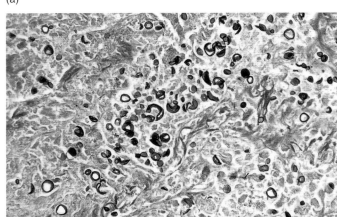

(b)

Figure 5.4.29 Blastomycosis. There is a neutrophil and giant cell reaction to *Blastomyces dermatitidis* yeasts, several of which have been ingested by giant cells. (a) Haematoxylin and eosin, (b) Grocott stain.

PARACOCCIDIOIDOMYCOSIS ('SOUTH AMERICAN BLASTOMYCOSIS')[171,172]

Epidemiology

Infection with *Paracoccidioides brasiliensis* is limited to Latin American countries from Mexico to Argentina but does not occur in all countries in this area. The endemic regions are the tropical and subtropical forests, particularly those of Brazil, Venezuela and Colombia. Paracoccidioidomycosis has not been proved to occur in any other part of the world. Cases reported from North America[173] and England[174] had all lived in South or Central America. The fungus is thought to live in the soil but its exact ecological niche is still unknown. Man is the only known naturally infected animal host. Person-to-person transmission is of little importance in the epidemiology of the disease, which is thought to be acquired by inhalation.

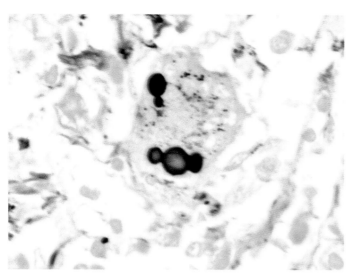

Figure 5.4.30 *Paracoccidioides brasiliensis.* The larger of the organisms illustrated is forming multiple buds. Grocott's methenamine silver stain. (Case provided by Dr PM Cury, Sao Jose do Rio Preto, Brazil.)

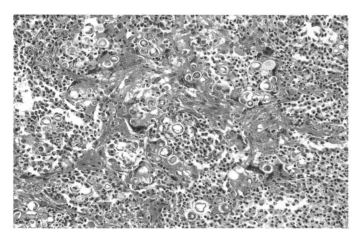

Figure 5.4.31 Paracoccidioidomycosis. There is a giant cell and neutrophil reaction to numerous spores of *Paracoccidioides brasiliensis.*

Mycology

P. brasiliensis is a dimorphic fungus that grows as a mould at ambient temperatures and as a yeast at 37°C. Infection is acquired by inhalation of conidia produced in the mycelial phase. Its tissue form is characterised by the development of multiple buds over the surface of the parent cell (Figs 5.4.30).

Clinicopathological features

Both pulmonary and disseminated forms of the disease are described.[171] After the establishment of a primary complex in the lung and hilar lymph nodes there may be haematogenous dissemination. Primary infection occurs in childhood and generally heals spontaneously. The sexes are affected equally in childhood but the development of the yeasts is inhibited by oestrogen and in adults the disease is largely limited to male agricultural workers. It is also described in patients with the acquired immune deficiency syndrome.[175] Disseminated disease tends to be acute and generalised in children and chronic and localised in adults. Chronic disseminated disease may take the form of lymphadenopathy, painful oropharyngeal ulceration or destruction of tissues such as the adrenal glands. Progressive pulmonary paracoccidioidomycosis is characterised by multiple cavities that mimic tuberculosis, or by progressive fibrosis of the lower lobes with traction bronchiectasis and paracicatricial emphysema in a bilaterally symmetrical distribution.[176] The tissue response is generally granulomatous but may be purulent (Fig. 5.4.31). Calcification is not a prominent feature. The diagnosis is established by recognising the spores in smears or culture of sputum or pus, or in tissue sections, or by serology. Biopsy is an excellent diagnostic procedure. The spores are best recognised with silver stains: the characteristic buds around the periphery of the parent spore have been likened to the handles of a ship's wheel but a better analogy is 'Mickey Mouse ears' (Fig. 5.4.30).

RARE PULMONARY MYCOSES

Fungi responsible for extrinsic allergic alveolitis are listed in Table 6.1.1 (p. 281) and the occurrence of intracavitary colonies of various fungi is mentioned on p. 228. Allergic bronchopulmonary candidosis, helminthosporiosis, penicilliosis and curvulariosis, similar to the more familiar allergic aspergillosis, have all been described on rare occasions.[91]

Pulmonary mycoses not dealt with above are rare and ordinarily occur as a result of lowering of the body's resistance by other diseases or their treatment.[177] Some examples are dealt with below. Others include infection by the common saprophytic mould *Geotrichum candidum, Trichosporon cutaneum,* the organism of white piedra (tinea alba),[178,179] *Chaetomium globosum,*[63] *Paecilomyces lilacinus,*[180] *Penicillium marneffei,*[181] *Dactylaria gallopava*[182] and *Ochroconis galloparvum.*[183] Chromomycosis (caused by species of *Phialophora* or *Cladosporium*) and rhinosporidiosis (caused by *Rhinosporidium seeberi*) are very occasionally found as infections of the lungs; in most cases such infection has spread, by the airways or in the blood, from a site elsewhere in the body.

Torulopsosis

Torulopsis glabrata, also known as *Candida glabrata,* is a common yeast on the body surface and is frequently isolated as a contaminant of urine cultures. Human infection is usually opportunistic, taking the form of pneumonia, septicaemia, pyelonephritis or endocarditis in debilitated or immunocompromised patients, particularly those with the acquired immune deficiency syndrome, advanced cancer or being treated with wide-spectrum antibiotics.[184,185] Pulmonary infection is often by aspiration. Unlike *Candida albicans* it does not form hyphae. Its cells are nearly invisible in haematoxylin-eosin sections but are easily seen in Grocott preparations. They are difficult to distinguish from those of *Histoplasma capsulatum* but are rounded rather than ovoid.

Sporotrichosis

Sporotrichosis is usually seen as an indurated ulcer of the finger acquired from the prick of a thorn. Pulmonary involvement is rare and when present is generally secondary to disseminated lymphocutaneous sporotrichosis. Primary pulmonary sporotrichosis (involvement of the lung in the absence of cutaneous disease) is distinctly unusual.[186-188] However, because it mimics tuberculosis, its incidence may be greater than is generally recognised. The causative agent, *Sporothrix schenckii* is a yeast-like fungus that occurs worldwide on decaying vegetation, contaminated soil and living plants, especially roses. Primary pulmonary sporotrichosis is acquired by inhalation of the spores and usually presents as a chronic, cavitary, bilateral, apical disease, most often in a clinical setting of alcoholism and chronic obstructive airway disease: less often it forms a solitary, necrotising, peripheral pulmonary nodule.[187] Fungal stains demonstrate many round or ovoid, budding yeast forms, 2–4 μm in size, in the areas of necrosis. Hyphae bearing sessile budding yeasts are found infrequently.

Adiaspiromycosis[189-195]

Adiaspiromycosis is caused by a remarkable fungus, *Chrysosporium (Emmonsia) crescens*, which is a soil saprophyte of worldwide distribution. The term adiaspiromycosis derives from the conidia of this fungus, the adiaconidia, which are quite small but exhibit the unique property of progressive enlargement, perhaps a million-fold in volume, without replication, at 37°C. The disease is ordinarily limited to wild rodents but has been seen exceptionally in man.

The disease, which is entirely pulmonary, is characterised by the formation of tuberculoid granulomas around the cells of the organism. The fungal cell is usually solitary and has a thick yellowish wall, up to about 8 μm in thickness, surrounding a central mass of amorphous cytoplasm in which there is a single nucleus. The fungal cells are remarkable for the great size that they may reach – as much as 600 μm in diameter. They are too large to be effectively mobilised by the host cells and since proliferation does not occur in human tissues, the granulomatous response maintains a bronchiolocentric distribution indicative of inhalational infection and dissemination does not occur. Diagnosis relies on recognition of the fungus in lung tissue as serology and culture are unreliable.

Light infection may result in a solitary adiaspiromycotic granuloma, which would only be found incidentally in an asymptomatic individual. Widespread adiaspiromycotic granulomas are indicative of heavy infection and patients so affected may complain of fever, cough and dyspnoea and show a diffuse, micronodular pattern on chest radiographs.[192] Death is very unusual.[193]

Malasseziosis

Malassezia furfur, the causative organism of tinea versicolor (pityriasis versicolor), is dependent for its growth on high concentrations of fatty acids and is normally limited to the skin. Systemic infection has however complicated prolonged lipid infusions through central venous catheters, in which circumstances the small yeast-like organisms have been noted infiltrating the walls of pulmonary arteries and in small pulmonary thromboemboli.[196,197] As is so often the case with fungi, identification of the species depends upon cultural characteristics.

Pseudallescheriosis (Monosporiosis)

Pseudallescheria boydii (syn. *Petriellidium boydii, Allescheria boydii*) is a fungus of worldwide distribution in soils and is of low pathogenicity. It is the commonest cause of mycetoma in Europe and North America, gaining access to the subcutaneous tissues through cuts and abrasions in the skin. Pulmonary involvement may occur through the inhalation of airborne spores but is rare: it may take the form of an intracavitary fungal ball,[98] comparable to an aspergilloma, or in conditions such as leukaemia it may be invasive and disseminate widely.[198-200] Allergic bronchopulmonary Pseudallescheriosis is also described.[90]

P. boydii usually grows in hyphal form within the body but within air-filled cavities conidia may develop. The conidial state is known as *Monosporium* (syn. *Scedosporium*) *apiospermum* and infection showing such growth may be termed Monosporiosis. The hyphae are slender, thin-walled and of fairly constant diameter with numerous septa and branching points. The hyphae are slightly indented at the septa. They are more slender and their branches less clearly dichotomous than those of aspergilli but the differences are insufficient to discriminate between them with confidence morphologically. This requires immunohistochemistry.[64] The distinction of these two fungi is important because their drug sensitivities differ.[200]

Penicillium marneffei infection

Penicillium marneffei is a dimorphic fungus endemic in southeast Asia.[201] At room temperature, it grows as a mould with red to black conidia, whereas in tissue it forms a 3–5 μm yeast-like cell that divides by binary fission. The yeasts therefore display clear central septation, unlike *H. capsulatum* and other fungi that divide by budding. Infection, which is highest after the rainy season, is by inhalation but the pulmonary changes are usually overshadowed by systemic features such as hepatosplenomegaly, skin lesions and bone marrow involvement. However, there may be diffuse infiltration, mass lesions or cavities in the lungs. While it can affect the immunocompetent, infection is mainly associated with AIDS, for which it is clinical marker in the endemic areas.[181]

REFERENCES

Pneumocystis

1. Watts JC, Chandler FW. Evolving concepts of infection by *Pneumocystis carinii*. Pathol Annu 1991; 26(Part 1):93–138.

2. Miller R, Huang L. Pneumocystis jirovecii infection. Thorax 2004; 59:731–733.

3. Dutz W, Jennings-Khodadad E, Post C, Kohout E, Nazarian I, Esmaili H. Marasmus and *Pneumocystis carinii* pneumonia in institutionalised infants. Observations during an endemic. Z Kinderheilk 1974; 117:241–258.

4. Vanek J, Jivorec O, Luckes J. Interstitial plasma cell pneumonia in infants. Ann Pediatr 1953; 180:1–21.

5. Lunseth JH, Kirmse TW, Prezyna AP, Gerth R. Interstitial plasma cell pneumonia. J Pediatr 1955; 46:137–145.

6. Haque A, Plattner SB, Cook RT, Hart MN. *Pneumocystis carinii*. Taxonomy as viewed by electron microscopy. Am J Clin Pathol 1987; 87:504–510.

7. Edman JC, Kovacs JA, Masur H, Santi DV, Elwood HJ, Sogin ML. Ribosomal RNA sequence shows *Pneumocystis carinii* to be a member of the fungi. Nature 1988; 334:519–522.

8. Sidhu GS, Cassa ND, Pei ZH. *Pneumocystis carinii*: An update. Ultrastruct Pathol 2003; 27:115–122.

9. Ham EK, Greenberg SD, Reynolds RC, Singer DB. Ultrastructure of *Pneumocystis carinii*. Exp Mol Pathol 1971; 14:362–372.

10. Campbell WG. Ultrastructure of Pneumocystis in human lung. Arch Pathol 1972; 93:312–324.

11. Sueishi K, Hisano S, Sumiyoshi A, Tanaka K. Scanning and transmission electron microscopic study of human pulmonary pneumocystosis. Chest 1977; 72:213–216.

12. Corrin B, Dewar A. Respiratory diseases. In: Papadimitriou JM, Henderson DW, Spagnolo DV, eds. Diagnostic Ultrastructure of Non-Neoplastic Diseases. Edinburgh: Churchill Livingstone; 1992:264–286.

13. Lanken PN, Minda M, Pietra GG, Fishman AP. Alveolar response to experimental *Pneumocystis carinii* pneumonia in the rat. Am J Pathol 1980; 99:561–588.

14. Yoneda K, Walzer PD. Mechanism of pulmonary alveolar injury in experimental *Pneumocystis carinii* pneumonia in the rat. Br J Exp Pathol 1981; 62:339–346.

15. Coker RJ, Clark D, Claydon EL, et al. Disseminated *Pneumocystis-carinii* infection in AIDS. J Clin Pathol 1991; 44:820–823.

16. Gryzan S, Paradis IL, Zeevi A, et al. Unexpectedly high incidence of *Pneumocystis carinii* infection after heart-lung transplantation. Implications for lung defense and allograft survival. Am Rev Respir Dis 1988; 137:1268–1274.

17. Varthalitis I, Aoun M, Daneau D, Meunier F. *Pneumocystis-carinii* pneumonia in patients with cancer – an increasing incidence. Cancer 1993; 71:481–485.

18. Pifer LL, Hughes WT, Stagno S, Woods D. *Pneumocystis carinii* infection: evidence for high prevalence in normal and immunosuppressed children. Pediatrics 1978; 61:35–41.

19. Peters SE, Wakefield AE, Sinclair K, Millard PJ, Hopkin JM. A search for latent *Pneumocystis carinii* infection in post-mortem lungs by DNA amplification. J Pathol 1991; 166:195–198.

20. Miller RF, Mitchell DM. AIDS and the lung - Update 1992 .1. *Pneumocystis-carinii* pneumonia. Thorax 1992; 47:305–314.

21. Young JA, Stone JW, McGonigle RJS, Adu D, Michael J. Diagnosing *Pneumocystis carinii* pneumonia by cytological examination of bronchoalveolar lavage fluid: report of 15 cases. J Clin Pathol 1986; 39:945–949.

22. Elvin KM, Bjorkman A, Linder E, Heurlin N, Hjerpe A. *Pneumocystis carinii* pneumonia: detection of parasites in sputum and bronchoalveolar lavage fluid by monoclonal antibodies. BMJ 1988; 297:381–384.

23. Wakefield AE, Pixley FJ, Banerji S, Miller RF, Moxon ER, et al. Detection of *Pneumocystis carinii* with DNA amplification. Lancet 1990; 336:451–453.

24. Lipschik GY, Gill VJ, Lundgren JD, et al. Improved diagnosis of *Pneumocystis carinii* infection by polymerase chain reaction on induced sputum and blood. Lancet 1992; 340:203–206.

25. Leigh TR, Gazzard BG, Rowbottom A, Collins JV. Quantitative and qualitative comparison of DNA amplification by PCR with immunofluorescence staining for diagnosis of *Pneumocystis carinii* pneumonia. J Clin Pathol 1993; 46:140–144.

26. Wakefield AE, Miller RF, Guiver LA, Hopkin JM. Granulomatous *Pneumocystis carinii* pneumonia: DNA amplification studies on bronchoscopic alveolar lavage samples. J Clin Pathol 1994; 47:664–666.

27. Eisen D, Ross BC, Fairbairn J, Warren RJ, Baird RW, Dwyer B. Comparison of *Pneumocystis carinii* detection by toluidine blue O staining, direct immunofluorescence and DNA amplification in sputum specimens from HIV positive patients. Pathology 1994; 26:198–200.

28. Armbuster CH, Pokieser L, Hassl A. Diagnosis of *Pneumocystis carinii* pneumonia by bronchoalveolar lavage in AIDS patients. Comparison of Diff-Quik, Fungifluor stain, direct immunofluorescence test and polymerase chain reaction. Acta Cytol 1995; 39:1089–1093.

29. Barrio JL, Suarez M, Rodriguez JL, Saldana MJ, Pitchenik AE. *Pneumocystis carinii* pneumonia presenting as cavitating and noncavitating solitary pulmonary nodules in patients with the acquired immunodeficiency syndrome. Am Rev Respir Dis 1986; 134:1094–1096.

30. Liu YC, Tomashefski JF, Tomford JW, Green H. Necrotising *Pneumocystis carinii* vasculitis associated with lung necrosis and cavitation in a patient with acquired immunodeficiency syndrome. Arch Pathol Lab Med 1989; 113:494–497.

31. Watts JC, Chandler FW. *Pneumocystis carinii* pneumonitis. The nature and diagnostic significance of the methenamine silver-positive 'intracystic bodies'. Am J Surg Pathol 1985; 9:744–751.

32. Mahan CT, Sale GE. Rapid methenamine silver stain for Pneumocystis and fungi. Arch Pathol 1978; 102:351–352.

33. Musto L, Flanigan M, Elbadawi A. Ten-minute silver stain for *Pneumocystis carinii* and fungi in tissue sections. Arch Pathol 1982; 106:292–294.

34. Shimono LH, Hartman B. A simple and reliable rapid methenamine silver stain for *Pneumocystis carinii* and fungi. Arch Pathol Lab Med 1986; 110:855–856.

35. Kim H-K, Hughes WT. Comparison of methods for identification of *Pneumocystis carinii* in pulmonary aspirates. Am J Clin Pathol 1973; 60:462–466.

36. Cameron RB, Watts JC, Kasten BL. *Pneumocystis carinii* pneumonia: an approach to rapid laboratory diagnosis. Am J Clin Pathol 1979; 72:90–93.

37. Amin MB, Mezger E, Zarbo RJ. Detection of *Pneumocystis-carinii* – comparative study of monoclonal antibody and silver staining. Am J Clin Pathol 1992; 98:13–18.

38. Kobayashi M, Urata T, Ikezoe T, et al. Simple detection of the 5S ribosomal RNA of *Pneumocystis carinii* using in situ hybridisation. J Clin Pathol 1996; 49:712–716.

39. LeGolvan DP, Heidelberger KP. Disseminated, granulomatous *Pneumocystis carinii* pneumonia. Arch Pathol 1973; 95:344–348.

40. Weber WR, Askin FB, Dehner LP. Lung biopsy in *Pneumocystis carinii* pneumonia. A histopathologic study of typical and atypical features. Am J Clin Pathol 1977; 67:11–19.

41. Askin FB, Katzenstein AA. Pneumocystis infection masquerading as diffuse alveolar damage. A potential source of diagnostic error. Chest 1981; 79:420–422.

42. Cupples JB, Blackie SP, Road JD. Granulomatous *Pneumocystis carinii* pneumonia mimicking tuberculosis. Arch Pathol Lab Med 1989; 113:1281–1284.

43. Travis WD, Pittaluga S, Lipschik GY, et al. Atypical pathologic manifestations of *Pneumocystis carinii* pneumonia in the acquired immune deficiency syndrome. Review of 123 lung biopsies from 76 patients with emphasis on cysts, vascular invasion, vasculitis and granulomas. Am J Surg Pathol 1990; 14:615–624.

44. Birley HDL, Buscombe JR, Griffiths MH, Semple SJG, Miller RF. Granulomatous *Pneumocystis carinii* pneumonia in a patient with the acquired immunodeficiency syndrome. Thorax 1990; 45:769–771.

45. Lee MM, Schinella RA. Pulmonary calcification caused by *Pneumocystis-carinii* pneumonia - a clinicopathological study of 13 cases in acquired immune deficiency syndrome patients. Am J Surg Pathol 1991; 15:376–380.

46. Foley NM, Griffiths MH, Miller RF. Histologically atypical *Pneumocystis-carinii* pneumonia. Thorax 1993; 48:996–1001.

47. Blumenfeld W, Basgoz N, Owen WF, Schmidt DM. Granulomatous pulmonary lesions in patients with the acquired immunodeficiency syndrome (AIDS) and *Pneumocystis carinii* infection. Ann Intern Med 1988; 109:505–507.

48. Nash G, Said JW, Nash SV, Degirolami U. The pathology of AIDS – bronchiectasis, pulmonary fibrosis with honeycombing, necrotising bacterial pneumonia, invasive fungal infection consistent with aspergillosis, cytomegalovirus pneumonia and healed pneumo-cystis pneumonia with pulmonary calcification. Mod Pathol 1995; 8:203–205.

49. Travis WD, Fox CH, Devaney KO, et al. Lymphoid pneumonitis in 50 adult patients infected with the human immunodeficiency virus – lymphocytic interstitial pneumonitis versus nonspecific interstitial pneumonitis. Hum Pathol 1992; 23:529–541.

50. Moran CA, Suster S, Pavlova Z, Mullick FG, Koss MN. The spectrum of pathological changes in the lung in children with the acquired immunodeficiency syndrome: an autopsy study of 36 cases. Hum Pathol 1994; 25:877–882.

51. Saldana MJ, Mones JM. Pulmonary pathology in AIDS: atypical *Pneumocystis carinii* infection and lymphoid interstitial pneumonia. Thorax 1994; 49:S46–S55.

52. Mariuz P, Raviglione MC, Gould IA, Mullen MP. Pleural *Pneumocystis carinii* infection. Chest 1991; 99:774–776.

53. Murry CE, Schmidt RA. Tissue invasion by *Pneumocystis-carinii* – a possible cause of cavitary pneumonia and pneumothorax. Hum Pathol 1992; 23:1380–1387.

54. Ferre C, Baguena F, Podzamczer D, et al. Lung cavitation associated with *Pneumocystis carinii* infection in the acquired immunodeficiency syndrome – a report of six cases and review of the literature. Eur Respir J 1994; 7:134–139.

55. Lazard T, Guidet B, Meynard JL, Capron F, Offenstadt G. Generalized air cysts complicated by fatal bilateral pneumothoraces in a patient with AIDS-related *Pneumocystis carinii* pneumonia. Chest 1994; 106:1271–1272.

56. Grimes MM, LaPook JD, Bar MH, Wasserman HS, Dwork A. Disseminated *Pneumocystis carinii* infection in a patient with acquired immunodeficiency syndrome. Hum Pathol 1987; 18:307–308.

57. Ragni MV, Dekker A, Derubertis FR, et al. *Pneumocystis-carinii* infection presenting as necrotising thyroiditis and hypothyroidism. Am J Clin Pathol 1991; 95:489–493.

58. Matsuda S, Urata Y, Shiota T, et al. Disseminated infection of *Pneumocystis carinii* in a patient with the acquired immunodeficiency syndrome. Virchows Arch A Pathol Anat Histopathol 1989; 414:523–527.

59. Deroux SJ, Adsay NV, Ioachim HL. Disseminated pneumocystosis without pulmonary involvement during prophylactic aerosolized pentamidine therapy in a patient with the acquired immunodeficiency syndrome. Arch Pathol Lab Med 1991; 115:1137–1140.

60. Fishman JA, Mattia AR, Lee MJ, Mark EJ, Davis BT. A 29-year-old man with AIDS and multiple splenic abscesses – disseminated *Pneumocystis carinii* infection and mycobacterium avium complex infection involving the spleen and liver. N Engl J Med 1995; 332:249–257.

60a. Shelburne SA, Hamill RJ. The immune reconstitution inflammatory syndrome. AIDS Rev 2003; 5:67–79.

61. Wang N-S, Huang S-N, Thurlbeck WM. Combined *Pneumocystis carinii* and cytomegalovirus infection. Arch Pathol 1970; 90:529–535.

Aspergillus

62. Verweij PE, Smedts F, Poot T, Bult P, Hoogkamp-Korstanje JAA, Meis JFGM. Immunoperoxidase staining for identification of aspergillus species in routinely processed tissue sections. J Clin Pathol 1996; 49:798–801.

63. Yeghen T, Fenelon L, Campbell CK, et al. Chaetomium pneumonia in a patient with acute myeloid leukaemia. J Clin Pathol 1996; 49:184–186.

64. Jensen HE, Salonen J, Ekfors TO. The use of immunohistochemistry to improve sensitivity and specificity in the diagnosis of systemic mycoses in patients with haematological malignancies. J Pathol 1997; 181:100–105.

65. Nime FA, Hutchins GM. Oxalosis caused by Aspergillus infection. Johns Hopkins Med J 1973; 133:183–194.

66. Bryan RL, Hubscher SG. Aspergillosis associated with calcinosis and hypocalcaemia following liver transplantation. J Pathol 1988; 155:353A.

67. Ghio AJ, Peterseim DS, Roggli VL, Piantadosi CA. Pulmonary oxalate deposition associated with Aspergillus-niger infection – an oxidant hypothesis of toxicity. Am Rev Respir Dis 1992; 145:1499–1502.

68. Lee SH, Barnes WG, Schaetzel WP. Pulmonary aspergillosis and the importance of oxalate crystal recognition in cytology specimens. Arch Pathol Lab Med 1986; 110:1176–1179.

69. Benoit G, de Chauvin MF, Cordonnier C, Astier A, Bernaudin J-F. Oxalic acid level in bronchoalveolar lavage fluid from patients with invasive pulmonary aspergillosis. Am Rev Respir Dis 1985; 132:748–751.

70. Nakajima M, Niki Y, Manabe T. False-positive antineutrophil cytoplasmic antibody in aspergillosis with oxalosis. Arch Pathol Lab Med 1996; 120:425–426.

71. Proia AD, Brinn NT. Identification of calcium oxalate crystals using alizarin red S stain. Arch Pathol Lab Med 1985; 109:186–189.

72. Kurrein F, Green GH, Rowles SL. Localized deposition of calcium oxalate around a pulmonary Aspergillus niger fungus ball. Am J Clin Pathol 1975; 64:556–563.

73. Soubani AO, Chandrasekar PH. The clinical spectrum of pulmonary aspergillosis. Chest 2002; 121:1988–1999.

74. Barth PJ, Rossberg C, Koch S, Ramaswamy A. Pulmonary aspergillosis in an unselected autopsy series. Pathol Res Pract 2000; 196(2):73–80.

75. Makker H, McConnochie K, Gibbs AR. Postirradiation pulmonary fibrosis complicated by aspergilloma and bronchocentric granulomatosis. Thorax 1989; 44:676–677.

76. Ein ME, Wallace Jr RJ, Williams Jr TW. Allergic bronchopulmonary aspergillosis-like syndrome consequent to aspergilloma. Am Rev Respir Dis 1979; 119:811–820.

77. McCarthy DS, Pepys J. Allergic bronchopulmonary aspergillosis. Clinical immunology:1 Clinical features. Clin Allergy 1971; 1:261–286.

78. Reich JM. Pneumothorax due to pleural perforation of a pseudocavity containing aspergillomas in a patient with allergic bronchopulmonary aspergillosis. Chest 1992; 102:652–653.

79. Hinson KFW, Moon AJ, Plummer NS. Broncho-pulmonary aspergillosis: a review and report of eight cases. Thorax 1952; 7:317–333.

80. Sanerkin NG, Seal RME, Leopold JG. Plastic bronchitis, mucoid impaction of the bronchi and allergic broncho-pulmonary aspergillosis and their relationship to bronchial asthma. Ann Allergy 1966; 24:586–594.

81. Bosken CH, Myers JL, Greenberger PA, Katzenstein A-LA. Pathologic features of allergic bronchopulmonary aspergillosis. Am J Surg Pathol 1988; 12:216–222.

81a. Zander DS. Allergic bronchopulmonary aspergillosis: an overview. Arch Pathol Lab Med 2005; 129:924–928.

82. Nelson LA, Callerame ML, Schwartz RH. Aspergillosis and atopy in cystic fibrosis. Am Rev Respir Dis 1979; 120:863–873.

83. Aubry MC, Fraser R. The role of bronchial biopsy and washing in the diagnosis of allergic bronchopulmonary aspergillosis. Modern Pathol 1998; 11:607–611.

84. Jelihovsky T. The structure of bronchial plugs in mucoid impaction, bronchocentric granulomatosis and asthma. Histopathology 1983; 7:153–167.

85. Benatar S, Allan B, Hewitson R, Don P. Allergic broncho-pulmonary stemphyliosis. Thorax 1980; 35:515–518.

86. Glancy JJ, Elder JL, McAleer R. Allergic bronchopulmonary fungal disease without clinical asthma. Thorax 1981; 36:345–349.

87. McAleer R, Kroenert D, Elder J, Froudist J. Allergic bronchopulmonary disease caused by Curvularia lunata and Drechslera hawaiiensis. Thorax 1981; 36:338–344.

88. Halwig JM, Brueske DA, Greenberger PA, Dreisin RB, Sommers HM. Allergic bronchopulmonary curvulariosis. Am Rev Respir Dis 1985; 132:186–189.

89. Backman KS, Roberts M, Patterson R. Allergic bronchopulmonary mycosis caused by Fusarium vasinfectum. Am J Respir Crit Care Med 1995; 152:1379–1381.

90. Miller MA, Greenberger PA, Amerian R, et al. Allergic bronchopulmonary mycosis caused by Pseudallescheria-boydii. Am Rev Respir Dis 1993; 148:810–812.

91. Travis WD, Kwonchung KJ, Kleiner DE, et al. Unusual aspects of allergic bronchopulmonary fungal disease – report of two cases due to Curvularia organisms associated with allergic fungal sinusitis. Hum Pathol 1991; 22:1240–1248.

92. Buchanan DR, Lamb D. Saprophytic invasion of infarcted pulmonary tissue by aspergillus species. Thorax 1982; 37:693–698.

93. Smith FB, Beneck D. Localized Aspergillus infestation in primary lung carcinoma – clinical and pathological contrasts with post-tuberculous intracavitary aspergilloma. Chest 1991; 100:554–556.

94. Mehrad B, Paciocco G, Martinez FJ, Ojo TC, Iannettoni MD, Lynch JP. Spectrum of aspergillus infection in lung transplant recipients. Case series and review of the literature. Chest 119, 169–175. 2001.

95. Nunley DR, Gal AA, Vega JD, Perlino C, Smith P, Lawrence EC. Saprophytic fungal infections and complications involving the bronchial anastomosis following human lung transplantation. Chest 2002; 122:1185–1191.

96. British Thoracic and Tuberculosis Association. Aspergilloma and residual tuberculous cavities - the results of a resurvey. Tubercle 1970; 51:227–245.

97. McGregor DH, Papasian CJ, Pierce PD. Aspergilloma within cavitating pulmonary adenocarcinoma. Am J Clin Pathol 1989; 91:100–103.

98. McCarthy DS, Longbottom JL, Riddell RW, Batten JC. Pulmonary mycetoma due to Allescheria boydii. Am Rev Respir Dis 1969; 100:213–216.

99. Kwon-Chung KJ, Schwartz IS, Rybak BJ. A pulmonary fungus ball produced by Cladosporium cladosporioides. Am J Clin Pathol 1975; 64:564–568.

100. Kirkpatrick MB, Pollock HM, Wimberley NE, Bass JB, Davidson JR, Boyd BW. An intracavitary fungus ball composed of Syncephalastrum. Am Rev Respir Dis 1979; 120: 943–947.

101. Iadarola P, Lungarella G, Martorana PA, et al. Lung injury and degradation of extracellular matrix components by Aspergillus fumigatus serine proteinase. Exp Lung Res 1998; 24:233–251.

102. Awe RJ, Greenberg SD, Mattox KL. The source of bleeding in pulmonary aspergillomas. Texas Medicine 1984; 80:58–61.

103. Denning DW, Follansbee SE, Scolaro M, Norris S, Edelstein H, Stevens DA. Pulmonary aspergillosis in the acquired immunodeficiency syndrome. N Engl J Med 1991; 324:654–662.

104. Hummel M, Schuler S, Hempel S, Rees W, Hetzer R. Obstructive bronchial aspergillosis after heart transplantation. Mycoses 1993; 36:425–428.

105. Williams AJ, Zardawi I, Walls J. Disseminated aspergillosis in high dose steroid therapy. Lancet 1983; i:1222.

106. Lake KB, Browne PM, Van Dyke JJ, Ayers L. Fatal disseminated aspergillosis in an asthmatic patient treated with corticosteroids. Chest 1983; 83:138–139.

107. Karam GH, Griffin FM. Invasive pulmonary aspergillosis in non immunocompromised non neutropenic hosts. Rev Infect Dis 1986; 8:357–363.

108. Gerson SL, Talbot GH, Hurwitz S, Strom BL, Lusk EJ, Cassileth PA. Prolonged granulocytopenia: the major risk factor for invasive pulmonary aspergillosis in patients with acute leukemia. Ann Intern Med 1984; 100:345–351.

109. Vaideeswar P, Prasad S, Deshpande JR, Pandit SP. Invasive pulmonary aspergillosis: A study of 39 cases at autopsy. J Postgrad Med 2004; 50:21–26.

110. Variwalla AG, Smith AP, Melville-Jones G. Necrotising aspergillosis complicating fulminating viral pneumonia. Thorax 1980; 35:215–216.

111. Lewis M, Kallenbach J, Ruff P, Zaltzman M, Abramowitz J, Zwi S. Invasive pulmonary aspergillosis complicating influenza A pneumonia in a previously healthy patient. Chest 1985; 87:691–693.

112. Ali ZA, Ali AA, Tempest ME, Wiselka MJ. Invasive pulmonary aspergillosis complicating chronic obstructive pulmonary disease in an immunocompetent patient. J Postgrad Med 2003; 49:78–80.

113. Pervez NK, Kleinerman J, Kattan M, et al. Pseudomembranous necrotising bronchial aspergillosis. A variant of invasive aspergillosis in a patient with haemophilia and acquired immune deficiency syndrome. Am Rev Respir Dis 1985; 131:961–963.

114. Marchevsky A, Rosen MJ, Chrystal G, Kleinerman J. Pulmonary complications of the acquired immunodeficiency syndrome: a clinicopathologic study of 70 cases. Hum Pathol 1985; 16:659–670.

115. Nash G, Irvine R, Kerschmann RL, Herndier B. Pulmonary aspergillosis in acquired immune deficiency syndrome: Autopsy study of an emerging pulmonary complication of human immunodeficiency virus infection. Hum Pathol 1997; 28:1268–1275.

116. Mylonakis E, Barlam TF, Flanigan T, Rich JD. Pulmonary aspergillosis and invasive disease in AIDS: Review of 342 cases. Chest 1998; 114:251–262.

117. Klapholz A, Salomon N, Perlman DC, Talavera W. Aspergillosis in the Acquired Immunodeficiency Syndrome. Chest 1991; 100:1614–1618.

118. Miller WT, Sais GJ, Frank I, Gefter WB, Aronchick JM. Pulmonary aspergillosis in patients with AIDS - clinical and radiographic correlations. Chest 1994; 105:37–44.

119. Cornet M, Mallat H, Somme D, et al. Fulminant invasive pulmonary aspergillosis in immunocompetent patients – a two-case report. Clin Microbiol Infect 2003; 9:1224–1227.

120. Przyjemski C, Mattii R. The formation of pulmonary mycetomata. Cancer 1980; 46:1701–1704.

121. Gefter W, Weingrad T, Ochs RH, Miller WT. ‘Semi-invasive’ pulmonary aspergillosis. A new look at the spectrum of Aspergillus infections of the lung. Radiology 1981; 140:313–321.

122. Binder RE, Faling LJ, Pugatch RD, Mahasaen C, Snider GL. Chronic necrotising pulmonary aspergillosis: a discrete clinical entity. Medicine (Baltimore) 1982; 61:109–124.

123. Slevin ML, Knowles GK, Phillips MJ, Stansfeld AG, Lister TA. The air crescent sign of invasive pulmonary aspergillosis in acute leukaemia. Thorax 1982; 37:554–555.

124. Kibbler CC, Milkins SR, Bhamra A, Spiteri MA, Noone P, Prentice HG. Apparent pulmonary mycetoma following invasive aspergillosis in neutropenic patients. Thorax 1988; 43:108–112.

125. Wiggins J, Clark TJH, Corrin B. Chronic necrotising pneumonia caused by Aspergillus niger. Thorax 1989; 44:440–441.

126. Yamaguchi M, Nishiya H, Mano K, Kunii O, Miyashita H. Chronic necrotising pulmonary aspergillosis caused by aspergillus niger in a mildly immunocompromised host. Thorax 1992; 47:570–571.

127. Yousem SA. The histological spectrum of chronic necrotising forms of pulmonary aspergillosis. Hum Pathol 1997; 28:650–656.

128. Kradin RL, Drucker EA, Malhotra A, Mark EJ, Schwartz DR. An 83-year-old woman with long-standing asthma and rapidly progressing pneumonia. Chronic necrotising pulmonary aspergillosis (Aspergillus fumigatus), with elements of bronchocentric granulomatosis. N Engl J Med 1998; 339:1228–1236.

128a. Hiltermann TJN, Bredius RGM, Gesink-vd Veer BJ, et al. Bilateral cavity pulmonary consolidations in a patient undergoing allogenic bone marrow transplantation for acute leukemia. Chest 2003; 123:929–934.

129. Hines DW, Haber MH, Yaremko L, Britton C, McLawhon RW, Harris AA. Pseudomembranous-tracheobronchitis caused by aspergillus. Am Rev Respir Dis 1991; 143:1408–1411.

130. Niimi T, Kajita M, Saito H. Necrotising bronchial aspergillosis in a patient receiving neoadjuvant chemotherapy for non-small-cell lung carcinoma. Chest 1991; 100:277–279.

131. Kramer MR, Denning DW, Marshall SE, et al. Ulcerative tracheobronchitis after lung transplantation. A new form of invasive aspergillosis. Am Rev Respir Dis 1991; 144:552–556.

132. Tait RC, O’Driscoll BR, Denning DW. Unilateral wheeze caused by pseudomembranous aspergillus tracheobronchitis in the immunocompromised patient. Thorax 1993; 48:1285–1287.

133. Nicholson AG, Sim KM, Keogh BF, Corrin B. Pseudomembranous necrotising bronchial aspergillosis complicating chronic airways limitation. Thorax 1995; 50:807–808.

134. Tron V, Churg A. Chronic necrotising pulmonary aspergillosis mimicking bronchocentric granulomatosis. Pathol Res Pract 1986; 181:621–626.

135. Tazelaar HD, Baird AM, Mill M, Grimes MM, Schulman LL, Smith CR. Bronchocentric mycosis occurring in transplant recipients. Chest 1989; 96:92–95.

Mucor

136. Brown RB, Lau SK, Gonzalez RG, Smith CH. A 59-year-old diabetic man with unilateral visual loss and oculomotor-nerve palsy. Invasive fungal

sinusitis and osteomyelitis due to mucormycosis (Diabetes mellitus). N Engl J Med 2001; 344:286–293.

137. Frater JL, Hall GS, Procop GW. Histologic features of zygomycosis: emphasis on perineural invasion and fungal morphology. Arch Pathol Lab Med 2001; 125: 375–378.

138. Matsushima T, Soejima R, Nakashima T. Solitary pulmonary nodule caused by phycomycosis in a patient without obvious predisposing factors. Thorax 1980; 35:877–878.

139. Murray HW. Pulmonary mucormycosis: one hundred years later. Chest 1977; 72:1–3.

140. Bigby TD, Serota ML, Tierney LM, Matthay MA. Clinical spectrum of pulmonary mucormycosis. Chest 1986; 89:435–439.

141. Harada M, Manabe T, Yamashita K, Okamoto N. Pulmonary mucormycosis with fatal massive hemoptysis. Acta Pathol Jpn 1992; 42:49–55.

Candida

142. Hopfer RL, Fainstein V, Luna MP, Bodey GP. Disseminated candidiasis caused by four different candida species. Arch Pathol Lab Med 1981; 105:454–455.

143. Knox WF, Hooton VN, Barson AJ. Pulmonary vascular candidiasis and use of central venous catheters in neonates. J Clin Pathol 1987; 40:559–565.

144. O'Driscoll BRC, Cooke RDP, Mamtora H, Irving MH, Bernstein A. Candida lung abscesses complicating parenteral nutrition. Thorax 1988; 43:418–419.

Cryptococcus

145. Campbell GD. Primary pulmonary cryptococcosis. Am Rev Respir Dis 1965; 94:236–243.

146. Torda A, Kumar RK, Jones PD. The pathology of human and murine pulmonary infection with Cryptococcus neoformans var gattii. Pathology 2001; 33:475–478.

147. Douketis JD, Kesten S. Miliary pulmonary cryptococcosis in a patient with the acquired immunodeficiency syndrome. Thorax 1993; 48:402–403.

148. Harding SA, Scheld WM, Feldman PS, Sande MA. Pulmonary infection with capsule-deficient Cryptococcus neoformans. Virchows Arch A Pathol Anat Histopathol 1979; 382:113–118.

149. Lazcano O, Speights VO, Strickler JG, Bilbao JE, Becker J, Diaz J. Combined histochemical stains in the differential diagnosis of Cryptococcus-neoformans. Mod Pathol 1993; 6:80–84.

150. Haugen RK, Baker RD. The pulmonary lesions in cryptococcosis with special reference to subpleural nodules. Am J Clin Pathol 1954; 24:1381–1390.

151. McDonnell JM, Hutchins GM. Pulmonary cryptococcosis. Hum Pathol 1985; 16:121–128.

152. Nash G, Said JW, Nash SV, Degirolami U. The pathology of AIDS – pulmonary cryptococcosis. Mod Pathol 1995; 8:202–203.

Histoplasma

153. Symmers W St C. Histoplasmosis contracted in Britain: a case of histoplasmic lymphadenitis following clinical recovery from sarcoidosis. BMJ 1956; 2:786–789.

154. Peterson MW, Pratt AD, Nugent KM. Pneumonia due to Histoplasma capsulatum in a bone marrow transplant recipient. Thorax 1987; 42:698–699.

155. Sathapatayavongs B, Batteiger BE, Wheat J, Slama TG, Wass JL. Clinical and laboratory features of disseminated histoplasmosis during two large urban outbreaks. Medicine 1983; 62:263–270.

156. Wheat LJ, Conolly-Stringfield PA, Baker RL, et al. Disseminated histoplasmosis in the acquired immune deficiency syndrome: clinical findings, diagnosis and treatment and review of the literature. Medicine 1990; 69:361–374.

157. Levitz SM, Mark EJ, Ko JP, Kretsinger K, Colvin RB, Caliendo AM. A 19-year-old man with the acquired immunodeficiency syndrome and persistent fever. Disseminated histoplasmosis. Acquired immunodeficiency syndrome. N Engl J Med 1998; 339:1835–1843.

158. Godwin RA, Nickell JA, Des Prez AM. Mediastinal fibrosis complicating healed primary histoplasmosis and tuberculosis. Medicine 51, 227–246. 1972.

Coccidioides

159. Bayer AS. Fungal pneumonias; pulmonary coccidioidal syndromes (Part 1). Chest 1981; 79:575–583.

160. Bayer AS. Fungal pneumonias: pulmonary coccidioidal syndromes (Part 2). Chest 1981; 79:686–691.

161. Feldman BS, Snyder LS. Primary pulmonary coccidioidomycosis. Semin Respir Infect 2001; 16:231–237.

162. Panackal AA, Hajjeh RA, Cetron MS, Warnock DW. Fungal infections among returning travelers. Clin Infect Dis 2002; 35:1088–1095.

163. Centers for Disease Control and Preventation. Coccidioidomycosis among persons attending the world championship of model airplane flying – Kern County, California, October 2001. JAMA 2002; 287:312.

164. Kirkland TN, Fierer J. Coccidioidomycosis: a reemerging infectious disease. Emerg Infect Dis 1996; 2:192–199.

Blastomyces

165. Bradsher RW, Chapman SW, Pappas PG. Blastomycosis. Infect Dis Clin North Am 2003; 17:21–40, vii.

166. Patel RG, Patel B, Petrini MF, Carter RR, III, Griffith J. Clinical presentation, radiographic findings and diagnostic methods of pulmonary blastomycosis: a review of 100 consecutive cases. South Med J 1999; 92:289–295.

167. Lemos LB, Guo M, Baliga M. Blastomycosis: organ involvement and etiologic diagnosis. A review of 123 patients from Mississippi. Ann Diagn Pathol 2000; 4:391–406.

168. Meyer KC, McManus EJ, Maki DG. Overwhelming pulmonary blastomycosis associated with the adult respiratory distress syndrome. N Engl J Med 1993; 329:1231–1236.

169. Guccion JG, Rohatgi PK, Saini NB, French A, Tavaloki S, Barr S. Disseminated blastomycosis and acquired immunodeficiency syndrome: a case report and ultrastructural study. Ultrastruct Pathol 1996; 20: 429–435.

170. Lemos LB, Baliga M, Guo M. Acute respiratory distress syndrome and blastomycosis: presentation of nine cases and review of the literature. Ann Diagn Pathol 2001; 5:1–9.

Paracoccidioides

171. Londero AT, Ramos CD. Paracoccidioidomycosis: a clinical and mycologic study of forty-one cases observed in Santa Maria, RS, Brazil. Am J Med 1972; 52:771–775.

172. Bethlem EP, Capone D, Maranhao B, Carvalho CR, Wanke B. Paracoccidioidomycosis. Curr Opin Pulm Med 1999; 5:319–325.

173. Murray HW, Littman ML, Roberts RB. Disseminated paracoccidioidomycosis (South American blastomycosis) in the United States. Am J Med 1974; 56:209–220.

174. Bowler S, Woodcock A, Da Costa P, Turner-Warwick M. Chronic pulmonary paracoccidioidomycosis masquerading as lymphangitis carcinomatosa. Thorax 1986; 41:72–73.

175. Goldani LZ, Martinez R, Landell GAM, Machado AA, Coutinho V. Paracoccidioidomycosis in a patient with acquired immunodeficiency syndrome. Mycopathologia 1989; 105:71–74.

176. Funari M, Kavakama J, Shikanai-Yasuda MA, et al. Chronic pulmonary paracoccidioidomycosis (South American blastomycosis): high-resolution CT findings in 41 patients. Am J Roentgenol 1999; 173:59–64.

Rare pulmonary mycoses

177. Huang S-N, Harris LS. Acute disseminated penicilliosis. Report of a case and review of pertinent literature. Am J Clin Pathol 1963; 39:167–174.

178. Saul SH, Khachatoorian T, Poorsattar A, et al. Opportunistic Trichosporon pneumonia. Arch Pathol Lab Med 1981; 105:456–459.

179. Ito T, Ishikawa Y, Fujii R, et al. Disseminated Trichosporon capitatum infection in a patient with acute leukaemia. Cancer 1988; 61:585–588.

180. Ono N, Sato K, Yokomise H, Tamura K. Lung abscess caused by Paecilomyces lilacinus. Respiration 1999; 66:85–87.

181. McShane H, Tang CM, Conlon CP. Disseminated Penicillium marneffei infection presenting as a right upper lobe mass in an HIV positive patient. Thorax 1998; 53:905–906.

182. Mazur JE, Judson MA. A case report of a dactylaria fungal infection in a lung transplant patient. Chest 2001; 119:651–653.

183. Odell JA, Alvarez S, Cvitkovich DG, Cortese DA, McComb BL. Multiple lung abscesses due to Ochroconis gallopavum, a dematiaceous fungus, in a nonimmunocompromised wood pulp worker. Chest 2000; 118:1503–1505.

184. Aisner J, Schimpff SC, Sutherland JC, Young VM, Wiernik MD. Torulopsis glabrata infections in patients with cancer. Increasing incidence and relationship to colonisation. Am J Med 1976; 61:23–28.

185. Srivastava S, Kleinman G, Manthous CA. Torulopsis pneumonia – a case report and review of the literature. Chest 1996; 110:858–861.

186. Beland JE, Mankiewicz E, MacIntosh DJ. Primary pulmonary sporotrichosis. Can Med Assoc J 1968; 99:813–816.

187. England DM, Hochholzer L. Primary pulmonary sporotrichosis. Am J Surg Pathol 1985; 9:193–204.

188. England DM, Hochholzer L. Sporothrix infection of the lung without cutaneous disease. Primary pulmonary sporotrichosis. Arch Pathol Lab Med 1987; 111:298–300.

189. Watts JC, Callaway CS, Chandler FW, Kaplan W. Human pulmonary adiaspiromycosis. Arch Pathol 1975; 99:11–15.

190. Schwarz J. Adiaspiromycosis. Pathol Annu 1978; 13:41–53.

191. Rippon JW. Medical mycology: the pathogenic fungi and the pathogenic actinomycetes. Philadelphia: W.B. Saunders, 1988; 718–721.

192. Filho JVB, Amato MBP, Deheinzelin D, Saldiva PHN, de Carvalho CRR. Respiratory failure caused by adiaspiromycosis. Chest 1990; 97:1171–1175.

193. Peres LC, Figueiredo F, Peinado M, Soares FA. Fulminant disseminated pulmonary adiaspiromycosis in humans. Am J Trop Med Hyg 1992; 46:146–150.

194. England DM, Hochholzer L. Adiaspiromycosis: an unusual fungal infection of the lung. Report of 11 cases. Am J Surg Pathol 1993; 17:876–886.

195. Nuorva K, Pitkanen R, Issakainen J, Huttunen NP, Juhola M. Pulmonary adiaspiromycosis in a two year old girl. J Clin Pathol 1997; 50:82–85.

196. Redline RW, Redline SS, Boxerbaum B, Dahms BB. Systemic Malassezia furfur infections in patients receiving intralipid therapy. Hum Pathol 1988; 16:852–854.

197. Shek YH, Tucker MC, Viciana AL, Manz HJ, Connor DH. Mallassezia furfur – Disseminated infection in premature infants. Am J Clin Pathol 1989; 92:595–603.

198. Tadros TS, Workowski KA, Siegel RJ, Hunter S, Schwartz DA. Pathology of hyalohyphomycosis caused by Scedosporium apiospermum (Pseudallescheria boydii): An emerging mycosis. Hum Pathol 1998; 29:1266–1272.

199. Nonaka D, Yfantis H, Southall P, Sun CC. Pseudallescheriasis as an aggressive opportunistic infection in a bone marrow transplant recipient. Arch Pathol Lab Med 2002; 126:207–209.

200. Raj R, Frost AE. Scedosporium apiospermum fungemia in a lung transplant recipient. Chest 2002; 121:1714–1716.

201. Deng Z, Ribas JL, Gibson DW, Connor DH. Infections caused by Penicillium marneffei in China and Southeast Asia: review of eighteen published cases and report of four more Chinese cases. Rev Infect Dis 1988; 10:640–652.

5

Infectious diseases

5.5

Parasitic infestations

This chapter describes infestation of the lungs by certain parasitic protozoa, helminths and arthropods, of which man may be either the natural or the accidental host.

Protozoal diseases of the lungs include toxoplasmosis and amoebic abscess, while severe malaria may be complicated by acute respiratory failure. The lungs may also be involved in generalised leishmaniasis but in this condition the pulmonary lesions are subsidiary (Fig. 5.5.1) and similar to those elsewhere in the body and will not be described here. However, note is taken of bronchopulmonary involvement by parasites usually confined to other organs being reported in AIDS patients (e.g. microsporidiosis).

Helminths of all three major classes may infest the lung. Trematodes include the blood flukes (genus *Schistosoma*), the lung flukes (genus *Paragonimus*) and certain liver flukes (genus *Opisthorchis*). The cestodes are represented by the larval forms of *Echinococcus* and *Taeni*, which are responsible for hydatid disease and cysticercosis, respectively, while nematodes found in the lung include immature forms of *Ascaris*, *Strongyloides*, *Ancylostoma*, *Necator*, *Wuchereria* and *Brugia* and the adult forms of heartworm (*Dirofilaria*) and gapeworm (*Syngamus*).

Arthropods include the ticks and mites (arachnids), adult forms of which may cause pulmonary acariasis. Pulmonary pentastomiasis is a manifestation of infestation by larvae of *Linguatula* or of *Armillifer*.

The mode of transmission is variable. Some of these parasites are transmitted by an insect bite, e.g. those causing tropical pulmonary eosinophilia, dirofilariasis and malaria; some penetrate the skin directly, e.g. *Strongyloides*, hookworms and schistosomes; others are ingested, e.g. *Paragonimus*, *Entamoeba* and *Echinococcus*.

The human lungs may be involved in the life cycle of these parasites in various ways:

1 The lungs may be the natural location of the parasite, for example *Paragonimus* and *Syngamus*.
2 The larval form of the parasite may encyst in the lungs, for example *Echinococcus*.

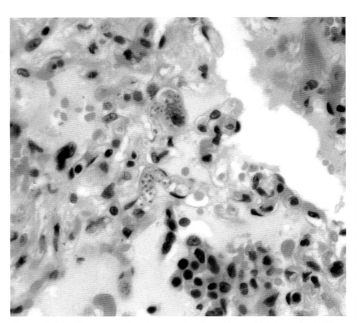

Figure 5.5.1 Pulmonary involvement in disseminated leishmaniasis. The protozoa are seen within macrophages in alveoli and capillaries. (Case provided by Dr J DeGaetano, Malta.)

3 The lung may be a migratory route for the larvae of the parasite; this includes most of the nematodes listed above and the larvae responsible for pentastomiasis.

4 The parasite may reach the lungs as an embolus. Most schistosomal ova and the dead adult canine heartworm, *Dirofilaria*, are examples of this.

5 The parasite may invade the lung through the diaphragm from the liver, for example *Entamoeba histolytica* and the liver fluke *Opisthorchis*.

6 The lungs may be involved in disseminated parasitosis, for example microsporidiosis in the acquired immune deficiency syndrome.

Although immunodeficient patients are particularly prone to parasitic infestation, most of these pulmonary parasites are capable of infecting and causing disease in the immunocompetent; only a few are opportunists (e.g. Cryptosporidium spp.). Many of them have a characteristic distribution, often in tropical or subtropical countries. In the developed world parasitic diseases of the lung mainly affect immigrants and tourists.

PROTOZOA

Toxoplasmosis

Toxoplasmosis represents infection with the coccidian parasite *Toxoplasma gondii*, this name deriving from the crescentic bow shape of the parasite's tachyzoites and its discovery in the gondi, a North African rodent used as a laboratory animal. The disease occurs in many species of wild and domestic birds and mammals throughout the world and these provide a ready

source of human infection. Ingestion of infected animal material is the usual route of infection of adults but neonatal disease generally reflects placental transmission. Toxoplasmosis is one of the most prevalent protozoal infections of man but the parasite rarely harms its host and the vast majority of human infections remain occult throughout life, causing damage only when cellular immunity is impaired. Gametogenesis and oocyst formation take place in the intestine of animals such as cats; outside the body, sporozoites are liberated which can infect other species, including man. Only asexual cysts containing dormant bradyzoites are formed in normal accidental hosts but if immunity fails the cysts liberate motile tachyzoites and it is these that swarm through the host tissues causing cell damage and inflammation.

Pulmonary toxoplasmosis is rare and most cases have been in patients suffering from generalised disease attributable to immunodeficiency from diseases such as lymphoma and AIDS. Transplant recipients are also liable to develop toxoplasmosis. Because many of these patients undergo toxoplasma seroconversion after they receive new organs, it is likely that the parasite is introduced in the donor tissues in which it presumably lay dormant. In lung transplant patients, recognition of the parasites in transbronchial biopsies is important in distinguishing infection from the changes of graft rejection. Because of the size of the parasite relative to the thickness of tissue sections, many laboratories involved in transplantation work cut serial sections through these small biopsies.

Pulmonary infection is initially non-specific. There is an interstitial infiltrate of lymphocytes and alveolar macrophages are increased. Hyaline membranes may develop, indicating necrosis of the alveolar epithelium and the changes are then those of diffuse alveolar damage. Alveoli adjacent to those lined by hyaline membranes show type II pneumocyte hyperplasia. Up to this stage the parasites are scanty but if immunity is sufficiently impaired, enormous numbers of tachyzoites develop. These cause necrosis on a major scale. Air spaces may be filled with necrotic debris or broad tracts of the lung undergo coagulative necrosis.[1–6] In one case macrophages filled with toxoplasma trophozoites formed a mass lesion.[7]

Individual tachyzoites are very difficult to recognise in histological sections but their identification is facilitated by immunocytochemistry,[5,6] which is superior to the Giemsa stain formerly used. The tachyzoites are crescentic in shape and measure within the range $4–7 \times 2–3\,\mu m$; the intracystic bradyzoites tend to be shorter and more rounded. Cysts and pseudocysts are easier to recognise but both are generally very rare. The cysts, which represent the latent form of the parasite, lie free in the intercellular tissues and provoke no inflammatory response (Fig. 5.5.2). They vary considerably in size but are commonly of the order of $60\,\mu m$ diameter. Although single tachyzoites are difficult to identify, they invade and proliferate within host cells to form distinctive collections known as pseudocysts. These resemble true cysts in size and appearance but are intracellular and lack an outer membrane.

Treatment with pyrimethamine and sulphonamides is effective if initiated promptly.[8] The mortality for toxoplasma

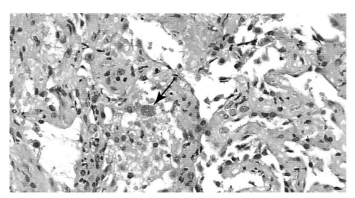

Figure 5.5.2 A toxoplasma cyst exciting little inflammatory reaction in the surrounding lung.

pneumonia is 55%, although survival is much better in the immunocompetent.[9]

Amoebiasis

Entamoeba histolytica, the causative organism of amoebic dysentery, is a protozoon with a trophozoite and a cystic stage that is endemic in much of sub-Saharan Africa, South America and southern Asia. Infection is acquired by the ingestion of food or water contaminated by amoebic cysts. Trophozoites develop in the small intestine and are carried to the large bowel, which they ulcerate. From there they may spread in the blood, giving rise to metastatic foci of infection. These are found most frequently in the liver, lungs and brain, in that order. Although the lesions in these organs are conventionally described as abscesses, they are not accompanied by suppuration unless there is secondary bacterial infection.

If there is amoebic ulceration of the lower part of the rectum, amoebae may reach the rectal venous plexus and, bypassing the liver, make their way directly in the systemic circulation to the lungs. More often, amoebic pulmonary abscesses are secondary to those in the liver: the amoebae pass though the diaphragm to infect the lungs and are therefore more common in the right lung. Whether the pleural cavity becomes infected in the course of this extension of the disease from liver to lung depends on whether adhesions have formed that bind the apposed pleural surfaces sufficiently to protect the cavity from invasion. Pleuropulmonary complications develop in less than 5% of patients with intestinal amoebiasis but in 50% of those with liver abscesses. They may include broncho-hepatic fistulas.[10]

An amoebic abscess in the lung, like one in the liver, is essentially a focus of localised destruction in which part of the lung is converted into a cavity filled with reddish-brown, viscous fluid. There is little inflammatory reaction in the surrounding tissues but amoebae with their characteristic ingested erythrocytes may be seen in the zone bordering the cavity or on aspiration cytology.[11] Often the area of destruction extends to involve one of the bronchi and much of the contents, often blood-stained, may then be expectorated. Should this happen, there may be secondary bacterial infection of the cavity. Metronidazole is the treatment of choice.[10]

Malaria

Severe *Plasmodium falciparum* malaria may be complicated by acute respiratory failure.[12–14] The clinical features are those of non-cardiogenic oedema or the acute respiratory distress syndrome, which as usual has diffuse alveolar damage as its pathological basis. This suggests that the various cytokines that have been identified in the blood in complicated forms of malaria[15–17] may be more important than the ischaemia occasioned by heavy erythrocyte parasite burdens rendering the red blood cells less deformable and so inclined to occlude capillaries. However, blood sludging undoubtedly takes place in the lungs as well as the brain and elsewhere. The pulmonary capillaries are engorged with parasitised erythrocytes, pigment-laden macrophages and neutrophils. This is contributed to by endothelial activation and increased expression of intercellular adhesion molecule-1[18] as well as the non-deformability of the parasitised cells. The parasites in the lung are largely early trophozoites or ring forms rather than the later schizonts that predominate in cerebral vessels, possibly because the higher oxygen levels in the lung inhibit plasmodium maturation.[19] Therapeutic measures resulting in fluid overload and oxygen toxicity may aggravate the respiratory distress. Even after treatment, altered pulmonary function in malaria is common, with airflow obstruction, impaired ventilation, impaired gas transfer and increased pulmonary phagocytic activity. This occurs in both vivax and falciparum malaria suggesting common underlying inflammatory mechanisms.[20]

Cryptosporidiosis

Cryptosporidia species cause diarrhoea in many species. In man, enteric cryptosporidiosis was first recognised in an immunodeficient patient and the disease has now become a serious problem in AIDS.[21] It also affects the immunocompetent and is a common cause of short-term diarrhoea in day nurseries and in travellers. Infection is by faecal-oral transmission of an encysted form and generally involves drinking water. A small number of immunocompromised patients show respiratory as well as enteric infection, complaining of cough and chest pain (Fig. 5.5.3).[22–25]

Cryptosporidia are extracellular protozoan parasites which adhere to the surface of lining epithelia. They are seen as faintly haematoxyphil dots measuring up to 5 μm arrayed along the mucosal surface. In the respiratory tract they have been identified on the surface and glandular epithelium of the trachea and bronchi and in the lung parenchyma, associated with extensive squamous metaplasia of the conductive airways.[23] The superficial location of cryptosporidia helps distinguish them from microsporidia, which are found within the cytoplasm of epithelial cells. Electron microscopy shows that cryptosporidia occupy a vacuole that communicates with the cell surface: they lie just beneath the level of cell membrane but are nevertheless extracellular.

There is no agreement on therapy but antiretroviral therapy has been shown to improve gastrointestinal symptoms, presumably through restoring immunity.[26]

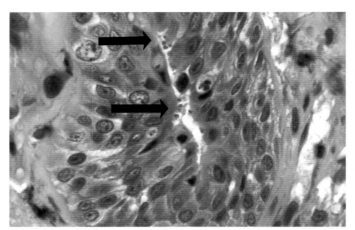

Figure 5.5.3 Cryptosporidia (arrows) are seen in the bronchial lumen of a patient suffering from AIDS. (Photomicrograph courtesy of Dr M Antoine, Paris, France.)

Microsporidiosis

Microsporidia are obligate intracellular protozoal parasites that infect many animals and have emerged as important opportunistic pathogens in AIDS. They are also being increasingly recognised in HIV-negative individuals.[27] Four microsporidian genera, *Enterocytozoon*, *Encephalitozoon*, *Pleistophora* and *Nosema* have been reported to infect man. Infection generally involves the gastrointestinal tract but may become generalised.[27,28] Pulmonary involvement is unusual but heavy infestation of the tracheobronchial mucosa is recorded.[29–32] The infected respiratory epithelium may show focal proliferation with little inflammation or there may be a lymphocytic infiltrate of the airway epithelium similar to that seen in the bowel; heavy infestations cause sloughing and ulceration of the tracheobronchial mucosa and severe subacute inflammation. In haematoxylin and eosin stained sections the parasite appears as a supranuclear 'blue body' but the staining is weak and it is easily overlooked, even when infestation is heavy. It is ovoid or spherical and measures approximately 2 μm in length and is Gram-positive. Immunocytochemistry, electron microscopy and *in situ* hybridisation are useful for confirming the diagnosis.[33]

As with cryptosporidiosis, antiretroviral therapy has been shown to improve gastrointestinal symptoms, presumably through restoring immunity,[26] and albendazole has also been effective in some patients.

HELMINTHS

Trematodes

Schistosomiasis[34,35]

Pulmonary schistosomiasis (bilharziasis) may be due to any of the three most important species of human blood fluke, *Schistosoma haematobium*, *S. mansoni* and *S. japonicum*. Although involvement of the lung is relatively infrequent as a cause of

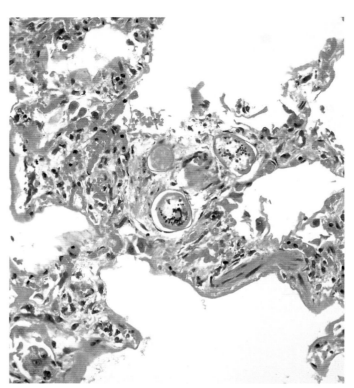

Figure 5.5.4 Schistosomiasis. Schistosomal ova are evident (centre) within the alveolar interstitium, which also shows a lymphocytic infiltrate.

clinical disease in comparison with the major locations of schistosomal infestation, it is recognised wherever schistosomiasis is endemic. However, with increased international travel, it seems that the non-endemic population have a higher incidence of pulmonary involvement once infected.[36,37] Specific changes are found in the lungs in a third of cases of clinically evident schistosomiasis in Egypt but contribute to death in only about 2% of these patients. The frequency of pulmonary involvement is least in the Far East where schistosomiasis is due to *S. japonicum*.

The schistosomal cercariae thrive in fresh water and penetrate the skin to transform into immature adults, which are transported in the blood to mature in venous plexuses around the bladder or rectum, where they reproduce. Pulmonary infestation generally comes from ova being carried to the lungs in the blood, either bypassing the portal venous circulation or having been produced by flukes inhabiting plexuses that drain directly into the inferior vena cava. Alternatively, if adult parasites are present within the pulmonary vasculature itself, ova are produced locally.

The ova, which measure from 70 to 170 μm in length by 50 to 70 μm in breadth, according to the species, are bound by their dimensions to lodge in blood vessels of corresponding calibre; local thrombosis and organisation result, with the formation of a characteristic tuberculoid granuloma round the egg itself (Figs 5.5.4, 5.5.5). Medial hypertrophy, intimal fibrosis, thrombosis and occasionally necrotizing angiitis and angiomatoid lesions (see p. 421) develop in the obstructed arteries.[38] Eosinophils may

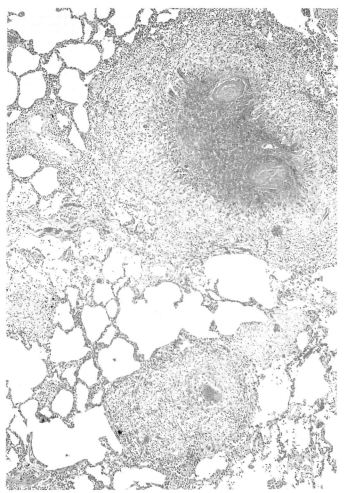

Figure 5.5.5 Schistosomiasis. Lodgement of the schistosomal eggs in the pulmonary microcirculation has provoked a vigourous granulomatous response.

be conspicuously numerous in the vicinity of the ova. It is uncertain whether the necrotizing arteritis and consequent angiomatoid lesions are attributable to vascular obstruction by the ova, to an allergic response to the parasite, or to the 'pipestem' hepatic fibrosis that is commonly found in schistosomiasis permitting vasoconstrictive substances that normally are metabolised in the liver to reach the pulmonary arteries.[38] Cor pulmonale may complicate pulmonary schistosomiasis and aneurysmal dilatation of the pulmonary trunk has been observed in long standing cases.

The ova also pass through the walls of the pulmonary arteries and initiate parenchymal lesions characterised by a similar granulomatous reaction and more widespread lymphocytic infiltrate and interstitial fibrosis. Although the ova may be much distorted during tissue processing, they are readily seen and recognised, particularly if they were viable at the time when the specimen was obtained (Fig. 5.5.4). Dead ova often become heavily calcified but may long retain identifiable traces of the contained embryo. Eosinophilic infiltration and necrotising angiitis are only seen in the presence of viable ova. The presence of eggs, viable or dead, is generally the clue to the diagnosis, but in some cases pulmonary arterial lesions, including thrombosis and arteritis, develop where no ova are demonstrable.

Occasionally, ova reach the respiratory bronchioles and cause a local tuberculoid bronchiolitis. Sometimes a tumour-like mass forms in the lungs, abutting and obstructing a bronchus: this proves to be a confluent growth of granulomatous tissue and scarring round great numbers of schistosome ova.

When adult flukes reach the lungs they appear to cause no reaction while alive, any associated lesions being caused by the presence of their ova. However, when the flukes die, thrombosis and arteritis result and there is commonly an accompanying focal consolidation of the adjacent parenchyma. This gives rise to nodules up to 1 cm and more in diameter that show as small 'coin' shadows in chest radiographs.

Katayama fever

As well as the classic chronic form of schistosomiasis described above, pulmonary symptoms such as cough feature in the severe form of acute schistosomiasis known as Katayama disease.[13] This systemic illness signifies seroconversion and develops about 3–6 weeks after penetration of the skin by water-borne cercariae. It is almost exclusively a disease of non-immune visitors to endemic areas and has been reported in several groups of tourists returning from such areas, especially those participating in water sports. The disease is self-limiting but recognition and treatment are important to avoid the sequelae of chronic infection.

Paragonimiasis

Infestation by lung flukes is endemic in the Far East and to a lesser extent in central Africa and parts of the Americas.[39–43] In its early stages the disease is characterised by chest pain or discomfort. Later, when it has become chronic, there is persistent cough and recurrent haemoptysis. Characteristic operculate eggs can then be found in the sputum; they are golden-brown and measure about 90 μm in length. In some cases the presence of the parasite is borne well; in others it leads to anorexia and debility. As long as the flukes remain in the lungs the disease is rarely fatal, but should they reach the brain, as happens in a minority of cases, the prognosis is grave. Occasionally the disease mimics lung cancer.[44] Rapid and reliable immunodiagnostic methods are now available and there are PCR techniques that distinguish individual species.[45,46]

The species most frequently responsible are *Paragonimus westermani* in the Far East and *P. kellicotti* in the Americas. Morphologically these differ from each other only slightly. The adults infest the lungs of many predatory animals: *P. westermani* in the dog, cat and pig and *P. kellicotti* in the mink. Small groups of them become sexually mature within the lung tissue, where necrosis and the formation of a fibrous capsule produce characteristic 'worm cysts' (abscess cavities) that eventually enlarge and break into the bronchial lumen (Fig. 5.5.6). The ova that

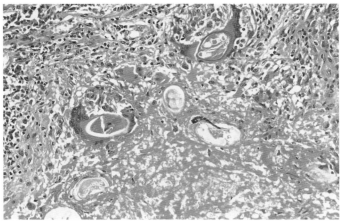

(a)

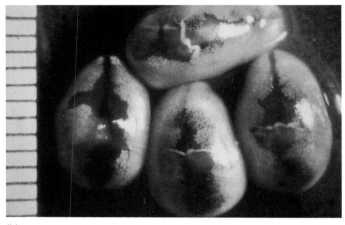

(b)

Figure 5.5.6 Paragonimiasis. (a) A 'worm cyst' including several Paragonimus eggs in the chronic inflammatory granulation tissue that borders the central necrosis. (b) Paragonimus eggs removed from the lung.

thus escape pass up the respiratory tract and are either expectorated or swallowed, to be eventually excreted in the stools. The life cycle of the fluke is a complex one: after several weeks in water or moist earth, the ovum hatches into a miracidium, a free-swimming form that eventually enters and parasitises water snails of the genus *Melania*. After its larval life in the snail, the fluke emerges as a cercaria, which in turn parasitises small fresh-water crabs and crayfish. It is through the consumption of these crustaceans, raw or insufficiently cooked, that man becomes infested. Pickling the crabs does not destroy the parasite. The disease may also be acquired by eating the flesh of another host, such as a pig, that has eaten infected crabs or crayfish. On reaching the duodenum of the human host, the parasite penetrates the gut wall and thence passes by way of the peritoneal cavity and diaphragm to the pleura and the lungs. It grows to a length of 12 mm and attains maturity about 5 weeks after reaching the lungs and so completing its life cycle.

In man, the flukes often lie singly in the connective tissue 'worm cysts' and the number of these rarely exceeds ten, each about 1–2 cm across. They may excite an eosinophilic pneumonia. Sometimes the young worms go astray and reach the liver, spleen, kidneys or brain. Occasionally dead worms in the lungs are associated with distant tissue reactions that probably have a hypersensitivity basis. The diagnosis is based on the demonstration of the eggs in bronchial secretions, pleural fluid or faeces.

Opisthorchiasis

Liver flukes generally remain within the hepatic bile ducts but in Thailand *Opisthorchis viverrini* has on rare occasions made its way from the liver through the diaphragm to the right lung.[47]

Cestodes

Hydatid disease (larval echinococcosis)

This disease has long been endemic in sheep-raising countries, notably Australia, New Zealand, Wales, parts of South Africa and South America and the Middle East.[48] Control measures are steadily lessening its incidence. The dog is the usual host of the mature tapeworm, *Echinococcus granulosus* and sheep the commonest host of its larval stage. The ova in the faeces of the dog reach sheep or man in contaminated food or water and, after hatching in the small intestine, larvae penetrate the gut wall and enter the portal circulation. Most are retained in the liver, but some negotiate the hepatic barrier to reach the systemic venous circulation and the lungs. The larval forms of this helminth thus tend to occur most frequently in the liver and the lungs. They take the form of hydatid cysts (Fig. 5.5.7). If a hydatid cyst is demonstrated in the lung, others are almost always present in the liver. Pulmonary hydatid cysts are usually solitary but bilateral instances are recorded.[48–50]

The wall of a hydatid cyst is formed of a semipermeable laminated capsule, which is composed of chitin and an inner germinal layer. Outside these is the pericyst, formed of a layer of chronic inflammatory granulation tissue or a fibrous capsule, these representing the host reaction to the parasite (Figs 5.5.8, 5.5.9). The germinal layer gives rise to brood capsules and from the germinal layer of these arise scolices. Free brood capsules and scolices form the hydatid 'sand' that can be seen as minute white grains in the otherwise clear cyst fluid (Fig. 5.5.10). When sheep tissues containing hydatid cysts are eaten by a dog, the scolices attach to the intestinal mucosa and develop into the adult worms, thus completing the life cycle. Scolices also have the potential to develop into secondary cysts if released by cyst rupture. They also form daughter cysts within the mother cyst, each daughter cyst being an exact true replica of the mother cyst. The daughter cysts may be packed together in the mother cyst or float freely in the mother cyst cavity. In older cysts, the contents degenerate into gelatinous material known as the matrix, which may be mistaken for pus. The cysts are usually bacteriologically sterile but they may become infected, resulting in true suppuration. Calcification commonly develops in the pericyst without affecting the

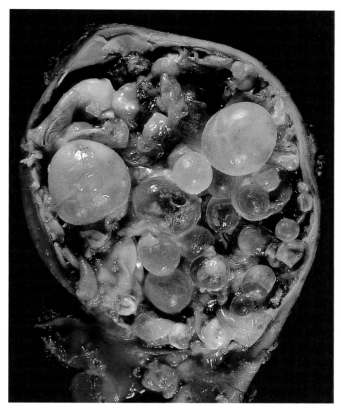

Figure 5.5.7 Hydatid cyst, the encysted larval form of the *Echinococcus granulosus* tapeworm, filled with numerous 'daughter' cysts.

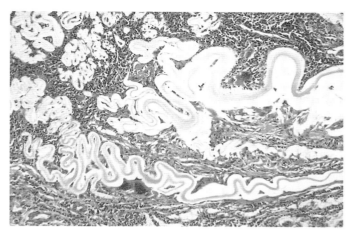

Figure 5.5.9 Hydatid cyst. The convoluted chitinous layer of a collapsed dead hydatid cyst.

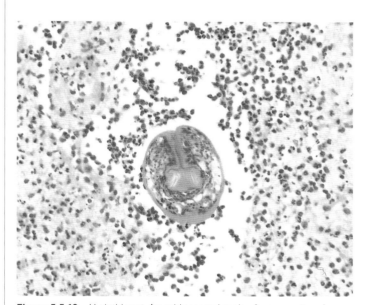

Figure 5.5.10 Hydatid cyst. An echinococcal scolex from a ruptured hydatid cyst is surrounded by pus.

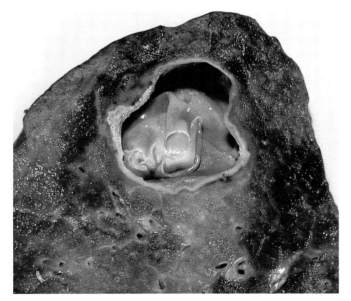

Figure 5.5.8 Hydatid cyst. The encysted larva of the *Echinococcus granulosus* tapeworm has died and the parasite's capsule has collapsed away from the fibrous capsule formed by its human host.

viability of the parasite but calcification of the endocyst indicates that it is dead.

Because the parasite has evolved mechanisms to avoid host immunity, the infection is often asymptomatic until a mechan-ical complication occurs.[51] Thus, most cases of pulmonary hydatid disease are discovered on routine chest radiography. Symptoms stem from compression, infection or rupture into a bronchus. The sudden escape of a large amount of its fluid con-tents may give rise to a grave, even fatal, anaphylactic reaction. Rupture of a hydatid cyst into a bronchus may also cause bron-chocentric granulomatosis[52] (see p. 463) or lymphoid hyperpla-sia (see p. 642). Aspiration of the cyst contents should not be undertaken because of the risk of spillage and a consequent hypersensitivity reaction. The treatment of choice for compres-sive cysts is surgical resection, with particular care being exer-cised to avoid rupture of the cyst, and postoperative drug therapy using albendazole.[53–55]

Cysticercosis (larval taeniasis)

Cysticercosis occurs when man becomes the intermediate host of the porcine tapeworm, *Taenium solium*, through the ingestion of the worm's eggs present in faecally contaminated water or food or on soiled hands, or by the eggs hatching within the intestine of those harbouring the adult worm.[56,57] The disease is common in Africa, China, south east Asia and South America. Once hatched, the embryo penetrates the intestinal wall and is disseminated by the bloodstream, giving rise to an encysted larva. Such cysticerci may form anywhere but the brain is particularly vulnerable. The lungs are seldom affected but may be the seat of either solitary or multiple lesions, the latter generally as part of disseminated disease, which probably reflects immune impairment.[57] The larva has an inverted scolex and lies within clear fluid bounded by a thin fibrous capsule. Little inflammation is induced while the larvae are alive but after their death a variable response is seen, often culminating in calcification.

Nematodes

Ascariasis ('larva migrans')

Although essentially an intestinal parasite, the large roundworm *Ascaris lumbricoides* passes through the lungs during one phase of its complex life cycle. Infection is endemic in much of Africa, Asia and South America. The infestation is acquired by ingesting food or water contaminated with ova passed in the faeces of an earlier host. The ova hatch in the small intestine, where the larvae quickly penetrate the mucosa and are carried either to the liver in the portal bloodstream or in lymph to the systemic veins, reaching the lungs about 5–6 days after ingestion of the eggs. In the lungs, the larvae pierce the alveolar wall to reach the air space, whence they are cleared to the pharynx to be swallowed. Maturation, copulation and ovulation occur in the small intestine.

Migration through the lungs may cause self-limiting pulmonary eosinophilia ('Löffler's syndrome', see p. 461) during which eosinophils and Charcot-Leyden crystals are often conspicuous in the sputum, although the larvae themselves are rarely seen. The illness is usually over within 3 weeks but in exceptional cases respiratory distress becomes so severe that the patient may die. Potentially fatal ascariasis pneumonitis may also complicate severe burns.[58]

Microscopical studies of the pulmonary lesions have been infrequent except in the rare fatal cases, or when the parasites are present by chance in lungs examined as a result of other disease. The larvae may be found in capillaries, the interstitial tissues, or air spaces, accompanied by eosinophils and neutrophils. When a larva dies, an intense reaction may develop, with dense local accumulation of eosinophils, lesser numbers of macrophages and neutrophils and fibrin. Identifiable remnants of larvae may be seen, sometimes in multinucleate giant cells. There may be local haemorrhage.

The larvae of *A. lumbricoides*, the ascarid parasite of man, are difficult to distinguish from those of other ascarids, such as species of *Toxocara*, that may also be found in human lung tissue. Morphological differentiation of these larvae in histological preparations is commonly beyond the ability even of professional parasitologists but investigation by means of specific immunocytochemical staining may be decisive. The larvae of the toxocarae have a greater tendency than those of *A. lumbricoides* to die in the lungs when they infest man; they then cause the development of tuberculoid granulomatous foci that eventually lead to fibrous encapsulation of the remains of the parasites.

Strongyloidiasis

Strongyloides stercoralis is another intestinal parasite that at one stage in its development passes through the lungs. Initial infection is through the skin but once established in the intestine infestation may persist for years by an endogenous cycle (autoinfection). The condition has been well described among individuals who were prisoners of the Japanese during the second world war: decades later, it affected a fifth of the survivors of those who worked on the notorious Burma railway.[59,60]

Most infestations cause at most a creeping skin eruption (larva migrans) or chronic diarrhoea but there is a real danger of fatal hyperinfestation if the individual becomes immunosuppressed. This may happen when corticosteroid drugs are administered, particularly in the treatment of unrelated conditions but also because of resistant asthma caused by unrecognised strongyloidiasis. In cases of such asthma the dose of corticosteroids may be progressively increased when the patient would have been better treated with anti-helminthic drugs.[61] Worsening asthma as the steroid dosage is increased should alert the clinician to the possibility of hyperinfestation. Heavy infestation is often associated with blood eosinophilia and fleeting pulmonary opacities that represent eosinophilic pneumonia but these features may be absent in those who are immunosuppressed. Other risk factors include advanced age, chronic lung disease and altered cellular immunity.[62]

The respiratory features in hyperinfestation may be those of the acute respiratory distress syndrome. At necropsy in such cases, the larvae are seen in huge numbers within the lumen and walls of airways of all sizes down to the alveoli and within interlobular septa (Fig. 5.5.11). They excite an inflammatory response, chiefly of plasma cells with smaller numbers of lymphocytes and eosinophils. Diffuse alveolar haemorrhage may be seen.[63] More chronic infestation may result in restrictive lung disease due to interlobular septal fibrosis or a mass lesion.[64,64a]

Hookworm infestation

The larval forms of the hookworms *Ancylostoma duodenale* and *Necator americanus*, like those of *Ascaris lumbricoides* and *Strongyloides stercoralis*, migrate through the heart, lungs and trachea to reach the intestine where they mature. On their way through the lungs, they may similarly cause fleeting eosinophilic pneumonia.

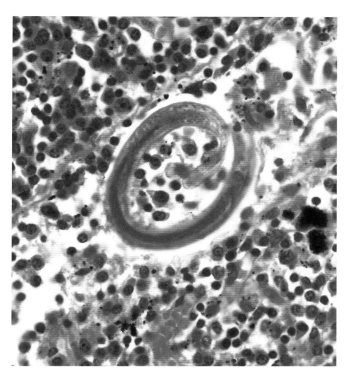

Figure 5.5.11 *Strongyloides stercoralis* filaria in the lung in a case of strongyloides superinfection. (Reproduced courtesy of the late Professor BE Heard, Brompton, UK.)

Filariasis: tropical eosinophilia

Filariasis is endemic in the tropics. The adult nematodes, *Wuchereria bancrofti*, *Brugia malayi*, *Brugia pahangi* and *Onchocerca volvulus* inhabit lymphatics where they produce eggs from which are released embryos known as microfilariae. These circulate in the blood and disseminate widely in the tissues, to be transmitted to others by mosquitoes.

Some of those infected present with 'tropical eosinophilia', a name that was given to a condition that was initially described from the coast of southern India but is now known to have a far wider distribution in the tropics.[65] The clinical signs are fever, loss of weight, dyspnoea and asthmatic attacks; there is marked blood eosinophilia and radiographs show nodular shadows in the lungs. The condition is benign and little is known of the changes in the lungs. Such reports as have been published describe whitish nodules 3–5 mm in diameter, scattered irregularly throughout the lungs. Histologically, the nodules are composed of groups of alveoli consolidated by eosinophils enmeshed in fibrin. In the centre of some of the nodules, the alveolar walls are destroyed and the area becomes an 'eosinophil abscess'. In others, a central collection of epithelioid cells becomes arranged in a palisade manner round deeply eosinophilic hyaline material that probably represents inspissated granules of eosinophil leukocytes. Giant cells and fibrosis are seen in some lesions and microfilariae are sometimes observed.[66,67] The condition is thought to represent an immunopathological response to the parasite rather than direct damage by the microfilariae because it is confined to those individuals who are highly sensitised to filarial antigens.

Tropical eosinophilia should be differentiated from pulmonary eosinophilia (see p. 459), which may be cryptogenic or due to drugs, asthma, allergic aspergillosis or the migratory larvae of *Ascaris*, *Strongyloides* or *Ankylostoma* (see above) and from Churg–Strauss granulomatosis (see p. 465). It is readily distinguished from all these forms of eosinophilia by the patient's history of residence in the tropics, by the presence of extraordinarily high levels of both serum IgE and antifilarial antibodies and by a dramatic therapeutic response to the filaricide diethylcarbamazine.

Dirofilariasis (heartworm infestation)

Pulmonary dirofilariasis occurs when man becomes an alternative host of the canine heartworm, *Dirofilaria immitis*, after being bitten by a mosquito or sandfly infested with the microfilariae. Early development occurs in a subcutaneous nodule, whence after a few weeks' development the young adult worm migrates to the right side of the heart and the pulmonary arteries. In man, the adult worm typically dies while it is immature and is carried from the heart to the lungs as a parasitic embolus to occlude a small pulmonary artery. This generally causes no symptoms. A necrotising granuloma forms about the dead worm and this is seen as an incidental 'coin' lesion in chest radiographs,[68] often prompting a needless thoracotomy as carcinoma is the principal differential diagnosis. The diagnosis is almost always made only when resected tissue is submitted to microscopy. The young adult worm is about 3 cm in length but the mature female measures up to 30 cm × 2 mm with the male about 20 cm × 2 mm. Very rarely an embolic tangle of worms results in major pulmonary infarction (Fig. 5.5.12a).

Heartworm is enzootic in the Gulf states of America but since the first report of human infestation in 1961 it has become recognised in dogs throughout the USA and in southern parts of Canada. Human cases have now been reported also from Japan, Australia, Brazil and various other countries.[69–74] The smaller *D. repens*, which is common in Italy, may result in a similar pulmonary nodule but the lung is a relatively rare locus for this species.[75]

The lesions in man are usually solitary, peripheral and lower lobar in distribution (Fig. 5.5.12b), but multiple bilateral nodules have been reported. They range in size from 1 to 4 cm. Most patients are asymptomatic but some complain of cough, chest pain, haemoptysis and fever, with up to 20% showing eosinophilia. Microscopically, a large central area of coagulative necrosis is surrounded by a thin band of chronic inflammatory granulomatous tissue containing occasional giant cells (Fig. 5.5.12c).[73,76,77] The diagnosis is made by identifying the dead worm within a thrombosed artery in the central area of necrosis (Fig. 5.5.12d). This may require step sections, which are therefore advisable when examining any necrobiotic nodule of obscure aetiology. Methenamine silver and elastin stains aid the

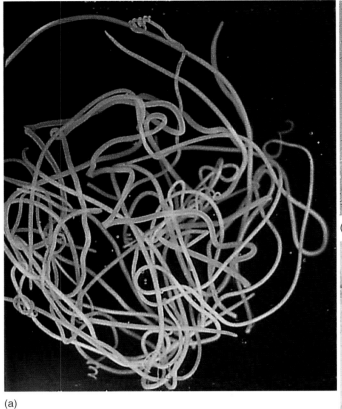

(a)

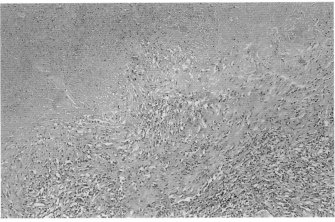

(c)

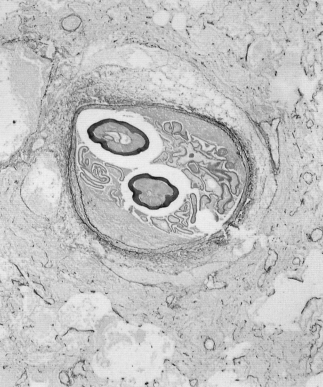

(d)

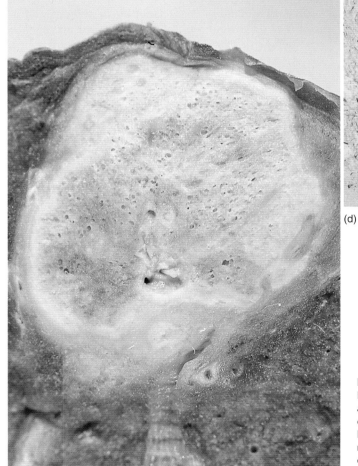

(b)

Figure 5.5.12 *Dirofilaria immitis*, the dog heartworm. (a) A tangle of Dirofilaria worms that was removed surgically from the pulmonary artery of a merchant seaman; it is not known where his infection was contracted. Magnification ×2 (Specimen provided by Professor F Ho, Hong Kong.) (b–d), *Dirofilaria immitis* causing a 3 cm, rounded, necrotizing nodule in the lung of a man who had lived rough in tropical countries. (b) Gross appearances, (c) microscopy, (d) elastin stain showing the worm situated within a pulmonary artery. (b–d reproduced courtesy of Dr M Jagusch, Auckland, New Zealand.)

identification and localisation of the parasite (5.5.12d), which has a thick cuticle and in man seldom measures more than 300 μm diameter. Non-specific fluorescent whitener stains are also recommended.[78]

Syngamiasis (gapeworm infestation)

Gapeworms of the Syngamidae family infest domestic mammals, rodents and birds, producing in domestic fowl a disease known as 'the gapes', which is characterised by dyspnoea and an asphyxial death due to the worms obstructing the bird's trachea and bronchi. Human infection is rare but isolated cases have been reported from the West Indies, Brazil, the Philippines and Korea.[79–82] Affected patients complain of dyspnoea, cough, wheeze and pain or a feeling of tightness in the chest. Ova and adult worms may be found in the sputum or on bronchoscopy. The adults live off the host's blood and are therefore bright red. The female measures up to 2 cm and the male one-quarter of this. They live in permanent copulation and since the vulva opens in the mid-region of the female's body, each pair forms a characteristic Y shape. It must be disconcerting to see the paired worms wriggling away from the bronchoscopy forceps.[79]

ARTHROPODS

Pulmonary acariasis

Adult ticks and mites are occasionally found in the sputum of those exposed to organic dust in tropical climates, probably representing bronchial saprophytes. This is known as pulmonary acariasis. Mites were found in the sputum of 5% of Chinese grain workers.[83]

Pentastomiasis

The upper or lower respiratory passages of some dogs, birds and snakes are inhabited by larvae that are of debatable taxonomic standing. These are the so-called pentastomes-*Linguatula* ('tongueworm') and *Armillifer* (*Porocephalus*).[84] The eggs of *Armillifer* may be transmitted to snake handlers in Africa and the Far East and those of *Linguatula* are transmitted to dog handlers worldwide, including western Europe. Larvae develop in the human intestine and penetrate the wall to reach many viscera, including the lungs, where in man, they die. A recognisable larva is occasionally encountered in human lungs but more often, barely recognisable parasitic remnants are observed within encapsulated, partly calcified, necrotic debris. Their identification from other metazoal remnants may be impossible, even for professional parasitologists. Involvement of the upper airways is also described in man, with worm like structures being recognised within nasal discharge.[85]

REFERENCES

Toxoplasma

1. Marchevsky A, Rosen MJ, Chrystal G, Kleinerman J. Pulmonary complications of the acquired immunodeficiency syndrome: a clinicopathologic study of 70 cases. Hum Pathol 1985; 16:659–670.
2. Tschirart D, Klatt EC. Disseminated toxoplasmosis in the acquired immunodeficiency syndrome. Arch Pathol Lab Med 1988; 112:1237–1241.
3. Bergin C, Murphy M, Lyons D, Gaffney E, Mulcahy FM. Toxoplasma pneumonitis – fatal presentation of disseminated toxoplasmosis in a patient with AIDS. Eur Respir J 1992; 5:1018–1020.
4. Artigas J, Grosse G, Niedobitek F. Anergic disseminated toxoplasmosis in a patient with the acquired immunodeficiency syndrome. Arch Pathol Lab Med 1993; 117:540–541.
5. Schurmann D, Ruf B. Extracerebral toxoplasmosis in AIDS. Histological and immunohistological findings based on 80 autopsy cases. Pathol Res Pract 1993; 189:428–436.
6. Nash G, Kerschmann RL, Herndier B, Dubey JP. The pathological manifestations of pulmonary toxoplasmosis in the acquired immunodeficiency syndrome. Hum Pathol 1994; 25:652–658.
7. Monso E, Vidal R, de Gracia X, Moragas A. Pulmonary toxoplasmoma presenting as obstructive pneumonia. Thorax 1986; 41:489–490.
8. Mariuz P, Bosler EM, Luft BJ. Toxoplasma pneumonia. Semin Respir Infect 1997; 12: 40–43.
9. Pomeroy C, Filice GA. Pulmonary toxoplasmosis: a review. Clin Infect Dis 1992; 14:863–870.

Amoeba

10. Lyche KD, Jensen WA. Pleuropulmonary amebiasis. Semin Respir Infect 1997; 12:106–112.
11. Bhambhani S, Kashyap V. Amoebiasis: diagnosis by aspiration and exfoliative cytology. Cytopathology 2001; 12:329–333.

Malaria

12. Taylor WR, White NJ. Malaria and the lung. Clin Chest Med 2002; 23:457–468.
13. Johnson S, Wilkinson R, Davidson RN. Acute tropical infections and the lung. Thorax 1994; 49:714–718.
14. Torres JR, Perez H, Postigo MM, Silva JR. Acute non-cardiogenic lung injury in benign tertian malaria. Lancet 1997; 350:31–32.
15. Kern P, Hemmer JC, Van Damme J, Gruss HJ, Dietrich M. Elevated tumour necrosis factor alpha and interleuki-6 serum levels as markers for complicated Plasmodium falciparum malaria. Am J Med 1989; 87:139–143.
16. Kwiatkowski D, Hill AVS, Sambou I, Twumasi P, Castracane J, Manogue KR. Tumour necrosis factor concentration in fatal cerebral, non-fatal cerebral and uncomplicated Plasmodium falciparum malaria. Lancet 1990; 336:1201–1204.
17. Davis TME, Sturm M, Yue-Rong Z, et al. Platelet-activating factor and lipid metabolism in acute malaria. J Infect 1993; 26:279–285.
18. Turner GDH, Morrison H, Jones M, et al. An immunohistochemical study of the pathology of fatal malaria – evidence for widespread endothelial activation and a potential role for intercellular adhesion molecule-1 in cerebral sequestration. Am J Pathol 1994; 145:1057–1069.
19. Macpherson GG, Warrell MJ, White NJ, Looareesuwan S, Warrell DA. Human cerebral malaria, a quantitative ultrastructural analysis of parasitised erythrocyte sequestration. Am J Pathol 1985; 119:385–401.
20. Anstey NM, Jacups SP, Cain T, et al. Pulmonary manifestations of uncomplicated falciparum and vivax malaria: cough, small airways obstruction, impaired gas transfer and increased pulmonary phagocytic activity. J Infect Dis 2002; 185:1326–1334.

Cryptospira and microsporidia

21. Chen XM, Keithly JS, Paya CV, LaRusso NF. Current concepts: Cryptosporidiosis. N Engl J Med 2002; 346:1723–1731.
22. Travis WD, Schmidt K, MacLowry JD, Masur H, Condron KS, Fojo AT. Respiratory cryptosporidiosis in a patient with malignant lymphoma.

Report of a case and review of the literature. Arch Pathol Lab Med 1990; 114:519–522.

23. Moore JA, Frenkel JK. Respiratory and enteric cryptosporidiosis in humans. Arch Pathol Lab Med 1991; 115:1160–1162.

24. Meynard JL, Meyohas MC, Binet D, Chouaid C, Frottier J. Pulmonary cryptosporidiosis in the acquired immunodeficiency syndrome. Infection 1996; 24:328–331.

25. Clavel A, Arnal AC, Sanchez EC, et al. Respiratory cryptosporidiosis: case series and review of the literature. Infection 1996; 24:341–346.

26. Maggi P, laRocca AM, Quarto M, et al. Effect of antiretroviral therapy on cryptosporidiosis and microsporidiosis in patients infected with human immunodeficiency virus type 1. Eur J Clin Microbiol Infect Dis 2000; 19:213–217.

27. Orenstein JM. Diagnostic pathology of microsporidiosis. Ultrastruct Pathol 2003; 27:141–149.

28. Tosoni A, Nebuloni M, Ferri A, et al. Disseminated microsporidiosis caused by Encephalitozoon cuniculi III (dog type) in an Italian AIDS patient: a retrospective study. Modern Pathol 2002; 15:577–583.

29. Schwartz DA, Bryan RT, Hewanlowe KO, et al. Disseminated microsporidiosis (Encephalitozoon-hellem) and Acquired Immunodeficiency Syndrome: autopsy evidence for respiratory acquisition. Arch Pathol Lab Med 1992; 116:660–668.

30. Weber R, Kuster H, Keller R, et al. Pulmonary and intestinal microsporidiosis in a patient with the acquired immunodeficiency syndrome. Am Rev Respir Dis 1992; 146:1603–1605.

31. Cowley GP, Miller RF, Papadaki L, Canning EU, Lucas SB. Disseminated microsporidiosis in a patient with acquired immunodeficiency syndrome. Histopathology 1997; 30:386–389.

32. Scaglia M, Sacchi L, Croppo GP, et al. Pulmonary microsporidiosis due to Encephalitozoon hellem in a patient with AIDS. J Infect 1997; 34:119–126.

33. Velasquez JN, Carnevale S, Labbe JH, Chertcoff A, Cabrera MG, Oelemann W. In situ hybridization: a molecular approach for the diagnosis of the microsporidian parasite Enterocytozoon bieneusi. Hum Pathol 1999; 30:54–58.

Schistosoma

34. Shaw AFB, Ghareeb AA. The pathogenesis of pulmonary schistosomiasis in Egypt with special reference to Ayerza's disease. J Pathol Bacteriol 1938; 46:401–423.

35. Cheever AW, Kamel IA, Elwi AM, Mosimann JE, Danner R, Sippel JE. Schistosoma mansoni and S haematobium infections in Egypt. Am J Trop Med Hyg 1978; 27:55–75.

36. Schwartz E, Rozenman J, Perelman M. Pulmonary manifestations of early schistosome infection among nonimmune travelers. Am J Med 2000; 109:718–722.

37. Schwartz E. Pulmonary schistosomiasis. Clin Chest Med 2002; 23:433–443.

38. Harris P, Heath D. The human pulmonary circulation Its form and function in health and disease. Edinburgh: Churchill Livingstone; 1986.

Paragonimus

39. Mariano EG, Borja SR, Vruno MJ. A human infection with Paragonimus kellicotti (lung fluke) in the United States. Am J Clin Pathol 1986; 86:685–687.

40. Rangdaeng S, Alpert LC, Khiyami A, Cottingham K, Ramzy I. Pulmonary paragonimiasis – report of a case with diagnosis by fine needle aspiration cytology. Acta Cytol 1992; 36:31–36.

41. Mukae H, Taniguchi H, Matsumuto L, et al. Clinicoradiologic features of pleuropulmonary Paragonimus westermani on Kyusyu Island, Japan. Chest 2001; 120:514–520.

42. DeFrain M, Hooker R. North American paragonimiasis – Case report of a severe clinical infection. Chest 2002; 121:1368–1372.

43. Castilla EA, Jessen R, Sheck DN, Procop GW. Cavitary mass lesion and recurrent pneumothoraces due to Paragonimus kellicotti infection – North American paragonimiasis. Am J Surg Pathol 2003; 27:1157–1160.

44. Watanabe S, Nakamura Y, Kariatsumari K, et al. Pulmonary paragonimiasis mimicking lung cancer on FDG-PET imaging. Anticancer Res 2003; 23:3437–3440.

45. Sugiyama H, Morishima Y, Kameoka Y, Kawanaka M. Polymerase chain reaction (PCR)-based molecular discrimination between Paragonimus westermani and P miyazakii at the metacercarial stage. Mol Cell Probes 2002; 16:231–236.

46. Nakamura-Uchiyama F, Mukae H, Nawa Y. Paragonimiasis: a Japanese perspective. Clin Chest Med 2002; 23:409–420.

Opsithorchis

47. Prijyanonda B, Tandhanand S. Opisthorchiasis with pulmonary involvement. Ann Intern Med 1961; 54:795–799.

Echinococcus

48. Tor M, Atasalihi A, Altuntas N, et al. Review of cases with cystic hydatid lung disease in a tertiary referral hospital located in an endemic region: A 10 years' experience. Respiration 2000; 67:539–542.

49. Scully RE, Mark EJ, McNeely WF, et al. A 34-year-old woman with one cystic lesion in each lung – Bilateral pulmonary echinococcal cysts. N Engl J Med 1999; 341:974–982.

50. Eroglu A, Kurkcuoglu C, Karaoglanoglu N. Bilateral multiple pulmonary hydatid cysts. Eur J Cardiothorac Surg 2003; 23:1053.

51. Baden LR, Elliott DD, Miseljic S, Ryan ET, Wain JC. Case 4–2003: A 42-year-old woman with cough, fever and abnormalities on thoracoabdominal computed tomography – Echinococcus granulosus infection. N Engl J Med 2003; 348:447–455.

52. Den Hertog RW, Wagenaar SjSc, Westermann CJJ. Bronchocentric granulomatosis and pulmonary echinococcosis. Am Rev Respir Dis 1982; 126:344–347.

53. Ayed AK, Alshawaf E. Surgical treatment and follow-up of pulmonary hydatid cyst. Med Princ Pract 2003; 12:112–116.

54. Dakak M, Genc O, Gurkok S, Gozubuyuk A, Balkanli K. Surgical treatment for pulmonary hydatidosis (a review of 422 cases). J R Coll Surg Edin 2002; 47:689–692.

55. Kabiri e, Caidi M, al Aziz S, el Maslout A, Benosman A. Surgical treatment of hydatidothorax. Series of 79 cases. Acta Chir Belg 2003; 103:401–404.

Cysticercosis

56. Walts AE, Nivatpumin T, Epstein A. Pulmonary cysticercus. Mod Pathol 1995; 8:299–302.

57. Mauad T, Battlehner CN, Bedrikow CL, Capelozzi VL, Saldiva PH. Case report: massive cardiopulmonary cysticercosis in a leukemic patient. Pathol Res Pract 1997; 193:527–529.

Ascaris

58. Heggers JP, Muller MJ, Elwood E, Herndon DN. Ascariasis pneumonitis: a potentially fatal complication in smoke inhalation injury. Burns 1995; 21:149–151.

Strongyloides

59. Gill V, Bell DR. Strongyloidiasis in ex-prisoners of war in south-east Asia. BMJ 1982; 280:1319.

60. Gill GV, Bell DR. Strongyloides stercoralis infection in Burma Star veterans. BMJ 1987; 294:1003–1004.

61. Higenbottam TW, Heard BE. Opportunistic pulmonary strongyloidiasis complicating asthma treated with steroids. Thorax 1976; 31:226–232.

62. Ting YM. Pulmonary strongyloidiasis – case report of 2 cases. Kaohsiung J Med Sci 2000; 16:269–274.

63. Kinjo T, Tsuhako K, Nakazato I, et al. Extensive intra-alveolar haemorrhage caused by disseminated strongyloidiasis. Int J Parasitol 1998; 28:323–330.

64. Lin AL, Kessimian N, Benditt JO. Restrictive pulmonary disease due to interlobular septal fibrosis associated with disseminated infection by strongyloides stercoralis. Am J Respir Crit Care Med 1995; 151:205–209.

64a. Mayayo E, Gomez-Aracil V, Azua-Blanco J, et al. Strongyloides stercolaris infection mimicking a malignant tumour in a non-immunocompromised patient. Diagnosis by bronchoalveolar cytology. J Clin Pathol 2005; 58:420–422.

Filaria

65. Udwadia FE. Tropical eosinophilia – a review. Respir Med 1993; 87:17–21.

66. Webb JGK, Job CK, Gault EW. Tropical eosinophilia: demonstration of microfilariae in lung, liver and lymph nodes. Lancet 1960; 1:835–842.

67. Danaraj TJ, Pacheco G, Shanmugaratnam K, Beaver PC. The etiology and pathology of eosinophilic lung (tropical eosinophilia). Am J Trop Med Hyg 1966; 15:183–189.

Dirofilaria

68. Kido A, Ishida T, Oka T, Tateishi M, Mitsudomi T, Sugimachi K. Pulmonary dirofilariasis causing a solitary lung mass and pleural effusion. Thorax 1991; 46:608–609.

69. Awe RJ, Mattox KL, Alvarez BA, Stork WJ, Estrada R, Greenberg SD. Solitary and bilateral pulmonary nodules due to Dirofilaria immitis. Am Rev Respir Dis 1975; 112:445–449.

70. Merrill JD, Otis J, Logan WD, Davis MB. The dog heartworm (Dirofilaria immitis) in man. An epidemic pending or in progress? JAMA 1980; 243:1066–1068.

71. Tsukayama C, Manabe T, Miura Y. Dirofilarial infection in human lungs. Acta Pathol Jpn 1982; 32:157–162.

72. Chesney TM, Martinez LC, Painter MW. Human pulmonary dirofilarial granuloma. Ann Thorac Surg 1983; 36:214–217.

73. Nicholson CP, Allen MS, Trastek VF, Tazelaar HD, Pairolero PC. Dirofilaria-immitis – a rare, increasing cause of pulmonary nodules. Mayo Clin Proc 1992; 67:646–650.

74. deCampos JRM, Barbas CSV, Filomeno LTB, et al. Human pulmonary dirofilariasis: Analysis of 24 cases from Sao Paulo, Brazil. Chest 1997; 112:729–733.

75. Pampiglione S, Rivasi F, Angeli G, et al. Dirofilariasis due to Dirofilaria repens in Italy, an emergent zoonosis: report of 60 new cases. Histopathology 2001; 38:344–354.

76. Flieder DB, Moran CA. Pulmonary dirofilariasis: A clinicopathologic study of 41 lesions in 39 patients. Hum Pathol 1999; 30:251–256.

77. Hiroshima K, Iyoda A, Toyozaki T, et al. Human pulmonary dirofilariasis: report of six cases. Tohoku J Exp Med 1999; 189:307–314.

78. Green LK, Ansari MQ, Schwartz MR, Ro JY, Alpert LC. Non-specific fluorescent whitener stains in the rapid recognition of pulmonary dirofilariasis: a report of 20 cases. Thorax 1994; 49:590–593.

Syngamus

79. Basden RDE, Jackson JW, Jones EI. Gapeworm infestation in man. Br J Dis Chest 1974; 68:207–209.

80. Grell GAC, Watty EI, Muller RL. Syngamus in a West Indian. BMJ 1978; 2:1464.

81. DeLara TDC, Barbosa MA, Deoliveira MR, Degodoy I, Queluz TT. Human syngamosis. Two cases of chronic cough caused by Mammomonogamus-laryngeus. Chest 1993; 103:264–265.

82. Kim HY, Lee SM, Joo JE, Na MJ, Ahn MH, Min DY. Human syngamosis: the first case in Korea. Thorax 1998; 53:717–718.

Acariasis and pentasomiasis

83. Li C, Li L. Human pulmonary ascariasis in Anhui Province: an epidemiological survey. Zhongguo Ji Sheng Chong Xue Yu Ji Sheng Chong Bing Za Zhi 1990; 8:41–44.

84. Guardia SN, Sepp H, Scholten T, Moravaprotzner I. Pentastomiasis in Canada. Arch Pathol Lab Med 1991; 115:515–517.

85. Morsy TA, El Sharkawy IM, Lashin AH. Human nasopharyngeal linguatuliasis (Pentasomida) caused by Linguatula serrata. J Egypt Soc Parasitol 1999; 29:787–790.

6

Diffuse parenchymal disease of the lung

Some diseases that affect the periphery of the lung largely involve the alveolar interstitium whereas others encroach upon, or preponderate within the alveolar lumen. Until the advent of modern imaging techniques this distinction was not fully appreciated by clinicians, with the result that many diseases have been termed interstitial, irrespective of the lung compartment predominantly involved. A recent classification corrects this anomaly by referring to them as the diffuse parenchymal lung diseases.[1]

The parenchyma of an organ is the part concerned with function. In most viscera, function resides in the epithelium, the interstitial connective tissue merely acting in a supporting role. This is not the case in the lungs. The function of the lungs is of course gas exchange, which takes place in the alveoli. It is unlikely that gas exchange could take place if any component of the alveolar wall were lacking. The lung parenchyma is therefore to be regarded as all the tissue of the gas exchanging region, which is that portion beyond the terminal bronchiole – the pulmonary acinus (see p. 4). It includes the alveolar interstitium and endothelium as well as its epithelium. Thus the term diffuse parenchymal lung disease is highly appropriate for a group of diseases that includes some which are truly interstitial and others that represent alveolar filling defects.

The idiopathic interstitial pneumonias form a major subgroup of the diffuse parenchymal lung diseases, and represent one in which there have been several recent advances. Histopathological patterns such as usual interstitial pneumonia (UIP) have been defined more precisely and separated from less specific patterns, leading to the introduction of terms such as non-specific interstitial pneumonia (NSIP). Considerable work has gone into correlating histopathological patterns with clinical course and radiological detail, as revealed by modern imaging techniques. The result has been an intensification of the usual clinicopathological correlation and a better appreciation of the likely clinical outcome.

The new classification concentrates upon the idiopathic interstitial pneumonias and in this area seeks to match disease diagnosis with predominant histological pattern so that there is often dual terminology (Table 6.1).[1] It brings together clinical, imaging and histological criteria and is of undoubted prognostic and therapeutic value. However, it is not above criticism,

Table 6.1 Classification of diffuse parenchymal lung disease[1]

1 Of known cause, e.g. drugs (Ch. 7.3) or of known association, e.g. collagen vascular disease (Ch. 10)

2 Idiopathic interstitial pneumonias

Diagnosis	*Predominant histological pattern*
Idiopathic pulmonary fibrosis (cryptogenic fibrosing alveolitis)	Usual interstitial pneumonia
Nonspecific interstitial pneumonia (provisional)[a]	Non-specific interstitial pneumonia
Desquamative interstitial pneumonia	Desquamative interstitial pneumonia
Respiratory bronchiolitis-associated interstitial lung disease	Respiratory bronchiolitis
Acute interstitial pneumonia	Diffuse alveolar damage
Cryptogenic organising pneumonia[b]	Organising pneumonia
Lymphoid interstitial pneumonia	Lymphoid interstitial pneumonia

3 Granulomatous eg sarcoidosis

4 Environmental or occupational (Chs 7.1 and 7.2)

5 Others, e.g. lymphangioleiomyomatosis, Langerhans cell histiocytosis

[a]A heterogenous group of diseases with poorly characterised clinical and radiological features that need further study.
[b]Synonymous with idiopathic bronchiolitis obliterans organising pneumonia.

particularly in its retention of terms such as interstitial pneumonia for a group of parenchymal diseases that may be either interstitial or intraalveolar. The term desquamative interstitial pneumonia (DIP) is retained although it is now well established that this process is not desquamative but exudative and has only a minor interstitial component. Cryptogenic organising pneumonia is a further condition listed under the idiopathic interstitial pneumonias despite it affecting the alveolar space rather than the interstitium. Furthermore, DIP and respiratory bronchiolitis (RB) are largely caused by smoking and are therefore not strictly idiopathic. Similarly, lymphoid interstitial pneumonia (LIP) is virtually never idiopathic and it is questionable whether it should be regarded as an interstitial pneumonia or a lymphoproliferative disease. The classification also uses the terms cryptogenic fibrosing alveolitis (CFA) and idiopathic pulmonary fibrosis (IPF) synonymously despite the former being introduced as an umbrella term for pulmonary fibrosis of uncertain aetiology occurring either in isolation or as part of a systemic disorder. This loses the useful distinction between lone and systemic CFA.

The prime reason for assembling the seven disparate entities listed in Table 6.1 as idiopathic interstitial pneumonias is that although they differ in their prognosis and treatment, they commonly enter the differential diagnosis of IPF at initial presentation.[1-7] The new classification provides pathological criteria that allow these patterns to be distinguished and it is encouraging that a recent assessment of the classification shows it to be fairly reproducible.[8] However, pathologists should be aware that some histological patterns may be seen in the same disease. This is illustrated by the occasional superimposition of diffuse alveolar damage on UIP,[9] the observation that in the same patient different lobes may concurrently show different histological patterns (e.g. UIP and NSIP)[10] and the occasional identification of different histological patterns in successive samples of the same lung.[11]

It is also worth noting that whereas a UIP pattern is largely confined to IPF, diffuse alveolar damage and NSIP patterns are seen in conditions other than IPF. Diffuse alveolar damage has many causes (see Box 4.1, p. 138) while NSIP is seen in a variety of unrelated conditions.[3] One review estimated that 68% of cases showing NSIP were idiopathic, 22% were associated with connective tissue disease, 8% represented atypical cases of extrinsic allergic alveolitis and 2% followed the acute respiratory distress syndrome.[12]

The terms AIP (acute interstitial pneumonia) and NSIP are relatively new and when the adjective 'usual' was originally introduced it was to contrast UIP with four other patterns of idiopathic interstitial pneumonia, namely DIP, LIP, a pattern occurring in association with bronchiolitis obliterans (BIP) and one marked by the presence of giant cells (GIP).[13] It was hoped that this histopathological classification would facilitate a better understanding of aetiology, pathogenesis and clinical features. This hope has been partly realised in that many cases of GIP are now known to be caused by hard metal alloys. The term BIP is no longer used, having been superseded initially by idiopathic bronchiolitis obliterans organising pneumonia and now by cryptogenic organising pneumonia.

Antedating all these terms, but now largely abandoned, are those applied by nineteenth century morbid anatomists who were evidently familiar with the pathological changes seen in IPF and applied graphic descriptive terms such as muscular cirrhosis of the lung[14] and cirrhosis cystica pulmonum.[15]

REFERENCES

1. American Thoracic Society/European Respiratory Society international multidisciplinary consensus classification of the idiopathic interstitial pneumonias. Am J Respir Crit Care Med 2002; 165:277–304.

2. Katzenstein ALA, Fiorelli RF. Nonspecific interstitial pneumonia/fibrosis – histologic features and clinical significance. Am J Surg Pathol 1994; 18:136–147.

3. Bjoraker JA, Ryu JH, Edwin MK, et al. Prognostic significance of histopathologic subsets in idiopathic pulmonary fibrosis. Am J Respir Crit Care Med 1998; 157:199–203.

4. Katzenstein ALA, Myers JL. Idiopathic pulmonary fibrosis: Clinical relevance of pathologic classification. Am J Respir Crit Care Med 1998; 157:1301–1315.

5. Nicholson AC, Colby TV, Dubois RM, Hansell DM, Wells AU. The prognostic significance of the histologic pattern of interstitial pneumonia in patients presenting with the clinical entity of cryptogenic fibrosing alveolitis. Am J Respir Crit Care Med 2000; 162:2213–2217.

6. King TE, Schwarz MI, Brown K, et al. Idiopathic pulmonary fibrosis. Relationship between histopathologic features and mortality. Am J Respir Crit Care Med 2001; 164:1025–1032.

7. Flaherty KR, Toews GB, Travis WD, et al. Clinical significance of histological classification of idiopathic interstitial pneumonia. Eur Resp J 2002; 19:275–283.

8. Nicholson AG, Addis BJ, Bharucha H, et al. Inter-observer variation between pathologists in diffuse parenchymal lung disease. Thorax 2004; 59:500–505.

9. Kondoh Y, Taniguchi H, Kawabata Y, Yokoi T, Suzuki K, Takagi K. Acute exacerbation in idiopathic pulmonary fibrosis – analysis of clinical and pathologic findings in three cases. Chest 1993; 103:1808–1812.

10. Flaherty KR, Travis WD, Colby TV, et al. Histopathologic variability in usual and nonspecific interstitial pneumonias. Am J Respir Crit Care Med 2001; 164:1722–1727.

11. Katzenstein ALA, Zisman DA, Litzky LA, Nguyen BT, Kotloff RM. Usual interstitial pneumonia – Histologic study of biopsy and explant specimens. Am J Surg Pathol 2002; 26:1567–1577.

12. Cottin V, Loire R, Chalabreyesse L, Thivolet F, Cordier JF. Pneumopathie interstitielle non specifique: une nouvelle entite anatomoclinique au sein des pneumopathies interstitielles diffuses idiopathiques. Rev Mal Respir 2001; 18:25–33.

13. Liebow AA. New concepts and entities in pulmonary disease. In: International Academy of Pathology, ed. Monograph No.8. The Lung. Baltimore: Williams & Wilkins; 1967:332–365.

14. Buhl vL. Muscular Zirrhose der Lungen. Lungenentzundung, Tuberkulose und Schwindsucht. Munich: Olderburg; 1873:169.

15. Rindfleisch GE. Ueber Cirrhosis Cystica Pulmonum. Zentralbl Pathol 1897; 8:864–865.

6

Diffuse parenchymal disease of the lung

6.1

Interstitial lung disease

The diseases described in this chapter predominantly involve the alveolar interstitium, which constitutes the connective tissue framework of the alveolar walls. Its boundaries are the epithelial and endothelial basement membranes (see p. 17 and Fig. 1.26, p. 15). Many of the diseases considered here involve the interstitial fibroblasts and progress to interstitial fibrosis and ultimately 'honeycombing' (see p. 271). They represent examples of restrictive lung disease, the other major cause of which is interstitial oedema, which is dealt with in Chapter 8.1 (p. 401). Lymphangioleiomyomatosis is an exception in that it progresses to severe cystic change without any appreciable degree of fibrosis.

USUAL INTERSTITIAL PNEUMONIA AND IDIOPATHIC PULMONARY FIBROSIS ('LONE' CRYPTOGENIC FIBROSING ALVEOLITIS)

Usual interstitial pneumonia (UIP) is the histological pattern predominantly encountered in idiopathic pulmonary fibrosis (IPF). However, although it is the commonest histological pattern of all the interstitial pneumonias and generally correlates clinically with IPF, it may also, on rare occasions, be encountered in drug reactions, collagen vascular diseases and hypersensitivity pneumonia. IPF can therefore only be diagnosed when these possibilities have been excluded.[1,2] Some regard UIP as the only acceptable pattern in IPF,[1] but others report fibrotic non-specific interstitial pneumonia (NSIP) in a minority of patients with this disease.[3-6] Occasionally, UIP is observed in one lobe and fibrotic NSIP in another, in which case it is the UIP that defines prognosis.[3,6] Although abundant macrophages may accompany UIP, desquamative interstitial pneumonia (DIP) is now considered to represent a separate process, which is dealt with on p. 310 in relation to alveolar filling defects.[4,7-10]

Epidemiology

IPF shows a wide age spectrum. A survey conducted in Britain in the 1990s reported the mean age at presentation to be 67

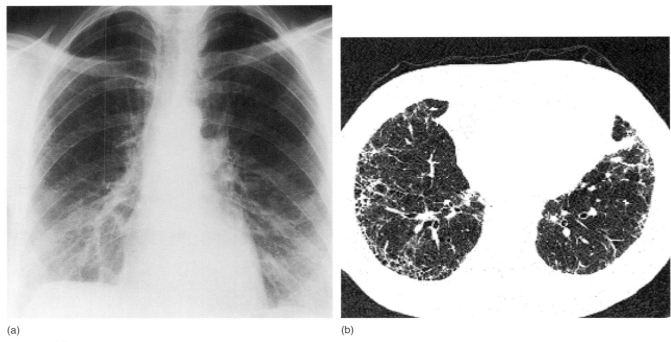

(a)   (b)

Figure 6.1.1 (a) Chest radiograph of a patient with idiopathic pulmonary fibrosis. Note the predominantly basal distribution with involvement of the costophrenic angles, which is characteristic of this disease. (b) HRCT of idiopathic pulmonary fibrosis. The lung bases show subpleural honeycombing.

years,[11] somewhat older than earlier studies that possibly included patients with DIP.[12,13] The disease affects twice as many men as women and about 75% of patients are current or ex-smokers.[11,13] Prevalence is between 1 and 5 per 100 000 population.[14] There is no predilection for specific countries, ethnic groups or urban/rural locations.[1] Occasionally, several members of a family are affected.[15]

Clinical features

Most patients with IPF complain of breathlessness on exertion, dry cough and loss of weight.[11] Bilateral basal crackles are heard on inspiration and digital clubbing is commonly found. Functional studies show a restrictive respiratory defect, the lungs being small and stiff. Chest radiographs may show a 'ground glass' pattern or fine linear mottling, predominantly affecting the subpleural region of the lung bases. Progressive elevation of the diaphragm and 'honeycombing' accompanies the shrinkage of the fibrotic lung tissue (Fig. 6.1.1a). On high resolution computed tomography (HRCT), the dominant pattern comprises irregular lines forming a reticular pattern, mainly involving the bases of the lungs. As the disease progresses, the reticular pattern becomes coarser and 'honeycombing' and 'traction bronchiectasis' develop (Fig. 6.1.1b). Serological abnormalities and changes detectable on bronchoalveolar lavage (outlined below under pathogenesis) contribute to a distinctive clinical picture. In the later stages, cyanosis and dyspnoea at rest presage death from respiratory failure, cardiac

failure or lung cancer, the latter being an important complication that is dealt with below.

The disease is generally diagnosed on the above clinical and imaging features; indeed, the diagnostic accuracy of HRCT in identifying patients with a UIP pattern and hence IPF is now such that patients seldom come to biopsy.[1] In Britain, only 40% of patients with IPF undergo any form of biopsy: 28% have a transbronchial biopsy and 12% a surgical lung biopsy.[11] Transbronchial biopsy may establish an alternative diagnosis, but a surgical biopsy is nearly always required to determine the pattern of interstitial pneumonia, and is now usually obtained at video-assisted thoracoscopy. In these instances, it is the presence of UIP that establishes the diagnosis of IPF and dictates prognosis.[16]

Course of the disease

Early studies from the Brompton Hospital showed that patients with 'lone cryptogenic fibrosing alveolitis' (CFA) had a mean survival of about 4 years,[13] but later studies limited to patients with UIP (as currently defined) showed a mean survival of about 2 years (Fig. 6.1.2).[4] This figure is in accord with other recent studies.[1,7,8,16] However, current smokers at the time of presentation appear to have a better prognosis than non-smokers.[17] Occasionally, an acute exacerbation is observed, often as a terminal event.[18–20]

Treatment is largely based on immunosuppression but is effective in only a minority of patients. It usually comprises

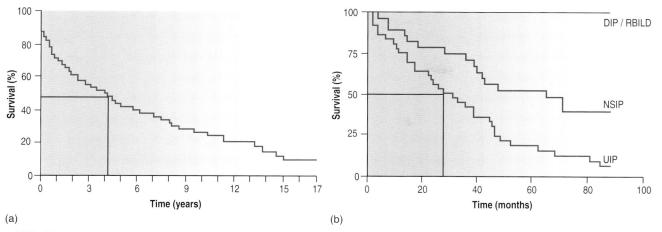

(a) (b)

Figure 6.1.2 The survival curve of two groups of patients treated for idiopathic pulmonary fibrosis at the Brompton Hospital. (a) In a group antedating the distinction of UIP and NSIP the median survival was about 4 years from the onset of symptoms whereas in a later group categorised according to their histological pattern (b) those with a UIP pattern had a median survival nearer to 2 years. (Redrawn from Nicholson et al.[4])

steroid therapy combined with other immunosuppressants such as azathioprine. However, trials of agents such as inter-feron-γ, N-acetyl cysteine, tumour necrosis factor-α antagonists, endothelin-1 receptor antagonists, and 5-lipo-oxygenase inhibitors are currently underway or are in the planning stages, these drugs reflecting recent advances in understanding the pathogenesis of the disease.[21,22a] Transplantation, often of a single lung, is increasingly being undertaken.

Morbid anatomy

In a typical case, the lungs are shrunken and firm when removed at autopsy or in preparation for transplantation. The lower lobes are most severely affected, with the pleura having a finely nodular 'cobblestone' pattern, resembling that of a cirrhotic liver (Fig. 6.1.3). Pleural fibrosis is uncommon, in contrast to asbestosis which IPF otherwise resembles macroscopically. The cut surface of the lung shows fibrosis and a variable degree of 'honeycombing', which is most marked beneath the pleura (Figs 6.1.4–6.1.6). The posterior basal segment is maximally affected and from here the process extends upwards, involving particularly the subpleural lung tissue. This rind of contracted fibrous tissue prevents the lungs from expanding and is an important factor contributing to the restrictive respiratory defect.

Histological changes

The cardinal features of UIP are presented in Box 6.1.1.[2] As noted above, the disease is most marked immediately beneath the pleura. A characteristic low power feature is that the changes are patchy. Areas of chronic interstitial inflammation and fibrosis alternate with foci of relatively normal lung (Fig. 6.1.7). Much of the fibrosis is well-established, consisting of poorly cellular hyaline collagen, but lying immediately adjacent

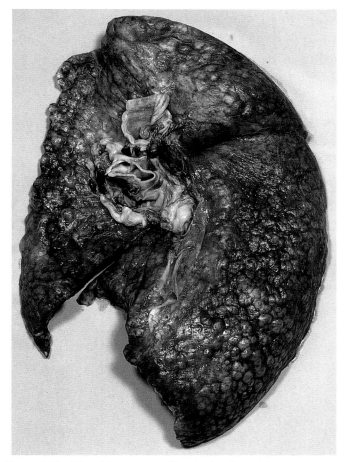

Figure 6.1.3 Idiopathic pulmonary fibrosis. The visceral pleura shows a 'cobblestone' pattern, reflecting changes in the underlying lung parenchyma. The pleura itself is not affected by the fibrotic process. (Specimen submitted by Dr RVP Dissanayake, Ilford, UK.)

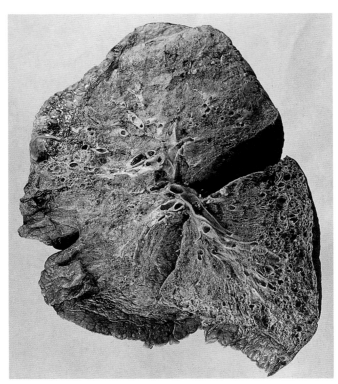

Figure 6.1.4 Idiopathic pulmonary fibrosis. The lung shows basal subpleural 'honeycombing'.

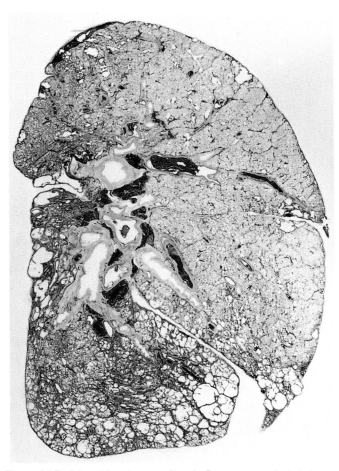

Figure 6.1.5 Idiopathic pulmonary fibrosis. Paper-mounted whole lung section. Note the predominance of the disease in the basal parts of the lung.

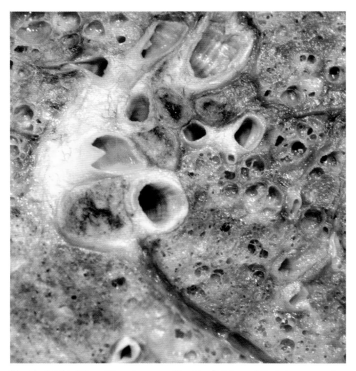

Figure 6.1.6 Idiopathic pulmonary fibrosis. Patches of fibrosis, some of which show honeycombing, alternate with areas of normal lung.

Box 6.1.1 Histological features of usual interstitial pneumonia[2]

Major features
Patchy parenchymal involvement
Subpleural and paraseptal predominance
Established fibrosis leading to loss of architecture
Honeycomb change
Fibroblastic foci adjacent to areas of established fibrosis
Mild to moderate interstitial chronic inflammation

Minor (or secondary) changes
Alveolar macrophage accumulation
Follicular hyperplasia
Smooth muscle hypertrophy/hyperplasia
Endarteritis
Alveolar neutrophil accumulation
Bronchiolar, bony, fatty and squamous metaplasia
Mild pleuritis and pleural fibrosis
Cholesterol clefts
Subpleural blebs
Prominent eosinophil accumulation
Focal alveolar fibrin

Pertinent negative features
Lack of inorganic dusts (e.g. asbestos)
Lack of granulomas
Lack of Langerhans cells

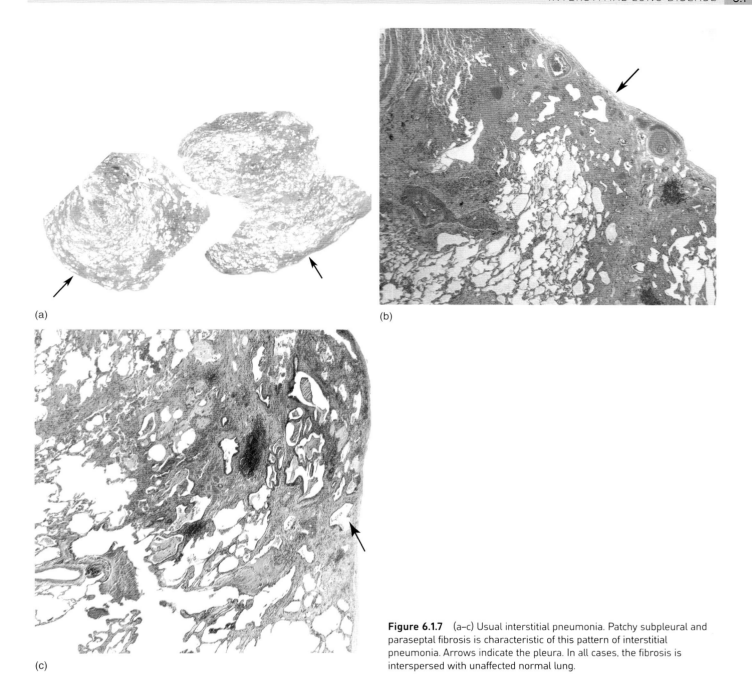

Figure 6.1.7 (a–c) Usual interstitial pneumonia. Patchy subpleural and paraseptal fibrosis is characteristic of this pattern of interstitial pneumonia. Arrows indicate the pleura. In all cases, the fibrosis is interspersed with unaffected normal lung.

to this older fibrous tissue are localised areas of granulation tissue consisting of plump fibroblasts set in a slightly haematoxyphilic myxoid stroma (Fig. 6.1.8). This variation in the age of the fibrosis is sometimes described as 'temporal heterogeneity'. The foci of immature fibrous tissue, termed 'fibroblastic foci', can be highlighted by staining the abundant acidic proteoglycans present in such granulation tissue with Alcian blue or Movat's stain (Fig. 6.1.8c). They are thought to represent the sites of repeated lung damage. The extent of these foci is associated with mortality and increased rate

of disease progression, whereas the more traditional feature of disease activity, interstitial mononuclear cell infiltration, is of lesser prognostic value.[23] Despite the term interstitial pneumonia, chronic inflammatory cell infiltration is generally only mild to moderate in intensity. Lymphoid follicles are not usually prominent in idiopathic disease and when present suggest collagen-vascular disease. As the process becomes more advanced, there is increased loss of alveolar architecture with remodelling and eventual formation of cysts separated by bands of fibrosis, so-called 'honeycombing' (Figs 6.1.4, 6.1.5, 6.1.6 and 6.1.9).

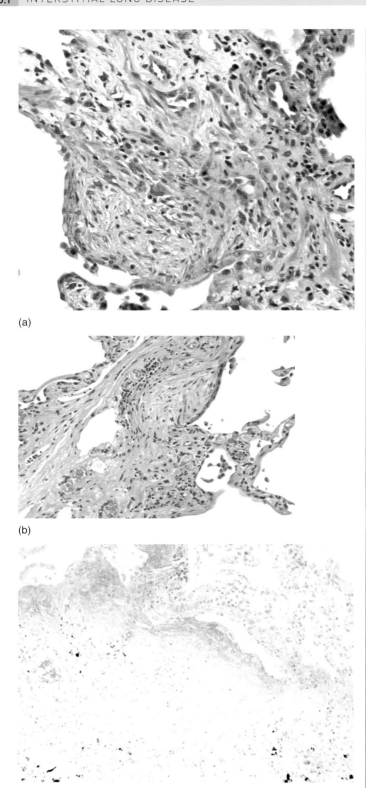

(a)

(b)

(c)

Figure 6.1.8 Usual interstitial pneumonia. (a) A fibroblastic focus consisting of granulation tissue adjacent to more collagenous interstitial fibrosis. (b) A fibroblastic focus showing a greater degree of collagenisation and overlying epithelialisation as it becomes incorporated into the interstitium. (c) Granulation tissue rich in alcianophilic proteoglycans (top) covers older, more fibrous tissue. (Alcian blue stain.)

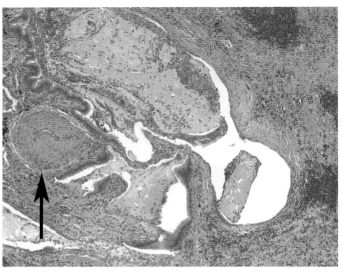

Figure 6.1.9 Idiopathic pulmonary fibrosis in an advanced stage. There is severe interstitial fibrosis with cystically dilated airspaces filled by mucus and inflammatory cell debris but only minor interstitial inflammation. A prominent thick-walled blood vessel is also evident (arrow).

Although widespread 'honeycombing' usually represents advanced IPF, attempts to differentiate end-stage UIP from end-stage NSIP have shown poor reproducibility[4] and it is preferable to classify these changes merely as end-stage lung rather than assign a particular histological pattern.[4,24] Such areas can often be avoided if the surgeon discusses the case with the radiologist and the pulmonologist before taking the biopsy to ascertain the probable sites of active disease.[2] Many centres now biopsy two sites to reduce the possibility of sampling error.[3,6]

A variety of secondary changes that are not specific to UIP and are of limited diagnostic value may also be observed:

- The residual airspaces are often lined by hyperplastic bronchiolar or cuboidal alveolar epithelium (Fig. 6.1.10a), sometimes showing squamous metaplasia (Fig. 6.1.10b) or goblet cell proliferation.
- The distorted air spaces often contain mucin, cellular debris, cholesterol crystal clefts, macrophages and other inflammatory cells (see Fig. 6.1.9).
- Blood vessel walls are usually thickened by intimal fibrosis in the affected areas but are normal elsewhere, unless there is secondary pulmonary hypertension (see Fig. 6.1.9, arrow).
- Reactive smooth muscle hyperplasia is often very marked (Fig. 6.1.10c), contributing to the archaic term 'muscular cirrhosis of the lung'. The hyperplastic muscle is probably derived from bronchioles and small blood vessels rather than the myofibroblasts of young fibrous tissue, but its origin is seldom evident.
- Occasionally, eosinophilic pneumonia-like areas may be seen.[25]

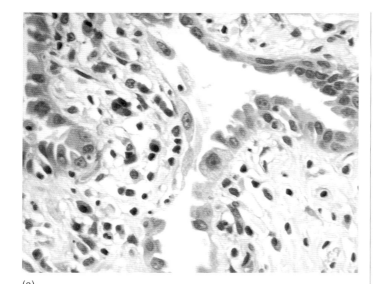

(a)

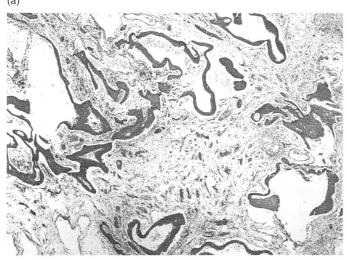

(b)

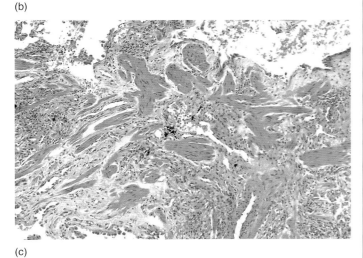

(c)

Figure 6.1.10 Secondary changes associated with usual interstitial pneumonia. (a) Type II cell hyperplasia (b) The regenerating alveolar epithelium has undergone marked squamous metaplasia. (c) An area of advanced interstitial fibrosis shows marked smooth muscle hyperplasia and hypertrophy.

- Other non-specific features include alveolar macrophage accumulation (sometimes mimicking DIP), mild pleuritis and pleural fibrosis, subpleural fatty metaplasia, dilated lymphatics, neutrophil accumulation (especially within areas of honeycomb change), osseous metaplasia, focal alveolar fibrin, and hyaline cytoplasmic inclusions in pneumocytes.[2] The cytoplasmic inclusions represent a tangle of cytokeratin filaments, similar to Mallory's hyalin found in the liver in alcoholic patients.[25a]

Electron microscopy

Ultrastructural studies support the view that the alveolar epithelium is the target tissue, identifying foci of bare epithelial basement membrane as an early feature of the disease (Fig. 6.1.11).[26–28]

Differential diagnosis

IPF was formerly categorised as either 'cellular' or 'fibrotic' and although this was of prognostic value,[13,29,30] the 'cellular' cases would now be recognised as having a different histological pattern (such as cellular NSIP, DIP or respiratory bronchiolitis (RB)), indicating a different clinicopathological diagnosis. It is important to distinguish UIP from these other patterns of interstitial pneumonia because its clinical correlate IPF differs radically from the other interstitial lung disease in its prognosis and treatment (see Fig. 6.1.2b). The most problematic area is the distinction of UIP from fibrotic NSIP.[31] The key features in this are a relatively diffuse pattern of interstitial fibrosis and an absence or dearth of fibroblastic foci (lack of temporal heterogeneity) in NSIP.[2] In reality, this can be very difficult and diagnostic confidence is often low.[31] In this instance especially, consideration of the clinical and imaging features may be of great help.

Sometimes there are abundant macrophages, resulting in a so-called DIP-like pattern, but attention to the interstitial changes reveals the characteristic and the presence of fibroblastic foci heterogeneity of UIP, represented by patchy fibrosis. Interstitial fibrosis, when present in DIP, is usually mild and diffuse with an absence of fibroblastic foci. Diffuse alveolar damage (DAD) is easily distinguished by its characteristic hyaline membranes but may be superimposed upon UIP in acute exacerbations of IPF (Fig. 6.1.12).[18,19] Organising pneumonia may progress to interstitial fibrosis and when the polypoid tufts of granulation tissue are closely applied to the alveolar wall, they may look identical to the fibroblastic foci of UIP, particularly in small biopsies. However, the subpleural distribution of UIP is not seen and the intraalveolar tufts of granulation tissue are generally evident elsewhere in the biopsy.

UIP differs from asbestosis primarily by the absence of asbestos bodies, from Langerhans cell histiocytosis by a lack of Langerhans cells, sarcoidosis by the absence of granulomas, and from lymphangioleiomyomatosis by the different nature of the smooth muscle, which is atypical and differs markedly from that seen as reactive hyperplasia in IPF (compare Figs 6.1.10c and 6.1.46). Extrinsic allergic alveolitis can also usually be excluded by the presence of granulomas, but chronic cases may

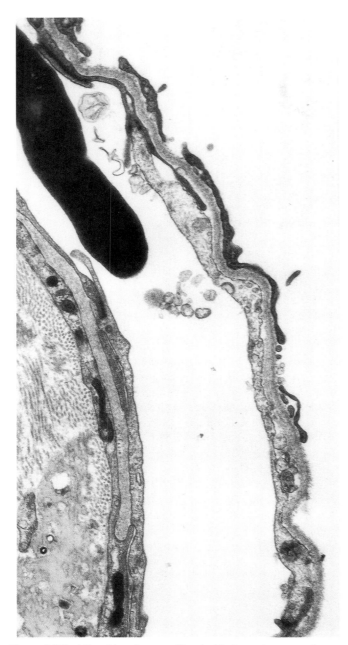

Figure 6.1.11 Idiopathic pulmonary fibrosis. Electron microscopy shows patchy loss of the alveolar epithelium (bottom right), remnants of which are shrunken and electron-dense (upper right). Between these cytoplasmic remnants, denuded epithelial basement membrane is exposed to alveolar air. (Reproduced from Corrin, Dewar, Rodriguez-Roisin and Turner-Warwick. Fine structural changes in cryptogenic fibrosing alveolitis and asbestosis. Journal of Pathology 1985; 147:107–119.[27] Copyright Pathological Society of Great Britain and Ireland. Reproduced with permission. Permission granted by John Wiley & Sons Ltd on behalf of PathSoc.)

exhibit a pattern of UIP.[32] This again emphasises the need to correlate the biopsy findings with clinical and imaging data.

If the vascular changes are so severe that primary pulmonary hypertension enters the differential diagnosis, attention should be paid to the vessels in the comparatively normal areas of the

biopsy, when it will generally be appreciated that the abnormal blood vessels are limited to areas of diseased parenchyma, unlike the generalised vascular hypertrophy seen in primary pulmonary hypertension.

Aetiology and pathogenesis

The histological features of IPF suggest that the disease results from repeated episodes of focal damage to the alveolar epithelium but provide no clue to the nature of the injurious agent. However, IPF has many features in common with the collagen vascular diseases and the concept of lone versus systemic CFA links the two.[33] Hyperglobulinaemia is common and circulating non-organ-specific autoantibodies such as rheumatoid factor and antinuclear factor are often present, even in lone CFA (which is synonymous with IPF).[30,34] In a national British survey of patients with lone CFA, rheumatoid factor was positive in 19% and antinuclear factor in 26%.[11] Antibodies directed against the alveolar epithelium have also been identified.[35,36] Immune complexes have been demonstrated in the serum[37] and occasionally in the wall of pulmonary capillaries, particularly in early cases.[38,39] It seems likely therefore that IPF has in part an autoimmune basis, with the alveolar epithelium being the target tissue. The initiating cause remains unknown although environmental and occupational pollutants,[11,40,41] gastric reflux,[42] viruses[43–48] and drugs[49] have all been incriminated from time to time. However, there is no firm evidence that any of these play a causative role.[50]

The fact that the disease is occasionally familial[15] suggests that genetic susceptibility may be important. There is evidence that in some families, susceptibility to the disease is inherited in an autosomal dominant manner.[51] The responsible gene is situated on chromosome 14q32, close to the alleles responsible for α_1-antitrypsin deficiency.[52] Rarely, several family members suffer from either IPF or α_1-antitrypsin deficiency.[53]

Following recognition of the alveolar epithelium as the site of initial injury, from which dysregulated repair and eventual fibrosis ensue, considerable attention has been paid to the cytokines associated with the regenerating epithelial cells. These cells express numerous profibrotic cytokines, including transforming growth factor-β (Fig. 6.1.13),[54–56] interleukin-10,[56] endothelin,[57] tumour necrosis factor-α,[58] insulin-like growth factor-1[59] and connective tissue growth factor.[60] Other factors identified in the regenerating epithelium include proteinases,[61] tenascin[55] and cytokines that inhibit cell migration and further re-epithelialisation, which may be important in that delayed or defective re-epithelialisation has been held responsible for fibroblast recruitment, activation and sustained proliferation.[62] Poor re-epithelialisation may be due in part to increased pneumocyte apoptosis, promoted by some of the above cytokines, for example, transforming growth factor-β.

Epithelial loss with resultant surfactant deficiency would also explain the focal collapse with apposition of bare basement membranes that has been described by electron microscopists, a change that is rendered permanent by regenerating epithelial

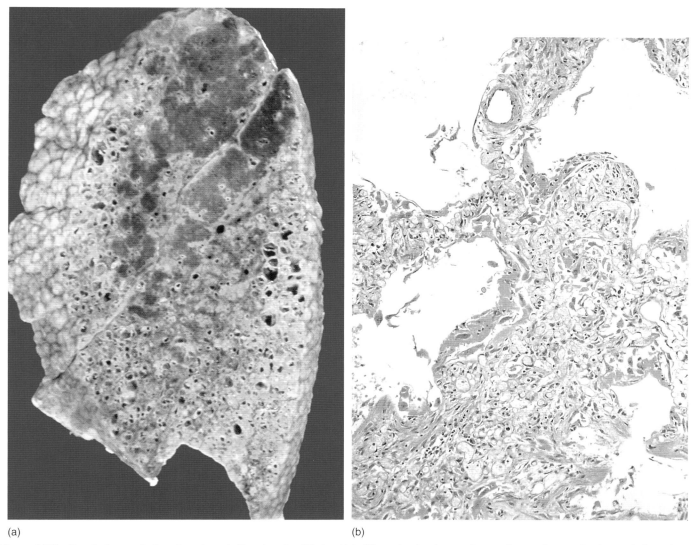

(a)　　　　　　　　　　　　　　　　　　　　　　　　(b)

Figure 6.1.12   Terminal exacerbation of cryptogenic fibrosing alveolitis in which diffuse alveolar damage is superimposed upon a background of usual interstitial pneumonia. (a) Extensive honeycombing affects the peripheral parts of the lung while the non-fibrotic central part is deeply congested. (b) Microscopically, the hyaline membranes that characterise diffuse alveolar damage are evident, superimposed upon the interstitial fibrosis. In hospitalised patients this change is usually attributable to respirator support with high oxygen concentrations but this was not the case in this patient: here the hyaline membranes are taken to indicate fresh auto-immune attach upon the alveolar epithelium.

cells bridging the mouths of collapsed alveoli (atelectatic induration).[28,63] This is at its most extreme in relation to acute exacerbations when hyaline membranes of diffuse alveolar damage are seen (Fig. 6.1.12).[64–67]

The fibrosis that follows the epithelial injury is initially fibroblastic and in advanced disease, the most recent injury is recognisable as foci of granulation tissue rich in these cells. The number of these fibroblastic foci correlates with the rate of disease progression and mortality.[23,68] The fibroblasts show an altered phenotype, typically myofibroblastic, that reflects activation and the production of extracellular matrix proteins. This is part of normal tissue repair but the persistence of an activated fibroblast phenotype probably contributes to the chronic progression to fibrosis and remodelling. This is enhanced by a reduced capacity for degradation of extracellular matrix proteins, through imbalances between matrix metallo-proteinases and their tissue inhibitors. Myofibroblasts also produce cytokines that induce epithelial cell apoptosis, thereby contributing to reduced re-epithelialisation.[62] Direct signalling between epithelial cells and fibroblasts may also be possible in view of the contacts that have been described between these cells through gaps in the epithelial basement membrane.[69,70] Eicosanoids, which are lipid metabolites that play a role in many inflammatory processes have also been suggested as

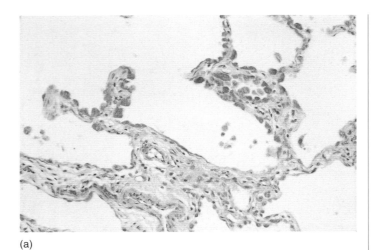

(a)

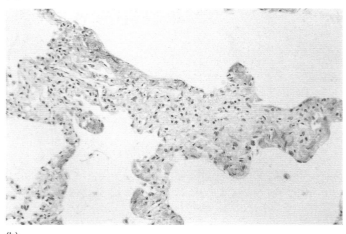

(b)

Figure 6.1.13 (a) Immunocytochemistry demonstrates the intracellular form of transforming growth factor-β within the hyperplastic alveolar epithelium. (From Corrin B, et al. Immunohistochemical localization of transforming growth factor-beta 1 in the lungs of patients with systemic sclerosis, cryptogenic fibrosing alveolitis and other lung disorders. Histopathology 1994; 24:145–150.[54] With permission from Blackwell Publishing Ltd.) (b) The extracellular form of transforming growth factor-β is seen within the alveolar interstitium immediately beneath the alveolar epithelium, compatible with it having been secreted by these cells.

playing a role in patients with IPF, with an imbalance of molecules leading to increased profibrotic leukotrienes and a decrease of the antifibrotic prostaglandin PGE2.[62] This has led to proposed trials of therapy with 5-lipooxygenase inhibitors.[22] Similarly, an imbalance of oxidants-antioxidants has led to trials of N-acetyl cysteine therapy, this being a precursor of the antioxidant glutathione, to protect the alveolar epithelium from further oxidant injury.[71]

It is noticeable from the above that the emphasis on pathogenesis has shifted from a process driven primarily by inflammation to one initiated by epithelial cell injury. However, it is likely that inflammatory cells still play a contributory role. Histological studies show that the severity of the interstitial inflammation correlates with disease progression,[23] and that the lymphocyte is the predominant interstitial inflammatory cell. Focal collections of B-lymphocytes cluster about the airways

while the diffuse infiltrate largely comprises T-lymphocytes, particularly of the suppressor/cytotoxic (T8) variety.[72,73] The alveolar epithelial cells show aberrant expression of HLA-DR antigen, suggesting that the epithelium may be recognised as autoantigenic by the cytotoxic T8 cells.[74,75] However, T4 (helper) lymphocytes are also found and a shift from their type I to type II cytokine profile may be important in the progression of inflammation to fibrosis, type II cytokine (IL-4 and IL-13) receptors being overexpressed in IPF[76] and type I cytokines, particularly interferon, being anti-fibrotic.[62]

Other inflammatory cells that may contribute to disease activity include macrophages and neutrophils, both of which are increased in lavage fluid in IPF (see Table A4, p. 742).[77] Suitably stimulated, these cells secrete a variety of proteases and toxic oxygen and hydroxyl radicals.[78–80] Proteases may so disturb the healing process as to perpetuate it, whilst the toxic radicals may be responsible for damage to the capillary endothelium and alveolar epithelium[78–80] that is evident on electron microscopy (Fig. 6.1.11).[26–28] Bronchoalveolar lavage also highlights a potential role for mast cells in IPF[81] and when mast cells are sought by appropriate staining in tissue sections they are seen to be numerous in the interstitial tissues of the lungs in this disease, and undergoing degranulation.[82] Electron microscopy demonstrates that they are frequently in close apposition to fibroblasts.[83] A variety of cytokines, including those that stimulate fibroblasts, are known to be released by mast cells.[84–85a]

Endothelial damage and interstitial oedema, which are evident on electron microscopy,[27] are probably also important since it is known that chronic interstitial oedema contributes to interstitial fibrosis in other circumstances, e.g. the 'brown induration' of the lungs seen in long-standing mitral stenosis.[86] Various mechanisms contributing to microvascular injury have been identified.[87] However, the exact role and relative importance of angiogenesis and vascular remodelling in IPF remain uncertain at present.[88]

In conclusion, a combination of environmental and genetic factors, age and other unknown agents appear to cause an initial injury to the alveolar epithelium that progresses to a state of persistent dysregulated repair eventually leading to irreversible architectural remodelling. The mechanisms involved in this process are represented diagrammatically in Figure 6.1.14.[62]

Scar cancer in IPF

A notable complication of IPF is the development of lung cancer, which has been reported in up to 13% of fatal cases.[89,90] When patients are matched for age and smoking habit, IPF is found to contribute a 14-fold increased risk of lung cancer.[91] The tumour may be of any histological type. Reports on the relative prevalence of the various histological types vary but overall their distribution does not appear to depart significantly from that found in the general population. The hyperplasia, metaplasia and dysplasia of alveolar lining cells found in IPF (Fig. 6.1.10) is thought to represent the starting point of the cancer. Muta-

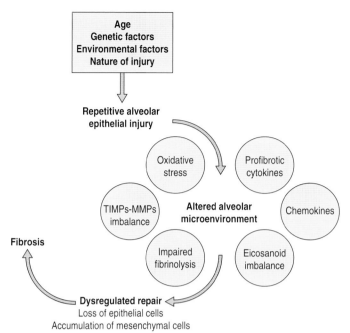

Figure 6.1.14 Progressive pulmonary fibrosis results from dynamic alterations in the alveolar microenvironment that eventually promote loss of alveolar epithelial cells and accumulation of activated fibroblasts/myofibroblasts. TIMPs, tissue inhibitors of matrix metalloproteinases; MMPs, matrix metalloproteinases. (Redrawn from Thannickal, Toews, White, Lynch and Martinez,[62] with permission from *The Annual Review of Medicine*, Volume 55 © 2004 by Annual Reviews, *www.annualreviews.org*.)

tions of the p53 oncogene have been demonstrated therein[92] and a high proportion of the cancers arise in the periphery of the lower lobes where the fibrosis and dysplasia are most severe.[90] The anatomical concordance of fibrosis and carcinoma is similar when the carcinoma complicates asbestosis. It can sometimes be difficult to decide whether alveolar epithelial atypia represents dysplasia or neoplasia, in which circumstance a decision has to be based on the degree of atypia. Non-small cell carcinoma complicating IPF may be resectable but operative mortality is high.[93] A few cases of pulmonary fibrosis have also been complicated by the development of pulmonary lymphoma.[94]

NON-SPECIFIC INTERSTITIAL PNEUMONIA

The term non-specific interstitial pneumonia (NSIP) was first used in the context of HIV-infection[95] and only later applied to a pattern of 'idiopathic' interstitial pneumonia that lacked specific features and could not be classified as one of the better defined subsets.[96] It is in this latter sense that the term is now used. The cause is unclear but clinical correlation suggests that it is multifactorial, some cases showing evidence of connective tissue disease, exposure to environmental allergens or previous

acute lung injury. This uncertainty is reflected in the ATS/ERS classification in that the diagnosis allocated to a histological pattern of NSIP is merely given as NSIP (provisional). However, the term is of value in that patients with a histological pattern of NSIP have consistently been shown to respond better to treatment and have a more favourable prognosis than patients with UIP (Fig. 6.1.2b).[2–4,7,8,96–98]

It remains uncertain what an NSIP pattern represents but some patients may have IPF as, on occasion, both NSIP and UIP are seen in the same patient and even in the same lobe.[3–5,99] In other cases, NSIP probably represents extrinsic allergic alveolitis in which there are insufficient defining histologic features. Alternatively, NSIP may represent connective tissue disorders that are not yet clinically manifest as such. Support for this comes from studies on interstitial pneumonia in the connective tissue disorders such as scleroderma[100] and polymyositis[101] ('systemic CFA'), which show a high incidence of NSIP. There is also indirect evidence that some cases of fibrotic NSIP may be smoking-related.[102] In the interim, a histologic pattern of NSIP should be viewed as a 'holding pattern' from which the clinician can return to the patient to look for such associations (Fig. 6.1.15), rather than a 'wastebasket' diagnosis.[99]

Clinical features

Symptoms and signs of NSIP are similar to those seen in IPF. The patients complain of breathlessness, cough and fever and are found to have crackles on auscultation. Clubbing is frequently evident. Some bronchoalveolar lavage (BAL) studies record increased numbers of lymphocytes,[103] but others have shown no difference from UIP in this respect.[104] HRCT shows ground-glass opacities and reticular changes which may be diffuse but mainly involve the lower lobes (Fig. 6.1.16).[105,106] Honeycombing is less prevalent than in UIP but may be seen on occasion.[105,106]

Histopathology

In contrast to UIP, NSIP is characterised by expansion of the interstitium by variable amounts of chronic inflammation and fibrosis. The distribution is more diffuse than in UIP, and usually lacks evidence of either bronchiolocentricity or a subpleural/paraseptal distribution (Fig. 6.1.17). Foci of organising pneumonia may be seen but they are not the dominant component. At high power, the inflammatory cell infiltrate is seen to comprise small lymphocytes with occasional plasma cells, whilst the fibrosis may be predominantly collagenous or fibroblastic in nature (Figs 6.1.18, 6.1.19). However, the fibrotic process is all of the same age (i.e. temporally homogenous) with fibroblastic foci being absent or, at most, scanty.[2]

NSIP was initially divided into inflammatory, mixed and fibrotic types (grades 1–3), but subsequent studies showed that the survival for the mixed and fibrotic patterns is similar.[4,8] NSIP is therefore now divided only into cellular and fibrotic, the latter having the worse prognosis (Box 6.1.2, Fig. 6.1.19).[2]

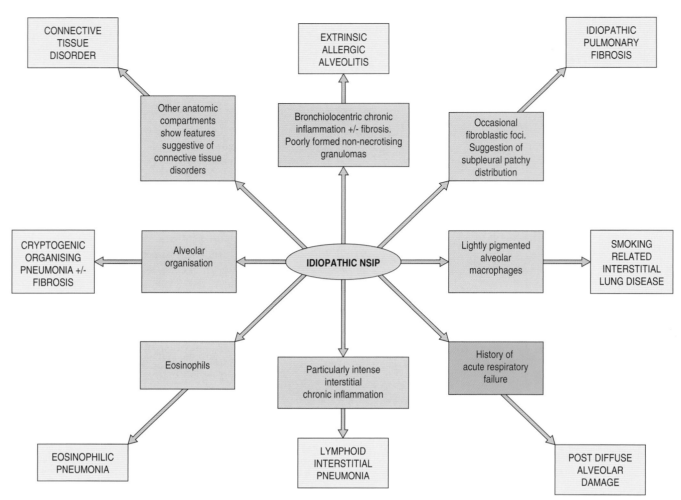

Figure 6.1.15 Clinical associations of non-specific interstitial pneumonia. Only a few cases with the histological appearances of non-specific interstitial pneumonia prove to be truly idiopathic (centre). Upon detailed clinical-radiological-pathological review, several clinical associations may be identified (yellow boxes). Certain histological features may help in this multidisciplinary process (blue boxes). For survivors of diffuse alveolar damage, clinical history provides the most relevant data (green box).

Differential diagnosis

The principal differential diagnosis is between fibrotic NSIP and UIP,[31] the key features of which are listed in Boxes 6.1.1 and 6.1.2.

The separation of cellular NSIP from DIP is facilitated by the relative dearth of alveolar macrophages in the former but rare cases of DIP may show mild to moderate fibrosis and overlap histologically with fibrotic NSIP. The exudative and organising phases of DAD are easily distinguishable from NSIP as neither hyaline membranes nor diffuse organising pneumonia are present, but in long-term survivors of DAD the histological features may be indistinguishable from those of fibrotic NSIP,[96] again emphasising the importance of clinical correlation. Extrinsic allergic alveolitis may also simulate fibrotic NSIP, in which case the presence of even a single granuloma or a suggestion of focal bronchiolocentricity should raise the suspicion of hypersensitivity. Distinction from lymphoid interstitial pneumonia

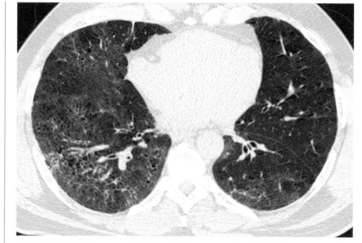

Figure 6.1.16 Non-specific interstitial pneumonia. HRCT shows ground-glass and faint reticular opacities.

(a)

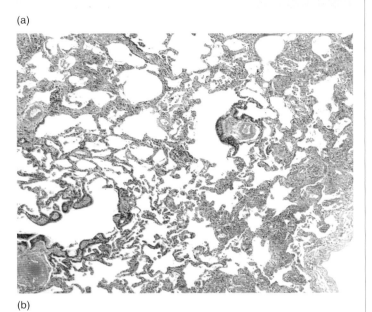

(b)

Figure 6.1.17 Non-specific interstitial pneumonia. (a) The changes are more diffuse than in UIP. (b) The cellular variant shows mild uniform expansion of the interstitium by a non-specific chronic inflammatory cell infiltrate.

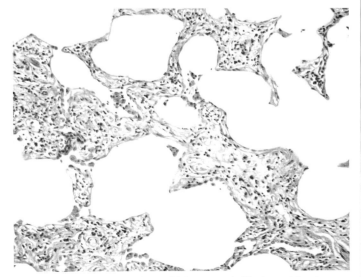

Figure 6.1.18 Non-specific interstitial pneumonia. The interstitium is infiltrated by lymphocytes, histiocytes and plasma cells, while the fibrosis is collagenous and lacks the fibroblastic foci of usual interstitial pneumonia.

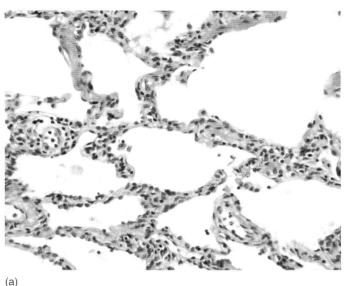

(a)

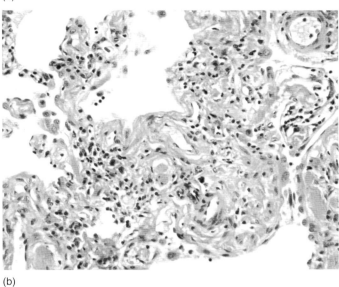

(b)

Figure 6.1.19 Non-specific interstitial pneumonia. (a) Cellular NSIP shows mild interstitial chronic inflammation without fibrosis. (b) Fibrotic NSIP shows interstitial chronic inflammation in association with established fibrosis.

(LIP, see p. 644) is subjective, being primarily based upon the intensity of the interstitial chronic inflammatory cell infiltrate, which is much more marked in LIP than in NSIP. Again imaging is of value as LIP more frequently shows cystic changes superimposed on the ground-glass opacities.

Prognosis

Patients with cellular NSIP show a good response to steroid therapy and have an excellent prognosis, their 5-year survival being close to 100%.[4,8,98] Data on fibrotic NSIP are less consistent but it is universally reported that 5-year survival is better than

Box 6.1.2 Histological features of non-specific interstitial pneumonia[2]

Cellular	Fibrotic
Major features	Major features
Mild to moderate interstitial chronic inflammation	Mild to moderate interstitial chronic inflammation
Diffuse involvement of affected parenchyma	Diffuse involvement of affected parenchyma
Preservation of alveolar architecture	Usually only mild to moderate loss of alveolar architecture
	Variable degree of interstitial fibrosis
	Lack or rarity of fibroblastic foci adjacent to areas of established fibrosis
Minor (or secondary) changes	Minor (or secondary) changes
Mild alveolar macrophage accumulation	Alveolar macrophage accumulation
Follicular hyperplasia	Follicular hyperplasia
Organising pneumonia	Organising pneumonia
Peribronchiolar fibrosis	Bronchiolar, bony, fatty and squamous metaplasia (less marked than UIP)
Mild chronic pleuritis	Smooth muscle hypertrophy/ hyperplasia (less marked than UIP)
Type II pneumocyte hyperplasia	Endarteritis
Focal alveolar fibrin	Mild chronic pleuritis and pleural fibrosis
	Type II pneumocyte hyperplasia
	Focal alveolar fibrin
Pertinent negative features	Pertinent negative features
Dense interstitial fibrosis	Lack or paucity of honeycomb change
Lack of inorganic dusts (e.g. asbestos)	Lack of inorganic dusts (e.g. asbestos)
Lack of granulomas	Lack of granulomas
Lack or paucity of eosinophils	Lack or paucity of eosinophils
Lack of organisms (e.g. viral inclusions)	Lack of organisms (e.g. viral inclusions)
	Lack of Langerhans cells

with UIP[2–4,7,8,96–98] though in the longer term the difference is less marked.[4,8]

Conclusion

Although there are still problems regarding aetiology and consistency of diagnosis, NSIP has gained acceptance in clinical, radiological and pathological fields. Application of agreed histological criteria should now allow more uniform cohorts to be studied, which should lead to a better understanding of the clinical conditions that may present with this histological pattern.

ACUTE INTERSTITIAL PNEUMONIA (IDIOPATHIC DIFFUSE ALVEOLAR DAMAGE)

Diffuse alveolar damage (DAD) is the histological pattern seen in the acute respiratory distress syndrome (ARDS). It is dis-

cussed in detail in Chapter 4 as a process of acute alveolar damage and repair of varied aetiology. However, although DAD has many well-recognised causes, it also constitutes one pattern of idiopathic interstitial pneumonia, when it is associated with an acute clinical syndrome known as acute interstitial pneumonia (AIP). As opposed to other interstitial lung diseases, AIP has an acute presentation and shows a rapid clinical progression.[107] The clinical features are very similar to those described by Hamman and Rich,[108–110] but minor differences have been described.[111] AIP starts with a flu-like episode, which is succeeded by rapidly progressive severe dyspnoea, often leading to death from respiratory failure. The age range is wide and, by definition, patients are previously healthy and have no underlying disease.[107,111] HRCT shows bilateral ground glass opacification, bronchial dilatation and dependent consolidation.

Histopathology

The histological features are those described in Chapter 4. DAD differs from UIP by its lack of established fibrosis and the presence of hyaline membranes in most cases, while long-term survivors lack the temporal heterogeneity of UIP although rare acute exacerbations of IPF may show DAD superimposed upon UIP (Fig. 6.1.12), often as a terminal event.[18,19,112] The organising phase of DAD may be indistinguishable from organising pneumonia due to other causes[113] and the late features may be indistinguishable from fibrotic NSIP.[96] It is important to exclude infection and special stains should be applied accordingly. Indeed, most biopsies come from the intensive care unit, with a view to confirming the presence of DAD and excluding infection, acute eosinophilic pneumonia and occult malignancy.

Prognosis

Mortality in AIP is reported as varying between 12 and 70%,[107,111] with survivors showing either complete recovery or residual fibrosis. Some patients experience repeated acute episodes and develop chronic progressive fibrosis.[114]

EXTRINSIC ALLERGIC ALVEOLITIS (HYPERSENSITIVITY PNEUMONITIS)

Extrinsic allergic alveolitis, which is also known as hypersensitivity pneumonia, is typically a granulomatous disease of the lungs that results from the inhalation of any of a wide variety of organic substances that are capable of acting as a foreign antigen and triggering a local hypersensitivity reaction.[115] Farmers' lung is the archetypal example but there are numerous different circumstances and allergens, frequently designated by exotic names such as paprika pod splitters' lung, maple bark strippers' lung and the like (Table 6.1.1).[116–118] The pathology is identical in them all and a more meaningful division is into those of sudden onset and those which come on gradually. Thus, the pigeon fancier with a large flock is likely to

Table 6.1.1 Some aetiological agents in extrinsic allergic alveolitis

Antigen	Source	Disease
Thermophilic bacteria		
Micropolyspora faeni	Mouldy hay	Farmers' lung
Thermoactinomyces vulgaris	Mouldy grain	Grain handlers' lung
M. faeni, T. vulgaris	Mushroom compost	Mushroom workers' lung
T. sacchari	Mouldy sugar cane (bagasse)	Bagassosis
T. vulgaris, T. thalpophilus	Contaminated water	Air conditioner lung
Other bacteria		
Bacillus subtilis	Biological washing powder	Detergent packers' lung
Fungi		
Cryptostroma corticale	Mouldy maple bark	Maple bark strippers' lung
Aspergillus clavatus	Mouldy malt or barley	Malt workers' lung
Aureobasidium pullulans	Mouldy redwood dust	Sequoiosis
Pencillium casei	Cheese mould	Cheese washers' lung
Pencillium frequentans	Mouldy cork dust	Suberosis
Trichosporon cutaneum	House dust, bird droppings	Summer-type pneumonitis[a]
Animal proteins		
Avian serum and excreta	Pigeons, budgerigars	Bird fanciers' lung[a]
Feathers, serum	Chickens, turkeys	Chicken/turkey handlers' lung
Rat urine and serum	Rats	Rodent handlers' lung
Sitophilus granaries	Infested wheat flour	Wheat weevil lung
Porcine or ovine protein	Pituitary snuff	Pituitary snuff-takers' lung
Drugs[b]		

[a]Budgerigar-fanciers' lung[117] and summer-type hypersensitivity pneumonitis[118] are the most common varieties of extrinsic alveolitis in Britain and Japan, respectively.
[b]Methotrexate, procarbazine, trimethoprim, sodium aurothiomalate in particular.

relate the onset of his symptoms to mucking out his loft a few hours previously, whereas the owner of a single budgerigar will probably not suspect that her gradually increasing breathlessness is attributable to the pet she has succoured without ill-effect for many years. In each case the allergen consists of avian protein in the birds' droppings.

Clinical features

Atopy is not a prerequisite for extrinsic allergic alveolitis. Anyone may develop this disease but certain alleles of the major histocompatibility complex appear to increase genetic susceptibility. Conversely, smoking appears to confer protection as the disease is unusual in smokers.[119] Patients with low constant exposure to the relevant allergen complain of slowly progressive breathlessness and are more likely to undergo lung biopsy than those with acute forms of the disease, which can generally be diagnosed from the occupational and clinical history.

The archetypal farmers' lung is liable to develop if hay has to be gathered when it is still damp, as often happens after a wet summer, in which circumstances various moulds grow on it during storage. Subsequent handling in late winter may raise a fine dust, which, if inhaled, can produce acute respiratory disease. This usually begins a few hours after exposure, with fever and a rigor, followed by cough, dyspnoea and, perhaps, expectoration of blood-stained sputum. About half such patients show transient pulmonary opacities on X-ray examination. Mild attacks clear up in two to three weeks but further

attacks may be more severe and protracted and recovery may never be complete. Occasional patients develop jejunal villous atrophy and suffer from intestinal malabsorption, as in coeliac disease.[120] The slowly progressive dyspnoea that results from constant low exposure is the result of a restrictive respiratory defect with decreased lung compliance and reduced gas diffusion.

Radiologically, acute disease is characterised by generalised ground-glass opacification with small centriacinar nodules whereas in chronic cases the process often affects the upper lobes and HRCT shows a reticular pattern, reflecting the development of fibrosis (Fig. 6.1.20).[121] A mosaic pattern of attenuation may also be seen reflecting the bronchiolitic component of the disease. As with many diffuse diseases of the pulmonary parenchyma the advent of HRCT has resulted in many cases being diagnosed without recourse to biopsy.

Bronchoalveolar lavage shows a lymphocytosis with a predominance of CD8 suppressor/cytotoxic T cells (see Table A4, p. 742). Skin tests and serology may provide further evidence in support of the diagnosis but there are many more antigens in nature than in the immunologist's armamentarium and often the responsible antigen is never identified.[32]

Histological appearances[32,122–124]

Lung biopsies taken during the first few months of extrinsic allergic alveolitis show poorly formed non-necrotizing granulomas. These are generally smaller and fewer than those seen in

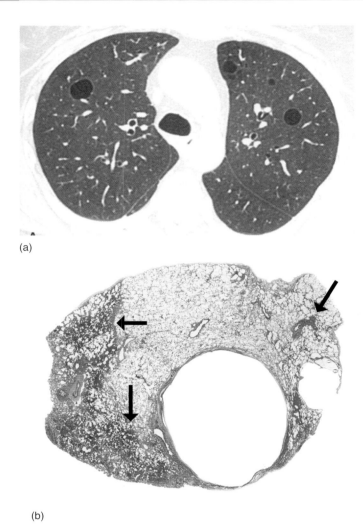

(a)

(b)

Figure 6.1.20 Extrinsic allergic alveolitis. (a) In the acute phase of the disease HRCT shows a generalised increase in the density of the lung parenchyma and faint nodularity. In this example, several thin-walled cystic air spaces are also evident, an occasional feature of the disease. (b) Biopsy in a chronic case shows cystic change and patchy bronchiolocentric inflammation (arrows).

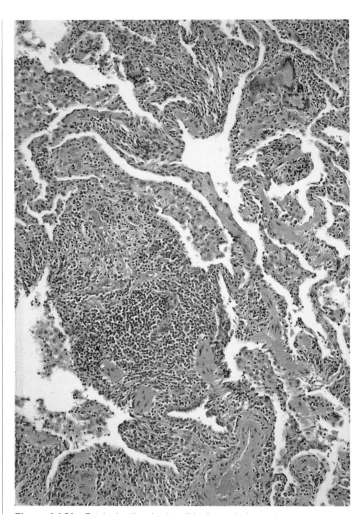

Figure 6.1.21 Extrinsic allergic alveolitis. A poorly formed non-necrotising giant cell granuloma (top right) is associated with widespread interstitial pneumonitis.

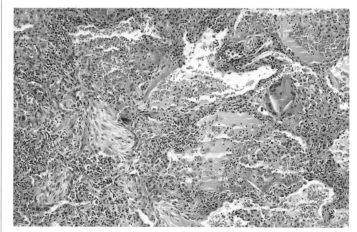

Figure 6.1.22 Extrinsic allergic alveolitis. A prominent giant cell contains two acicular crystal clefts while tufts of granulation tissue representing organisation of luminal exudates are also seen.

sarcoidosis (see Fig. 6.1.28, p. 287) and are accompanied by widespread thickening of the alveolar walls by a diffuse lymphocytic infiltrate (Fig. 6.1.21). No fungal elements are found, but small fragments of foreign material may be present. Schaumann bodies may also be observed. Isolated giant cells with cytoplasmic clefts are frequently observed: these are suggestive of the diagnosis but not specific (Fig. 6.1.22). In contrast to sarcoidosis, the hilar lymph nodes are unaffected. The diffuse background interstitial inflammation is another feature distinguishing the condition from sarcoidosis as it is only seen in the latter if biopsy is undertaken very early in the course of the disease. A further difference is the presence of knots of granulation tissue within alveoli and respiratory bronchioles (Fig.

6.1.22), evidence of organisation of luminal exudates that are responsible for the accumulation of lipid-laden macrophages (endogenous lipid pneumonia) which may also be evident.

The granulomas tend to resolve with time but the diagnosis may still be suggested by the inflammatory process being peribronchiolar (Fig. 6.1.23 and see Fig. 6.1.20b), these airways being the portal of entry of the aetiological agent. The peribronchiolar distribution of the inflammation also helps to distinguish extrinsic allergic alveolitis from non-specific interstitial pneumonia and lymphoid interstitial pneumonia (Fig. 6.1.15). The latter is a condition that may also show poorly formed granulomas but it is characterised by a more diffuse, intense infiltrate that is seldom accompanied by any appreciable degree of fibrosis.

These features are summarised in Table 6.1.2 and contrasted with those of sarcoidosis and lymphoid interstitial pneumonia in Table 6.1.3. Although they are characteristic of extrinsic allergic alveolitis and permit a confident histological diagnosis, exhaustive environmental and serological investigations quite commonly fail to identify the cause.[32]

The lung is seldom biopsied in the acute forms of the disease and there are consequently few descriptions of the pathological features in these patients but the authors have encountered prominent necrotizing granulomas in such a case. Others have reported capillaritis in an early acute fatal case[125] and following provocation tests.[126]

Progression and distribution of the lesions within the lungs

The granulomas resolve within about six months, unless there is further exposure, but the inflammation frequently progresses to irreversible scarring that may show histological patterns of either UIP or fibrotic NSIP.[32] In advanced cases, the lungs show end-stage features such as honeycombing. The upper lobes are affected more than the bases, although in acute cases chest radiographs show a basal preponderance. Whereas UIP is basal and affects a peripheral subpleural rim of lung, chronic extrinsic allergic alveolitis may affect the upper lobes more than the lower and is patchy and irregular in its distribution, with central portions affected as much as the periphery (Fig. 6.1.24). Also, the fibrosis is often more exclusively bronchiolocentric in distribution, rather than being predominantly subpleural and paraseptal as in UIP.

Aetiology[127,128]

The role of an inhaled agent in provoking extrinsic allergic alveolitis has been demonstrated with inhalation tests. For example, extracts of mouldy hay produced characteristic reactions in 12 of 15 patients with farmers' lung compared with none of 20 control individuals,[129] but such testing would now be regarded as unethical due to the danger of permanent lung damage.

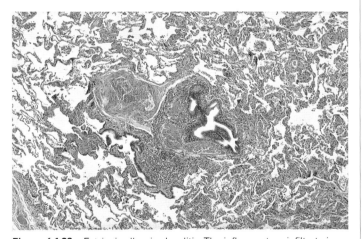

Figure 6.1.23 Extrinsic allergic alveolitis. The inflammatory infiltrate is maximal around bronchioles.

Table 6.1.2 Biopsy findings in 60 patients with farmers' lung

	n	(%)
Interstitial pneumonitis	60	100
Interstitial fibrosis	39	66
Intra-alveolar fibrosis	39	66
Foam cells	39	66
Bronchiolitis obliterans	30	50
Granulomas	42	70
Solitary giant cells	32	53
Vasculitis	0	
From Reyes, Wenzel, Lawton and Emanuel.[123]		

Table 6.1.3 A comparison of the histological features of pulmonary sarcoidosis, extrinsic allergic alveolitis and lymphoid interstitial pneumonia

	Sarcoidosis	*Extrinsic allergic alveolitis*	*Lymphoid interstitial pneumonia*
Granulomas	Persistent, well-formed	Evanescent, poorly-formed	Persistent, poorly-formed
Interstitial pneumonitis	Inconspicuous	Prominent, peribronchiolar	Very prominent, diffuse
Intraluminal fibrosis	Minimal	Moderate	Absent
Lymph node involvement	Prominent	Absent	Absent
Fibrosis	Dense in advanced cases	Dense in advanced cases	Slight

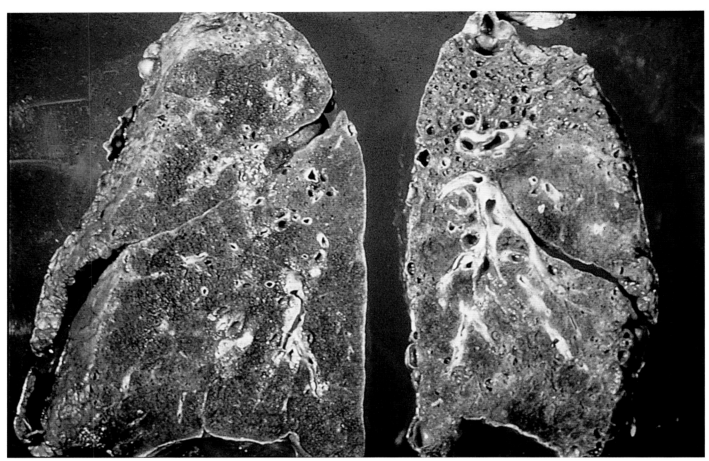

Figure 6.1.24 Farmers' lung. Irregular pale areas of fibrosis are seen in the centre of the lung as well as the subpleural regions: the base is not affected. (Photograph provided by Dr RME Seal, Cardiff, UK.)

A feature of all forms of extrinsic allergic alveolitis is the presence of serum precipitins against extracts of the substances known to produce symptoms of the disease and because of this the disease is widely believed to represent an immune complex disorder, with the antigen/antibody complexes forming locally rather than being filtered from the circulation. The precipitins are well demonstrated by double diffusion (Ochterlony) testing or by immunoelectrophoresis, whereby, for example, avian antigens give a pattern of precipitin arcs with serum from cases of bird fanciers' lung (Fig. 6.1.25). However, it should be noted that many exposed persons have circulating precipitins but show no evidence of disease. In support of an immune complex aetiology, biopsies from patients with farmers' lung subjected to provocation tests have shown immunoglobulin and complement around blood vessels.[126] The peribronchiolar/periarterial preponderance is explained by the antigen diffusing from the airways meeting antibodies diffusing from the blood at this site. Although granulomas are better known in cellular hypersensitivity states, they are quite compatible with immune complex disease as it has been shown that they form when antigen and antibody are present in a particular ratio that renders them insoluble.[130]

On the other hand, there is considerable evidence to support cellular immune mechanisms playing an important role in extrinsic allergic alveolitis. In addition to the granulomas, most of the lymphocytes recovered by alveolar lavage are T-suppressor/cytotoxic cells (see Table A4, p. 742). Furthermore, in a study of symptomatic and asymptomatic pigeon breeders, lymphocyte stimulation by pigeon serum extracts was only obtained in the first group, regardless of the presence or absence of precipitins, thus supporting a direct role of T-cell-mediated immunity in the aetiology of pigeon breeders' disease.[131] Further support for this comes from experiments producing hypersensitivity pneumonitis in athymic mice.[132]

Thus there is evidence that immune complexes and cellular hypersensitivity are both involved[115] and it is probably naive to conceive of any immune process as being wholly humoral or wholly cellular. Furthermore, non-immunological mechanisms involving activation of complement by the alternate pattern have also been implicated in the pathogenesis of extrinsic allergic alveolitis.[127] Impaired lung immunity may explain the apparent protection against extrinsic allergic alveolitis observed in smokers.[119]

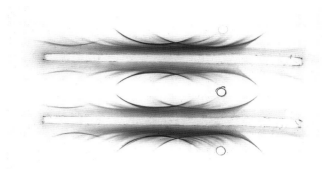

Figure 6.1.25 Extrinsic allergic alveolitis. Immunoelectrophoresis showing precipitation arcs where antibodies from the patient's serum have encountered the test antigen. (Photograph provided by Dr J Longbottom, Brompton, UK.)

SARCOIDOSIS

Sarcoidosis is a multisystem granulomatous disease of unknown cause that is characterised by enhanced cellular hypersensitivity at sites of involvement. Elsewhere in the body cellular hypersensitivity is depressed so that reactions to common allergens such as tuberculin are consistently negative.

The lesions of sarcoidosis may be confined to one organ or disseminated widely. Autopsy studies show that asymptomatic sarcoidosis is much commoner than is realised clinically.[133] Lymph nodes, the lungs, liver, spleen, skin and eyes are the organs most commonly affected but virtually any part of the body may be involved. The distribution of the lesions is consistent with the lungs being the portal entry of the unknown causative agent, the lymph nodes being affected by lymphatic spread from the lungs, and other organs being involved by a combination of lymphatic and blood spread, a situation entirely analogous with that in tuberculosis.

The minimal criteria for the diagnosis of sarcoidosis[134] are:

1 Histological evidence of non-necrotising epithelioid cell granulomas
2 Consistent clinical features
3 Exclusion of agents known to cause granulomatous disease, but the diagnosis may be made in biopsy-negative patients if there are appropriate clinical features and other supportive investigations.

The Kveim test, which was formerly used in diagnosis, has been abandoned because of fears of prion transmission, the inoculum consisting of supposedly sterilised ground human splenic tissue affected by sarcoidosis. It was often difficult to interpret histologically due to solid particles in the inoculum inciting either foreign body granulomas or nondescript clusters of epithelioid cells that did not quite amount to granulomas.

Epidemiology

Sarcoidosis occurs worldwide but appears to be more prevalent in the higher latitudes, with Scandinavia, other northern European countries and North America being particularly badly affected. In Britain the prevalence rate is about 30 per 100 000. The incidence and severity of the disease varies considerably between different racial groups living in the same geographical area. West Indian and Asian immigrants living in London have a 10-fold higher incidence than the native white population.[135] Similarly, black Americans have more sarcoidosis than whites, while the disease is quite rare in native Americans. It is also rare in Eskimos, Arabs and Chinese. Negroes are affected more acutely and more severely than other races.

Aetiology

The aetiology of sarcoidosis is obscure; no single factor is known. The racial differences referred to above have been attributed to genetic factors.[136–139] Associations have been shown with the major histocompatibility gene complex (MHC), in particular the class II MHC alleles, several of which confer susceptibility (HLA DR11,12,14,15,17), while others appear to be protective (HLA DR1, DR4 and possibly HLA DQ*0202).[140–142] Familial sarcoidosis has been described and generally also ascribed to genetic factors[143,144] rather than person-to-person transmission of a communicable agent or shared exposure to an environmental agent.[145,146] Certain polymorphisms have been shown to be associated with different patterns of disease, an example being the C-C chemokine receptor 2 gene being associated with those patients presenting with Stage I disease (Löfgren's syndrome).[147] This suggests that there are genetic differences between those patients with mild remitting disease and those with chronic persistent disease.[140]

Other evidence points to the uptake and processing of as yet unknown antigens, particularly by the respiratory system. Granulomas are of course found in a variety of conditions, notably tuberculosis, some fungal infections and chronic berylliosis. They may also be found in the vicinity of tumours. The granulomas of primary biliary cirrhosis resemble those of sarcoid and occasional patients have features of both these diseases.[148] Similar changes in the lungs have also been reported in HIV-infected patients receiving antiretroviral therapy[149] and in leukaemic patients being treated with interferon-α.[150]

Some authors regard sarcoidosis as an anomalous form of tuberculosis for occasional cases seem to swing from one of these conditions to the other and back again.[151,152] Acid fast bacterial L forms have been cultured from the blood of patients with sarcoidosis,[153] and the application of molecular probes for mycobacterial nucleic acids to granulomatous tissue from patients with sarcoidosis has given positive results in a variable proportion of cases.[154,155] However, positive cultures are very rare, antituberculous treatment is ineffective and there are notable differences in the distribution of the two diseases: for example, there is a high incidence of uveitis in sarcoidosis that is not seen in tuberculosis. Another bacterium for which there is similar genomic but negative cultural evidence in sarcoid tissue is *Propionibacterium acnes*.[156,157]

As noted above, sarcoidosis is characterised by anomalous immunological reactions. For example, the intracutaneous tuberculin reaction is generally negative, despite contact with tubercle bacilli, a phenomenon known as anergy. An explanation for this is provided by study of T-lymphocyte subsets.[158] In the blood, the suppressor-cell (CD8):helper-cell (CD4) ratio is increased in sarcoidosis whereas in bronchoalveolar lavage fluid the ratio alters in the opposite direction (see Table A4, p. 742). Analysis of lymphocyte subsets within the granuloma (see below) are in accordance with the lavage findings. The increase in CD4 helper T cells is seen especially in acute disease. When suitably stimulated these cells show a type I cytokine response, releasing cytokines such as IL-2, interferon-γ and IL-16 that attract other mononuclear cells into the granulomas. Cytokine profiles also correlate with disease progression. For example, increased IL-2 secretion is associated with a poor prognosis, while TGF-β is associated with spontaneous remission.[159]

Clinical features

Sarcoidosis usually appears early in adult life. It affects the sexes equally. Cigarette smokers appear to be less likely to develop sarcoidosis.[160] About one-third of patients develop erythema nodosum and this may be the presenting feature. Other extrapulmonary features include visual disturbances, neurological manifestations, arthralgia, parotid enlargement, hepatomegaly and cardiac dysrhythmia. Serum levels of calcium, angiotensin converting enzyme and gamma globulin levels are often elevated.

In the lungs, a multiplicity of small nodules comparable in size to large miliary tubercles develop. As with other granulomatous diseases of the lungs, the upper lobes are more severely affected than the lower. Occasionally, large tumour-like masses develop, so-called nodular sarcoid (Fig. 6.1.26).[161] The mediastinal lymph nodes often form large masses readily detectable by chest radiograph. On rare occasions, the disease is centred on the airways and the patient has obstructive rather than restrictive respiratory impairment.[162]

Course and prognosis

The course of the disease is unpredictable. In about 60% of cases the lesions regress over a period of 2–5 years and the patient recovers. After spontaneous improvement, relapse is unusual. Sometimes, however, the lungs become progressively infiltrated. When this happens, widespread fibrosis and bronchiectasis may follow. Based on the radiographic changes, four stages of thoracic sarcoidosis have been described:

1 Bilateral hilar lymphadenopathy (Löfgren's syndrome)
2 Bilateral hilar lymphadenopathy and lung involvement
3 Lung involvement without hilar lymphadenopathy
4 Irreversible pulmonary fibrosis.

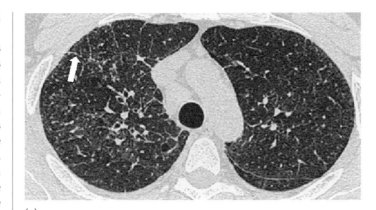

(a)

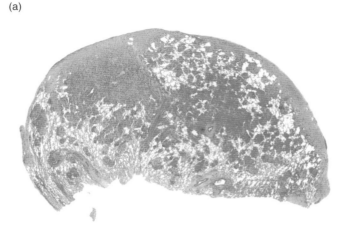

(b)

Figure 6.1.26 Sarcoidosis. (a) HRCT shows numerous small nodules, some of which involve the interlobular septa (arrow). Note the enlarged lymph node immediately anterior to the trachea. (b) Tissue section showing the lung to be studded by numerous small nodules. On the left the nodules have coalesced to form a mass lesion while the right side shows discrete nodules in a more typical lymphatic distribution.

An acute onset with erythema nodosum or asymptomatic bilateral hilar lymphadenopathy usually heralds a self-limiting course, whereas an insidious onset, especially with multiple extrapulmonary lesions, is more likely to be followed by relentless pulmonary fibrosis. Older patients and blacks do less well than the young and whites. Advanced pulmonary sarcoidosis may be complicated by life-threatening saprophytic aspergillosis (Fig. 6.1.27). An increased risk of pulmonary lymphoma and carcinoma has been identified in some studies[163,164] but not others.[165]

Because limited disease often resolves spontaneously, the decision to treat must be weighed against the risks of drug side-effects. In those patients that require therapy, corticosteroids are the drugs of choice. Patients with progressive disease may require additional therapy with drugs such as chloroquine, azathioprine and cyclophosphamide. Drugs that suppress tumour necrosis factor-α may also be of benefit, but have yet to be of proven efficacy.[142]

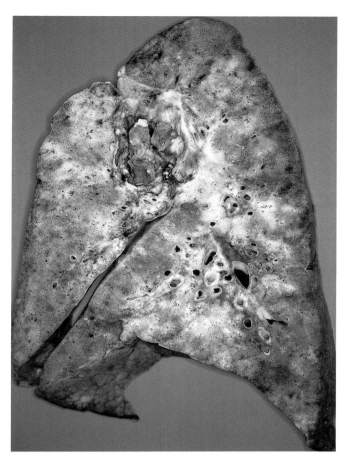

Figure 6.1.27 Pulmonary sarcoidosis complicated by saprophytic aspergillosis. An irregular fungus ball occupies a cavity just above the interlobar fissure. Elsewhere the lung shows irregular pale fibrosis, the result of longstanding sarcoidosis.

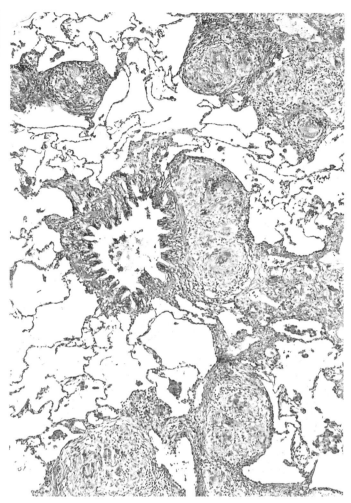

Figure 6.1.28 Pulmonary sarcoidosis. The lung is studded with discrete non-necrotising epithelioid and giant cell granulomas. Intervening alveolar walls are unaffected. Two granulomas are closely applied to a bronchiole.

The disease carries a mortality of about 5%. Half the deaths are attributable to cardiac involvement while in most of the remainder pulmonary fibrosis causing respiratory failure is responsible.[166] Rare causes of death include chronic renal failure due to nephrosclerosis and the cerebral effects of meningovascular sarcoidosis. If transplantation is undertaken the disease may develop in the new lungs.[167]

Pathological findings[168,169]

The histological hallmark of sarcoidosis is the granuloma, many of which are generally seen scattered throughout otherwise unremarkable lung tissue (Figs 6.1.26b and 6.1.28). The granulomas are preceded by a lymphocytic infiltrate[170] but this is transient and is seldom evident by the time lung biopsy is undertaken. Indeed, in contrast to extrinsic allergic alveolitis, the histopathology of pulmonary sarcoidosis is generally notable in that it lacks a diffuse lymphocytic infiltrate.

Sarcoid granulomas closely resemble early tubercles microscopically; they differ from tubercles in that they do not undergo caseation, although a little central necrosis is occa-

sionally seen microscopically (Fig. 6.1.29). Epithelioid cells and multinucleate giant cells, similar to the Langerhans cells of tuberculosis, are found in the centres of the granulomas. The giant cells often contain Schaumann and asteroid bodies (Figs 6.1.30, 6.1.31) but these are not pathognomonic of sarcoidosis, for they may be found in other forms of granulomatous inflammation. Schaumann bodies represent calcified lysosomal residual bodies,[170a,170b] while asteroid bodies are aggregates of vimentin microfilaments and microtubules derived from the cytosphere, the radial arrangement of which determines the bodies' stellate form.[171] Lymph nodes draining sarcoid tissue often contain small brown Hamazaki–Wesenberg bodies, which represent lysosomal ceroid pigment formed through the oxidation and polymerisation of unsaturated fatty acids. More often the follicular architecture of the hilar lymph nodes is completely effaced by numerous non-necrotising sarcoid granulomas.

Epithelioid cells are derived from macrophages but such is the transformation they undergo during this development that

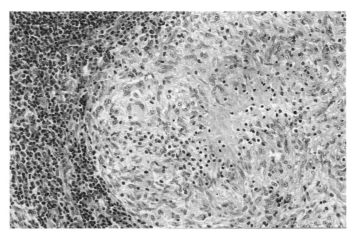

Figure 6.1.29 Sarcoid granulomas occasionally show a little central necrosis.

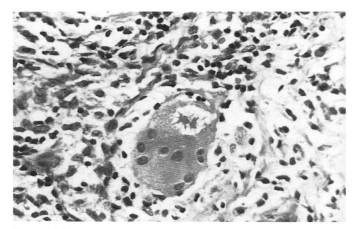

Figure 6.1.30 Pulmonary sarcoid, showing an asteroid body within a giant cell.

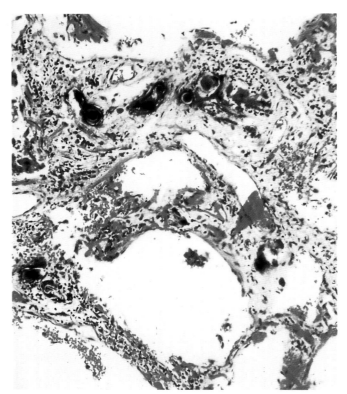

Figure 6.1.31 Pulmonary sarcoidosis in an advanced stage. The granulomas have healed, leaving only the central calcified Schaumann bodies and extensive fibrosis that has distorted the pulmonary parenchyma.

for the final hydroxylation and hence activation of vitamin D,[180] thereby accounting for the hypercalcaemia that is so frequently found in sarcoidosis.[181]

Closely associated with the centrally situated epithelioid cells are T-helper lymphocytes. T-suppressor lymphocytes are fewer in number and more peripherally situated.[182,183] Cytokine studies suggest that the T-helper lymphocytes are mainly of the Th1 phenotype, producing interleukin-2 and interferon-γ.[184,185] A switch to predominantly Th2 lymphocytes may underlie a change from healing by resolution to healing by fibrosis. Antigen-presenting reticular cells are found at the periphery of the granulomas and B-lymphocytes between the granulomas.[186]

At first sight the granulomas appear to be scattered haphazardly in the lung but in fact they are most numerous along the lymphatics and are therefore particularly well seen in relation to the centriacinar bronchiolo-arterial bundles (Fig. 6.1.33) and in the interlobular septa. They are very well developed in the main airways, including the mucosa, so this is a condition in which small fibre-optic bronchial biopsies frequently provide sufficient tissue for diagnostic purposes.[187] Also, because of their distribution along lymphatics, the granulomas come very close to arteries and veins and quite frequently involve all coats of these vessels in a granulomatous angiitis (Fig. 6.1.33).[169,188] All sizes of vessel, from large elastic arteries to venules and lym-

there are few ultrastructural similarities: gone are the phagosomes and lysosomes of a macrophage, replaced by cytoplasmic organelles more in keeping with a secretory cell. The immature epithelioid cell is rich in rough endoplasmic reticulum, as seen in cells synthesising a proteinaceous secretion; Golgi apparatus and storage vesicles then appear, and in the mature epithelioid cell these organelles predominate (Fig. 6.1.32).[172] These cells secrete a variety of proinflammatory cytokines and fibrogenic cytokines, for example, transforming growth factor-β, tumour necrosis factor-α, RANTES and nitric oxide synthase.[173–178] The enzyme dipeptidyl carboxypeptidase (EC3.4.15.1), which acts as a kininase but is best known by its trivial name angiotensin-converting enzyme, has been localised to the cytoplasm of the epithelioid cells,[179] which would therefore appear to be the source of the high serum levels of this enzyme that characterise granulomatous disease in general and sarcoidosis in particular. The granulomas are also responsible

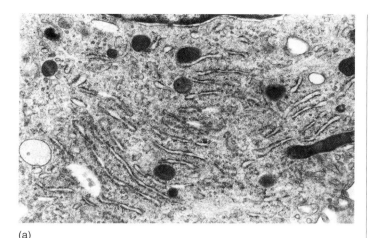

(a)

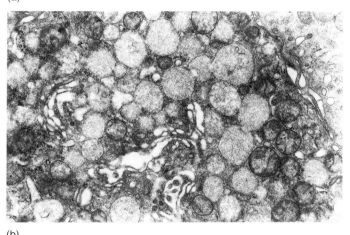

(b)

Figure 6.1.32 Electron micrographs of epithelioid cells in a pulmonary sarcoid granuloma. (a) An immature epithelioid cell showing abundant rough endoplasmic reticulum. The lysosomal dense bodies that characterise a macrophage are not evident. The electron-dense structures are mitochondria. (b) A mature epithelioid cell showing an abundance of vesicles and Golgi apparatus. (Illustrations provided by Dr C Danel and Miss A Dewar, Brompton, UK.)

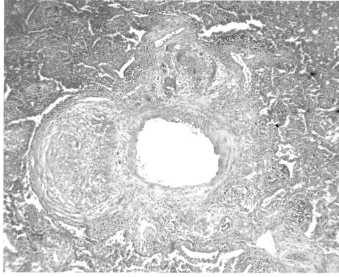

(a)

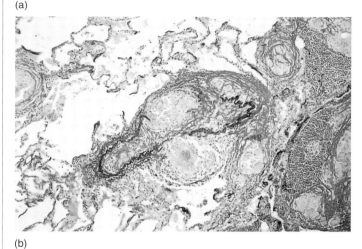

(b)

Figure 6.1.33 Pulmonary sarcoidosis. (a) The granulomas are clustered around small pulmonary blood vessels, where lymphatics are found. (b) Granulomas within and alongside a small vein, the lumen of which is occluded and the wall partly destroyed. (Elastin-van Gieson stain.)

phatics, may be affected, but veins are most commonly involved.[188] Right heart strain has been attributed to this vascular involvement,[189] although it is not a particularly common feature of sarcoidosis.[190] However, some degree of pulmonary hypertension develops in the majority of patients with advanced disease.[190a] Rarely, sarcoidosis is combined with disseminated visceral giant cell angiitis (see p. 445).

The granulomas may be so numerous that they become confluent, and rarely, large masses of sarcoid tissue are formed, the so-called nodular form of sarcoidosis (see 6.1.26b).[161] Sarcoid granulomas heal by progressive hyalinisation and Schaumann bodies may provide the only indication that extensive scarring is the result of granulomatous disease (Fig. 6.1.31). However, active and healed granulomas are often seen together, suggesting that the unknown stimulus to the disease is a continuing

one. Furthermore, early clinical disease may show fibrosis histologically, indicating that the disease may be quite advanced before it causes symptoms. As the granulomas heal there is increasing fibrosis, often with 'honeycombing' (Figs 6.1.34, 6.1.35).

Differential diagnosis

Sarcoid granulomas are a well-known phenomenon in lymph nodes draining tumours. They may also be seen close to a tumour in organs such as the lung and may even mask the tumour. Overlooking lymphoma in a lymph node showing florid secondary granulomas is a notorious trap for the unwary.

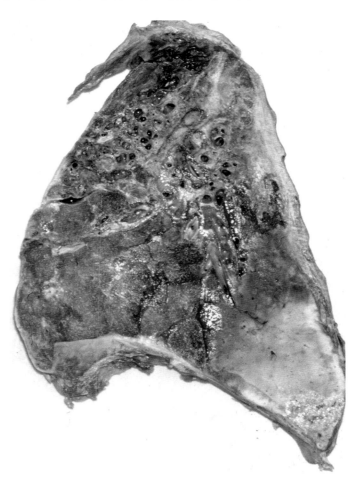

Figure 6.1.34 Late stage pulmonary sarcoidosis. A whole lung slice, showing fibrosis maximal in the upper lobe. (Reproduced by permission of Dr N Gubbay, Cheltenham, UK.)

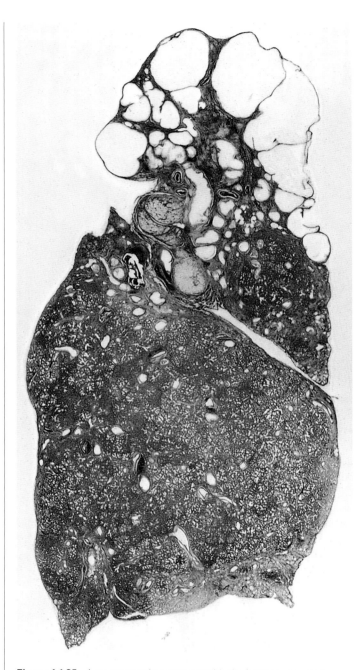

Figure 6.1.35 Late stage pulmonary sarcoidosis. A paper-mounted whole lung section showing fibrosis and 'honeycombing' maximal at the apex of the lung. Solid nodules at the upper end of the interlobar fissure are enlarged hilar lymph nodes, also involved by sarcoidosis.

Reports of sarcoidosis being associated with lymphoma should only be accepted if the two diseases affect anatomically distinct sites and the appropriate clinical, radiographic and biochemical features of each disease are present.[191]

Necrotising sarcoid granulomatosis differs from nodular sarcoid in showing large tracts of necrosis (see p. 444). Sarcoid-like granulomas may characterise extrinsic allergic alveolitis but the granulomas are generally more poorly formed, scanty, and seen on a background of diffuse chronic interstitial pneumonia, in contrast to sarcoidosis in which well-formed granulomas are usually studded throughout otherwise normal alveolar tissue. Even in very late sarcoidosis, lesions are generally recognisable as burnt-out granulomas, whereas in extrinsic allergic alveolitis the granulomas resolve without trace within a few months of last exposure to the responsible antigen. In both conditions, lymphocytes are increased in broncho-alveolar lavage fluid but in sarcoid the helper-cell:suppressor-cell ratio is high whereas in extrinsic allergic alveolitis it is low (see Table A4, p. 742).

PULMONARY LANGERHANS CELL HISTIOCYTOSIS (PULMONARY HISTIOCYTOSIS X, EOSINOPHILIC GRANULOMA OF THE LUNG)[192–196]

During the 1940s, it became clear that three previously described clinical conditions, Hand–Schüller–Christian disease, Letterer–Siwe disease and eosinophilic granuloma had much in

Table 6.1.4 The different forms of Langerhans cell histiocytosis

Clinical form	Age	Organs commonly involved	Prognosis
Generalised diffuse (Letterer–Siwe disease)	Infancy	Bone, bone marrow, skin, lymph nodes, liver, spleen, thymus, lung	Usually lethal
Generalised multifocal (Hand–Schuller–Christian disease)	Childhood, young adults	Bone, skin, lung	Chronic disabling disease
Localised (eosinophilic granuloma of bone)	Childhood, young adults	Bone	Variable. May stabilise or remit
Localised (eosinophilic granuloma of lung)	Young adult smokers	Lung	Variable. May stabilise or remit

common pathologically, and in 1953 the term histiocytosis X was introduced to encompass all three.[197] This grouping derived support from the electron microscopic identification of a distinctive cytoplasmic marker organelle in all forms of the disease, the Birbeck granule (Fig. 6.1.36).[198] In normal tissues, this marker organelle has been described only in Langerhans cells, the implication of this being that histiocytosis X represents a pathological proliferation of Langerhans cells. Accordingly, the term Langerhans cell histiocytosis (or granulomatosis) is now preferred (Table 6.1.4). However, a distinction is drawn between pulmonary and extrapulmonary Langerhans cell histiocytosis. The latter mainly affects children and is thought to be neoplastic, whereas pulmonary Langerhans cell histiocytosis is largely confined to young adult cigarette smokers and is thought to be reactive despite evidence of clonality in some of the pulmonary nodules.[199,200]

Langerhans cells are a constant feature of the normal epidermis and are occasionally found in the dermis. They are believed to be involved in delayed hypersensitivity reactions, particularly the transport of antigen from the skin to the draining lymph nodes. Langerhans cells are rarely identified in completely normal lung but they appear there in response to cigarette smoke.[201] They have also been observed in the lung in various pulmonary diseases, both reactive[202] and neoplastic.[203] Epithelial hyperplasia and metaplasia induced by tobacco smoke are particularly likely to be targeted by Langerhans cells,[201,204] which appear to be attracted by the altered airway epithelium expressing granulocyte-macrophage colony stimulating factor.[205] Interleukin-2 has an inhibitory effect on Langerhans cells and it is notable that tobacco smoke constituents impair interleukin-2 production.[206,207] In pulmonary Langerhans cell histiocytosis, electron microscopy shows that the Langerhans cells are in close contact with lymphocytes that have been previously characterised as T-helper cells: it is therefore suggested that the disease represents a hyperimmune response in which the Langerhans cells serve as accessory cells.[208]

Langerhans cells and their pathological counterpart have a moderate amount of light eosinophilic cytoplasm that is devoid of pigment, and a single nucleus with an indented cerebriform outline and a finely dispersed chromatin pattern. They carry surface receptors for Fc and C_3 but are poorly phagocytic. Electron microscopy shows that they have few lysosomes but contain elongated pentilaminar structures of constant width (40–45 nm) with a longitudinal periodicity (10 nm) in their central laminae, the Birbeck granules (Fig. 6.1.36).[198,209] Inter-

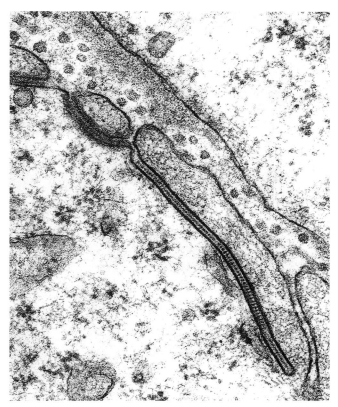

Figure 6.1.36 The ultrastructural marker organelle of the Langerhans cell (the Birbeck granule) is a pentilaminar structure with regularly spaced cross striations. It is occasionally observed communicating with the cell surface, as depicted here. (Electron micrograph provided by Miss A. Dewar, Brompton, UK)

digitating dendritic cells are functionally related and morphologically similar to Langerhans cells but lack this marker organelle.[198] Both these cells express S100 protein but CD1a and fascin are specific immunocytochemical markers of Langerhans cells.[210–212]

Clinical features

The lungs may be involved in the disseminated forms of Langerhans cell histiocytosis but they are most often affected in isolation. Young adults are affected most frequently but there is a wide age distribution. The great majority of patients are cig-

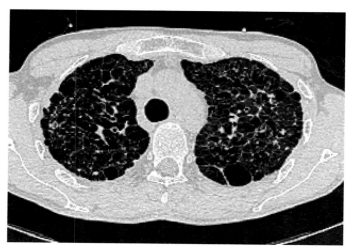

Figure 6.1.37 Langerhans cell histiocytosis. HRCT shows irregular cystic changes and scattered nodules.

Table 6.1.5 Evolution of the disease in 67 patients with pulmonary Langerhans cell histiocytosis		
Evolution	*No. of patients*	*(%)*
Improved	9	14
Stabilised	27	40
Deteriorated	14	21
Died	17	25
From Basset, Corrin and Spencer.[192]		

arette smokers.[160,213] Males outnumber females in most series but the more recent literature suggests a trend to a more equal sex distribution, reflecting the increasing number of women who smoke.

Non-specific chest complaints such as cough and dyspnoea are often accompanied by multiple pneumothoraces and sometimes by general symptoms such as weight loss and fever.[192] Some patients are asymptomatic despite radiographic evidence of lung disease. One previously asymptomatic patient presented with bilateral pneumothoraces due to advanced disease and rapidly succumbed. Chest radiographs typically show bilateral reticulonodular shadowing, most marked in the mid-zones[214] with sparing of the costophrenic angles, this last forming a useful point of distinction from idiopathic interstitial fibrosis. HRCT shows features that reflect the stage of disease, ranging from nodules to cysts, again sparing the costophrenic angles (Fig. 6.1.37). In a smoker, these features are highly specific and often obviate the need for biopsy. Rarely, the disease may present as a solitary pulmonary nodule or even tracheal obstruction.[215,215a] With advancing disease, cystic changes appear and all zones of the lung become involved. Lung function tests usually show a restrictive impairment. Blood eosinophilia is never found and, if present, should suggest alternative diagnoses such as eosinophilic pneumonia. Extra-pulmonary involvement occurs in up to 15% of cases, when features such as lytic bone lesions or diabetes insipidus may give a clue to the diagnosis.

Course of the disease and response to therapy

The natural history of Langerhans cell histiocytosis of the lungs varies considerably (Table 6.1.5).[192,216–218] A few patients follow a rapidly downhill course and die early, while others improve spontaneously and become symptom-free with disappearance of the radiological changes. Others experience spontaneous remissions and relapses and slowly deteriorate, but the disease

may arrest at any stage. Such patients are left with residual functional incapacity but suffer no further progression of the disease. Unfavourable prognostic features include generalised multisystem disease, prolonged fever and weight loss, widespread involvement of the lungs, multiple pneumothoraces and extremes of age.[192,216]

Cytotoxic drugs have only been beneficial in Letterer–Siwe disease. Claims that steroids are beneficial are not substantiated in other series.[192] Generalised disease has been treated by bone marrow transplantation[219] and advanced pulmonary disease by lung transplantation, but some patients undergoing lung transplantation have developed the disease in their new lungs.[220] It seems sensible to advise patients with pulmonary Langerhans cell histiocytosis to stop smoking and there is anecdotal evidence that this is helpful. An infant with osseous Langerhans cell histiocytosis is reported to have responded well to interleukin-2 therapy, the relevance of which to Langerhans cell proliferation is referred to above.[206]

Rare cases have been reported in which Langerhans cell histiocytosis has been associated with malignant lymphoma or leukaemia, the association following various patterns.[221] The basis of this association is unclear and may be multifactorial.[195] A hypothetical relationship between Langerhans cell histiocytosis of the lung and pulmonary carcinoma may be explained by the sharing of an aetiological agent, such as cigarette smoking, rather than as a direct cause and effect relationship.[222]

Pathological findings[192,193,223–225]

Microscopically, early lesions show a focal interstitial infiltrate of mitotically-active Langerhans cells intermingled with eosinophils (Fig. 6.1.38). The lesions are centred on the bronchioles (Fig. 6.1.39, 6.1.40), which are often weakened so that small cavities develop (Fig. 6.1.41). The cavitation may ultimately progress to gross cystic change (Fig. 6.1.42), which is responsible for the repeated pneumothoraces that are such a prominent clinical feature of the disease.

As the lesions heal, their appearances alter and they assume the form of stellate fibrous scars (Fig. 6.1.43, 6.1.44) in which Langerhans cells and eosinophils are no longer readily apparent, having been replaced by pigment-laden macrophages, lymphocytes, plasma cells and fibroblasts. The pigment in the macrophages is partly exogenous, this largely derived from the cigarette smoke to which these patients have almost always

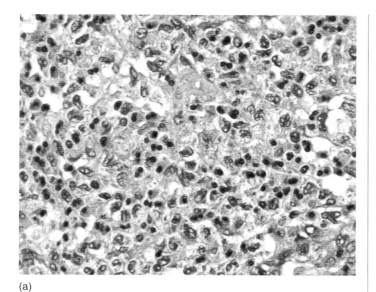

(a)

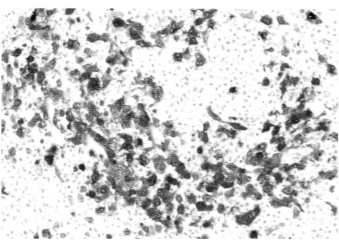

(b)

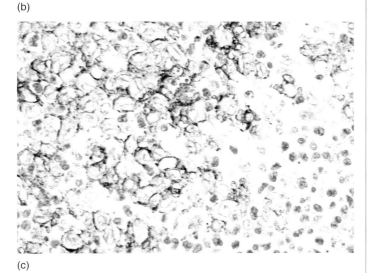

(c)

Figure 6.1.38 Langerhans cell histiocytosis. (a) The Langerhans cells have vesicular nuclei and a moderate amount of pale cytoplasm that is devoid of phagocytosed material. Numerous eosinophils are also present. Staining for S-100 (b) and CD1a (c) highlight the Langerhans cells.

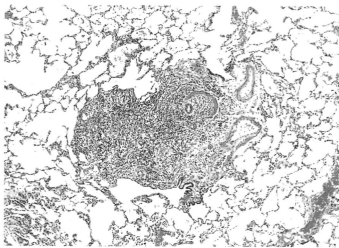

Figure 6.1.39 Langerhans cell histiocytosis. The lesions are focal, peribronchiolar and interstitial.

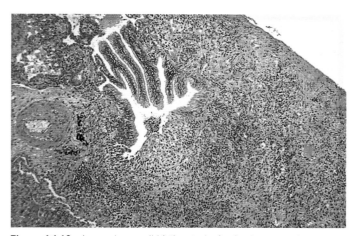

Figure 6.1.40 Langerhans cell histiocytosis. A mixed mononuclear interstitial infiltrate has destroyed part of the bronchiolar wall. (Reproduced from Corrin and Basset.[193])

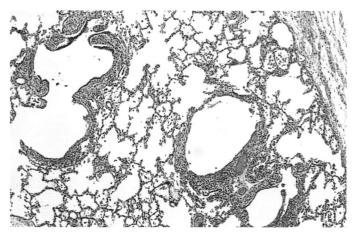

Figure 6.1.41 Langerhans cell histiocytosis showing microcystic change.

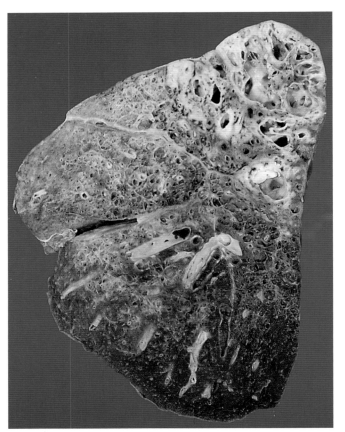

Figure 6.1.42 Langerhans cell histiocytosis of the lung at autopsy. Severe fibrocystic change is seen at the apex of the upper lobe.

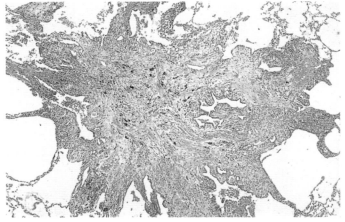

Figure 6.1.43 Pulmonary Langerhans cell histiocytosis. Older lesions often have a characteristically stellate outline.

been exposed, and partly endogenous, this component generally being weakly Perls and periodic acid-Schiff positive and diastase-resistant. Old and active lesions are often found in the same specimen. At autopsy, interstitial fibrosis is widespread and there may be marked 'honeycombing': nevertheless, the predilection for the mid- and upper-zones with sparing of the

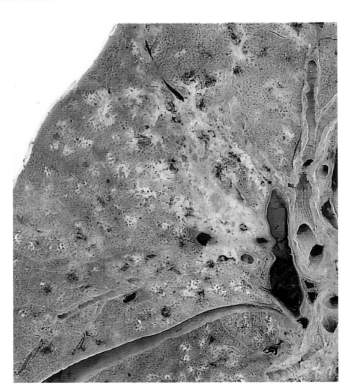

Figure 6.1.44 Pulmonary Langerhans cell histiocytosis. Small stellate scars on the cut surface represent healed lesions.

costophrenic angles, evident in life radiographically, is often still apparent after death (Fig. 6.1.42). The fibrosis may be attributable to fibroblast-stimulating cytokines such as platelet derived growth factor, transforming growth factor-β, tumour necrosis factor-α and interleukin-1[54,226,227] and the cavitation to collagenolytic activity mediated by matrix metalloproteinases,[228,229] all of which have been demonstrated in Langerhans cells within active lesions.

Differential diagnosis

Differential pathological diagnoses include eosinophilic pneumonia (see p. 461), reactive eosinophilic pleuritis (see p. 695) and various patterns of idiopathic interstitial pneumonia. The interstitial rather than intraluminal location of the eosinophils should indicate Langerhans cell histiocytosis (eosinophilic granuloma) rather than eosinophilic pneumonia, whereas an associated blood eosinophilia would favour the latter condition. HRCT patterns for these two disorders are also notably different. Reactive eosinophilic pleuritis is caused by pneumothorax and is limited to the pleura and subpleural lung tissue. Idiopathic pulmonary fibrosis/usual interstitial pneumonia and fibrotic non-specific interstitial pneumonia lack the focal centriacinar distribution of the lesions of eosinophilic granuloma. When Langerhans cell histiocytosis is completely inactive and the lung has reached an end stage of widespread 'honeycombing' common to many diseases, a definite histological diagno-

Table 6.1.6 A comparison of pulmonary lymphangioleiomyomatosis and tuberous sclerosis

	Tuberous sclerosis	Pulmonary lymphangioleiomyomatosis
Family history	Common	Absent
Sex incidence	Equal[b]	Exclusively female
Cerebral 'gliomas'[a]	Present[b]	Absent
Facial angiofibromas[a]	Frequent	Absent
Cardiac rhabdomyomas	Occasional	Absent
Angiomyolipomas	Frequent	Frequent (47–57%[249,250])
Lymph node angioleiomyomatosis	Occasional	Occasional
Pulmonary lymphangioleiomyomatosis	Occasional[b]	Present
Multifocal type II cell hyperplasia	Occasional	Absent

[a]Features regarded as diagnostic of tuberous sclerosis.
[b]If attention is concentrated on those cases of tuberous sclerosis with pulmonary involvement, neurological disorders are rare and the sex incidence is overwhelmingly female. Clinically evident pulmonary lymphangioleiomyomatosis is found in 2.3% of patients with tuberous sclerosis[251] but may be detected by computed tomography in 34–39% of women with tuberous sclerosis who are devoid of respiratory symptoms.[252,253] It accounts for 10% of deaths[245] in tuberous sclerosis.

sis may no longer be possible but the focal distribution and stellate outline of the scars are very suggestive of burnt-out Langerhans cell histiocytosis.

The immunocytochemical demonstration of CD1a, S100 protein or fascin may be used to augment routine light microscopy[210–212] but positive results are only of significance in the right pathological setting (Fig. 6.1.38). Langerhans cells and the related S100-positive interdigitating dendritic cells are widely distributed and increased in a variety of reactive and neoplastic diseases:[202,230] CD1a and fascin are more specific than S-100 and can be detected in paraffin sections.[210–212]

The diagnosis has been made on transbronchial biopsy but surgical lung biopsy is generally required for a definite tissue diagnosis. Histological diagnosis is most difficult in the healing phase when Langerhans cells are poorly represented. At this stage immunocytochemistry is least helpful. The optimal applications of immunocytochemistry are probably in the examination of small fibreoptic specimens, in which the valuable architectural features evident in a surgical lung biopsy cannot be assessed, and in the evaluation of bronchoalveolar lavage cells.[231,232] Electron microscopy may also be used to identify Langerhans cells in lavage specimens but immunocytochemistry is more suited to the enumeration of lavage cells that is necessary for diagnosis. Patients with pulmonary Langerhans cell histiocytosis have an increased but variable number of Langerhans cells in their lavage fluid (1 to 25%) compared with normal non-smokers (fewer than 1%) and to normal smokers and patients with other interstitial lung diseases (up to 3%) (see Table A4, p. 742).[231,232]

LYMPHANGIOLEIOMYOMATOSIS

Lymphangioleiomyomatosis is a rare but distinctive disease that in its fully developed state combines widespread proliferation of unusual smooth muscle in the lungs with lymphangioleiomyomas in thoracoabdominal lymph nodes.[233] However, either the lungs or the lymph nodes may be affected in isola-

tion. Lymphangioleiomyomatosis may occur sporadically or as a manifestation of the hereditary disease tuberous sclerosis. A notable feature is that it is largely confined to women in the reproductive years. Onset is not recorded before the menarche and is rare after the menopause.[234,235] Until 2000, it could be safely affirmed that the disease was exclusively confined to women but in that year the first case involving a man was reported.[236] A further male patient was reported in 2003.[237] We are also aware of lymphangioleiomyomatosis developing in a patient with the XXY chromosomal abnormality of Klinefelter's syndrome.

Aetiology

The fact that lymphangioleiomyomatosis is largely confined to women in the reproductive years suggests that it has a hormonal basis and this is supported by reports of exacerbations of the disease during pregnancy[238,239] and the menses,[240] and following oestrogen therapy.[241,242] Oestrogen or progesterone receptors have been identified in the diseased lung tissue.[243] Many women in the reproductive age group take oral contraceptives but a UK national case control study found no evidence that these caused the disease. In the same study, no differences were identified between the patients and their age and sex matched controls in regard to age of menarche, menstrual history, smoking, or the presence of uterine leiomyomas, but the patients had experienced fewer pregnancies.[244]

Lymphangioleiomyomatosis has an intriguing relationship to tuberous sclerosis (see also p. 488). The pulmonary changes are identical[233,245,246] and renal angiomyolipomas (one of the extracerebral features of tuberous sclerosis) are found in 60% of patients with lymphangioleiomyomatosis.[247] Not surprisingly therefore, it has been suggested that lymphangioleiomyomatosis is a *forme fruste* of tuberous sclerosis,[248] but there are notable differences in the natural history of these two conditions (Table 6.1.6).[245,249–253] Whereas lymphangioleiomyomatosis is almost exclusively confined to women, tuberous sclerosis affects both sexes, and whereas tuberous sclerosis is an autosomal dominant condition showing a familial tendency, no such hereditary pattern is evident in pulmonary lymphangioleiomyomatosis. Nevertheless, in tuberous sclerosis the pulmonary lesions are largely limited to adult females who have only minor cerebral disease.[254] Furthermore, the genes responsible for tuberous sclerosis (TSC1 and 2, located on chromosomes 9 and 16, respectively[255–257]) show high penetrance but variable expression so that it is difficult to identify all affected family members. Also, about 60% of tuberous sclerosis patients appear to have developed their disease because of spontaneous mutation.[258]

Molecular studies have identified mutation of the TSC2 gene in the pulmonary lesions of lymphangioleiomyomatosis.[259–261] However, there is as yet no record of a woman suffering from sporadic pulmonary lymphangioleiomyomatosis giving birth to a child with the stigmata of tuberous sclerosis, suggesting that in these patients the mutation is confined to certain somatic cells. The cells concerned are unusual in that they show features of both smooth muscle and melanocytes, with some of them at least carrying oestrogen or progesterone receptors. The TSC2 gene product, tuberin, acts as a tumour suppressor and it is therefore not surprising that TSC2 mutation is associated with cellular proliferation.

The demonstration of identical TSC2 mutations in the pulmonary and renal lesions of a patient with sporadic lymphangioleiomyomatosis indicated that their constituent cells were derived from the same source and led to the suggestion that those comprising the pulmonary lesions had metastasised from the renal angiomyolipoma.[259] Metastatic spread also appears to be the explanation for recurrent lymphangioleiomyomatosis in some cases in which identical mutations were identified in the native and donor lungs;[262,263] metastasis from lung to lung was suggested in one case as renal angiomyolipoma was excluded at autopsy.[263] However, in another case, sex chromosomal analysis showed that the recurrent smooth muscle proliferation was of donor origin.[264]

Clinical features

Patients with pulmonary lymphangioleiomyomatosis present at an average age of 32–34 years.[235,265–268] They complain of breathlessness of insidious onset and are liable to develop any of three complications: repeated pneumothoraces, chylous effusions and pulmonary haemorrhage, all of which are satisfactorily explained by the pathological features of the disease, as outlined below.[233] The functional features are variable and may indicate obstructive, restrictive or mixed disease, generally with markedly reduced diffusing capacity, and a normal or mildly increased total lung capacity.[247,267,269–272] Bronchoalveolar lavage typically recovers haemosiderin-laden macrophages. Radiographically, the lungs show a reticular pattern but unlike fibrotic lungs they appear enlarged and ultimately show gross cystic change.[270] Septal lines (Kerley B) may be seen as a result of the lymphatic obstruction. The appearance on computed tomography is virtually diagnostic in the appropriate clinical context.[247,273] Thin-walled cysts with well-defined walls and of

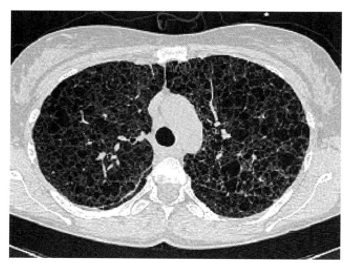

Figure 6.1.45 Pulmonary lymphangioleiomyomatosis. HRCT shows thin-walled cystic spaces with no zonal distribution and no accompanying nodules.

fairly uniform size are evenly distributed throughout all lung zones (Fig. 6.1.45).

Course of the disease and prognosis

The natural course of the disease is one of inexorable decline in respiratory function over a period of several years, inevitably culminating in death except in patients who reach the menopause, when the clinical state stabilizes.[233,265,274] However, survival figures have progressively improved, probably due to a combination of improved patient management and early radiographic identification of the disease in asymptomatic women. Thus, 10-year survival figures of 20% were reported in 1975, 40% in 1995 and 79% in 1999.[233,239,275] Severe cystic change indicates advanced disease and a correspondingly worse prognosis.[275] Conversely, those patients in whom the lungs are spared and only extrapulmonary lymphatics are affected have a relatively good prognosis.[274,276]

Pathological findings

The essential pathological feature is a proliferation of unusual smooth muscle cells that involves all parts of the lungs,[233,269,270] often in a focal manner. The smooth muscle nature of the cells may not be immediately apparent and they may be mistaken for fibroblasts. They are generally plump and spindle-shaped with pale eosinophilic cytoplasm (Fig. 6.1.46) but the cytoplasm may be clear and the cells polygonal in outline so that they appear epithelioid. Electron microscopy shows them to have all the features of smooth muscle.[277] Immunostaining is in accord with this, both cell types being strongly positive for smooth muscle actin.[278] However, an unusual feature is that 17–67%

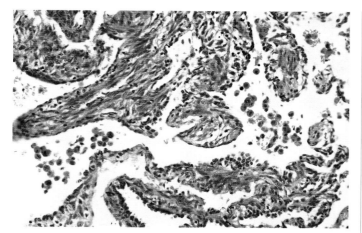

Figure 6.1.46 Pulmonary lymphangioleiomyomatosis. Spindle cells infiltrate the alveolar walls.

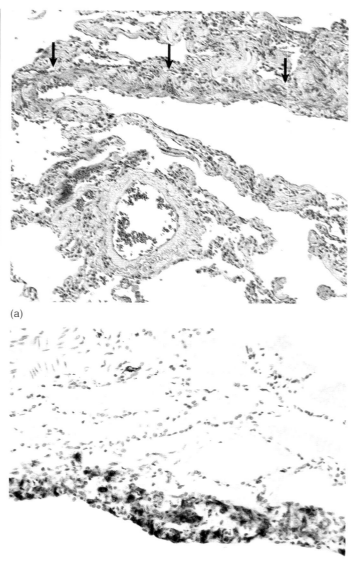

(a)

(b)

Figure 6.1.47 Pulmonary lymphangioleiomyomatosis. (a) Spindle cells evident in the walls of cystic spaces (arrows) stain for HMB-45 (b). (Case of Dr D Snead, Coventry, UK.)

of the proliferating cells react for the melanoma-related marker human melanin black-45 (HMB-45) (Fig. 6.1.47).[247,279–283] Electron microscopy shows the HMB-45 immunoreactivity to be localised to cytoplasmic inclusions similar to premelanosomes.[279] HMB-45 reactivity is a feature that lymphangioleiomyomatosis shares with the angiomyolipomas of tuberous sclerosis and benign clear cell tumour of the lung (see p. 613). The term perivascular epithelioid cell has been applied to the essential constituent of lymphangioleiomyoma, angiomyolipoma and benign clear cell tumour; it is described as a mesenchymal cell that is either spindle-shaped or has a plump, glycogen-rich epithelioid phenotype, and co-expresses actin and HMB-45.[246,284,285] It is reported that HMB-45 and the receptors for oestrogen and progesterone are confined to the plump epithelioid cells whereas metalloproteases and proliferating-cell nuclear antigen are confined to the spindle cells[246,279,286,287] but this is not invariably the case.

The alveolar walls are infiltrated by the unusual smooth muscle cells and consequently thickened, sometimes in nodular fashion. The walls of bronchioles are similarly affected, with consequent air trapping.[233] The interstitial connective tissue is structurally abnormal,[277,288] probably due to the protease activity exhibited by the spindle cells.[287,289] Coupled with valvular bronchiolar obstruction, this leads to focal cystic change, which ultimately culminates in gross 'honeycombing' throughout the lungs (Fig. 6.1.48). It has been shown that airway collapse consequent upon the cystic change is the principal mechanism contributing to airflow limitation.[290] Rupture of the cysts explains the frequent pneumothoraces which are one of the distinctive complications of this disease. A histological score based on the severity of the cystic change and the degree of smooth muscle infiltration has been shown to be of prognostic value.[291]

The proliferating cells also infiltrate blood vessels and the use of elastic stains demonstrates that small veins are often totally obliterated (Fig. 6.1.49).[233] This veno-occlusive process causes pulmonary haemorrhage, so explaining the haemoptyses that complicate the breathlessness. It also causes haemosiderosis (Fig. 6.1.50) and occasionally this is sufficiently severe to encrust the elastic laminae of pulmonary blood vessels with iron and calcium. Fragmentation of the encrusted elastin elicits a foreign body giant cell reaction, as in pulmonary veno-occlusive disease (see pp. 427, 450).

Involvement of lymphatics in the myoproliferative process and the development of lymphangioleiomyomas in mediastinal lymph nodes explain the frequent chylothoraces.[233,292]

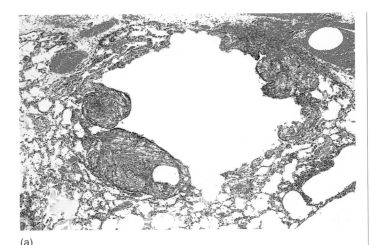

(a)

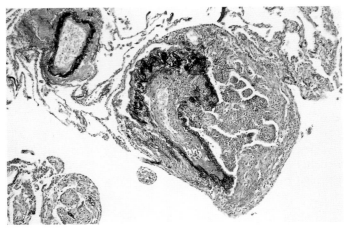

Figure 6.1.49 Pulmonary lymphangioleiomyomatosis. Elastin staining reveals that small post-capillary blood vessels are infiltrated and their lumen markedly narrowed.

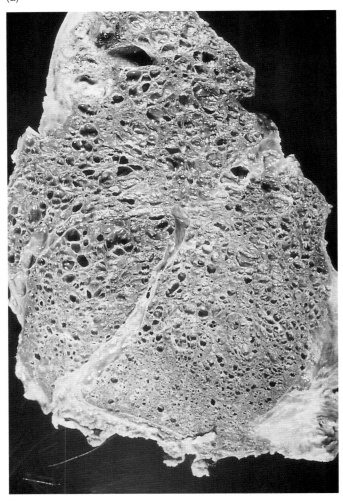

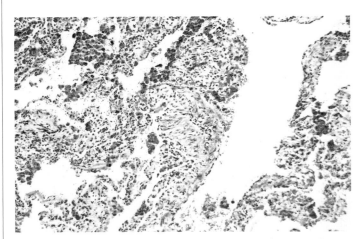

Figure 6.1.50 Pulmonary lymphangioleiomyomatosis. Occlusion of post-capillary blood vessels results in capillary rupture and haemosiderosis.

(b)

Figure 6.1.48 Pulmonary lymphangioleiomyomatosis. Infiltration of the alveolar walls weakens them, causing focal cystic change (a) and ultimately (b) gross honeycombing (b; Reproduced by courtesy of the late Dr AA Liebow, San Diego, USA.)

Chyloptysis, chylous ascites and even chyluria may also develop.[240] It is largely because the disease involves extrapulmonary lymphatics that the excess smooth muscle in the lung is believed to be derived from pulmonary lymphatics. Only in early cases can a close relationship to pulmonary lymphatics be appreciated.[246]

Occasionally, pulmonary lymphangioleiomyomatosis is associated with micronodular type II pneumocyte hyperplasia (see p. 689) but this is to be regarded as an independent manifestation of tuberous sclerosis rather than a component of lymphangioleiomyomatosis.

Differential diagnosis

One of the conditions that histologically enters the differential diagnosis is idiopathic pulmonary fibrosis showing reactive hyperplasia of bronchiolar and vascular smooth muscle (so-called 'muscular cirrhosis of the lung'). However, the reactive smooth muscle hyperplasia that accompanies fibrosis is quite mature and readily recognisable as smooth muscle, whereas this is not the case in lymphangioleiomyomatosis. Idiopathic pulmonary fibrosis also has an inflammatory component, which is not seen in lymphangioleiomyomatosis. If doubt remains, HRCT will probably establish the diagnosis. Indeed, few cases now come to biopsy because of the high specificity of the imaging features, those that do often being smokers with a differential diagnosis of emphysema, which may co-exist with lymphangioleiomyomatosis.

A further condition to be distinguished is that of so-called benign metastasising leiomyomas (see p. 676).[293,294] This also affects women in the reproductive years and both conditions are to some extent hormonally dependent. However, the metastasising leiomyomas form distinct tumours: sharply outlined spherical masses that usually exceed two centimetres in diameter. Histologically, they exactly reproduce the appearances of benign myometrial fibroids, containing smooth muscle that is readily recognisable as such, unlike the immature cells of lymphangioleiomyomatosis. Leiomyomas are also HMB-45-negative and the patients either have uterine fibroids or have had them removed. Although immature, lymphangioleiomyomatosis cells lack the atypia of a sarcoma, which was the diagnosis in what was probably the first report of the condition.[295] Lymphangiomatosis (see p. 621) is distinguished from lymphangioleiomyomatosis by being evidently vascular and lacking the distinctive HMB-45-positive cells. Emphysema also lacks these cells, as do the metastases of endometrial stromal sarcoma,[296,297] two further conditions that have been mistaken for lymphangioleiomyomatosis.

Treatment

Because the disease is largely confined to women in the reproductive years attempts have been made to arrest the condition[266] by oophorectomy, ovarian ablation with X-rays and hormonal manipulation.[298–303] Response has been varied and sometimes unrelated to sex steroid receptor analysis.[304] The oestrogen antagonist, tamoxifen, has often been employed but is probably best avoided as it may have agonist activity. After an analysis of 30 previously reported patients treated with eight different regimens, a combination of oophorectomy and progesterone was recommended.[305] A retrospective review of 32 patients noted progression despite oophorectomy but a more favourable course with progesterone, and recommended that all asymptomatic patients with lymphangioleiomyomatosis should receive at least a 1-year trial of medroxyprogesterone acetate (at a dose of 400–800 mg intramuscularly per month).[265] In this series, the overall prognosis was much better than in earlier publications, with 25 of 32 (78%) patients still living 8 years after the onset of disease, whereas previous investigators found that most patients died within 4 years[274] or within 10 years.[233] In a comparison of untreated patients and others treated with tamoxifen and progesterone, oestrogen and progesterone receptors could

only be demonstrated on the lymphangioleiomyomatosis cells in the untreated group, suggesting that the treatment had suppressed the receptors.[287] If hormonal therapy is unsuccessful, lung transplantation offers an alternative treatment. It has been successfully performed in several patients[306] but recurrence in the allograft has been encountered, even with lungs obtained from male donors.[307,308]

Concern that children born to affected patients may suffer from tuberous sclerosis appears to be unwarranted and genetic counselling is not currently considered necessary, although pregnancy itself may be inadvisable because of reports of the lung disease being exacerbated during childbearing. An informative patient support group may be consulted at http://lam.uc.

REFERENCES

Usual interstitial pneumonia

1. American Thoracic Society/European Respiratory Society. Idiopathic pulmonary fibrosis: diagnosis and treatment. International consensus statement. Am J Respir Crit Care Med 2000; 161:646–664.
2. American Thoracic Society/European Respiratory Society. International multidisciplinary consensus classification of the idiopathic interstitial pneumonias. Am J Respir Crit Care Med 2002; 165:277–304.
3. Flaherty KR, Travis WD, Colby TV, et al. Histopathologic variability in usual and nonspecific interstitial pneumonias. Am J Respir Crit Care Med 2001; 164:1722–1727.
4. Nicholson AG, Colby TV, Dubois RM, Hansell DM, Wells AU. The prognostic significance of the histologic pattern of interstitial pneumonia in patients presenting with the clinical entity of cryptogenic fibrosing alveolitis. Am J Respir Crit Care Med 2000; 162:2213–2217.
5. Katzenstein ALA, Zisman DA, Litzky LA, Nguyen BT, Kotloff RM. Usual interstitial pneumonia – Histologic study of biopsy and explant specimens. Am J Surg Pathol 2002; 26:1567–1577.
6. Monaghan H, Wells AU, Colby TV, et al. Prognostic implications of histologic patterns in multiple surgical lung biopsies from patients with idiopathic interstitial pneumonias. Chest 2004; 125:522–526.
7. Bjoraker JA, Ryu JH, Edwin MK, et al. Prognostic significance of histopathologic subsets in idiopathic pulmonary fibrosis. Am J Respir Crit Care Med 1998; 157:199–203.
8. Travis WD, Matsui K, Moss J, Ferrans VJ. Idiopathic nonspecific interstitial pneumonia: Prognostic significance of cellular and fibrosing patterns. Survival comparison with usual interstitial pneumonia and desquamative interstitial pneumonia. Am J Surg Pathol 2000; 24:19–33.
9. Hartman TE, Primack SL, Kang EY, et al. Disease progression in usual interstitial pneumonia compared with desquamative interstitial pneumonia: assessment with serial CT. Chest 1996; 110:378–382.
10. Akira M, Yamamoto S, Hara H, Sakatani M, Ueda E. Serial computed tomographic evaluation in desquamative interstitial pneumonia. Thorax 1997; 52:333–337.
11. Johnston IDA, Prescott RJ, Chalmers JC, Rudd RM. British Thoracic Society study of cryptogenic fibrosing alveolitis: current presentation and initial management. Thorax 1997; 52:38–44.
12. Carrington CB, Gaensler EA, Coutu RE, FitzGerald MX, Gupta RG. Natural history and treated course of usual and desquamative interstitial pneumonia. N Engl J Med 1978; 298:801–809.
13. Turner-Warwick M, Burrows B, Johnson A. Cryptogenic fibrosing alveolitis: clinical features and their influence on survival. Thorax 1980; 35:171–180.
14. Hubbard R, Johnston I, Coultas DB, Britton J. Mortality rates from cryptogenic fibrosing alveolitis in seven countries. Thorax 1996; 51:711–716.

15. Marshall RP, Puddicombe A, Cookson WOC, Laurent GJ. Adult familial cryptogenic fibrosing alveolitis in the United Kingdom. Thorax 2000; 55:143–146.

16. Flaherty KR, Thwaite EL, Kazerooni EA, et al. Radiological versus histological diagnosis in UIP and NSIP: survival implications. Thorax 2003; 58:143–148.

17. King TE, Tooze JA, Schwarz MI, Brown KR, Cherniack RM. Predicting survival in idiopathic pulmonary fibrosis: Scoring system and survival model. Am J Respir Crit Care Med 2001; 164:1171–1181.

18. Rice AJ, Wells AU, Bouros D, et al. Terminal diffuse alveolar damage in relation to interstitial pneumonias. An autopsy study. Am J Clin Pathol 2003; 119:709–714.

19. Akira M. Computed tomography and pathologic findings in fulminant forms of idiopathic interstitial pneumonia. J Thorac Imaging 1999; 14:76–84.

20. Ambrosini V, Cancellieri A, Chilosi M, et al. Acute exacerbation of idiopathic pulmonary fibrosis: report of a series. Eur Resp J 2003; 22:821–826.

21. Honore I, Nunes H, Groussard O, et al. Acute respiratory failure after interferon-gamma therapy of end-stage pulmonary fibrosis. Am J Respir Crit Care Med 2003; 167:953–957.

22. Selman M, Thannickal VJ, Pardo A, et al. Idiopathic pulmonary fibrosis: pathogenesis and therapeutic approaches. Drugs 2004; 64:405–430.

22a. Bajwa EK, Ayas NT, Schulzer M, et al. Interferon-γ1b therapy in idiopathic pulmonary fibrosis. Chest 2005; 128:203–206.

23. Nicholson AG, Fulford LG, Colby TV, et al. The relationship between individual histologic features and disease progression in idiopathic pulmonary fibrosis. Am J Respir Crit Care Med 2002; 166:173–177.

24. Katzenstein ALA, Myers JL. Idiopathic pulmonary fibrosis: Clinical relevance of pathologic classification. Am J Respir Crit Care Med 1998; 157:1301–1315.

25. Yousem SA. Eosinophilic pneumonia-like areas in idiopathic usual interstitial pneumonia. Mod Pathol 2000; 13:1280–1284.

25a. Warnock ML, Press M, Churg A. Further observations on cytoplasmic hyaline in the lung. Hum Pathol 1980; 11:59–65.

26. Coalson JJ. The ultrastructure of human fibrosing alveolitis. Virchows Arch A Pathol Anat Histopathol 1982; 395:181–199.

27. Corrin B, Dewar A, Rodriguez-Roisin R, Turner-Warwick M. Fine structural changes in cryptogenic fibrosing alveolitis and asbestosis. J Pathol 1985; 147:107–119.

28. Katzenstein A-LA. Pathogenesis of 'fibrosis' in interstitial pneumonia: an electron microscopic study. Hum Pathol 1985; 16:1015–1024.

29. Scadding JG, Hinson KFW. Diffuse fibrosing alveolitis (diffuse interstitial fibrosis of the lungs): correlation of histology at biopsy with prognosis. Thorax 1967; 22:291–304.

30. Stack BHR, Choo-Kang YFJ, Heard BE. The prognosis of cryptogenic fibrosing alveolitis. Thorax 1972; 27:535–542.

31. Nicholson AG, Addis BJ, Bharucha H, et al. Inter-observer variation between pathologists in diffuse parenchymal lung disease. Thorax 2004; 59:500–505.

32. Coleman A, Colby TV. Histologic diagnosis of extrinsic allergic alveolitis. Am J Surg Pathol 1988; 12:514–518.

33. Scadding JG. Fibrosing alveolitis. BMJ 1964; 2:686.

34. Turner-Warwick M, Doniach D. Auto-antibody studies in interstitial pulmonary fibrosis. BMJ 1965; 1:886–891.

35. Wallace WAH, Roberts SN, Caldwell H, et al. Circulating antibodies to lung protein(s) in patients with cryptogenic fibrosing alveolitis. Thorax 1994; 49:218–224.

36. Wallace WAH, Schofield JA, Lamb D, Howie SEM. Localisation of a pulmonary autoantigen in cryptogenic fibrosing alveolitis. Thorax 1994; 49:1139–1145.

37. Haslam PL, Thompson B, Mohammed I, et al. Circulating immune complexes in patients with cryptogenic fibrosing alveolitis. Clin Exp Immunol 1979; 37:381–390.

38. Schwarz MI, Dreisin RB, Pratt DS, Stanford RE. Immunofluorescent patterns in the idiopathic interstitial pneumonias. J Lab Clin Med 1978; 91:929–938.

39. Fox B, Shousha S, James KR, Miller GC. Immunohistological study of human lungs by immunoperoxidase technique. J Clin Pathol 1982; 35:144–150.

40. Hubbard R, Lewis S, Richards K, Johnston I, Britton J. Occupational exposure to metal or wood dust and aetiology of cryptogenic fibrosing alveolitis. Lancet 1996; 347:284–289.

41. Hubbard R. Occupational dust exposure and the aetiology of cryptogenic fibrosing alveolitis. Eur Resp J 2001; 32:119S–121S.

42. Tobin RW, Pope CE, Pellegrini CA, et al. Increased prevalence of gastroesophageal reflux in patients with idiopathic pulmonary fibrosis. Am J Respir Crit Care Med 1998; 158:1804–1808.

43. Meliconi R, Andreone P, Fasano L, et al. Incidence of hepatitis C virus infection in Italian patients with idiopathic pulmonary fibrosis. Thorax 1996; 51:315–317.

44. Kuwano K, Nomoto Y, Kunitake R, et al. Detection of adenovirus E1A DNA in pulmonary fibrosis using nested polymerase chain reaction. Eur Resp J 1997; 10:1445–1449.

45. Yonemaru M, Kasuga I, Kusumoto H, et al. Elevation of antibodies to cytomegalovirus and other herpes viruses in pulmonary fibrosis. Eur Resp J 1997; 10:2040–2045.

46. Tsukamoto K, Hayakawa H, Sato A, et al. Involvement of Epstein–Barr virus latent membrane protein 1 in disease progression in patients with idiopathic pulmonary fibrosis. Thorax 2000; 55:958–961.

47. Bando M, Ohno S, Oshikawa K, et al. Infection of TT virus in patients with idiopathic pulmonary fibrosis. Resp Med 2001; 95:935–942.

48. Kelly BG, Lok SS, Hasleton PS, Egan JJ, Stewart JP. A rearranged form of Epstein-Barr virus DNA is associated with idiopathic pulmonary fibrosis. Am J Respir Crit Care Med 2002; 166:510–513.

49. Hubbard R, Venn A, Smith C, et al. Exposure to commonly prescribed drugs and the etiology of cryptogenic fibrosing alveolitis: A case-control study. Am J Respir Crit Care Med 1998; 157:743–747.

50. Britton J, Hubbard R. Recent advances in the aetiology of cryptogenic fibrosing alveolitis. Histopathology 2000; 37:387–392.

51. Musk AW, Zilko PJ, Manners P, Kay PH, Kamboh MI. Genetic studies in familial fibrosing alveolitis. Possible linkage with immunoglobulin allotypes (Gm). Chest 1986; 89:206–210.

52. Geddes DM, Webley M, Brewerton DA, et al. alpha 1-antitrypsin phenotypes in fibrosing alveolitis and rheumatoid arthritis. Lancet 1977; 2:1049–1051.

53. Lane KB, Marney A, Phillips JA, et al. Familial interstitial pulmonary fibrosis and linkage to chromosome 14. Chest 2001; 120:75S–76S.

54. Corrin B, Butcher D, McAnulty BJ, et al. Immunohistochemical localization of transforming growth factor- beta^1 in the lungs of patients with systemic sclerosis, cryptogenic fibrosing alveolitis and other lung disorders. Histopathology 1994; 24:145–150.

55. Wallace WAH, Howie SEM. Upregulation of tenascin and TGF beta production in a type II alveolar epithelial cell line by antibody against a pulmonary auto-antigen. J Pathol 2001; 195:251–256.

56. Bergeron A, Soler P, Kambouchner M, et al. Cytokine profiles in idiopathic pulmonary fibrosis suggest an important role for TGF-beta and IL-10. Eur Resp J 2003; 22:69–76.

57. Giaid A, Michel RP, Stewart DJ, et al. Expression of endothelin-1 in lungs of patients with cryptogenic fibrosing alveolitis. Lancet 1993; 341:1550–1554.

58. Nash JRG, McLaughlin PJ, Butcher D, Corrin B. Expression of tumour necrosis factor-alpha in cryptogenic fibrosing alveolitis. Histopathology 1993; 22:343–347.

59. Uh ST, Inoue Y, King TE, et al. Morphometric analysis of insulin-like growth factor-I localization in lung tissues of patients with idiopathic pulmonary fibrosis. Am J Respir Crit Care Med 1998; 158:1626–1635.

60. Pan LH, Yamauchi K, Uzuki M, et al. Type II alveolar epithelial cells and interstitial fibroblasts express connective tissue growth factor in IPF. Eur Resp J 2001; 17:1220–1227.

61. Fukuda Y, Ishizaki M, Kudoh S, Kitaichi M, Yamanaka N. Localization of matrix metalloproteinases-1, -2, and -9 and tissue inhibitor of metalloproteinase-2 in interstitial lung diseases. Lab Invest 1998; 78:687–698.

62. Thannickal VJ, Toews GB, White ES, Lynch JP. III, Martinez FJ. Mechanisms of pulmonary fibrosis. Annu Rev Med 2004; 55:395–417.

63. Burkhardt A. Alveolitis and collapse in the pathogenesis of pulmonary fibrosis. Am Rev Respir Dis 1989; 140:513–524.

64. Basset F, Ferrans VJ, Soler P, et al. Intraluminal fibrosis in interstitial lung disorders. Am J Pathol 1986; 122:443–461.

65. Kondo A, Saiki S. Acute exacerbation in idiopathic interstitial pneumonia. In: Harasawa M, Fukuchi Y, Morinari H, eds. Interstitial Pneumonia of Unknown Etiology. Tokyo: University of Tokyo Press; 1989:33–42.

66. Shimabukuro DW, Sawa T, Gropper MA. Injury and repair in lung and airways. Crit Care Med 2003; 31:S524–31.

67. Fukuda Y, Basset F, Ferrans VJ, Yamanaka N. Significance of early intra-alveolar fibrotic lesions and integrin expression in lung biopsy specimens from patients with idiopathic pulmonary fibrosis. Hum Pathol 1995; 26:53–61.

68. King TE, Schwarz MI, Brown K, et al. Idiopathic pulmonary fibrosis. Relationship between histopathologic features and mortality. Am J Respir Crit Care Med 2001; 164:1025–1032.

69. Brody AR, Craighead JE. Interstitial associations of cells lining air spaces in human pulmonary fibrosis. Virchows Arch A Pathol Anat Histopathol 1976; 372:39–49.

70. Adamson IYR, Hedgecock C, Bowden DH. Epithelial cell-fibroblast interactions in lung injury and repair. Am J Pathol 1990; 137:385–392.

71. Mastruzzo C, Crimi N, Vancheri C. Role of oxidative stress in pulmonary fibrosis. Monaldi Arch Chest Dis 2002; 57:173–176.

72. Kradin RL, Divertie MB, Colvin RB, et al. Usual interstitial pneumonitis is a T cell alveolitis. Clin Immunol Immunopathol 1986; 40:224–235.

73. Wells AU, Lorimer S, Majumdar S, et al. Fibrosing alveolitis in systemic sclerosis: increase in memory T-cells in lung interstitium. Eur Respir J 1995; 8:266–271.

74. Kallenberg CGM, Schilizzi BM, Beaumont F, Leij L De, Poppema S. The TH. Expression of class II major histocompatibility complex antigens on alveolar epithelium in interstitial lung disease: relevance to pathogenesis of idiopathic pulmonary fibrosis. J Clin Pathol 1987; 40:725–733.

75. Komatsu T, Yamamoto M, Shimokata K, Nagura H. Phenotypic characterization of alveolar capillary endothelial cells, alveolar epithelial cells and alveolar macrophages in patients with pulmonary fibrosis with special reference to MHC class II antigens. Virchows Arch A Pathol Anat Histopathol 1989; 415:79–90.

76. Jakubzick C, Choi ES, Kunkel SL, et al. Augmented pulmonary IL-4 and IL-13 receptor subunit expression in idiopathic interstitial pneumonia. J Clin Pathol 2004; 57:477–486.

77. Obayashi Y, Yamadori I, Fujita J, et al. The role of neutrophils in the pathogenesis of idiopathic pulmonary fibrosis. Chest 1997; 112:1338–1343.

78. Martin WJ. Neutrophils kill pulmonary endothelial cells by a hydrogen-peroxide-dependent pathway. An in vitro model of neutrophil-mediated lung injury. Am Rev Respir Dis 1984; 130:209–213.

79. Ayars GH, Altman LC, Rosen H, Doyle T. The injurious effect of neutrophils on pneumocytes in vitro. Am Rev Respir Dis 1984; 130:964–973.

80. Donaldson K, Slight J, Brown GM, Bolton RE. The ability of inflammatory bronchoalveolar leucocyte populations elicited with microbes or mineral dust to injure alveolar epithelial cells and degrade extracellular matrix in vitro. Br J Exp Pathol 1988; 69:327–338.

81. Chanez P, Lacoste JY, Guillot B, et al. Mast cells' contribution to the fibrosing alveolitis of the scleroderma lung. Am Rev Respir Dis 1993; 147:1497–1502.

82. Hunt LW, Colby TV, Weiler DA, Sur S, Butterfield JH. Immunofluorescent staining for mast cells in idiopathic pulmonary fibrosis – quantification and evidence for extracellular release of mast cell tryptase. Mayo Clin Proc 1992; 67:941–948.

83. Heard BE, Dewar A, Corrin B. Apposition of fibroblasts to mast cells and lymphocytes in normal human lung and in cryptogenic fibrosing alveolitis – ultrastructure and cell perimeter measurements. J Pathol 1992; 166:303–310.

84. Inoue Y, King TE, Tinkle SS, Dockstader K, Newman LS. Human mast cell basic fibroblast growth factor in pulmonary fibrotic disorders. Am J Pathol 1996; 149:2037–2054.

85. Inoue Y, King TE, Barker E, Daniloff E, Newman LS. Basic fibroblast growth factor and its receptors in idiopathic pulmonary fibrosis and lymphangioleiomyomatosis. Am J Respir Crit Care Med 2002; 166:765–773.

85a. Garbuzenko E, Puxeddu I, Levi-Schaffer F, et al. Mast cells induce activation of human lung fibroblasts in vitro. Exp Lung Res 2004; 30:705–721.

86. Spencer H. Interstitial pneumonia. Ann Rev Med 1967; 18:423–442.

87. Magro CM, Allen J. PopeHarman A et al. The role of microvascular injury in the evolution of idiopathic pulmonary fibrosis. Am J Clin Pathol 2003; 119:556–567.

88. Renzoni EA. Neovascularization in idiopathic pulmonary fibrosis: too much or too little? Am J Respir Crit Care Med 2004; 169:1179–1180.

89. Hubbard R, Venn A, Lewis S, Britton J. Lung cancer and cryptogenic fibrosing alveolitis. A population-based cohort study. Am J Respir Crit Care Med 2000; 161:5–8.

90. Park J, Kim DS, Shim TS, et al. Lung cancer in patients with idiopathic pulmonary fibrosis. Eur Resp J 2001; 17:1216–1219.

91. Turner-Warwick M, Lebowitz M, Burrows B, Johnston A. Cryptogenic fibrosing alveolitis and lung cancer. Thorax 1980; 35:496–499.

92. Hojo S, Fujita J, Yamadori I, et al. Heterogeneous point mutations of the p53 gene in pulmonary fibrosis. Eur Resp J 1998; 12:1404–1408.

93. Kumar P, Goldstraw P, Yamada K, et al. Pulmonary fibrosis and lung cancer: risk and benefit analysis of pulmonary resection. J Thorac Cardiovasc Surg 2003; 125:1321–1327.

94. Nicholson AG, Wotherspoon AC, Jones AL, et al. Pulmonary B-cell non-Hodgkin's lymphoma associated with autoimmune disorders: a clinicopathological review of six cases. Eur Respir J 1996; 9:2022–2025.

Non-specific interstitial pneumonia

95. Ognibene FP, Masur H, Rogers P, et al. Nonspecific interstitial pneumonitis without evidence of pneumocystis carinii in asymptomatic patients infected with human immunodeficiency virus (HIV). Ann Intern Med 1988; 109:874–879.

96. Katzenstein ALA, Fiorelli RF. Nonspecific interstitial pneumonia/fibrosis – histologic features and clinical significance. Am J Surg Pathol 1994; 18:136–147.

97. Daniil ZD, Gilchrist FC, Nicholson AG, et al. A histologic pattern of nonspecific interstitial pneumonia is associated with a better prognosis than usual interstitial pneumonia in patients with cryptogenic fibrosing alveolitis. Am J Respir Crit Care Med 1999; 160:899–905.

98. Nagai S, Kitaichi M, Itoh H, et al. Idiopathic nonspecific interstitial pneumonia/fibrosis: comparison with idiopathic pulmonary fibrosis and BOOP. Eur Resp J 1998; 12:1010–1019.

99. Nicholson AG, Wells AU. Nonspecific interstitial pneumonia – Nobody said it's perfect. Am J Respir Crit Care Med 2001; 164:1553–1554.

100. Bouros D, Wells AU, Nicholson AG, et al. Histopathologic subsets of fibrosing alveolitis in patients with systemic sclerosis and their relationship to outcome. Am J Respir Crit Care Med 2002; 165:1581–1586.

101. Douglas WW, Tazelaar HD, Hartman TE, et al. Polymyositis-dermatomyositis-associated interstitial lung disease. Am J Respir Crit Care Med 2001; 164:1182–1185.

102. Craig PJ, Wells AU, Doffman S, et al. Desquamative interstitial pneumonia, respiratory bronchiolitis and their relationship to smoking. Histopathology 2004; 45:275–282.

103. Cottin V, Donsbeck AV, Revel D, Loire R, Cordier JF. Nonspecific interstitial pneumonia. Individualization of a clinicopathologic entity in a series of 12 patients. Am J Respir Crit Care Med 1998; 158:1286–1293.

104. Veeraraghavan S, Latsi PI, Wells AU, et al. BAL findings in idiopathic nonspecific interstitial pneumonia and usual interstitial pneumonia. Eur Resp J 2003; 22:239–244.

105. MacDonald SL, Rubens MB, Hansell DM, et al. Nonspecific interstitial pneumonia and usual interstitial pneumonia: comparative appearances at and diagnostic accuracy of thin-section CT. Radiology 2001; 221:600–605.

106. Akira M, Inoue G, Yamamoto S, Sakatani M. Non-specific interstitial pneumonia: findings on sequential CT scans of nine patients. Thorax 2000; 55:854–859.

Acute interstitial pneumonia

107. Katzenstein A-LA, Myers JL, Mazur MT. Acute interstitial pneumonia. A clinicopathologic, ultrastructural, and cell kinetic study. Am J Surg Pathol 1986; 10:256–267.
108. Hamman L, Rich AR. A clinico-pathological conference. Internat Clin 1933; 1:197.
109. Hamman L, Rich AR. Fulminating diffuse interstitial fibrosis of the lungs. Trans Am Clin Climatol Assn 1935; 51:154.
110. Hamman L, Rich AR. Acute diffuse interstitial fibrosis of the lungs. Bull Johns Hopkins Hosp 1944; 74:177–212.
111. Olson J, Colby TV, Elliott CG. Hamman-Rich syndrome revisited. Mayo Clin Proc 1990; 65:1538–1548.
112. Kondoh Y, Taniguchi H, Kawabata Y, et al. Acute exacerbation in idiopathic pulmonary fibrosis - analysis of clinical and pathologic findings in three cases. Chest 1993; 103:1808–1812.
113. Colby TV. Pathologic aspects of bronchiolitis obliterans organizing pneumonia. Chest 1992; 102:S38–S43.
114. Vourlekis JS, Brown KK, Cool CD, et al. Acute interstitial pneumonitis. Case series and review of the literature. Medicine (Baltimore) 2000; 79:369–378.

Extrinsic allergic alveolitis

115. Bourke SJ, Dalphin JC, Boyd G, McSharry C, Baldwin CI, Calvert JE. Hypersensitivity pneumonitis: current concepts. Eur Resp J 2001; 32:81S–92S.
116. Hapke EJ, Seal RME, Thomas GO, Hayes M, Meek JC. Farmer's lung. Thorax 1968; 23:451–468.
117. Hendrick DJ, Faux JA, Marshall R. Budgerigar-fancier's lung: the commonest variety of allergic alveolitis in Britain. BMJ 1978; 2:81–84.
118. Ando M, Arima K, Yoneda R, Tamura M. Japanese summer-type hypersensitivity pneumonitis – geographic distribution, home environment, and clinical characteristics of 621 cases. Am Rev Respir Dis 1991; 144:765–769.
119. Warren CPW. Extrinsic allergic alveolitis: a disease commoner in non-smokers. Thorax 1977; 32:567–569.
120. Godfrey RC, Evans CC. A national survey of bird fanciers' lung: including its possible association with jejunal villous atrophy. Br J Dis Chest 1984; 78:75–88.
121. Franquet T, Hansell DM, Senbanjo T, Remy-Jardin M, Muller NL. Lung cysts in subacute hypersensitivity pneumonitis. J Comput Assist Tomogr 2003; 27:475–478.
122. Seal RME, Hapke EJ, Thomas GO, Meek JC, Hayes M. The pathology of the acute and chronic stages of farmer's lung. Thorax 1968; 23:469–489.
123. Reyes CN, Wenzel FJ, Lawton BR, Emanuel DA. The pulmonary pathology of farmer's lung disease. Chest 1982; 81:142–146.
124. Kawanami O, Basset F, Barrios R, et al. Hypersensitivity pneumonitis in man. Light- and electron-microscopic studies of 18 lung biopsies. Am J Pathol 1983; 110:275–289.
125. Barrowcliff DF, Arblaster PG. Farmer's lung: a study of an early acute fatal case. Thorax 1968; 23:490–493.
126. Ghose T, Landrigan P, Killeen R, Dill J. Immunopathological studies in patients with farmer's lung. Clin Allergy 1974; 4:119–129.
127. Pepys J. Clinical and therapeutic significance of patterns of allergic reactions of the lungs to extrinsic agents. Am Rev Respir Dis 1977; 116:573–588.
128. Roberts RC, Moore VL. Immunopathogenesis of hypersensitivity pneumonitis. Am Rev Respir Dis 1977; 116:1075–1090.
129. Williams JV. Inhalation and skin tests with extracts of hay and fungi in patients with farmer's lung. Thorax 1963; 18:182–196.
130. Spector WG, Heesom N. The production of granulomata by antigen-antibody complexes. J Pathol 1969; 98:31–39.
131. Hansen PJ, Penny R. Pigeon-breeder's disease. Study of the cell-mediated immune response to pigeon antigens by the lymphocyte culture technique. Int Arch Allergy Appl Immunol 1974; 47:498–507.
132. Takizawa H, Ohta K, Horiuchi T, et al. Hypersensitivity pneumonitis in athymic nude mice – additional evidence of T-cell dependency. Am Rev Respir Dis 1992; 146:479–484.

Sarcoidosis

133. Hagerstrand I, Linell F. The prevalence of sarcoidosis in the autopsy material from a Swedish town. Acta Med Scand 1964; 425:171.
134. Statement on sarcoidosis. Joint Statement of the American Thoracic Society (ATS), the European Respiratory Society (ERS) and the World Association of Sarcoidosis and Other Granulomatous Disorders (WASOG) adopted by the ATS Board of Directors and by the ERS Executive Committee. J Respir Crit Care Med 1999; 160:736–755.
135. Edmondstone WM, Wilson AR. Sarcoidosis in caucasians, blacks and Asians in London. Br J Dis Chest 1985; 79:27–36.
136. Luisetti M, Beretta A, Casali L. Genetic aspects in sarcoidosis. Eur Resp J 2000; 16:768–780.
137. Schurmann M, Reichel P, Muller-Myhsok B, et al. Results from a genome-wide search for predisposing genes in sarcoidosis. Am J Respir Crit Care Med 2001; 164:840–846.
138. Verleden GM, Dubois RM, Bouros D, et al. Genetic predisposition and pathogenetic mechanisms of interstitial lung diseases of unknown origin. Eur Resp J 2001; :17S–29S.
139. Moller DR, Chen ES. Genetic basis of remitting sarcoidosis - Triumph of the trimolecular complex? Am J Respir Cell Molec Biol 2002; 27:391–395.
140. Grutters JC, Sato H, Welsh KI, Dubois RM. The importance of sarcoidosis genotype to lung phenotype. Am J Respir Cell Molec Biol 2003; 29: S59–S62.
141. Grunewald J, Eklund A, Olerup O. Human leukocyte antigen class I alleles and the disease course in sarcoidosis patients. Am J Respir Crit Care Med 2004; 169:696–702.
142. Baughman RP. Lower EE, du Bois RM. Sarcoidosis Lancet 2003; 361:1111–1118.
143. McGrath DS, Daniil Z, Foley P, et al. Epidemiology of familial sarcoidosis in the UK. Thorax 2000; 55:751–754.
144. Rybicki BA, Iannuzzi MC, Frederick MM, et al. Familial aggregation of sarcoidosis - A Case-Control Etiologic Study of Sarcoidosis (ACCESS). Am J Respir Crit Care Med 2001; 164:2085–2091.
145. Parkes SA, Baker SBD, Bourdillon RE, Murray CRH, Rakshit M. Epidemiology of sarcoidosis in the Isle of Man – 1: A case controlled study. Thorax 1987; 42:420–426.
146. Hills SE, Parkes SA, Baker SBD. Epidemiology of sarcoidosis in the Isle of Man – 2: Evidence for space-time clustering. Thorax 1987; 42:427–430.
147. Spagnolo P, Renzoni EA, Wells AU, et al. C-C chemokine receptor 2 and sarcoidosis: association with Lofgren's syndrome. Am J Respir Crit Care Med 2003; 168:1162–1166.
148. Fagan EA, Moore-Gillon JC, Turner-Warwick M. Multiorgan granulomas and mitochondrial antibodies. N Engl J Med 1983; 308:572–575.
149. Naccache JM, Antoine M, Wislez M, et al. Sarcoid-like pulmonary disorder in human immunodeficiency virus-infected patients receiving antiretroviral therapy. Am J Respir Crit Care Med 1999; 159:2009–2013.
150. Pietropaoli A, Modrak J, Utell M. Interferon-alpha therapy associated with the development of sarcoidosis. Chest 1999; 116:569–572.
151. Scadding JG. Mycobacterium tuberculosis in the aetiology of sarcoidosis. BMJ 1960; 2:1617–1623.
152. Wong CF, Yew WW, Wong PC, Lee J. A case of concomitant tuberculosis and sarcoidosis with mycobacterial DNA present in the sarcoid lesion. Chest 1998; 114:626–629.
153. Almenoff PL, Johnson A, Lesser M, Mattman LH. Growth of acid fast L forms from the blood of patients with sarcoidosis. Thorax 1996; 51:530–533.
154. Wilsher ML, Menzies RE, Croxson MC. Mycobacterium tuberculosis DNA in tissues affected by sarcoidosis. Thorax 1998; 53:871–874.
155. Ikonomopoulos JA, Gorgoulis VG, Zacharatos PV, et al. Multiplex polymerase chain reaction for the detection of mycobacterial DNA in cases of tuberculosis and sarcoidosis. Mod Pathol 1999; 12:854–862.
156. Eishi Y. [Sarcoidosis and Propionibacterium acnes]. Nippon Naika Gakkai Zasshi 2003; 92:1182–1189.
157. Eishi Y, Suga M, Ishige I, et al. Quantitative analysis of mycobacterial and propionibacterial DNA in lymph nodes of Japanese and European patients with sarcoidosis. J Clin Microbiol 2002; 40:198–204.

158. Hunninghake GW, Crystal RG. Pulmonary sarcoidosis. A disorder mediated by excess helper T-lymphocyte activity at sites of disease activity. N Engl J Med 1981; 305:429–434.

159. Ziegenhagen MW, Muller-Quernheim J. The cytokine network in sarcoidosis and its clinical relevance. J Intern Med 2003; 253:18–30.

160. Hance AJ, Basset F, Saumon G, et al. Smoking and interstitial lung disease. The effect of cigarette smoking on the incidence of pulmonary histiocytosis X and sarcoidosis. Ann N Y Acad Sci 1986; 465:643–656.

161. Abramowicz MJ, Ninane V, Depierreux M, Defrancquen P, Yernault JC. Tumour-like presentation of pulmonary sarcoidosis. Eur Respir J 1992; 5:1286–1287.

162. McCann BG, Harrison BDW. Bronchiolar narrowing and occlusion in sarcoidosis - correlation of pathology with physiology. Respir Med 1991; 85:65–67.

163. Askling J, Grunewald J, Eklund A, Hillerdal G, Ekbom A. Increased risk for cancer following sarcoidosis. Am J Respir Crit Care Med 1999; 160:1668–1672.

164. Bouros D, Hatzakis K, Labrakis H, Zeibecoglou K. Association of malignancy with diseases causing interstitial pulmonary changes. Chest 2002; 121:1278–1289.

165. Seersholm N, Vestbo J, Viskum K. Risk of malignant neoplasms in patients with pulmonary sarcoidosis. Thorax 1997; 52:892–894.

166. Perry A, Vuitch F. Causes of death in patients with sarcoidosis: a morphologic study of 38 autopsies with clinicopathologic correlations. Arch Pathol Lab Med 1995; 119:167–172.

167. Johnson BA, Duncan SR, Ohori NP, et al. Recurrence of sarcoidosis in pulmonary allograft recipients. Am Rev Respir Dis 1993; 148: 1373–1377.

168. Mitchell DN, Scadding JG, Heard BE. Hinson KFW. Sarcoidosis: histopathological definition and clinical diagnosis. J Clin Pathol 1977; 30:395–408.

169. Rosen Y, Vuletin JC, Pertschuk LP, Silverstein E. Sarcoidosis : from the pathologist's vantage point. Pathol Annu 1979; 14:405–439.

170. Rosen Y, Athanassiades TJ, Moon S, Lyons HA. Nongranulomatous interstitial pneumonitis in sarcoidosis. Relationship to development of epithelioid granulomas. Chest 1978; 74:122–125.

170a. Reid JD, Andersen ME. Calcium oxalate in sarcoid granulomas. With particular reference to the small ovoid body and a note on the finding of dolomite. Am J Clin Pathol 1988; 90:545–558.

170b. Visscher D, Churg A, Katzenstein AL. Significance of crystalline inclusions in lung granulomas. Mod Pathol 1988; 1:415–419.

171. Cain H, Kraus B. Immunofluorescence microscopic demonstration of vimentin filaments in asteroid bodies of sarcoidosis. Comparison with electron microscopic findings. Virchows Arch B Cell Pathol 1983; 42:213–226.

172. Vos R De, Wolf-Peeters C de, Facchetti F, Desmet V. Plasmacytoid monocytes in epithelioid cell granulomas: ultrastructural and immunoelectron microscopic study. Ultrastruct Pathol 1990; 14:291–302.

173. Mornex JF, Leroux C, Greenland T, Ecochard D. From granuloma to fibrosis in interstitial lung diseases - molecular and cellular interactions. Eur Respir J 1994; 7:779–785.

174. Myatt N, Coghill G, Morrison K, Jones D, Cree IA. Detection of tumour necrosis factor alpha in sarcoidosis and tuberculosis granulomas using in situ hybridisation. J Clin Pathol 1994; 47:423–426.

175. Petrek M, Pantelidis P, Southcott AM, et al. The source and role of RANTES in interstitial lung disease. Eur Resp J 1997; 10:1207–1216.

176. Tolnay E, Kuhnen C, Voss B, Wiethege T, Muller KM. Expression and localization of vascular endothelial growth factor and its receptor flt in pulmonary sarcoidosis. Virchows Arch 1998; 432:61–65.

177. Shigehara K, Shijubo N, Hirasawa M, Abe S, Uede T. Immunolocalization of extracellular matrix proteins and integrins in sarcoid lymph nodes. Virchows Arch 1998; 433:55–61.

178. Facchetti F, Vermi W, Fiorentini S, et al. Expression of inducible nitric oxide synthase in human granulomas and histiocytic reactions. Am J Pathol 1999; 154:145–152.

179. Pertschuk LP, Silverstein E, Friedland J. Immunohistologic diagnosis of sarcoidosis. Detection of angiotensin-converting enzyme in sarcoid granulomas. Am J Clin Pathol 1981; 75:350–354.

180. Adams JS, Sharma OP, Glacad MA, Singer FR. Metabolism of 25-hydroxyvitamin D3 by cultured pulmonary alveolar macrophages in sarcoidosis. J Clin Invest 1983; 72:1856–1860.

181. Papapoulos SE, Frahjer LJ, Sandler LM, et al. 1,25-dihydroxycholecalciferol in the pathogenesis of the hypercalcemia of sarcoidosis. Lancet 1979; ii:627–630.

182. Oord JJ van den, Wolf-Peeters C de, Fachetti F, Desmet VJ. Cellular composition of hypersensitivity-type granulomas: immunohistochemical analysis of tuberculous and sarcoidal lymphadenitis. Hum Pathol 1984; 15:559–565.

183. Maarsseven ACMT van, Mullink H, Alons CL, Stam J. Distribution of T-lymphocyte subsets in different portions of sarcoid granulomas: Immunohistologic analysis with monoclonal antibodies. Hum Pathol 1986; 17:493–500.

184. Baumer I, Zissel G, Schlaak M. MullerQuernheim J. Th1/Th2 cell distribution in pulmonary sarcoidosis. Am J Respir Cell Molec Biol 1997; 16:171–177.

185. Minshall EM, Tsicopoulos A, Yasruel Z, et al. Cytokine mRNA gene expression in active and nonactive pulmonary sarcoidosis. Eur Resp J 1997; 10:2034–2039.

186. Fazel SB, Howie SEM, Krajewski AS, Lamb D. Lymphocyte-B accumulations in human pulmonary sarcoidosis. Thorax 1992; 47:964–967.

187. Hsu RM, Connors AF, Tomashefski JF. Histologic, microbiologic, and clinical correlates of the diagnosis of sarcoidosis by transbronchial biopsy. Arch Pathol Lab Med 1996; 120:364–368.

188. Takemura T, Matsui Y, Saiki S, Mikami R. Pulmonary vascular involvement in sarcoidosis – a report of 40 autopsy cases. Hum Pathol 1992; 23:1216–1223.

189. Battesi JP, Georges R, Basset F, Saumon G. Chronic cor pulmonale in pulmonary sarcoidosis. Thorax 1978; 33:76–84.

190. Rodman DM, Lindenfeld JA. Successful treatment of sarcoidosis-associated pulmonary hypertension with corticosteroids. Chest 1990; 97:500–502.

190a. Shorr AF, Helman DL, Davies DB, Nathan SD. Pulmonary hypertension in advanced sarcoidosis: epidemiology and clinical characteristics. Eur Respir J 2005; 25:783–788.

191. Karakantza M, Matutes E, Maclennan K, et al. Association between sarcoidosis and lymphoma revisited. J Clin Pathol 1996; 49:208–212.

Langerhans cell histiocytosis

192. Basset F, Corrin B, Spencer H. Pulmonary histiocytosis X. Am Rev Respir Dis 1978; 118:811–820.

193. Corrin B, Basset F. A review of histiocytosis X with particular reference to eosinophilic granuloma of the lung. Invest Cell Pathol 1979; 2:137–146.

194. Tazi A, Soler P, Hance AJ. Adult pulmonary Langerhans' cell histiocytosis. Thorax 2000; 55:405–416.

195. Vassallo R, Ryu JH, Colby TV, Hartman T, Limper AH. Medical progress: Pulmonary Langerhans'-cell histiocytosis. N Engl J Med 2000; 342:1969–1978.

196. Sundar KM, Gosselin MV, Chung HL, Cahill BC. Pulmonary Langerhans cell histiocytosis: Emerging concepts in pathobiology, radiology, and clinical evolution of disease. Chest 2003; 123:1673–1683.

197. Lichtenstein L, Histiocytosis X. Integration of eosinophilic granuloma of bone, 'Letterer–Siwe disease' and 'Schuller–Christian disease' as related manifestations of a single nosologic entity. Arch Pathol 1953; 56:84–102.

198. Birbeck MS, Breathnach AS, Everall JD. An electron microscopic study of basal melanocytes and high level clear cells (Langerhans' cell) in vitiligo. J Invest Derm 1961; 37:51.

199. Yousem SA, Colby TV, Chen YY, Chen WG, Weiss LM. Pulmonary Langerhans' cell histiocytosis - Molecular analysis of clonality. Am J Surg Pathol 2001; 25:630–636.

200. Weiss LM, Grogan TM, Muller-Hermelink HK, et al. Langerhans cell histiocytosis. World Health Organization Classification of Tumours: Tumours of haematopoietic and lymphoid tissue. Lyons: IARC Press; 2001:280–282.

201. Casolaro MA, Bernaudin J-F, Saltini C, Ferrans VJ, Crystal RG. Accumulation of Langerhans' cells on the epithelial surface of the lower respiratory tract in normal subjects in association with cigarette smoking. Am Rev Respir Dis 1988; 137:406–411.

202. Kawanami O, Basset F, Ferrans VJ, Soler P, Crystal RG. Pulmonary Langerhans' cells in patients with fibrotic lung disorders. Lab Invest 1981; 44:227.

203. Furukawa T, Watanabe S, Kodama T, et al. T-zone histiocytes in adenocarcinoma of the lung in relation to postoperative prognosis. Cancer 1985; 56:2651–2656.

204. Soler P, Moreau A, Basset F, Hance AJ. Cigarette smoking-induced changes in the number and differentiated state of pulmonary dendritic cells/Langerhans cells. Am Rev Respir Dis 1989; 139:1112–1117.

205. Tazi A, Bonay M, Bergeron A, et al. Role of granulocyte-macrophage colony stimulating factor (GM- CSF) in the pathogenesis of adult pulmonary histiocytosis X. Thorax 1996; 51:611–614.

206. Hirose M, Saito S, Yoshimoto T, Kuroda Y. Interleukin-2 therapy of Langerhans cell histiocytosis. Acta Paediatr 1995; 84:1204–1206.

207. Rajagopol J, Shepard JAO, Mark EJ, Malhotra A. A 58-year-old man with interstitial pulmonary disease. Eosinophilic granuloma, late (Burned-out) stage. N Engl J Med 2002; 347:1262–1268.

208. Tazi A, Bonay M, Gransaigne M, et al. Surface phenotype of Langerhans cells and lymphocytes in granulomatous lesions from patients with pulmonary histiocytosis-X. Am Rev Respir Dis 1993; 147:1531–1536.

209. Robb IA, Jimenez CL, Carpenter BF. Birbeck granules or Birbeck junctions – intercellular zipper-like lattice junctions in eosinophilic granuloma of bone. Ultrastruct Pathol 1992; 16:423–428.

210. Krenacs L, Tiszalvicz L, Krenacs T, Boumsell L. Immunohistochemical detection of CD1A antigen in formalin-fixed and paraffin-embedded tissue sections with monoclonal antibody 010. J Pathol 1993; 171:99–104.

211. Emile JF, Wechsler J, Brousse N, et al. Langerhans' cell histiocytosis: definitive diagnosis with the use of monoclonal antibody 010 on routinely paraffin-embedded samples. Am J Surg Pathol 1995; 19:636–641.

212. Pinkus GS, Lones MA, Matsumura F, et al. Langerhans cell histiocytosis – Immunohistochemical expression of fascin, a dendritic cell marker. Am J Clin Pathol 2002; 118:335–343.

213. Lieberman PH, Jones CR, Steinman RM, et al. Langerhans cell (eosinophilic) granulomatosis: a clinicopathologic study encompassing 50 years. Am J Surg Pathol 1996; 20:519–552.

213a. Nakhla H, Jumbelic MI. Sudden death of a patient with pulmonary Langerhans cell histiocytosis. Arch Pathol Lab Med 2005; 129:798–799.

214. Lacronique J, Roth C, Battesti J-P, Basset F, Chretien J. Chest radiological features of pulmonary histiocytosis X: a report based on 50 adult cases. Thorax 1982; 37:104–109.

215. Fichtenbaum CJ, Kleinman GM, Haddad RG. Eosinophilic granuloma of the lung presenting as a solitary pulmonary nodule. Thorax 1990; 45:905–906.

215a. Fridlender ZG, Glazer M, Amir G, Berkman N. Obstructing tracheal pulmonary Langerhans cell histiocytosis. Chest 2005; 128:1057–1058.

216. Delobbe K, Durieu J, Duhamel A, Wallaert B. Determinants of survival in pulmonary Langerhans' cell granulomatosis (histiocytosis X). Eur Respir J 1996; 9:2002–2006.

217. Tazi A, Montcelly L, Bergeron A, et al. Relapsing nodular lesions in the course of adult pulmonary Langerhans cell histiocytosis. Am J Respir Crit Care Med 1998; 157:2007–2010.

218. Vassallo R, Ryu JH, Schroeder DR, Decker PA, Limper AH. Clinical outcomes of pulmonary Langerhans'-cell histiocytosis in adults. N Engl J Med 2002; 346:484–490.

219. Stoll M, Freund M, Schmid H, et al. Allogeneic bone marrow transplantation for Langerhans' cell histiocytosis X. Cancer 1990; 66:284–288.

220. Habib SB, Congleton J, Carr D, et al. Recipient Langerhans cell histiocytosis recurring following bilateral lung transplantation. Thorax 1998; 53:323–325.

221. Li SY, Borowitz MJ. CD79a⁺ T-cell lymphoblastic lymphoma with coexisting Langerhans cell histiocytosis – A short case report and review of the literature. Arch Pathol Lab Med 2001; 125:958–960.

222. Sadoun D, Vaylet F, Valeyre D, et al. Bronchogenic carcinoma in patients with pulmonary histiocytosis-X. Chest 1992; 101:1610–1613.

223. Sakuma N, Kamei T, Ohta M, et al. Immunohistochemical and ultrastructural examination of histiocytosis-X in pulmonary eosinophilic granuloma. Acta Pathol Jpn 1992; 42:719–726.

224. Travis WD, Borok Z, Roum JH, et al. Pulmonary Langerhans cell granulomatosis (histiocytosis-X) – a clinicopathologic study of 48 cases. Am J Surg Pathol 1993; 17:971–986.

225. Kambouchner M, Basset FO, Marchal L, et al. Three-dimensional characterization of pathologic lesions in pulmonary Langerhans cell histiocytosis. Am J Respir Crit Care Med 2002; 166:1483–1490.

226. Asakura S, Colby TV, Limper AH. Tissue localization of transforming growth factor-beta 1 in pulmonary eosinophilic granuloma. Am J Respir Crit Care Med 1996; 154:1525–1530.

227. Graaf JH de, Tamminga RYJ, Dam-Meiring A, Kamps WA, Timens W. The presence of cytokines in Langerhans' cell histiocytosis. J Pathol 1996; 180:400–406.

228. Rousseau-Merck MF, Barbey S, Mouly H, Bazin S, Nezelof C. Collagenolytic activity of eosinophilic granuloma in vitro. Experientia 1979; 35:1226–1227.

229. Hayashi T, Rush WL, Travis WD, et al. Immunohistochemical study of matrix metalloproteinases and their tissue inhibitors in pulmonary Langerhans' cell granulomatosis. Arch Pathol Lab Med 1997; 121:930–937.

230. Shimizu S, Yoshinouchi T, Ohtsuki Y, et al. The appearance of S-100 protein-positive dendritic cells and the distribution of lymphocyte subsets in idiopathic nonspecific interstitial pneumonia. Resp Med 2002; 96:770–776.

231. Danel C, Israelbiet D, Costabel U, Rossi GA, Wallaert B. The clinical role of BAL in pulmonary histiocytosis-X. Eur Respir J 1990; 3:949–950.

232. Auerswald U, Barth J, Magnussen H. Value of CD-1-positive cells in bronchoalveolar lavage fluid for the diagnosis of pulmonary histiocytosis-X. Lung 1991; 169:305–309.

Lymphangioleiomyomatosis

233. Corrin B, Liebow AA, Friedman PJ. Pulmonary lymphangiomyomatosis. Am J Pathol 1975; 79:347–382.

234. Baldi S, Papotti M, Valente ML, et al. Pulmonary lymphangioleiomyomatosis in postmenopausal women: report of two cases and review of the literature. Eur Respir J 1994; 7:1013–1016.

235. Johnson SR, Tattersfield AE. Clinical experience of lymphangioleiomyomatosis in the UK. Thorax 2000; 55:1052–1057.

236. Aubry MC, Myers JL, Ryu JH, et al. Pulmonary lymphangioleiomyomatosis in a man. Am J Respir Crit Care Med 2000; 162:749–752.

237. Kim NR, Chung MP, Park CK, Lee KS, Han JH. Pulmonary lymphangioleiomyomatosis and multiple hepatic angiomyolipomas in a man. Pathol Int 2003; 53:231–235.

238. Hughes E, Hodder RV. Pulmonary lymphangiomyomatosis complicating pregnancy. A case report. J Reprod Med 1987; 32:553.

239. Urban T, Lazor R, Lacronique J, et al. Pulmonary lymphangioleiomyomatosis. A study of 69 patients. Groupe d'Etudes et de Recherche sur les Maladies 'Orphelines' Pulmonaires (GERM'O'P). Medicine (Baltimore) 1999; 78:321–337.

240. Gray SR, Carrington CB. Cornog JL. Lymphangiomyomatosis. Report of a case with ureteral involvement and chyluria. Cancer 1975; 35:490–498.

241. Shen A, Iseman ID, Waldron JA, King TE. Exacerbation of pulmonary lymphangioleiomyomatosis by exogenous estrogens. Chest 1987; 91:782–785.

242. Yano S. Exacerbation of pulmonary lymphangioleiomyomatosis by exogenous oestrogen used for infertility treatment. Thorax 2002; 57:1085–1086.

243. Berger U, Khaghani A, Pomerance A, Yacoub MH, Coombes RC. Pulmonary lymphangioleiomyomatosis and steroid receptors. An immunocytochemical study. Am J Clin Pathol 1990; 93:609–614.

244. Wahedna I, Cooper S, Williams J, et al. Relation of pulmonary lymphangioleiomyomatosis to use of the oral contraceptive pill and fertility in the UK: a national case control study. Thorax 1994; 49:910–914.

245. Shepherd CW, Gomez MR, Lie JT, Crowson CS. Causes of death in patients with tuberous sclerosis. Mayo Clin Proc 1991; 66:792–796.

246. Bonetti F, Chiodera P. The lung in tuberous sclerosis. In: Corrin B, ed. Pathology of Lung Tumors. Edinburgh: Churchill Livingstone; 1997:225–240.

247. Chu SC, Horiba K, Usuki J, et al. Comprehensive evaluation of 35 patients with lymphangioleiomyomatosis. Chest 1999; 115:1041–1052.

248. Valensi QJ. Pulmonary lymphangiomyoma, a probable forme fruste of tuberous sclerosis: a case report and survey of the literature. Am Rev Respir Dis 1973; 108:1411–1415.

249. Bernstein SM, Newell JD, Adamczyk D, et al. How common are renal angiomyolipomas in patients with pulmonary lymphangiomyomatosis? Am J Respir Crit Care Med 1995; 152:2138–2143.

250. Maziak DE, Kesten S, Rappaport DC, Maurer J. Extrathoracic angiomyolipomas in lymphangioleiomyomatosis. Eur Respir J 1996; 9:402–405.

251. Castro M, Shepherd CW, Gomez MR, Lie JT, Ryu JH. Pulmonary tuberous sclerosis. Chest 1995; 107:189–195.

252. Franz DN, Brody A, Meyer C, et al. Mutational and radiographic analysis of pulmonary disease consistent with lymphangioleiomyomatosis and micronodular pneumocyte hyperplasia in women with tuberous sclerosis. Am J Respir Crit Care Med 2001; 164:661–668.

253. Moss J, Avila NA, Barnes PM, et al. Prevalence and clinical characteristics of lymphangioleiomyomatosis (LAM) in patients with tuberous sclerosis complex. Am J Respir Crit Care Med 2001; 164:669–671.

254. Lie JT, Miller RD, Williams DE. Cystic disease of the lungs in tuberous sclerosis. Clinicopathologic correlation, including body plethysmographic lung function tests. Mayo Clin Proc 1980; 55:547–553.

255. Fryer AE, Chalmers A, Connor JM, et al. Evidence that the gene for tuberous sclerosis is on chromosome 9. Lancet 1987; 1:659–661.

256. European chromosome 16 consortium. Identification and characterization of the tuberous sclerosis gene on chromosome 16. Cell 1993; 75:1305–1315.

257. Menchine M, Emelin JK, Mischel PS, et al. Tissue and cell-type specific expression of the tuberous sclerosis gene, TSC2, in human tissues. Mod Pathol 1996; 9:1071–1080.

258. Sampson JR, Scahill SJ, Stephenson JBP, Mann L, Connor JM. Genetic aspects of tuberous sclerosis in the west of Scotland. J Med Genet 1989; 26:28–31.

259. Carsillo T, Astrinidis A, Henske EP. Mutations in the tuberous sclerosis complex gene TSC2 are a cause of sporadic pulmonary lymphangioleiomyomatosis. Proc Natl Acad Sci USA 2000; 97:6085–6090.

260. Maruyama H, Seyama K, Sobajima J, et al. Multifocal micronodular pneumocyte hyperplasia and lymphangioleiomyomatosis in tuberous sclerosis with a TSC2 gene. Mod Pathol 2001; 14:609–614.

261. Yu J, Astrinidis A, Henske EP. Chromosome 16 loss of heterozygosity in tuberous sclerosis and sporadic lymphangiomyomatosis. Am J Respir Crit Care Med 2001; 164:1537–1540.

262. Bittmann I, Rolf B, Amann G, Lohrs U. Recurrence of lymphangioleiomyomatosis after single lung transplantation: New insights into pathogenesis. Hum Pathol 2003; 34:95–98.

263. Karbowniczek M, Astrinidis A, Balsara BR, et al. Recurrent lymphangiomyomatosis after transplantation – Genetic analyses reveal a metastatic mechanism. Am J Respir Crit Care Med 2003; 167:976–982.

264. Bittmann I, Dose TB, Muller C. Dienemann H. Lymphangioleiomyomatosis: Recurrence after single lung transplantation. Hum Pathol 1997; 28:1420–1423.

265. Taylor JR, Ryu J, Colby TV. Raffin TA. Lymphangioleiomyomatosis. Clinical course in 32 patients. N Engl J Med 1990; 323:1254–1260.

266. Johnson S. Rare diseases – 1 – Lymphangioleiomyomatosis: clinical features, management and basic mechanisms. Thorax 1999; 54:254–264.

267. Sullivan EJ. Lymphangioleiomyomatosis – A review. Chest 1998; 114:1689–1703.

268. Oh YM, Mo EK, Jang SH, et al. Pulmonary lymphangioleiomyomatosis in Korea. Thorax 1999; 54:618–621.

269. Vadas G, Pare JAP, Thurlbeck WM. Pulmonary and lymph node myomatosis: review of the literature and report of a case. Can Med Assoc J 1967; 96:420–424.

270. Carrington CB, Cugell DW, Gaensler EA, et al. Lymphangioleiomyomatosis. Physiologic-pathologic-radiologic correlations. Am Rev Respir Dis 1977; 116:977–995.

271. Burger CD, Hyatt RE, Staats BA. Pulmonary mechanics in lymphangioleiomyomatosis. Am Rev Respir Dis 1991; 143:1030–1033.

272. Crausman RS, Jennings CA, Irvin CG. King TE. Lymphangioleiomyomatosis: the pathophysiology of diminished exercise capacity. Am J Respir Crit Care Med 1996; 153:1368–1376.

273. Aberle DR, Hansell DM, Brown K. Tashkin DP. Lymphangiomyomatosis: CT, chest radiographic, and functional correlations. Radiology 1990; 176:381–387.

274. Silverstein EF, Ellis K, Wolff M, Jaretzki A. Pulmonary lymphangiomyomatosis. AJR Am J Roentgenol 1974; 120:832–850.

275. Kitaichi M, Nishimura K, Itoh H, Izumi T. Pulmonary lymphangioleiomyomatosis: a report of 46 patients including a clinicopathologic study of prognostic factors. Am J Respir Crit Care Med 1995; 151:527–533.

276. Bhattacharyya AK, Balogh K. Retroperitoneal lymphangioleiomyomatosis. Cancer 1985; 56:1144–1146.

277. Basset F, Soler P, Marsac J, Corrin B. Pulmonary lymphangiomyomatosis. Three new cases studied with electron microscopy. Cancer 1976; 38:2357–2366.

278. Matthews TJ, Hornall D, Sheppard MN. Comparison of the use of antibodies to alpha-smooth muscle actin and desmin in pulmonary lymphangiomyomatosis. J Clin Pathol 1993; 46:479–480.

279. Bonetti F, Chiodera PL, Pea M, et al. Transbronchial biopsy in lymphangiomyomatosis of the lung - HMB45 for diagnosis. Am J Surg Pathol 1993; 17:1092–1102.

280. Hoon V, Thung SN, Kaneko M, Unger PD. HMB-45 reactivity in renal angiomyolipoma and lymphangioleiomyomatosis. Arch Pathol Lab Med 1994; 118:732–734.

281. Chan JKC, Tsang WYW, Pau MY, et al. Lymphangiomyomatosis and angiomyolipoma: closely related entities characterized by hamartomatous proliferation of HMB-45-positive smooth muscle. Histopathology 1993; 22:445–455.

282. Tanaka H, Imada A, Morikawa T, et al. Diagnosis of pulmonary lymphangioleiomyomatosis by HMB45 in surgically treated spontaneous pneumothorax. Eur Respir J 1995; 8:1879–1882.

283. Kalassian KG, Doyle R, Kao P, Ruoss S. Raffin TA. Lymphangioleiomyomatosis: new insights. Am J Respir Crit Care Med 1997; 155:1183–1186.

284. Bonetti F, Pea M, Martignoni G, et al. Clear cell ('sugar') tumor of the lung is a lesion strictly related to angiomyolipoma - the concept of a family of lesions characterized by the presence of the perivascular epithelioid cells (PEC). Pathology 1995; 26:230–236.

285. Pea M, Martignoni G, Zamboni G, Bonetti F. Perivascular epithelioid cell. Am J Surg Pathol 1996; 20:1149–1153.

286. Matsumoto Y, Horiba K, Usuki J, et al. Markers of cell proliferation and expression of melanosomal antigen in lymphangioleiomyomatosis. Am J Respir Cell Molec Biol 1999; 21:327–336.

287. Matsui K, Takeda K, Yu ZX, et al. Downregulation of estrogen and progesterone receptors in the abnormal smooth muscle cells in pulmonary lymphangioleiomyomatosis following therapy – An immunohistochemical study. Am J Respir Crit Care Med 2000; 161:1002–1009.

288. Fukuda Y, Kawamoto M, Yamamoto A, et al. Role of elastic fiber degradation in emphysema-like lesions of pulmonary lymphangiomyomatosis. Hum Pathol 1990; 21:1252–1261.

289. Hayashi T, Fleming MV, Stetler-Stevenson WG, et al. Immunohistochemical study of matrix metalloproteinases (MMPs) and their tissue inhibitors (TIMPs) in pulmonary lymphangioleiomyomatosis (LAM). Hum Pathol 1997; 28:1071–1078.

290. Sobonya RE, Quan SF, Fleishman JS. Pulmonary lymphangioleiomyomatosis: quantitative analysis of lesions producing airflow limitation. Hum Pathol 1985; 16:1122–1128.

291. Matsui K, Beasley MB, Nelson WK, et al. Prognostic significance of pulmonary lymphangioleiomyomatosis histologic score. Am J Surg Pathol 2001; 25:479–484.

292. Matsui K, Tatsuguchi A, Valencia J, et al. Extrapulmonary lymphangioleiomyomatosis (LAM): Clinicopathologic features in 22 cases. Hum Pathol 2000; 31:1242–1248.

293. Steiner PE. Metastasizing fibroleiomyoma of the uterus - report of a case and review of the literature. Am J Pathol 1939; 15:89–109.

294. Spiro RH, McPeak CJ. On the so-called metastasizing leiomyoma. Cancer 1966; 19:544–548.

295. Burrel LST, Ross JM. A case of chylous effusion due to leiomyosarcoma. Br J Tuberc Dis Chest 1937; 31:38–39.

296. Itoh T, Mochizuki M, Kumazaki S, Ishihara T, Fukayama M. Cystic pulmonary metastases of endometrial stromal sarcoma of the uterus, mimicking lymphangiomyomatosis: A case report with immunohistochemistry of HMB45. Pathol Int 1997; 47:725–729.

297. Mahadeva R, Stewart S, Wallwork J. Metastatic endometrial stromal sarcoma masquerading as pulmonary lymphangioleiomyomatosis. J Clin Pathol 1999; 52:147–148.

298. Svendsen TL, Viskum K, Hansborg N, Thorpe SM, Nielsen NC. Pulmonary lymphangioleiomyomatosis: a case of progesterone receptor positive lymphangioleiomyomatosis treated with medroxyprogesterone, oophorectomy and tamoxifen. Br J Dis Chest 1984; 78:264–271.

299. Westermann CJJ, Oostveen ACM. Wagenaar SSc et al. Pulmonary tuberous sclerosis treated with tamoxifen and progesterone. Thorax 1986; 41:892–893.

300. Kitzsteiner KA, Mallen RG. Pulmonary lymphangiomyomatosis: treatment with castration. Cancer 1980; 46:2248–2249.

301. Banner A, Carrington CB, Emory WB, et al. Efficacy of oophorectomy in lymphangioleiomyomatosis and benign metastasizing leiomyoma. N Engl J Med 1981; 305:204–209.

302. Adamson D, Heinrichs WL, Raybin DM, Raffin TA. Successful treatment of pulmonary lymphangioleiomyomatosis with oophorectomy and progesterone. Am Rev Respir Dis 1985; 132:916–921.

303. Urban T, Kuttenn F, Gompel A, Marsac J, Lacronique J. Pulmonary lymphangiomyomatosis – follow-up and long-term outcome with antiestrogen therapy - a report of 8 cases. Chest 1992; 102:472–476.

304. Dishner W, Cordasco EM, Blackburn J, et al. Pulmonary lymphangiomyomatosis. Chest 1984; 85:796–799.

305. Eliasson AH, Phillips YY, Tenholder MF. Treatment of lymphangioleiomyomatosis. A meta-analysis. Chest 1989; 196:1352–1355.

306. Boehler A, Speich R, Russi EW, Weder W. Lung transplantation for lymphangioleiomyomatosis. N Engl J Med 1996; 335:1275–1280.

307. Nine JS, Yousem SA, Paradis IL, Keenan R, Griffith BP. Lymphangioleiomyomatosis recurrence after lung transplantation. J Heart Lung Transplant 1994; 13:714–719.

308. O'Brien JD, Lium JH, Parosa JF, et al. Lymphangiomyomatosis recurrence in the allograft after single-lung transplantation. Am J Respir Crit Care Med 1995; 151:2033–2036.

6

Diffuse parenchymal disease of the lung

6.2

Alveolar filling defects

CRYPTOGENIC ORGANISING PNEUMONIA (IDIOPATHIC BRONCHIOLITIS OBLITERANS ORGANISING PNEUMONIA)

The first description of this alveolar-filling defect should probably be attributed to Liebow,[1] who used the title interstitial pneumonia with bronchiolitis obliterans (BIP) despite the predominant involvement of airspaces rather than the interstitium. Subsequent workers drew attention to the steroid-sensitivity of the condition[2,3] and the terms cryptogenic organising pneumonia (COP)[4] and bronchiolitis obliterans organising pneumonia (BOOP)[5] followed, the latter covering both the idiopathic variety and those of known causation. The emphasis on bronchiolar involvement in the term BOOP inevitably led to confusion with constrictive obliterative bronchiolitis characterised by airflow obstruction. While it is true that the luminal fibrosis of organising pneumonia extends proximally into alveolar ducts, respiratory bronchioles and even membranous bronchioles, it remains limited to relatively peripheral airspaces and the functional deficit is restrictive rather than obstructive. An appreciation of the geometry of the airways (see Table 1.2, p. 4) helps in understanding the different functional and clinical effects of proximal and distal airway obliteration.

The steroid-sensitivity of cryptogenic organising pneumonia is probably attributable to its collagen being of type III (newly formed, flexible and susceptible to enzymatic digestion), rather than the more mature type I and the abundance of proteolytic enzymes within the Masson bodies.[6] This steroid-sensitivity probably applies to organising pneumonia irrespective of the cause of the initial exudate.

Clinical features

Cryptogenic organising pneumonia presents a distinct clinico-pathological syndrome, recognition of which is important because of its steroid-responsiveness.[2-4] Men and women are affected about equally and most are in the 40–60-year age group. Persistent cough, shortness of breath and malaise are

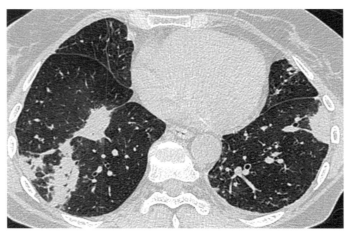

Figure 6.2.1 Cryptogenic organising pneumonia. HRCT shows patchy bilateral airspace consolidation with a predominantly subpleural distribution. Focal ground-glass shadows are also seen in the left lower lobe.

Table 6.2.1 Conditions resulting in organising pneumonia

Condition	Suggestive histological features
Bacterial pneumonia	Neutrophilia, organisms on special stains
Bronchial obstruction, chronic bronchiolitis	
Diffuse alveolar damage (organising phase)	More diffuse low power distribution, exudative foci
Radiation	
Aspiration pneumonia	Foreign material
Fume and toxin exposure	
Connective tissue disease	Other manifestations of such disease (e.g. rheumatoid nodules)
Extrinsic allergic alveolitis	Bronchocentricity, granulomas
Pulmonary eosinophilia	Eosinophils
Drug reactions	Eosinophils
Transplantation (bone marrow, lung, kidney)	
Inflammatory bowel disease	
Adjacent disease, e.g.	
Abscess	
Wegener's granulomatosis	Vasculitis, granulomas
Neoplasms	Tumour
Langerhans cell histiocytosis	Langerhans cells
Cryptogenic organising pneumonia	

common complaints. The onset is insidious. Chest radiographs show widespread blotchy opacities, which regress in some places whilst progressing in others and developing anew elsewhere.[7] HRCT scans typically show bilateral consolidation, which has a predominantly subpleural and peribronchial distribution (Fig. 6.2.1). Reticular changes, localised nodules and ground-glass opacification are less common. The changes wax and wane, unlike those of bronchioloalveolar carcinoma, which cryptogenic organising pneumonia may otherwise resemble. Pulmonary function tests generally show a predominantly restrictive ventilatory defect but some patients have a mixed obstructive and restrictive pattern. The erythrocyte sedimentation rate is elevated but no evidence of infection can be detected, either by culture or serologically. Bronchoalveolar lavage shows a lymphocytosis with a low T-helper/suppressor cell ratio (see Table A4, p. 742).[8,9]

Some patients are affected each spring and in these there is an intriguing association with cholestasis.[10] Circulating immune complexes have been identified in some patients.[11] Another intriguing observation is that post-irradiation organising pneumonia appears to 'prime' the non-irradiated areas of the lungs as these may subsequently develop the same changes,[12–14] a point of difference from the usual form of radiation pneumonitis which is generally confined to the irradiated area of lung. One woman suffered self-limited attacks a few days before each menstrual period.[15]

The prognosis is usually excellent, particularly with steroid therapy, but rare patients have unusually severe disease and deteriorate rapidly despite treatment. Autopsy in such cases has shown interstitial fibrosis rather than the intraalveolar fibrosis seen on biopsy.[16]

Histopathology and differential diagnosis[4,5,17]
Various conditions cause organising pneumonia (Table 6.2.1) but whatever its aetiology, biopsy shows micropolypoid buds of granulation tissue (bourgeons conjonctifs or Masson bodies)

in the air spaces (Fig. 6.2.2a–d). The buds may extend from one alveolus to the next through the pores of Kohn, which were first identified by this process. Alveoli are mainly affected but the process also involves respiratory bronchioles and the more peripheral membranous bronchioles. Occasionally, residual fibrin is seen in or near the connective tissue buds, which also contain small numbers of lymphocytes, plasma cells and neutrophils in addition to macrophages and fibroblasts. The inflammatory cells tend to cluster in the centres of the buds. Chronic inflammation and interstitial fibrosis of the alveolar walls may also be seen but the predominant change is that within the air spaces (Fig. 6.2.2a–d). The alveoli are often lined by reactive type II cells. Electron microscopy shows evidence of acute alveolar epithelial injury.[18]

Only occasionally is the cause of organising pneumonia evident histologically (Fig. 6.2.3) but a striking histological feature of the cryptogenic condition is its temporal homogeneity, which gives the impression of damage occurring at a single moment. This contrasts with usual interstitial pneumonia (UIP) where fibroblastic foci lie adjacent to areas of well established interstitial fibrosis. However, in time, the intraalveolar granulation tissue of organising pneumonia may be incorporated into the alveolar wall by an accretive process, resulting in interstitial fibrosis and a similarity to UIP, with a correspondingly worse prognosis.[16,19] In such cases, HRCT may reveal more typical features elsewhere in the lungs. Cryptogenic organising pneumonia (COP) is distinguished from the exudative phase of diffuse alveolar damage by an absence of hyaline membranes but the organising phase of diffuse alveolar damage may resemble COP and only be separable by review of clinical data. Features that

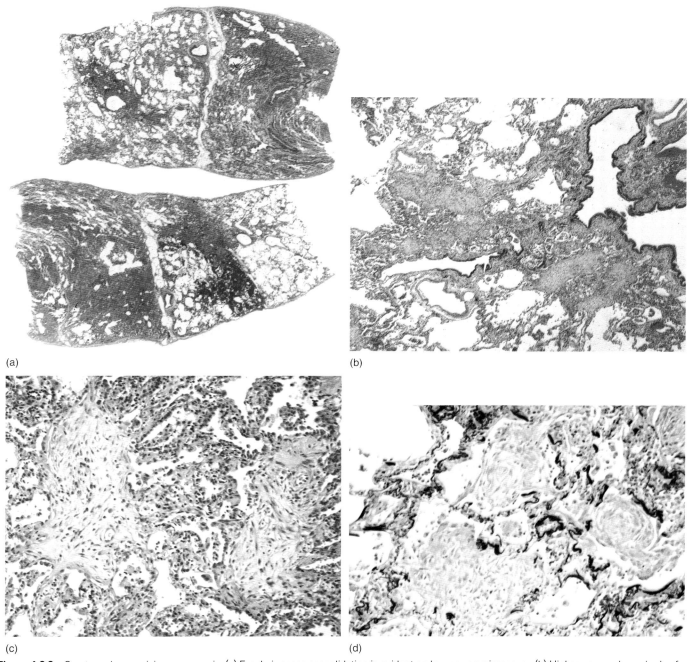

(a)

(b)

(c)

(d)

Figure 6.2.2 Cryptogenic organising pneumonia. (a) Focal air space consolidation is evident on low power microscopy. (b) Higher power shows buds of granulation tissue with alveoli adjacent to a bronchovascular bundle. (c) Partial epithelialisation of the granulation tissue may occur. (d) An elastin stain highlights the intra–alveolar rather than interstitial location.

favour COP over organising diffuse alveolar damage include a patchy peribronchiolar distribution and relatively little expansion of the interstitium by oedematous fibro-inflammatory tissue.

Pathologists conducting necropsies on patients dying of bronchopneumonia will be familiar with the histological pattern of organising pneumonia but before dismissing it in a biopsy as yet another example of healing bacterial pneumonia

they should ask themselves why a condition that is usually diagnosed without such recourse should be so investigated. Consultation with the clinician may lead to a diagnosis of cryptogenic organising pneumonia and successful treatment with corticosteroids. Many causes of organising pneumonia are only identifiable clinically. Without clinical input, a reasonable pathological conclusion is 'organising pneumonia, aetiology not apparent'.

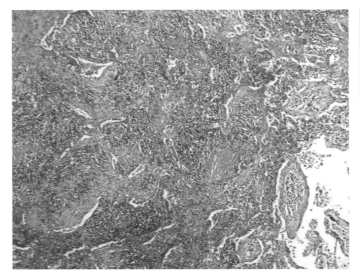

(a)

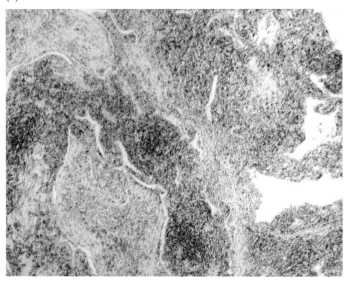

(b)

Figure 6.2.3 Organising pneumonia secondary to non-Hodgkin lymphoma. (a) At low power, the dominant feature is organising pneumonia, but compared to Fig. 6.2.2 the background lymphoid infiltrate is more prominent. (b) CD20 staining reveals a diffuse B-cell infiltrate. Clinicopathological correlation confirmed the presence of a non-Hodgkin lymphoma.

Acute fibrinous and organising pneumonia

On occasion, organising pneumonia may be associated with prominent knots of fibrin, resulting in a histological pattern that has been termed acute fibrinous and organising pneumonia (Fig. 6.2.4).[20] The clinical features and course of the disease are those of acute alveolar injury but the hyaline membranes of diffuse alveolar damage are not evident and there is no eosinophilia. Imaging shows bilateral basal opacities that are either diffuse or reticulonodular. The prognosis is poor, similar to that seen in relation to other causes of diffuse alveolar damage.

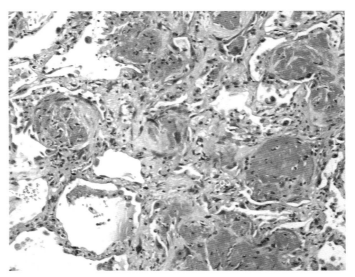

Figure 6.2.4 Acute fibrinous and organising pneumonia. The alveoli contain both fibrin and buds of granulation tissue.

DESQUAMATIVE INTERSTITIAL PNEUMONIA

Desquamative interstitial pneumonia (DIP) is characterised by an excess of alveolar macrophages so marked that the alveoli are practically filled by these cells. This is accompanied by only a mild degree of chronic interstitial inflammation so that the alveolar walls are only slightly thickened, if at all. The adjective 'interstitial' therefore puts the wrong emphasis on what is essentially an alveolar filling defect (Fig. 6.2.5). Furthermore, the term 'desquamative' is quite inappropriate. It was introduced[21] in the belief that the free cells were exfoliated (desquamated) alveolar epithelial cells, a misconception that is easy to understand when only routinely stained sections are examined (Fig. 6.2.6): the true nature of the free cells was shown first by electron microscopy[22,23] and then by immunocytochemistry (Fig. 6.2.7), which demonstrate that they are macrophages. Nevertheless, although the term 'alveolar macrophage pneumonia' has been suggested, the consensus view is to continue with the more familiar, if histogenetically incorrect, term of desquamative interstitial pneumonia.[24]

Aetiology

The nature of DIP is not well understood but its recognised associations suggest that it is a pathological response to a variety of pulmonary insults rather than a specific disease. In adults it mainly affects cigarette smokers and in these individuals it may be regarded merely as an excessive macrophage response to inhaled smoke.[24a] DIP is also seen in workers exposed to exceptionally dusty environments.[23,25,26] Others apparently develop DIP in response to relatively low levels of atmospheric pollution, presumably being hypersensitive to dust.[27] Long-term therapy with drugs such as nitrofurantoin may also result in DIP.[28] A minority of patients have collagen

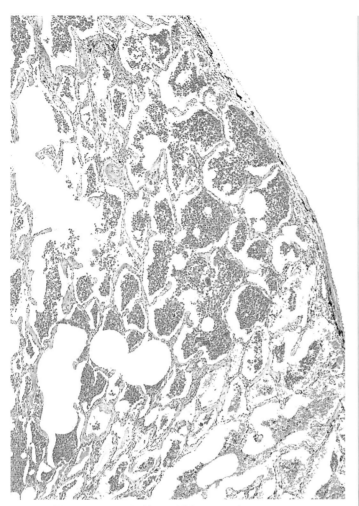

Figure 6.2.5 'Desquamative' interstitial pneumonia represents an alveolar filling defect rather than an interstitial disease.

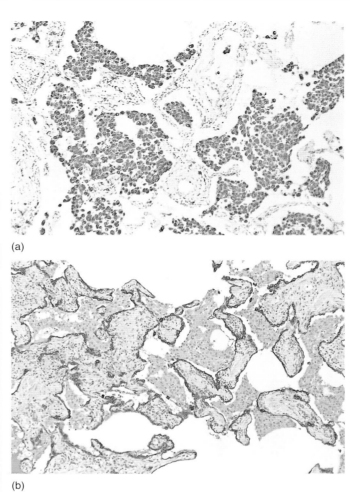

(a)

(b)

Figure 6.2.7 'Desquamative' interstitial pneumonia. Immunostaining for (a) the macrophage marker CD68 and (b) the epithelial (cytokeratin) marker MNF116 shows that the cells filling the alveoli are macrophages rather than desquamated epithelial cells.

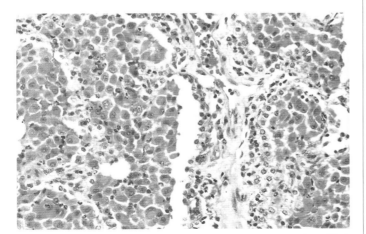

Figure 6.2.6 'Desquamative' interstitial pneumonia. The alveoli are filled by mononuclear cells that morphologically resemble the adjacent hyperplastic alveolar type II epithelial cells and it is easy to imagine a desquamative process.

vascular disease or the autoantibodies that characterise such disease suggesting that in these individuals the changes represent a particularly cellular (or 'luminal') pattern of cryptogenic fibrosing alveolitis.[29] However, all these patients were smokers and the association between connective tissue diseases and DIP may therefore be tenuous. There remains a small group of patients, who despite all clinical investigations, have no evidence of any potential causative association and may therefore be regarded as having idiopathic DIP.[30]

DIP is also encountered in children, sometimes as a manifestation of surfactant apoprotein B deficiency. Other children with DIP have had lipid storage diseases and it is possible that unrecognised metabolic defects may be responsible for other cases.

Clinical features

Most patients with DIP are middle-aged cigarette smokers who complain of breathlessness and cough of insidious onset. HRCT shows hazy 'ground-glass' opacification of the lower lung

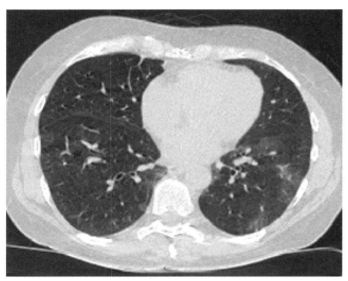

Figure 6.2.8 'Desquamative' interstitial pneumonia. HRCT shows patchy peripheral ground-glass shadowing.

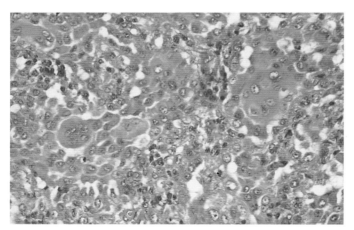

Figure 6.2.9 'Desquamative' interstitial pneumonia. The macrophages that fill the alveoli include multinucleate forms.

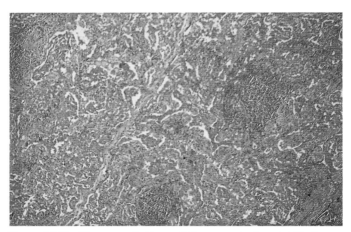

Figure 6.2.10 'Desquamative' interstitial pneumonia. Lymphoid foci representing follicular bronchiolitis stand out against the general consolidation.

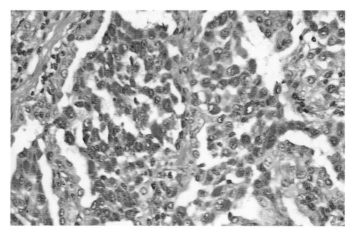

Figure 6.2.11 'Desquamative' interstitial pneumonia. Endogenous cytoplasmic pigment granules are strongly stained by the periodic acid-Schiff reaction.

fields, sometimes accompanied by reticular markings (Fig. 6.2.8).[31,32] Pulmonary function tests show a restrictive pattern with a reduction in diffusing capacity. Hypoxaemia is often evident on blood gas analysis. Most patients respond well to corticosteroids,[32–34] especially if they quit smoking. They may recover completely, or stabilise, but relapse many years later is recorded,[35,36] even after lung transplantation.[37] In a minority of patients the disease progresses slowly to interstitial fibrosis,[30,38] ultimately proving fatal after, on average, 12 years.[32] The outcome is worse in children, especially in infants and those with familial disease, probably reflecting a different aetiology (see Chapter 2, p. 48).

Pathological features
The principal histopathological feature is consolidation of the lung by large numbers of alveolar macrophages, which may be multinucleate (Figs 6.2.6 and 6.2.9). This is accompanied by an interstitial lymphocytic infiltrate and fibrosis, both of which are usually mild. There is often also follicular bronchiolitis, the scattered lymphoid follicles contrasting with the diffuse macrophage accumulation (Fig. 6.2.10). The macrophages have abundant eosinophilic cytoplasm, which often contains brown granules that stain with both Perls and periodic acid-Schiff reagents (Fig. 6.2.11). Eosinophils may be evident (Fig. 6.2.12)[30] and centriacinar emphysema may be seen as an independent smoking-related condition.

Differential diagnosis
As well as being a response to extrinsic stimuli such as smoke, dust and drugs, DIP, or an appearance very like it, often accompanies other lung diseases, which it may mask.[39] For example, the small, focal lesions of Langerhans cell histiocytosis are often accompanied by an excess of alveolar macrophages and may consequently be overlooked. Similarly, alveolar macrophages are often considerably increased near a tumour and may be the

only abnormality evident in a small biopsy: if a neoplasm is suspected clinically but only an excess of macrophages is found, a further biopsy should be advised rather than proffering a diagnosis of DIP. In resolving eosinophilic pneumonia, eosinophils may be scanty and macrophages numerous so that the appearances simulate DIP.

The frequent association of DIP with cigarette smoking is also seen in respiratory bronchiolitis-associated interstitial lung disease (RB-ILD) (see below), which it closely resembles histologically, the principal differences being the centriacinar concentration of the macrophages and the mild peribronchiolar fibrosis of the latter condition. The term smoking related-interstitial lung disease has been proposed to encompass DIP, respiratory bronchiolitis-associated interstitial lung disease and Langerhans cell histiocytosis,[40] but there are differences in the spectrum of associated clinical disorders.[24]

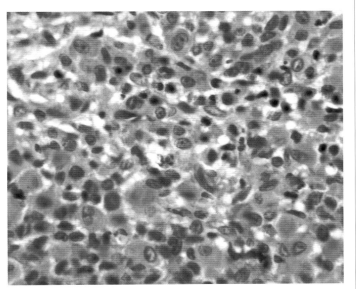

Figure 6.2.12 'Desquamative' interstitial pneumonia. Eosinophils may be amongst the macrophages.

UIP may be associated with considerable numbers of alveolar macrophages and therefore resemble DIP but the latter is more uniform in its distribution and appearance: the patchy subpleural preponderance of UIP is not seen in DIP. These two processes are compared in Table 6.2.2 (see also Fig. 6.1.2b). Any fibrosis that develops in DIP is diffuse and temporally uniform, resembling NSIP more than UIP and possibly representing a further effect of smoking.[30]

If multinucleate macrophages are prominent, the giant cell interstitial pneumonia of cobalt workers may be considered but the multinucleate epithelial cells that characterise this condition are not evident in DIP.

A lipidosis may result in a pattern resembling DIP. Cytoplasmic vacuolation of the alveolar macrophages favours such a diagnosis, especially if there is no evidence of airway obstruction.

Lastly, DIP may be mimicked by an unusual pattern of carcinomatous spread in the lungs, one in which the neoplastic cells are poorly cohesive and fill rather than destroy the alveoli (see Fig. 12.6.7, p. 673). Immunostaining for epithelial and macrophage markers (cytokeratin and CD67, respectively) readily distinguishes the two.[41]

RESPIRATORY BRONCHIOLITIS-ASSOCIATED INTERSTITIAL LUNG DISEASE

Respiratory bronchiolitis (RB) and its clinical correlate respiratory bronchiolitis-associated interstitial lung disease (RBILD)[42] are considered in this chapter rather than that preceding, because they affect the airspaces more than the interstitium and need to be considered in conjunction with DIP. In both these conditions the predominant change is an excess of alveolar macrophages but in RB the changes are centriacinar, the excess macrophages filling alveoli around the terminal and respiratory bronchioles rather than being diffusely distributed throughout the acinus (Fig. 6.2.13). The macrophages also fill the lumina of the respiratory bronchioles. As in DIP the macrophages contain an abundance of brown smoke particles (see Fig. 1.33)

Table 6.2.2 Comparison of UIP and DIP*[33,33a,33b]

	UIP	DIP
Peak age (years)	60–70	30–50
Current cigarette smokers	<15%	About 90%
Lung function	Restrictive. Decrease in DL_{CO}	Restrictive. Decrease in DL_{CO}
Chest radiograph	Basal predominant, reticular abnormality Volume loss	Ground-glass opacity
HRCT	Reticular, honeycombing, traction bronchiectasis Architectural distortion, focal ground-glass	Ground-glass opacity, reticular lines
Response to therapy (steroids +/– immunosuppressive therapy)	Poor	Usually good**
Mortality at 5 years	~20%	~100%
Median survival (years)	2–3	>10

*UIP/DIP: Usual and desquamative patterns of interstitial pneumonia.
**May include smoking cessation.

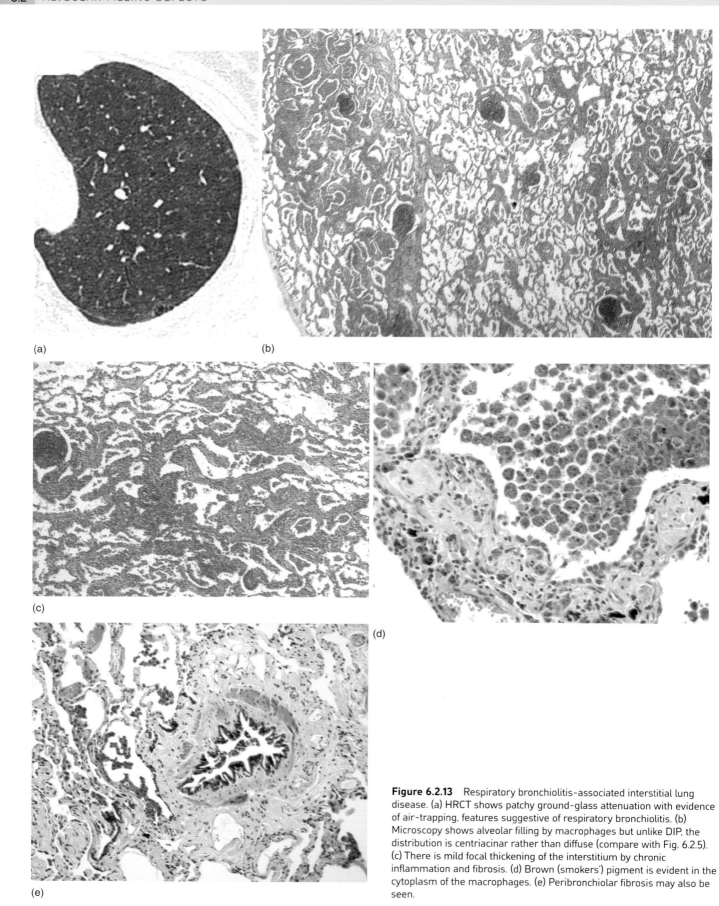

Figure 6.2.13 Respiratory bronchiolitis-associated interstitial lung disease. (a) HRCT shows patchy ground-glass attenuation with evidence of air-trapping, features suggestive of respiratory bronchiolitis. (b) Microscopy shows alveolar filling by macrophages but unlike DIP, the distribution is centriacinar rather than diffuse (compare with Fig. 6.2.5). (c) There is mild focal thickening of the interstitium by chronic inflammation and fibrosis. (d) Brown (smokers') pigment is evident in the cytoplasm of the macrophages. (e) Peribronchiolar fibrosis may also be seen.

and the affected patients are almost universally heavy cigarette smokers.[24a] The interstitial component of the disease is less marked, consisting of a mild-to-moderate degree of chronic inflammation and fibrosis around the bronchioles and involving the walls of adjacent alveoli. The peripheral pulmonary parenchyma is usually normal but may show independent smoking-related changes such as emphysema.[43] 'Honeycombing' is not a feature and if present suggests that the RB is an incidental finding. Distinction from other patterns of interstitial pneumonia is the same as for DIP.

Patients with respiratory bronchiolitis-associated interstitial lung disease are often asymptomatic and unaware that there is anything amiss with their lungs. Others complain of cough and breathlessness.[42,44] Other symptoms include chest pain, weight loss and, rarely, fever and haemoptysis. Clubbing is unusual. Radiologically, there may be linear opacities suggestive of interstitial lung disease. HRCT shows varying degrees of patchy ground glass opacity and centrilobular nodules,[43] and considerable overlap with the appearances of DIP (Fig. 6.2.13a). Similar but less extensive findings are seen in many asymptomatic smokers.[42–45] Lung function tests may be normal or show a mild restrictive defect. RBILD may be considered a peripheral extension of small airway disease (see p. 97), which is well described in young cigarette smokers, coupled with features of DIP concentrated at the centres of the lung acini. It is notable that most patients with DIP are also cigarette smokers (see Table 6.2.2) and it may be that DIP is a particularly florid form of RBILD.[34,44] Many cases formerly identified as DIP would now be regarded as showing RB and the two may merely be regarded as different aspects of 'smoking-related interstitial lung disease'.[40]

EXOGENOUS LIPID PNEUMONIA

Exogenous lipid pneumonia results from the aspiration or inhalation of oils, which may be animal, vegetable or mineral. A common example is liquid paraffin, which gains access to the lungs via the trachea when it is taken orally as a lubricant for constipation and inadvertently aspirated,[46–51] or when it is used as a vehicle for drugs administered by a nasal spray. It is not very irritative and the patient is often unaware that aspiration is occurring. Aspiration of the ingested oil occurs during sleep and is especially likely if there is achalasia of the cardia or hiatus hernia with reflux.[49] Aspiration of petroleum jelly applied to the nose has also led to exogenous lipid pneumonia.[52] Examples of animal or vegetable fat being aspirated include milk[53] or fatty dietary supplements such as ghee[54] entering the lungs of debilitated children with feeding difficulties. The aspiration of vegetable oil also occurred in the past from the use of menthol in olive oil for the treatment of tuberculous laryngitis and occasionally from the use of iodinated vegetable oils for bronchography.[55,56] Unusual causes of exogenous lipid pneumonia include occupational exposure to oil mists[57] and the smoking of blackfat tobacco (see p. 377).[58]

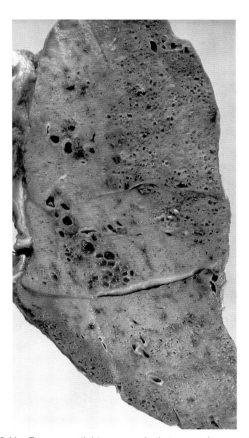

Figure 6.2.14 Exogenous lipid pneumonia that was only recognised post mortem. Subsequent enquiries established that, unknown to her medical attendants, the patient had been ingesting massive amounts of liquid paraffin to counter constipation. (Specimen provided by the late Dr R. Salm, London, UK.)

In the lungs, the oil gives rise to a chronic granulomatous lesion that radiologically may simulate a carcinoma and in some such cases lobectomy has been undertaken unnecessarily.[46] The term 'paraffinoma' is often applied to localised tumour-like lesions caused by the aspiration of liquid paraffin. In other cases, a widespread 'pneumonia' has proved fatal, its true nature only being recognised *post mortem* (Fig. 6.2.14).[48]

Histologically, droplets of oil are surrounded by macrophages and foreign body giant cells. The droplets may form a fine sieve-like pattern, but adjoining droplets tend to coalesce, with the result that many alveoli are filled by a single large globule (Fig. 6.2.15a). Since the oil is dissolved out in histological processing, the alveoli appear empty and may be mistakenly thought to have contained air rather than lipid. Attention may then be concentrated on the relatively minor interstitial changes and the alveolar filling overlooked. On closer examination, however, multinucleated giant cells are evident stretched around the globules and this should suggest the true diagnosis. If reserve tissue is available, frozen sections may be stained for fat (Fig. 6.2.15b).

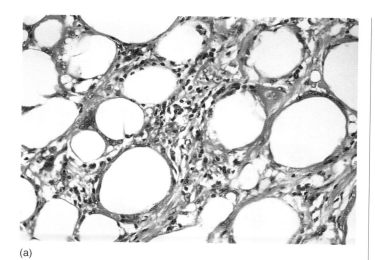

(a)

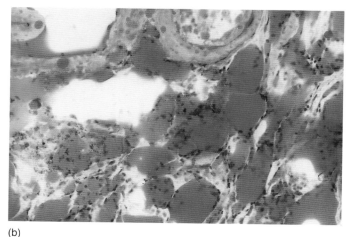

(b)

Figure 6.2.15 Exogenous lipid pneumonia. (a) What might appear at first sight to be airspaces actually represent dissolved globules of liquid paraffin; multinucleate foreign body giant cells stretched around the globules provide a clue to the diagnosis. (b) Oil red O fat stain performed on frozen section shows that the spaces contain lipid rather than air.

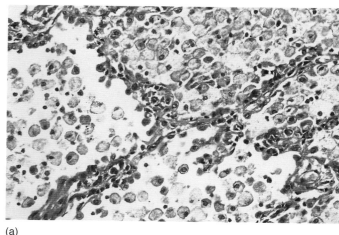

(a)

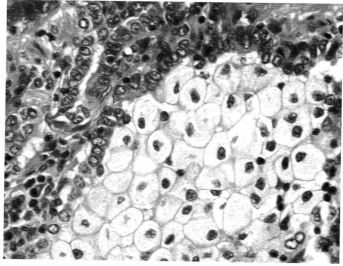

(b)

Figure 6.2.16 Endogenous lipid pneumonia due to bronchial obstruction. The clearance of lung lipids, chiefly spent surfactant, is impaired and foamy macrophages fill the alveoli (a). (b) In contrast to exogenous lipoid pneumonia the cytoplasm shows fine vacuolation.

In contrast to the relatively inactive long chain saturated hydrocarbons of mineral derivation, animal oils may cause intense inflammation and even necrosis. This is caused by injurious free fatty acids, which may be present in the oil itself, or released by enzymatic action within the lungs.

Most animal and vegetable oils contain unsaturated lipids, which are osmiophilic, whereas mineral oils such as liquid paraffin that are fully saturated do not stain with osmic acid. Halogenated hydrocarbons such as the bronchography medium lipiodol (iodised poppy seed oil) can be differentially stained with brilliant cresyl blue.[59] In a few cases, infrared spectrophotometry has been used to identify the nature of the oils.[47,49,50]

In infants, the presence of foamy macrophages in the sputum or bronchoalveolar lavage is often taken to indicate gastric reflux and poorly defined respiratory problems are then ascribed to the aspiration of gastric material,[60,61] but this cannot go unchallenged as macrophage clearance is one of the ways

the lung normally rids itself of spent surfactant, resulting in lipid-laden foamy macrophages.

ENDOGENOUS LIPID PNEUMONIA (OBSTRUCTIVE PNEUMONITIS)

The lung generates considerable amounts of lipid to reduce alveolar surface tension. Much of this lipid is recycled by the alveolar epithelium but some is cleared via the airways and if these are obstructed, for example, by a tumour, then the spent surfactant accumulates in alveolar macrophages. These cells often increase in number and size and take on the usual appearance of lipophages, developing a voluminous foamy cytoplasm (Fig. 6.2.16). The alveoli become filled with these cells and macroscopically the affected area shows yellow consolidation,

Table 6.2.3   Comparison of exogenous and endogenous lipid pneumonia

	Exogenous	Endogenous
Foamy macrophages	Intra-alveolar and interstitial	Usually intra-alveolar
Giant cells	Around droplets	Absent (except around cholesterol crystals)
Extracellular fat droplets	Many and varied in size	Absent
Obstructing lesion	Absent	Sometimes present
Lipid	Usually mineral (saturated and therefore non-osmiophilic)	Animal (unsaturated and therefore osmiophilic)

Table 6.2.4   Causes of endogenous lipoid pneumonia

Localised	Airway obstruction (usually tumour)
	Successful tumour ablation
Bronchocentric	Diffuse panbronchiolitis
Diffuse	Drug reaction (e.g. amiodarone)
	Inborn error of metabolism (e.g. Niemann–Pick)

sometimes referred to as golden or obstructive pneumonia.[62,63] Similar changes develop when the alveolar architecture is disrupted, impairing the clearance of lung lipids, as in diffuse fibrosis. In long-standing cases foamy macrophages may distend the interstitium rather than the airspaces and the appearances simulate those of diffuse panbronchiolitis (see p. 122). Endogenous and exogenous lipid are compared in Table 6.2.3.

Chronic interstitial pneumonia generally develops and if the obstruction is not relieved, infection is almost inevitable, causing acute pneumonia, which may progress to abscess formation or bronchiectasis. Occasionally granulomatous inflammation destroys the walls of airways beyond the obstruction, closely simulating the appearances of bronchocentric granulomatosis.[64] Sometimes the foamy macrophages disintegrate to release their charge of ingested lipid and the accumulation of this material may closely simulate the appearances of alveolar lipoproteinosis, which is described next, even to the extent of including cholesterol crystals. Endogenous lipid pneumonia may also develop without airway obstruction in lipidoses such as Niemann–Pick disease[65] and in response to amphiphilic drugs such as amiodarone (Table 6.2.4).

ALVEOLAR LIPOPROTEINOSIS

Alveolar lipoproteinosis is a rare condition characterised by finely granular eosinophilic material filling the air spaces. It was first named and is still generally known as pulmonary alveolar proteinosis,[66] but lipoproteinosis reflects better the chemical composition of the alveolar material. The nature of the lipoprotein varies and several causes are now recognised. Since its initial description in 1958, over 400 cases have been reported.[67]

Aetiology and pathogenesis
Alveolar lipoproteinosis has long been regarded as representing a failure of the alveolar macrophages to rid the lungs of spent surfactant[68–71] and it is now recognised that this defect

generally has an autoimmune basis. In most cases the condition is attributable to the development of autoantibodies that neutralise granulocyte-macrophage colony-stimulating factor and so impair macrophage function.[72–74] An alveolar CD4 lymphocytosis is evident once the alveoli have been cleared of the lipoproteinaceous material.[75]

In other patients the condition is secondary to heavy dust exposure.[76–80] Here it appears to be due to hypersecretion of surfactant exceeding the capability of the normal clearance mechanism. Evidence for this derives from animal dusting experiments leading to alveolar lipoproteinosis in which it was found that surfactant synthesis trebled whereas macrophage clearance only doubled.[81,82] Such experiments also show that the condition evolves through a stage of endogenous lipid pneumonia characterised by the accumulation of large lipid-laden macrophages that eventually break down to release their burden of spent surfactant.[83,84] At first the released material is loosely floccular and weakly staining but it gradually condenses to assume the characteristic staining properties of alveolar lipoproteinosis described below.[85] Some patients exhibit both alveolar lipoproteinosis and endogenous lipid pneumonia.[86]

In a further animal model, rats given high doses of amphiphilic drugs such as chlorphentermine, iprindole and amiodarone over long periods developed endogenous lipid pneumonia[87–89] and occasionally this progressed to alveolar lipoproteinosis.[90] These drugs block lysosomal sphingomyelinase and phospholipase and the material that accumulates in the alveoli of these animals represents the accumulated substrate of these lipases. The process here is analogous to the lipid storage disorders, except that the lysosomal deficiency is acquired rather than inborn.

Alveolar lipoproteinosis has also been reported in children with various enzyme defects, notably one that results in deficiency of surfactant protein B (see p. 45).[91–96] It seems likely that in these children the alveolar lipoproteinosis represents a compensatory hypersecretion of surfactant. Again there is an initial stage of endogenous lipid pneumonia, representing macrophage ingestion of the excess surfactant. Alveolar lipoproteinosis has also been reported in patients with lysinuric protein intolerance, appearing first in either childhood[97,98] or adult life.[99] These patients are therefore also presumed to have a defect in surfactant synthesis. Other children with alveolar lipoproteinosis show mutation of the gene responsible for the β-chain of the granulocyte-macrophage colony-stimulating factor receptor.[100]

Other patients with alveolar lipoproteinosis have leukaemia, lymphoma or other diseases characterised by immunosup-

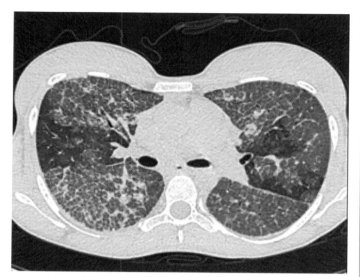

Figure 6.2.17 Alveolar lipoproteinosis. HRCT shows a 'crazy paving' pattern of opacification.

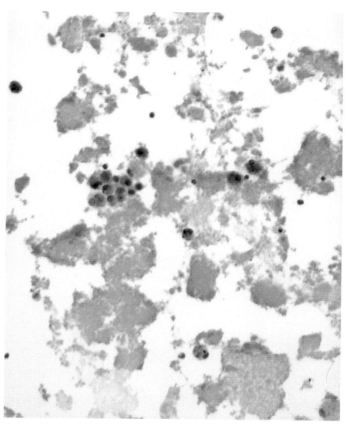

Figure 6.2.18 Alveolar lipoproteinosis. Lung lavage shows clumps of acellular proteinaceous debris with very few inflammatory cells (Papanicolau stain).

pression,[101–104] In these patients surfactant is only weakly represented in the alveolar material[105,106] and there is also interstitial pneumonia or fibrosis.[107] The pathogenesis in these patients is poorly understood but the lipoprotein may represent autophagosomal residual bodies extruded from degenerate alveolar cells.[108] A similar mechanism may operate in the rare cases that complicate pulmonary infection[109] or lung transplantation.[110]

Appearances very similar to those of alveolar lipoproteinosis may result from bronchial obstruction, as described above under endogenous lipid pneumonia. They have also been described in association with a surfactant-secreting bronchioloalveolar cell carcinoma.[111]

One conclusion to be drawn from these varied observations is that alveolar lipoproteinosis represents a clinico-pathological syndrome of multiple causation rather than a single disease.

Clinical features

Alveolar lipoproteinosis may affect patients of any age, but the majority are between 30 and 50 years, with men outnumbering women by 4 to 1 and there being an increased incidence in smokers.[112,113] However, the genetic defects referred to above generally manifest themselves in childhood. Rare familial cases have been reported.[114,115] The main symptom is slowly increasing dyspnoea. Radiographically, alveolar lipoproteinosis is often characterised by patches of consolidation alternating with normal lung although in the first case to be described there were perihilar feathery opacities that suggested oedema.[66] However, no cause for oedema was apparent and no evidence of oedema is ever found on auscultation. HRCT is characteristic, showing a 'crazy paving' pattern of alveolar 'ground-glass' consolidation with interlobular septal thickening (Fig. 6.2.17).[113,116,117] The diagnosis may be established by bronchoalveolar lavage (Fig. 6.2.18),[112,118–120] while the identification of autoantibodies against

granulocyte macrophage colony-stimulating factor is diagnostic in those cases in which these antibodies play a causative role.[121]

Spontaneous remission occurs in about a third of patients, a further third stabilise and the remainder progress.[122] These last patients formerly died of the disease but therapeutic lung lavage[118,123–125] has transformed the prognosis and more recently the subcutaneous injection of granulocyte-macrophage colony-stimulating factor has been introduced as a further treatment option.[75,126] The regulatory relationship between interleukin-10 and GM-CSF suggest that levels of IL-10 and anti-GM-CSF titres are indicative of response to GM-CSF therapy.[125,127,128]

Therapeutic lavage is performed under general anaesthesia, one lung being washed out at a time with up to 30 l of saline introduced through a cuffed double lumen tube that permits respiration to continue in the other lung.[118,123] The recovered lavage fluid is milky white and with time white flocculent material precipitates out (Fig. 6.2.19). Residual saline is rapidly absorbed.[129] Lavage may be repeated if the disease recurs and ultimately this treatment generally proves effective. Some patients have undergone lung transplantation but recurrent alveolar lipoproteinosis is recorded, even following double lung transplantation.[130]

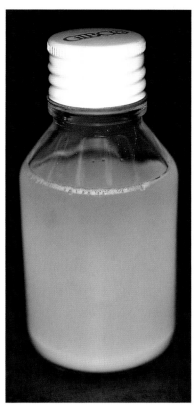

Figure 6.2.19 Alveolar lipoproteinosis. Therapeutic bronchoalveolar lavage recovers an opalescent, white fluid.

Pathological features

Chemical analysis of material washed from patients' lungs shows considerable amounts of lipids, including those that normally lower the alveolar surface tension. The lavage material is deficient in such physical properties, perhaps due to lysosomal activity within alveolar macrophages, but its surface activity can be restored by ethanol.[131]

Histologically, the alveoli are filled with a finely granular acellular deposit that is eosinophilic and generally periodic acid-Schiff positive and diastase-resistant (Fig. 6.2.20a,b).[66,101] The staining with periodic acid-Schiff reagents is explained by the presence of large amounts of surfactant apoprotein, which is heavily glycosylated. The surfactant apoprotein can also be demonstrated immunohistochemically (Fig. 6.2.20c).[105,106] Electron microscopy shows that the alveolar deposit consists of innumerable osmiophilic lamellar bodies consistent with denatured surfactant (Fig. 6.2.21).[118] Foamy macrophages and cholesterol crystal clefts are often found within the granular material. The alveolar walls are generally unremarkable and the condition is essentially an alveolar-filling defect. However, those cases in which the disease complicates immunosuppression differ in that surfactant apoprotein is only weakly represented[106] and there is also interstitial pneumonia or fibrosis.[106–108]

At autopsy, the lungs are heavy, firm and yellow on the cut surface (Fig. 6.2.22).

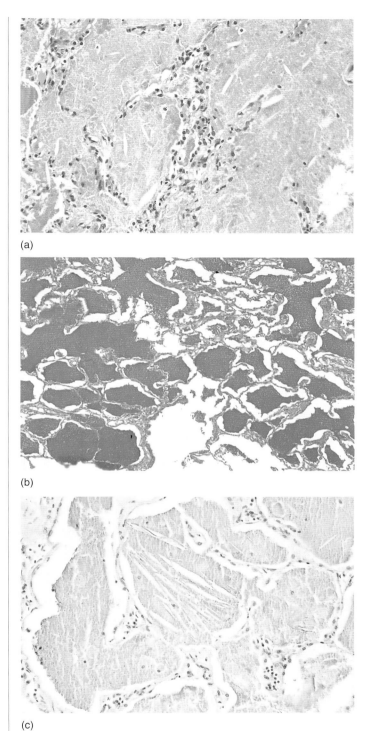

(a)

(b)

(c)

Figure 6.2.20 Alveolar lipoproteinosis. The alveoli are filled by eosinophilic amorphous or finely granular material in which there are the acicular clefts of dissolved cholesterol. The alveolar walls are unremarkable. (a) Haematoxylin and eosin stain. (b) Periodic acid-Schiff stain. (c) Immunoperoxidase stain for surfactant apoprotein.

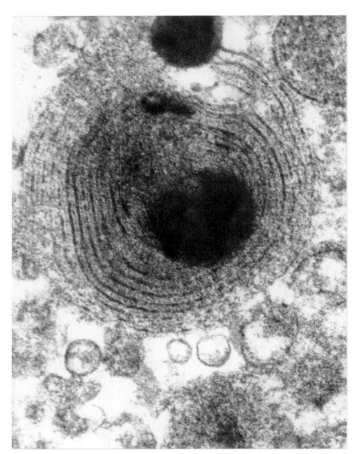

Figure 6.2.21 Alveolar lipoproteinosis. Electron microscopy of the alveolar material recovered in lung washings. The granular material is lamellar and osmiophilic. The appearances are those of a complex lipid and are consistent with the material representing denatured surfactant.

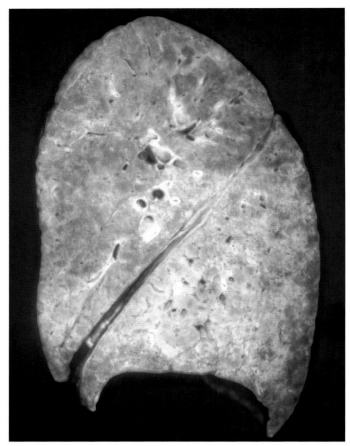

Figure 6.2.22 Alveolar lipoproteinosis. At autopsy the lungs are heavy, firm and yellow on the cut surface.

Differential diagnosis

The differential diagnosis of alveolar lipoproteinosis is from Pneumocystis pneumonia and pulmonary oedema, but the alveolar material is granular rather than foamy or amorphous and is associated with cholesterol crystal clefts and foamy macrophages that are not found in either of these conditions.

Complications

Opportunistic infections represent the major complication of alveolar lipoproteinosis. Nocardia and fungi are mainly involved but mycobacteriosis may also develop.[132–134] It is notable that the growth of these microbes is enhanced *in vitro* if their culture medium is enriched with the lipoproteinaceous material obtained at lavage.[135] Infection is also promoted by abnormalities in surfactant apoprotein and poor macrophage function impairing host defence.[68–70]

CHOLESTEROL PNEUMONITIS

Cholesterol accumulation in the lung is manifest in paraffin sections as sheaves of acicular crystal clefts in both the alveolar spaces and interstitium (Fig. 6.2.23). The cholesterol crystals are frequently attended by foreign body giant cells and a non-specific chronic inflammatory infiltrate. Large numbers of cholesterol crystals may be seen in obstructive pneumonitis and also without recognised cause.[136] Disruption of the alveolar architecture, as in diffuse fibrosis, impairs the clearance of lung lipids and leads to the accumulation of surfactant, which may be manifest as focal alveolar lipoproteinosis and cholesterol pneumonitis. Diffuse pulmonary fibrosis is often accompanied by type II cell hyperplasia and the metabolic activity of these surfactant synthesising cells may also contribute to the accumulation of cholesterol and other lipids.[137]

Scanty cholesterol crystal clefts are often a feature of extrinsic allergic alveolitis and are occasionally seen in other granulomatous conditions, for example, sarcoid. They are also recorded in pulmonary hypertension,[138,139] and localised collections are found in necrotic foci such as chronic tuberculous lesions and progressive massive fibrosis of coal-workers.

A review[140] of idiopathic cholesterol pneumonitis identified it as a disease of the elderly, particularly men who were heavy smokers, but the disease is also encountered in children, sometimes in siblings. In children it may sometimes co-exist with or progress to alveolar lipoproteinosis (Figs 6.2.22, 6.2.23).[141] The

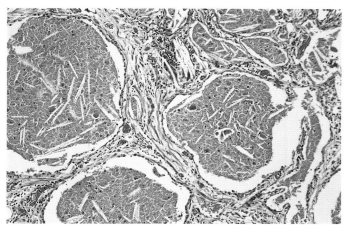

Figure 6.2.23 Cholesterol pneumonitis. Numerous elongated clefts of dissolved cholesterol crystals are evident in this lung biopsy of a young girl who within 4 years had died of alveolar lipoproteinosis (shown in Fig. 6.2.22).

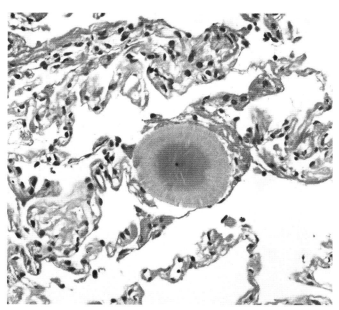

Figure 6.2.24 Corpora amylacea. These structures are sometimes found incidentally in the lungs. This one has a central black particle, which has possibly acted as the starting point on which the body has formed.

relationship of cholesterol pneumonitis to alveolar lipoproteinosis is also demonstrated by the development of either condition in patients with errors in surfactant synthesis and lysinuric protein intolerance.[97–99]

Changes resembling those of cholesterol pneumonitis are found in alkane lipogranulomatosis but this is a generalised storage disorder that affects many other organs as well as the lungs (see p. 492).

CORPORA AMYLACEA

Corpora amylacea identical to those more commonly seen in the prostate were first described in the lungs by Friedrich in 1856.[142] They are an incidental finding, more common in the elderly and on occasion they may be observed in the sputum.[143] They are round, intra-alveolar structures, 50–150 µm diameter, which stain uniformly with both eosin and Congo red (Fig. 6.2.24). With the latter stain, polarisers show both the birefringence and dichroism of amyloid,[143] which immunocytochemically is shown to be derived from β-2 macroglobulin.[144] Polarising filters also show both radial striations and circumferential lamellae,[143] the latter representing periodic precipitation zones (Liesegang rings) that occur spontaneously in colloidal solutions.[145] Electron microscopy[143] shows that the bodies consist largely of sheaves of microfibrils, possibly representing cytokeratin derived from alveolar epithelial cells. Elongated macrophages occasionally adhere to the surface of the bodies. Occasionally a central black spherule is evident, suggesting that a dust particle has provided a nidus on which alveolar secretions of cellular components may have precipitated (Fig. 6.2.24).[143,146] Corpora amylacea are merely microscopic curiosities that have no clinical importance, unless they are mistaken for fungal spores or parasitic ova.

ALVEOLAR MICROLITHIASIS

Alveolar microlithiasis is a rare condition of unknown aetiology characterised by extensive alveolar accumulation of calcified microliths in the absence of any recognised abnormality of calcium metabolism. It was first described in 1918[147] and received its current designation in 1933.[148] Over 400 cases have now been reported, 269 sporadic and 155 familial, the latter probably reflecting autosomal recessive inheritance.[149–152] Virtually any age group may be affected but the third and fourth decades are most frequently involved.[149,150,153,154] Males outnumber females in the sporadic cases whereas the reverse is true when the disease is familial. There is a wide geographical distribution but exceptionally high numbers are reported from Turkey, Italy and the USA.[155,156]

The disease is characterised by a distinctive fine micronodular calcification in the lungs that is heaviest basally or around the hila but may be so extensive as to produce almost complete radiographic opacification. Lymph nodes are not enlarged. The condition may be symptomless and discovered by chance on routine chest radiography. HRCT shows dense alveolar calcification with a perilobular and bronchovascular distribution at the level of the secondary pulmonary lobule.[157] The disease may stabilise at any time but more often over a period of many years it progressively restricts lung movement and impairs gas diffusion until it eventually leads to severe dyspnoea and death from respiratory and cardiac failure.[150,158,159] No effective medical treatment has yet been reported except for regression of the opacification in one patient treated with disodium editronate, an agent that inhibits the microcrystalline growth of hydroxyapatite.[160] Lung transplantation has proved successful in some cases.[161]

Many cases have been diagnosed at necropsy, when the lungs are rock-hard and extremely heavy, a band saw generally being needed to cut them into slices. However, with greater recognition of the disorder, diagnosis is now usually made on either transbronchial biopsy or bronchoalveolar lavage. Indeed, HRCT alone may be sufficient in when other family members are affected.[156] In decalcified sections, enormous numbers of wavy concentrically laminate microliths, up to 300 μm in diameter can be seen filling the alveoli (Fig. 6.2.25). The alveolar walls surrounding them may undergo fibrosis. In less advanced areas, only occasional microliths are scattered among otherwise normal air spaces. Rarely, the microliths are also present in the alveolar interstitium and bronchial mucosa.[162] Sometimes they are identified in the sputum,[150,163] where they are to be distinguished from the larger 'liths' that derive from a focus of dystrophic calcification eroding a bronchus.[164,165] Analysis shows them to consist of calcium and phosphorus salts in the form of carboxyapatite.[154,166,167]

CALCOSPHERITES (CONCHOIDAL BODIES)

The term calcospherite or conchoidal body is applied to certain laminated calcified structures found in either the air spaces or the tissues of the lung, where they are respectively known as blue bodies and Schaumann bodies.

'Blue bodies'

Blue bodies are laminated intra-alveolar structures that are usually found in focal collections (Fig. 6.2.26).[168–170] Individually, they measure 15–40 μm diameter and are hence smaller than microliths or corpora amylacea. The name blue body derives from their weak haematoxyphilia. Calcium carbonate in a mucopolysaccharide matrix is the major component but there is also an outer rim of iron. Blue bodies are most frequently found when there is an excessive number of alveolar macrophages, as in desquamative interstitial pneumonia; they probably represent the extruded residual bodies of lysosomes. They are a histopathological curio of no clinical importance, unless mistaken for life-threatening conditions such as alveolar microlithiasis (see above).[171]

Schaumann bodies

Schaumann bodies are found within connective tissue rather than the air spaces but will be dealt with here as they are similar to blue bodies. They are commonly found in granulomas and like blue bodies, they probably represent the residuum of lysosomal activity. They may be found in large numbers in the scars of healed sarcoidosis or berylliosis (see Fig. 6.1.31). They are larger than blue bodies, measuring up to 80 μm in diameter and are more distinctly laminate and calcific. Similar calcospherites

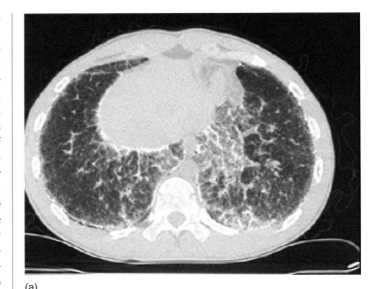

(a)

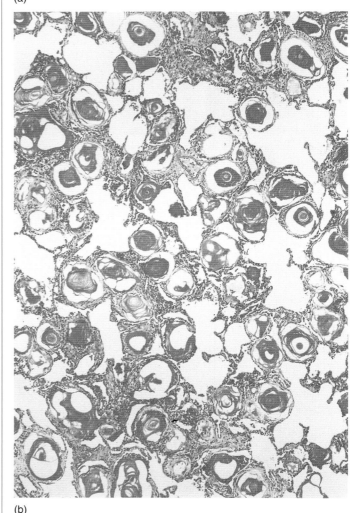

(b)

Figure 6.2.25 Alveolar microlithiasis. (a) HRCT shows patchy alveolar shadowing with dense subpleural and septal opacification. (b) The alveoli are filled by innumerable heavily calcified lamellar bodies of wavy configuration.

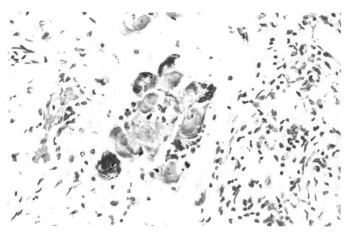

Figure 6.2.26 Alveolar calcospherites. These structures probably derive from alveolar macrophage lysosomal activity, being found in conditions marked by increased numbers of these cells. Their haematoxyphilia is responsible for their colloquial name of 'blue bodies'.

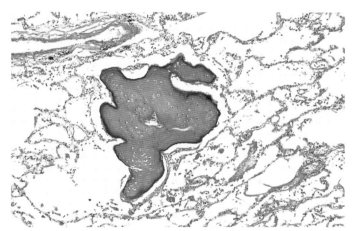

Figure 6.2.27 Osseous metaplasia. An incidental finding in the lungs of a man dying of unrelated causes.

are sometimes found within the stroma of papillary tumours, both in the lung and other organs.

ALVEOLAR OSSIFICATION

Dystrophic ossification is common in the lung but is interstitial and is therefore dealt with elsewhere (see p. 145). This section deals with isolated foci of laminated bone that are found on occasion within alveoli of otherwise normal appearance (Fig. 6.2.27).[172,173] This form of ossification is commonest in the elderly and particularly in association with prolonged pulmonary congestion or thromboembolism. It is therefore likely to represent a form of acquired metaplasia rather than a congenital heterotopia. It is generally an incidental finding of no clinical consequence.

REFERENCES

Cryptogenic organizing pneumonia

1. Liebow AA, Carrington CB. The interstitial pneumonias. In: Simon M, ed. Frontiers of Pulmonary Radiology New York: Grune & Stratton; 1969:102–141.
2. Otto H, Mieth I. Morphology and therapeutic chances of interstitial lung disease. Respiration 1979; 38:171–176.
3. Grinblat J, Mechlis S, Lewitus Z. Organising pneumonia-like process. An unusual observation in steroid responsive cases with features of chronic interstitial pneumonia. Chest 1981; 80:259–263.
4. Davison AG, Heard BE, McAllister WAC, Turner-Warwick MEH. Cryptogenic organising pneumonitis. Q J Med 1983; 52:382–394.
5. Epler GR, Colby TV, McLoud TC, Carrington CB, Gaensler EA. Bronchiolitis obliterans organising pneumonia. N Engl J Med 1985; 312:152–158.
6. Fukuda Y, Ishizaki M, Kudoh S, Kitaichi M, Yamanaka N. Localization of matrix metalloproteinases-1, –2 and –9 and tissue inhibitor of metalloproteinase-2 in interstitial lung diseases. Lab Invest 1998; 78:687–698.
7. King TE. BOOP: an important cause of migratory pulmonary infiltrates? Eur Respir J 1995; 8:193–195.
8. Costabel U, Teschler H, Guzman J. Bronchiolitis obliterans organising pneumonia (BOOP) - the cytological and immunocytological profile of bronchoalveolar lavage. Eur Respir J 1992; 5:791–797.
9. Cordier JF. Organising pneumonia. Thorax 2000; 55(4):318–328.
10. Spiteri MA, Klenerman P, Sheppard MN, Padley S, Clark TJK, Newman-Taylor A. Seasonal cryptogenic organising pneumonia with biochemical cholestasis – a new clinical entity. Lancet 1992; 340:281–284.
11. Miyagawa Y, Nagata N, Shigematsu N. Clinicopathological study of migratory lung infiltrates. Thorax 1991; 46:233–238.
12. Crestani B, Kambouchner M, Soler P, et al. Migratory bronchiolitis obliterans organising pneumonia after unilateral radiation therapy for breast carcinoma. Eur Respir J 1995; 8:318–321.
13. Bayle JY, Nesme P, Bejui-Thivolet F, Loire R, Guerin JC, Cordier JF. Migratory organising pneumonitis 'primed' by radiation therapy. Eur Respir J 1995; 8:322–326.
14. Stover DE, Milite F, Zakowski M. A newly recognized syndrome – Radiation related bronchiolitis obliterans and organising pneumonia. Respiration 2001; 68:540–544.
15. Yigla M, BenItzhak O, Solomonov A, Guralnik L, Oren I. Recurrent, self-limited, menstrual-associated bronchiolitis obliterans organising pneumonia. Chest 2000; 118(1):253–256.
16. Cohen AJ, King TEJr, Downey GP. Rapidly progressive bronchiolitis obliterans with organising pneumonia. Am J Respir Crit Care Med 1994; 149:1670–1675.
17. Colby TV. Pathologic aspects of bronchiolitis obliterans organising pneumonia. Chest 1992; 102:S38–S43.
18. Myers JL, Katzenstein A-LA. Ultrastructural evidence of alveolar epithelial injury in idiopathic bronchiolitis obliterans-organising pneumonia. Am J Pathol 1988; 132:102–109.
19. Yousem SA, Lohr RH, Colby TV. Idiopathic bronchiolitis obliterans organising pneumonia/cryptogenic organising pneumonia with unfavorable outcome: Pathologic predictors. Modern Pathol 1997; 10:864–871.
20. Beasley MB, Franks TJ, Galvin JR, Gochuico B, Travis WD. Acute fibrinous and organising pneumonia – A histologic pattern of lung injury and possible variant of diffuse alveolar damage. Arch Pathol Lab Med 2002; 126:1064–1070.

Desquamative interstitial pneumonia

21. Liebow AA. Definition and classification of interstitial pneumonias in human pathology. Prog Resp Res 1975; 8:1–33.
22. Leroy EP. Desquamative interstitial pneumonia. Virchows Arch A Pathol Anat Histopathol 1969; 348:117–130.

23. Corrin B, Price AB. Electron microscopic studies in desquamative interstitial pneumonia associated with asbestos. Thorax 1972; 27:324–331.

24. American Thoracic Society/European Respiratory Society international multidisciplinary consensus classification of the idiopathic interstitial pneumonias. Am J Respir Crit Care Med 2002; 165:277–304.

24a. Ryu JH, Myers JL, Capizzi SA, et al. Desquamative interstitial pneumonia and respiratory bronchiolitis-associated interstitial lung disease. Chest 2005; 127:178–184.

25. Herbert A, Sterling G, Abraham J, Corrin B. Desquamative interstitial pneumonia in an aluminum welder. Hum Pathol 1982; 13:694–699.

26. Freed JA, Miller A, Gordon RE, Fischbein A, Kleinerman J, Langer AM. Desquamative interstitial pneumonia associated with chrysotile asbestos fibres. Br J Ind Med 1991; 48:332–337.

27. Abraham JL, Hertzberg MA. Inorganic particulates associated with desquamative interstitial pneumonia. Chest 1981; 80S:67S–70S.

28. Bone RC, Wolfe J, Sobonya RE, et al. Desquamative interstitial pneumonia following long-term nitrofurantoin therapy. Am J Med 1976; 60:697–701.

29. Tubbs RR, Benjamin SP, Reich NE, McCormack LJ, van Ordstrand HS. Desquamative interstitial pneumonitis: cellular phase of fibrosing alveolitis. Chest 1977; 72:159–165.

30. Craig PJ, Wells AU, Doffman S et al. Desquamative interstitial pneumonia, respiratory bronchiolitis and their relationship to smoking. Histopathology 2004; 45; 275–282.

31. Hartman TE, Primack SL, Kang EY, et al. Disease progression in usual interstitial pneumonia compared with desquamative interstitial pneumonia: assessment with serial CT. Chest 1996; 110:378–382.

32. Akira M, Yamamoto S, Hara H, Sakatani M, Ueda E. Serial computed tomographic evaluation in desquamative interstitial pneumonia. Thorax 1997; 52:333–337.

33. Carrington CB, Gaensler EA, Coutu RE, FitzGerald MX, Gupta RG. Natural history and treated course of usual and desquamative interstitial pneumonia. N Engl J Med 1978; 298:801–809.

33a. Nicholson AG, Colby TV, du Bois RM, et al. The prognostic significance of the histologic pattern of interstitial pneumonia in patients presenting with clinical entity of cryptogenic fibrosing alveolitis. Am J Respir Crit Care Med 2000; 162:2213–2217.

33b. American Thoracic Society/European Respiratory Society International Multidisciplinary Consensus Classification of the Idiopathic Interstitial Pneumonias. Am J Respir Crit Care Med 2002; 165:277–304.

34. Turner-Warwick M, Burrows B, Johnson A. Cryptogenic fibrosing alveolitis: clinical features and their influence on survival. Thorax 1980; 35:171–180.

35. Hunter AM, Lamb D. Relapse of fibrosing alveolitis (desquamative interstitial pneumonia) after twelve years. Thorax 1979; 34:677–679.

36. Lipworth BJ, Woodcock A, Addis B, Turner-Warwick M. Late relapse of desquamative interstitial pneumonia. Am Rev Respir Dis 1987; 136:1253–1255.

37. Verleden GM, Sels F, VanRaemdonck D, Verbeken EK, Lerut T, Demedts M. Possible recurrence of desquamative interstitial pneumonitis in a single lung transplant recipient. Eur Resp J 1998; 11:971–974.

38. McCann BG, Brewer DB. A case of desquamative interstitial pneumonia progressing to 'honeycomb lung'. J Pathol 1974; 112:199–202.

39. Bedrossian CWM, Kuhn C, Luna MA, Conklin RH, Byrd RB, Kaplan PD. Desquamative interstitial pneumonia-like reaction accompanying pulmonary lesions. Chest 1977; 72:166–169.

40. Ryu JH, Colby TV, Hartman TE, Vassallo R. Smoking-related interstitial lung diseases: a concise review. Eur Resp J 2001; 17:122–132.

41. Mutton AE, Hasleton PS, Curry A, et al. Differentiation of desquamative interstitial pneumonia (DIP) from pulmonary adenocarcinoma by immunocytochemistry. Histopathology 1998; 33:129–135.

Respiratory bronchiolitis-associated interstitial lung disease

42. Myers JL, Veal CF, Shin MS, Katzenstein A-LA. Respiratory bronchiolitis causing interstitial lung disease. A clinicopathological study of six cases. Am Rev Respir Dis 1987; 135:880–884.

43. Moon J, Dubois RM, Colby TV, Hansell DM, Nicholson AG. Clinical significance of respiratory bronchiolitis on open lung biopsy and its relationship to smoking related interstitial lung disease. Thorax 1999; 54:1009–1014.

44. Yousem SA, Colby TV, Gaensler EA. Respiratory bronchiolitis-associated interstitial lung disease and its relationship to desquamative interstitial pneumonia. Mayo Clin Proc 1989; 64:1373–1380.

45. Heyneman LE, Ward S, Lynch DA, Remy-Jardin M, Johkoh T, Muller NL. Respiratory bronchiolitis, respiratory bronchiolitis-associated interstitial lung disease and desquamative interstitial pneumonia: different entities or part of the spectrum of the same disease process? Am J Roentgenol 1999; 173:1617–1622.

Exogenous lipid pneumonia

46. Wagner JC, Adler DI, Fuller DN. Foreign body granulomata of the lungs due to liquid paraffin. Thorax 1955; 10:157–170.

47. Elston CW. Pneumonia due to liquid paraffin: with chemical analysis. Arch Dis Child 1966; 41:428–434.

48. Salm R, Hughes EW. A case of chronic paraffin pneumonitis. Thorax 1970; 25:762–768.

49. Fox B. Liquid paraffin pneumonia – with chemical analysis and electron microscopy. Virchows Arch A Pathol Anat Histopathol 1979; 382:339–346.

50. Corrin B, Crocker PR, Hood BJ, Levison DA, Parkes WR. Paraffinoma confirmed by infrared spectrophotometry. Thorax 1987; 42:389–390.

51. Midulla F, Strappini PM, Ascoli V, et al. Bronchoalveolar lavage cell analysis in a child with chronic lipid pneumonia. Eur Resp J 1998; 11:239–242.

52. Brown AC, Slocum PC, Putthoff SL, Wallace WE, Foresman BH. Exogenous lipoid pneumonia due to nasal application of petroleum jelly. Chest 1994; 105:968–969.

53. Gibson JB. Infection of the lungs by 'saprophytic' mycobacteria in achalasia of the cardia, with report of a fatal case showing lipoid pneumonia due to milk. J Pathol Bacteriol 1953; 65:239–251.

54. Annobil SH, Morad NA, Khurana P, Kameswaran M, Ogunbiyi O, Almalki T. Reaction of human lungs to aspirated animal fat (ghee): a clinicopathological study. Virchows Arch 1995; 426:301–305.

55. Felton WL. The reaction of pulmonary tissue to lipiodol. J Thorac Surg 1953; 25:530–542.

56. Greenberg SD, Spjut HJ, Hallman GL. Experimental study of bronchographic media on lung. Arch Otolaryngol Head Neck Surg 1966; 83:276–282.

57. Skorodin MS, Chandrasekhar AJ. An occupational cause of exogenous lipoid pneumonia. Arch Pathol Lab Med 1983; 107:610–611.

58. Miller GJ, Ashcroft MT, Beadnell HMSG, Wagner JC, Pepys J. The lipoid pneumonia of blackfat tobacco smokers in Guyana. Q J Med 1971; 40:457–470.

59. Felton WL. A method for the identification of lipiodol in tissue sections. Lab Invest 1952; 1:364–367.

60. Nussbaum E, Maggi JC, Mathis R, Galant SP. Association of lipid-laden alveolar macrophages and gastroesophageal reflux in children. J Pediatr 1987; 110:190–194.

61. Moran JR, Block SM, Lyerly AD, Brooks LE, Dillard RG. Lipid-laden alveolar macrophages and lactose assay as markers of aspiration in neonates with lung disease. J Pediatr 1988; 112:643–645.

Endogenous lipid pneumonia

62. De Navasquez SJ, Trounce JR, Wayte AB. Lipoid pneumonia (non-inhalation) in carcinoma of the lung treated by radiotherapy. Lancet 1951; 1:1206–1208.

63. De Navasquez SJ, Haslewood GAD. Endogenous lipoid pneumonia with special reference to carcinoma of the lung. Thorax 1954; 9:35–37.

64. Clee MD, Lamb D, Clark RA. Bronchocentric granulomatosis: a review and thoughts on pathogenesis. Br J Dis Chest 1983; 77:227–234.

65. Nicholson AG, Wells AU, Hooper J, Hansell DM, Kelleher A, Morgan C. Successful treatment of endogenous lipoid pneumonia due to Niemann-Pick type B disease with whole-lung lavage. Am J Respir Crit Care Med 2002; 165:128–131.

Alveolar lipoproteinosis

66. Rosen SH, Castleman B, Liebow AA. Pulmonary alveolar proteinosis. N Engl J Med 1958; 258:1123–1142.

67. Seymour JF, Presneill JJ. Pulmonary alveolar proteinosis – Progress in the first 44 years. Amer J Respir Crit Care Med 2002; 166:215–235.

68. Golde DW, Territo M, Finley TN, Cline MJ. Defective lung macrophages in pulmonary alveolar proteinosis. Ann Intern Med 1976; 85:304–309.

69. Nugent KM, Pesanti EL. Macrophage function in pulmonary alveolar proteinosis. Am Rev Respir Dis 1983; 127:780–781.

70. Gonzalez-Rothi RJ, Harris JO. Pulmonary alveolar proteinosis. Further evaluation of abnormal alveolar macrophages. Chest 1986; 90:656:661.

71. Trapnell BC, Whitsett JA, Nakata K. Pulmonary alveolar proteinosis. N Engl J Med 2003; 349(26):2527–2539.

72. Dranoff G, Crawford AD, Sadelain M, et al. Involvement of granulocyte-macrophage colony-stimulating factor in pulmonary homeostasis. Science 1994; 264:713–716.

73. Seymour JF, Begley CG, Dirksen U, et al. Attenuated hematopoietic response to granulocyte-macrophage colony-stimulating factor in patients with acquired pulmonary alveolar proteinosis. Blood 1998; 92:2657–2667.

74. Kitamura T, Tanaka N, Watanabe J, et al. Idiopathic pulmonary alveolar proteinosis as an autoimmune disease with neutralizing antibody against granulocyte/macrophage colony-stimulating factor. J Exp Med 1999; 190:875–880.

75. Schoch OD, Schanz U, Koller M, et al. BAL findings in a patient with pulmonary alveolar proteinosis successfully treated with GM-CSF. Thorax 2002; 57:277–280.

76. Buechner HA, Ansari A. Acute silico-proteinosis. Dis Chest 1969; 55:274–284.

77. Xipell JM, Ham KN, Price CG, Thomas DP. Acute silicolipoproteinosis. Thorax 1977; 32: 104–111.

78. Suratt PM, Winn WC, Brody AR, Bolton WK, Giles RD. Acute silicosis in tombstone sandblasters. Am Rev Respir Dis 1977; 115:521–529.

79. Miller RR, Churg AM, Hutcheon M, Lam S. Case report: pulmonary alveolar proteinosis and aluminum dust exposure. Am Rev Respir Dis 1984; 130:312–315.

80. McDonald JW, Alvarez F, Keller CA. Pulmonary alveolar proteinosis in association with household exposure to fibrous insulation material. Chest 2000; 117:1813–1817.

81. Heppleston AG, Fletcher K, Wyatt I. Changes in the composition of lung lipids and the 'turnover' of dipalmitoyl lecithin in experimental alveolar lipo-proteinosis induced by inhaled quartz. Br J Exp Pathol 1974; 55:384–395.

82. Miller BE, Bakewell WE, Katyal SL, Singh G, Hook GE. Induction of surfactant protein (SP-A) biosynthesis and SP-A mRNA in activated type II cells during acute silicosis in rats. Am J Respir Cell Mol Biol 1990; 3:217–226.

83. Gross P, DeTreville RTP. Alveolar proteinosis. Its experimental production in rodents. Arch Pathol 1968; 86:255–261.

84. Corrin B, King E. Experimental endogenous lipid pneumonia and silicosis. J Pathol 1969; 97:325–330.

85. Corrin B, King E. Pathogenesis of experimental pulmonary alveolar proteinosis. Thorax 1970; 25:230–236.

86. McDonald JW, Roggli VL, Bradford WD. Coexisting endogenous and exogenous lipoid pneumonia and alveolar proteinosis in a patient with neurodevelopmental disease. Pediatr Pathol 1993; 14:505–511.

87. Heath D, Smith P, Hasleton PS. Effects of chlorphentermine on the rat lung. Thorax 1973; 28:551–558.

88. Vijeyaratnam GS, Corrin B. Fine structural alterations in the lungs of iprindole-treated rats. J Pathol 1974; 114:233–239.

89. Costa-Jussa FR, Corrin B, Jacobs JM. Amiodarone lung toxicity: a human and experimental study. J Pathol 1984; 144:73–79.

90. Vijeyaratnam GS, Corrin B. Pulmonary alveolar proteinosis developing from desquamative interstitial pneumonia in long term toxicity studies of iprindole in the rat. Virchows Arch A Pathol Anat Histopathol 1973; 358:1–10.

91. Nogee LM, Demello DE, Dehner LP, Colten HR. Brief report – deficiency of pulmonary surfactant protein-B in congenital alveolar proteinosis. N Engl J Med 1993; 328:406–410.

92. Demello DE, Nogee LM, Heyman S, et al. Molecular and phenotypic variability in the congenital alveolar proteinosis syndrome associated with inherited surfactant protein B deficiency. J Pediatr 1994; 125:43–50.

93. Nogee L, Garnier G, Dietz H, Singer L, Murphy A, DeMello D. A mutation in the surfactant protein B gene responsible for fatal neonatal respiratory disease in multiple kindreds. J Clin Invest 1994; 93:1860–1863.

94. Demello DE, Heyman S, Phelps DS, et al. Ultrastructure of lung in surfactant protein B deficiency. Am J Respir Cell Mol Biol 1994; 11:230–239.

95. Ball R, Chetcuti PAJ, Beverley D. Fatal familial surfactant protein B deficiency. Arch Dis Child 1995; 73:F53.

96. Mildenberger E, Demello DE, Lin ZW, Kossel H, Hoehn T, Versmold HT. Focal congenital alveolar proteinosis associated with abnormal surfactant protein B messenger RNA. Chest 2001; 119:645–647.

97. Parto K, Kallajoki M, Aho H, Simell O. Pulmonary alveolar proteinosis and glomerulonephritis in lysinuric protein intolerance: case reports and autopsy findings of four pediatric patients. Hum Pathol 1994; 25:400–407.

98. McManus DT, Moore R, Hill CM, Rodgers C, Carson DJ, Love AHG. Necropsy findings in lysinuric protein intolerance. J Clin Pathol 1996; 49:345–347.

99. Parto K, Maki L, Pelliniemi LJ, Simell O. Abnormal pulmonary macrophages in lysinuric protein intolerance: ultrastructural, morphometric and X-ray microanalytic study. Arch Pathol Lab Med 1994; 118:536–541.

100. Dirksen U, Nishinakamura R, Groneck P, et al. Human pulmonary alveolar proteinosis associated with a defect in GM- CSF/IL-3/IL-5 receptor common beta chain expression. J Clin Invest 1997; 100:2211–2217.

101. Williams GE, Medley DRK, Brown R. Pulmonary alveolar proteinosis. Lancet 1960; i:1385–1388.

102. Carnovale R, Zornoza J, Goldman AM, Luna M. Pulmonary alveolar proteinosis: its association with hematologic malignancy and lymphoma. Radiology 1977; 122:303–306.

103. Bedrossian CWM, Luna MA, Conklin RH, Miller WC. Alveolar proteinosis as a consequence of immunosuppression. A hypothesis based on clinical and pathologic observations. Hum Pathol 1980; 11(Suppl):527–535.

104. Ruben FL, Talamo TS. Secondary pulmonary alveolar proteinosis occurring in two patients with acquired immune deficiency syndrome. Am J Med 1986; 80:1187–1190.

105. Singh G, Katyal SL. Surfactant apoprotein in nonmalignant pulmonary disorders. Am J Pathol 1980; 101:51–62.

106. Singh G, Katyal SL, Bedrossian CWM, Rogers RM. Pulmonary alveolar proteinosis. Chest 1983; 83:82–86.

107. Hudson AR, Halprin GM, Miller JA, Kilburn KH. Pulmonary interstitial fibrosis following alveolar proteinosis. Chest 1974; 65:700–702.

108. Jacobovitz-Derks D, Corrin B. Degenerative processes in the pathogenesis of pulmonary alveolar lipoproteinosis. Virchows Arch A Pathol Anat Histopathol 1977; 376:165–174.

109. Butnor KJ, Sporn TA. Human parainfluenza virus giant cell pneumonia following cord blood transplant associated with pulmonary alveolar proteinosis. Arch Pathol Lab Med 2003; 127:235–238.

110. Yousem SA. Alveolar lipoproteinosis in lung allograft recipients. Hum Pathol 1997; 28:1383–1386.

111. Vazquez M, Sidhu GS. Surfactant production by neoplastic type II pneumocytes. Ultrastruct Pathol 1988; 12:605–612.

112. du Bois RM, McAllister WAC, Branthwaite MA. Alveolar proteinosis: diagnosis and treatment over a 10 year period. Thorax 1983; 38:360–363.

113. Shah PL, Hansell D, Lawson PR, Reid KBM, Morgan C. Pulmonary alveolar proteinosis: clinical aspects and current concepts on pathogenesis. Thorax 2000; 55:67–77.

114. Webster JR, Battifora H, Furey C, Harrison RA, Shapiro B. Pulmonary alveolar proteinosis in two siblings with decreased immunoglobulin A. Am J Med 1980; 69:786–789.

115. Teja K, Cooper PH, Squires JE, Schnatterly PT. Pulmonary alveolar proteinosis in four siblings. N Engl J Med 1981; 305:1390–1392.

116. Rossi SE, Erasmus JJ, Volpacchio M, Franquet T, Castiglioni T, McAdams HP. 'Crazy-paving' pattern at thin-section CT of the lungs: radiologic-pathologic overview. Radiographics 2003; 23:1509–1519.

117. Holbert JM, Costello P, Li W, Hoffman RM, Rogers RM. CT features of pulmonary alveolar proteinosis. Am J Roentgenol 2001; 176:1287–1294.

118. Costello JF, Moriarty DC, Branthwaite MA, Turner-Warwick M, Corrin B. Diagnosis and management of alveolar proteinosis: the role of electron microscopy. Thorax 1975; 30:121–132.

119. Milleron BJ, Costabel U, Teschler H, et al. Bronchoalveolar lavage cell data in alveolar proteinosis. Am Rev Respir Dis 1991; 144:1330–1332.

120. Mikami T, Yamamoto Y, Yokoyama M, Okayasu I. Pulmonary alveolar proteinosis: diagnosis using routinely processed smears of bronchoalveolar lavage fluid. J Clin Pathol 1997; 50:981–984.

121. Bonfield TL, Russell D, Burgess S, Malur A, Kavuru MS, Thomassen MJ. Autoantibodies against granulocyte macrophage colony-stimulating factor are diagnostic for pulmonary alveolar proteinosis. Am J Respir Cell Molec Biol 2002; 27:481–486.

122. Larson RK, Gordinier R. Pulmonary alveolar proteinosis: report of six cases, review of the literature and formulation of a new theory. Ann Intern Med 1965; 62:292–312.

123. Danel C, Israel-Biet D, Costabel U, Klech H. Therapeutic applications of bronchoalveolar lavage. Eur Respir J 1992; 5:1173–1175.

124. Beccaria M, Luisetti M, Rodi G, et al. Long-term durable benefit after whole lung lavage in pulmonary alveolar proteinosis. Eur Resp J 23, 526–531. 2004.

125. Morgan C. The benefits of whole lung lavage in pulmonary alveolar proteinosis. Eur Respir J 2004; 23:503–505.

126. Barraclough RM, Gillies AJ. Pulmonary alveolar proteinosis: a complete response to GM-CSF therapy. Thorax 2001; 56:664–665.

127. Bonfield TL, Kavuru MS, Thomassen MJ. Anti-GM-CSF titer predicts response to GM-CSF therapy in pulmonary alveolar proteinosis. Clin Immunol 2002; 105:342–350.

128. Thomassen MJ, Raychaudhuri B, Bonfield TL, et al. Elevated IL-10 inhibits GM-CSF synthesis in pulmonary alveolar proteinosis. Autoimmunity 2003; 36:285–290.

129. Chesnutt MS, Nuckton TJ, Golden J, Folkesson HG, Matthay MA. Rapid alveolar epithelial fluid clearance following lung lavage in pulmonary alveolar proteinosis. Chest 2001; 120:271–274.

130. Parker LA, Novotny DB. Recurrent alveolar proteinosis following double lung transplantation. Chest 1997; 111:1457–1458.

131. McClenahan JB, Mussenden R. Pulmonary alveolar proteinosis. Arch Intern Med 1974; 133:284–287.

132. Burbank B, Morrione TG, Cutler SS. Pulmonary alveolar proteinosis and nocardiosis. Am J Med 1960; 28:1002–1007.

133. Summers JE. Pulmonary alveolar proteinosis. Review of the literature with follow-up studies and report of two new cases. Calif Med 1966; 104:428–436.

134. Reyes JM, Putong PB. Association of pulmonary alveolar lipoproteinosis with mycobacterial infection. Am J Clin Pathol 1980; 74:478–485.

135. Ramirez-R J, Savard EV, Hawkins JE. Biological effects of pulmonary washings from cases of alveolar proteinosis. Am Rev Respir Dis 1966; 94:244–246.

Cholesterol pneumonitis

136. Waddell WR, Sniffen RC, Sweet RH. Chronic pneumonitis: its clinical and pathologic importance. Report of ten cases showing interstitial pneumonitis and unusual cholesterol deposits. J Thorac Surg 1949; 18:707–737.

137. Kay JM, Heath D, Hasleton PS, Littler WA. Aetiology of pulmonary cholesterol-ester granulomas. Br J Dis Chest 1970; 64:55–57.

138. Fischer EG, Marek JM, Morris A, Nashelsky MB. Cholesterol granulomas of the lungs associated with microangiopathic hemolytic anemia and thrombocytopenia in pulmonary hypertension - A case report and review of the literature. Arch Pathol Lab Med 2000; 124:1813–1815.

139. Nolan RL, McAdams HP, Sporn TA, Roggli VL, Tapson VF, Goodman PC. Pulmonary cholesterol granulomas in patients with pulmonary artery hypertension: chest radiographic and CT findings. Am J Roentgenol 1999; 172:1317–1319.

140. Lawler W. Idiopathic cholesterol pneumonitis. Histopathology 1977; 1:385–395.

141. Sato K, Takahashi H, Amano H, Uekusa T, Dambara T, Kira S. Diffuse progressive pulmonary interstitial and intra-alveolar cholesterol granulomas in childhood. Eur Respir J 1996; 9:2419–2422.

Corpora amylacea

142. Friedreich N. Corpora amylacea in den Lungen. Arch Path Anat 1856; 9:613–618.

143. Michaels L, Levene C. Pulmonary corpora amylacea. J Path Bact 1957; 74:49–56.

144. Rocken C, Linke RP, Saeger W. Corpora amylacea in the lung, prostate and uterus - a comparative and immunohistochemical study. Pathol Res Pract 1996; 192:998–1006.

145. Tuur SM, Nelson AM, Gibson DW, et al. Liesegang rings in tissue. How to distinguish Liesegang rings from the giant kidney worm, Dioctophyma renale. Am J Surg Pathol 1987; 11:598–605.

146. Hollander DH, Hutchins GM. Central spherules in pulmonary corpora amylacea. Arch Pathol Lab Med 1978; 102:629–630.

Alveolar microlithiasis

147. Harbitz F. Extensive calcification of the lungs as a distinct disease. Arch Intern Med 1918; 21:139–146.

148. Puhr L. Mikrolithiasis alveolaris pulmonum. Virchows Arch A Pathol Anat Histopathol 1933; 290:156–160.

149. Sosman MC, Dodd GD, Jones WD. The familial occurrence of pulmonary alveolar microlithiasis. Am J Roentgenol 1957; 77:947–1012.

150. Prakash UBS, Barham SS, Rosenow EC, Brown ML, Payne WS. Pulmonary alveolar microlithiasis: a review including ultrastructural and pulmonary function studies. Mayo Clin Proc 1983; 58:290–300.

151. Mariotta S, Guidi L, Mattia P, et al. Pulmonary microlithiasis – report of two cases. Respiration 1997; 64:165–169.

152. Senyigit A, Yaramis A, Gurkan F, et al. Pulmonary alveolar microlithiasis: A rare familial inheritance with report of six gases in a family – Contribution of six new cases to the number of case reports in Turkey. Respiration 2001; 68(2):204–209.

153. Volle E, Kaufmann HJ. Pulmonary alveolar microlithiasis in pediatric patients. Review of the world literature and two new observations. Pediatr Radiol 1987; 17:439–442.

154. Moran CA, Hochholzer L, Hasleton PS, Johnson FB, Koss MN. Pulmonary alveolar microlithiasis: A clinicopathologic and chemical analysis of seven cases. Arch Pathol Lab Med 1997; 121:607–611.

155. Lauta VM. Pulmonary alveolar microlithiasis: an overview of clinical and pathological features together with possible therapies. Resp Med 2003; 97(10):1081–1085.

156. Castellana G, Lamorgese V. Pulmonary alveolar microlithiasis. World cases and review of the literature. Respiration 2003; 70:549–555.

157. Cluzel P, Grenier P, Bernadac P, Laurent F, Picard JD. Pulmonary alveolar microlithiasis: CT findings. J Comput Assist Tomogr 1991; 15:938–942.

158. Balikian JP, Fuleihan FJD, Nucho CN. Pulmonary alveolar microlithiasis. Report of five cases with special reference to roentgen manifestations. Am J Roentgenol 1968; 103:509–518.

159. O'Neil RP, Cohn JE, Pellegrino ED. Pulmonary alveolar microlithiasis. A family study. Ann Intern Med 1967; 67:957–967.

160. Ozcelik U, Gulsun M, Gocmen A, et al. Treatment and follow-up of pulmonary alveolar microlithiasis with disodium editronate: radiological demonstration. Pediatr Radiol 2002; 32:380–383.

161. Edelman JD, Bavaria J, Kaiser LR, Litzky LA, Palevsky HI, Kotloff RM. Bilateral sequential lung transplantation for pulmonary alveolar microlithiasis. Chest 1997; 112:1140–1144.

162. Sears MR, Chang AR, Taylor AJ. Pulmonary alveolar microlithiasis. Thorax 1971; 26:704–711.

163. Tao LC. Microliths in sputum specimens and their relationship to pulmonary alveolar microlithiasis. Am J Clin Pathol 1978; 69:482–485.

164. Pritzker KPH, Desai SD, Patterson MC, Cheng P-T. Calcite sputum lith. Characterization by analytic scanning electron microscopy and X-ray diffraction. Am J Clin Pathol 1981; 75:253–257.

165. Samson IM, Rossoff LJ. Chronic lithoptysis with multiple bilateral broncholiths. Chest 1997; 112:563–565.

166. Barnard NJ, Crocker PR, Blainey AD, Davies RJ, Ell SR, Levison DA. Pulmonary alveolar microlithiasis. A new analytical approach. Histopathology 1987; 11:639–645.

167. Pracyk JB, Simonson SG, Young SL, Chio AJ, Roggli VL, Piantadosi CA. Composition of lung lavage in pulmonary alveolar microlithiasis. Respiration 1996; 63:254–260.

Calcospherites
168. Dail D, Liebow AA. Intraalveolar conchoidal bodies. Am J Pathol 1976; 82:43–44a.
169. Gardiner IT, Uff JS. 'Blue bodies' in a case of cryptogenic fibrosing alveolitis (desquamative type) – an ultra-structural study. Thorax 1978; 33:806–813.
170. Koss MN, Johnson FB, Hochholzer L. Pulmonary blue bodies. Hum Pathol 1981; 12:258–266.

171. Ratjen FA, Schoenfeld B, Wiesemann HG. Pulmonary alveolar microlithiasis and lymphocytic interstitial pneumonitis in a 10 year old girl. Eur Respir J 1992; 5:1283–1285.

Alveolar ossification
172. Green JD, Harle TS, Greenberg SD, Weg JG, Nevin H, Jenkins DE. Disseminated pulmonary ossification. A case report with demonstration of electron-microscopic features. Am Rev Respir Dis 1970; 101:293–298.
173. Gortenuti G, Portuese A. Disseminated pulmonary ossification. Eur J Radiol 1985; 5:14.

7

Occupational, environmental and iatrogenic lung disease

7.1

Occupational lung disease

This chapter deals with the pneumoconioses, occupational asthma, occupational fevers and the effects of toxic fume and gases. Occupational diseases of the lung considered elsewhere include the effects of atmospheric pressure changes (see p. 369), extrinsic allergic alveolitis (see p. 280), carcinoma of the lung (see pp. 527–582) and asbestos-induced pleural disease (see pp. 698–713).

PNEUMOCONIOSIS: GENERAL FEATURES

Definition of pneumoconiosis

The term pneumoconiosis is an abbreviation (and etymological corruption) of Zenker's pneumonokoniosis,[1] which derives from *pneumon* (lung) and *konis* (dust) and therefore translates as dusty lung; in practice the term is confined to the effects of mineral dust on the lungs. Diseases caused by organic dusts are not included among the pneumoconioses and, in medico-legal practice at least, the presence of dust alone is insufficient to indicate pneumoconiosis: for compensation to be considered, the mineral dust must alter the structure of the lung and cause disability. The British Industrial Injuries Advisory Council defined pneumoconiosis as 'permanent alteration of lung structure due to the inhalation of mineral dust and the tissue reactions of the lung to its presence, excluding bronchitis and emphysema'.[2] Parkes recommends that cancer and asthma caused by mineral dust should also be excluded from the definition.[3]

Dust deposition in the lung

To reach the lung, dust particles have to be very small. Particle density and shape also affect the aerodynamic properties of dust. Host factors such as airflow characteristics, airway

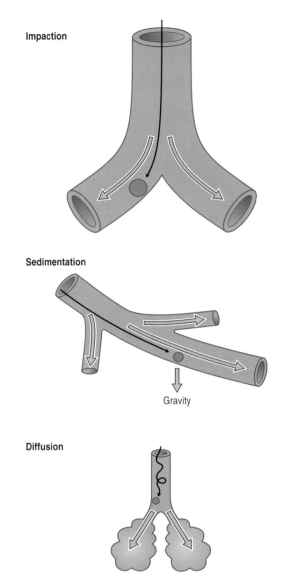

Figure 7.1.1 Mechanisms of particle deposition in the respiratory tract.

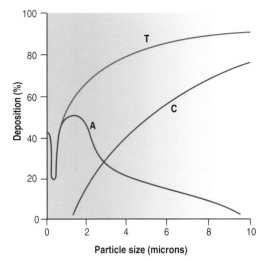

Figure 7.1.2 Percentage dust deposition in the respiratory tract according to particle diameter. T, total dust deposition; C, deposition on the ciliated epithelium; A, alveolar deposition.

branching patterns and airway disease also affect dust deposition. Three deposition mechanisms are recognised (Fig. 7.1.1):

1 Inertial impaction. When airstreams change direction or velocity, the inertia of the entrained particles causes them to maintain their original direction for a distance that depends upon their density and the square of their diameter.

2 Sedimentation (gravitational settlement). Under the influence of gravity, particles settle with a speed that is proportional to their density and the square of their diameter.

3 Diffusion. Very small air-borne particles acquire a random motion as a result of bombardment by the surrounding gas molecules.

Inhaled dust particles are liable to sediment out in the alveoli if they have a diameter in the range 1–5 μm, are roughly spherical in shape, and in density approximate to that of water. Larger

or denser particles impact or precipitate on the walls of the conductive airways and are rapidly removed by ciliary action. Smaller particles may reach the alveoli but do not sediment so readily and many are therefore exhaled. Very small particles are deposited on the walls of alveoli by diffusion but because they are so small the total amount of dust deposited in this way is insignificant compared with that deposited by sedimentation (Fig. 7.1.2). Direct measurement shows that most lung dust (96%) has a particle diameter less than 2.5 μm.[4]

Fibrous dust particles behave differently. Fibres over 100 μm in length may reach the alveoli if they are very thin and remain aligned with the airstream. Fibre penetration is inversely related to path length and the number of bifurcations.[5]

Slightly more dust is deposited in the right lung than the left, probably because the right main bronchus is more in line with the trachea, is broader and shorter than the left, and carries 55% of the inhaled air.[6,7]

Dust clearance from the lung

Inhaled dust that settles in the conductive airways is removed within a day or two by ciliary action. Only dust that reaches the alveoli is liable to cause pneumoconiosis and much of this is also removed, but the clearance rate here is much slower: many coal miners continue to expectorate mine dust years after retirement. Alveolar clearance is largely effected by macrophages, principally via the airways to the pharynx but also via lymphatics to the regional lymph nodes. The airway and interstitial routes interconnect at the bronchiolar level[8] where some dust-laden macrophages leave the interstitium for the air space.[9] This interconnection is probably the route utilised by circulating macrophages clearing other parts of the body of endogenous or exogenous particulate matter via the lung.[10] Long asbestos fibres present a particular problem to macrophage clearance.

Some minerals, notably chrysotile asbestos, undergo slow physicochemical dissolution in the lungs.

Only a small fraction of the inhaled dust gains access to the interstitium, a necessary step if it is to cause pneumoconiosis. Some free dust enters through the bronchus associated lymphoid tissue[8,9] and some is taken up by, or pierces, the alveolar epithelium (see Fig. 1.32, p. 19).[11–13] Some of this is transported within hours to the hilar lymph nodes.[14] So rapid is this translocation that it is thought not to involve phagocytes, although interstitial macrophages are undoubtedly important in continuing the transportation of dust to the nodes. Ultrafine dust particles are particularly liable to be transported across the alveolar epithelium.[8] The integrity of the alveolar epithelium is very important to dust translocation from the air spaces to the interstitium. Much more dust reaches the interstitium if the epithelium is damaged.[15,16]

It is widely thought that macrophages that have left the interstitium for the alveolar space never return,[14,17] but this is probably untrue.[18] Heavily laden macrophages accumulate in alveoli bordering the terminal and respiratory bronchioles, eventually filling them completely. Erosion of the alveolar epithelium permits re-entry of these macrophages into the interstitium,[19] very close to foci of bronchial mucosa-associated lymphoid tissue (MALT), which are found near the terminal bronchioles.[20] These aggregates guard the mouths of lymphatics, which commence at this point; alveoli are devoid of lymphatics. Dust-laden interstitial macrophages accumulate in and around the bronchial MALT, which Macklin therefore referred to as dust sumps.[21] Most pneumoconiotic lesions are found in the region of the dust sumps and are therefore focal. Asbestosis is diffuse rather than focal because the long asbestos fibres are not readily mobilised and cannot be concentrated in the centriacinar dust sumps. This is also seen on occasion with platy non-fibrous dusts such as talc, mica, kaolinite and feldspar.[22–30] Within the dust sumps the dust particles are not static. They are constantly being freed and re-ingested by interstitial macrophages and because these cells are mobile, successively inhaled dusts soon become intimately mixed.[31] Macrophages play an important role in pneumoconiosis and if the dust is fibrogenic the repeated phagocytosis of indestructible mineral particles results in constant fibroblast stimulation.

The zonal distribution of pneumoconiosis

Pneumoconiosis affects both lungs but seldom evenly and some pneumoconioses show characteristic patterns of lung involvement. In most, the lesions are more numerous and better developed in the upper lobes than the bases but the reverse is true of asbestosis. The reasons for this are complex and poorly understood but undoubtedly involve the dust deposition:clearance ratio for the effect of the dust will depend upon both its amount and the duration of its stay in the lungs. There are well recognised regional differences in the distribution and clearance of inhaled material, which in turn are dependent upon man's upright posture, the consequent gravitational forces being maximal at the apices.[32] When standing at rest, the apices of the

lungs are hardly perfused, so that lymph formation and clearance are much better at the bases.[33–35] Similarly, the apices are relatively less well aerated, alveoli in the lower lobes receiving more air than those in the upper lobes.[34,36] The greater respiratory excursions at the bases are thought to promote macrophage mobility there. It is to be expected therefore that the bases would both receive and clear more dust than the apices, rendering it difficult to predict on theoretical grounds which parts of the lungs carry the heaviest dust burden. In fact, more dust of all types is found in the upper lobes, the part most severely affected by every type of pneumoconiosis except asbestosis.[37,38] The predilection of asbestos to affect the periphery of the lower lobes is attributed to the dangerous long asbestos fibres preponderating there, a consequence of their special aerodynamic properties.[38,39]

Pulmonary reactions to mineral dust

The main tissue reaction to mineral dust is fibrosis. Silica is highly fibrogenic and is therefore very likely to cause pneumoconiosis. Carbon is non-fibrogenic and therefore, unless there are complications, coal pneumoconiosis causes little disability. Tin too is harmless, and stannosis therefore unimportant, although the chest radiograph is highly abnormal because tin is very radio-opaque. Stannosis is one of several terms that specify pneumoconiosis due to a particular mineral, the best known being silicosis, asbestosis and anthracosis. Table 7.1.1 summarises the various pulmonary reactions to mineral dust.

Identification of the dust

The blackness of carbon and red-brown colour of iron (Fig. 7.1.3) give ample evidence, both naked eye and microscopically, of the type and amount of these dusts when they are present in

Table 7.1.1 Pulmonary reactions to mineral dust	
Pulmonary reaction	*Examples*
Macrophage accumulation with a little reticulin deposition	Anthracosis
	Siderosis
	Stannosis
	Baritosis
	Coal pneumoconiosis (macules)
	Aluminium pneumoconiosis (granular aluminium)
Nodular or massive fibrosis	Silicosis
	Mixed dust pneumoconiosis
	Coal pneumoconiosis (nodules)
Diffuse fibrosis	Asbestosis
	Hard metal pneumoconiosis
	Aluminium pneumoconiosis (aluminium fume and stamped aluminium)
Epithelioid and giant cell granulomas	Chronic berylliosis
Alveolar lipoproteinosis	'Acute' silicosis, but also seen with heavy exposure to other dusts (see p. 338)
Small airway disease	Various dusts (see p. 97)

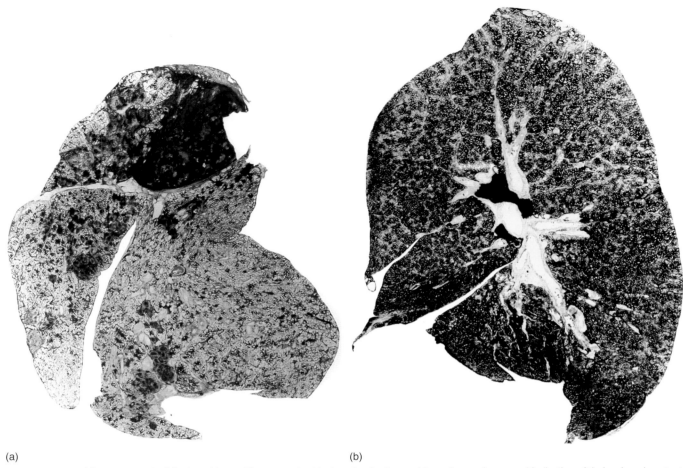

(a)
(b)

Figure 7.1.3 Coal (a) and haematite (b) miners' lungs. The respective black and red colours of these lungs give a good indication of their mineral content. (Illustrations of paper-mounted whole lung sections provided by WGJ Edwards, London, UK.)

the lung, but other inorganic dust may be more difficult to identify. However, a flick-out substage condenser and Polaroid® filters to test for refractility and birefringence respectively are useful adjuncts, which are too often neglected by the histopathologist. It should be noted that crystalline silica is traditionally regarded as being only weakly birefringent, in contrast to silicates which generally show up brightly with simple crossed Polaroid® filters.[40] However, some workers report that with modern microscope lamps both silica and silicates are birefringent,[41] demonstrating the importance when using Polaroid® filters of working with the light source at high intensity. Mineralogists use polarising microscopy for analysis, but only by studying large polished crystals with controlled orientation of the light. The small dust particles found in tissue sections are too small to permit analysis by this technique but it is nevertheless very useful for detecting their presence (Fig. 7.1.4).

Particle shape gives a useful indication of mineral type but appearances are sometimes deceptive: the plate-like crystals of talc are seldom observed as such, usually being viewed edge on when they appear to be needle-shaped. Occasionally, stains can be used to identify minerals, e.g. a modified Perls' reaction for

inhaled iron, and Irwin's aluminon stain for aluminium, but these too have largely been replaced by modern analytical techniques.

Microincineration combined with darkfield microscopy can also be used to demonstrate small particles. Incombustible mineral particles that cannot be seen with brightfield or polarising microscopy are rendered visible by this technique and their position on the slide can be compared with tissue reactions evident in a serial section that has not been incinerated. Microincineration has, however, also been largely replaced by modern analytical techniques that will now be considered.

Analytical electron microscopy is now proving very helpful in identifying minerals, whether applied to lung digests or tissue sections.[42–45] Scanning electron microscopy permits the examination of thicker sections than does transmission electron microscopy but does not detect very small particles. However, scanning electron microscopy allows more tissue to be examined and avoids the difficulty of cutting mineral particles with an ultramicrotome.

Particles in a 5 μm thick deparaffinised section can be recognised in a scanning electron microscope set to collect the back scattered electrons.[43] The instrument can then be focussed on

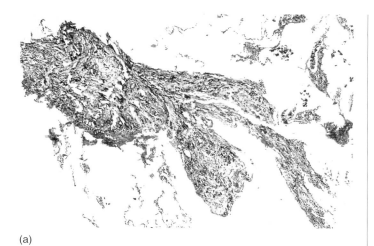

(a)

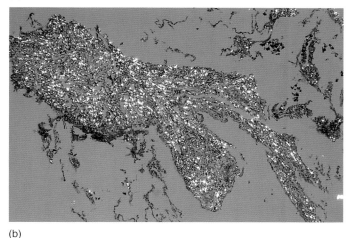

(b)

Figure 7.1.4 Talc pneumoconiosis. Only carbon is evident when the lesions are viewed with (a) non-polarised light, whereas the abundant talc particles are readily seen when (b) polarised light is employed.

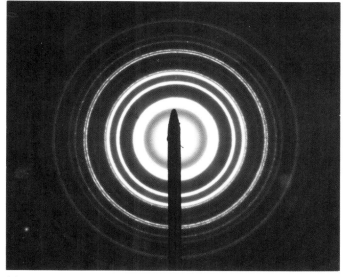

(a)

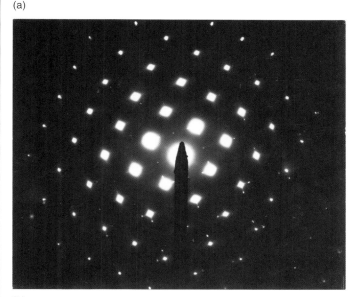

(b)

Figure 7.1.5 Electron diffraction patterns of gold, used for calibration purposes. The ring pattern (a) indicates that the material is polycrystalline and the spot pattern (b) indicates that it is a single crystal: amorphous materials give no regular pattern. The spacing of the rings gives information on crystalline structure and can be usefully applied to distinguish the various crystalline forms of silica (quartz, tridymite, cristobalite) for example. (Illustration provided by Dr M Wineberg, London, UK.)

points of potential interest and switched to X-ray analysis. X-ray diffraction patterns provide information on crystal structure (Fig. 7.1.5) while elemental analysis is available from either energy dispersive or wavelength dispersive X-ray spectroscopy. With energy dispersive X-ray spectroscopy, all elements of atomic number above 11 that are present in the area under examination are identified, while with the latter the section can be scanned for one particular element. With energy dispersive spectroscopy different elements are shown graphically as individual peaks, the heights of which are proportional to the amounts of the different elements within the particle studied, thereby giving information on probable molecular formula (Fig. 7.1.6 and see Box 7.1.4, p. 349). Thus, different silicates can be distinguished from each other and also from silica, which registers as pure silicon, oxygen (atomic number 8) not being detected. The fact that the elements of low atomic number that constitute organic chemicals are not detected means that any minerals present (except beryllium, atomic number 4) can be recognised easily in tissue sections. Only particles can be analysed however: elements present in only molecular amounts cannot be detected.

Trace amounts of substances such as beryllium require bulk chemical analysis or techniques such as atomic absorption spectrometry, neutron activation analysis and microprobe mass spectrometry based on either focused laser or ion beam irradiation.[46] The last of these techniques can also provide molecular (as opposed to elemental) analysis of organic as well as inorganic particles.[47] Another promising analytical technique is microscopic infrared spectroscopy which provides data on the compound nature of microscopic particles in tissue sections

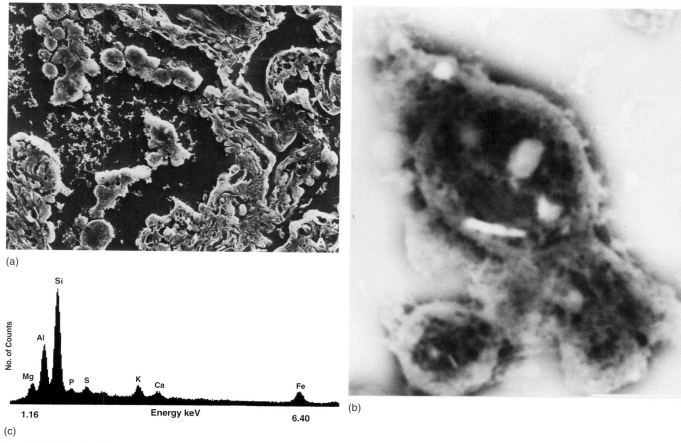

(a)

(b)

(c)

Figure 7.1.6 Dust particles in the lung: electron-microprobe analysis. (a) The secondary (scanning) electron microscopic image of a deparaffinised 5 μm thick section of lung showing clumps of macrophages in an alveolar lumen. (b) Back-scattered scanning electron microscopic image showing three of the macrophages at higher power: several bright particles worthy of further attention are evident. (c) X-ray energy spectrum of one of the particles showing it to be a silicate. The section had been transferred from a glass to a perspex slide to avoid background signals from the siliceous nature of glass. Each element emits a unique energy pattern when bombarded by electrons while the number of counts is in proportion to the amount of the particular element that is present in the particle. (Illustration provided by Professor DA Levison, Dundee, UK.)

(Fig. 7.1.7). Micro-Raman spectroscopy is also useful in this respect.

Radiological grading of pneumoconiosis

A scheme for grading pneumoconiosis radiologically by comparison with standard radiographs has been adopted by the International Labour Organisation and is widely used.[48] Small opacities (up to 1 cm diameter) are graded by their profusion, 1, 2 and 3 indicating increasing numbers, and by their size, increasing through p, q and r if rounded and s, t and u if irregular. Type p opacities are described as punctiform and measure up to 1.5 mm in diameter; larger lesions up to 3 mm in diameter (type q) are described as micronodular or miliary; and those over 3 mm and up to 1 cm in diameter (type r) are described as nodular. Irregular opacities cannot be sized so accurately, s, t and u indicating fine, medium and coarse respectively. Large opacities (over 1 cm diameter) are graded by their combined size, increasing through A – an opacity measuring between 1 and 5 cm in diameter, B – one or more opacities whose combined

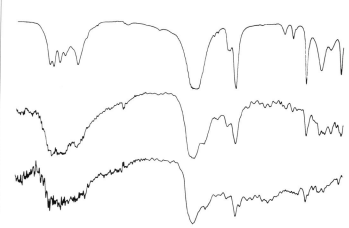

Figure 7.1.7 Infrared spectra of calcium oxalate. Top, reference standard; centre and bottom, crystals in human tissue sections. (Illustration provided by Professor DA Levison, Dundee, UK.)

area does not exceed the equivalent of one-third of the area of the right lung field (when they are regrouped in the mind's eye or measured with a transparent ruler) and C – one or more opacities whose combined area exceeds one-third of the area of the right lung field (when similarly regrouped). In coal workers, small opacities (up to 1 cm diameter) correspond to simple coal workers' pneumoconiosis and large opacities (over 1 cm diameter) to complicated coal workers' pneumoconiosis, which is also known as progressive massive fibrosis (see Fig. 7.1.16, p. 343).

SILICOSIS[40]

Mineralogy

Silicosis is caused by the inhalation of silica (silicon dioxide, SiO_2), which is to be distinguished from the silicates, these being more complex compounds in which silicon and oxygen form an anion combined with cations such as aluminium and magnesium: talc for example is a hydrated magnesium silicate with the formula $Mg_3Si_4O_{10}(OH)_2$. The element silicon is also to be distinguished from the synthetic organic polymer silicone, used in implants.

Crystalline silica is highly fibrogenic whereas amorphous silica and silicates other than asbestos are relatively inert. Silica exists in several crystalline forms, of which quartz, cristobalite and tridymite are the most important: tridymite is the most fibrogenic and cristobalite more so than quartz.[40,49]

Occupations at risk

Silicotic lesions have been identified in the lungs of Egyptian mummies, and the injurious effects on the lungs of inhaling mine dust have been recognised for more than 400 years. As long ago as the sixteenth century in Joachimsthal, Bohemia (now Jachymov, Czech Republic), diseases of miners' lungs were attributed to the dust the miners breathed. Silicosis, tuberculosis and lung cancer are all now known to have been prevalent among the miners in this region, the cancer being largely attributable to the high level of radioactivity in the mines.

Silicosis was recognised in Britain soon after the discovery in 1720 that the addition of calcined flint to the clay from which china is made produced a finer, whiter and tougher ware. The preparation and use of this flint powder was highly dangerous, causing the condition known as potters' rot, one of the first of the many trade names by which silicosis has since been known. Aluminium oxide (alumina) now provides a safe, effective substitute for flint in this industry. In 1830, it was noted that Sheffield fork grinders who used a dry grindstone died early, and among other preventive measures it was recommended that the occupation should be confined to criminals: fortunately for them, the substitution of carborundum (silicon carbide) for sandstone was effective enough. However, silicosis still occurs in some miners, tunnellers, quarrymen, stone dressers and metal workers.

Silica in one form or another is used in many trades – in the manufacture of glass and pottery, in the moulds used in iron foundries, as an abrasive in grinding and sandblasting, and as a furnace lining that is refractory to high temperatures. Rocks such as granite and sandstone are siliceous and their dusts are encountered in many mining and quarrying operations. In coal mining in the UK, the highest incidence of the disease was in pits where the thinness of the coal seams required the removal of a large amount of siliceous rock, a process known as 'hard heading'. In South Africa, silicosis causes a high mortality among the gold miners on the Witwatersrand, where the metallic ore is embedded in quartz. Slate is a metamorphic rock that contains both silica and silicates, and slate workers develop both silicosis and mixed dust pneumoconiosis (see p. 340).[50,51] Nor are rural industries immune from the disease, particularly if ventilation is inadequate, as it is in certain African huts where stone implements are used to pound meal and the occupants develop mixed dust pneumoconiosis.[52] Silicosis and mixed dust pneumoconiosis have also been reported in dental technicians.[53]

Desert sand is practically pure silica but the particles are generally too large to reach the lungs. However, silicosis has been reported in inhabitants of the Sahara, Libyan and Negev deserts and those living in windy valleys high in the Himalayan mountains,[54-60] while in California the inhalation of dust raised from earth has led to silicate pneumoconiosis in farm workers,[61] horses[62] and a variety of zoo animals.[63]

The silica in rocks such as granite, slate and sandstone is largely in the form of quartz and this is therefore the type of silica encountered in most of the industries considered above. Cristobalite and tridymite, which are possibly even more fibrogenic than quartz, are more likely to be encountered in the ceramic, refractory and diatomaceous earth industries where processing involves high temperatures.

Clinical features

Many workers with silicosis are asymptomatic. As a general rule, exposure to silica dust extends over many years, often 20 or more, before the symptoms of silicosis first appear: by the time the disease becomes overt clinically, much irreparable damage has been inflicted on the lungs. The initial symptoms are cough and breathlessness. From then onwards, respiratory disability progresses, even if the patient is no longer exposed to silica dust. Ultimately, there may be distressing dyspnoea with even the slightest exercise.

Silicosis sometimes develops more rapidly, perhaps within a year or so of first exposure. Such 'acute silicosis' was observed in the scouring powder industry in the 1930s when these cleansing agents consisted of ground sandstone mixed with a little soap and washing soda.[64,65] The additives were considered to have rendered the silica in the sandstone more dangerous but it is possible that the rapidity of onset of the disease merely reflected the intensity of the dust cloud to which the packers were exposed. Confusingly, the term 'acute silicosis' has since been applied to a further effect of heavy dust exposure in tunnellers, sand blasters and silica flour workers, namely pulmonary alveolar lipoproteinosis (see below),[66,67] while the terms 'accelerated silicosis' or 'cellular phase silicosis' have been substituted for 'acute silicosis' in referring to the rapid development of early cellular lesions.[40,68]

The time from first exposure to the development of symptoms (the latency period) would appear to be inversely proportional to the exposure level. Furthermore, it is evident that a certain amount of silica can be tolerated in the lungs without fibrosis developing, indicating either a time factor in the pathogenetic process or a threshold dust load that has to be reached before fibrosis develops.

Pathological findings

Silica particles that are roughly spherical in shape and of a diameter in the range of 1–5 μm sediment out in the alveoli and are concentrated within macrophages at Macklin's dust sumps, as explained previously (see pp. 27, 331). Early lesions, as seen in so-called accelerated or cellular phase silicosis, consist of collections of macrophages separated by only an occasional wisp of collagen. The early lesions have been likened to granulomas and on occasion have been mistaken for Langerhans cell histiocytosis or a storage disorder, but Langerhans cells are scanty and the histiocytes contain dust particles rather than accumulated lipid or polysaccharide. The macrophages of the early lesion are gradually replaced by fibroblasts and collagen is laid down in a characteristic pattern. The mature silicotic nodule is largely acellular and consists of hyaline collagen arranged in a whorled pattern, the whole lesion being well demarcated (Fig. 7.1.8) and sometimes calcified. Small numbers of birefringent crystals are generally evident within the nodules when polarising filters are used, but these mainly represent silicates such as mica and talc, inhaled with the silica. Silica particles are generally considered to be only weakly birefringent,[40] although this is disputed (see above).[41]

The silicotic nodules are situated in the centres of the pulmonary acini and are more numerous in the upper zones than the bases (Fig. 7.1.9). They measure up to 5 mm across and are hard and easily palpable. They are grey if caused by relatively pure silica but black in coal miners and red in haematite miners.

Silicotic nodules develop first in the hilar lymph nodes and are generally better developed there than in the lungs.[69–71] Indeed, silicotic nodules are occasionally found in the hilar lymph nodes of persons who have no occupational history of exposure to silica and whose lungs are free of such lesions, the silica in the nodes being presumed to represent inhaled particles derived from quartz-rich soil.[72] Severely affected lymph nodes often calcify peripherally, giving a characteristic eggshell-like radiographic pattern. This is sometimes the only radiological abnormality.[71] Such enlarged lymph nodes may occasionally press upon and obstruct adjacent large bronchi[73] or result in a left recurrent laryngeal nerve palsy,[74] so simulating malignancy.[75] Sometimes the nodules develop within the walls of major bronchi, occasionally causing a middle lobe syndrome (see p. 89).[76] Silicotic nodules are also found along the lines of the pleural lymphatics[70,77] where they have been likened to drops of candle wax on the visceral pleura. Very rarely, silica-induced fibrosis is more pronounced in the pleura than in the lungs.[78]

Lung tissue between the nodules is often quite normal and not until the process is very advanced is there any disability. In

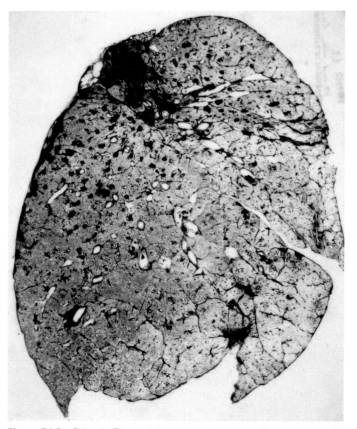

Figure 7.1.9 Silicosis. The nodules are most numerous in the upper part of the lung where there is a conglomerate silicotic mass at one point. Paper-mounted whole lung section.

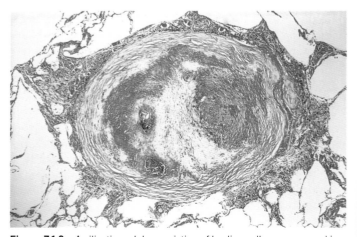

Figure 7.1.8 A silicotic nodule consisting of hyaline collagen arranged in a whorled pattern.

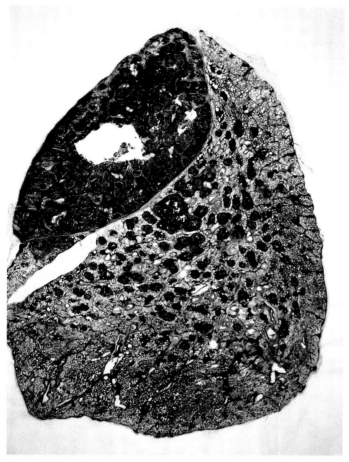

Figure 7.1.10 Silicosis. The nodules are larger than in Fig. 7.1.9 and have fused together. Cavitating conglomerate silicosis destroys most of the upper lobe. Paper-mounted whole lung section.

severe cases large masses of fibrous tissue are formed (Fig. 7.1.10).[79] On close inspection it is evident that these consist of conglomerations of many silicotic nodules closely packed together. In such severe cases cor pulmonale develops. Occasionally, silicotic nodules develop in the abdominal as well as the thoracic lymph nodes, and in the liver, spleen, peritoneum and bone marrow.[80–84]

In about 10% of cases, the typical pulmonary nodules that predominantly affect the upper lobes are accompanied by diffuse fibrosis that is maximal in the lower lobes.[24,30,85–87] The latter may show 'honeycombing' and closely resemble cryptogenic fibrosing alveolitis. The association is too common to be explained by chance and the diffuse fibrosis is therefore regarded as a further manifestation of the pneumoconiosis, possibly due to an interaction between the dust and the immunological factors discussed below.

Pathogenesis

The pathogenesis of silicosis has excited much interest and many different theories have been advanced over the years. An early theory held that the hardness of the silica was respon-

sible, but this was discounted by the observation that silicon carbide (carborundum) is harder than silica but is non-fibrogenic. Theories based on the piezoelectric property and on the solubility of silica were successively abandoned although the latter had a long period of popularity. It gained support from Kettle's experiments, which showed that fibrosis developed about chambers placed in an animal's peritoneal cavity if the chambers contained silica powder sealed in by a collodion membrane through which solutes such as silicic acid could pass. However, it was later shown that the pores in a collodion membrane were quite irregular in size and when the experiments were repeated using chambers guarded by millipore membranes, no fibrosis developed, despite solutes being able to diffuse out.[88] The solubility theory also fails to take account of the differing fibrogenicity of the various forms of silica despite them being of similar solubility.[49] Furthermore, if the outer, more soluble layer of the particles is removed by etching, fibrogenicity is increased although solubility is decreased. In line with this, freshly-fractured crystalline silica is more pathogenic in every respect than its aged equivalent,[89] which may partly explain the severity of silicosis in trades such as sandblasting. These observations suggest that the fibrogenicity of silica is connected with its surface configuration.

It is now known that uptake of the silica by macrophages is necessary for silicosis to develop. If silica and macrophages are enclosed together in peritoneal millipore chambers, a soluble product of the macrophages diffuses out and causes fibrosis. This observation led to the realisation that the fibrogenicity of the various crystalline forms of silica correlated well with their toxicity to macrophages and for a time macrophage death was thought to be necessary.[90] It is now considered that before the macrophages are killed by the ingested silica, they are stimulated to secrete factors that both damage other constituents of the lung and promote fibrosis.[91–97] Transforming growth factor-β is one fibrogenic factor that has been implicated in the pathogenesis of silicosis.[98–100]

Toxic damage to macrophages is due to silica particles injuring the phagolysosomal membranes, so releasing acid hydrolases into the cytoplasm.[90] It is important in the pathogenesis of the disease indirectly because when the macrophage crumbles, the silica particles are taken up by fresh macrophages and the fibrogenic process continues. It has been suggested that early involvement of the hilar lymph nodes in the fibrogenic process promotes the development of the disease in the lung by delaying dust clearance.[69]

Immunological aspects of silicosis

Immunological factors have been implicated in the pathogenesis of silicosis because many patients with silicosis have polyclonal hypergammaglobulinaemia, rheumatoid factor or antinuclear antibodies, and because there is a well-recognised association between autoimmune diseases such as systemic sclerosis and rheumatoid disease and exposure to silica.[40,101–104] The relation of immunity to dust exposure appears to be a reciprocal one: on the one hand, the presence of dust results in rheumatoid lesions in the lungs being more florid (see Caplan's syndrome, p. 344), while on the other, non-specific immunisation of rabbits with horse serum results in experimental silicotic lesions being larger and more collagenous.[105] It is doubtful whether pneumoconiosis and autoimmune disease play a causative role in each other but one seems to aggravate the other and may lead to its earlier development.

Tuberculosis complicating silicosis (silicotuberculosis)

One of the most common and most feared complications of silicosis is chronic respiratory tuberculosis.[104] Once this infection has been added to the silicosis, the prognosis rapidly worsens. It is thought that in the presence of silica, the tubercle bacilli proliferate more rapidly because the ingested silica particles damage phagolysosomal membranes and thereby interfere with the defensive activity of the macrophages. The synergistic action of silica dust has long been held responsible for the inordinately high incidence of respiratory tuberculosis in mining communities. Many former South African gold miners now have AIDS as well as silicosis and tuberculosis has consequently reached almost epidemic proportions among these men. Phagocyte damage by ingested dust particles may also account for some cases of chronic necrotising aspergillosis complicating pneumoconiosis.[106]

Silica-induced lung cancer

A series of studies suggesting that there might be a link between silica inhalation and lung cancer was reviewed by the International Agency for Research on Cancer in 1987, leading to the conclusion that the evidence for carcinogenicity of crystalline silica in experimental animals was sufficient, while in man it was limited.[107] Subsequent epidemiological publications were reviewed in 1996, when it was concluded that the epidemiological evidence linking exposure to silica to the risk of lung cancer had become somewhat stronger but that in the absence of lung fibrosis remained scanty.[108] The pathological evidence in man is also weak in that premalignant changes around silicotic nodules are seldom evident.[109] Nevertheless, on this rather insubstantial evidence, lung cancer in the presence of silicosis (but not coal- or mixed dust pneumoconiosis) has been accepted as a prescribed industrial disease in the UK since 1992.[110] Some subsequent studies have provided support for this decision.[111] In contrast to the sparse data on classic silicosis, the evidence linking carcinoma of the lung to the rare diffuse pattern of fibrosis attributed to silica and mixed dusts is much stronger and appears incontrovertible.[30,87]

Alveolar lipoproteinosis in response to heavy dust exposure

A further complication of exposure to silica is the development of alveolar lipoproteinosis (see p. 317).[66,67,112,113] Very heavy experimental exposure to silica, and indeed other dusts, stimu-

lates hypersecretion of alveolar surfactant to such an extent that the normal clearance mechanism is overwhelmed.[114–120] Alveolar macrophages are enlarged by numerous phagolysosomes distended by lamellar bodies that represent ingested surfactant. The alveoli are filled by such cells and, having a foamy cytoplasm, they produce the appearances of endogenous lipid pneumonia, similar to that more usually encountered as part of an obstructive pneumonitis distal to a bronchial tumour (see p. 316). The macrophages gradually disintegrate and the free denatured surfactant slowly becomes compacted, during which time its staining with both eosin and the periodic acid-Schiff reagents intensifies until the appearances are finally those of alveolar lipoproteinosis. This process prevents the aggregation and concentration of the dust in the usual foci and thereby hinders the development of silicosis. Lipoproteinosis and silicosis may be seen in conjunction but, more often, different areas of the lung show one or the other. The lipoproteinosis has its own severe impact on lung function, but, unlike silicosis, is potentially reversible (by massive alveolar lavage).

Silica-induced renal disease

Occasional patients exposed to silica develop renal disease.[121–124] Two mechanisms appear to operate. First, translocation of silica particles from the lungs leads to their deposition in the renal interstitium with resultant nephrotoxicity. Second, silica stimulates an autoimmune response characterised by the formation of various antibodies, notably rheumatoid factor and antinuclear antibodies, which leads to the development of immune complex-mediated glomerulonephritis.[123,124]

Amorphous silica

Man-made submicron forms of silica, variously known as amorphous, vitreous, colloidal, synthetic or precipitated silica, are widely used in industry. They consist of pure non-crystalline silicon dioxide. Particle sizes range from 5 to 200 nm but aggregates of the particles measure from 1 to 10 μm. Industrial surveys suggest that inhalation of such dust is harmless, observations that are in accord with the results of animal experiments.[49]

Diatomaceous earth (*kieselguhr*)

An amorphous silica is the principal component of the fossilised remains of diatoms that constitute the sedimentary rock, diatomite (Fig. 7.1.11). This is generally obtained by open cast mining, following which the rock is crushed and calcined. The calcined product is used in filters, insulation material and as a filler. Being amorphous, the silica in diatomite is harmless, but calcining (>1000°C) results in its conversion to crystalline forms of silica. Diatomaceous earth pneumoconiosis is unusual and its risk appears to be related to the amount of cristobalite and tridymite (two forms of crystalline silica) produced in the calcining process.[125]

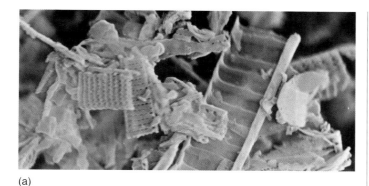

(a)

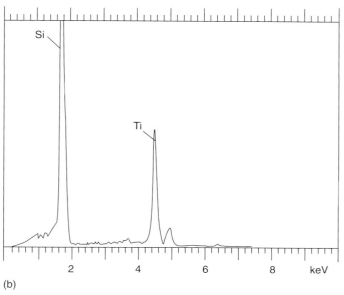

(b)

Figure 7.1.11 Diatomaceous earth. (a) Scanning electron micrograph showing the calcified diatoms. (b) Electron microprobe analysis shows only silicon (Si), the oxygen with which silicon is combined in silica (silicon dioxide, SiO_2) is of too low an atomic number to register. The titanium (Ti) peak derives from the sample holder. (Illustration provided by Dr D Dinsdale, Leicester, UK and Professor B Nemery, Leuven, Belgium.)

SILICATES

The silicates[40] are complex compounds in which silicon and oxygen form an anion combined with cations such as aluminium and magnesium: talc for example is a hydrated magnesium silicate with the formula $Mg_3Si_4O_{10}(OH)_2$. Silicates include fibrous forms (asbestos and the zeolites), plate-like forms (talc and mica), and clays (kaolinite and Fuller's earth). In histological sections, the platy talc and mica particles are generally cut tangentially and therefore appear needle-shaped (Fig. 7.1.4). They are strongly birefringent whereas the clays are only weakly so. Talc particles in the lung exceeding $5\mu m$ in length should arouse suspicion of intravenous drug abuse.[126]

Of the fibrous silicates, zeolite is used as a building material in certain communities, notably in central Turkey. Pneumoco-

niosis is not a problem but zeolites are of medical interest because, like asbestos, they present a mesothelioma risk (see p. 702). Asbestosis is dealt with separately (see p. 345).

Pneumoconiosis has been described with various non-fibrous silicates, notably in the rubber industry, which uses talc and less commonly mica as lubricants. Other occupations posing a risk include the extraction of kaolinite from china clay (kaolin),[24,127,128] and in the open-cast and underground mining of Fuller's earth (montmorillonite, bentonite and attapulgite clays, which were originally used in 'fulling' (de-greasing) wool).[22,129] However, all these substances are commonly contaminated with silica, asbestos, or both, and it has been questioned whether in pure state they are at all fibrogenic. The modifying effect of inert substances such as iron on that of silica is well known (see mixed dust pneumoconiosis, below) and it has been suggested that talc, mica and Fuller's earth act in a similar way in regard to their more fibrogenic contaminants, the pneumoconioses attributed to them in reality representing mixed dust pneumoconiosis or asbestosis. Contrary evidence comes from reports of pulmonary fibrosis in persons heavily exposed to pure talc, mica or kaolin.[29]

All these silicates are evident in the tissues as plate-like birefringent crystals, which often provoke a foreign body giant cell reaction (Fig. 7.1.4) and may result in fibrotic nodules. Large focal lesions resembling the progressive massive fibrosis of coal workers (see p. 343) may be produced, and also a diffuse 'asbestosis-like' form of pneumoconiosis, the latter attributed to poor macrophage mobilisation of the plate-like particles.[22,24–29,127–132] It would appear therefore that silicates are indeed fibrogenic if enough is inhaled; they appear to vary in the fibrogenicity but in all cases they are less fibrogenic than silica.

INERT DUSTS

Inert dusts are non-fibrogenic and therefore of little clinical consequence although elements of high atomic number can give rise to a striking chest radiograph.[133] It should be noted however that inert or lowly fibrogenic materials may be associated with substances of medical importance, for example, kaolin, bentonite and barytes (barite) may all be contaminated with silica[24,129,134] and talc may be contaminated with tremolite asbestos.

The best known of the inhaled inert mineral dusts is carbon but because this forms the basis of coal it is considered separately (see below). Of the remainder, iron is the most widespread. Others include tin and barium. With all these dusts, particles retained in the lung are gathered at Macklin's dust sumps by heavily-laden macrophages which are lightly bound together there by a few reticulin fibres. Collagen is not formed and the worker suffers no ill-effects. The lungs take on the colour of the dust and, in siderosis, assume a deep brick-red hue.

Iron dust in the lungs was first described by Zenker in 1867, when he also introduced the terms siderosis and pneumonokoniosis.[1] Zenker was describing a woman who coloured paper with iron oxide powder ('rouge'), which substance is still encountered by some workers engaged in polishing silver, glass, stone and cutlery. Siderosis is also found in welders (see p. 357), iron foundry fettlers, steel workers, boiler scalers and haematite miners and crushers (see Fig. 7.1.3b). Iron dust particles are reddish-brown but in the lung may be masked by carbon:[135] when evident, or revealed by microincineration, they resemble haemosiderin and generally give a positive Perls' reaction, but particularly with haematite, heat (60–80°C) and concentrated (12N) hydrochloric acid may be necessary.[136]

Haematite miners in both Britain (Cumbria) and France (Lorraine) have an increased risk of bronchial carcinoma, but radon gas rather than haematite is the suspected carcinogen. Radon is a decay product of uranium. Minute amounts are present in all rocks but local concentrations occur and these are liable to build up in mines if ventilation is limited.

Silver, as well as iron, is found in the lungs of silver polishers, where it stains elastin in alveolar walls and pulmonary vessels grey. Such argyro-siderosis is as harmless as siderosis.

Tin miners are subject to silicosis but not stannosis because the ore, which is found in association with siliceous rocks, contains only low concentrations of the metal. Tin smelters, on the other hand, and factory workers exposed to high concentrations of tin dust or fume, are liable to inhale large amounts of this inert metal and develop the striking chest radiograph of stannosis. They remain in good health however for tin is completely non-fibrogenic. Tin particles in the lung resemble carbon but are strongly birefringent and remain after microincineration: microprobe analysis provides positive identification.

Other inert dusts include barium, which also has a high atomic number and is therefore radio-opaque,[133] and minerals of low radiodensity such as limestone, marble and cement (all chiefly composed of calcium carbonate) and gypsum (hydrated calcium sulphate). However, the extraction of barium ore (almost entirely in the form of barium sulphate, which is known as barytes in Europe and barite in the USA) may entail exposure to silica and silicates. Pure baritosis resembles stannosis and siderosis.

MIXED DUST PNEUMOCONIOSIS

The term 'mixed dust pneumoconiosis' refers to the changes brought about by inhaling a mixture of silica and some other less fibrogenic substance such as iron, carbon, kaolin or mica.[135] The proportion of silica is usually less than 10%. Typical occupations include foundry work and welding and the mining of coal, haematite, slate, shale and china clay.

The action of the silica is modified and although fibrotic nodules are formed, they lack the well-demarcated outline and concentric pattern of classical silicosis. The lesions are found in a centriacinar position and are stellate in outline with adjacent scar emphysema. They are firm and generally measure no more than 5 mm in diameter. They closely resemble the fibrotic nodules of simple coal pneumoconiosis (see below). Confluent

lesions also occur on occasions. These resemble the progressive massive fibrosis of coal workers and appear to represent a single large lesion rather than a conglomeration of individual nodules, as in advanced silicosis. Abundant dust is generally evident in lesions of all sizes; this consists of black carbon or brown iron mixed with crystals of varying degrees of birefringence, silicates generally being strongly birefringent and silica weakly so. Calcification is unusual. Mixed dust pneumoconiosis carries an increased risk of pulmonary tuberculosis, but not to the same degree as silicosis. In some cases the stellate nodules are accompanied by diffuse fibrosis, as in silicosis and again possibly involving interactions between the dust and immunological factors (see p. 337).

COAL PNEUMOCONIOSIS[137]

The term anthracosis was initially applied to changes observed in a coal miner's lung[138] but is now often extended to include the common carbon pigmentation of city dwellers' lungs, and the term coal pneumoconiosis is more appropriate to a special form of pneumoconiosis to which coal workers are subject, particularly those who work underground. The principal constituent of coal, carbon, is non-fibrogenic, so suspicion has naturally fallen on the ash content of mine dust, some of which derives from the coal, some from adjacent rock strata and some from stone dust laid in the roadways to minimise the risk of coal dust explosions. Coal itself appears to be the responsible agent because coal-trimmers, working in the docks and not exposed to rock dust, also develop the disease.[139] Coal miners encountering siliceous rock are, of course, also liable to develop silicosis like other underground workers.

Mineralogy

Coal consists largely of elemental carbon, oxygen and hydrogen with traces of iron ore and clays such as kaolinite, muscovite and illite, but no silica. The mineral content varies with the type and rank (calorific value) of the coal. All coal derives from peat, the youngest type being lignite and the oldest anthracite, with bituminous (house) coal in between. As it ages, the oxygen and mineral constituents diminish and the coal hardens. Lignite is soft and said to be of low rank, anthracite hard and of high rank, with bituminous coal intermediate.

Although high rank coal is of low mineral content, its dust is more toxic to macrophages *in vitro* and is cleared more slowly *in vivo*. This observation may explain why, in Britain, high rank coal is associated with a higher prevalence of coal pneumoconiosis.

The low mineral content of high rank coal is reflected in the mineral content of the lungs of those who hew such coal in Britain, but in the Ruhr, in Germany, and in Pennsylvania, in the USA, anthracite miners' lungs contain more silica than those who hew bituminous coal, the silica presumably deriving from other sources. Not surprisingly, the presence of silica is reflected in the tissue reaction to the inhaled dust, resulting in a more fibrotic reaction very analogous to mixed dust pneumoconiosis. A spectrum of changes is therefore encountered in coal miners' lungs, ranging from coal pneumoconiosis through mixed dust pneumoconiosis to silicosis, the findings in any individual depending upon the nature of the coal being mined and the type of work undertaken.

In high rank British collieries the development of coal pneumoconiosis appears to depend on the total mass of dust inhaled, whereas in low rank British collieries the mineral content of the lung dust appears to be more important.[140] This may explain apparently contrary data drawn from different coalfields – data based on coals of different composition that are not strictly comparable. Some workers have stressed the importance of silica in the dust whereas others, particularly in the high rank coalfields of South Wales, have been unable to detect any association between silica and the level of pneumoconiosis. Both findings may be correct – but only for the particular group of miners examined in each case.[141]

Pathology

The lesions of coal pneumoconiosis are generally focal and fall into one of two major types: simple and complicated, depending upon whether the lesions measure up to or over 1 cm; 'simple' corresponds to categories 1 to 3 of the International Labour Organisation (ILO) grading system (see p. 334) and 'complicated', which is also known as progressive massive fibrosis, to ILO categories A to C. More diffuse interstitial fibrosis has been reported in about 16% of Welsh and West Virginian coal miners, usually involving those carrying a particularly heavy dust burden; it runs a more benign course than non-occupational interstitial fibrosis (idiopathic pulmonary fibrosis).[142] Similar findings have been reported from France.[143]

Simple coal pneumoconiosis consists of focal dust pigmentation of the lungs, which may be associated with a little fibrosis and varying degrees of emphysema. Its clinical effects are relatively minor. Some degree of black pigmentation (anthracosis) of the lungs is common in the general urban population, especially in industrial areas, but much denser pigmentation is seen in coal miners, whose lungs at necropsy are black or slate-grey (see Fig. 7.1.3a). Black pigment is evident in the visceral pleura along the lines of the lymphatics and on the cut surface where it outlines the interlobular septa and is concentrated in Macklin's centriacinar dust sumps (Fig. 7.1.12). The dust is generally more plentiful in the upper parts of the lungs and in the hilar lymph nodes,[143] possibly due to poorer perfusion and consequently poorer lymphatic drainage there.

Two forms of coal dust foci are recognised, macules and nodules, the former being soft and impalpable and the latter hard, due to substantial amounts of collagen. Both lesions are typically stellate but the more fibrotic the nodules, the more rounded they become, until it is difficult to distinguish them macroscopically from those of silicosis. In these circumstances reliance has to be placed on the whorled pattern of the collagen that is evident microscopically in silicosis. The stellate nodules are analogous to those seen in mixed dust pneumoconiosis

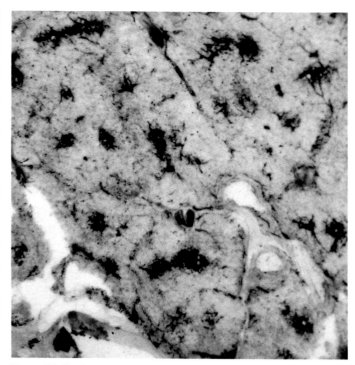

Figure 7.1.12 A coal miner's lung showing heavy dust deposition in the centres of the acini. On palpation the dust deposits felt soft and were consequently described as macules rather than nodules. Despite the heavy dust deposition, there is minimal pneumoconiosis. Paper-mounted whole lung section.

caused by mixtures of silica and inert dusts other than carbon (see p. 340). With polarising filters, small numbers of birefringent crystals may be seen in both macules and nodules, usually representing mica or kaolinite derived from rock that bordered the coal.

Macules consist of closely-packed dust particles, free or within heavily laden macrophages, so that the lesion appears black throughout (Fig. 7.1.13). Appropriate stains show that the dust-laden macrophages and free dust are lightly bound by reticulin. Very little collagen is evident. Although striking in their appearance, dust macules are thought to have little effect on lung function.

Nodules contain substantial amounts of collagen and are thought to have an adverse, but limited, effect on respiration. They vary from a heavily pigmented, stellate lesion, which apart from its collagen content resembles the dust macule (Fig. 7.1.14), to one that is less pigmented and more circumscribed. The stellate, heavily-pigmented type of nodule is seen in lungs that have a relatively low ash content while the more rounded and less pigmented nodule is seen in lungs with relatively high ash loads.[144]

Radiologically (see p. 334), p type opacities correspond to macules, q type opacities to the stellate nodules that resemble those of mixed dust pneumoconiosis, and r type opacities to the rounded nodules that resemble those of silicosis.[48,145] Thus, the radiological changes of simple coal workers' pneumoconiosis

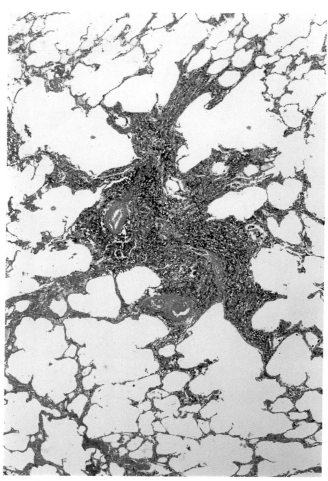

Figure 7.1.13 Coal macule. A centriacinar dust deposit of stellate outline consisting of macrophages heavily-laden with coal dust and bound together by only a little reticulin. Collagen is not well represented.

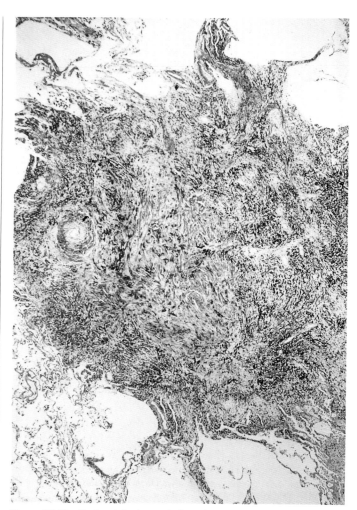

Figure 7.1.14 Coal nodule. A centriacinar dust nodule of stellate outline in which coal dust-laden macrophages are mixed with moderate amounts of collagen.

are due to the dust and the small amount of collagen present and do not reflect any emphysema that may also be present. However, pulmonary dust foci are often associated with emphysema (Fig. 7.1.15) and the severity of the emphysema appears to correlate with the dust load. The prevalence of chronic bronchitis and emphysema is high in the coal industry and it has long been debated whether occupation or cigarette smoking is the major factor contributing to emphysema in coal miners.[146–149] As well as mineral dust, nitrous fumes from shot-firing form another occupational hazard of coal mining.

Heppleston made a special study of the emphysema found in coal miners, claiming that it differs from centriacinar emphysema, as seen in smokers in the general population, and attributing it to the dust.[150] He introduced the term focal emphysema of coal workers to describe this special process. Others find it very difficult to identify any convincing difference between the emphysema of coal workers and that encountered outside the industry but Heppleston based his claims on the study of serial sections. By this means he showed that although

both forms affect respiratory bronchioles, the focal emphysema of coal workers affects more proximal orders of these airways and is not associated with the bronchiolitis seen with centriacinar emphysema. Furthermore, focal emphysema is a dilatation lesion whereas centriacinar emphysema involves destruction of adjacent alveolar walls. By definition, therefore, focal emphysema is not a true emphysema at all (see p. 105). However, it has been shown that mineral dusts cause elastin and collagen breakdown in the rat lung.[151] Focal emphysema may progress to the destructive centriacinar form and this has strengthened claims that mine dust plays a causal role in centriacinar emphysema.[152–156] In the UK, these claims have been accepted and chronic bronchitis and emphysema in coal miners and metal production workers have been accepted as prescribed industrial diseases since 1992.[157] In Germany too, chronic obstructive pulmonary disease is now compensatable as an occupational disease. The conditions for compensation in Britain were initially:

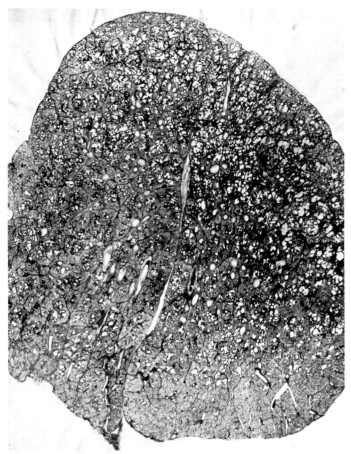

Figure 7.1.15 Coal workers' pneumoconiosis – simple type, consisting of coal macules and nodules associated with focal emphysema. Paper-mounted whole lung section.

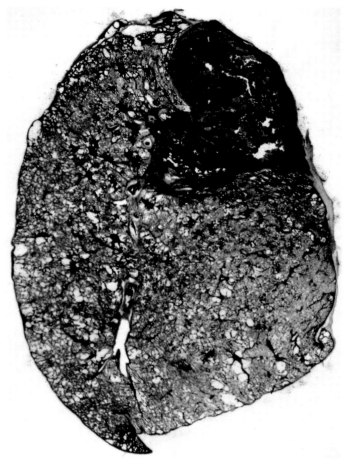

Figure 7.1.16 Coal pneumoconiosis – complicated type. In addition to the focal dust deposits there is a large area of progressive massive fibrosis in the upper lobe. Paper-mounted whole lung section.

- Underground coal mining for a minimum of 20 years in aggregate
- Forced expiratory volume in 1 second at least 1 litre below that expected or less than 1 litre in total
- Radiological category of at least 1/1 (see p. 334)

but the last of these criteria has now been dropped. The inclusion of a time element and the omission of some estimate of dust load (such as radiological category) have been criticised with some justification.[158] As with lung cancer caused by chromates benefit is paid irrespective of smoking habits.

Whereas simple coal pneumoconiosis, particularly the macular variety, has little effect on lung function, complicated coal pneumoconiosis, also known as progressive massive fibrosis, can have very serious consequences. Particularly when the lesions are large, it is associated with productive cough, breathlessness, significant impairment of lung function and premature death. The major factor accounting for the development of progressive massive fibrosis appears to be the sheer bulk of coal dust in the lung, rather than coal rank or the silica content of the mine dust.[159] Progressive massive fibrosis has occasionally been recorded in dockers loading silica-free coal into the holds

of ships[139] and in workers exposed to pure carbon in the manufacture of carbon black and carbon electrodes.[160–162]

Progressive massive fibrosis is characterised by large (over 1 cm) black masses, situated anywhere in the lungs but most common in the upper lobes. The lesions may be solitary or multiple and very large, occupying most of the lobe and even crossing an interlobar fissure to involve an adjacent lobe (Fig. 7.1.16). They cut fairly easily, often with the release from a central cavity of black fluid flecked by cholesterol crystals. For many years, it was believed that the condition was the result of synergism between mycobacterial infection and dust but the failure of the attack rate to decrease as tuberculosis declined negated this view.[163] Today, more emphasis is placed on total dust load for the lesions tend to affect lungs that carry an unduly heavy dust burden. If the remainder of the lung shows little evidence of dust accumulation, the possibility of the masses representing Caplan-type lesions (see below) should be considered.

Microscopically, the lesions consist of dust and connective tissue intermixed in a random fashion. Central necrosis and cavitation commonly occur. The necrosis is thought to be ischaemic.[164] It is amorphous or finely granular, and eosinophilic apart from abundant dust particles and cholesterol crystal clefts. The fibrotic component in a complicated pneumoconiotic lesion is rich in fibronectin, with collagen only more abundant at the periphery.[165] Two types of progressive massive fibrosis are recognisable, corresponding to the two types of nodule described in simple coal pneumoconiosis.[144] The first appears to have arisen by enlargement of a single nodule, whereas the second is a conglomeration of individual lesions, each of which corresponds to the more circumscribed type of nodule seen in simple coal pneumoconiosis. The ash content of the lungs bearing these two types of progressive massive fibrosis varies in the same way as with the two types of simple pneumoconiotic nodules, the enlarged single lesion being found in lungs with a relatively low ash content, and the conglomerate lesion in lungs with a relatively high ash content. The second type resembles the conglomerate nodules of large silicotic lesions but lacks the characteristic whorled pattern of the latter.

The diffuse interstitial fibrosis found in a minority of coal workers is associated with heavy dust deposition. It may progress to honeycombing but as with the focal forms and unlike idiopathic interstitial fibrosis it is better developed in the upper zones, the reasons for which are discussed above (see the zonal distribution of pneumoconiosis, p. 331).

Pathogenesis

The pathogenesis of coal pneumoconiosis has much in common with that of silicosis, and indeed many other pneumoconioses. It involves the promotion of fibrogenic factor synthesis and release by cells phagocytosing the inhaled dust. Several such factors have now been identified, the degree of fibrosis produced varying with the amount of dust inhaled and the ability of its constituents to promote the production of the responsible cytokines. These include platelet-derived growth factor, insulin-like growth factors 1 and 6, transforming growth factor-β and tumour necrosis factor-α.[96,166,167] As with other minerals, the indestructability of the dust perpetuates the process.

As in silicosis, immunological factors appear to be involved, for there is an increased prevalence of rheumatoid arthritis[168] and of circulating autoantibodies[169–171] in miners with coal pneumoconiosis. Rheumatoid factor has also been demonstrated within the lung lesions.[172] These abnormalities are generally more pronounced in miners with complicated pneumoconiosis but are also found in those with the simple variety. It is also possibly pertinent to the immunological basis of coal pneumoconiosis that some of the pulmonary manifestations of rheumatoid disease are more pronounced in coal miners. This was first pointed out by Caplan and will now be considered.

PNEUMOCONIOSIS AND RHEUMATOID DISEASE (CAPLAN'S SYNDROME)

Caplan described distinctive radiographic opacities in the lungs of coal miners with rheumatoid disease,[173] and it is now recog-

nised that similar lesions may develop in rheumatoid patients exposed to siliceous dusts. The development of such rheumatoid pneumoconiosis does not correlate with the extrapulmonary or serological activity of the rheumatoid process. Nor is there a strong relation to dust burden: Caplan lesions are characteristically seen in chest radiographs that show little evidence of simple coal pneumoconiosis.

Pathologists recognise the lesions as particularly large necrobiotic nodules similar to those seen in rheumatoid patients who are not exposed to dust. However, because of their large size (up to 5 cm diameter) they may be confused with progressive massive fibrosis undergoing central ischaemic necrosis (see above) or silicosis complicated by caseating tuberculosis. Such errors will be less likely if the radiological evolution of the lesions is considered for they tend to cavitate and undergo rapid remission, only to be succeeded by others. They are also well demarcated radiologically. Pathologically, they resemble rheumatoid nodules in showing peripheral palisading but differ in their large size and the presence of dust.[174] The dust accumulates in circumferential bands or arcs within the necrotic centres of the lesion (Fig. 7.1.17), an arrangement that suggests periodic episodes of inflammatory activity. Caplan lesions differ from tuberculosis in lacking satellite lesions and tubercle bacilli, and from progressive massive fibrosis in showing characteristic bands of dust pigmentation (Table 7.1.2).

Table 7.1.2 Histological features of Caplan lesions, silicotuberculosis and progressive massive fibrosis

	Caplan lesions	Silicotuberculosis	Progressive massive fibrosis
Palisading	+	−	−
Dust banding	+	−	−
Satellite tubercles	−	+	−
Necrosis	+	+	+
Cholesterol crystals	+	±	+
Calcification	+	+	±

+, present; ±, poorly represented; −, absent

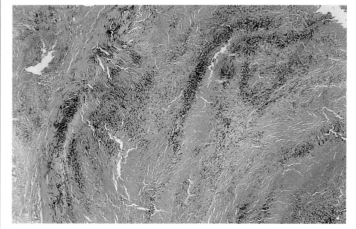

Figure 7.1.17 A Caplan lesion, characterised by successive bands of dust within the centre of a large necrobiotic nodule.

ASBESTOSIS

Asbestosis is limited to pulmonary fibrosis caused by asbestos. It does not include asbestos-induced carcinoma of the lung or asbestos-induced pleural disease. The development of asbestosis depends on the presence of fairly large dust burdens: this is in contrast to mesothelioma and other forms of asbestos-induced pleural disease, which although also dose-related, follow the inhalation of far smaller amounts of asbestos.

Asbestos types and production

Asbestos is a generic term for more than 30 naturally occurring fibrous silicates, fibre being defined as an elongated particle with a length to breadth (aspect) ratio of at least three. Asbestos fibres have a high aspect ratio, generally over eight. Based on their physical configuration they can be divided into two major groups: serpentine and amphibole. The physical dimensions and configuration of asbestos fibres are strongly linked to their pathogenicity.

Chrysotile (white asbestos) is the only important serpentine form. It accounts for most of the world production of asbestos of all types.[175] Being a serpentine mineral, chrysotile consists of long, curly fibres that can be carded, spun and woven like cotton (Fig. 7.1.18). The curly chrysotile fibres are carried into the lungs less readily than the straight amphibole asbestos

fibres, and once there undergo physico-chemical dissolution and are cleared more readily. Chrysotile is thought to be the least harmful type of asbestos in respect of all forms of asbestos-induced pleuropulmonary disease,[176–178] but nevertheless causes pulmonary fibrosis if sufficient is inhaled.[179,180]

The main amphibole forms of asbestos of commercial importance are amosite (brown asbestos) and crocidolite (blue asbestos). These consist of straight rigid fibres. Crocidolite, reputedly the most dangerous in regard to all forms of asbestos-related disease, was formerly mined in Western Australia (Wittenoom) and South Africa (Cape Province and the Transvaal); it was the principal amphibole used in Great Britain. Amosite, the name of which derives from the acronym for the former Asbestos Mines of South Africa company in the Transvaal, was the principal amphibole used in North America. Amphiboles are no longer imported by the developed countries but much remains in old lagging and presents a considerable dust hazard when this is removed. Tremolite, a further amphibole asbestos, contaminates the Quebec chrysotile deposits and many forms of commercial (non-cosmetic) talc and is responsible for much of the asbestos-related disease in chrysotile miners and millers.[181] Another amphibole asbestos, anthophyllite, was formerly mined in Finland. It causes pleural plaques (see p. 700) but not lung disease, possibly because its fibres are relatively thick (Fig. 7.1.19).[182]

Asbestos use and exposure

Exposure to asbestos occurs in countries where it is extracted (Box 7.1.1), which is mostly by the open-cast method, and in those countries that formerly imported or continue to use this mineral (Box 7.1.2). The developed nations have largely ceased to use asbestos but countries keen to develop their industrial base and less concerned with health issues continue to use considerable amounts in a vast range of trades. Asbestos is used particularly for fireproofing, in heat and sound insulation and for strengthening plastics and cement. Thus, unless adequate precautions are taken, exposure is experienced by dockers unloading asbestos in the close confines of a ship's hold, by thermal insulation workers (laggers and strippers) in shipyards, power stations, train maintenance depots, factories and other large buildings, by construction workers such as carpenters cutting asbestos building panels, and by workers making

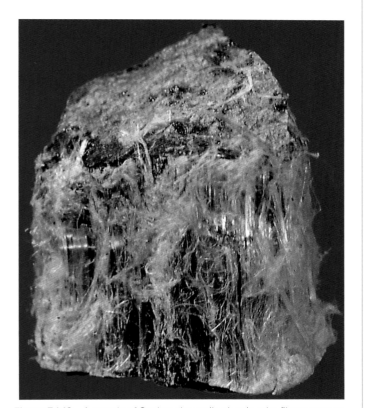

Figure 7.1.18 A sample of Quebec chrysotile showing the fibrous nature of the ore.

Box 7.1.1 Asbestos production by country, 2000[175]	
Country	**Tons p.a.**
Russia	752 000
China	350 000
Canada	320 000
Brazil	209 000
Kazakhstan	179 000
Zimbabwe	152 000
Others	88 000

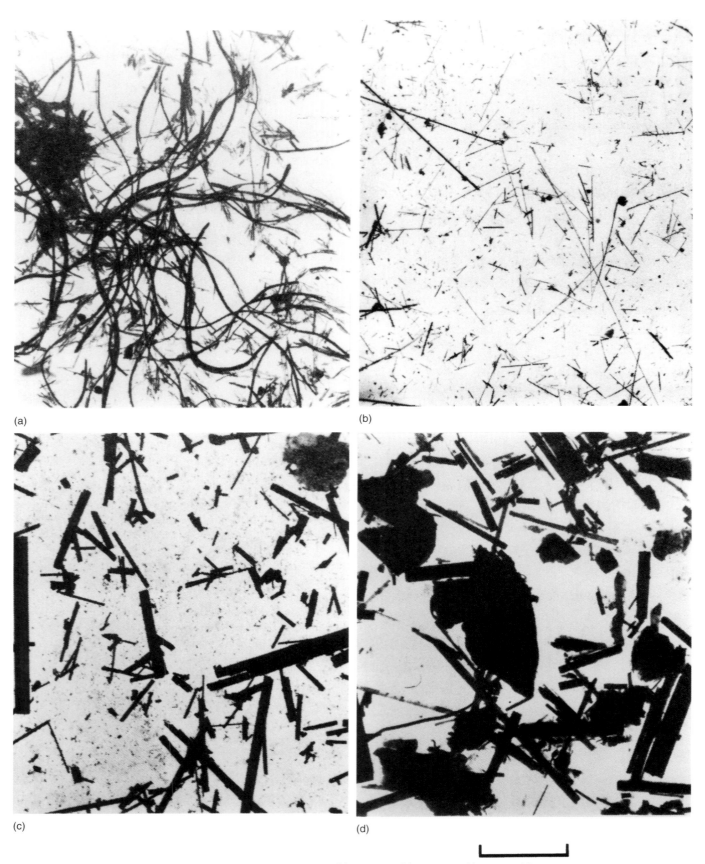

(a)

(b)

(c)

(d)

Figure 7.1.19 Electron micrographs of dispersed samples of asbestos. (a) Chrysotile, (b) crocidolite, (c) amosite, (d) anthophyllite, all × 2800, the bar representing 10 μm. (Reproduced from Wagner JC, Berry G, Pooley FD. Carcinogenesis and mineral fibres. British Medical Bulletin 1980; 36:53–56,[182] by permission of Oxford University Press and Professor FD Pooley.)

Box 7.1.2 Asbestos consumption by country, 2000[175]

Country	Tons	kg/capita/year
Russia	447 000	3.4
China	410 000	0.4
Brazil	182 000	1.3
India	125 000	0.2
Thailand	121 000	3.0
Japan	99 000	1.5
Indonesia	55 000	0.3
South Korea	29 000	1.9
Mexico	27 000	0.4
Others	178 000	

Box 7.1.3 Circumstances in which asbestos fibre counts are desirable

Quantitation desirable	Quantitation unnecessary
Mesothelioma if exposure is disputed and asbestos bodies are not evident	Mesothelioma if there is a history of exposure or asbestos bodies are evident
Pulmonary fibrosis (with or without carcinoma of the lung) in an asbestos worker but asbestos bodies are not evident	If there is obvious asbestosis
	Carcinoma of the lung in an asbestos worker if there is no fibrosis*

*Disputed. See Table 7.1.5, p. 352.

asbestos products such as fire-proof textiles, brake and clutch linings and specialised cement.

As well as such direct exposure, exposure may also be:

- indirect, as experienced by the families of asbestos workers
- para-occupational, as experienced by those working alongside an asbestos worker
- neighbourhood, as experienced by those living downwind of an asbestos works or mine
- ambient, as experienced by those living or working in a building containing asbestos.

Exposure to asbestos incorporated in the structure of a building carries a negligible health risk if the asbestos material is well maintained to prevent shedding of dust. Stripping asbestos out is more dangerous than maintaining it *in situ*, but maintenance is sometimes neglected. The near indestructibility of asbestos accentuates the health problems that its ubiquity poses and much remains in industrial countries that no longer import the ore.

Asbestos bodies

Because of their aerodynamic properties, fibres of 100 μm or more in length may reach the finer bronchioles and alveoli. Once impacted, the asbestos fibres become coated with a film of protein that is rich in iron. The coating is thickest at the ends of the fibres, giving a dumb-bell appearance. In time, a distinctive segmentation of this outer layer develops (Fig. 7.1.20). These coated structures are termed 'asbestos bodies'. Because other fibres may gain a similar coat, the non-specific term 'ferruginous body' has been advocated. However, coated carbon fibres (so-called coal bodies) are easily recognised as such by their black core.[183] In practice, ferruginous bodies with the appearance of asbestos bodies almost always prove to have an asbestos core.[184] Long fibres are more likely to be coated than short ones, which are cleared more quickly. In one study, few fibres less than 5 μm in length were coated and few fibres over 40 μm in length were uncoated.[185] Amphiboles form bodies more readily than chrysotile. A comparison of light and electron microscopic fibre counts found that 0.14% of chrysotile, 5% of crocidolite and 26.5% of amosite formed bodies.[186] Nevertheless,

sufficient chrysotile fibres are coated to permit recognition of asbestosis by standard histological criteria (diffuse fibrosis and asbestos bodies), even if chrysotile is the only asbestos present.[187] Despite the biodegradability of chrysotile, asbestos body numbers do not materially diminish with time.[188]

There is evidence that alveolar macrophages are involved in the coating of asbestos fibres to form asbestos bodies and that the bodies are less harmful to the macrophages than uncoated fibres.[189] Asbestos bodies give a Prussian blue reaction for iron when stained by Perls' method and their yellow-brown colour makes them easily recognisable in unstained films of sputum or in unstained histological sections. Sections may be cut 30 μm thick to increase the yield and help identify bodies that lie at an angle to the microtome blade. There is a good correlation between the numbers of asbestos bodies seen in lung sections and those in tissue digests.[190,191] The bodies may be found singly or in irregular clumps or stellate clusters. They are unevenly distributed but in well-established asbestosis they are easily found. If they are not evident, asbestos burden may be assessed quantitatively in tissue digests (see below). Their presence in lung tissue, sputum or broncho-alveolar lavage fluid merely confirms exposure, not the presence of disease. However, the number of asbestos bodies in lavage fluid correlates well with lung asbestos burden[192,193] and the number in sputum correlates with the duration and intensity of exposure.[192-194]

Fibre counts[195–200]

Quantitation is desirable in certain circumstances (Box 7.1.3), in which case it is best effected on tissue digests. These may be obtained by using caustic soda or bleach, or by ashing,[196] following which the fibres may be collected on a millipore membrane or viewed in suspension in a red blood cell counting chamber. If phase contrast optics are used to examine digests, both coated and uncoated fibres can be assessed.[195] Alternatively, dark ground illumination can be used to demonstrate uncoated fibres.[197] However, electron microscopy detects far more fibres than are visible by light microscopy and can provide information on fibre type.

Ambient fibres are generally shorter than 5 μm and some workers therefore confine their counts to fibres that are at least

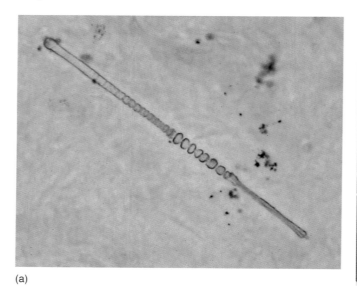

(a)

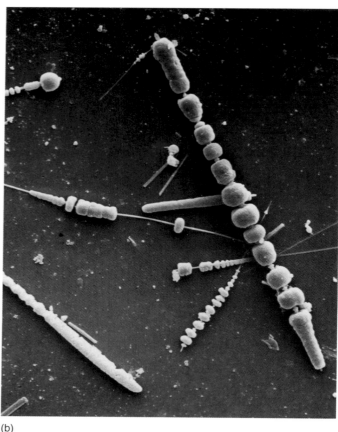

(b)

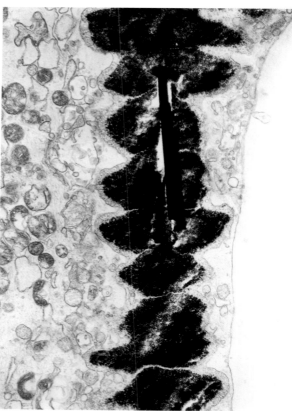

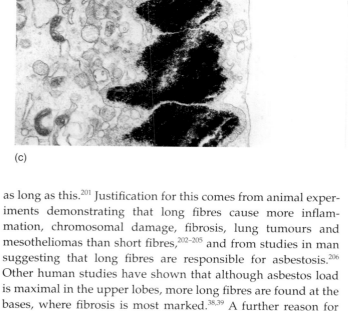

(c)

Figure 7.1.20 Asbestos bodies seen by light microscopy in an unstained 30 μm thick paraffin section (a), by scanning electron microscopy in the digest of an asbestos worker's lung (b) and by transmission electron microscopy in lung tissue (c). The asbestos fibres have acquired the iron-protein coating that characterises an asbestos body. In most places the coating has become segmented, giving rise to bead-like formations, a change accompanying ageing of the bodies. (Fig (b) is reproduced by permission of Dr B Fox, London, UK and (c) by permission of Miss A Dewar, Brompton, UK.)

as long as this.[201] Justification for this comes from animal experiments demonstrating that long fibres cause more inflammation, chromosomal damage, fibrosis, lung tumours and mesotheliomas than short fibres,[202–205] and from studies in man suggesting that long fibres are responsible for asbestosis.[206] Other human studies have shown that although asbestos load is maximal in the upper lobes, more long fibres are found at the bases, where fibrosis is most marked.[38,39] A further reason for limiting attention to the longer fibres is that the shorter ones are

cleared more easily and their number therefore varies with the time lapsed since last exposure. Most long fibres are coated.[185]

Values are best expressed as fibres/g dry lung. By light microscopy, normal values range up to 50 000: over 20 000 is seen with mesotheliomas, and over 1 000 000 in asbestosis (Table 7.1.3).[192,201,207, 208] However, compared with electron microscopy, light microscopy is relatively insensitive, showing only 26.5% of the amosite, 5% of the crocidolite and 0.14% of the chrysotile.[186] Light microscopic counts correlate poorly with

Table 7.1.3   Lung asbestos fibre counts per gram of dried lung

	Light microscopy	Electron microscopy
Normal city dwellers	Up to 20 000	Up to 2 000 000
Mesothelioma	Over 20 000	Over 2 000 000
Asbestosis (minimal)	Over 100 000	Over 10 000 000
Asbestosis (established)	Over 1 000 000	Over 100 000 000

The light microscopic counts include total fibres (coated and uncoated). The electron microscopic counts include only amphibole asbestos. Results from different laboratories vary and these figures, derived from several sources,[192,207,208] provide only a general guide. Reliable results depend upon counts being made regularly and the normal range from that laboratory being ascertained. Ratios of counts obtained by electron and light microscopy vary greatly but approximate to 100.

Box 7.1.4 Molecular formulae of various forms of asbestos. When subjected to microprobe analysis, the total counts recorded for each element (Fig. 7.1.6c) are proportional to the numbers of their atoms in the molecule. Thus, with tremolite the silicon peak would be four times as high as that for calcium

Chrysotile	$Mg_3(Si_2O_5)(OH)_4$
Crocidolite	$Na_2Fe_5(Si_8O_{22})(OH)_2$
Amosite	$(Fe,Mg)_7(Si_8O_{22})(OH)_2$
Tremolite	$Ca_2Mg_5(Si_8O_{22})(OH)_2$

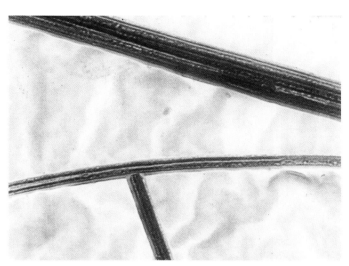

Figure 7.1.21   At high magnification chrysotile fibres are seen to be tubular. Transmission electron micrograph × 51 000. (Reproduced by permission of Miss A Dewar, Brompton, UK.)

severity of asbestosis[195] and electron microscopy is better in this respect.[176–178] By transmission electron microscopy, values may range up to 5 000 000 in controls, with asbestosis generally above 100 000 000 and mesotheliomas found at any level down to 1 000 000, all these figures representing amphibole fibres/g dried lung (Table 7.1.3).[192,207,208] It should be noted that counts from different parts of the same lung may vary widely;[39,207–211] caution should therefore be exercised in interpreting a count obtained on a single sample. There is also wide discrepancy between laboratories, even when analysing the same sample.[210] Results obtained in an individual case therefore have to be evaluated against a standard set of values unique to that laboratory.

Electron microscopy also provides valuable information on the type of fibre. Chrysotile differs physically from the amphiboles in two respects: its fibres are both curved and hollow (Figs 7.1.19a, 7.1.21). With an electron microscope equipped for microprobe analysis, the various forms of asbestos may also be distinguished from other fibres and from each other (Box 7.1.4),[212,213] an important point as it is being increasingly recognised that the amphibole forms of asbestos are far more dangerous than chrysotile.[176–178]

Non-asbestos fibres commonly found in the lung include mullite, which derives from fly ash. This may constitute 25 to 50% of the total fibre burden and is thought to be harmless. There is no firm evidence that man-made fibres present a health hazard,[214] but in certain localities natural non-asbestos mineral fibres, zeolites for example, are important causes of mesothelioma (see p. 702).

Clinical and radiological features

Asbestosis causes a restrictive respiratory deficit. Breathlessness develops slowly,[215,216] as in silicosis, and as in that disease, the pulmonary fibrosis may be followed in the course of years by right heart strain. However, radiographs of the lungs are very different, showing linear basal opacities in asbestosis whereas in silicosis there are nodules, which are better developed in the upper lobes.

Morbid anatomy

When the lungs from a patient with asbestosis are seen at necropsy, pleural fibrosis is often found, and although this may also be attributable to asbestos exposure it is to be regarded as an independent process and not part of the asbestosis.

Slicing the lung affected by asbestosis shows a fine subpleural fibrosis, especially of the lower lobes (Fig. 7.1.22). In severe cases the fibrosis often extends upwards to involve the middle lobe and lingula, and sometimes the upper lobes also. Microcystic change associated with the fibrosis develops in advanced cases and in severe disease there may be cysts over 1 cm diameter. However, these classic changes are seldom seen in Britain today. Following decades of dust suppression in asbestos factories, current patients have mild to moderate asbestosis and are dying of related cancer or of non-pulmonary disease.[217] In some of these cases the asbestosis is only detectable microscopically. Fixation of the lungs through the bronchi and the use of Heard's barium sulphate impregnation technique facilitate demonstration of the fibrosis (see Fig. 7.1.22 and p. 738). The mild degree of asbestosis currently encountered is of little functional significance but is often critical in determining whether an associated carcinoma of the lung should be attributed to asbestos exposure (see below).

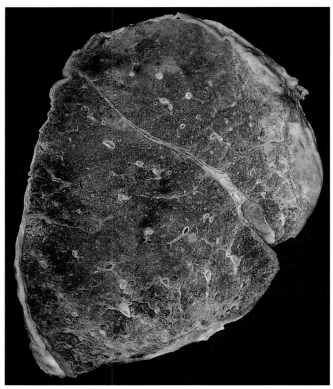

Figure 7.1.22 Asbestosis. Fine interstitial fibrosis is evident beneath the pleura at the base of the lung. Barium sulphate impregnated specimen.

Box 7.1.5 Criteria for grading asbestosis (with an indication of the numbers of asbestos bodies likely to be found in each grade, grading being based solely on the extent and severity of the fibrosis)[218,219]

Extent

A	None
B	Less than 25% of the lung substance involved.
C	25–50% of the lung affected.
D	More than 50% of the lung diseased.

Severity

0 (None)	No fibrosis
1 (Minimal)	Slight focal fibrosis around respiratory bronchioles (prolonged search reveals occasional asbestos bodies, on average one or less per section)
2 (Slight)	The fibrosis is found around the respiratory bronchioles and alveolar ducts of scattered acini, extending into the walls of adjacent airspaces (asbestos bodies average 1 to 3 per section)
3 (Moderate)	A further increase and condensation of the peribronchiolar fibrosis with early widespread interstitial fibrosis (asbestos bodies are easily found and occasionally form clumps)
4 (Severe)	Widespread diffuse fibrosis in which few alveoli are recognisable and bronchioles are distorted (asbestos bodies are numerous and often form clumps)

The widely accepted view that the fibrosis should be diffuse would exclude grade 1 and possibly grade 2.

Histological appearances

It is generally considered that asbestosis begins about the respiratory bronchioles and alveolar ducts where most of the asbestos fibres impact.[12] Alveolar walls attached to these bronchioles show fine interstitial fibrosis. However, this early lesion has to be interpreted with caution because it is not specific to asbestos, being found with other inhaled mineral dusts and even in many cigarette smokers who have not been so exposed. It more likely represents a non-specific reaction to a variety of inhaled particles. It may cause mild airflow obstruction but is not associated with the radiographic, clinical or restrictive changes of classic asbestosis.

As the disease progresses, the focal changes join up so that the basal subpleural regions show widespread interstitial fibrosis and eventually complete destruction of the alveolar architecture. In severe cases there may be honeycombing and metaplastic changes in the alveolar and bronchiolar epithelium. Some widely quoted criteria for grading asbestosis (Box 7.1.5) include early changes that do not amount to the diffuse fibrosis envisaged in current definitions of asbestosis (see below).[218,219] Apart from the presence of asbestos bodies the changes resemble those of non-specific interstitial pneumonia, or more rarely usual interstitial pneumonia. There is often an increase in alveolar macrophages but the desquamative interstitial pneumonia that has been reported in association with asbestos[220,221] is not to be regarded as a variant of asbestosis;[222] concomitant smoking is a more likely cause. A variety of other non-specific inflammatory processes such as organising pneumonia have been reported in asbestos workers and if localised some have been suspected of representing malignancy until biopsied.[223]

In well-established asbestosis, asbestos bodies are numerous and easy to find, aggregates of them sometimes forming clumps (Fig. 7.1.23). In earlier lesions a detailed search may be necessary, in which case the examination of unstained or Perls-stained sections facilitates their identification. Minimum criteria for a diagnosis of asbestosis have been variably defined. A North American committee recommended peribronchiolar (grade 1) fibrosis and the presence of asbestos bodies (number not specified)[219] whereas the more recent Helsinki criteria require the identification of diffuse interstitial fibrosis in well inflated lung tissue remote from a lung cancer or other mass lesion and the presence of either two or more asbestos bodies in tissue with a section area of $1\,cm^2$ or a count of uncoated asbestos fibres that falls in the range recorded for asbestosis by the same laboratory.[222] The minimum Helsinki criterion of diffuse interstitial fibrosis is being increasingly accepted although it equates with grade 3 of the older classification shown in Box 7.1.5.

Some workers report that there is a good correlation between asbestos body score and fibrosis grade,[188] but others have found the reverse,[191,195] although identifying a good correlation between asbestos body numbers in sections and asbestos fibre

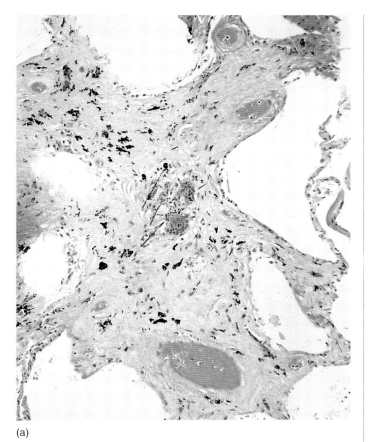

(a)

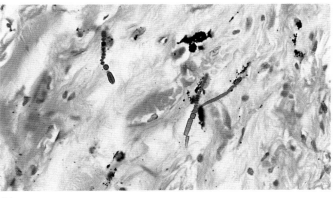

(b)

Figure 7.1.23 Asbestosis. Interstitial fibrosis is associated with many asbestos bodies (a), which are shown in detail in (b).

burden.[191] No matter how many asbestos bodies are found, by themselves they merely indicate exposure. Conversely, if an asbestos worker has interstitial fibrosis but no asbestos bodies are evident despite careful scrutiny of several sections it would be exceptional for analysis of lung digests to reveal substantial amounts of asbestos.[224] There are marked variations in the concentration of asbestos fibres between samples from the same lung[192,211] and it is therefore recommended that at least three areas be sampled, the apices of the upper and lower lobes and the base of the lower lobe.[200]

The equivalent of Mallory's alcoholic hyalin of the liver has been described in the lungs in asbestosis,[225] and subsequently in other pulmonary conditions.[226] It is seen as small eosinophilic cytoplasmic inclusions within hyperplastic type II alveolar epithelial cells. Electron microscopy shows that the inclusions consist of a tangle of tonofilaments and by immunocytochemistry a positive reaction is obtained with antibodies to cytokeratin, both these features being typical of Mallory's hyalin in the liver.

Differential diagnosis

The differential diagnosis of asbestosis includes pulmonary fibrosis due to many other causes, any of which may of course affect an asbestos worker as much as members of the general population. However, the principal differential diagnosis is from cryptogenic fibrosing alveolitis. The proportion of diffuse pulmonary fibrosis in asbestos workers that is not attributable to asbestos has been estimated to be as high as 5% and likely to rise as the risk of asbestosis diminishes with better industrial hygiene.[224] Both diseases affect the bases and periphery of the lungs predominantly. In the late stages, cystic change is more evident in cryptogenic fibrosing alveolitis but this criterion is not totally reliable. Nor is the presence of pleural fibrosis although it is usually present in asbestosis and is seldom found in cryptogenic fibrosing alveolitis. Asbestosis seldom progresses or does so very slowly after exposure ceases[215,216] whereas cryptogenic fibrosing alveolitis typically proves fatal within 3–4 years from onset. Very often the distinction of these two diseases has to be based on the amount of asbestos in the lung and if asbestos bodies are either not readily identifiable this has to depend on fibre counts (see above). Errors are made both by overlooking substantial numbers of asbestos bodies completely and by ascribing undue importance to scanty bodies. If considering the possibility of minimal asbestosis (which would justify attributing carcinoma of the lung to asbestos), it should be remembered that a little peribronchiolar fibrosis is also characteristic of centriacinar emphysema.[227] As described above, at least two asbestos bodies/cm^2 in the presence of fibrosis distant from any lung cancer or other mass lesion is required for a diagnosis of asbestosis.[222]

Pathogenesis

Although the causes of asbestosis and cryptogenic fibrosing alveolitis are very different, they resemble each other in several ways, suggesting that similar pathogenetic mechanisms may operate.[100,228–230] In both these diseases there is degeneration of the alveolar epithelium and capillary endothelium, with patchy loss of the former,[228] and bronchoalveolar lavage shows neutrophil leukocytes and an increase in macrophages, inflammatory cells that might perpetuate the damage by releasing lysosomal enzymes, nitric oxide and hydroxyl radicals.[229,231–233] Both diseases are also characterised by an increased prevalence of circulating non-organ specific autoantibodies.[234] Experimentally, asbestos exposure leads to the activation of a variety of inflammatory and fibrogenic cytokines at sites of lung injury.[100,235–240]

Inhaled asbestos activates a complement-dependent chemoattractant for macrophages[241] and macrophage stimulation involves the secretion of fibroblast stimulating factors,[242–244] asbestos being intermediate between haematite and silica in regard to macrophage mediated fibrogenicity.[245] The epithelial damage could be mediated directly by the needle-like asbestos fibres or indirectly through enhanced phagocyte generation of free radicals (which is much greater with amphibole asbestos than with either chrysotile or silica).[240,246] Fibrogenic cytokines released by activated pulmonary phagocytes and regenerating alveolar epithelial cells in asbestosis include tumour necrosis factor-α and transforming growth factor-β,[240] as in cryptogenic fibrosing alveolitis (see p. 274).

Asbestos-induced lung cancer

As a result of better industrial hygiene, asbestosis is less severe today than in earlier years when it followed much heavier exposure, with the consequence that death from respiratory failure and cor pulmonale is less common and sufferers are surviving longer. There is therefore a greater risk of them eventually developing asbestos-related cancer. Asbestos exposure predisposes to two varieties of malignant neoplasm, carcinoma of the lung and mesothelioma of the pleura and peritoneum. In one group of men with asbestosis, 39% died of pulmonary carcinoma, 10% of mesothelioma and 19% of other respiratory diseases.[217] Although there were many earlier reports, the link with carcinoma of the lung may be considered to have been firmly established by 1955,[247] that between crocidolite asbestos and mesothelioma by 1960,[248] and that between amosite asbestos and mesothelioma by 1972.[249] Mesothelioma is considered on p. 701.

In regard to carcinoma of the lung, asbestos is not such a potent pulmonary carcinogen as cigarette smoke but together their effects are multiplicative rather than additive (Table 7.1.4).[250,251] It is uncertain[109] whether the increased risk of pulmonary carcinoma is caused by the asbestos[222,252–257] or the asbestosis.[258–265a] The general view inclines to the latter but there is increasing advocacy of the former (Table 7.1.5).[222] In the UK, industrial compensation is unlikely to be awarded to an asbestos worker for carcinoma of the lung unless there is also asbestosis (or diffuse pleural fibrosis – see p. 699). Compensa-

tion standards for asbestos-associated lung cancer in different countries are shown in Box 7.1.6.[257]

As a complication of asbestosis, carcinoma is traditionally thought to arise from foci of alveolar epithelial hyperplasia,

Table 7.1.5 Requirements for attributing carcinoma of the lung to asbestos

The traditional view that the carcinoma complicates asbestosis	The Helsinki criteria[222] which are based upon substantial exposure
1 Asbestosis. It is not stipulated how this should be recognised but pathological corroboration of appropriate clinico-radiological features is desirable *And* 2 A minimum lag-time of 20 years.	1 Asbestosis diagnosed clinically, radiologically or histologically *Or* A minimum count of 5000 asbestos bodies per gram dry lung tissue (/g dry), or an uncoated asbestos fibre burden of 2 million amphibole fibres more than 5 μm in length/g dry, or 5 million amphibole fibres more than 1 μm in length/g dry *Or* Estimated cumulative exposure to asbestos of at least 25 fibres/ml-years *Or* An occupational history of one year of heavy exposure to asbestos (e.g. manufacture of asbestos products, asbestos spraying) or 5–10 years of moderate exposure (e.g. construction or shipbuilding) *And* 2 A minimum lag-time of 10 years

Box 7.1.6 Compensation standards for asbestos-associated lung cancer in different countries[257]

Government standards vary considerably and in the civil courts claims are often based on lesser evidence. Some examples of government standards are:

UK: Either asbestosis or bilateral diffuse pleural fibrosis is required.
USA: The requirements are the presence of asbestos-related bilateral pleural plaques or asbestos-related bilateral pleural thickening and occupational exposure and a lag time of at least 12 years.
Germany: Compensation is based on the presence of asbestosis or pleural plaques or diffuse pleural thickening or fibre-years of exposure.
Denmark: Only fibre-years of exposure are taken into account.
Finland: Exposure, at least 10 years latency and asbestos-related pleural or parenchymal changes are required.
Sweden: Asbestosis is not required but smoking is taken into consideration.
Norway: Attempts are made to quantify separately the attributability to asbestos, smoking and other factors (e.g. radon).

Table 7.1.4 Excess mortality from carcinoma of the lung attributable to asbestos exposure and cigarette smoking in insulation workers.[250] Together, these factors have a multiplicative rather than additive effect

Group	Mortality ratio
Non-smoking controls	1
Non-smoking asbestos workers	5
Cigarette smoking controls	11
Cigarette smoking asbestos workers	53

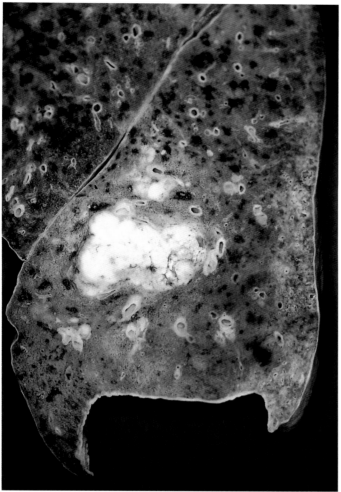

Figure 7.1.24 Asbestosis associated with carcinoma of the lung. The asbestosis has been highlighted by barium sulphate impregnation and is seen as a grey subpleural band to the right of the picture. Although the carcinoma has arisen in the same lobe as the asbestosis it has not obviously arisen in an area affected by asbestosis.

which are common in interstitial fibrosis, with dysplasia representing an intermediate stage in the process. A wholly comparable situation appertains in cryptogenic fibrosing alveolitis (see p. 276). The increased risk involves carcinomas of all the histological types encountered in the lung, although adenocarcinoma is disproportionately over-represented. Most arise in the bronchi rather than the alveolar tissue, but there are more in the sites worst affected by asbestosis, the lower lobes and the periphery of the lung, than is seen in the general population (Fig. 7.1.24).[217,218,266–270] There is usually a latent period in excess of 20 years between first exposure to asbestos and the development of lung cancer and the risk increases the greater the cumulative exposure.

Asbestos-induced airway disease

Although asbestosis causes a restrictive respiratory defect, airflow limitation is also seen in this disease. Much of the airflow limitation is attributable to cigarette smoking but it is also seen in non-smoking asbestos workers and is worse in those with asbestosis.[271] The pathological basis of this appears to be small airways disease (see p. 97)[272] or fibrosis about the respiratory bronchioles.[273] It is possibly a non-specific reaction to inhaled dust or cigarette smoke and its recognition casts doubt on the theory that small airway abnormalities are the earliest form of asbestosis.[273] Because it is not established that this lesion progresses to diffuse interstitial fibrosis (asbestosis) the term 'asbestos airways disease' is suggested.[273] It should also be noted that although emphysema is considered to be a destructive rather than fibrotic condition, a little focal fibrosis is generally evident in this common condition[227] and does not necessarily indicate early asbestosis.

ALUMINIUM PNEUMOCONIOSIS

Aluminium holds a paradoxical position in regard to lung disease. In certain industries it has caused very severe pulmonary fibrosis, yet in others it has proved harmless. Indeed, at one time, Canadian miners breathed aluminium dust before work, in the belief that this would reduce the danger of silica in the mine dust[274] and more recently silicosis has been treated by such means in France.[275] It is questionable whether this practice is effective but it at least appears to cause no harm. The explanation for these contradictory observations probably lies in differing methods of manufacture of aluminium powder.

Aluminium metal appears to be an inert substance but this is only because it has a high affinity for oxygen and the surface layer of aluminium oxide so formed is very firmly bound to the underlying metal, unlike ferric oxide which permits further rusting of iron. Granular aluminium powders, produced in a ball mill or from a jet of molten aluminium, therefore acquire a protective coat of surface oxide. With stamped aluminium powders, however, surface oxidation is prevented by lubricants added to aid the separation of these flake-like particles. The usual lubricant (stearin) contains stearic acid and this polar compound combines with the underlying metal, which is thereby protected from both atmospheric oxidation and the action of body fluids when such dust is inhaled. In certain circumstances, however, non-polar lubricants in the form of mineral oils have been substituted for stearin. This happened in Germany during the Second World War, when stearin was difficult to obtain,[276,277] and in Britain in the 1950s for commercial reasons.[278] *In vitro*, oil-coated stamped aluminium powder reacts with water to produce aluminium hydroxide, which affords the underlying metal no protection against further attack, so that aluminium hydroxide continues to be formed.[279] This substance is a protein denaturant, once used in the tanning industry, and it is believed that this property underlies the very exceptional cases of severe pulmonary fibrosis that have occurred in connection with stamped aluminium powder produced with mineral oil rather than stearin.[279,280] The fibrosis has a very characteristic pattern, similar to that described in bauxite smelters exposed to aluminium and silica fume (Shaver's disease)[281] and in welders exposed to aluminium fume.[282]

Aluminium pneumoconiosis is a severe diffuse fibrosis, predominantly affecting the upper lobes.[278] It progresses rapidly, the interval from onset of symptoms to death being as short as two years. There is marked shrinkage of the lungs with gross elevation of the diaphragm and buckling of the trachea. The lungs are grey in colour; microscopically, numerous small black jagged particles are seen. These can be shown to contain aluminium with Irwin's aluminon stain or by microprobe analysis.[283]

What appears to be a different pathological effect of aluminium dust on the lungs is the rare development of granulomatous disease resembling sarcoidosis and berylliosis.[284,285] Other pulmonary abnormalities reported include desquamative interstitial pneumonia in an aluminium welder.[283]

RARE EARTH (CERIUM) PNEUMOCONIOSIS

Elements with atomic numbers from 57 (lanthanum) to 71 (lutetium) are known as the lanthanides or rare earth metals. They are used in many manufacturing processes, including the production of high temperature ceramics and the grinding of optical lenses. Carbon arc lamps used in reproduction photography emit appreciable quantities of oxidised lanthanides, particularly cerium oxide, and there are reports of pneumoconiosis in exposed individuals.[286] The pathological changes reported have varied from granulomatous nodules to diffuse interstitial fibrosis indistinguishable from the idiopathic variety except for the presence of rare earth elements (usually cerium) detected by polarising light microscopy and electron microprobe analysis.[286]

HARD METAL DISEASE (COBALT LUNG)

Hard metal is a tungsten alloy containing small amounts of cobalt, titanium, molybdenum and nickel. It is exceptionally tough and once formed can only be worked with diamond. It is used in the tips of drill bits, on abrasive wheels and discs, and in armaments. Interstitial lung disease is liable to arise in its manufacture or in those using hard metal as an abrasive.[287] Experimental work suggests that cobalt is the dangerous constituent[288] but this element is soluble and unless industrial contact has been recent analysis of lung tissue usually shows tungsten and titanium but no cobalt. The role of cobalt is also indicated by the development of similar interstitial lung disease in diamond polishers using high-speed polishing discs made with a diamond-cobalt surface that lacked tungsten carbide and the other constituents of hard metal.[289,290]

Hard metal lung disease and cobalt lung take two forms, an industrial asthma and interstitial fibrosis. The latter has a diffuse lower zonal distribution and the appearances mimic cryptogenic fibrosing alveolitis. However, an unusual feature is the presence of moderate, or perhaps only small numbers, of giant cells (Fig. 7.1.25a,b).[287,291] Not only are there multinucleate alveolar macrophages but syncytial cell forms develop in the alveolar epithelium. Electron microscopy confirms that these are multinucleate type II pneumocytes (Fig. 7.1.25c).[287] Such epithelial changes are well known in measles pneumonia but the viral inclusion bodies that characterise this infection are not found in hard metal pneumoconiosis. The changes are those initially described as a particular pattern of idiopathic interstitial pneumonia termed giant cell interstitial pneumonia or GIP. Elemental analysis shows that many, but not all, cases of GIP represent hard metal disease. The exceptions seldom give a history of cobalt exposure and must be presumed to represent true idiopathic cases. Conversely epithelial giant cells are not always found in hard metal pneumoconiosis and so their presence, although highly characteristic, is neither totally specific nor totally sensitive.

BERYLLIOSIS

Beryllium compounds may cause contact dermatitis, conjunctivitis, or acute or chronic pulmonary disease.[292–294] The acute lung damage represents chemical injury (see pp. 137, 358) but the other diseases associated with beryllium are allergic in nature. Beryllium is also classified as a probable pulmonary carcinogen,[295] but this is controversial.

Uses of beryllium and occupations at risk

Chronic beryllium-induced lung disease was first reported in Germany in 1933[296] and was soon recognised as a cause of considerable disability and mortality in the fluorescent lamp industry. Mainly because of the danger they posed, beryllium compounds have been replaced by other substances in this application but the metal has since proved to be of great value in the nuclear, electronic, computer and aerospace industries. Its mechanical strength, high melting point, good thermal conductivity and lightness give beryllium metal many advantages. A further use therefore is in the production of refractory materials and crucibles that are to be subjected to particularly high temperatures. The alloys of beryllium are now widely used, especially those with copper, on which it confers elasticity and resistance to fatigue. Alloy manufacture and the machining of beryllium alloys are further industries that entail a risk of berylliosis.

Inhalation of beryllium dust or fumes is now known to be exceedingly dangerous. Those who worked with beryllium compounds before precautionary measures were taken suffered a high morbidity and mortality. Sometimes, the escape of dangerous fumes from the factories was on such a scale that people living nearby, downwind from the places in which these materials were being worked, contracted and occasionally died from berylliosis ('neighbourhood cases'). Alternatively, contamination of a beryllium worker's clothes might lead to berylliosis in a relative.[297] Seemingly innocuous occupations such as dental laboratory technician have also led to chronic berylliosis.[298]

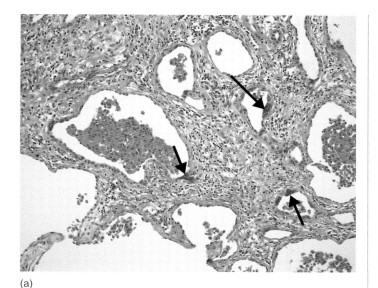

(a)

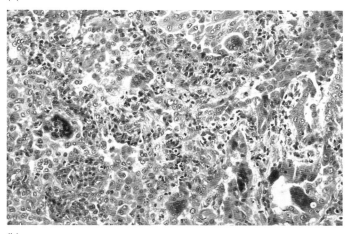

(b)

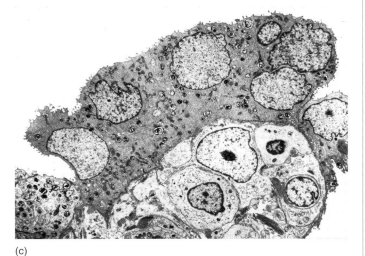

(c)

Figure 7.1.25 Giant cell interstitial pneumonia in hard metal workers. (a) There is interstitial pneumonia and fibrosis and several alveolar epithelial cells are multinucleate (arrows). (b) Higher magnification shows a light lymphocytic infiltrate, numerous alveolar macrophages and several multinucleate giant cells. (c) Electron microscopy confirms that the multinucleate epithelial cells are type II pneumocytes recognisable from their osmiophilic lamellar inclusions and microvilli.

Pathogenesis

There are good grounds for regarding chronic berylliosis as an allergic condition. Many of those affected react strongly to skin tests with dilute solutions of beryllium salts, although skin tests in suspected cases must be undertaken with care for occasionally in a highly sensitised person even so small an exposure may evoke a systemic reaction. *In vitro* lymphocyte transformation testing[297,299] is safe, but not wholly reliable and indicates only sensitisation, rather than berylliosis. As in sarcoidosis, bronchoalveolar lavage demonstrates an excess of T-helper lymphocytes[300,301] and a positive transformation test given by these lymphocytes is a more reliable indicator of disease.

Susceptibility to berylliosis varies widely from person to person and it is notable that chronic pulmonary disease is strongly associated with the HLA antigen DPβ1, the gene for which encodes for glutamate in the 69 position.[302,303] The importance of genetic factors is supported by a report of the disease in identical twins.[300]

Pathological changes

Should beryllium enter the subcutaneous tissues through a cut or abrasion, as often happened in the earlier days of fluorescent lamp manufacture, a sarcoid-like granuloma soon appears at the site; in time, the overlying epidermis may break down to form an ulcer.

Even more serious are the lesions produced in the lungs. Pulmonary berylliosis occurs in two forms. One is an acute chemical pneumonia manifest as diffuse alveolar damage (see p. 137). The other, more common form, is a widespread granulomatous pneumonia with a histological picture identical to that of sarcoidosis (Fig. 7.1.26a). Both berylliosis and sarcoidosis affect the upper lobes more than the lower (Fig. 7.1.26b) and in both diseases the granulomas are preferentially distributed along lymphatics and may involve adjacent blood vessels. In neither condition is there widespread necrosis but in both diseases the granulomas occasionally display a little central necrosis or hyalinisation. As in sarcoidosis, the hilar lymph nodes may be involved but unlike sarcoidosis, not in isolation.

Over a period of many years, the sarcoid-like granulomas gradually undergo progressive fibrosis, with consequent impairment of pulmonary function. In the later stages, when the disease has become chronic, dispersal of beryllium from its site of initial absorption may lead to generalisation of the disease and to the appearance of similar granulomas elsewhere, particularly in the liver, kidneys, spleen and skin, but this is unusual.

Clinical features

Chronic berylliosis is characterised by the gradual onset of cough, shortness of breath, chest pain, night sweats and fatigue. These symptoms may develop within few weeks of exposure or many years later. Once the worker is exposed, the beryllium is retained in the tissues and there is a life-long risk of disease. Progression often entails alternating exacerbations and remissions, long after exposure has ceased.

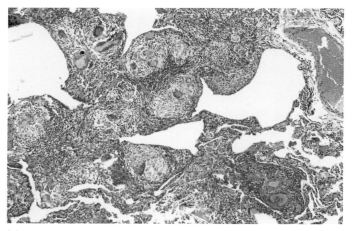

(a)

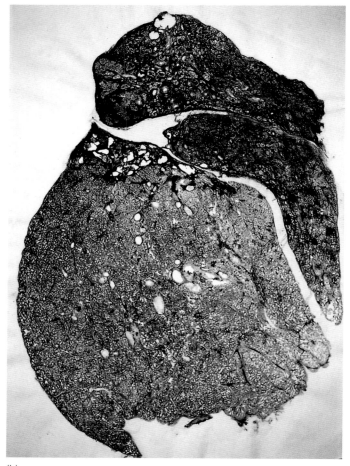

(b)

Figure 7.1.26 Chronic berylliosis. (a) Numerous non-necrotising epithelioid and giant cell granulomas are seen in the lungs. (b) The upper and middle lobes and the apex of the lower lobe are contracted by extensive fibrosis. Paper mounted whole lung section.

Analysis

In keeping with the view that berylliosis is a hypersensitivity reaction, very little beryllium is necessary to cause the disease. Particulate beryllium is so scanty in the affected tissues and the atomic number of beryllium so low that electron microprobe analysis is unsuitable for its detection. Until recently, chemical analysis of bulk tissue has been required, but ion or laser microprobe mass spectroscopy can detect very small amounts of beryllium in tissue sections.[46,300,304,305]

Differential diagnosis

The differential diagnosis of berylliosis[306,307] is from sarcoidosis, which berylliosis closely resembles morphologically. However, as noted above, it is unusual for berylliosis to cause significant hilar lymphadenopathy in the absence of pulmonary disease, which is a common feature of sarcoidosis. Extrathoracic granulomas, erythema nodosum and uveitis, which are all common in sarcoidosis, are unusual in berylliosis. An occupational history, evidence of hypersensitivity to beryllium and tissue analysis may all provide evidence of exposure.

POLYVINYL CHLORIDE PNEUMOCONIOSIS

Although polyvinyl is not a mineral and the reaction of the lungs to its presence is therefore not a true pneumoconiosis, it is generally so termed and is dealt with here for convenience. Workers are exposed to polyvinyl chloride dust in the milling and bagging of this plastic and micronodular opacities may be detected in their lungs radiologically. However, the material is non-fibrogenic and histology merely shows a foreign body reaction to the dust particles.[308] The radiological opacities may abate when exposure ceases.[309] Nevertheless, one polyvinyl chloride worker developed systemic sclerosis,[310] which is a recognised complication of silicosis (see p. 337). Polyvinyl chloride is produced from vinyl chloride monomer, which has a causal association with angiosarcoma of the liver and probably other forms of cancer, including carcinoma of the lung (see p. 530).

FLOCK WORKER'S LUNG

In the late 1990s, a characteristic lung disease was identified in workers at several North American factories producing plush fabric by spraying nylon flock onto an adhesive backing material.[311–313] A further case involving polyethylene flock has since been reported from Spain.[314] The flock fibres are too large to be inspired but may be mixed with smaller nylon shards of respirable size. The workers complained of cough and breathlessness and were found to have a restrictive ventilatory defect with interstitial markings on radiography. Their symptoms improved on removal from the workplace but relapsed on return to work. Pathologically, there was lymphocytic bronchiolitis and peribronchiolitis with widespread lymphoid hyperplasia represented by lymphoid aggregates. Granulomas were not identified. The histological appearances suggest a severe immunological reaction and raise possibilities such as rheumatoid disease and Sjögren's syndrome but consideration of the clinical and serological setting and the occupation should permit recognition of the cause.

POPCORN WORKER'S LUNG

In 2000, eight former workers at a popcorn packaging plant were found to have obstructive airway disease. Biopsy showed peribronchiolar fibrosis and granulomas.[315] Air sampling identified many volatile organic compounds but diacetyl, a ketone added to give the popcorn a buttery flavour, is suspected of being responsible for the bronchiolitis.

PAINT SPRAYING

It is difficult to continue paint spraying (air brushing, aerographics) without adequate respiratory protection but in the early 1990s several small aerographic factories operated in the neighbourhood of Alicante, south-eastern Spain without any concern for the workers' health. The workers were required to paint patterns on textiles using a hand-held spray gun. The atmospheric pollution was intense but complaints of respiratory difficulties were met with reassurances and the workers urged to continue. This they did because of the otherwise poor economy, often returning to work when disabling breathlessness had settled down. A change in paint formulation (to Acramin F) may have contributed because the worst affected workers were employed at two plants that had made this switch. Their illness has been described as the Ardystil syndrome after the name of one of these factories. Some workers were left with permanent respiratory disability. One required a lung transplant and 6 others died.[316–319] Transbronchial biopsy showed organising pneumonia, which in the fatal cases had progressed to irreversible interstitial fibrosis. A similar outbreak of respiratory disease was subsequently reported in Algerian textile factories where Acromin F was applied by the same technique.[320,321]

MINERAL OILS AND PETROLEUM

Workers in engineering workshops may be exposed to the prolonged inhalation of fine sprays or mists of the longer chain hydrocarbons that constitute many mineral oils. This may result in exogenous lipid pneumonia,[322] which is described on p. 315. The vapour of shorter chain hydrocarbons such as paraffin oil (kerosene: $C_{10–16}$) and petrol (gasoline: $C_{4–12}$) and gaseous hydrocarbons such as propane may act as acute asphyxiants or central nervous system depressants but have negligible pulmonary tox-

Table 7.1.6 Principal respiratory risks of welding

Source	Derivative	Effect
Metals being welded	Iron	Siderosis
	Zinc	Metal fume fever
	Beryllium	Berylliosis (acute or chronic)
	Chrome, nickel	Asthma
	Cadmium, manganese	Diffuse alveolar damage
	Chrome, nickel, arsenic	Lung cancer
Burning of adjacent surfaces	Isocyanates	Asthma
	Phosgene	Bronchitis, bronchiolitis
	Tetrafluoroethylene	Polymer fume fever
	Oxides of nitrogen	Bronchitis
Electrode insulation; protective clothes	Asbestos	Mesothelioma
Gas used to prevent oxidation	Carbon dioxide	Asphyxia
Combustive gas	Carbon monoxide	Carbon monoxide poisoning
Ultraviolet light	Ozone	Bronchitis
Various	Silica, silicates	Silicosis, mixed dust pneumoconiosis

icity. However, if they are ingested or aspirated in their liquid form they are acutely toxic to the lungs, producing a chemical pneumonitis with the features of diffuse alveolar damage (see p. 131). Ingestion may be accidental or deliberate (see Fig. 4.18, p. 138), whereas aspiration is generally inadvertent, occurring in siphoning accidents, such as those experienced by fairground operatives who 'breath or eat fire' ('fire-eaters lung').[323,324] Animal experiments involving the intratracheal injection of kerosene resulted in acute pulmonary exudates, which cleared except for residual bronchiolitis.[325]

WELDING

Welders' pneumoconiosis, first recognised in 1936,[326] essentially represents the fairly harmless deposition of iron in the lungs (siderosis – see p. 340). However, welders may suffer various ill-effects from the inhalation of substances other than iron (Table 7.1.6). Some of these are para-occupational risks, that is, encountered by welders because they work near another process and are inadvertently exposed: thus, shipyard welders may be exposed to asbestos,[327] and those in foundries to silica. Welders may therefore develop a mixed dust pneumoconiosis (see p. 340), rather than just siderosis. However, one analytical investigation identified excess amounts of iron alone in association with pulmonary fibrosis, the silicon content not differing from that in controls.[328]

More directly, welders may be exposed to asbestos insulation that they themselves use, while welders of special steel alloys run the risk of metal-induced asthma, metal fume fever, polymer fume fever and the consequences of toxic metal fume inhalation,[329] all of which are described separately in this chapter. Chronic bronchitis has been attributed to the inhalation of low concentrations of irritants such as ozone and nitrogen dioxide by welders but this risk is unproven and the subject of much controversy. Welders may also inhale carcinogenic hexavalent chromium compounds in the course of their work and therefore develop lung cancer. The term welders' lung is often applied indiscriminately to any of these diseases and, as it has no specific meaning, is best avoided.

TOXIC FUMES AND GASES

Dust, fume and gas are some of the terms used to describe different physical forms of respirable agents. They are defined in Box 7.2.1 on p. 373. The parts of the respiratory tract at which they exert their maximal effect is influenced by particle size and solubility, as outlined on p. 372 and in Table 7.2.1, p. 373.

Toxic metal fume[330]

The finely divided fume of several metals is highly toxic to the lungs and capable of producing severe acute and chronic damage to both the conductive airways and the alveoli, resulting in acute tracheobronchitis and bronchiolitis, diffuse alveolar damage, obliterative bronchiolitis and pulmonary fibrosis. Important metal fumes in this respect include aluminium, which is released together with silica fume in bauxite smelting (Shaver's disease[281]), cadmium from welding or cutting special steels, chromium from cutting its alloys or in the manufacture of chromates, cobalt released in the production and use of its alloys (see hard metal disease above), mercury released in various industries and in the home,[331] nickel carbonyl released during the purification of metallic nickel or the manufacture of nickel alloys,[332] and beryllium (see above).

Toxic gases

Many irritant gases cause severe acute and chronic damage to both the conductive airways and alveoli. The changes are non-specific and similar to those wrought by toxic metal fumes (see above) and viruses among other agents. They consist of acute tracheobronchitis and bronchiolitis, obliterative bronchiolitis, diffuse alveolar damage and pulmonary fibrosis.

The gases liable to produce such damage include oxides of nitrogen, sulphur dioxide, ozone, phosgene, chlorine, ammonia and various constituents of smoke, notably acrolein. Some of these are also touched upon in Chapter 7.2 because they are of general as well as occupational importance, although there is no rigid difference between general and occupational pollution.

Ozone, sulphur dioxide and nitrogen dioxide are oxidising gases that may be found together as industrial atmospheric pollutants. Each is capable of producing diffuse alveolar damage by means of its oxidising properties and the release of free active radicals. In addition, they cause damage to distal airways,

particularly terminal and respiratory bronchioles, with resulting bronchiolitis.

Oxides of nitrogen may be encountered with fatal consequences by farmhands seeking to free a blockage in a silo when they encounter pockets of gas that have accumulated on top of the fermenting silage: the term silo-fillers' disease is generally applied to the obliterative bronchiolitis that develops in those who survive the initial acute bronchiolitis.[333–336] Other farmhands have suffered from the inhalation of toxic gases, and bacteria, when handling liquid manure.[337–340] Welding, which is considered above, may also involve exposure to toxic gases such as oxides of nitrogen.

Ozone, the principal oxidant gas of photochemical smog, produces pulmonary changes at ambient levels and may be encountered at higher concentrations in various industries. Potentially dangerous levels of ozone are produced from atmospheric oxygen by ultraviolet radiation given off in welding while ozone is used in industry to sterilise water, bleach paper, flour and oils and mask the odour of organic effluents. The damage wrought by ozone is predominantly centriacinar in distribution, affecting terminal and respiratory bronchiolar epithelium and proximal alveolar epithelium.[341–343] There is loss of cilia and necrosis of centriacinar alveolar type I epithelial cells. The changes are dose dependent and, in one study, the youngest animals were most sensitive.[344] In long-term experiments, hyperplastic bronchiolar Clara and ciliated cells extended peripherally to line alveolar ducts.[345] The role of granulocytes is stressed in some experimental studies[346] and it is notable that neutrophil migration is prominent when the human lungs are damaged by ozone.[347]

Aldehydes such as acetaldehyde, formaldehyde and acrylic aldehyde (acrolein) are widely used in the plastics and chemical industries. The first is a liquid and the others are water-soluble gases. Pathologists are of course familiar with formaldehyde solution from its use as a disinfectant and histological fixative. All these aldehydes are intensely irritant and their acute effects generally prevent prolonged exposure to high concentrations. Chronic effects include skin sensitivity and asthma, and in rats nasal carcinoma. However, the doses to which these experimental animals were exposed far exceed any that are likely to be encountered by man, in whom there is no convincing evidence of aldehyde-induced cancer.[348]

Ammonia gas is extensively used in industry as a raw material, notably in the manufacture of nitrogenous products such as fertilisers and plastics. It is highly soluble and its acute irritative effects are mainly felt in the eyes, nose and throat, but high levels affect the major airways, possibly leading to them being blocked by exudates. Survival usually brings full recovery but bronchiectasis and obliterative bronchiolitis have been described.

Chlorine gas is widely used in the chemical industry. It is transported and stored under pressure in liquid form. Heavy exposure through its accidental release or use as a war gas has proved fatal through its acute toxicity causing exudative airway occlusion and pulmonary oedema. Survivors usually recover completely but as with nitrogen dioxide and ammonia there is a risk of obliterative bronchiolitis.

Phosgene (carbonyl chloride) is a poisonous, colourless gas that was responsible for thousands of deaths during the First World War, when it was used in chemical warfare. It is used industrially in the preparation of some organic chemical compounds and is formed, perhaps inadvertently, by the combustion of methylene chloride in products such as paint strippers.[349] Phosgene causes injury to terminal bronchioles and alveoli, with resulting oedema and hyaline membrane formation. The mechanism of cell damage is uncertain but it may depend on inactivation of intracellular enzymes by the gas. Long-term problems are rare but chronic bronchitis and emphysema have been described in survivors.

Thionyl chloride is used in the manufacture of lithium batteries where it is liable to result in the release of sulphur dioxide and hydrochloric acid fumes. Workers in such factories have developed lung injury varying from mild, reversible interstitial disease to severe obliterative bronchiolitis.[350]

ANOXIC ASPHYXIA

The danger of asphyxia from the inhalation of gases devoid of oxygen is fairly widespread in industry.[351] It generally arises from the use of inert gases, which, being non-toxic give a false sense of security. Pockets of these gases tend to form in confined spaces. Anoxic death from the accumulation of methane is well known in mines and has also occurred in slurry pits and sewers. Anoxic asphyxia in both diving and anaesthesia has resulted from the incorrect connection of gas cylinders or failure to notice that a mixed gas contains insufficient oxygen. Deaths have occurred in welding, when argon or carbon dioxide has been used to shield the weld and prevent oxidation of the metals at the high temperatures employed. Deaths have also resulted from inadvertent entry to discharged oil tanks filled with nitrogen to reduce the risk of explosions, or from the formation of pockets of nitrogen gas applied in liquid form to freeze the contents of damaged pipes so that they can be repaired without the necessity to drain down.

The respiration of a gas devoid of oxygen causes loss of consciousness within seconds because it not only fails to provide oxygen but removes that present in the pulmonary arterial blood. The changes at autopsy are those common to cellular hypoxia whatever the cause, whether it be carbon monoxide poisoning or a foreign body obstructing the airway: petechial haemorrhages are found in the brain and on the serosal surfaces and the lungs may show oedema and haemorrhage.

OCCUPATIONAL ASTHMA

Occupational asthma is the commonest cause of work-related respiratory disease in the UK (Table 7.1.7).[352] It occurs in many industries (Table 7.1.8)[353] and occupational factors can be identified as contributing to asthma in about 2% of adult cases. Over 250 aetiological agents have been identified.[354] In the UK a third are organic, a third chemical, 6% metallic and the rest miscella-

Table 7.1.7 Work related respiratory disease in the UK[352]

Disease	Estimated annual number of cases
Occupational asthma	941
Non-malignant pleural disease	730
Mesothelioma	644
Pneumoconiosis	341
Inhalation accidents	280
Lung cancer	70
Infectious disease	59
Extrinsic allergic alveolitis	46
Bronchitis	38
Byssinosis	1
Other diagnoses	117
Total	3207

Table 7.1.8 Agents that cause occupational asthma and examples of the occupations involved[353]

Causative agent	Occupations involved
High molecular weight agents (patients are usually atopic)	
Laboratory animals	Laboratory animal handling
Flour and grain	Baking, milling, farming
Enzymes	Detergent and drug manufacture, baking
Seafoods	Food processing
Gums	Carpet and drug manufacture
Low molecular weight agents (patients are not necessarily atopic)	
Isocyanates	Foam and plastic manufacture, spray painting, insulation
Anhydrides	Plastic and epoxy resin handling
Wood dusts	Forestry, carpentry
Soldering fluxes	Electronics
Formaldehyde, glutaraldehyde	Histopathology, nursing, radiography
Amines	Shellac and lacquer handling, soldering
Chloramine	Cleaning
Dyes	Textiles
Acrylates	Adhesive application
Metals	Solderers, refiners
Drugs	Pharmaceutical work

neous. The commonest, in descending order, are isocyanates, flour and grain, laboratory animals, glutaraldehyde, solder or colophony (pine resin) and hardening agents.[355]

Atopy appears to predispose to occupational asthma when the allergen is of high molecular weight but not when it is of low molecular weight. For example, atopic individuals are particularly prone to develop asthma if employed in the manufacture of biological detergents, whereas atopy does not increase the risk of asthma from sensitisation to toluene diisocyanate, which is a serious health problem in the manufacture of polyurethane. Similarly, platinum salts are such potent sensitising agents that nearly all those who are exposed to them develop asthma. Asthma-provoking metals other than platinum include chromium, cobalt, nickel and vanadium, all of which are used in steel alloys. Other asthma-inducing factors encountered in industry include grain and flour dust, certain wood dusts, soldering fluxes containing colophony, epoxy resin hardeners such as phthalic anhydride, isocyanate-containing foams and paints, formaldehyde and the excreta of laboratory animals. Contaminated humidifiers may cause occupational asthma as well as humidifier fever and extrinsic allergic alveolitis.[356] Pathologically, occupational asthma is identical to non-occupational asthma (see p. 106).

Byssinosis

Byssinosis is a further form of occupational asthma,[357] one encountered in the cotton industry. The sensitising agent is a component of the cotton bract, which is the part of the cotton harvest other than the cotton fibre. Bract consists of dried leaf, other plant debris and soil particles and contains a variety of fungal and bacterial residues, including lipopolysaccharide endotoxin, but the exact nature of the sensitising agent remains unknown.[358] The endotoxin is unlikely to be responsible for byssinosis but may be the cause of so-called mill fever, a self-limiting illness characterised by malaise, fever and leukocytosis that is experienced by many people on first visiting a cotton mill.

Dust levels and the risk of byssinosis are particularly high in the carding rooms where the raw cotton is teased out before it is spun. Affected workers are worse when they return to work after the weekend break, a feature attributed to antibody levels having built up during this brief respite from the cotton dust. There is no link with atopy and the fluctuating antibodies are precipitins of the immunoglobulin G class. Complement activation by both arms of the complement cascade has been reported.[359,360]

When the Lancashire economy was largely cotton-based, necropsies on workers suffering from byssinosis generally showed gross emphysema, and this came to be accepted as evidence of byssinosis. However, it is now realised that in this heavily industrialised part of England, emphysema is as common in the general population as in cotton workers and it can no longer be considered a component of byssinosis. Other findings in byssinosis are more commensurate with asthma, namely an increase in bronchial muscle and mucous cells.[361] No granulomas or other evidence of extrinsic allergic alveolitis are found.

OCCUPATIONAL FEVERS

Fever may be the predominant feature in a variety of occupational illnesses and the unifying term inhalation fever has been proposed.[362] However, the individual occupations are of interest and these conditions will therefore be considered separately. Mill fever has been mentioned above under byssinosis.

Humidifier fever[363]

Humidifier fever is an acute illness characterised by malaise, fever, myalgia, cough, tightness in the chest and breathlessness, all of which are worse on Monday mornings if the humidifier

responsible is at work rather than home. The chest complaints, and their aggravation on return to work after the weekend, are features shared with byssinosis (see above) but the general complaints fit better with extrinsic allergic alveolitis. Humidifier fever develops in circumstances that also lead to the development of a form of extrinsic allergic alveolitis, and not surprisingly the same name has been extended to this latter condition, with inevitable confusion. Both diseases are caused by microbiological contamination of humidifiers or air conditioners so that a fine spray of micro-organisms is emitted into the office, factory or home. Investigations have generally shown the baffle plates of the air conditioner to be covered with a slime of bacteria, fungi or protozoa (mainly amoeba and ciliates), and extracts of this have been used to identify precipitins in the patients' sera, as in extrinsic allergic alveolitis. However, unlike extrinsic allergic alveolitis, humidifier fever resolves within a day and leaves no permanent injury. For this reason there is seldom the opportunity to study the tissue changes, and partly for this reason it remains unclear whether the disease is mediated by immune complexes, as in extrinsic allergic alveolitis, or by endotoxins derived from the contaminants.

Pulmonary mycotoxicosis

A febrile illness occurring in precipitin-negative farm-workers after heavy exposure to fungi in their silos was attributed to inhaled fungal toxins and named pulmonary mycotoxicosis.[364] It is also known as precipitin test negative farmers' lung and organic dust toxic syndrome.[365] The condition is generally self-limiting and is seldom biopsied but desquamative interstitial pneumonia and diffuse alveolar damage have been reported.[366,367]

Metal fume fever

This is a self-limiting acute illness characterised by fever, sweating, myalgia, chest pain, headache and nausea, that comes on Monday mornings when occupational exposure is experienced after a weekend's respite, as with byssinosis and humidifier fever: during the week tolerance develops.[330,368] The disease involves the release of cytokines such as tumour necrosis factor and is presumed to have an allergic basis.[369] The metals involved are chiefly zinc, copper and magnesium, and to a lesser extent, aluminium, antimony, iron, manganese and nickel. Occupations at risk include any that generate such metal fumes, but particularly welding. It is most commonly associated with welding zinc-coated surfaces. If the symptoms persist, alternative diagnoses, such as acute cadmium poisoning and other specific toxic metal fume diseases, should be suspected: these are not self-limiting and may cause severe bronchiolitis or diffuse alveolar damage (see above).

Polymer fume fever

This illness resembles metal fume fever except that it occurs without regard to previous exposure: no tolerance develops and there is therefore no particular susceptibility on Mondays. The polymers concerned are quite inert, except when heated to produce fume: polytetrafluorethylene (PTFE, Teflon, Fluon, Halon) is a notable example. As with other self-limiting diseases, little is known of the tissue changes.

REFERENCES

Pneumoconiosis: general references

1. Meiklejohn A. The origin of the term 'pneumonokoniosis'. Br J Ind Med 1960; 17:155–160.
2. Industrial Injuries Advisory Council. Pneumoconiosis and byssinosis. London: HMSO; 1973:1.
3. Parkes WR, ed. Aerosols, their deposition and clearance. In: Occupational Lung Disorders. Oxford: Butterworth-Heinemann; 1994:35.
4. Churg A, Brauer M. Human lung parenchyma retains PM2.5. Am J Respir Crit Care Med 1997; 155:2109–2111.
5. Pinkerton KE, Plopper CG, Mercer RR, et al. Airway branching patterns influence asbestos fiber location and the extent of tissue injury in the pulmonary parenchyma. Lab Invest 1986; 55:688–695.
6. Schlesinger MR, Lippman M. Particle deposition in casts of the human upper tracheobronchial tree. Am Ind Hyg Assoc J 1972; 33:237–250.
7. Pityn P, Chamberlain MJ, King ME, Morgan WKC. Differences in particle deposition between the two lungs. Respir Med 1995; 89:15–19.
8. Ferin J, Oberdorster G, Penney DP. Pulmonary retention of ultrafine and fine particles in rats. Am J Respir Cell Mol Biol 1992; 6:535–542.
9. Brundelet PJ. Experimental study of the dust-clearance mechanism of the lung. Acta Path Microbiol Scand 1965; 175(Suppl):7–141.
10. Cordingley JL, Nicol T. The lung: an excretory route for macromolecules and particles. J Physiol (London) 1967; 190:197.
11. Corrin B. Phagocytic potential of pulmonary alveolar epithelium with particular reference to surfactant metabolism. Thorax 1970; 25:110–115.
12. Brody AR, Hill LH, Adkins B, O'Connor RW. Chrysotile asbestos inhalation in rats: deposition pattern and reaction of alveolar epithelium and pulmonary macrophages. Am Rev Respir Dis 1981; 123:670–678.
13. Churg A. The uptake of mineral particles by pulmonary epithelial cells. Am J Respir Crit Care Med 1996; 154:1124–1140.
14. Lehnert BE, Valdez YE, Stewart CC. Translocation of particles to the tracheobronchial lymph nodes after lung deposition: kinetics and particle-cell relationships. Exp Lung Res 1986; 10:245–266.
15. Adamson IYR, Hedgecock C. Patterns of particle deposition and retention after instillation to mouse lung during acute injury and fibrotic repair. Exp Lung Res 1995; 21:695–709.
16. Adamson IYR, Prieditis H. Silica deposition in the lung during epithelial injury potentiates fibrosis and increases particle translocation to lymph nodes. Exp Lung Res 1998; 24:293–306.
17. Gross P, Westrick M. The permeability of lung parenchyma to particulate matter. Am J Pathol 1954; 30:195–207.
18. Corry D, Kulkarni P, Lipscomb MF. The migration of bronchoalveolar macrophages into hilar lymph nodes. Am J Pathol 1984; 115:321–328.
19. Policard A, Collet A, Pregermain S, Reuet C. Etude au microscope electronique du granulome pulmonaire silicotique experimental. Presse Med 1957; 65:121–124.
20. Emery JL, Dinsdale F. The postnatal development of lymphoreticular aggregates and lymph nodes in infants' lungs. J Clin Pathol 1973; 26:539–545.
21. Macklin CS. Pulmonary sumps, dust accumulations, alveolar fluid and lymph vessels. Acta Anat 1955; 23:1–33.
22. Sakula A. Pneumoconiosis due to Fuller's earth. Thorax 1961; 16:176–179.
23. Pintar K, Funahashi A, Siegesmund KA. A diffuse form of pulmonary silicosis in foundry workers. Arch Pathol Lab Med 1976; 100:535–538.
24. Wagner JC, Pooley FD, Gibbs A, et al. Inhalation of china stone and china clay dusts: relationship between mineralogy of dust retained in the lungs and pathological changes. Thorax 1986; 41:190–196.

25. Kleinfeld M, Giel CP, Majeranowski JF, Messite J. Talc pneumoconiosis. A report of six patients with postmortem findings. Arch Env Health 1963; 7:101–115.
26. Ruttner JR, Spycher MA, Sticher H. Diffuse 'asbestosis-like' interstitial fibrosis of the lung. Pathol Microbiol 1972; 38:250–257.
27. Vallyathan NV, Craighead JE. Pulmonary pathology in workers exposed to nonasbestiform talc. Hum Pathol 1981; 12:28–35.
28. Davies D, Cotton R. Mica pneumoconiosis. Br J Ind Med 1983; 40:22–27.
29. Gibbs AE, Pooley FD, Griffiths DM, et al. Talc pneumoconiosis - a pathologic and mineralogic study. Hum Pathol 1992; 23:1344–1354.
30. Honma K, Chiyotani K. Diffuse interstitial fibrosis in nonasbestos pneumoconiosis - a pathological study. Respiration 1993; 60:120–126.
31. Heppleston AG. The disposal of coal and haematite dusts inhaled successively. J Pathol Bacteriol 1958; 75:113–126.
32. Glazier JB, Hughes JMB, Maloney JE, West JB. Vertical gradient of alveolar size in lungs of dogs frozen intact. J Appl Physiol 1967; 23:694–705.
33. Dock W. Apical localization of phthisis. Am Rev Tuberc 1946; 53:297–305.
34. West JB, Dollery CT. Distribution of blood flow and ventilation perfusion ratio in the lung, measured with radioactive CO_2. J Appl Physiol 1960; 15:405–410.
35. Goodwin RA, Des Prez RM. Apical localization of pulmonary tuberculosis, chronic pulmonary histoplasmosis, and progressive massive fibrosis of the lung. Chest 1983; 83:801–805.
36. Bake B, Wood L, Murphy B, Macklem PT, Milic-Emili J. Effect of inspiratory flow rate on the regional distribution of inspired gas. J Appl Physiol 1974; 37:8–17.
37. Davson J, Susman W. Apical scars and their relationship to siliceous dust accumulation in non-silicotic lungs. J Path Bact 1937; 45:597–612.
38. Sebastien P, Fondimare A, Bignon J, et al. Topographic distribution of asbestos fibres in human lung in relation to occupational and non-occupational exposure. In: Walton WH, ed. Inhaled Particles IV. Oxford: Pergamon Press; 1977:435–446.
39. Churg A. The distribution of amosite asbestos in the periphery of the normal human lung. Br J Ind Med 1990; 47:677–681.
40. Silicosis and Silicate Disease Committee. Diseases associated with exposure to silica and nonfibrous silicate minerals. Arch Pathol Lab Med 1988; 112:673–720.
41. McDonald JW, Roggli VL. Detection of silica particles in lung tissue by polarizing light microscopy. Arch Pathol Lab Med 1995; 119:242–246.
42. Crocker PR, Doyle DV, Levison DA. A practical method for the identification of particulate and crystalline material in paraffin-embedded tissue specimens. J Pathol 1980; 131:165–173.
43. Crocker PR, Toulson E, Levison DA. Particles in paraffin sections demonstrated in the backscattered electron image [BEI]. Micron 1982; 13:437–446.
44. Abraham JL, Burnett BR. Quantitative analysis of inorganic particulate burden in situ in tissue sections. Scanning Electron Microsc 1983; II:681–696.
45. Levison DA. Microanalysis in histopathology. J Pathol 1989; 157:95–97.
46. Abraham JL, Rossi R, Marquez N, Wagner RM. Ion microprobe mass analysis of beryllium in situ in human lung: preliminary results. Scanning Electron Microsc 1976; III:501–506.
47. DeNollin S, Poels K, VanVaeck L, et al. Molecular identification of foreign inclusions in inflammatory tissue surrounding metal implants by Fourier transform laser microprobe mass spectrometry. Pathol Res Pr 1997; 193:313–318.
48. Vallyathan V. Brower PS, Green FHY, Attfield MD. Radiographic and pathologic correlation of coal workers' pneumoconiosis. Am J Respir Crit Care Med 1996; 154:741–748.

Silicosis

49. King EJ, Mohanty GP, Harrison CV, Nagelschmidt G. The action of different forms of pure silica on the lungs of rats. Br J Ind Med 1953; 10:9–17.
50. Gibbs AR, Craighead JE, Pooley FD, Wagner JC. The pathology of slate workers' pneumoconiosis in North Wales and Vermont. Ann Occup Hyg 1988; 32(Suppl 1):273–278.

51. Craighead JE, Emerson RJ, Stanley DE. Slateworker's pneumoconiosis. Hum Pathol 1992; 23:1098–1105.

52. Palmer PES, Daynes G. Transkei silicosis. S Afr Med J 1967; 41:1182–1188.

53. Selden A, Sahle W, Johansson L, Sorenson S, Persson B. Three cases of dental technician's pneumoconiosis related to cobalt-chromium-molybdenum dust exposure: diagnosis and follow-up. Chest 1996; 109:837–842.

54. Policard A, Collet A. Deposition of silicosis dust in the lungs of the inhabitants of the Sahara regions. Arch Ind Hyg Occup Med 1952; 5:527–534.

55. Fossati C. Sulla possibilita e sulla frequenza della silicosi pulmonare tra gli abitanti del deserto libico. Med Lav 1969; 60:144–149.

56. Hirsch M, Bar-Ziv J, Lehmann E, Goldberg GM. Simple siliceous pneumoconiosis of Bedouin females in the Negev desert. Clin Radiol 1974; 25:507–510.

57. Bar-Ziv J, Goldberg G. Simple siliceous pneumoconiosis in Negev Bedouins. Arch Environ Health 1974; 29:121–126.

58. Fennerty A, Hunter AM, Smith AP, Pooley FD. Silicosis in a Pakistani farmer. BMJ 1983; ii:648.

59. Norboo T, Angchuk PT, Yahya M, et al. Silicosis in a Himalayan village population – role of environmental dust. Thorax 1991; 46:341–343.

60. Saiyed HN, Sharma YK, Sadhu HG, et al. Non-occupational pneumoconiosis at high altitude villages in central Ladakh. Br J Ind Med 1991; 48:825–829.

61. Sherwin RP, Barman ML, Abraham JL. Silicate pneumoconiosis of farm workers. Lab Invest 1979; 40:576–582.

62. Schwartz LW, Knight HD, Malloy RL, Abraham JL, Tyler NK. Silicate pneumoconiosis and pulmonary fibrosis in horses from the Monterey-Carmel peninsula. Chest 1981; 80:82S–85S.

63. Brambilla C, Abraham J, Brambilla E, Benirschke K, Bloor C. Comparative pathology of silicate pneumoconiosis. Am J Pathol 1979; 96:149–170.

64. MacDonald G, Piggot AP, Gilder FW. Two cases of acute silicosis – with a suggested theory of causation. Lancet 1930; 2:846–848.

65. Chapman EM. Acute silicosis. JAMA 1932; 98:1439–1441.

66. Vincent M, Arthaud Y, Crettet G, et al. Silicose aigue fatale par inhalation volontaire de poudre a recurer. Rev Mal Resp 1995; 12:499–502.

67. Suratt PM, Winn WC, Brody AR, Bolton WK, Giles RD. Acute silicosis in tombstone sandblasters. Am Rev Respir Dis 1977; 115:521–529.

68. Seaton A, Legge JS, Henderson J, Kerr KM. Accelerated silicosis in Scottish stonemasons. Lancet 1991; 337:341–344.

69. Murray J, Webster I, Reid G, Kielkowski D. The relation between fibrosis of hilar lymph glands and the development of parenchymal silicosis. Br J Ind Med 1991; 48:267–269.

70. Hessel PA, Sluis-Cremer GK, Lee SL. Distribution of silicotic collagenization in relation to smoking habits. Am Rev Respir Dis 1991; 144:297–301.

71. Baldwin DR, Lambert L, Pantin CFA, Prowse K, Cole RB. Silicosis presenting as bilateral hilar lymphadenopathy. Thorax 1996; 51:1165–1167.

72. Tosi P, Franzinelli A, Miracco C, et al. Silicotic lymph node lesions in non-occupationally exposed lung carcinoma patients. Eur J Respir Dis 1986; 68:362–369.

73. Kampalath BN, McMahon JT, Cohen A, Tomashefski JF, Kleinerman J. Obliterative central bronchitis due to mineral dust in patients with pneumoconiosis. Arch Pathol Lab Med 1998; 122:56–62.

74. Lardinois D, Gugger M, Balmer MC, Ris HB. Left recurrent laryngeal nerve palsy associated with silicosis. Eur Resp J 1999; 14:720–722.

75. Argani P, Ghossein R, Rosai J. Anthracotic and anthracosilicotic spindle cell pseudotumors of mediastinal lymph nodes: Report of five cases of a reactive lesion that simulates malignancy. Hum Pathol 1998; 29:851–855.

76. Chien HP, Lin TP, Chen HL, Huang TW. Right middle lobe atelectasis associated with endobronchial silicotic lesions. Arch Pathol Lab Med 2000; 124:1619–1622.

77. Rashid AMH, Green FHY. Pleural pearls following silicosis: a histological and electronmicroscopic study. Histopathology 1995; 26:84–87.

78. Zeren EH, Colby TV, Roggli VL. Silica-induced pleural disease: An unusual case mimicking malignant mesothelioma. Chest 1997; 112:1436–1438.

79. Ng TP, Chan SL. Factors associated with massive fibrosis in silicosis. Thorax 1991; 46:229–232.

80. Lynch KM. Silicosis of systemic distribution. Am J Pathol 1942; 18:313–331.

81. Langlois SLEP, Sterrett GF, Henderson DW. Hepatosplenic silicosis. Australas Radiol 1977; 21:143–149.

82. Carmichael GP, Targoff C, Pintar K, et al. Lewin KJ. Hepatic silicosis. Am J Clin Pathol 1980; 73:720–722.

83. Eide J, Gylseth B, Skaug V. Silicotic lesions of the bone marrow: histopathology and microanalysis. Histopathology 1984; 8:693–703.

84. Miranda RN, McMillan PN, Pricolo VE, Finkelstein SD. Peritoneal silicosis. Arch Pathol Lab Med 1996; 120:300–302.

85. Harding HE, McLaughlin AIG. Pulmonary fibrosis in non-ferrous foundry workers. Br J Ind Med 1955; 12:92–99.

86. Cockcroft AE, Wagner JC, Seal EM, Lyons JP, Campbell MJ. Irregular opacities in coalworkers' pneumoconiosis–correlation with pulmonary function and pathology. Ann Occup Hyg 1982; 26:767–787.

87. Katabami M, Dosakaakita H, Honma K, et al. Pneumoconiosis-related lung cancers - Preferential occurrence from diffuse interstitial fibrosis-type pneumoconiosis. Am J Respir Crit Care Med 2000; 162:295–300.

88. Rowsell EV, Nagelschmidt G, Curran RC. The effects of dusts on peritoneal cells within diffusion chambers. J Pathol Bacteriol 1960; 80:337–344.

89. Vallyathan V, Castranova V, Pack D, et al. Freshly fractured quartz inhalation leads to enhanced lung injury and inflammation: potential role of free radicals. Am J Respir Crit Care Med 1995; 152:1003–1009.

90. Allison AC, Harington JS, Birbeck M. An examination of the cytotoxic effects of silica on macrophages. J Exp Med 1966; 124:141–154.

91. Heppleston AG, Styles JA. Activity of macrophage factor in collagen formation by silica. Nature 1967; 214:521–522.

92. Aalto M, Kulonen E. Fractionation of connective-tissue-activating factors from the culture medium of silica-treated macrophages. Acta Path Microbiol Scand Sect C 1979; 87:241–250.

93. Aalto M, Turakainen H, Kulonen E. Effect of SiO2-liberated macrophage factor on protein synthesis in connective tissue in vitro. Scand J Clin Lab Invest 1979; 39:205–213.

94. Lugano EM, Dauber JH, Elias JA, et al. The regulation of lung fibroblast proliferation by alveolar macrophages in experimental silicosis. Am Rev Respir Dis 1984; 129:767–771.

95. Donaldson K, Slight J, Brown GM, Bolton RE. The ability of inflammatory bronchoalveolar leucocyte populations elicited with microbes or mineral dust to injure alveolar epithelial cells and degrade extracellular matrix in vitro. Br J Exp Pathol 1988; 69:327–338.

96. Vanhee D, Gosset P, Boitelle A, Wallaert B, Tonnel AB. Cytokines and cytokine network in silicosis and coal workers' pneumoconiosis. Eur Respir J 1995; 8:834–842.

97. Claudio E, Segade F, Wrobel K, Ramos S, Lazo PS. Activation of murine macrophages by silica particles in vitro is a process independent of silica-induced cell death. Am J Respir Cell Mol Biol 1995; 13:547–554.

98. Mariani TJ, Roby JD, Mecham RP, et al. Localization of type I procollagen gene expression in silica- induced granulomatous lung disease and implication of transforming growth factor-beta as a mediator of fibrosis. Am J Pathol 1996; 148:151–164.

99. Jagirdar J, Begin R, Dufresne A, et al. Transforming growth factor-beta (TGF-beta) in silicosis. Am J Respir Crit Care Med 1996; 154:1076–1081.

100. Mossman BT, Churg A. Mechanisms in the pathogenesis of asbestosis and silicosis. Am J Respir Crit Care Med 1998; 157:1666–1680.

101. Erasmus LD. Scleroderma in gold-miners on the Witwatersrand with particular reference to pulmonary manifestations. S Afr J Lab Clin Med 1957; 3:209–231.

102. Vigliani EC, Pernis B. Immunological factors in the pathogenesis of the hyaline tissue of silicosis. Br J Ind Med 1958; 15:8–14.

103. Scheule RK, Holian A. Mini-review - immunologic aspects of pneumoconiosis. Exp Lung Res 1991; 17:661–685.

104. Beckett W, Abraham J, Becklake M, et al. Adverse effects of crystalline silica exposure. Am J Respir Crit Care Med 1997; 155:761–768.

105. Powell DEB, Gough J. Experimental silicosis. Br J Exp Pathol 1959; 40:40–43.

106. Kato T, Usami I, Morita H, et al. Chronic necrotizing pulmonary aspergillosis in pneumoconiosis – clinical and radiologic findings in 10 patients. Chest 2002; 121:118–127.

107. International Agency for Research on Cancer (Lyons). Silica and some silicates. Mono Eval Carcinogenic Risks to Humans 1987; 42.

108. Weill H, McDonald JC. Occupational lung disease: 1. exposure to crystalline silica and risk of lung cancer: the epidemiological evidence. Thorax 1996; 51:97–102.

109. Craighead JE. Do silica and asbestos cause lung cancer? Arch Pathol Lab Med 1992; 116:16–20.

110. Department of Social Security. Lung cancer in relation to occupational exposure to silica. Report by the Industrial Injuries Advisory Council in accordance with Section 171 of the Social Security Administration Act. London: HMSO; 1992:1–5.

111. Checkoway H, Hughes JM, Weill H, Seixas NS, Demers PA. Crystalline silica exposure, radiological silicosis, and lung cancer mortality in diatomaceous earth industry workers. Thorax 1999; 54:56–59.

112. Buechner HA, Ansari A. Acute silico-proteinosis. Dis Chest 1969; 55:274–284.

113. Xipell JM, Ham KN, Price CG, Thomas DP. Acute silicolipoproteinosis. Thorax 1977; 32:104–111.

114. Heppleston AG. Atypical reaction to inhaled silica. Nature 1967; 213:199.

115. Gross P, DeTreville RTP. Alveolar proteinosis. Its experimental production in rodents. Arch Pathol 1968; 86:255–261.

116. Corrin B, King E. Experimental endogenous lipid pneumonia and silicosis. J Pathol 1969; 97:325–330.

117. Corrin B, King E. Pathogenesis of experimental pulmonary alveolar proteinosis. Thorax 1970; 25:230–236.

118. Heppleston AG, Fletcher K, Wyatt I. Changes in the composition of lung lipids and the 'turnover' of dipalmitoyl lecithin in experimental alveolar lipo-proteinosis induced by inhaled quartz. Br J Exp Pathol 1974; 55:384–395.

119. Miller RR, Churg AM, Hutcheon M, Lam S. Case report: pulmonary alveolar proteinosis and aluminum dust exposure. Am Rev Respir Dis 1984; 130:312–315.

120. Miller BE, Bakewell WE, Katyal SL, Singh G, Hook GE. Induction of surfactant protein (SP-A) biosynthesis and SP-A mRNA in activated type II cells during acute silicosis in rats. Am J Respir Cell Mol Biol 1990; 3:217–226.

121. Hauglustaine D, Damme B Van, Daenens P, Michielsen P. Silicon nephropathy: a possible occupational hazard. Nephron 1980; 26:219–224.

122. Bolton WK, Suratt PM, Strugill BC. Rapidly progressive silicon nephropathy. Am J Med 1981; 71:823–828.

123. Osorio AM, Thun MJ, Novak RF, Cura EJ Van, Avner ED. Silica and glomerulonephritis: case report and review of the literature. Am J Kidney Dis 1987; 9:224–230.

124. Sherson D, Jorgensen F. Rapidly progressive crescenteric glomerulonephritis in a sandblaster with silicosis. Br J Ind Med 1989; 46:675–676.

125. Dutra FR. Diatomaceous earth pneumoconiosis. Arch Env Health 1965; 11:613–619.

Silicates

126. Abraham JL, Brambilla C. Particle size for differentiation between inhalation and injection pulmonary talcosis. Environ Res 1980; 21:94–96.

127. Lapenas DJ, Gale PN. Kaolin pneumoconiosis. A case report. Arch Pathol Lab Med 1983; 107:650–653.

128. Lapenas D, Gale P, Kennedy T, Rawlings W Jr, Dietrich P. Kaolin pneumoconiosis. Radiologic, pathologic and mineralogic findings. Am Rev Respir Dis 1984; 130:282–288.

129. Phibbs BP, Sundin RE, Mitchell RS. Silicosis in Wyoming bentonite workers. Am Rev Respir Dis 1971; 103:1–17.

130. Wells IP, Dubbins PA, Whimster WF. Pulmonary disease caused by the inhalation of cosmetic talcum powder. Br J Radiol 1979; 52:586–588.

131. Berner A, Gylseth B, Levy F. Talc dust pneumoconiosis. Acta Path Microbiol Scand 1981; 89:17–21.

132. Landas SK, Schwartz DA. Mica-associated pulmonary interstitial fibrosis. Am Rev Respir Dis 1991; 144:718–721.

Dusts

133. Doig AT. Baritosis: a benign pneumoconiosis. Thorax 1976; 31:30–39.

134. Seaton A, Ruckley VA, Addison J, Rhind Brown W. Silicosis in barium miners. Thorax 1986; 41:591–595.

135. McLaughlin AIG, Harding HE. Pneumoconiosis and other causes of death in iron and steel foundry workers. Arch Ind Health 1956; 14:350–378.

136. Highman B. Histochemical study of certain iron ore dusts. Bull Internat Assoc Med Mus 1951; 32:97–99.

Coal pneumoconiosis

137. Green FHY, Laqueur WA. Coal workers' pneumoconiosis. Pathol Annu 1980; 15:333–410.

138. Stratton TML. Edin Med Surg J 1838; 49:490.

139. Gough J. Pneumoconiosis in coal trimmers. J Pathol Bacteriol 1940; 51:277–285.

140. Douglas AN, Robertson A, Chapman JS, Ruckley VA. Dust exposure, dust recovered from the lung, and associated pathology in a group of British coalminers. Br J Ind Med 1986; 43:795–801.

141. Davis JMG. The relationship between the mass and composition of coal mine dust and the development of pneumoconiosis. In: Rom WN, Archer VE, eds. Health implication of new energy technologies. Ann Arbor: Butterworths; 1980:283–292.

142. McConnochie K, Green FHY, Vallyathan V, et al. Interstitial fibrosis in coal miners – experience in Wales and West Virginia. Ann Occup Hyg 1988; 32:553–560.

143. Remy-Jardin M, Degreef JM, Beuscart R, Voisin C, Remy J. Coal worker's pneumoconiosis: CT assessment in exposed workers and correlation with radiographic findings. Radiology 1990; 177:363–371.

144. Davis JMG, Chapman J, Collings P, et al. Variations in the histological patterns of the lesions of coal workers' pneumoconiosis in Britain and their relationship to lung dust content. Am Rev Respir Dis 1983; 128:118–124.

145. Ruckley VA, Fernie JM, Chapman JS, et al. Comparison of radiographic appearances with associated pathology and lung dust content in a group of coalworkers. Br J Ind Med 1984; 41:459–467.

146. Churg A, Wright JL, Wiggs B, Pare PD, Lazar N. Small airways disease and mineral dust exposure. Prevalence, structure and function. Am Rev Respir Dis 1985; 131:139–143.

147. Morgan WKC. Coal mining, emphysema, and compensation revisited. Br J Ind Med 1993; 50:1051–1052.

148. Seaton A. Coal mining, emphysema, and compensation revisited – reply. Br J Ind Med 1993; 50:1052–1053.

149. Coggon D, Taylor AN. Coal mining and chronic obstructive pulmonary disease: a review of the evidence. Thorax 1998; 53:398–407.

150. Heppleston AG. The pathogenesis of simple pneumokoniosis in coal workers. J Path Bact 1954; 67:51–63.

151. Li K, Keeling B, Churg A. Mineral dusts cause elastin and collagen breakdown in the rat lung: a potential mechanism of dust-induced emphysema. Am J Respir Crit Care Med 1996; 153:644–649.

152. Ryder R, Lyons JP, Campbell H, Gough J. Emphysema in coal workers' pneumoconiosis. BMJ 1970; 3:481–487.

153. Lyons JP, Ryder R, Campbell H, Gough J. Pulmonary disability in coal workers' pneumoconiosis. BMJ 1972; :713–716.

154. Leigh J, Outhred KG, McKenzie HI, Glick M, Wiles AN. Quantified pathology of emphysema, pneumoconiosis, and chronic bronchitis in coal workers. Br J Ind Med 1983; 40:258–263.

155. Ruckley VA, Gauld SJ, Chapman JS, et al. Emphysema and dust exposure in a group of coal workers. Am Rev Respir Dis 1984; 129:528–532.

156. Oxman AD, Muir DCF, Shannon HS, et al. Occupational dust exposure and chronic obstructive pulmonary disease – a systematic overview of the evidence. Am Rev Respir Dis 1993; 148:38–48.

157. Department of Social Security. Chronic bronchitis and emphysema. Report by the Industrial Injuries Advisory Council in accordance with Section 171 of the Social Security Administration Act. London: HMSO; 1992:1.

158. Seaton A. The new prescription: industrial injuries benefits for smokers? Thorax 1998; 53:335–336.

159. Hurley JF, Alexander WP, Hazledine DJ, Jacobsen M, Maclaren WM. Exposure to respirable coalmine dust and incidence of progressive massive fibrosis. Br J Ind Med 1987; 44:661–672.

160. Watson AJ, Black J, Doig AT, Nagelschmidt G. Pneumoconiosis in carbon electrode makers. Br J Ind Med 1959; 16:274.

161. Miller AA, Ramsden F. Carbon pneumoconiosis. Br J Ind Med 1961; 18:103–113.

162. Gaensler EA, Cadigan JB, Sasahara AA, Fox EO, MacMahon HE. Graphite pneumoconiosis of electrotypers. Am J Med 1966; 41:864–882.

163. Cochrane AL. The attack rate of progressive massive fibrosis. Br J Ind Med 1962; 19:52–64.

164. Theodos PA, Cathcart RT, Fraimow W. Ischemic necrosis in anthracosilicosis. Arch Env Health 1961; 2:609–619.

165. Wagner JC, Wusterman FS, Edwards JH, Hill RJ. The composition of massive lesions in coal miners. Thorax 1975; 30:382–388.

166. Vanhee D, Gosset P, Wallaert B, Voisin C, Tonnel AB. Mechanisms of fibrosis in coal workers' pneumoconiosis increased production of platelet-derived growth factor, insulin-like growth factor type I, and transforming growth factor beta and relationship to disease severity. Am J Respir Crit Care Med 1994; 150:1049–1055.

167. Vanhee D, Gosset P, Marquette CH, et al. Secretion and mRNA expression of TNF alpha and IL-6 in the lungs of pneumoconiosis patients. Am J Respir Crit Care Med 1995; 152:298–306.

168. Caplan A, Payne RB, Withey JL. A broader concept of Caplan's syndrome related to rheumatoid factors. Thorax 1962; 17:205–212.

169. Ball J. Differential agglutination test in rheumatoid arthritis complicated by pneumoconiosis. Ann Rheum Dis 1955; 14:159–161.

170. Soutar CA, Turner-Warwick M, Parkes WR. Circulating antinuclear antibody and rheumatoid factor in coal pneumoconiosis. BMJ 1974; 3:145–152.

171. Pearson DJ, Mentnech MS, Elliott JA, et al. Serologic changes in pneumoconiosis and progressive massive fibrosis of coal workers. Am Rev Respir Dis 1981; 124:696–699.

172. Wagner JC, McCormick JN. Immunological investigations of coalworkers' disease. J R Coll Physicians Lond 1967; 2:49–56.

Caplan's syndrome

173. Caplan A. Certain unusual radiological appearances in the chest of coal-miners suffering from rheumatoid arthritis. Thorax 1953; 8:29–37.

174. Gough J, Rivers D, Seal RME. Pathological studies of modified pneumoconiosis in coal-miners with rheumatoid arthritis (Caplan's syndrome). Thorax 1955; 10:9–18.

Asbestosis

175. LaDou J. The asbestos cancer epidemic. Environ Health Perspect 2004; 112:285–290.

176. Wagner JC, Pooley FD, Berry G, et al. A pathological and mineralogical study of asbestos-related deaths in the United Kingdom in 1977. Ann Occup Hyg 1982; 26:423–431.

177. Wagner JC, Moncrieff CB, Coles R, Griffiths DM, Munday DE. Correlation between fibre content of the lungs and disease in naval dockyard workers. Br J Ind Med 1986; 43:391–395.

178. Wagner JC, Newhouse ML, Corrin B, Rossiter CER, Griffiths DM. Correlation between fibre content of the lung and disease in east London asbestos factory workers. Br J Ind Med 1988; 45:305–308.

179. Wagner JC, Berry G, Skidmore JW, Timbrell V. The effects of the inhalation of asbestos in rats. Br J Cancer 1974; 29:252–269.

180. Davis JMG, Beckett ST, Bolton RE, Collings P, Middleton AP. Mass and number of fibres in the pathogenesis of asbestos related lung disease in rats. Br J Cancer 1978; 37:673–688.

181. Churg A, Wright JL, Vedal S. Fiber burden and patterns of asbestos-related disease in chrysotile miners and millers. Am Rev Respir Dis 1993; 148:25–31.

182. Wagner JC, Berry G, Pooley FD. Carcinogenesis and mineral fibres. Br Med Bull 1980; 36:53–56.

183. Dodson RF, O'Sullivan M, Corn CJ, et al. Analysis of ferruginous bodies in bronchoalveolar lavage from foundry workers. Br J Ind Med 1993; 50:1032–1038.

184. Warnock ML. Analysis of the cores of ferruginous (asbestos) bodies from the general population. Lab Invest 1979; 40:622–626.

185. Morgan A, Holmes A. Concentrations and dimensions of coated and uncoated asbestos fibres in the human lung. Br J Ind Med 1980; 37:25–32.

186. Pooley FD, Ranson DL. Comparison of the results of asbestos fibre dust counts in lung tissue obtained by analytical electron microscopy and light microscopy. J Clin Pathol 1986; 39:313–317.

187. Holden J, Churg A. Asbestos bodies and the diagnosis of asbestosis in chrysotile workers. Environ Res 1986; 39:232–236.

188. Johansson LG, Albin MP, Jakobsson KM, et al. Ferruginous bodies and pulmonary fibrosis in dead low to moderately exposed asbestos cement workers: histological examination. Br J Ind Med 1987; 44:550–558.

189. McLemore TL, Roggli V, Marshall MV, et al. Comparison of phagocytosis of uncoated versus coated asbestos fibers by cultured human pulmonary alveolar macrophages. Chest 1981; 80:39S–42S.

190. Roggli VL, Pratt PC. Numbers of asbestos bodies on iron-stained tissue sections in relation to asbestos body counts in lung tissue digests. Hum Pathol 1983; 14:355–361.

191. Roggli VL, Pratt PC, Brody AR. Asbestos content of lung tissue in asbestos associated diseases: a study of 110 cases. Br J Ind Med 1986; 43:18–28.

192. Gibbs AR, Pooley FD. Analysis and interpretation of inorganic mineral particles in 'lung' tissues. Thorax 1996; 51:327–334.

193. Karjalainen A, Piipari R, Mantyla T, et al. Asbestos bodies in bronchoalveolar lavage in relation to asbestos bodies and asbestos fibres in lung parenchyma. Eur Respir J 1996; 9:1000–1005.

194. Paris C. GalateauSalle F, Creveuil C et al. Asbestos bodies in the sputum of asbestos workers: correlation with occupational exposure. Eur Respir J 2002; 20:1167–1173.

195. Ashcroft T, Heppleston AG. The optical and electron microscopic determination of pulmonary asbestos fibre concentration and its relation to human pathology reaction. J Clin Pathol 1973; 26:224–234.

196. Davis JMG, Glyseth B, Morgan A. Assessment of mineral fibres from human lung tissue. Thorax 1986; 41:167–175.

197. James KR, Bull TB, Fox B. Detection of asbestos fibres by dark ground microscopy. J Clin Pathol 1987; 40:1259–1260.

198. Churg A. Analysis of lung asbestos content. Br J Ind Med 1991; 48:649–652.

199. Churg A. Fiber counting and analysis in the diagnosis of asbestos-related disease. Hum Pathol 1982; 13:381–392.

200. Vuyst P De, Karjalainen A, Dumortier P, et al. Guidelines for mineral fibre analyses in biological samples: report of the ERS Working Group. Eur Resp J 1998; 11:1416–1426.

201. Whitwell F, Scott J, Grimshaw M. Relationship between occupations and asbestos-fibre content of the lungs in patients with pleural mesothelioma, lung cancer, and other diseases. Thorax 1977; 32:377–386.

202. Donaldson K, Brown GM, Brown DM, Bolton RE, Davis JMG. Inflammation-generating potential of long and short-fibre amosite asbestos samples. Br J Ind Med 1989; 46:271–276.

203. Donaldson K, Li XY, Dogra S, Miller BG, Brown GM. Asbestos-stimulated tumour necrosis factor release from alveolar macrophages depends on fibre length and opsonization. J Pathol 1992; 168:243–248.

204. Davis JMG, Addison J, Bolton RE, et al. The pathogenicity of long versus short fibre amosite asbestos administered to rats by inhalation and intra-peritoneal injection. Br J Exp Pathol 1986; 67:415–430.

205. Donaldson K, Golyasnya N. Cytogenetic and pathogenic effects of long and short amosite asbestos. J Pathol 1995; 177:303–307.

206. Green FHY, Harley R, Vallyathan V, et al. Exposure and mineralogical correlates of pulmonary fibrosis in chrysotile asbestos workers. Occup Environ Med 1997; 54:549–559.

207. Gibbs AR, Stephens M, Griffiths DM, Blight BJN, Pooley FD. Fibre distribution in the lungs and pleura of subjects with asbestos related diffuse pleural fibrosis. Br J Ind Med 1991; 48:762–770.

208. Dawson A, Gibbs AR, Pooley FD, Griffiths DM, Hoy J. Malignant mesothelioma in women. Thorax 1993; 48:269–274.

209. Churg A, Wood P. Observations on the distribution of asbestos fibres in human lungs. Environ Res 1983; 31:374–380.

210. Gylseth B, Churg A, Davis JMG, et al. Analysis of asbestos fibres and asbestos bodies in tissue samples from human lung: an international interlaboratory trial. Scand J Work Environ Health 1985; 11:107–110.

211. Morgan A, Holmes A. Distribution and characteristics of amphibole asbestos fibres in the left lung of an insulation worker measured with the light microscope. Br J Ind Med 1983; 40:45–50.

212. Pooley FD. The identification of asbestos dust with an electron microprobe analyser. Ann Occup Hyg 1975; 13:181–186.

213. Pooley FD, Clark NJ. Quantitative assessment of inorganic fibrous particulates in dust samples with an analytical transmission electron microscope. Ann Occup Hyg 1979; 22:253–271.

214. Doll R. Symposium on man-made mineral fibres, Copenhagen, October 1986: overview and conclusions. Ann Occup Hyg 1987; 31:805–820.

215. Berry G. Mortality of workers certified by pneumoconiosis medical panels as having asbestosis. Br J Ind Med 1981; 38:130–137.

216. Jones RN, Diem JE, Ziskand MM, Rodriguez M, Weill H. Radiographic evidence of asbestos effects in American marine engineers. J Occup Med 1984; 26:281–284.

217. Coutts II, Gilson JC, Kerr IH, Parkes WR, Turner-Warwick M. Mortality in cases of asbestosis diagnosed by a pneumoconiosis medical panel. Thorax 1987; 42:111–116.

218. Hinson KFW, Otto H, Webster I, Rossiter CE. Criteria for the diagnosis and grading of asbestosis. In: Bogovski P, Gilson JC, Timbrell V, Wagner JC, ed. Biological effects of asbestos. I.A.R.C.Lyon. Scientific publications no.8. Oxford: Pergamon Press; 1973:54–57.

219. Craighead JE, Abraham JL, Churg A, et al. The pathology of asbestos-associated diseases of the lung and pleural cavities: diagnostic criteria and proposed grading schema. Report of the Pneumoconiosis Committee of the College of American Pathologists and the National Institute for Occupational Safety and Health. Arch Pathol Lab Med 1982; 106:544–596.

220. Corrin B, Price AB. Electron microscopic studies in desquamative interstitial pneumonia associated with asbestos. Thorax 1972; 27:324–331.

221. Freed JA, Miller A, Gordon RE, et al. Desquamative interstitial pneumonia associated with chrysotile asbestos fibres. Br J Ind Med 1991; 48:332–337.

222. Asbestos. asbestosis, and cancer: the Helsinki criteria for diagnosis and attribution Scand. J Work Environ Health 1997; 23:311–316.

223. Hammar SP, Hallman KO. Localized inflammatory pulmonary disease in subjects occupationally exposed to asbestos. Chest 1993; 103:1792–1799.

224. Gaensler EA, Jederlinic PJ, Churg A. Idiopathic pulmonary fibrosis in asbestos-exposed workers. Am Rev Respir Dis 1991; 144:689–696.

225. Kuhn C, Kuo TT. Cytoplasmic hyalin in asbestosis. Arch Pathol 1973; 95:190–194.

226. Warnock ML, Press M, Churg A. Further observations on cytoplasmic hyaline in the lung. Hum Pathol 1980; 11:59–65.

227. Thurlbeck WM. Morphology of emphysema and emphysema-like conditions. In: Thurlbeck WM, ed. Chronic Airflow Obstruction in Lung Disease. Philadelphia, PA: Saunders; 1976:98–99.

228. Corrin B, Dewar A, Rodriguez-Roisin R, Turner-Warwick M. Fine structural changes in cryptogenic fibrosing alveolitis and asbestosis. J Pathol 1985; 147:107–119.

229. Gadek J, Hunninghake G, Schoenberger C, Fells G, Crystal R. Pulmonary asbestosis and idiopathic pulmonary fibrosis: pathogenetic parallels. Chest 1981; 80:63S–64S.

230. Adamson IYR, Bowden DH. Crocidolite-induced pulmonary fibrosis in mice. Cytokinetic and biochemical studies. Am J Pathol 1986; 122:261–267.

231. Schapira RM, Ghio AJ, Effros RM, et al. Hydroxyl radicals are formed in the rat lung after asbestos instillation in vivo. Am J Respir Cell Mol Biol 1994; 10:573–579.

232. Thomas G, Ando T, Verma K, Kagan E. Asbestos fibers and interferon-gamma up-regulate nitric oxide production in rat alveolar macrophages. Am J Respir Cell Mol Biol 1994; 11:707–715.

233. Kinnula VL. Oxidant sand antioxidant mechanisms of lung disease caused by asbestos fibres. Eur Resp J 1999; 14:706–716.

234. Turner-Warwick M, Haslam P. Antibodies in some chronic fibrosing lung diseases. Clin Allergy 1971; 1:83–95.

235. Janssen YMW, Driscoll KE, Howard B, et al. Asbestos causes translocation of p65 protein and increases NF- kappa B DNA binding activity in rat lung epithelial and pleural mesothelial cells. Am J Pathol 1997; 151:389–401.

236. Liu JY, Morris GF, Lei WH, et al. Rapid activation of PDGF-A and -B expression at sites of lung injury in asbestos-exposed rats. Am J Respir Cell Molec Biol 1997; 17:129–140.

237. Lasky JA, Tonthat BH, Liu JY, Friedman M, Brody AR. Upregulation of the PDGF-alpha receptor precedes asbestos- induced lung fibrosis in rats. Am J Respir Crit Care Med 1998; 157:1652–1657.

238. Liu JY, Brass DM, Hoyle GW, Brody AR. TNF-alpha receptor knockout mice are protected from the fibroproliferative effects of inhaled asbestos fibers. Am J Pathol 1998; 153:1839–1847.

239. Tsuda A, Stringer BK, Miljailovich SM, et al. Alveolar cell stretching in the presence of fibrous particles induces interleukin-8 responses. Am J Respir Cell Molec Biol 1999; 21:455–462.

240. Kamp DW, Weitzman SA. The molecular basis of asbestos induced lung injury. Thorax 1999; 54:638–652.

241. Warheit DB, George G, Hill LH, Snyderman R, Brody AR. Inhaled asbestos activates a complement-dependent chemoattractant for macrophages. Lab Invest 1985; 52:505–514.

242. Lemaire I, Beaudoin H, Masse S, Grondin C. Alveolar macrophage stimulation of lung fibroblast growth in asbestos-induced pulmonary fibrosis. Am J Pathol 1986; 122:205–211.

243. Rom WN, Travis WD, Brody AR. Cellular and molecular basis of the asbestos-related diseases. Am Rev Respir Dis 1991; 143:408–422.

244. Liu JY, Morris GF, Lei WH, Corti M, Brody AR. Up-regulated expression of transforming growth factor-α in the bronchiolar-alveolar duct regions of asbestos-exposed rats. Am J Pathol 1996; 149:205–217.

245. Bateman ED, Emerson RJ, Cole PJ. A study of macrophage-mediated initiation of fibrosis by asbestos and silica using a diffusion chamber technique. Br J Exp Pathol 1982; 63:414–425.

246. Vallyathan V, Mega JF, Shi XL, Dalal NS. Enhanced generation of free radicals from phagocytes induced by mineral dusts. Am J Respir Cell Mol Biol 1992; 6:404–413.

247. Doll R. Mortality from lung cancer in asbestos workers. Br J Ind Med 1955; 12:81–86.

248. Wagner JC, Sleggs CA, Marchand P. Diffuse pleural mesotheliomas and asbestos exposure in Northwestern Cape Province. Br J Ind Med 1960; 17:260–271.

249. Selikoff IJ, Hammond EC, Churg J. Carcinogenicity of amosite asbestos. Arch Env Health 1972; 25:183–186.

250. Hammond EC, Selikoff IJ, Seidman H. Asbestos exposure, cigarette smoking and death rates. Ann N Y Acad Sci 1979; 330:473–490.

251. de Klerk NH, Musk AW, Armstrong BK, Hobbs MST. Smoking, exposure to crocidolite, and the incidence of lung cancer and asbestosis. Br J Ind Med 1991; 48:412–417.

252. Martischnig KM, Newell DJ, Barnsley WC, et al. Unsuspected exposure to asbestos and bronchogenic carcinoma. BMJ 1977; 1:746–749.

253. Vos Irvine H De, Lamont DW, Hole DJ, Gillis CR. Asbestos and lung cancer in Glasgow and the west of Scotland. BMJ 1993; 306:1503–1506.

254. Mark EJ, Shin D-H. Asbestos and the histogenesis of lung carcinoma. Semin Diagn Pathol 1992; 9:110–116.

255. Klerk NH de, Musk AW, Eccles JL, Hansen J, Hobbs MS. Exposure to crocidolite and the incidence of different histological types of lung cancer. Occup Environ Med 1996; 53:157–159.

256. Rudd R. Asbestos and lung cancer. Thorax 1997; 52:306.

257. Henderson DW, Klerk NH de, Hammar SP, et al. Asbestos and lung cancer: is it attributable to asbestosis or to asbestos fibre burden? In: Corrin B ed. Pathology of Lung Tumors. Edinburgh, UK: Churchill Livingstone; 1997:83–118.

258. Browne K. Is asbestos or asbestosis the cause of the increased risk of lung cancer in asbestos workers? Br J Ind Med 1986; 43:145–149.

259. Browne K. Asbestos related malignancy and the Cairns hypothesis. Br J Ind Med 1991; 48:73–76.

260. Sluis-Cremer GK, Bezuidenhout BN. Relation between asbestosis and bronchial cancer in amphibole asbestos miners. Br J Ind Med 1989; 46:537–540.

261. Hughes JM, Weill H. Asbestosis as a precursor of asbestos related lung cancer - results of a prospective mortality study. Br J Ind Med 1991; 48:229–233.

262. Jones RN, Hughes JM, Weill H. Asbestos exposure, asbestosis, and asbestos-attributable lung cancer. Thorax 1996; 51:S9–S15.

263. Jones RN. Asbestos and lung cancer – Reply. Thorax 1997; 52:306.

264. Asbestosis WW. A marker for the increased risk of lung cancer among workers exposed to asbestos. Chest 1999; 115:536–549.

264a. Hessel PA, Gamble JF, McDonald JC. Asbestos, asbestosis, and lung cancer: a critical assessment of the epidemiological evidence. Thorax 2005; 60:433–436.

265. Cagle PT. Criteria for attributing lung cancer to asbestos exposure. Am J Clin Pathol 2002; 117:9–15.

266. Whitwell F, Newhouse ML, Bennett DR. A study of the histological cell types of lung cancer in workers suffering from asbestosis in the United Kingdom. Br J Ind Med 1974; 31:298–303.

267. Churg A. Lung cancer cell type and asbestos exposure. JAMA 1985; 253:2984–2985.

268. Johansson L, Albin M, Jakobsson K, Mikoczy Z. Histological type of lung carcinoma in asbestos cement workers and matched controls. Br J Ind Med 1992; 49:626.

269. Raffn E, Lynge E, Korsgaard B. Incidence of lung cancer by histological type among asbestos cement workers in Denmark. Br J Ind Med 1993; 50:85–89.

270. Raffn E, Villadsen E, Engholm G, Lynge E. Lung cancer in asbestos cement workers in Denmark. Occup Environ Med 1996; 53:399–402.

271. Begin R, Cantin A, Berthiaume Y, et al. Airway function in lifetime-nonsmoking older asbestos workers. Am J Med 1983; 75:631–638.

272. Wright JL, Churg A. Severe diffuse small airways abnormalities in long term chrysotile asbestos miners. Br J Ind Med 1985; 42:556.

273. Wright JL, Churg A. Morphology of small-airway lesions in patients with asbestos exposure. Hum Pathol 1984; 15:68–74.

Aluminium pneumoconiosis

274. Crombie DW, Blaischell JL, MacPherson G. The treatment of silicosis by aluminum powder. Can Med Assoc J 1944; 50:318–328.

275. Duchange L, Brichet A, Lamblin C, et al. Silicose aigue. Caracteristiques cliniques, radiologiques, fonctionnelles et cytologiques du liquide broncho-alveolaire. A propos de 6 observations. Rev Mal Resp 1998; 15:527–534.

276. Goralewski G. Jaeger R. Zur Klinik, Pathologie and Pathogenesis der Aluminiumlunge. Arch Gewerbepath Hyg 1941; 11:102–105.

277. Goralewski G. Die Aluminiumlunge – eine neue Gewerbeerkrankung. Z. f. d. ges. Inn Med 1947; 2(21/22):665–673.

278. Mitchell J, Manning GB, Molyneux M, Lane RE. Pulmonary fibrosis in workers exposed to finely powdered aluminium. Br J Ind Med 1961; 18:10–20.

279. Corrin B. Aluminium pneumoconiosis I in vitro comparison of stamped aluminium powders containing different lubricating agents and a granular aluminium powder. Br J Ind Med 1963; 20:264–267.

280. Corrin B. Aluminium pneumoconiosis II. Effect on the rat lung of intratracheal injections of stamped aluminium powders containing different lubricating agents and of a granular aluminium powder. Br J Ind Med 1963; 20:268–276.

281. Shaver CG, Riddell AR. Lung changes associated with the manufacture of alumina abrasives. Am J Med Sci 1947; 29:145–157.

282. Hull MJ, Abraham JL. Aluminum welding fume-induced pneumoconiosis. Hum Pathol 2002; 33:819–825.

283. Herbert A, Sterling G, Abraham J, Corrin B. Desquamative interstitial pneumonia in an aluminum welder. Hum Pathol 1982; 13:694–699.

284. Vuyst P, Dumortier P, Schandene L, et al. Sarcoidlike lung granulomatosis induced by aluminum dusts. Am Rev Respir Dis 1987; 135:493–497.

285. Chen W-J, Monnat RJ, Chen M, Mottet NK. Aluminum induced pulmonary granulomatosis. Hum Pathol 1978; 9:705–711.

Rare earth pneumoconiosis

286. McDonald JW, Ghio AJ, Sheehan CE, Bernhardt PF, Roggli VL. Rare earth (cerium oxide) pneumoconiosis: analytical scanning electron microscopy and literature review. Mod Pathol 1995; 8:859–865.

287. Davison AG, Haslam PL, Corrin B, et al. Interstitial lung disease and asthma in hard-metal workers: bronchoalveolar lavage, ultrastructural, and analytical findings and results of bronchial provocation tests. Thorax 1983; 38:119–128.

288. Schepers GWH. The biological action of tungsten carbide and cobalt: studies on experimental pulmonary histopathology. Arch Ind Health 1955; 12:140–146.

289. Demedts M, Gheysens B, Nagels J, et al. Cobalt lung in diamond polishers. Am Rev Respir Dis 1984; 130:130–135.

290. Nemery B, Nagels J, Verbeken E, Dinsdale D, Demedts M. Rapidly fatal progression of cobalt lung in a diamond polisher. Am Rev Respir Dis 1990; 141:1373–1378.

291. Rolfe MW, Paine R, Davenport RB, Strieter RM. Hard metal pneumoconiosis and the association of tumor necrosis factor-alpha. Am Rev Respir Dis 1992; 146:1600–1602.

Berylliosis

292. Williams WJ. Beryllium disease. Postgrad Med J 1988; 64:511–516.

293. Kriebel D, Brain JD, Sprince NL, Kazemi H. The pulmonary toxicity of beryllium. Am Rev Respir Dis 1988; 137:464–473.

294. Meyer KC. Beryllium and lung disease. Chest 1994; 106:942–946.

295. International Agency for Research on Cancer. An evaluation of carcinogenic risk to humans. Overall evaluation of carcinogenicity: an updating of IARC monographs, Vols 1–42, Supplement 7. Lyons: IARC; 1987.

296. Weber HH, Englehardt WE. Uber eine Apparatur zur Erzeugung niedriger Staubkonzentrationen von grosser Konstanz und eine Methode zur mikrogravinctrischen Staubbestemmung. Anwendung bei der Untersuchung von Stauben aus der Berylliumsgewinnung. Zentbl GewHyg Unfallerhut 1933; 10:41–47.

297. Newman LS, Kreiss K. Nonoccupational beryllium disease masquerading as sarcoidosis – identification by blood lymphocyte proliferative response to beryllium. Am Rev Respir Dis 1992; 145:1212–1214.

298. Kotloff RM, Richman PS, Greenacre JK, Rossman MD. Chronic beryllium disease in a dental laboratory technician. Am Rev Respir Dis 1993; 147:205–207.

299. Jones Williams W, Williams WR. Value of beryllium lymphocyte transformation test in chronic beryllium disease and in potentially exposed workers. Thorax 1983; 38:41–44.

300. McConnochie K, Williams WR, Kilpatrick GS, Williams WJ. Beryllium disease in identical twins. Br J Dis Chest 1988; 82:431–435.

301. Saltini C, Winestock K, Kirby M, Pinkston P, Crystal RG. Maintenance of alveolitis in patients with chronic beryllium disease by beryllium-specific helper T cells. N Engl J Med 1989; 320:1103–1109.

302. Richeldi L, Sorrentino R, Saltini C. HLA-DPB1 glutamate 69: a genetic marker of beryllium disease. Science 1993; 262:242–248.

303. Saltini C, Amicosante M, Franchi A, Lombardi G, Richeldi L. Immunogenetic basis of environmental lung disease: lessons from the berylliosis model. Eur Resp J 1998; 12:1463–1475.

304. Williams WJ, Kelland D. New aid for diagnosing chronic beryllium disease [CBD]: Laser Ion Mass Analysis [LIMA]. J Clin Pathol 1986; 39:900–901.

305. Jones-Williams W, Wallach ER. Laser probe mass spectrometry (LAMMS) analysis of beryllium, sarcoidosis and other granulomatous diseases. Sarcoidosis 1991; 6:111–117.

306. Jones Williams W. Diagnostic criteria for chronic beryllium disease (CBD) based on the UK Registry 1945–1991. Sarcoidosis 1993; 10:41–43.

307. Jones Williams W. United Kingdom beryllium registry: mortality and autopsy study. Environ Health Perspect 1996; 104:949–951.

Polyvinyl chloride pneumoconiosis

308. Arnaud A, Pommier Santi P de, Garbe L, Payan H, Charpin J. Polyvinyl chloride pneumoconiosis. Thorax 1978; 33:19–25.

309. White NW, Ehrlich RI. Regression of polyvinylchloride polymer pneumoconiosis. Thorax 1997; 52:748–749.

310. Studnicka MJ, Menzinger G, Drlicek M, Maruna H, Neumann MG. Pneumoconiosis and systemic sclerosis following 10 years of exposure to polyvinyl chloride dust. Thorax 1995; 50:583–585.

Flock workers' and popcorn workers' lung

311. Eschenbacher WL, Kreiss K, Lougheed MD, et al. Nylon flock-associated interstitial lung disease. Am J Respir Crit Care Med 1999; 159:2003–2008.

312. Boag AH, Colby TV, Fraire AE, et al. The pathology of interstitial lung disease in nylon flock workers. Am J Surg Pathol 1999; 23:1539–1545.

313. Kern DG, Kuhn C, Ely EW, et al. Flock worker's lung: broadening the spectrum of clinicopathology, narrowing the spectrum of suspected etiologies [see comments]. Chest 2000; 117:251–259.

314. Barroso E, Ibanez MD, Aranda FI, Romero S. Polyethylene flock-associated interstitial lung disease in a Spanish female. Eur Resp J 2002; 20:1610–1612.

315. Kreiss K, Gomaa A, Kullman G, et al. Clinical bronchiolitis obliterans in workers at a microwave-popcorn plant. N Engl J Med 2002; 347: 330–338.

Paint spraying, mineral oils and petroleum

316. Sanz P, Prat A. Toxicity in textile air-brushing in Spain. Lancet 1993; 342: 240.

317. Moya C, Anto JM, Taylor AJN, et al. Outbreak of organising pneumonia in textile printing sprayers. Lancet 1994; 344:498–502.

318. Sole A, Cordero PJ, Morales P, et al. Epidemic outbreak of interstitial lung disease in aerographics textile workers – the 'Ardystil syndrome': a first year follow up. Thorax 1996; 51:94–95.

319. Romero S, Hernandez L, Gil J, Aranda I, Martin C. SanchezPaya J. Organizing pneumonia in textile printing workers: a clinical description. Eur Resp J 1998; 11:265–271.

320. Kadi OF, Mohammed-Brahim B, Fyad A, Lellou S, Nemery B. Outbreak of pulmonary disease in textile dye sprayers in Algeria. Lancet 1994; 344: 962–963.

321. Kadi FO, Abdesslam T, Nemery B. Five-year follow-up of Algerian victims of the 'Ardystil syndrome'. Eur Resp J 1999; 13:940–941.

322. Skorodin MS, Chandrasekhar AJ. An occupational cause of exogenous lipoid pneumonia. Arch Pathol Lab Med 1983; 107:610–611.

323. Brander PE, Taskinen E, Stenius-Aarniala B. Fire-eater's lung. Eur Respir J 1992; 5:112–114.

324. Gentina T, Tillie-Leblond I, Birolleau S, et al. Fire-eater's lung: seventeen cases and a review of the literature. Medicine (Baltimore) 2001; 80:291–297.

325. Scharf SM, Prinsloo I. Pulmonary mechanics in dogs given different doses of kerosene intratracheally. Am Rev Respir Dis 1982; 126:695–700.

Welding

326. Doig MB, McLaughlin ALG. X-ray appearance of the lungs of electric arc welders. Lancet 1936; i:771–775.

327. McMillan GH. The health of welders in naval dockyards: the risk of asbestos-related diseases occuring in welders. J Soc Occup Med 1983; 25: 727–730.

328. Funahashi A, Schlueter DP, Pintar K, Bemis EL, Siegesmund KA. Welders' pneumoconiosis: tissue elemental microanalysis by energy dispersive X ray analysis. Br J Ind Med 1988; 45:14–18.

329. Sferlazza SJ, Beckett WS. The respiratory health of welders. Am Rev Respir Dis 1991; 143:1134–1148.

Toxic fumes and gases

330. Nemery B. Metal toxicity and the respiratory tract. Eur Respir J 1990; 3: 202–219.

331. Asano S, Eto K, Kurisaki E, et al. Acute inorganic mercury vapor inhalation poisoning. Pathol Int 2000; 50:169–174.

332. Sunderman FW, Kincaid JF. Nickel poisoning II. Studies on patients suffering from acute exposure to vapors of nickel carbonyl. JAMA 1954; 155:889–894.

333. Lowry T, Schuman LM. Silo-filler's disease – a syndrome caused by nitrogen dioxide. JAMA 1956; 162:153.

334. Ramirez-R J, Dowell AR. Silo-filler's disease: nitrogen dioxide-induced lung injury. Ann Intern Med 1971; 74:569–576.

335. Douglas WW, Hepper NGG, Colby TV. Silo filler's disease. Mayo Clin Proc 1989; 64:291–304.

336. Zwemer FL, Pratt DS, May JJ. Silo-filler's disease in New York state. Am Rev Respir Dis 1992; 146:650–653.

337. Osbern L, Crapo R. Dung lung: a report of toxic exposure to liquid manure. Ann Intern Med 1981; 95:312–314.

338. Morse DL, Woodbury MA, Rentmeester K, Farmer D. Death caused by fermenting manure. JAMA 1981; 245:63–64.

339. Donham KJ, Knapp LW, Monson R, Gustafson K. Acute toxic exposure to gases from liquid manure. J Occup Med 1982; 24:142–145.

340. Fahy JV, Walley T, Gibney RTN, McCabe M, FitzGerald MX. Slurry lung: a report of three cases. Thorax 1991; 46:394–395.

341. Plopper CG, Dungworth DL, Tyler WS. Pulmonary lesions in rats exposed to ozone. Am J Pathol 1973; 71:375–394.

342. Pratt PC. Pathology of adult respiratory distress syndrome. In: Thurlbeck WM, Abell MR, eds. The Lung. Baltimore, MD: Williams & Wilkins; 1978: 43–57.

343. Harkema JR, Plopper CG, Hyde DM, et al. Response of macaque bronchiolar epithelium to ambient concentrations of ozone. Am J Pathol 1993; 143:857–866.

344. Bils RF. Ultrastructural alterations of alveolar tissue of mice. Arch Env Health 1970; 20:468–480.

345. Pinkerton KE, Dodge DE, Cederdahl-Demmler J, et al. Differentiated bronchiolar epithelium in alveolar ducts of rats exposed to ozone for 20 months. Am J Pathol 1993; 142:947–956.

346. Hyde DM, Hubbard WC, Wong V, et al. Ozone-induced acute tracheobronchial epithelial injury – relationship to granulocyte emigration in the lung. Am J Respir Cell Mol Biol 1992; 6:481–497.

347. Aris RM, Christian D, Hearne PQ, et al. Ozone-induced airway inflammation in human subjects as determined by airway lavage and biopsy. Am Rev Respir Dis 1993; 148:1363–1372.

348. Gardner MJ, Pannett B, Winter PD, Cruddas AM. A cohort study of workers exposed to formaldehyde in the British chemical industry – an update. Br J Ind Med 1993; 50:827–834.

349. Snyder RW, Mishel HS, Christensen GC. Pulmonary toxicity following exposure to methylene chloride and its combustion product, phosgene. Chest 1992; 102:1921

350. Konichezky S, Schattner A, Ezri T, Bokenboim P, Geva D. Thionyl-chloride-induced lung injury and bronchiolitis obliterans. Chest 1993; 104: 971–973.

351. James PB, Calder IM. Anoxic asphyxia – a cause of industrial fatalities: a review. J R Soc Med 1991; 84:493.

Occupational asthma

352. Ross DJ, Sallie BA, McDonald JC. SWORD '94: surveillance of work-related and occupational respiratory disease in the UK. Occup Med 1995; 45:175–178.

353. Sallie BA, Ross DJ, Meredith SK, McDonald JC. SWORD '93: surveillance of work-related and occupational respiratory disease in the UK. Occup Med 1994; 44:177–182.

354. Chanyeung M, Malo JL. Aetiological agents in occupational asthma. Eur Respir J 1994; 7:346–371.

355. McDonald JC, Keynes HL, Meredith SK. Reported incidence of occupational asthma in the United Kingdom, 1989–1997. Occup Environ Med 2000; 57:823–829.

356. Burge PS, Finnegan M, Horsefield N et al. Occupational asthma in a factory with a contaminated humidifier. Thorax 1985; 40:248–254.

357. Rooke GB. The pathology of byssinosis. Chest 1981; 79:67S–71S.

358. Niven RM. Pickering CAC. Byssinosis: a review. Thorax 1996; 51: 632–637.

359. Mundie TG, Boackle RJ, Ainsworth SK. In vitro alternative and classical activation of complement by extracts of cotton mill dust: a possible mechanism in the pathogenesis of byssinosis. Environ Res 1983; 32: 47–56.

360. Kutz SA, Olenchock SA, Elliot JA, Pearson DJ, Major PC. Antibody independent complement activation by card-room cotton dust. Environ Res 1979; 19:405–14.

361. Edwards C, Macartney J, Rooke G, Ward F. The pathology of the lung in byssinotics. Thorax 1975; 30:612–623.

Occupational fevers

362. Raskandersen A, Pratt DS. Inhalation fever – a proposed unifying term for febrile reactions to inhalation of noxious substances. Br J Ind Med 1992; 49:40.

363. Symposium MRC. Humidifier fever. Thorax 1977; 32:653–663.

364. Emanuel DA, Wenzel FJ, Lawton BR. Pulmonary mycotoxicosis. Chest 1975; 67:293–297.

365. May JJ, Stallones L, Darrow D, Pratt DS. Organic dust toxicity [pulmonary mycotoxicosis] associated with silo unloading. Thorax 1986; 41:919–923.

366. Lougheed MD, Roos JO, Waddell WR, Munt PW. Desquamative interstitial pneumonitis and diffuse alveolar damage in textile workers: potential role of mycotoxins. Chest 1995; 108:1196–1200.

367. Perry LP, Iwata M, Tazelaar HD, Colby TV, Yousem SA. Pulmonary mycotoxicosis: A clinicopathologic study of three cases. Mod Pathol 1998; 11:432–436.

368. Vogelmeier C, Konig G, Bencze K, Fruhmann G. Pulmonary involvement in zinc fume fever. Chest 1987; 92:946–948.

369. Blanc PD, Boushey HA, Wong H, Wintermeyer SF, Bernstein MS. Cytokines in metal fume fever. Am Rev Respir Dis 1993; 147:134–138.

7

Occupational, environmental and iatrogenic lung disease

7.2

Environmental lung disease

ATMOSPHERIC PRESSURE CHANGES

The body is vulnerable to both increases and decreases in pressure and it is the lungs that often bear the brunt of the damage. Increased pressure may result in blast injury or crushing of the chest while decreased pressure may result in the lungs literally bursting or dissolved gases being released within the blood (Caisson disease), or the vascular alterations that underlie mountain sickness. Some of these pressure changes entail a risk of pneumothorax and it is essential that this is properly investigated post-mortem by the chest being opened under a water seal.

Blast injury

Explosions may cause injury by the body being violently thrown against a less moveable object, by objects being thrown against the body, or by the blast wave hitting the body. These mechanisms often act together but sometimes there is only blast injury, to which the lungs are particularly vulnerable. For a time it was considered that the damage was direct, the blast wave travelling down the airways to injure the lungs. However, at the start of the second world war, experiments conducted in Britain showed that the lungs were injured indirectly, the blast wave being transmitted to them through the chest wall: pulmonary blast injury is worst on the side of the body towards the explosion, and can be reduced by protective clothing.[1] Underwater explosions are particularly dangerous because water is incompressible. There may be severe internal injury but no external evidence of damage other than a trickle of blood from the mouth or nose. This is because the injury is rate dependent. Quite small thoracic deformation may produce severe pulmonary damage if peak compression is attained very quickly, typically in less than 5 ms. Conversely, severe chest wall distortion may produce only minor pulmonary contusion if this time is extended beyond 20 ms.[2]

At necropsy, the lungs are contused, with blood evident in the airways and parenchyma. Depending on the force of the blast, the haemorrhage may be pinpoint, patchy or confluent. It tends to follow the lines of the ribs and may be accompanied by pleuropulmonary lacerations having the same distribution. In this case there will also be haemothorax, pneumothorax and possibly air embolism. Patchy pulmonary haemorrhages cuff the blood vessels.[3] In patients who survive for a few days, the lungs resemble the liver macroscopically and histologically show chronic interstitial inflammation and fibrosis as well as haemorrhage.[4] Other injuries are often present and fat embolism, aspiration pneumonia, fluid overload and infection may all be added to the effects of the blast wave.

Chest squeeze

'Chest squeeze' is another form of barotrauma caused by high pressure but here the body is compressed rather than subject to a sudden wave of pressure as in blast injury. It is experienced by divers who descend very deeply, thereby subjecting their bodies to such high pressure that their chest walls are literally crushed, so that their ribs break and their lungs are severely compressed. More common mishaps experienced by divers include drowning and decompression sickness, both of which are dealt with below, and neurological syndromes such as nitrogen narcosis.[5]

Burst lung[6]

'Burst lung' is the most acute form of decompression sickness. It is experienced by divers and submariners making rapid ascents from depth and by aviators who ascend too rapidly in unpressurised aeroplanes, experience failure of a plane's pressure system or have to eject at high altitudes. Injury to the lung is caused by trapped alveolar gas expanding so rapidly that it exceeds total lung capacity before it can escape through the trachea. The lungs literally burst: the alveolar walls rupture and blood mixes directly with alveolar air. The victim experiences chest pain and there may be bloodstained froth at the mouth or frank haemoptysis. Air may enter the alveolar walls to cause interstitial emphysema (see p. 105). Diving mammals such as porpoises and whales are protected from such dangers of peripheral air-trapping by cartilage extending far out into the finest conductive airways so that these passages never close, even at the end of full expiration (Fig. 7.2.1).[7,8]

Patients requiring positive pressure artificial respiration are also at risk of burst lung, but the complications of the resultant interstitial emphysema differ from those experienced by divers. In divers, the chest wall is buttressed by the surrounding water

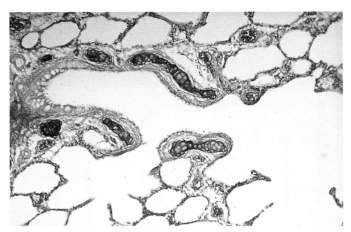

Figure 7.2.1 Sea lion lung. The smallest airways of deep-diving mammals such as the sea lion are buttressed by cartilage to ensure that all air is evacuated from the lungs when the animal is at depth to prevent the lungs bursting on rapid ascent. In man there are several generations of airways that lack cartilage (the bronchioles). This is normally of no consequence but it poses a danger of the lungs bursting if ascent is rapid, whether in the sea or by air. (Illustration provided by Professor D Denison, Brompton, UK.)

and air in the interstitium is liable to track towards the hilum of the lungs and enter pulmonary veins, with resultant cerebral and coronary air embolism, either of which may prove fatal.[9] Iatrogenic burst lung, on the other hand, takes place in patients whose chest wall is not so buttressed, and then outward rupture of the interstitial air is more likely, resulting in pneumothorax. Extension of the interstitial emphysema to the mediastinum, neck and chest wall is also more likely in such patients, resulting in surgical emphysema at these sites. However, there are exceptional cases marked by both cerebral embolism and extensive air tracking.[10]

Decompression sickness (caisson disease)[6]

The same circumstances that lead to burst lung may also cause decompression sickness, which is also known as caisson disease. In this condition there is a sudden release of nitrogen gas that has gone into solution in the lipids of adipose tissue and of myelinated nervous tissue at the higher pressure: the released nitrogen gains access to the blood stream in which it forms bubbles.[11] Doppler ultrasound techniques show that this is quite customary when divers ascend from depth, but the lungs generally provide an effective filter so that there are no untoward systemic effects, although there may be sudden chest pain on deep inspiration (*the chokes*). Gradual decompression permits the nitrogen to diffuse across the alveolar membranes and be exhaled. If, however, substantial amounts of nitrogen are released from solution, sufficient pulmonary arteries may be blocked to cause pulmonary hypertension, with resultant opening of arteriovenous communications or a patent foramen ovale, so permitting the gas to enter the systemic circulation. This is often followed by limb pains (*the bends*) and perhaps cerebral symptoms. Fatal cases are characterised by gas bubbles within blood vessels throughout the body and froth in the heart chambers. Delayed effects include ischaemic necrosis of bones and other tissues.[12]

Mountain sickness

Mountain sickness is due to reduced atmospheric pressure brought about more slowly than that responsible for decompression sickness. It may be acute or chronic.

Acute mountain sickness[13] is likely to be experienced by anyone who ascends above 3000 to 4000 m without a period of acclimatisation at intermediate levels. Symptoms are as liable to occur in people born at high altitude who return after a few weeks spent at sea level as in those who go to the mountains for the first time: acclimatisation is obviously short-lived and is therefore necessary whenever an ascent is to be made. The ill-effects are commonly precipitated by exercise. In the susceptible, acute mountain sickness commonly appears within 3 days of ascent.

The basis of acute mountain sickness is tissue hypoxia. It results in deteriorating intellectual and psychological function, headache, nausea, vomiting, and more rarely pulmonary and cerebral oedema. High altitude pulmonary oedema is characterised by increasing dyspnoea, cyanosis and a dry cough, and later the production of copious, frothy sputum, which sometimes becomes blood-stained.[14] The pulmonary artery pressure is markedly raised but wedge pressures are normal, indicating that the left side of the heart is unaffected and that pulmonary venous constriction is unlikely to be an important contributory factor.

The pulmonary oedema fluid has a high protein content[15] and the condition has been characterised as a non-cardiogenic high permeability oedema associated with excessive pulmonary hypertension.[16,17] Hypoxia is a well known cause of pulmonary arteriolar constriction but in acute mountain sickness the vascular response appears to be exaggerated for the pulmonary artery pressure is considerably higher than is usual for the altitude. An association with certain HLA complexes (HLA-DR6 and HLA-DQ4) suggests that this has a genetic basis.[18] Although arteriolar constriction would only tend to protect the pulmonary capillaries, it could explain the oedema if the process was patchy – as is the resultant oedema – for patchy arteriolar constriction would subject the rest of the lung to abnormally high pressures and lead to capillary stress failure in these areas (see p. 402).[19,20] Measurements of capillary pressure suggest that this is indeed the case.[21] Furthermore, vasodilators such as calcium channel blocking agents[16,22] and inhaled nitric oxide gas[23] have been used with success to counter acute mountain sickness, supporting the idea that hypoxic vasoconstriction plays a central role.

Autopsy shows the lungs to be heavy and firm. The cut surface weeps oedema fluid, which is usually blood stained, but a striking feature is the patchy distribution of the changes. Areas of haemorrhagic oedema alternate with others that contain clear oedema fluid and others that are normal apart

from overinflation. Pulmonary arterial thrombi are commonly found. Microscopy confirms the presence of haemorrhagic oedema and may show neutrophils and hyaline membranes in the alveoli. The alveolar capillaries are congested and may contain thrombi. There may also be an increase in mast cells and rarely pulmonary infarction. The right ventricle is commonly dilated whereas the left ventricle is normal. Highlanders generally show right ventricular hypertrophy and increased muscle in their pulmonary arteries but these changes are not apparent in lowlanders.[24,25]

Prolonged residence at high altitude leads to hypoxic pulmonary hypertension (see p. 425) and an increase in red cell mass. A small minority of permanent residents in the Andes develop these changes to a marked degree and are said to suffer from *chronic mountain sickness or Monge's disease*.[26] The basis of this is alveolar hypoventilation, which leads to a progressive fall in systemic arterial oxygen saturation and elevation of haemoglobin concentration. The latter averages about 25 g/dl, which exceeds even the 20 g/dl found in healthy high altitude residents. Patients with Monge's disease are so deeply cyanosed that their lips are virtually black. Their pulmonary artery resistance is also markedly raised. The cause of the alveolar hypoventilation is uncertain but the only cases of Monge's disease that have come to necropsy had conditions such as kyphoscoliosis that predispose to alveolar hypoxia.

DROWNING

Drowning is defined as suffocation by submersion, usually in water. It is the most common cause of accidental death among divers, but 96% of drowning accidents do not involve deep descents. Falling into quite shallow water is a particularly common cause of drowning in young children. Amongst adults dying from drowning, men outnumber women by 4 to 1. More people die in fresh water than the sea, not because it is more hazardous to the lungs than seawater, but because unguarded inland waters and swimming pools are visited more frequently. Alcohol consumption contributes to many deaths by drowning.

Drowning is not simply a matter of being unable to keep one's head above water. This may be merely a secondary event. For example, the entry dive may result in underwater head injury, or the exertion of swimming may precipitate a heart attack. Furthermore, the struggling swimmer going down for the third time ('drowning not waving') is the exception: most drowning is characterised by the swimmer failing to surface or quietly dropping beneath the surface without anyone noticing.

Swimming underwater can be extremely hazardous if it is preceded by hyperventilation, a danger that needs to be more widely appreciated. Hyperventilation results in undue loss of carbon dioxide so that instead of hypercapnia forcing the swimmer to surface to breathe, progress under water may be continued until hypoxia causes sudden loss of consciousness.

Panic contributes to many swimming accidents and is often precipitated by the inadvertent aspiration of just a little water. Most people are naturally buoyant, but only slightly so. With the lungs fully expanded the average adult has a positive buoyancy of about 2.5 kg, which is sufficient to keep the head out of the water if the rest of the body is submerged. If an arm (weight about 3 kg) is raised to wave for help, the head will go down. If the swimmer shouts, exhalation reduces buoyancy to neutral at normal end-expiration and to negative at residual volume. Buoyancy cannot be regained when the head is submerged and unless able to swim to the surface, the person will continue to sink.

Autopsy generally shows that the lungs are full of water, but some victims die of 'dry drowning' due to laryngospasm. Events may also be modified by the temperature of the water. Sudden immersion in cold water may result in tachycardia, hypertension and hyperventilation, making it difficult for the victim to keep the airways free of water. It may also result in sudden death due to ventricular fibrillation. Even a good swimmer loses consciousness within an hour of immersion in very cold water. Drowning is then inevitable unless a correctly fitted life jacket is worn, in which case there is a danger of death from hypothermia. However, as in open heart surgery, cold prolongs the interval before there is irreversible brain damage.

If the person is rescued, water in the lungs is quickly absorbed, even if it is saline, and therefore hyperosmolar: aspirated seawater is quickly equilibrated by pure water joining it from the blood but the alveolar epithelial barrier remains impermeable to protein and once osmotic equilibrium is reached, all is quickly reabsorbed.[27,28] Fresh water is absorbed even more quickly. It is unnecessary to tip the patient to hasten this process. Any water recovered in this way comes from the stomach and time that should be devoted to mouth-to-mouth breathing and cardiac massage is lost. These resuscitative efforts may need to be prolonged as fresh water in particular inactivates alveolar surfactant, leading to alveolar collapse, which persists until the surfactant is replenished. Very few victims who are resuscitated on site fail to survive, and very few who cannot be resuscitated on site recover later.

Interchange of fluid between the blood and air spaces may cause major fluctuations in plasma volume with consequent changes in ionic concentrations and haemolysis. Hypervolaemia may cause circulatory problems but hyperkalaemia consequent upon the haemolysis is not thought to be so important as was formerly believed: ventricular fibrillation following submersion is more likely to be a complication of hypothermia than of electrolyte imbalance.

Circulatory collapse may ensue shortly after rescue. This is due to loss of the circulatory support provided by the pressure the water exerts on the body, which results in a considerable increase in cardiac output while the body is immersed. On leaving the water, the loss of this support results in a tendency to venous pooling. Although this is countered by baroreceptor responses, these are reduced by prolonged immersion in cold water. Circulatory collapse is believed to be the cause of death in many persons who perish within minutes of rescue. To counter this effect, patients should be lifted out of the water in the prone position.

It can be seen that in fatal cases, the pathologist is faced with several possibilities. Thus, death may have been due to:

- natural causes before the body entered the water
- unnatural causes before entry, the body merely being disposed of in the water
- natural causes in the water
- injuries received in the water from impact with rocks, a boat or a ship's propeller, or in tropical waters from predators such as a crocodile or a shark (any of which may also be incurred after death, as may disfigurement by fish and rats)
- 'dry drowning'
- true drowning
- hypothermia
- circulatory failure after rescue.

True drowning is indicated by froth in the airways and heavy water-filled lungs. Both fresh and salt water contain numerous microscopic algae known as diatoms and those representative of the water in which the drowning occurred are found in the lungs. Unless death occurred before submersion, diatoms are also found in other viscera because these tiny life-forms easily enter the circulation. Thus, the presence of diatoms in digests of organs such as the kidneys, liver, brain and bone marrow suggests that death was due to drowning. Because they have a siliceous capsule, diatoms are resistant to putrefaction as well as digestion and can be identified in the body long after death. However, a positive test is not always accepted as proof of drowning and a negative test does not exclude drowning.

INHALED TOXIC AGENTS

The various physical forms in which respirable environmental agents may be encountered are defined in Box 7.2.1. Some effects of inhalant lung injury are recognised as distinct disease entities and are dealt with elsewhere: for example, the pneumoconioses on p. 329, extrinsic allergic alveolitis on p. 280, chronic bronchitis on p. 94 and lung cancer on p. 528. Other respirable agents, such as lead fume and carbon monoxide gas, exert their harmful effects elsewhere in the body and will not be considered further. This section is concerned with toxic substances that may be inhaled by the general public. Those that are more likely to be encountered in the workplace are considered on p. 358.

The lungs have a rather stereotyped pattern of response to inhaled toxins, displaying degenerative changes and inflammation of varying degree, the former sometimes amounting to necrosis. In general, the site of maximal absorption or injury is related to solubility (for gases and vapours) and particle size (for aerosols such as dusts, fog, fumes, mists, smog and smoke): the less water soluble and the smaller the particle size, the further down the respiratory tract the agent will penetrate (Table 7.2.1).[29,30] Thus, ammonia produces intense congestion of the upper respiratory passages and laryngeal oedema whereas

---

Box 7.2.1 Definitions of respirable agents by physical form

Gas	A formless compressible fluid in which all molecules of the agent move freely at room temperature (25°C) and standard pressure (760 mmHg) to fill the space available
Vapour	Gaseous state of an agent which is normally liquid or solid at room temperature and standard pressure
Aerosol	Dispersion of solid or liquid particles of microscopic size in a gaseous medium. The following are all examples:
Dust	Dispersion of solid particles. Those of respirable size are not readily seen with the naked eye unless they are bathed in bright light
Fog	Dispersion of liquid particles generated by condensation from the vapour state
Fume	Dispersion of solid particles generated by condensation from the vapour state
Mist	Dispersion of liquid particles generated by condensation or mechanical means (e.g. nebulisation). The droplets are generally larger than those of a fog and may be visible individually to the naked eye
Smog	Mixture of smoke and fog: the former being the result of industrial pollution, the latter of natural climatic factors
Smoke	Dispersion of small particles (usually less than 0.1 μm diameter) resulting from incomplete combustion of organic substances

---

Table 7.2.1 Relation of solubility of an inhaled gas to its major site of absorption or toxicity[30]

Gas	Henry's constant	Major site of absorption or toxicity
Ammonia	0.0011	Upper respiratory tract
Sulphur dioxide	0.05	Upper respiratory tract and bronchi
Formaldehyde	0.56	Upper respiratory tract
Ozone	6.4	Tracheobronchial and centriacinar
Nitrogen dioxide	8.8	Tracheobronchial and pulmonary
Oxygen	42	Pulmonary
Nitrogen	77	Pulmonary

Henry's constant: moles/l (air)/moles/l (water) at 37°C

---

phosgene has little effect on these sites but causes pulmonary oedema.[29]

Air pollution

The toxic (as opposed to allergenic) air pollutants thought to pose the greatest threat to the lungs comprise smoke particles, sulphur dioxide, oxides of nitrogen, various aldehydes and ozone.[31–35] Smoke and sulphur dioxide derive particularly from the combustion of fossil fuels in domestic fires and power stations, nitrogen dioxide is an important car exhaust and domestic gas appliance pollutant and ozone is the principal photochemical product of smog. Aldehydes such as formaldehyde and acrylic aldehyde (acrolein) also contribute to general air pollution because they are released in the combustion of diesel oil and petrol. Collectively, these pollutants are now attracting much attention as they have been incriminated (but not proved) to exacerbate (rather than cause) asthma, predispose to respiratory infection and result in airway inflammation and hypersecretion.[36,37] Their effect on children is of particular concern because development of the lungs is known to continue well into childhood and damage to the lungs before their growth is complete is likely to be irreparable. At the other extreme of life episodes of severe air pollution are known to hasten the deaths of many patients with chronic airway disease. Particularly high concentrations of the agents responsible for air pollution may be encountered in industry and their effects are therefore also considered in the chapter covering occupational diseases of the lung. Many of the polycyclic hydrocarbons found in polluted air are carcinogenic and it is therefore not surprising that urban air pollution has been found to be associated with excess mortality from lung cancer.[38] Volcanic ash (tephra) irritates the eyes, skin and respiratory tract and in some eruptions (e.g. Monserrat) may contain much free silica or be associated with the release of radon gas (e.g. the Azores).[39]

Allergenic air pollutants are dealt with in detail in the sections on asthma and extrinsic allergic alveolitis. Allergenic air pollution is generally occupational or domestic but periodic widespread air pollution was responsible for the epidemics of asthma seen in Barcelona in the 1980s, which were eventually traced to ships discharging cargoes of soya flour.[39a]

Tobacco smoke

Smoking-related diseases figure large throughout this book and in this section they are merely summarised collectively. Of the greatest importance, both in the number of patients they affect and in their clinical effects on the individual, are the various forms of chronic obstructive lung disease and lung cancer, but there are many other respiratory diseases associated with smoking, and a few that are less common in smokers (Box 7.2.2).[40] Not surprisingly, these diseases are often encountered in combination and sometimes one may obscure another. For example, the focal lesions of Langerhans cell histiocytosis may be overlooked if there is also desquamative interstitial pneumonia. The term smoking-related interstitial lung disease has been introduced to cover a spectrum of interstitial diseases related to smoking.[40,41] Smoking is also associated with disease of other organs (e.g. carcinoma of the oesophagus and bladder) but these are outwith the remit of this text.

Cigarette smokers are at greater risk of lung disease than cigar and pipe smokers, probably because they inhale more deeply. They do this because cigarette smoke is more acidic than cigar and pipe smoke and its nicotine content is therefore absorbed more easily through the lungs than the buccal mucosa. Smokers obviously put their own health at greatest risk but the lesser hazards of passive smoking are now well recognised (see p. 528). Passive smoking involves both the smoke exhaled by others and that coming from smouldering tobacco between

---

Box 7.2.2 Diseases related to smoking

Respiratory diseases caused by smoking
Carcinoma
Chronic obstructive lung disease
Chronic bronchitis
'Small airways disease'
Emphysema
Respiratory bronchiolitis
Desquamative interstitial pneumonia

Respiratory diseases that are more common or worse in smokers
Adult respiratory distress syndrome
Respiratory infections
  Common cold
  Influenza
  Varicella pneumonia
  Bacterial pneumonia
  Tuberculosis
Pneumothorax
Cryptogenic fibrosing alveolitis
Langerhans cell histiocytosis
Asbestosis
Goodpasture's disease

Respiratory diseases that are less common or less severe in smokers
Extrinsic allergic alveolitis
Sarcoidosis

Box 7.2.3 Possible pulmonary insults in burned patients, arranged in approximate sequential order

Blast injury
Asphyxia
Poisoning by combustion products (e.g. carbon monoxide, cyanide)
Direct thermal injury (largely limited to the trachea)
Irritant smoke, fume and gas (e.g. oxides of nitrogen, ammonia, acrolein, sulphur dioxide)
Hypovolaemic shock secondary to skin loss
Septicaemic shock from:
  infected skin burns
  infected central lines
Secondary viral and bacterial pneumonia
Fluid overload
Tracheostomy complications including tracheobronchitis, pneumonia and barotrauma
Oxygen toxicity
Absorption of toxic topical disinfectants
Thromboembolism
Uraemia

---

puffs, the latter being known as sidestream smoke. The harmful effects of maternal smoking on the unborn child also come in this category. They include increased airway responsiveness and reduced lung function during the neonatal period and an increased risk of sudden infant death syndrome. Reduced numbers of alveolar attachment points have been demonstrated in such infants.[42]

Burns and smoke inhalation

The lungs may be injured in burned patients in many ways (Box 7.2.3),[43,44] but an important consideration when a body is recovered from a fire is whether death was due to the fire or took place beforehand, the latter raising the possibility of foul play. A vital reaction to the skin burns and the presence of soot in the lower airways provide evidence that death occurred in the fire but an absence of soot from the airways may be due to death occurring rapidly, from asphyxia or poisoning by gases released in the conflagration. Soot is cleared rapidly and if the patient survives a few days an absence of soot from the airways is to be expected.[43]

The effects of heat alone were seen in men exposed to steam escaping from a fractured boiler pipe.[45] Those dying immediately showed coagulative necrosis of the respiratory mucosa down to the level of the alveolar ducts and alveolar congestion and oedema, while those surviving a little longer exhibited diffuse alveolar damage. The diffuse alveolar damage possibly represents a manifestation of shock from their extensive cutaneous scalding whereas the mucosal necrosis is directly attributable to heat.

The ubiquity of plastics today means that smoke contains numerous irritants, including isocyanates, aldehydes and fluorinated organic chemicals. Irritant smoke products have two principal effects. First, they cause an immediate painful stimulation of the eyes and respiratory tract, which at low concentrations may prevent escape and at high concentrations may cause laryngeal spasm and death. Second, they cause bronchopulmonary injury some hours after exposure. Burned patients dying within 4 to 12 days often show tracheobronchial necrosis and diffuse alveolar damage with prominent hyaline membranes.[43,44,46] Secondary herpes virus infection is often present.[47,48]

The respiratory changes caused by heat and smoke are nonspecific and careful consideration of the many causes of lung injury in burned patients listed (see Box 7.2.3) and of the clinical circumstances and management is generally required. Often it will be concluded that the cause of the lung injury is multifactorial. Long-term consequences of smoke inhalation include bronchiectasis and obliterative bronchiolitis.[49]

Methyl isocyanate, the chemical released at Bhopal

The Bhopal catastrophe of 1984 was caused by the accidental release of 30 tons of methyl isocyanate gas (CH_3-N=C=O) from a pesticide plant.[50] Over 200 000 people were exposed, of whom 2500 died, mostly within hours of exposure, and 60 000 were seriously injured. The victims complained of intense ocular and respiratory irritation. Some survivors were left with persistent respiratory impairment.[51,52] Twenty years later the local water table is still polluted by toxic chemicals from the factory.

Methyl isocyanate is an extremely potent respiratory irritant, destroying the epithelium throughout the conducting airways, with comparatively less parenchymal injury. In survivors, epithelial regeneration, often involving squamous metaplasia, quickly commences, but not before endobronchial granulation tissue projections have developed, resulting in obliterative bronchiolitis.

INGESTED TOXIC AGENTS

Toxins reaching the lungs via the blood stream include drugs, food contaminants, metabolites produced elsewhere in the body, and chemicals ingested intentionally or accidentally, either in the home or the workplace.

The lungs are selectively damaged by certain bloodborne toxins for a variety of reasons. For example, the herbicide paraquat is preferentially taken up by the lungs because of its molecular homology with certain endogenous substances. As detailed below, the type I alveolar epithelial cells are the cells that bear the brunt of the damage in paraquat poisoning. On the other hand, the alveolar capillary endothelium has its own selective uptake mechanisms (see Metabolic functions of the pulmonary endothelium, p. 23) which may be responsible for it being selectively damaged by other chemicals.

The bronchiolar Clara cells are selectively injured by some ingested chemicals because they are equipped to deal with inhaled xenobiotics, but occasionally this activity results in metabolites that are extremely toxic. An example of this from veterinary medicine is provided by the furan-derivative 4-ipomeanol, which is found in mouldy sweet potatoes and results in acute pulmonary oedema in cattle fed such a diet. When this chemical is injected into mice, the bronchioles are denuded of Clara cells whereas the intervening ciliated cells are completely unaffected. The selective damage to the bronchiolar Clara cells appears to stem from the oxidative efficiency of their P-450 cytochromes,[53] which is much higher than those of the liver. Chemicals having a similarly selective effect on bronchiolar Clara cells include 3-methylfuran, carbon tetrachloride, naphthalene and 1,1-dichloroethylene, the last of which is a volatile compound that is widely used in the plastics industry. Procarcinogens may be activated in the airways by similar mechanisms.

Paraquat

Paraquat is a dipyridylium compound that is widely used in agriculture as a herbicide. It kills all green plants but is inactivated on contact with the soil. It is applied as a spray and if the manufacturer's instructions are followed there is no danger to the health. Most fatal cases of paraquat poisoning, both accidental and suicidal, have been due to ingestion of the 20% aqueous solution Gramoxone®. The less concentrated granular form Weedol® is unlikely to be ingested accidentally but may be taken suicidally:[54] in 2005 it was withdrawn from sale

Figure 7.2.2 Formulae of paraquat and the endogenous oligoamines putrescine, spermine and spermidine showing the molecular similarities. The name paraquat derives from the chemical's para-methyl groups and its quaternary nitrogen atoms.

throughout the European Union. Paraquat is not absorbed by the intact skin but repeated or prolonged application so damages the epidermis that absorption into the blood stream with consequent systemic effects is possible, but rare.[55]

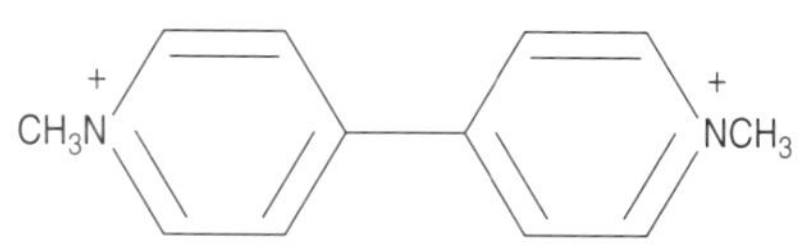

Although paraquat has toxic effects on the liver, kidneys and myocardium, these are transient and attention has centred on the pulmonary changes, which are usually fatal. Following suicidal ingestion of large amounts of paraquat, death from multiorgan failure and pulmonary haemorrhage occurs within a few days, whereas most victims of accidental paraquat poisoning die from progressive pulmonary fibrosis between 10 and 14 days after ingestion. In those who survive longer, a honeycomb pattern of pulmonary fibrosis may be apparent.[56]

Paraquat is a powerful oxidant and owes its toxicity to the production of active oxygen radicals. The lungs are particularly susceptible because paraquat is concentrated there by an active uptake mechanism in the alveolar epithelium. The inadvertent uptake of paraquat probably stems from a similarity between the molecular arrangement of its quaternary nitrogen atoms and the amine groups of endogenous oligoamines such as putrescine, spermidine and spermine, which are concerned in alveolar epithelial cell division and differentiation (Fig. 7.2.2).[57] This results in paraquat levels being six to ten times higher in the lung than in the plasma. Once taken up by the lung, paraquat is not metabolised but participates in redox cycling so that superoxide radicals are constantly produced. Epithelial injury is proportional to the concentration of paraquat, while it is lessened by hypoxia and antioxidants such as superoxide dismutase and potentiated by increased concentrations of oxygen.[58–61] The high concentration of oxygen in the alveoli is a further reason why the lungs are particularly vulnerable to paraquat.

Knowledge of the toxic effects of paraquat comes from observations on autopsy series[54,62,63] and from experimental studies that have enabled the sequence of pulmonary changes to be observed.[64–67] In accordance with paraquat being taken up by the alveolar epithelium, electron microscopy shows that these cells suffer more profound damage than the endothelium.[64] Type I epithelial cells swell and undergo necrosis (Fig. 7.2.3),[68] while type II cells, although remaining capable of proliferation, show ultrastructural evidence of damage with derangement of

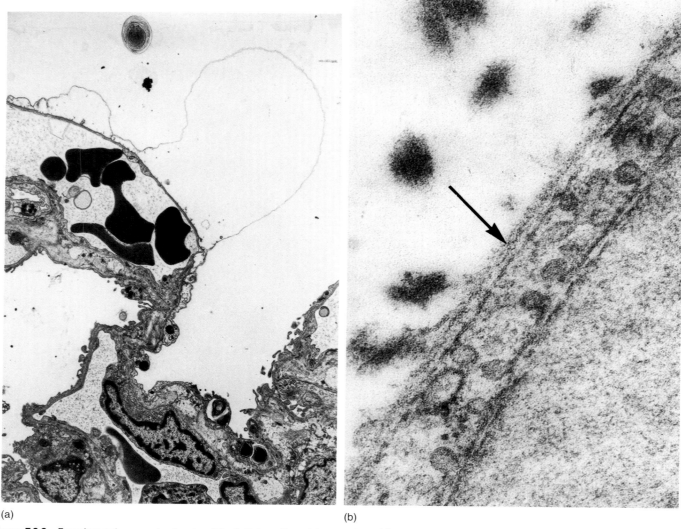

(a)   (b)

Figure 7.2.3 Experimental paraquat poisoning. After initial swelling of the cytoplasm (a) the type I alveolar epithelial cells proceed to complete necrosis (b), exposing the basement membrane (arrow) they share with the alveolar capillary endothelium to alveolar air. Flecks of fibrin are seen in the alveolus. Intact endothelium and part of an erythrocyte are seen beneath the denuded basement membrane. (Reproduced from Vijeyaratnam and Corrin. Experimental paraquat poisoning. Journal of Pathology 1971; 103:123–129[64] and Corrin and Vijeyaratnam. Experimental models of interstitial pneumonia: paraquat, iprindole. Prog Resp Res 1975; 8:107–120.[68] Copyright Pathological Society of Great Britain and Ireland. Permission granted by John Wiley & Sons on behalf of PathSoc.)

cell organelles.[64,65] Histological changes in the lungs follow the pattern of diffuse alveolar damage, with a characteristic feature of the early exudative phase being intense vascular congestion and alveolar haemorrhage.[54,62,69] Hyaline membranes are most clearly seen by about 5 days (Fig. 7.2.4) and epithelial proliferation and fibrosis are conspicuous by about 14 days.

The pattern of pulmonary fibrosis in paraquat poisoning has been disputed. Some authors have stressed its interstitial position, whereas others have clearly demonstrated that it is intra-alveolar.[63,67,69–72] However, as described on p. 143, it generally assumes an obliterative pattern of intra-alveolar fibrosis in which the lumina of several adjacent alveoli are totally effaced, rendering them completely airless (see Fig. 4.23, p. 143).

Toxic oil syndrome

A new multisystem disease appeared abruptly in the environs of Madrid in 1981.[73–75] Over 20 000 people were affected and about 1 in 60 died. The disease was initially thought to be mycoplasma pneumonia but was soon found to be associated with the use of adulterated oil sold illicitly by door-to-door salesmen. Although it was sold for culinary purposes the oil had been produced for industrial use in steel manufacture. It consisted of rapeseed and olive oil mixed with liquified animal fat, aniline and other organic chemicals. It has not been possible to identify the exact chemical responsible for the disease or to reproduce the changes in other species but the later induction

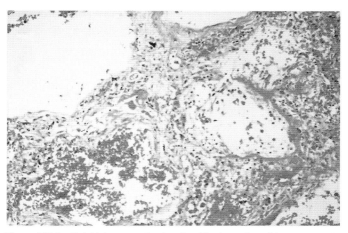

Figure 7.2.4 Suicidal paraquat poisoning. The ingestion of large amounts of the chemical has led to death from pulmonary haemorrhage and diffuse alveolar damage within 3 days. Note the hyaline membrane formation and early interstitial fibrosis. (Material provided by Dr D Melcher, Brighton, UK.)

of similar pathological changes by another substance contaminated with an aniline derivative is possibly relevant (see L-tryptophan-induced eosinophilia-myalgia syndrome, p. 389).[76] Some clinical and pathological features of the disease suggest that immune mechanisms may also be involved.

The initial clinical features included fever, respiratory distress, cough, haemoptysis, skin eruptions and marked eosinophilia. Radiographs suggested pulmonary oedema and sometimes showed pleural effusion. About 5% of patients died at this stage but most recovered quickly. However, within a few weeks many were re-admitted to hospital with nausea, vomiting, diarrhoea and abdominal pain. About a quarter then proceeded to develop weakness, myalgia, weight loss, scleroderma-like skin signs and pulmonary hypertension.[77,78] Many of these patients died after a long, wasting illness or are permanently disabled with neurological and hepatic disorders.

In the early phase the lungs showed the most severe changes, which consisted of a combination of diffuse alveolar damage, eosinophilic infiltrates and arterial lumenal narrowing by endothelial swelling and vacuolation, intimal foam cell infiltration and a non-necrotizing vasculitis.[74,77,79] There was also capillary thrombosis, which later extended into arteries and veins, culminating in fibrosing obliteration of these blood vessels. In some patients dying of haemoptysis, dilated thin-walled blood vessels were identified in the mucosa of major blood-filled airways. Late features in the lungs included plexogenic arteriopathy (see p. 421), possibly secondary to changes in the liver. Similar inflammatory and vascular changes were seen in many other tissues. Notable extrapulmonary features included fasciitis, vasculitis, neuronal degeneration, perineuritis, hepatic injury and tissue eosinophilia.

Sauropus androgynus

Sauropus androgynus is a vegetable that is widely cultivated for the table in many south-eastern Asian countries. It is apparently harmless when cooked but recently there has been a vogue in Taiwan for consuming large amounts of its unprocessed juice, blended with that of guavas or pineapple, because of its supposed efficacy as a slimming aid and in blood pressure control. Coincident with this fad there has been an upsurge in patients with symptoms of obstructive lung disease. Within a 4-month period more than 60 such patients were seen at one hospital.[80–82] They had four features in common: recent consumption of uncooked *S.androgynus* juice, fixed ventilatory obstruction, radiological evidence of bilateral bronchiectasis and an absence of any previous chronic respiratory disease. Four patients agreed to undergo open lung biopsy. This showed chronic bronchiolitis or obliterative bronchiolitis of constrictive pattern. The lymphocytes were mainly T cells but immunofluorescent and electron microscopy showed no evidence of an immune process. Four patients underwent single lung transplantation. The excised lungs showed sclerotic obliteration of bronchial arteries in the walls of bronchi 4–5 mm in diameter with segmental necrosis of bronchi 2–4 mm in diameter. The changes were considered to fit best with segmental ischaemic necrosis of bronchi at the water-shed zone of the bronchial and pulmonary vasculature.[83] Further patients have required lung transplantation but public education of the dangers of this herbal medicine now appears to have been successful.[84]

RECREATIONAL DRUGS

Alcohol and nicotine outstrip all other recreational drugs in popularity and their effects are of course well known. Those of tobacco smoking are summarised above and dealt with in detail in the chapters on obstructive lung disease and carcinoma of the lung. Less well known is the lung disease that results from smoking *blackfat tobacco*, a practice popular with Guyanese Indians. 'Blackfat' is the trade name of a type of tobacco that is flavoured with mineral oil, some of which vapourises and is inhaled when the tobacco is smoked, to cause exogenous lipid pneumonia (see Ch. 6.2, p. 315).[85] In recent years the smoking of two other substances, marijuana and cocaine, has gained in popularity. It would not be surprising if the long-term effects of smoking these substances were similar to those of cigarette smoking but as yet it is too early to judge. However, the short-term effects are similar to those of tobacco smoking and this bodes badly for their ultimate effects.

Marijuana

Marijuana consists of the dried leaves of the cannabis plant, also known as hemp, as opposed to hashish, which is the plant's resin. Cannabis alkaloids have psychoactive effects but marijuana smoking exposes the lungs to many of the same respiratory irritants that are found in tobacco smoke. Initial exposure to marijuana smoke often results in coughing and habitual smokers produce black sputum. Bronchial biopsy shows inflammation and squamous metaplasia and bronchoalveolar lavage demonstrates increased numbers of cells, which are predominantly macrophages but also include neutrophils.[86–89] These changes are virtually identical to the short-term effects of tobacco smoke and are therefore likely to be similarly followed by the development of chronic bronchitis and emphysema and possibly lung cancer. Indeed the dangers of smoking marijuana are possibly greater than those of smoking tobacco, as compared with which, it is associated with a 5-fold greater increase in blood carboxyhaemoglobin and a 3-fold increase in the amount of tar inhaled.[90] It is estimated that three cannabis cigarettes result in the same degree of bronchial damage as 20 tobacco cigarettes.[91] As yet there has been insufficient time for the necessary epidemiological studies but individual cases of lung injury attributed to marijuana smoking are already being reported.[92] There is also evidence that the effects of smoking marijuana and tobacco are additive.[93]

Barotrauma is a further complication of smoking marijuana (or cocaine). Inhalation of these substances involves deep, sustained inspiratory effort, which may be enhanced by a partner applying positive ventilatory pressure by mouth-to-mouth contact. This occasionally results in interstitial emphysema, surgical emphysema and pneumothorax (Fig. 7.2.5).[94]

Cocaine

Cocaine hydrochloride is a fine white powder derived from the leaves of the plant *Erythroxolon coca* by a complex chemical process. It is heat-labile and therefore cannot be smoked. Users inject it intravenously or inhale it unheated through the nose, the latter practice being known as 'snorting'. However, a heat-stable free-base form that can be smoked is easily prepared from the hydrochloride with baking powder and a solvent such as ether. This process results in a crystalline deposit that is known as 'rock' because of its appearance or 'crack' because of the crackling sound it emits when heated. When smoked, the cocaine is readily absorbed and an intense surge of euphoria is experienced within 8 seconds. The intravenous route takes twice as long and 'snorting' several minutes. The hard addict therefore prefers to smoke 'crack'.

A variety of pulmonary complications of smoking free-base cocaine has been reported.[93,95–104] Acute effects include cough, shortness of breath, chest pain and haemoptysis. Asthma may be aggravated, black sputum is produced and pneumothorax and interstitial emphysema have resulted from Valsalva manoeuvres undertaken in the belief that they promote even more rapid absorption. Biopsy has shown pulmonary congestion and oedema, organising pneumonia, haemorrhage, haemosiderosis, diffuse alveolar damage and interstitial pneumonia or fibrosis. Less common effects include eosinophilic pneumonia, extrapulmonary eosinophilic angiitis, medial thickening of pulmonary arteries and the barotrauma described above (Fig. 7.2.5). Severe burning of the airways has also been

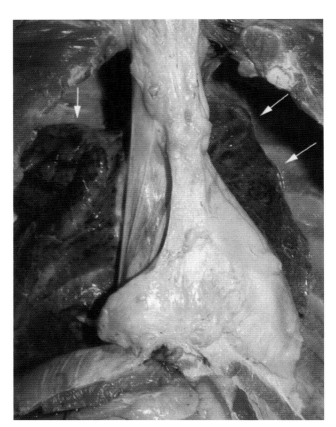

Figure 7.2.5 Bilateral pneumothoraces in a 23-year-old man who died suddenly while smoking marijuana. The collapsed lungs (arrows) have retracted towards the mediastinum. (From Tomashefski JF Jr, Felo JA. The pulmonary pathology of illicit drug and substance abuse. Current Diagnostic Pathology 2004; 10:413–426.[94] With permission from Elsevier Ltd.)

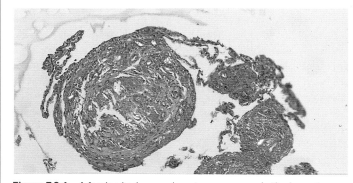

Figure 7.2.6 A foreign body granulomatous response in the lungs to cellulose filler inhaled by a cocaine sniffer. Section viewed by partially polarised light microscopy.

seen due to 'crack' being smoked before all the ether used in its preparation has evaporated.

'Snorting' unheated cocaine has its own complications: substances such as cellulose or talc with which the drug is 'cut' (mixed as a diluent) are liable to provoke a foreign body giant cell reaction in the lungs (Fig. 7.2.6).[105] However, particles of foreign material larger than those in the usual respirable range (allowing for the fibrous shape of substances such as cellulose) should suggest intravenous use (see 'filler embolism' below).

Heroin

Heroin is usually injected, but it may be smoked, when, as with marijuana, it is liable to lead to a very pronounced macrophage response (Fig. 7.2.7). Intravenous heroin abuse sometimes causes the sudden onset of a potentially fatal high permeability pulmonary oedema (Fig. 7.2.8). Intravenous abuse of heroin and other drugs is also liable to cause 'filler embolism', which will now be considered.

'Filler embolism'

'Filler embolism' is the result of illicit drug usage in which compounds designed for oral use are injected intravenously to heighten their effects. Oral preparations consist largely of fillers such as talc or starch and this insoluble particulate matter accumulates in the pulmonary capillaries. It provokes a foreign body giant cell reaction, thrombosis and fibrosis and may cause pulmonary hypertension (Fig. 7.2.9 and see Fig. 8.1.12, p. 412).[106–113] The various materials may be distinguished by their morphology, staining characteristics (Fig. 7.2.9 and Table 7.2.2) and

elemental composition, as studied by X-ray diffraction (see p. 333).

4-methyl-aminorex

This 'designer' drug, taken for its central stimulant activity (street names 'ice' or 'U-4-E-uh' pronounced euphoria), is related to the appetite suppressor aminorex discussed on p. 390 and has similarly been associated with pulmonary hypertension.[114]

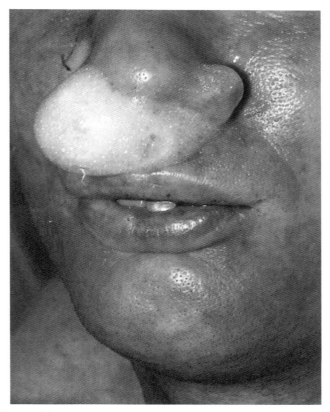

Figure 7.2.8 Frothy oedema fluid protrudes from the nostrils of a person who died while injecting heroin intravenously. Similar froth filled the whole respiratory tract. (From Tomashefski JF Jr, Felo JA. The pulmonary pathology of illicit drug and substance abuse. Current Diagnostic Pathology 2004; 10:413–426.[94] With permission from Elsevier Ltd.)

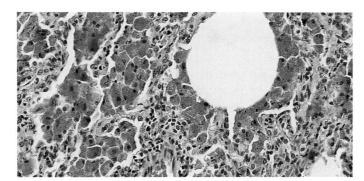

Figure 7.2.7 Numerous brown macrophages fill the alveoli of an addict who smoked heroin.

Table 7.2.2	Tablet filler materials			
Filler	*Shape*	*Size*	*Polarisation*	*Histochemistry*
Starch	Round	8–12 μm	Maltese cross	d-PAS, Ag
Talc	Platy but seen edge-on as needles	5–15 μm	Strong	None
Cellulose	Fibrous	25–200 μm	Strong	Ag, PAS, Congo red
Crospovidone	Globular or coral-like	100 μm	Negative	Mucicarmine, Congo red
Magnesium stearate	Irregular	5–10 μm	Positive	None
Silica	Irregular	10–20 μm	Positive	None

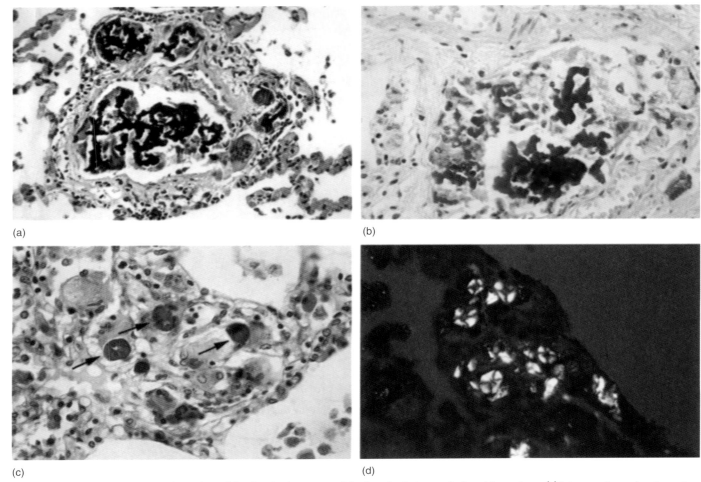

(a)

(b)

(c)

(d)

Figure 7.2.9 Tablet filler materials in the lungs following the intravenous injection of substances designed for oral use. (a) Intravascular and perivascular deposits of the tablet dispersant crospovidone eliciting a foreign body giant cell reaction. (b) A crospovidone granuloma stained with mucicarmine. (c) A starch granuloma stained with periodic acid Schiff reagents. (d) The Maltese cross birefringence of starch viewed by polarised light. (From Tomashefski JF Jr, Felo JA. The pulmonary pathology of illicit drug and substance abuse. Current Diagnostic Pathology 2004; 10:413–426.[94] With permission from Elsevier Ltd.)

REFERENCES

Atmospheric pressure changes

1. Zuckerman S. Experimental study of blast injuries to the lungs. Lancet 1940; 2:219–224.

2. Cooper GJ, Taylor DEM. Biophysics of impact injury to the chest and abdomen. J R Army Med Corps 1989; 135:58–67.

3. Tsokos M, Paulsen F, Petri S, et al. Histologic, immunohistochemical, and ultrastructural findings in human blast lung injury. Am J Respir Crit Care Med 2003; 168(5):549–555.

4. Brown RFR, Cooper GJ, Maynard RL. The ultrastructure of rat lung following acute primary blast injury. Int J Exp Pathol 1993; 74:151–162.

5. Nadel JA, Denison D. Disorders associated with diving. In: Murray JF, Nadel JA, eds. Textbook of Respiratory Medicine. Philadelphia, PA: Saunders; 1994:2099–2116.

6. Kidd DJ, Elliott DH. Decompression disorders in divers. In: Bennett PB, Elliott DH, eds. The physiology and medicine of diving and compressed air work. London: Balliere Tindall; 1975:471–495.

7. Denison DM, Warrell DA, West JB. Airway structure and alveolar emptying in the lungs of sea lions and dogs. Respir Physiol 1971; 13:253–260.

8. Denison DM, Kooyman GL. The structure and function of the small airways in pinniped and sea otter lungs. Respir Physiol 1973; 17:1–10.

9. Cooperman EM, Hogg J, Thurlbeck WM. Mechanisms of death in shallow-water scuba diving. Can Med Assoc J 1968; 99:1128–1131.

10. Broome CR, Jarvis LJ, Clark RJ. Pulmonary barotrauma in submarine escape training. Thorax 1994; 49:186–187.

11. Elliott DH, Hallenbeck JM. The pathophysiology of decompression sickness. In: Bennett PB, Elliott DH, eds. The Physiology and Medicine of Diving and Compressed Air Work. London: Balliere Tindall; 1975: 435–455.

12. McCallum RI. Dysbaric osteonecrosis: aseptic necrosis of bone. In: Bennett PB, Elliott DH, eds. The Physiology and Medicine of Diving and Compressed Air Work. London: Balliere Tindall; 1975:504–521.

13. Hackett PH, Roach RC. Current concepts: High-altitude illness. N Engl J Med 2001; 345:107–114.

14. Bartsch P. High altitude pulmonary edema. Respiration 1997; 64:435–443.

15. Schoene RB, Hackett PH, Henderson WR, et al. High altitude pulmonary oedema; characteristics of lung lavage fluid. JAMA 1986; 256:63–69.

16. Bartsch P, Maggiorini M, Ritter M, et al. Prevention of high-altitude pulmonary edema by nifedipine. N Engl J Med 1991; 325:1284–1289.

17. Naeije R. Pulmonary circulation at high altitude. Respiration 1997; 64:429–434.

18. Hanaoka M, Kubo K, Yamazaki Y, et al. Association of high-altitude pulmonary edema with the major histocompatibility complex. Circulation 1998; 97:1124–1128.

19. West JB, Colice GL, Lee YJ, et al. Pathogenesis of high-altitude oedema: direct evidence of stress failure of pulmonary capillaries. Eur Respir J 1995; 8:523–529.

20. Hultgren HN. High-altitude pulmonary edema: current concepts. Annu Rev Med 1996; 47:267–284.

21. Maggiorini M, Melot C, Pierre S, et al. High-altitude pulmonary edema is initially caused by an increase in capillary pressure. Circulation 2001; 103:2078–2083.

22. Reeves JT, Schoene RB. When lungs on mountains leak – studying pulmonary edema at high altitudes. N Engl J Med 1991; 325:1306–1307.

23. Scherrer U, Vollenweider L, Delabays A, et al. Inhaled nitric oxide for high-altitude pulmonary edema. N Engl J Med 1996; 334:624–629.

24. Hultgren HN, Wilson R, Kosek JC. Lung pathology in high-altitude pulmonary edema. Wilderness Environ Med 1997; 8:218–220.

25. Droma Y, Hanaoka M, Hotta J, et al. Pathological features of the lung in fatal high altitude pulmonary edema occurring at moderate altitude in Japan. High Alt Med Biol 2001; 2:515–523.

26. Harris P, Heath D. The Human Pulmonary Circulation. Its Form and Function in Health and Disease. Edinburgh, UK: Churchill Livingstone; 1986.

Drowning

27. Cohen DS, Matthay MA, Cogan MG, Murray JF. Pulmonary edema associated with salt water near-drowning – new insights. Am Rev Respir Dis 1992; 146:794–796.

28. Folkesson HG, Kheradmand F, Matthay MA. The effect of salt water on alveolar epithelial barrier function. Am J Respir Crit Care Med 1994; 150:1555–1563.

Inhaled toxic agents

29. Haggard HW. Action of irritant gases upon the respiratory tract. J Indust Hyg 1924; 5:390.

30. Miller FJ, Overton JH, Kimbell JS, Russell ML. Regional respiratory tract absorption of inhaled reactive gases. In: Gardner DE, Crapo JD, McClellan RO, eds. Toxicology of the Lung. New York, NY: Raven Press; 1993.

31. Bascom R, Bromberg PA, Hill C, et al. Health effects of outdoor air pollution. Am J Respir Crit Care Med 1996; 153(3):477–498.

32. Committee of the Environmental and Occupational Health Assembly. Health effects of outdoor air pollution. Committee of the Environmental and Occupational Health Assembly of the American Thoracic Society. Am J Respir Crit Care Med 1996; 153:3–50.

33. Committee of the Environmental and Occupational Health Assembly. Health effects of outdoor air pollution. Part 2. Committee of the Environmental and Occupational Health Assembly of the American Thoracic Society. J Respir Crit Care Med 1996; 153:477–498.

34. Samet JM, Dominici F, Curriero FC, Coursac I, Zeger SL. Fine particulate air pollution and mortality in 20 US Cities, 1987–1994. N Engl J Med 2000; 343:1742–1749.

35. Sydbom A, Blomberg A, Parnia S, et al. Health effects of diesel exhaust emissions. Eur Resp J 2001; 17(4):733–746.

36. Souza MB, Saldiva PHN, Pope CA, Capelozzi VL. Respiratory changes due to long-term exposure to urban levels of air pollution: A histopathologic study in humans. Chest 1998; 113:1312–1318.

37. Sherwin RP, Richters V, Everson RB, Richters A. Chronic glandular bronchitis in young individuals residing in a metropolitan area. Virchows Arch 1998; 433:341–348.

38. Dockery DW, Pope CA, Xu XP, et al. An association between air pollution and mortality in 6 United States cities. N Engl J Med 1993; 329:1753–1759.

39. Weinstein P, Cook A. Human health impacts of volcanic activity. Histopathology 2002; 41:329–333.

39a. Picado C. Barcelona's asthma epidemics: clinical aspects and intriguing findings. Thorax 1992; 47:197–200.

40. Ryu JH, Colby TV, Hartman TE, Vassallo R. Smoking-related interstitial lung diseases: a concise review. Eur Resp J 2001; 17(1):122–132.

41. Nagai S, Hoshino Y, Hayashi M, Ito I. Smoking-related interstitial lung diseases. Curr Opin Pulm Med 2000; 6:415–419.

42. Elliot JG, Carroll NG, James AL, Robinson PJ. Airway alveolar attachment points and exposure to cigarette smoke in utero. Am J Respir Crit Care Med 2003; 167:45–49.

43. Foley FD, Moncrief JA, Mason AD. Pathology of the lung in fatally burned patients. Ann Surg 1968; 167:251–264.

44. Toor AH, Tomashefski JF, Kleinerman J. Respiratory tract pathology in patients with severe burns. Hum Pathol 1990; 21:1212–1220.

45. Brinkmann B, Puschel K. Heat injuries to the respiratory system. Virchows Arch A Pathol Anat Histopathol 1978; 379:299–311.

46. Nash G, Foley FD, Langlinais PC. Pulmonary interstitial edema and hyaline membranes in adult burn patients. Hum Pathol 1975; 5:149–160.

47. Hayden FG, Himel HN, Heggers JP. Herpesvirus infections in burn patients. Chest 1994; 106:S15–S21.

48. Byers RJ. Hasleton PS, Quigley A, et al. Pulmonary herpes simplex in burns patients. Eur Respir J 1996; 9:2313–2317.

49. Tasaka S, Kanazawa M, Mori M, et al. Long-term course of bronchiectasis and bronchiolitis obliterans as late complication of smoke inhalation. Respiration 1995; 62:40–42.

50. Weill H. Disaster at Bhopal: the accident, early findings and respiratory health outlook in those injured. Bull Eur Physiopath Resp 1987; 23: 587–590.

51. Vijayan VK, Sankaran K, Sharma SK, Misra NP. Chronic lung inflammation in victims of toxic gas leak at Bhopal. Respir Med 1995; 89:105–111.

52. Cullinan P, Acquilla S, Ramana Dhara V. Respiratory morbidity 10 years after the Union Carbide gas leak at Bhopal: a cross sectional survey. BMJ 1997; 314:338–342.

Ingested toxic agents

53. Boyd MR. Evidence for the Clara cell as a site of cytochrome P450-dependent mixed-function oxidase activity in lung. Nature 1977; 269:713–715.

54. Rebello G, Mason JK. Pulmonary histological appearances in fatal paraquat poisoning. Histopathology 1977; 2:53–66.

55. Papiris SA, Maniati MA, Kyriakidis V, Constantopoulos SH. Pulmonary damage due to paraquat poisoning through skin absorption. Respiration 1995; 62:101–103.

56. Hudson M, Patel SB, Ewen SWB, Smith CC, Friend JAR. Paraquat induced pulmonary fibrosis in three survivors. Thorax 1991; 46:201–204.

57. Hoet PHM, Dinsdale D, Lewis CPL, et al. Kinetics and cellular localisation of putrescine uptake in human lung tissue. Thorax 1993; 48:1235–1241.

58. Fisher HK, Clements JA, Wright RR. Enhancement of oxygen toxicity by the herbicide paraquat. Am Rev Respir Dis 1973; 107:246–252.

59. Rhodes ML, Zavala DC, Brown D. Hypoxic protection in paraquat poisoning. Lab Invest 1976; 35:496–500.

60. Raffin TA, Simon LM, Douglas WHJ, Theodore J, Robin ED. The effects of variable O_2 tension and of exogenous superoxide dismutase on type II pneumocytes exposed to paraquat. Lab Invest 1980; 42:205.

61. Skillrud DM, Martin WJ. Paraquat-induced injury of type II alveolar cells. Am Rev Respir Dis 1984; 129:995–999.

62. Parkinson C. The changing pattern of paraquat poisoning in man. Histopathology 1980; 4:171–183.

63. Takahashi T, Takahashi Y, Nio M. Remodeling of the alveolar structure in the paraquat lung of humans: a morphometric study. Hum Pathol 1994; 25:702–708.

64. Vijeyaratnam GS, Corrin B. Experimental paraquat poisoning. J Pathol 1971; 103:123–129.

65. Smith P, Heath D, Kay JM. The pathogenesis and structure of paraquat-induced pulmonary fibrosis in rats. J Pathol 1974; 114:57–67.

66. Sykes BI, Purchase IFH, Smith LL. Pulmonary ultrastructure after oral and intravenous dosage of paraquat to rats. J Pathol 1977; 121:233–241.

67. Fukuda Y, Ferrans VJ, Schoenberger CI, Rennard SI, Crystal RG. Patterns of pulmonary structural remodeling after experimental paraquat toxicity. Am J Pathol 1985; 118:452–475.

68. Corrin B, Vijeyaratnam GS. Experimental models of interstitial pneumonia: paraquat, iprindole. Prog Resp Res 1975; 8:107–120.

69. Toner PG, Vetters JM, Spilg WGS, Harland WA. Fine structure of the lung lesion in a case of paraquat poisoning. J Pathol 1970; 102:182–183.

70. Copland GM, Kolin A, Shulman HS. Fatal pulmonary intra-alveolar fibrosis after paraquat ingestion. N Engl J Med 1974; 291:290–292.

71. Smith P, Heath D. Paraquat lung: a reappraisal. Thorax 1974; 29:643–653.

72. Hara H, Manabe T, Hayashi T. An immunohistochemical study of the fibrosing process in paraquat lung injury. Virchows Arch A Pathol Anat Histopathol 1989; 415:357–366.

73. Tabuenca JM. Toxic-allergic syndrome caused by ingestion of rapeseed oil denatured with aniline. Lancet 1981; 2:567–568.

74. Martinez-Tello FJ, Navas-Palacios JJ, Ricoy JR, et al. Pathology of a new toxic syndrome caused by ingestion of adulterated oil in Spain. Virchows Arch A Pathol Anat Histopathol 1982; 397:261–285.

75. Kilbourne EM, Rigaue-Perez JG, Heath CW, et al. Clinical epidemiology of toxic oil syndrome. N Engl J Med 1983; 309:1408–1414.

76. Mayeno AN, Belongia EA, Lin F, Lundy SK, Gleich GJ. 3-(phenylamino)alanine, a novel aniline-derived amino acid associated with the eosinophilia-myalgia syndrome – a link to the toxic oil syndrome. Mayo Clin Proc 1992; 67:1134–1139.

77. Gomez-Sanchez MA, Juan MJM de, Gomez-Pajuelo C, et al. Pulmonary hypertension due to toxic oil syndrome. A clinicopathologic study. Chest 1989; 95:325–331.

78. Cheng TO. Pulmonary hypertension in patients with eosinophilia-myalgia syndrome or toxic oil syndrome. Mayo Clin Proc 1993; 68:823.

79. Fernandez-Segoviano P, Esteban A, Martinez-Cabruja R. Pulmonary vascular lesions in the toxic oil syndrome in Spain. Thorax 1983; 38:724–729.

80. Lai R-S, Chiang AA, Wu M-T, et al. Outbreak of bronchiolitis obliterans associated with consumption of Sauropus androgynus in Taiwan. Lancet 1996; 348:83–85.

81. Chang H, Wang JS, Tseng HH, Lai RS, Su JM. Histopathological study of Sauropus androgynus-associated constrictive bronchiolitis obliterans: a new cause of constrictive bronchiolitis obliterans. Am J Surg Pathol 1997; 21:35–42.

82. Wang JS, Tseng HH, Lai RS, Hsu HK, Ger LP. Sauropus androgynus-constrictive obliterative bronchitis/ bronchiolitis – histopathological study of pneumonectomy and biopsy specimens with emphasis on the inflammatory process and disease progression. Histopathology 2000; 37:402–410.

83. Chang YL, Yao YT, Wang NS, Lee YC. Segmental necrosis of small bronchi after prolonged intakes of Sauropus androgynus in Taiwan. Am J Respir Crit Care Med 1998; 157:594–598.

84. Wang JS, Tseng HH, Lai RS. Sauropus bronchiolitis – Reply. Am J Surg Pathol 1998; 22:380–381.

Recreational drugs

85. Miller GJ, Ashcroft MT, Beadnell HMSG, Wagner JC, Pepys J. The lipoid pneumonia of blackfat tobacco smokers in Guyana. Q J Med 1971; 40:457–470.

86. Hyashi M, Sornberger GC, Huber GL. A morphometric analysis of the male and female tracheal epithelium after experimental exposure to marijuana smoke. Lab Invest 1980; 42:65–69.

87. Barbers RG, Gong H, Tashkin DP, Oishi J, Wallace JM. Differential examination of bronchoalveolar lavage cells in tobacco cigarette and marijuana smokers. Am Rev Respir Dis 1987; 135:1271–1275.

88. Gong H, Fligiel S, Tashkin DP, Barbers RG. Tracheobronchial changes in habitual, heavy smokers of marijuana with and without tobacco. Am Rev Respir Dis 1987; 136:142–149.

89. Roth MD, Arora A, Barsky SH, et al. Airway inflammation in young marijuana and tobacco smokers. Am J Respir Crit Care Med 1998; 157:928–937.

90. Wu TC, Tashkin DP, Djahed B, Rose JE. Pulmonary hazards of smoking marijuana as compared with tobacco. N Engl J Med 1988; 318:347–351.

91. British Lung Foundation. A smoking gun? www.lunguk.org/news/index.html. 2003.

92. Johnson MK, Smith RP, Morrison D, Laszlo G, White RJ. Large lung bullae in marijuana smokers. Thorax 2000; 55:340–342.

93. Fligiel SEG, Roth MD, Kleerup EC, et al. Tracheobronchial histopathology in habitual smokers of cocaine, marijuana, and/or tobacco. Chest 1997; 112:319–326.

94. Tomashefski JF Jr., Felo JA. The pulmonary pathology of illicit drug and substance abuse. Curr Diagn Pathol 2004; 10:413–426.

95. Ettinger NA, Albin RJ. A review of the respiratory effects of smoking cocaine. Am J Med 1989; 87:664–668.

96. Jentzen J. Medical complications of cocaine abuse. Am J Clin Pathol 1993; 100:475–476.

97. Greenebaum E, Copeland A, Grewal R. Blackened bronchoalveolar lavage fluid in crack smokers - a preliminary study. Am J Clin Pathol 1993; 100:481–487.

98. Bailey ME, Fraire AE, Greenberg SD, Barnard J, Cagle PT. Pulmonary histopathology in cocaine abusers. Hum Pathol 1994; 25:203–207.

99. Haim DY, Lippmann ML, Goldberg SK, Walkenstein MD. Pulmonary complications of crack cocaine: a comprehensive review. Chest 1995; 107:233–240.

100. Orriols R, Munoz X, Ferrer J, Huget P, Morell F. Cocaine-induced Churg–Strauss vasculitis. Eur Respir J 1996; 9:175–177.

101. Murray RJ, Smialek JE, Golle M, Albin RJ. Pulmonary artery medial hypertrophy in cocaine users without foreign particle microembolization. Chest 1989; 96:1050–1053.

102. Forrester JM, Steele AW, Waldron JA, Parsons PE. Crack lung: an acute pulmonary syndrome with a spectrum of clinical and histopathologic findings. Am Rev Respir Dis 1990; 142:462–467.

103. Tashkin DP, Kleerup EC, Hoh CK, et al. Effects of 'crack' cocaine on pulmonary alveolar permeability. Chest 1997; 112:327–335.

104. Perez GMGR, Bragado FG, Gil AMP. Pulmonary hemorrhage and antiglomerular basement membrane antibody-mediated glomerulonephritis after exposure to smoked cocaine (crack): A case report and review of the literature. Pathol Int 1997; 47:692–697.

105. Cooper CB, Bai TR, Heyderman E, Corrin B. Cellulose granulomas in the lungs of a cocaine sniffer. BMJ 1983; 286:2021–2022.

106. Arnett EN, Battle WE, Russo JV, Roberts WC. Intravenous injection of talc-containing drugs intended for oral use. A cause of pulmonary granulomatosis and pulmonary hypertension. Am J Med 1976; 60:711–718.

107. Gross EM. Autopsy findings in drug addicts. Pathol Annu 1978; 13:35–67.

108. Pare JAP, Fraser RG, Hogg JC, Howlett JG, Murphy SB. Pulmonary 'mainline' granulomatosis: talcosis of intravenous methadone abuse. Medicine (Baltimore) 1979; 58:229–239.

109. Waller BF, Brownlee WJ, Roberts WC. Self induced pulmonary granulomatosis. A consequence of intravenous injection of drugs intended for oral use. Chest 1980; 78:90–94.

110. Tomashefski JFJr. Hirsch CS. The pulmonary vascular lesions of intravenous drug abuse. Hum Pathol 1980; 11:133–145.

111. Tomashefski JF, Hirsch CS, Jolly PN. Microcrystalline cellulose pulmonary embolism and granulomatosis. Arch Pathol Lab Med 1981; 105:89–93.

112. Farber HW, Fairman RP, Glauser FL. Talc granulomatosis: laboratory findings similar to sarcoidosis. Am Rev Respir Dis 1982; 125:258–261.

113. Rajs J, Harm T, Ormstad K. Postmortem findings of pulmonary lesions of older datum in intravenous drug addicts. A forensic-pathologic study. Virchows Arch A Pathol Anat Histopathol 1984; 402:405–414.

114. Gaine SP, Rubin LJ, Kmetzo JJ, Palevsky HI, Traill TA. Recreational use of Aminorex and pulmonary hypertension. Chest 2000; 118:1496–1500.

7

Occupational, environmental and iatrogenic lung disease

7.3

Iatrogenic lung disease

ADVERSE DRUG REACTIONS

It is estimated that 5% of all hospital admissions are due to effects of therapeutic drugs, that 10–18% of inpatients experience a drug reaction and that 3% of deaths in hospital may be related to drug therapy.[1-4] The lungs are often involved in these adverse reactions.

A useful scheme for assessing whether a particular clinical manifestation represents an adverse drug reaction considers previous experience with the drug, alternative aetiological agents, the timing of events, drug levels and the effect of withdrawing the drug and re-challenge with the drug.[5] It is worth bearing in mind that:

- One drug may cause several patterns of disease
- One pattern of disease may be produced by a variety of drugs
- A drug reaction may develop long after the drug has been withdrawn
- A drug reaction may develop suddenly even though the dose of the drug has not been altered
- Drug effects may be augmented by factors such as age, previous radiotherapy and elevated oxygen levels
- Drug reactions may be localized.

The mechanism of a drug reaction may be based on overdosage, intolerance, a side-effect, a secondary effect, hypersensitivity or idiosyncrasy.[6] Drug reactions may be further classified according to the type of drug (Box 7.3.1)[7] or, as will be followed here, the pattern of disease (Box 7.3.2). It is often helpful to consult a pharmacist for details of adverse reactions to specific drugs. Alternatively, up-to-date information on the long list of

---

Box 7.3.1 Principal therapeutic agents known to cause pulmonary disease[7]

Chemotherapeutic drugs	Analgesics
Azathioprine	Diamorphine (heroin)
Bleomycin	Ethchlorvynol
Busulphan	Methadone
Chlorambucil	Naloxone
Cyclophosphamide	Propoxyphene
Etoposide	Salicylates
Ifosfamide	
Melphalan	**Cardiovascular drugs**
Mitomycin	*Amiodarone*
Nitrosoureas	*Angiotensin-converting enzyme*
Procarbazine	*inhibitors*
Vinblastine	Anticoagulants
Cytosine arabinoside	β-antagonists
Methotrexate	
Procarbazine	**Fibrinolytic agents**
	Protamine
Antibiotics	Tocainide
Amphotericin B	
Nitrofurantoin	**Inhalants**
Sulfasalazine	*Aspirated mineral oil*
Sulfonamides	Oxygen
Pentamidine	
	Intravenous agents
Anti-inflammatory drugs	Ethanolamine oleate (sodium
Acetylsalicylic acid (aspirin)	morrhuate)
Gold	Iodised oil (lymphangiography)
Methotrexate	Fat emulsion
Nonsteroidal	
anti-inflammatory agents	**Miscellaneous**
Penicillamine	Bromocriptine
	Dantrolene
Immunosuppressive drugs	Hydrochlorothiazide
Cyclosporin	Methysergide
Interleukin-2	Oral contraceptives
	Tocolytic agents
	Tricyclics
	L-tryptophan
	X-irradiation

Particularly common offenders are italicised.

Box 7.3.2 Pathological patterns of drug-induced lung disease

Pathological pattern	Prototypic drug(s)
Cytotoxicity	Chemotherapy
Diffuse alveolar damage	
Interstitial fibrosis (NSIP, UIP, mixed)	
Organising pneumonia	
Phospholipidosis	Amiodarone
Alveolar proteinosis	Chemotherapy
Eosinophilic pneumonia	Nitrofurantoin
Eosinophilia-myalgia	L-tryptophan
syndrome	
Granulomatous alveolitis	Methotrexate
Aspiration lesions	Liquid paraffin
Pulmonary vascular disease	
Hypertension	Aminorex
Thromboembolism	Oestrogen
Haemorrhage	Anticoagulants
Opportunistic infection	Immunosuppressive agents
Metastatic calcification	Vitamin D
Carcinoma of the lung	Arsenicals
Pleural disease	Practolol

potentially pneumotoxic drugs may be obtained at *http://www.pneumotox.com*.

Reduced respiratory drive

Central depression of respiration occurs as a side-effect of barbiturates, morphine and its derivatives, and even mild sedatives, and may be particularly troublesome in patients suffering from chronic obstructive lung disease. Ventilation in such patients may be largely dependent on hypoxic respiratory drive and treatment with oxygen may therefore also have an adverse effect on respiration by lowering the degree of hypoxia and so diminishing the stimulation of the respiratory centre. Peripheral impairment of the respiratory drive may be brought about by aminosides and other antibiotics, while steroids may result in a myopathy affecting the respiratory muscles. Other iatrogenic hazards affecting the peripheral nerves controlling respiration include nerve root disease complicating immunisation and surgical damage to the spinal and phrenic nerves.

Drug-induced bronchospasm

Asthmatic patients are particularly susceptible to exacerbations of their disease by drugs (Box 7.3.3). This effect may occur either as a predictable pharmacological side-effect of the drug, or as an idiosyncratic allergic response. Examples of the former include β-adrenergic antagonists and cholinergic agents while examples of the latter include sensitivity to the colouring agent tartrazine, for which reason many manufacturers have eliminated tartrazine from their red, orange and yellow tablets. Allergic bronchoconstriction also forms part of generalised anaphylactic reactions induced by vaccines and antisera and occurs as a localised response to penicillin, iodine-containing contrast media, iron dextran and other medicaments. Bronchospasm may also be initiated by the non-specific irritant effect of inhaling nebulized drugs if they are prepared as a hypotonic solution, a side-effect that is prevented by using isotonic solutions.

Aspirin-induced asthma has been recognised for many years and more recently, several of the newer anti-inflammatory drugs have been found to exacerbate asthma in certain sensitive individuals. The basis for this is uncertain but the likelihood of an individual anti-inflammatory drug provoking an asthmatic response is related to its potency as an inhibitor of prostaglandin cyclo-oxygenase pathway, resulting in production of leukotrienes formerly known as the slow reacting substance of anaphylaxis.[8-10]

As well as asthma being exacerbated by drugs, the disease has been caused by occupational exposure in the pharmaceutical industry to certain drugs that can be inhaled during manufacture, notably penicillin, cephalosporin, methyldopa, cimetidine and piperazine.

Box 7.3.3 Drugs known to cause or aggravate bronchoconstriction

Non-specific
  Hypotonic nebulized preparations
Pharmacological
  β-sympathetic antagonists
  Cholinergic agents e.g. pilocarpine
Idiosyncratic
  Penicillin
  Iodine-containing contrast media
  Iron dextran
  Tartrazine
Prostaglandin potentiation
  Aspirin and other non-steroidal anti-inflammatory agents
Occupational allergy
  Penicillin
  Cephalosporin

Obliterative bronchiolitis

Constrictive obliterative bronchiolitis (see p. 119) has been reported with penicillamine[11] and gold[12,13] but in many cases it is possibly the underlying condition rather than the drug that is responsible. This is often rheumatoid disease, which is sometimes complicated by obliterative bronchiolitis whether the patient is under treatment or not.[14]

Organising pneumonia extending into peripheral bronchioles may be seen with a variety of drugs but results in a restrictive rather than obstructive lung defect and is to be regarded as a cytotoxic effect of the drug acting primarily at the alveolar level (see below).

Cytotoxic effects of drugs

The cytotoxic effects of drugs may be acute or chronic, leading to changes as varied as pulmonary oedema, diffuse alveolar damage, pulmonary haemorrhage and haemosiderosis, organising pneumonia, interstitial pneumonitis and interstitial fibrosis.[15] Some of the most severe acute effects are seen with the chemotherapeutic agents used in malignant disease but they are also recorded with drugs that are not traditionally thought to be cytotoxic, e.g. desferrioxamine administered as a prolonged intravenous infusion in acute iron poisoning.[16]

Pulmonary toxicity due to busulfan was first described in 1961,[17] and has been the subject of several subsequent studies.[18–21] It remains the mainstay of treatment for chronic myeloid leukaemia. Like other alkylating agents, it acts by cross-linking DNA strands. Clinical estimates of the incidence of pulmonary toxicity vary around 4% but subclinical damage is thought to be much more common. Although not strictly dose-dependent, toxicity is rarely seen with a total cumulative dose of less than 500 mg. Synergy with radiation and other cytotoxic drugs occurs.[22] Similar effects have been reported for most cytotoxic agents, particularly bleomycin.[23] Pulmonary toxicity is seen less commonly with other alkylating agents, such as cyclophosphamide and melphalan.[24–27]

Bleomycin is a cytotoxic antibiotic derived from *Streptomyces* species. It is widely used in the treatment of neoplasms such as lymphomas and germ cell tumours, and is thought to produce its therapeutic and toxic effects by altering the normal balance between oxidants (active oxygen radicals) and antioxidant systems.[23] Bleomycin produces superoxide radicals when incubated with oxygen and iron *in vitro*. Oxygen enhances its effects,[28] a fact well known to anaesthetists who accordingly take care to limit concentrations of inspired oxygen to 30% in patients on bleomycin who are undergoing surgery.[29–31] Radiotherapy and cytotoxic agents such as bleomycin are also synergistic. Bleomycin is preferentially concentrated in the lungs and pulmonary fibrosis can be produced in animals when it is administered intravenously, intraperitoneally or by intratracheal instillation. Electron microscopy shows that the early changes consist of swelling and vesiculation of endothelial cells, interstitial oedema and type I epithelial cell necrosis.[32,33] The reported incidence of bleomycin toxicity varies from 2 to 40% depending on the type of patient being treated and on dosage. In general, toxic effects increase with age and cumulative dose: above a total dose of about 500 units they rise significantly.

The acute morphological changes attributable to drugs include pulmonary oedema and diffuse alveolar damage. Acute pulmonary oedema is seen in heroin addicts who die while injecting themselves intravenously (see Fig. 7.2.8, p. 379) but it is also seen in patients administered a variety of drugs therapeutically, for example hydrochlorothiazide, salicylate, opiates, vinorelbine and desferrioxamine. The oedema is of the high permeability type, rich in protein and is occasionally haemorrhagic or accompanied by the hyaline membranes of diffuse alveolar damage.

Diffuse alveolar damage has alveolar epithelial necrosis as its basis (Figs 7.3.1, 7.3.2). However, the continuing action of many cytotoxic drugs affects the regeneration process so that atypical type II epithelial cells develop, a characteristic feature that was first described with busulfan and subsequently with bleomycin.[18,34] These two drugs differ chemically but both act (by different mechanisms) on DNA. The atypical cells have abundant deeply eosinophilic or amphophilic cytoplasm and large nuclei, which may be multiple but are usually single. The nuclei measure up to 12 μm and are densely stained throughout or contain either large homogeneous deeply eosinophilic inclusions or clear vacuoles (Fig. 7.3.3). Electron microscopy distinguishes the inclusions from nucleoli and shows them to consist of tubular aggregates derived from the internal nuclear membrane.[34] Airway epithelium shows similar nuclear changes and often undergoes squamous metaplasia. The presence of such cells in sputum specimens submitted for cytology can lead to a misdiagnosis of malignancy.

Fibrosis may follow diffuse alveolar damage or develop insidiously, perhaps many years after drug therapy ceased (Fig. 7.3.4).[35] It may be both interstitial and intra-alveolar. The interstitial component is often accompanied by a non-specific chronic inflammatory infiltrate. The proportions of inflammation, which is potentially reversible, and fibrosis, which when

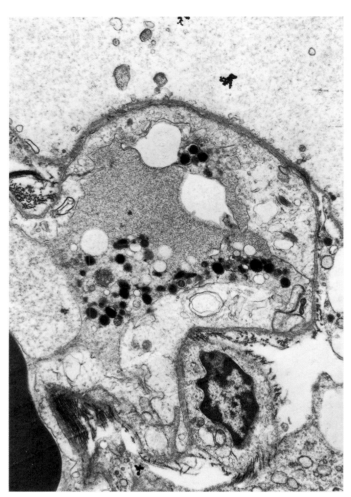

Figure 7.3.1 Drug toxicity. A cancer patient administered a cocktail of cytotoxic drugs developed acute respiratory distress and biopsy showed loss of the type I alveolar epithelial cells when examined by electron microscopy. The alveolar basement membrane is bare on its alveolar aspect (above). Capillary endothelial cells show cytoplasmic swelling. (Electron micrograph provided by Miss A Dewar, Brompton, UK.)

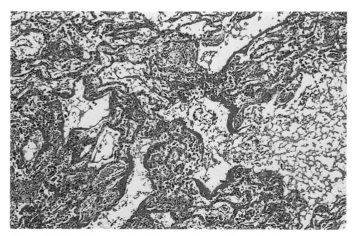

Figure 7.3.2 Amiodarone toxicity resulting in diffuse alveolar damage characterised by hyaline membrane formation.

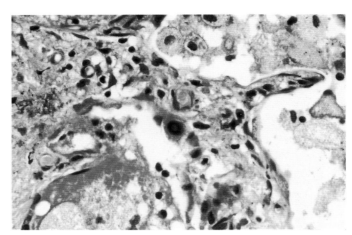

Figure 7.3.3 Busulfan toxicity. The alveoli are lined by regenerating epithelial cells and the central cell has a very prominent nucleus.

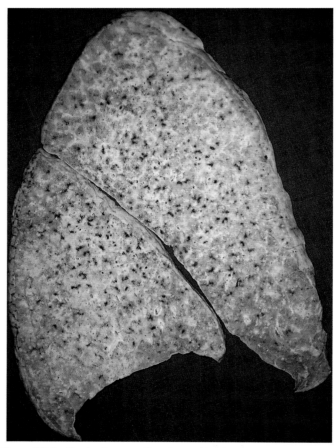

Figure 7.3.4 Fatal pulmonary fibrosis resulting from busulfan therapy, which had been administered for two years several years previously.

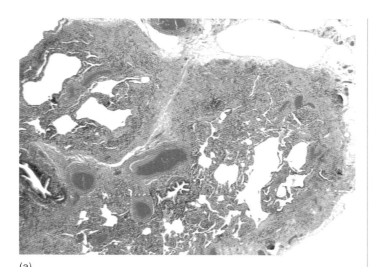

(a)

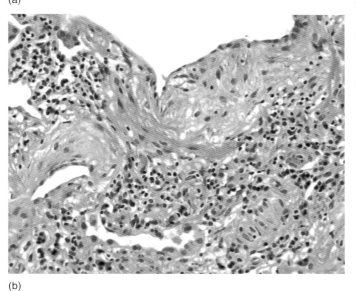

(b)

Figure 7.3.5 Nitrofurantoin toxicity. The lung shows patchy subpleural fibrosis (a) with fibroblastic foci (b), features typical of usual interstitial pneumonia. However, lung function improved after withdrawal of the drug.

collagenous is irreversible, obviously bear on the prognosis. However, most case reports antedate the recent classification of interstitial pneumonia described in Chapter 6 and it is uncertain how their pathological appearances would now be classified. The majority appear to lack the classic features of UIP and fibrotic NSIP and this alone should arouse suspicion that a drug may have been responsible. However, there are drugs that undoubtedly cause a usual interstitial pneumonia pattern, for example the chemotherapeutic agents and nitrofurantoin (Fig. 7.3.5), while others, for example the statins, are recorded as having induced a non-specific interstitial pneumonia pattern.[36] A drug history is therefore imperative when assessing any patient with diffuse parenchymal lung disease.

Organising pneumonia similar to the cryptogenic condition described on pp. 307–310, and probably similarly reversible with steroids, has been encountered with a variety of drugs including amiodarone, sulfasalazine and pencillamine.[37] Penicillamine has also been incriminated in the development of both diffuse alveolitis and obliterative bronchiolitis, but both these changes could well be due to the underlying rheumatoid disease for which the penicillamine is administered.[14] In busulfan lung there may be an organising intra-alveolar fibrinous exudate,[18] which at its most extreme results in irreversible effacement of the alveolar architecture by sheets of loose connective tissue (see Fig. 4.23, p. 143).

Some cytotoxic drugs result in pulmonary changes by more than one mechanism: for example, methotrexate may produce hypersensitivity reactions with granuloma formation[38–41] or pulmonary eosinophilia[42] as well as diffuse alveolar damage. Pulmonary toxicity is also occasionally seen in patients undergoing treatment with gold salts for rheumatoid disease: in addition to diffuse alveolar damage, there may be eosinophilia and dermatitis in these cases, again indicating possible hypersensitivity.[43] Nitrofurantoin is another example of a drug resulting in a variety of patterns of alveolar injury: diffuse alveolar damage, desquamative interstitial pneumonia, giant cell interstitial pneumonia, organising pneumonia, usual interstitial pneumonia and eosinophilic pneumonia have all been recorded in association with this drug.[44–46]

It should also be noted that in patients with neoplastic disease, clinical features suggestive of a pulmonary drug reaction may be due to factors other than drugs. In leukaemic patients, for example, these include direct infiltration of the lungs by leukaemic cells, opportunist infection and, if bone marrow transplantation has been undertaken, the effects of irradiation and possibly graft-versus-host disease.

Phospholipidosis

Phospholipidosis is encountered with drugs such as the antidysrhythmic agent amiodarone,[47] which block lysosomal enzymes involved in the breakdown of complex lipids. This leads to their accumulation throughout the body but the effect is most marked in tissues that take up the drug and contain cells rich in lysosomes. The lung fulfils both these requirements through its rich complement of alveolar macrophages. These cells accumulate the enzyme substrate (phospholipid) in their cytoplasm with the result that large foam cells fill the alveoli (Fig. 7.3.6). The appearances are those of endogenous lipid pneumonia, similar to that seen in obstructive pneumonitis. However, with amiodarone cytoplasmic vacuolation is also seen in epithelial and interstitial cells. The phospholipid inclusions contained within the vacuoles are particularly well seen in unstained frozen sections viewed by polarised light.[48] Identical changes to those induced by amiodarone were seen in the lungs of rats exposed to very high levels of the antidepressant drug iprindole[49] and the anorectic drug chlorphentermine.[50] These three compounds, iprindole, chlorphentermine and amiodarone, all belong to the amphiphilic group of drugs which block lysosomal phospholipase and sphingomyelinase. Although their pharmacological actions are very different, a molecular homology is apparent (Fig. 7.3.7).

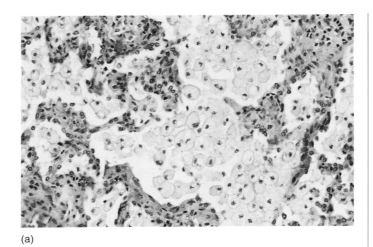

(a)

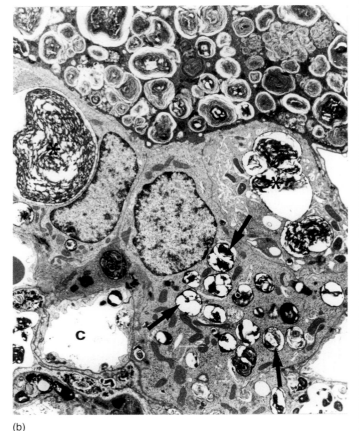

(b)

Figure 7.3.6 Phospholipidosis due to prolonged amiodarone administration. Amiodarone blocks lysosomal phospholipases, leading to the accumulation of phospholipids in many organs. In the lung this is manifest as endogenous lipid pneumonia. (a) By light microscopy the alveoli are filled with foamy macrophages. (b) Electron micrograph showing an alveolar macrophage (top) packed with osmiophilic lamellar bodies. The macrophage covers several type II pneumocytes that in addition to their normal surfactant inclusions (arrows) contain large lamellated drug-induced inclusions (asterisks), which are also seen in capillary endothelial cells. C, capillary. (Reproduced from Costa-Jussa FR, et al. Amiodarone lung toxicity: a human and experimental study. Journal of Pathology 1984; 144:73–79.[47] Copyright Pathological Society of Great Britain and Ireland. Reproduced with permission. Permission granted by John Wiley & Sons Ltd on behalf of PathSoc.)

Figure 7.3.7 Formulae of several amphiphilic drugs, all of which block lysosomal phospholipases and cause endogenous lipid pneumonia. The pharmacological actions of these drugs differ but a molecular homology is evident.

It is likely that all patients receiving substantial amounts of amiodarone develop phospholipidosis throughout the body, but this is generally well tolerated. Only a minority experience respiratory impairment and in these there is also evidence of pulmonary inflammation and fibrosis, which is possibly mediated immunologically.[51] These patients generally have a restrictive lung deficit, the onset of which may be acute or chronic. Bronchoalveolar lavage shows foamy macrophages but these cells indicate exposure to the drug rather than drug toxicity. Lymphocytes of suppressor type may also be detected on lavage.[51] Histologically, amiodarone toxicity is diagnosed on a combination of phospholipidosis and interstitial pneumonia and fibrosis. Occasionally the hyaline membranes of diffuse alveolar damage are superimposed on the interstitial changes (Fig. 7.3.2).[52–54] In some patients the fibrosis is intra-alveolar rather than interstitial and the appearances are those of organising pneumonia.[55]

Amiodarone toxicity is probably dose-dependent but there is considerable individual variation in the amount required,[56,57] which appears to be under genetic control.[58] Amiodarone toxicity is uncommon in patients taking daily doses of 200 mg or less, whereas the prevalence of the disease exceeds 50% in patients treated with doses of 1200 mg/day. Duration is also important: it may require 2–3 years for a patient on 200 mg/day to develop symptoms but only 10 months for one on 400 mg/day. The drug has a long half-life and may take weeks to clear the body completely. Previous pulmonary injury renders the lung unduly sensitive to amiodarone. Acute toxicity has been encountered in patients on moderate doses who have experienced recent or even concomitant pulmonary procedures such as intubation, lobectomy or ventilation with high concentrations of oxygen.[59]

Alveolar proteinosis

With continued experimental administration of the drug iprindole mentioned above, the phospholipidosis it produced gradually evolved into alveolar proteinosis (more properly called lipoproteinosis – see p. 317),[60] but this mechanism has not been reported to cause alveolar proteinosis in man. Alveolar proteinosis has however been recognised in a number of patients receiving chemotherapy for conditions such as leukaemia. The mechanism here is probably based on the cytotoxic action of the drug and the material filling the alveoli may represent the detritus of degenerate alveolar cells rather than excess pulmonary surfactant, as in the primary idiopathic form of alveolar proteinosis, or phospholipid, as with iprindole.

Eosinophilic pneumonia

Eosinophilic pneumonia, the pathology of which is described on p. 461, may be caused by several drugs, including nitrofurantoin, para-aminosalicylic acid, sulfasalazine, phenylbutazone, gold compounds, aspirin and penicillin (see Box 9.3, p. 460).[61,62] It may also follow radiation to the chest.[63] The tissue eosinophilia is generally accompanied by a rise in the number of eosinophils in the blood. The clinical picture varies from transient asymptomatic opacities on a chest radiograph, to a life threatening illness with severe respiratory distress and hypoxaemia, so-called acute eosinophilic pneumonia (see Ch. 9, p. 463). The reaction is often associated with a florid rash. Withdrawal of the drug may be all that is required to effect resolution but steroids are usually given as they produce a marked improvement.

Churg–Strauss syndrome

This syndrome of necrotising granulomatosis, vasculitis and eosinophilia in asthmatic patients, which is described more fully on p. 465, has been reported when leukotriene receptor antagonists have been used to treat asthma. However, it is likely that the syndrome has been merely unmasked by the antileukotriene permitting a reduction in corticosteroid dose rather than representing a direct effect of the antileukotriene.[64,65] Vasculitis has also been attributed to mesalazine used to treat inflammatory bowel disease.[66]

Eosinophilia-myalgia syndrome

The eosinophilia-myalgia syndrome was identified in the USA in 1989 and quickly recognised as being due to the ingestion of L-tryptophan from one particular Japanese supplier. Withdrawal of this substance led to the virtual elimination of the disease, but not before 2000 patients had been affected, 1 in 60 fatally.[67–71] Cases were subsequently described in Europe where there were further fatalities.

L-tryptophan is an essential amino acid that is freely available to the public: its purchase does not require a medical prescription. It has been promoted as a dietary supplement and as an agent against insomnia and pre-menstrual tension. Women in the reproductive years preponderated in the patients affected by the resultant eosinophilia-myalgia. The clinico-pathological features of the syndrome bear some resemblance to those of the Spanish toxic oil syndrome (see p. 376), differing more in degree than type. The discovery of an aniline-derived contaminant in the tryptophan-induced condition is a further link connecting these two syndromes.[72] An immune basis is suggested by the identification of T-lymphocytes activated against fibroblasts in the eosinophilia-myalgia syndrome.[73]

The illness is a multi-system disorder and besides blood eosinophilia and myalgia there may be arthralgia, fever, rash and involvement of the lungs, liver and central nervous system. As in the toxic oil syndrome, there is fasciitis, wasting and muscle pain associated with blood and tissue eosinophilia. The lungs are affected in 60% of cases. Pulmonary symptoms have included cough, dyspnoea and chest pain. Radiographs have shown diffuse bilateral infiltrates and pulmonary hypertension has been documented in a few cases.[74]

Histology of the lungs shows an oedematous myxoid intimal thickening affecting small pulmonary blood vessels and a diffuse interstitial lymphocytic and eosinophilic infiltrate.[67,68,70,71,75] These cells may also been seen within the walls of the thickened blood vessels (Fig. 7.3.8).[67,71] Massive ingestion of L-tryptophan has resulted in the appearances of an organising pneumonia.[76]

Granulomatous alveolitis

As an adverse drug reaction, granulomatous alveolitis is best exemplified by the extrinsic allergic alveolitis of pituitary snuff takers, but it is also encountered on rare occasions with cytotoxic and other drugs, including methotrexate, BCG immunisation, interferon, ciprofloxacin and antiviral therapy.[39–41,45,77–80] Interferons have been implicated in the pathogenesis of sarcoidosis and it is therefore perhaps not surprising that granulomatous alveolitis has occasionally followed the administration of interferon-α to treat leukaemia.[81,82]

Aspiration lesions

Exogenous lipid pneumonia may result from the unintentional aspiration of various fat-based medicaments such as liquid paraffin, oily nose drops and petroleum jelly or of fat-rich dietary supplements in the form of ghee.[83–89] The consumption of liquid paraffin as an aperient is common in some countries and may be taking place without the knowledge of the patient's medical practitioner. Regurgitation and aspiration of ingested oil is especially likely to happen during sleep in the presence of a hiatus hernia or when the oesophagus fails to empty completely into the stomach because of achalasia of the cardia. The

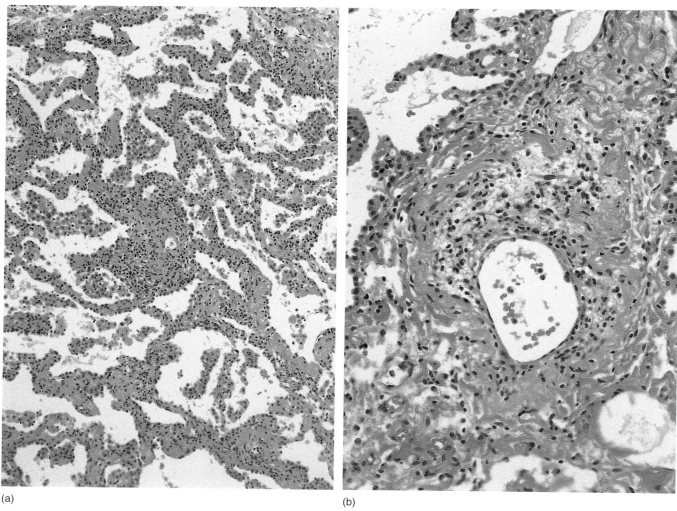

(a)

(b)

Figure 7.3.8   L–tryptophan toxicity. (a) There is a diffuse interstitial infiltrate of lymphocytes with smaller numbers of eosinophils. (b) The same infiltrate involves pulmonary blood vessels. (Section provided by Dr TV Colby, Scottsdale, USA.)

aspiration of vegetable oil occurred in the past from the use of menthol in olive oil for the treatment of tuberculous laryngitis, and occasionally from the use of iodinated vegetable oils for bronchography.[90–93] The pathology of exogenous lipid pneumonia is described in Ch. 6.2, p. 315. Other medicines may also be aspirated unwittingly, for example a ferrous sulphate tablet may cause brown iron staining and necrosis of the bronchus at the point of impact, progressing to bronchial stenosis.[94–96] Distal infection is then likely, as with any foreign body. Barium sulphate aspiration may complicate gastrointestinal radiography.[97] Large amounts may impair ventilation but being inert there is no permanent injury to the lungs although the striking changes are evident on the chest radiograph.

Pulmonary vascular disease

An outbreak of pulmonary hypertension affecting many Swiss, Austrian and German patients in the period 1966–1968 was probably due to the anorectic drug aminorex,[98] which was accordingly withdrawn. The pathology in these patients was identical to that of primary pulmonary hypertension, namely plexogenic arteriopathy (see p. 421). It proved impossible to reproduce the condition in laboratory animals but there is very strong epidemiological evidence that aminorex was to blame. Fenfluramine and phentermine, further anorectic drugs that are chemically similar to aminorex, have also been associated with plexogenic pulmonary hypertension,[99–103] and with fibroproliferative plaque on the tricuspid valve and pulmonary arteries.[104]

Pulmonary veno-occlusive disease, which may also produce severe pulmonary hypertension, has sometimes complicated the use of cytotoxic chemotherapeutic agents[105] or followed bone marrow transplantation.[106]

The older high-oestrogen contraceptive drugs carried a slight risk of thromboembolism but this is not seen with the newer preparations. Pulmonary thromboembolism has also occurred with a drug-induced lupus syndrome associated with anti-cardiolipin antibodies. Chemotherapeutic drugs such as mitomycin may cause widespread small vessel thrombosis

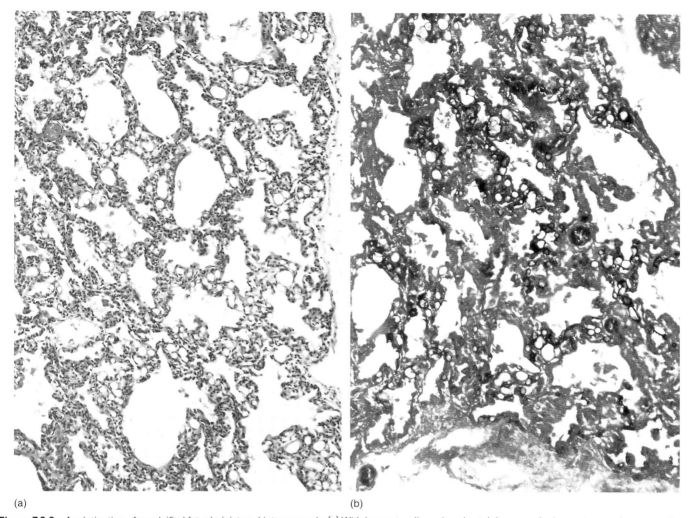

(a)   (b)

Figure 7.3.9 Agglutination of emulsified fat administered intravenously. (a) With haematoxylin and eosin staining, seemingly empty vacuoles appear to occupy the alveolar capillaries. (b) The agglutinated fat has not been dissolved in processing and can be demonstrated by Sudan black. (Sections provided by Dr G Hulman, Nottinghamshire, UK.)

resulting in the haemolytic-uraemia (thrombotic microangiopathic) syndrome. There is prominent involvement of pulmonary vessels and the patients often suffer from respiratory as well as renal insufficiency, and pulmonary hypertension. The syndrome can develop during treatment or up to several months after the drug has been withdrawn. Pulmonary thromboembolism is also recorded as a complication of immunoglobulin infusion.[107]

Non-traumatic fat embolism has resulted from the agglutination or 'creaming' of fat emulsions administered intravenously as a source of calories to debilitated patients.[108–113] The agglutinated liposomes occlude fine blood vessels throughout the body, causing such effects as priapism, osteonecrosis and pancreatitis. They may be demonstrated in the pulmonary capillaries but the lungs have considerable vascular reserve and it is uncertain what effect the vascular occlusion has on pulmonary function. Agglutination of these fat emulsions is particularly common in severely ill patients and this has been

attributed to the elevated blood levels of acute phase proteins, especially C-reactive protein, that are found in the very ill. The agglutination is also induced by calcium and may be brought about by administering calcium and other mineral supplements through the same venous line as the fat. Once agglutinated, the fat is less soluble and may be demonstrated in paraffin sections. Sudan black is especially useful for this purpose (Fig. 7.3.9). Microvascular crystal embolism is a further risk of parenteral nutrition, the crystals representing various calcium salts that may precipitate in the circulation.[114]

Transient diffusion abnormalities attributed to oil embolism are very common in patients undergoing lymphangiography but serious respiratory impairment is limited to those patients with pre-existing lung disease or in whom substantial amounts of contrast medium are injected rapidly.[115–118]

Other emboli of an iatrogenic nature described in pulmonary arteries include the broken-off ends of intravenous catheters and cannulas, particles from dialysis tubing,[119] prosthetic implants of substances such as Teflon and silicone[82,120–123] and various materials injected to occlude abnormal blood vessels.[124,125]

Pulmonary haemorrhage may result from interference with the clotting mechanism by anticoagulants[126] or from widespread pulmonary capillaritis, the latter reported in leukaemic patients treated with retinoic acid.[127] Pulmonary haemorrhage has also been reported as an idiosyncratic reaction to lymphangiography media[128] and as a complication of immunoglobulin infusion.[129]

Opportunistic infection

Infection is a common pulmonary hazard in any patient receiving steroids, chemotherapy or any other immunosuppressant drug. Viral, bacterial, fungal and protozoal infections, often in combination, may all develop in the lungs of such patients and tissue reactions may be atypical. *Pneumocystis jeroveci* for example may elicit a granulomatous reaction or cause diffuse alveolar damage rather than the usual foamy alveolar exudate (see p. 222).

Metastatic calcification

Metastatic calcification, described on p. 489, may result from any drug causing hypercalcaemia, e.g. high doses of vitamin D, calcium and inorganic phosphate or excessive alkali intake in the treatment of peptic ulceration.

Carcinoma of the lung

Carcinoma of the lung may be promoted by drugs. Arsenicals cause squamous metaplasia of the bronchi and occasionally squamous carcinoma, while peripheral scar cancers, usually adenocarcinomas, have developed in lungs showing diffuse fibrosis due to drugs such as busulfan.

Pleural disease

Drugs may result in a variety of pleural diseases.[130] Common examples include effusions, chronic inflammation and fibrosis. These are usually encountered in isolation but may be associated with chronic interstitial pneumonia or fibrosis. Sometimes there is also serological evidence of systemic lupus erythematosus: many drugs, including hydantoin, practolol, procainamide, hydralazine and sulphonamides, are associated with the development of a syndrome resembling systemic lupus erythematosus that includes pleural disease. Whether the drugs are directly responsible for the syndrome or merely promote the development of latent natural disease is uncertain.

Ergotamine derivatives such as methysergide and bromocriptine are notable for the production of pleural fibrosis associated with mediastinal and retroperitoneal fibrosis, but sometimes occurring alone: large amounts or prolonged treatment are generally required to produce this effect.[131–133] In patients given practolol, pleural thickening has become evident several years after the drug was discontinued. This shows the need for a careful drug history in any patient with unexplained pleural fibrosis.

MISCELLANEOUS IATROGENIC LUNG INJURY

Radiation injury

Reports of radiation-induced lung damage began to appear soon after ionising radiation became widely used in the treatment of malignant disease.[134–136] Despite refinements in radiotherapy techniques it is often impossible to avoid irradiating small areas of lung when treating cancer of the lung, breast, spine, thymus and oesophagus. Parts of the lungs are also included in 'mantle' irradiation of mediastinal lymph nodes affected by lymphoma. Occasionally, the whole of both lungs is irradiated, as in the treatment of widespread pulmonary metastases or as part of whole body irradiation prior to marrow transplantation for the treatment of leukaemia. Radiation pneumonitis, usually localised, is estimated to affect 5–15% of patients.[137]

Radiation may also be environmental, occupational or employed as a weapon of war. Nuclear explosions cause significant acute and long-term damage to the victims. The immediate mortality is high and in such cases it is difficult to separate the direct effects of radiation from those of thermal injury and the secondary effects of bone marrow failure. Nevertheless, by studying the victims of the atomic bombs dropped on Japan in 1945 much was learnt of the effects of large doses of whole body irradiation. The lungs of victims dying within 2 weeks showed focal collapse and oedema, while those dying between 2 and 6 weeks after exposure had centriacinar areas of necrosis and haemorrhage; and those dying more than 6 weeks afterwards showed broader areas of necrosis with a heavy infiltrate of neutrophils.[138]

Therapeutic irradiation is given as divided doses over several weeks in order to minimise damage to adjacent tissue. The effects of such fractionated treatment are cumulative. In the lungs an early exudative phase soon passes and progressive damage becomes apparent only after months or even years.[137,139] The changes are generally confined to the area of lung that is irradiated but are widespread when the whole body is irradiated prior to bone marrow transplantation or there is accidental whole body irradiation. However, localised irradiation of the lung has been followed by abnormalities in non-irradiated areas. These include bilateral alveolar exudates, migratory organising pneumonia affecting both lungs and fulminant bilateral interstitial pneumonia.[140–143] The likelihood of lung injury is increased by the simultaneous use of cytotoxic drugs.[144] Furthermore, chemotherapy following irradiation may result in exacerbation of the injury in areas previously irradiated, a phenomenon termed 'recall pneumonitis'.[145,146] In the long term, irradiation also results in an increased incidence of lung carcinoma. This was seen in patients given therapeutic irradiation to the spine for ankylosing spondylitis[147] and is still encountered on occasion following irradiation for breast cancer.[148]

Pathogenesis

Radiation generates free radicals in the tissues and its effects are potentiated by the presence of oxygen. Free radicals result in DNA damage and chromosomal abnormalities.[137] At the cellular level, alveolar capillary endothelial cells and type I epithelial cells are most susceptible.

Endothelial injury is believed to be of prime importance in radiation pneumonitis.[149] Severe or prolonged endothelial damage disturbs the normal endothelial-mesenchymal relationships and allows uncoordinated fibroblast proliferation. Endothelial changes are detectable within days of exposure. In rats they are seen within 48 h after 1100 rads and within 5 days after 650 rads.[150] Endothelial cells become swollen and vacuolated and separate from the basement membrane, resulting in increased capillary permeability and interstitial oedema. Adhesion of platelets to the denuded basement membrane initiates thrombosis and occlusion of the vascular lumen. Proliferation of endothelial cells follows and endothelial basement membrane is reduplicated.[137,150,151] By light microscopy the early vascular changes are evident as thrombosis, which is followed by cellular intimal thickening or even complete occlusion of small arteries and arterioles. In the later fibrotic stage vessels are thick-walled and hyaline.[135]

Epithelial cell damage is also well described in radiation injury. Within 10 days of exposure type I cells become swollen and undergo necrosis and sloughing with the formation of hyaline membranes. Type II cells proliferate and appear swollen and vacuolated.[151] Pleomorphism of regenerating alveolar lining cells is apparent and similar changes are seen in bronchial and bronchiolar epithelium.[136] In many respects therefore the appearances closely resemble those due to cytotoxic drugs (see above).

Pathology

Early changes in human lung include oedematous thickening of the alveolar walls, hyperplasia and swelling of type II cells, and alveolar exudates. Fibrosis develops later and is typically interstitial. Type II cells and fibroblasts are often atypical, with large nuclei and prominent nucleoli. Blood vessels are sclerosed and the vasculature consequently reduced. Unusual reactions involving non-irradiated areas of the lung have been mentioned above. Irradiation also impairs the bactericidal properties of pulmonary macrophages and predisposes to infection. In the pleura, radiation causes fibrinous effusions and adhesions. Chronic eosinophilic pneumonia is an unusual complication of radiation therapy for breast cancer.[63]

Respirator lung and oxygen toxicity

Patients requiring mechanical ventilation are liable to suffer lung injury in a number of ways. In addition to such effects of barotrauma as pneumothorax and surgical emphysema, they often develop diffuse alveolar damage. The high oxygen tension that is often combined with mechanical ventilation is a major factor[152–154] but mechanical forces other than the high pressures responsible for barotrauma can also contribute to this form of lung injury, notably by resulting in excessive end-expiratory stretch and repeated collapse/recruitment of the alveolar walls.[155,156]

Although oxygen is necessary to life, it is cytotoxic in high concentrations. Severe hyperoxia damages DNA, inhibits cellular proliferation and ultimately kills cells. Its toxicity is thought to be due to the intracellular production of active oxygen radicals, some of which derive from activated neutrophils attracted to the site of injury.[157–160] Under normal conditions most of the oxygen is reduced to water by cytochrome oxidase, and any active radicals produced are eliminated by superoxide dismutase, catalase and other antioxidants. However, these defence mechanisms may prove inadequate when active radicals are produced in excess.[161]

Problems are likely to arise in clinical practice when lung disease necessitates the concentration of oxygen in the inspired air being raised in order to maintain normal blood levels of oxygen and prevent cerebral hypoxia.[162–164] A 'safe' level for oxygen administration is not firmly established and because of species differences in susceptibility to oxygen, caution is needed in extrapolating from animal studies. However, animal experiments have shown that previous damage to the lungs renders them unduly sensitive to oxygen[165,166] and conversely that prior exposure to high levels of oxygen confers some resistance to subsequent oxygen exposure.[167] Clinical studies suggest that less than 50% oxygen (at atmospheric pressure) can be tolerated for long periods without ill effect. Little, if any, serious lung damage results from administration of 100% oxygen for up to 48 h but concentrations between 50% and 100% carry a risk of damage if this period is exceeded.[161,168] Extracorporeal oxygenation of the blood circumvents the problem but if it is to be prolonged it becomes a major undertaking that poses its own hazards; it is therefore generally reserved for patients who remain hypoxaemic despite other measures.[169] Intravenous blood oxygenators are employed to minimise the supplementation of inspired oxygen and partial liquid ventilation utilising perfluorocarbon has also been used.[170] At the experimental level, disruption of CD40 binding to reduce the release of proinflammatory cytokines has shown promising results in blunting oxygen-induced lung injury.[171]

None of the morphological changes attributable to oxygen toxicity is specific.[164] The earliest ultrastructural change in experimental oxygen poisoning is swelling of endothelial cells, the cytoplasm of which becomes grossly oedematous and vacuolated. Swelling and fragmentation of type I epithelial cells follows and these cells become separated from their basement membrane, which is then coated by thin strands of protein.[168] This coating is replaced by proliferating type II cells by the twelfth day. With recovery in room air the lungs practically return to normal.[172] The full clinical picture of oxygen poisoning is the acute respiratory distress syndrome and the corresponding pathological changes are those of diffuse alveolar damage,[164] as described on p. 131.

Blood transfusion

Patients with hypovolaemic shock or undergoing major surgery often require massive blood transfusions and this provides another possible cause of pulmonary damage. Although hypervolaemia is the commonest cause of pulmonary oedema after blood transfusion, transfusion-related acute lung injury is more often fatal. Platelet and white cell aggregates are known to develop in stored blood, but a relationship between the number of microaggregates transfused and the degree of respiratory impairment has not been convincingly demonstrated. Leukocyte antibodies are a more likely cause of lung injury in these patients. Such antibodies are often found in multiparous female donors as a result of sensitisation by fetal white cells during pregnancy. Alternatively, the recipient may have developed them during pregnancy or as a result of previous blood transfusions. The implicated antibodies are thought to initiate alveolar capillary damage within hours of transfusion by stimulating granulocyte aggregation.[173,174] Electron microscopy has shown capillary endothelial damage with activated granulocytes in contact with alveolar basement membranes.[175]

Cardiopulmonary bypass

Cardiopulmonary bypass entails oxygenation and circulation of the blood by extracorporeal devices, so permitting major heart surgery. In the early days of such surgery it was not unusual for patients to develop fatal respiratory insufficiency in the postoperative period. This led to the term 'post-perfusion lung'. Electron microscopic studies showed alveolar damage with degranulation of neutrophils in pulmonary capillaries.[176,177] The syndrome is now less common but infants remain susceptible.[178]

The most likely explanation is that the synthetic materials with which blood comes into contact during the bypass procedure are able to activate complement. This is mediated by Hageman factor (factor XII) and the alternative pathway. Aggregation of neutrophils leads to their sequestration in the lungs and damage results from their release of lysosomal enzymes and active radicals.[178–180] The process is delayed by hypothermia.[179]

Complications of tracheal manipulations[181,182]

Tracheotomy entails a small immediate risk of haemorrhage from damaged sub-thyroidal arteries, while an endotracheal tube predisposes to infection, as with all foreign bodies. Infection is also promoted by the filtering action of the upper respiratory air passages being bypassed. The latter factor also necessitates humidification of the inspired air and on occasion the humidifier or ventilator has become contaminated so that an aerosol of bacteria is introduced directly into the lower respiratory tract.[183] High pressure ventilation may also lead to

interstitial emphysema, pneumothorax and surgical emphysema.

Asphyxia may follow an endotracheal tube becoming blocked by secretions or through it being badly positioned. Secretions need to be constantly removed yet repeated suctioning to achieve this has led to cardiac dysrhythmia and even cardiac arrest.[184]

If the balloon on the endotracheal tube is too near the tracheostomy it may act as a fulcrum, causing the tip of the tube to press into the tracheal wall. Pressure necrosis and perforation may follow, leading to mediastinitis, tracheo-oesophageal fistula or erosion of a large blood vessel. These are also complications of tracheobronchial laser therapy.

Pressure from the balloon may lead to a tracheal diverticulum and after the tube is withdrawn the trachea may become narrowed at either the site of the incision or further down where the balloon on the tracheal tube causes pressure. Small, shallow ulcers generally heal quickly but deeper ulcers cause necrosis of the tracheal cartilage, and healing is then often accompanied by fibrous stenosis (Fig. 7.3.10) or web formation. This results in wheezing and dyspnoea but not before the trachea has narrowed to 30% of its original size, which may take months. Earlier narrowing may be caused by a fibrinous pseudomembrane.[185] Sometimes the stenosis takes the form of a large mass of granulation tissue at the tracheostomy site, a so-called 'granuloma ball'. In children especially, intubation may lead to tracheomalacia so that after the tube is removed the airway collapses.[186] Necrotising sialometaplasia is a further complication of prolonged intubation.[187] The incidence of such post-tracheostomy complications can be minimised by careful placement of the stoma and tube, avoidance of large apertures and high cuff pressures, elimination of heavy connecting equipment and meticulous care of the tracheostomy.

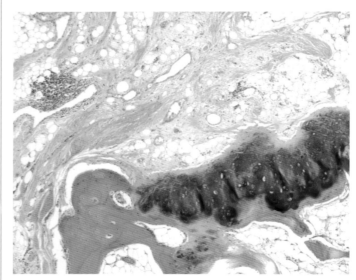

Figure 7.3.10 Tracheal stenosis following prolonged intubation. The tracheal wall shows fibrosis while the tracheal cartilage is dysplastic and shows osseous metaplasia, appearances similar to those seen in relapsing polychondritis (compare with Fig. 3.4, p. 91).

Nasogastric feeding tubes may of course lead to aspiration lesions in the lungs and even fatal asphyxia if they are inadvertently allowed to enter the trachea rather than the oesophagus.

Complications of thoracic drainage tubes

The pleural cavity is intubated in the treatment of pneumothorax and pleural effusions, being placed anteriorly to drain air and posteriorly to drain fluid. Complications include laceration of an intercostal artery or vein, the lung, the diaphragm and the heart.

Complications of central vascular cannulation

Central venous cannulation (*syn* catheterisation) is widely used in treating seriously ill patients and may give rise to serious complications. The commonest early complications related to the respiratory tract are caused by local trauma: they include pneumothorax, subcutaneous emphysema, haemothorax and air embolism. Infection occurs later, causing endocarditis, septic emboli and lung abscesses.[188] Thrombosis is another common late complication, one autopsy study of patients with central venous lines showing that 15% had major pulmonary emboli and 65% had microscopic emboli in their pulmonary arteries.[189] Pulmonary artery cannulation, for example with a Swan–Ganz catheter, may result in pulmonary infarction or any of the traumatic complications of central venous catheterisation mentioned above.

Complications of cardiac injury

A post-cardiac injury syndrome develops after a variety of myocardial or pericardial injuries: it has been described after cardiac surgery (postpericardiotomy syndrome), myocardial infarction (Dressler's syndrome), blunt trauma to the chest, percutaneous puncture of the heart and implantation of a pacemaker.[190] There is a delay of anything between a few days and a few months between the cardiac injury and the onset of symptoms, which comprise chest pain, breathlessness, dyspnoea and fever. Examination usually reveals haemorrhagic pleural or pericardial effusions and pulmonary infiltrates. The syndrome usually resolves spontaneously and few pathological studies have therefore been conducted. However, the changes of diffuse alveolar damage have been reported, principally hyaline membrane formation and type II pneumocyte hyperplasia.[191] The pathogenesis is obscure. Antibodies reacting with myocardial antigens often develop after cardiac surgery but there is no relationship between these and the development of the syndrome.[191–193]

Pneumonectomy[194]

Pneumonectomy has been practiced since the 1930s, since when the mortality associated with this operation has dropped from over 50% to near zero in the best hospitals. Risk factors include underlying lung disease, other medical conditions and more extensive procedures such as pleuropneumonectomy and pneumonectomy combined with chest wall resection.

The anatomic changes after pneumonectomy have been extensively studied by radiologists who describe the air-filled post-pneumonectomy space gradually filling with fluid and contracting as the mediastinum shifts and the ipsilateral dome of the diaphragm rises.[195] Much of the space is filled by fluid within 2 weeks but complete opacification may take up to 6 months. Rapid filling in the immediate postoperative period suggests haemorrhage or chylothorax. However, fluid accumulation is rapid after pleuropneumonectomy and may compromise the function of the other lung. A reduction in fluid accompanied by mediastinal shift towards the other lung suggests that a bronchopleural fistula has developed. Pathologists conducting autopsies long after the operation may find complete fibrous obliteration of the postpneumonectomy space, coupled with mediastinal shift and elevation of the hemidiaphragm, but often there is persistent brown fluid, which may be clear, cloudy or occasionally purulent.[196] The remaining lung is generally enlarged, with its volume greater than predicted. Animal studies have shown that if one lung is excised early in life the enlargement is partly due to enhanced growth but later it represents only dilatation of existing airspaces. Hepatocyte growth factor is thought to be involved in the proliferation of residual lung cells following pneumonectomy.[197]

Pulmonary complications include those typically seen after other thoracic procedures, such as collapse and infection, and those unique to the postpneumonectomy state, namely postpneumonectomy pulmonary oedema and a so-called postpneumonectomy syndrome. The pathogenesis of postpneumonectomy pulmonary oedema is probably multifactorial but apart from factors such as fluid overload and high inspired oxygen concentrations there may be an element of alveolar wall injury, possibly induced by oxidant generation secondary to surgical trauma.[198,199] The post-pneumonectomy syndrome follows severe shift of the heart and mediastinum, which is more common in children and young adults in whom the tissues are more compliant.[200–203] The condition is commoner following excision of the right lung when severe herniation of the left lung into the post-pneumonectomy space stretches the trachea and left main bronchus and the latter is compressed between the left pulmonary artery in front and the arch of the aorta behind. The compression can result in bronchomalacia and post-obstructive bronchiectasis.

REFERENCES

Adverse drug reactions

1. Shapiro S, Slone D, Lewis GP, Jick H. Fatal drug reactions among medical inpatients. JAMA 1971; 216:467–472.
2. Roughead EE, Gilbert AL, Primrose JG, Sansom LN. Drug-related hospital admissions: a review of Australian studies published 1988-1996. Med J Aust 1998; 168:405–408.
3. Lazarou J, Pomeranz BH, Corey PN. Incidence of adverse drug reactions in hospitalized patients: a meta-analysis of prospective studies [see comments]. JAMA 1998; 279:1200–1205.

4. Wilson RM, Runciman WB, Gibberd RW, et al. The quality in Australian health care study. Med J Aust 1995; 163:458–471.

5. Hutchinson TA, Leventhal JM, Kramer MS, et al. An algorithm for the operational assessment of adverse drug reactions. II. Demonstration of reproducibility and validity. JAMA 1979; 242:633–638.

6. Rosenheim ML, Moulton R. Sensitivity reactions to drugs. Oxford: Blackwell Science; 1958.

7. Rosenow EC, Myers JL, Swensen SJ, Pisani RJ. Drug-induced pulmonary disease – an update. Chest 1992; 102:239–250.

8. Arsdel PP Van. Aspirin idiosyncrasy and tolerance. J Allergy Clin Immunol 1984; 73:431–434.

9. Ameisen JC, Capron A, Joseph M, et al. Aspirin-sensitive asthma: abnormal platelet response to drugs inducing asthmatic attacks; diagnostic and physiopathological implications. Int Arch Allergy Appl Immunol 1985; 78:438–448.

10. Lee TH. Mechanism of aspirin sensitivity. Am Rev Respir Dis 1992; 145:S34–S36.

11. Epler GR, Snider GL, Gaensler EA, Cathcart ES. FitzGerald MX, Carrington CB. Bronchiolitis and bronchitis in connective tissue disease. A possible relationship to the use of penicillamine. JAMA 1979; 242:528–532.

12. Schwartzman KJ, Bowie DM, Yeadon C, et al. Constrictive bronchiolitis obliterans following gold therapy for psoriatic arthritis. Eur Respir J 1995; 8:2191–2193.

13. Tomioka H, King TE. Gold-induced pulmonary disease: Clinical features, outcome, and differentiation from rheumatoid lung disease. Am J Respir Crit Care Med 1997; 155:1011–1020.

14. Geddes DM, Corrin B, Brewerton DA, Davies RJ, Turner-Warwick M. Progressive airway obliteration in adults and its association with rheumatoid disease. Q J Med 1977; 46:427–444.

15. Camus P, Foucher P, Bonniaud P, Ask K. Drug-induced infiltrative lung disease. Eur Resp J 2001; 18:93S–100S.

16. Tenenbein M, Kowalski S, Sienko A, Bowden DH, Adamson IYR. Pulmonary toxic effects of continuous desferrioxamine administration in acute iron poisoning. Lancet 1992; 339:699–701.

17. Oliner H, Schwartz R, Rubio R, Damashek W. Interstitial pulmonary fibrosis following busulfan therapy. Am J Med 1961; 31:134–139.

18. Heard BE, Cooke RA. Busulphan lung. Thorax 1968; 23:187–193.

19. Burns WA, McFarland W, Matthews MJ. Busulphan-induced pulmonary disease. Report of a case and review of the literature. Am Rev Respir Dis 1970; 101:408–413.

20. Podoll LN, Winkler SS. Busulfan lung: report of two cases and review of the literature. AJR Am J Roentgenol 1974; 120:151–156.

21. Elias AD, Mark EJ, Trotman-Dickenson B. A 60-year-old man with pulmonary infiltrates after a bone marrow transplantation – Busulfan pneumonitis. N Engl J Med 1997; 337:480–489.

22. Cooper JAD, White DA, Matthay RA. Drug-induced pulmonary disease. Am Rev Respir Dis 1986; 133:321–340.

23. Moseley PL, Shasby DM, Brady M, Hunninghake GW. Lung parenchymal injury induced by bleomycin. Am Rev Respir Dis 1984; 130:1082–1086.

24. Slavin RE, Millan JC, Mullins CM. Pathology of high dose intermittent cyclophosphamide therapy. Hum Pathol 1975; 6:693–709.

25. Mark GJ, Lehimgar-Zaden A, Ragsdale BD. Cyclophosphamide pneumonitis. Thorax 1978; 33:89–93.

26. Taetle R. Dickman PS, Feldman PS. Pulmonary histopathologic changes associated with melphalan therapy. Cancer 1978; 42:1239–1245.

27. Goucher G, Rowland V, Hawkins J. Melphalan-induced pulmonary interstitial fibrosis. Chest 1980; 77:805–806.

28. Tryka AF, Skornik WA, Godlaski JJ, Brain JD. Potentiation of bleomycin-induced lung injury by exposure to 70% oxygen. Am Rev Respir Dis 1982; 126:1074–1079.

29. Goldiner PL, Carlon GC, Cvitkovik E, Schweizer O, Howland WS. Factors influencing postoperative morbidity and mortality in patients treated with bleomycin. BMJ 1978; i:1664–1667.

30. Alan SC, Riddell GS, Butchart EG. Bleomycin therapy and anaesthesia. Anaesthesia 1981; 36:60–63.

31. Hulbert JC, Grossman JE, Cummings KB. Risk factors of anesthesia and surgery in bleomycin-treated patients. J Urol 1983; 130:163–164.

32. Adamson IYR, Bowden DH. The pathogenesis of bleomycin-induced pulmonary damage in mice. Am J Pathol 1974; 77:185–197.

33. Bedrossian CWM, Greenberg SD, Yawn DH, O'Neal RM. Experimentally induced bleomycin sulfate toxicity. Arch Pathol Lab Med 1977; 101: 248–254.

34. Gyorkey F, Gyorkey P, Sinkovics JG. Origin and significance of intranuclear tubular inclusions in type II pulmonary alveolar epithelial cells of patients with bleomycin and busulfan toxicity. Ultrastruct Pathol 1980; 1:211–221.

35. Hasleton PS, O'Driscoll BR, Lynch P et al. Late BCNU lung – a light and ultrastructural study on the delayed effect of BCNU on the lung parenchyma. J Pathol 1991; 164:31–36.

36. Lantuejoul S, Brambilla E, Brambilla C, Devouassoux G. Statin-induced fibrotic nonspecific interstitial pneumonia. Eur Resp J 2002; 19:577–580.

37. Camus P, Lombard JN, Perrichon M, et al. Bronchiolitis obliterans organizing pneumonia during treatment with acebutolol and amiodarone. Thorax 1989; 44:711–715.

38. Sastman HD, Matthay RA, Putman CE. Methotrexate-induced pneumonitis (Baltimore). Medicine (Baltimore) 1976; 55:371–388.

39. White DA, Rankin JA, Stover DE, Gellene RA, Gupta S. Methotrexate pneumonitis. Bronchoalveolar lavage findings suggest an immunologic disorder. Am Rev Respir Dis 1989; 139:18–21.

40. Leduc D, Devuyst P, Lheureux P, et al. Pneumonitis complicating low-dose methotrexate therapy for rheumatoid arthritis – discrepancies between lung biopsy and bronchoalveolar lavage findings. Chest 1993; 104:1620–1623.

41. Imokawa S, Colby TV, Leslie KO, Helmers RA. Methotrexate pneumonitis: review of the literature and histopathological findings in nine patients. Eur Resp J 2000; 15:373–381.

42. Ginsberg SJ, Comis RL. The pulmonary toxicity of antineoplastic agents. Semin Oncol 1982; 9:34–35.

43. Scott DL, Bradby GVH, Aitman TJ, Zaphiropoulos GC, Hawkins CF. Relationship of gold and penicillamine therapy to diffuse interstitial lung disease. Proc Soc Exp Biol Med 1981; 40:136–141.

44. Bone RC, Wolfe J, Sobonya RE, et al. Desquamative interstitial pneumonia following long-term nitrofurantoin therapy. Am J Med 1976; 60:697–701.

45. Magee F, Wright JL, Chan N, et al. Two unusual pathological reactions to nitrofurantoin: case reports. Histopathology 1986; 10:701–706.

46. Cameron RJ, Kolbe J, Wilsher ML, Lambie N. Bronchiolitis obliterans organising pneumonia associated with the use of nitrofurantoin. Thorax 2000; 55:249–251.

47. Costa-Jussa FR, Corrin B, Jacobs JM. Amiodarone lung toxicity: a human and experimental study. J Pathol 1984; 144:73–79.

48. Jacobson W, Stewart S, Gresham GA, Goddard MJ. Effect of amiodarone on the lung shown by polarized light microscopy. Arch Pathol Lab Med 1997; 121:1269–1271.

49. Vijeyaratnam GS, Corrin B. Fine structural alterations in the lungs of iprindole-treated rats. J Pathol 1974; 114:233–239.

50. Heath D, Smith P, Hasleton PS. Effects of chlorphentermine on the rat lung. Thorax 1973; 28:551–558.

51. Akoun GM, Gauthier-Rahman S, Milleron BJ, Perrot JY, Mayaud CM. Amiodarone-induced hypersensitivity pneumonitis. Evidence of an immunological cell-mediated mechanism. Chest 1984; 85:133–135.

52. Darmanata JI, Zandwijk N van, Duren DR, et al. Amiodarone pneumonitis: three further cases with a review of published reports. Thorax 1984; 39:57–64.

53. Dean PJ, Groshart KD, Porterfield JG, Iansmith DH, Golden EB Jr. Amiodarone-associated pulmonary toxicity. A clinical and pathologic study of eleven cases. Am J Clin Pathol 1987; 87:7–13.

54. Myers JL, Kennedy JI, Plumb VJ. Amiodarone lung: pathologic findings in clinically toxic patients. Hum Pathol 1987; 18:349–354.

55. Oren S, Turkot S, Golzman B, et al. Amiodarone-induced bronchiolitis obliterans organizing pneumonia (BOOP). Respir Med 1996; 90:167–169.

56. Polkey MI, Wilson POG, Rees PJ. Amiodarone pneumonitis: no safe dose. Respir Med 1995; 89:233–235.

57. Hargreaves MR, Benson MK. Amiodarone pneumonitis: no safe dose. Respir Med 1996; 90:119.

58. Wilson BD, Lippmann ML. Susceptibility to amiodarone-induced pulmonary toxicity: relationship to the uptake of amiodarone by isolated lung cells. Lung 1996; 174:31–41.

59. Handschin AE, Lardinois D, Schneiter D, Bloch K, Weder W. Acute amiodarone-induced pulmonary toxicity following lung resection. Respiration 2003; 70:310–312.

60. Vijeyaratnam GS, Corrin B. Pulmonary alveolar proteinosis developing from desquamative interstitial pneumonia in long term toxicity studies of iprindole in the rat. Virchows Arch A Pathol Anat Histopathol 1973; 358:1–10.

61. Allen JN, Davis WB. Eosinophilic lung diseases. Am J Respir Crit Care Med 1994; 150:1423–1438.

62. Tanigawa K, Sugiyama K, Matsuyama H, et al. Mesalazine-induced eosinophilic pneumonia. Respiration 1999; 66:69–72.

63. Cottin V, Frognier R, Monnot H, et al. Chronic eosinophilic pneumonia after radiation therapy for breast cancer. Eur Resp J 2004; 23:9–13.

64. Wechsler ME, Finn D, Gunawardena D, et al. Churg–Strauss syndrome in patients receiving montelukast as treatment for asthma. Chest 2000; 117:708–713.

65. LeGall C, Pham S, Vignes S, et al. Inhaled corticosteroids and Churg–Strauss syndrome: a report of five cases. Eur Resp J 2000; 15:978–981.

66. Faller M, Gasser B, Massard G, Pauli G, Quoix E. Pulmonary migratory infiltrates and pachypleuritis in a patient with Crohn's disease. Respiration 2000; 67:459–463.

67. Tazelaar HD, Myers JL, Drage CW, et al. Pulmonary disease associated with L-tryptophan-induced eosinophilic myalgia syndrome. Clinical and pathologic features. Chest 1990; 97:1032–1036.

68. Flannery MT, Wallach PM, Espinoza LR, Dohrenwend MP, Moscinski LC. A case of the eosinophilia-myalgia syndrome associated with use of an L-tryptophan product. Ann Intern Med 1990; 112:300–301.

69. Belongia EA, Hedberg CW, Gleich GJ, et al. An investigation of the cause of the eosinophilia-myalgia syndrome associated with tryptophan use. N Engl J Med 1990; 323:357–365.

70. Herrick MK, Chang Y, Horoupian DS, Lombard CM, Adornato BT. L-tryptophan and the eosinophilia-myalgia syndrome: pathologic findings in eight patients. Hum Pathol 1991; 22:12–21.

71. Winkelmann RK, Connolly SM, Quimby SR, Griffing WL, Lie JT. Histopathologic features of the L-tryptophan-related eosinophilia-myalgia (fasciitis) syndrome. Mayo Clin Proc 1991; 66:457–463.

72. Mayeno AN, Belongia EA, Lin F, Lundy SK, Gleich GJ. 3-(phenylamino)alanine, a novel aniline-derived amino acid associated with the eosinophilia-myalgia syndrome – a link to the toxic oil syndrome. Mayo Clin Proc 1992; 67:1134–1139.

73. Illa I, Dinsmore S, Dalakas MC. Immune-mediated mechanisms and immune activation of fibroblasts in the pathogenesis of eosinophilia-myalgia syndrome induced by L- tryptophan. Hum Pathol 1993; 24:702–709.

74. Cheng TO. Pulmonary hypertension in patients with eosinophilia-myalgia syndrome or toxic oil syndrome. Mayo Clin Proc 1993; 68:823.

75. Tazelaar HD, Myers JL, Strickler JG, Colby TV, Duffy J. Tryptophan-induced lung disease – an immunophenotypic, immunofluorescent, and electron microscopic study. Mod Pathol 1993; 6:56–60.

76. Mar KE, Sen P, Tan K, Krishnan R, Ratkalkar K. Bronchiolitis obliterans organizing pneumonia associated with massive L-tryptophan ingestion. Chest 1993; 104:1924–1926.

77. Clarysse AM, Cathey WJ, Cartwright GE, Wintrobe MM. Pulmonary disease complicating intermittent therapy with methotrexate. JAMA 1969; 209:1861–1864.

78. Hasan FM, Mark EJ. Case records of the Massachusetts General Hospital. A 28-year-old man with increasing dyspnea, dry cough, and fever after chemotherapy for lymphoma. N Engl J Med 1990; 323:737–747.

79. Dekerviler E, Tredaniel J, Revlon G, et al. Fluoxetin-induced pulmonary granulomatosis. Eur Respir J 1996; 9:615–617.

80. Steiger D, Bubendorf L, Oberholzer M, Tamm M, Leuppi JD. Ciprofloxacin-induced acute interstitial pneumonitis. Eur Resp J 2004; 23:172–174.

81. Pietropaoli A, Modrak J, Utell M. Interferon-alpha therapy associated with the development of sarcoidosis. Chest 1999; 116:569–572.

82. Vavricka SR, Wettstein T, Speich R, Gaspert A, Bachli EB. Pulmonary granulomas after tumour necrosis factor alpha antagonist therapy. Thorax 2003; 58:278–279.

83. Elston CW. Pneumonia due to liquid paraffin: with chemical analysis. Arch Dis Child 1966; 41:428–434.

84. Salm R, Hughes EW. A case of chronic paraffin pneumonitis. Thorax 1970; 25:762–768.

85. Fox B. Liquid paraffin pneumonia – with chemical analysis and electron microscopy. Virchows Arch A Pathol Anat Histopathol 1979; 382:339–346.

86. Corrin B, Crocker PR, Hood BJ, Levison DA, Parkes WR. Paraffinoma confirmed by infrared spectrophotometry. Thorax 1987; 42:389–390.

87. Wagner JC, Adler DI, Fuller DN. Foreign body granulomata of the lungs due to liquid paraffin. Thorax 1955; 10:157–170.

88. Brown AC, Slocum PC, Putthoff SL, Wallace WE, Foresman BH. Exogenous lipoid pneumonia due to nasal application of petroleum jelly. Chest 1994; 105:968–969.

89. Annobil SH, Morad NA, Khurana P, et al. Reaction of human lungs to aspirated animal fat (ghee): a clinicopathological study. Virchows Arch 1995; 46:301–305.

90. Rayl JE. Clinical reactions following bronchography. Ann Otol Rhinol Laryngol 1965; 74:1120–1132.

91. Felton WL. The reaction of pulmonary tissue to lipiodol. J Thorac Surg 1953; 25:530–542.

92. Greenberg SD, Spjut HJ, Hallman GL. Experimental study of bronchographic media on lung. Arch Otolaryngol Head Neck Surg 1966; 83:276–282.

93. Felton WL. A method for the identification of lipiodol in tissue sections. Lab Invest 1952; 1:364–367.

94. Lamaze R, Trechot P, Martinet Y. Bronchial necrosis and granuloma induced by the aspiration of a tablet of ferrous sulphate. Eur Respir J 1994; 7:1710–1711.

95. Lee P, Culver DA, Farver C, Mehta AC. Syndrome of iron pill aspiration. Chest 2002; 121:1355–1357.

96. Sundar KM, Elliott CG, Thomsen GE. Tetracycline aspiration – Case report and review of the literature. Respiration 2001; 68:416–419.

97. Tamm I, Kortsik C. Severe barium sulfate aspiration into the lung: Clinical presentation, prognosis and therapy. Respiration 1999; 66:81–84.

98. Kay JM, Smith P, Heath D. Aminorex and the pulmonary circulation. Thorax 1971; 26:262–270.

99. Douglas JG, Munro JF, Kitchin AH, Muir AL, Proudfoot AT. Pulmonary hypertension and fenfluramine. BMJ 1981; 283:881–883.

100. McMurray J, Bloomfield P, Miller HC. Irreversible pulmonary hypertension after treatment with fenfluramine. BMJ 1986; 292:239–240.

101. Kay JM. Dietary pulmonary hypertension. Thorax 1994; 49:S33–S38.

102. Abenhaim L, Moride Y, Brenot F, et al. Appetite-suppressant drugs and the risk of primary pulmonary hypertension. N Engl J Med 1996; 335:609–616.

103. Mark EJ, Patalas ED, Chang HT, Evans RJ, Kessler SC. Fatal pulmonary hypertension associated with short-term use of fenfluramine and phentermine. N Engl J Med 1997; 337:602–606.

104. Tomita T, Zhao Q. Autopsy findings of heart and lungs in a patient with primary pulmonary hypertension associated with use of fenfluramine and phentermine. Chest 2002; 121:649–652.

105. Lombard CM, Churg A, Winokur S. Pulmonary veno-occlusive disease following therapy for malignant neoplasms. Chest 1987; 92:871–876.

106. Williams LM, Fussell S, Veith RW, Nelson S, Mason CM. Pulmonary veno-occlusive disease in an adult following bone marrow transplantation: case report and review of the literature. Chest 1996; 109:1388–1391.

107. Alliot C, Rapin JP, Besson M, Bedjaoui F, Messouak D. Pulmonary embolism after intravenous immunoglobulin. J R Soc Med 2001; 94:187–188.

108. Barson AJ, Chiswick ML, Doig CM. Fat embolism in infancy after intravenous fat infusions. Arch Dis Child 1978; 53:218–223.

109. Levene MI, Wigglesworth JS, Desai R. Pulmonary fat accumulation after intralipid infusion in the preterm infant. Lancet 1980; II:815–818.

110. Hulman G, Levene M. Intralipid microemboli. Arch Dis Child 1986; 61:702–703.

111. Hulman G. The pathogenesis of fat embolism. J Pathol 1995; 176:3–9.

112. Kitchell CC, Balogh K. Pulmonary lipid emboli in association with long-term hyperalimentation. Hum Pathol 1986; 17:83–85.

113. Lekka ME, Liokatis S, Nathanail C, Galani V, Nakos G. The impact of intravenous fat emulsion administration in acute lung injury. Am J Respir Crit Care Med 2004; 169:638–644.

114. Reedy JS, Kuhlman JE, Voytovich M. Microvascular pulmonary emboli secondary to precipitated crystals in a patient receiving total parenteral nutrition – A case report and description of the high-resolution CT findings. Chest 1999; 115:892–895.

115. Gough JH, Gough MH, Thomas ML. Pulmonary complications following lymphangiography with a note on technique. Br J Radiol 1964; 37: 416–421.

116. Fraimow W, Wallace S, Lewis P, Greening RR, Cathcart RT. Changes in pulmonary function due to lymphangiography. Radiology 1965; 85:231–241.

117. Davidson JW. Pulmonary complications of lymphangiography. N Engl J Med 1971; 285:237.

118. Silvestri RC, Hyseby JS, Rughani I, Thorning D, Culver BH. Respiratory distress syndrome from lymphangiography contrast medium. Am Rev Respir Dis 1980; 122:543–549.

119. Leong AS-Y, Disney APS, Gove DW. Spallation and migration of silicone from blood-pump tubing in patients on hemodialysis. N Engl J Med 1982; 306:135–140.

120. Chastre J, Basset F, Viau F, et al. Acute pneumonitis after subcutaneous injections of silicone in transsexual men. N Engl J Med 1983; 308:764–767.

121. Robinson MJ, Nestor M, Rywlin AM. Pulmonary granulomas secondary to embolic prosthetic valve material. Hum Pathol 1981; 12:759–762.

122. Mittleman RE, Marraccini JV. Pulmonary Teflon granulomas following periurethral Teflon injection for urinary incontinence. Arch Pathol Lab Med 1983; 107:611–612.

123. Lai YF, Chao TY, Wong SL. Acute pneumonitis after subcutaneous injections of silicone for augmentation mammaplasty. Chest 1994; 106:1152–1155.

124. Fairfax AJ, Ball J, Batten JC, Heard BE. A pathological study following bronchial artery embolization for haemoptysis in cystic fibrosis. Br J Dis Chest 1980; 74:345–352.

125. Coard K, Silver MD, Perkins G, Fox AJ, Vinuela EV. Isobutyl-2-cyanoacrylate pulmonary emboli associated with occlusive embolotherapy of cerebral arteriovenous malformations. Histopathology 1984; 8:917–926.

126. Lena H, Desrues B, Quinquenel ML, et al. Hemorragie alveolaire diffuse secondaire a l'utilisation d'anticoagulants oraux. Rev Mal Resp 1995; 12:496–498.

127. Nicolls MR, Terada LS, Tuder RM, Prindiville SA, Schwarz MI. Diffuse alveolar hemorrhage with underlying pulmonary capillaritis in the retinoic acid syndrome. Am J Respir Crit Care Med 1998; 158:1302–1305.

128. Wiertz LM, Gagnon JH, Anthonisen NR. Intrapulmonary hemorrhage with anemia after lymphangiography. N Engl J Med 1971; 285:1364–1365.

129. Kalra S, Bell MR, Rihal CS. Alveolar hemorrhage as a complication of treatment with abciximab. Chest 2001; 120:126–131.

130. Morelock SY, Sahn SA. Drugs and the pleura. Chest 1999; 116:212–221.

131. Pfitzenmeyer P, Foucher P, Dennewald G, et al. Pleuropulmonary changes induced by ergoline drugs. Eur Respir J 1996; 9:1013–1019.

132. Comet R, Domingo C, Such JJ, et al. Pleuropulmonary disease as a side-effect of treatment with bromocriptine. Resp Med 1998; 92:1172–1174.

133. Danoff SK, Grasso ME, Terry PB, Flynn JA. Pleuropulmonary disease due to pergolide use for restless legs syndrome. Chest 2001; 120:313–316.

Miscellaneous iatrogenic lung injury

134. Hines LE. Fibrosis of the lung following roentgen-ray treatments for tumor. JAMA 1922; 79:720–722.

135. Warren S, Spencer J. Radiation reaction in the lung. AJR Am J Roentgenol 1940; 43:682–701.

136. Warren S, Gates O. Radiation pneumonitis: experimental and pathologic observations. Arch Pathol Lab Med 1940; 30:440–460.

137. Gross NJ. The pathogenesis of radiation-induced lung damage. Lung 1981; 159:115–125.

138. Liebow AA, Warren S, DeCowsey E. Pathology of atomic bomb casualties. Am J Pathol 1949; 25:853–940.

139. Chandler Smith J. Radiation pneumonitis: a review. Am Rev Respir Dis 1963; 87:647–655.

140. Fulkerson WJ, McLendon RE, Proznitz LR. Adult respiratory distress syndrome after limited thoracic radiotherapy. Cancer 1986; 57:1941–1946.

141. Crestani B, Kambouchner M, Soler P, et al. Migratory bronchiolitis obliterans organizing pneumonia after unilateral radiation therapy for breast carcinoma. Eur Respir J 1995; 8:318–321.

142. Bayle JY, Nesme P, Bejui-Thivolet F, et al. Migratory organizing pneumonitis 'primed' by radiation therapy. Eur Respir J 1995; 8:322–326.

143. Wharton SP, Rogers TK. Hamman–Rich syndrome 'primed' by radiation? Resp Med 1999; 93:136–137.

144. Ma LD, Taylor GA, Wharam MD. Wiley JM. 'Recall' pneumonitis: adriamycin potentiation of radiation pneumonitis in two children. Radiology 1993; 187:465–467.

145. Thomas PS, Agrawal S, Gore M, Geddes DM. Recall lung pneumonitis due to carmustine after radiotherapy. Thorax 1995; 50:1116–1118.

146. Movsas B, Raffin TA, Epstein AH, Link CJ Jr. Pulmonary radiation injury. Chest 1997; 111:1061–1076.

147. Court-Brown WM, Doll R. Mortality from cancer and other causes after radiotherapy for ankylosing spondylitis. BMJ 1965; 2:1327–1332.

148. Neugut AI, Murray T, Santos J, et al. Increased risk of lung cancer after breast cancer radiation therapy in cigarette smokers. Cancer 1994; 73:1615–1620.

149. Adamson IYR, Bowden DH. Endothelial injury and repair in radiation-induced pulmonary fibrosis. Am J Pathol 1983; 112:224–230.

150. Adamson IYR, Bowden DH, Wyatt JP. A pathway to pulmonary fibrosis: an ultrastructural study of mouse and rats following radiation to the whole body and hemithorax. Am J Pathol 1970; 58:481–498.

151. Madrazo A, Suzuki Y, Churg J. Radiation pneumonitis: ultrastructural changes in the pulmonary alveoli following high doses of radiation. Arch Pathol Lab Med 1973; 96:262–268.

152. Nash G, Bowen JA, Langlinais PC. Respirator lung – a misnomer. Arch Pathol Lab Med 1972; 21:234–238.

153. Pratt PC. Pathology of adult respiratory distress syndrome. In: Thurlbeck WM, Abell MR, eds. The Lung. Baltimore, MD: Williams & Wilkins; 1978:43–57.

154. Pratt PC, Vollmer RT, Shelburne JD, Crapo JD. Pulmonary morphology in a multihospital collaborative extracorporeal membrane oxygenation project. Am J Pathol 1979; 95:191–214.

155. Slutsky AS. Lung injury caused by mechanical ventilation. Chest 1999; 116:9S–15S.

156. Ricard JD, Dreyfuss D, Saumon G. Ventilator-induced lung injury. Eur Resp J 2003; 22:2S–9S.

157. Sacks T, Moldow CF, Craddock PR, Bowers TK, Jacob HS. Oxygen radicals mediate endothelial cell damage by complement-stimulated granulocytes. J Clin Invest 1978; 61:1161–1167.

158. Johnson KJ, Fantone JC, Daplan J, Ward PA. In vitro damage of rat lungs by oxygen metabolites. J Clin Invest 1981; 67:983–993.

159. Wegner CD, Wolyniec WW, Laplante AM, et al. Intercellular adhesion molecule-1 contributes to pulmonary oxygen toxicity in mice – role of leukocytes revised. Lung 1992; 170:267–279.

160. Kang BH, Crapo JD, Wegner CD, Letts LG, Chang LY. Intercellular adhesion molecule-1 expression on the alveolar epithelium and its modification by hyperoxia. Am J Respir Cell Mol Biol 1993; 9:350–355.

161. Deneke SM, Fanburg BL. Normobaric oxygen toxicity of the lung. N Engl J Med 1980; 303:76–86.

162. Kapanci Y, Tosco R, Eggermann J, Gould VE. Oxygen pneumonitis in man. Chest 1972; 62:162–169.

163. Pratt PC. Pathology of pulmonary oxygen toxicity. Am Rev Respir Dis 1974; 110 (Suppl):51–57.

164. Katzenstein A-LA, Bloor CM, Liebow AA. Diffuse alveolar damage – the role of oxygen, shock and related factors. Am J Pathol 1976; 85:210–222.

165. Haschek WM, Brody AR, Klein-Szanto AJP, Witschi H. Diffuse interstitial pulmonary fibrosis. Pulmonary fibrosis in mice induced by treatment

with butylated hydroxytoluene and oxygen. Am J Pathol 1981; 105: 334–335.

166. Witschi HR, Haschek WM, Klein-Szanto AJP, Hakkinen PJ. Potentiation of diffuse lung damage by oxygen: determining values. Am Rev Respir Dis 1981; 123:98–103.

167. Yamamoto E, Wittner M, Rosenbaum RM. Resistance and susceptibility to oxygen toxicity by cell types of the gas-blood barrier of the rat lung. Am J Pathol 1970; 59:409–436.

168. Gould VE, Tosco R, Wheelis RF, Gould NF, Kapanci Y. Oxygen pneumonitis in man. Ultrastructural observations on the development of the alveolar lesions. Lab Invest 1972; 26:499–508.

169. Peek GJ, Moore HM, Moore N, Sosnowski AW, Firmin RK. Extracorporeal membrane oxygenation for adult respiratory failure. Chest 1997; 112:759–764.

170. Bruch LA, Flint A, Hirschl RB. Pulmonary pathology of patients treated with partial liquid ventilation. Mod Pathol 1997; 10:463–468.

171. Adawi A, Zhang Y, Baggs R, Finkelstein J, Phipps RP. Disruption of the CD40-CD40 ligand system prevents an oxygen-induced respiratory distress syndrome. Am J Pathol 1998; 152:651–657.

172. Kapanci Y, Weibel ER, Kaplan HP, Robinson FR. Pathogenesis and reversibility of the pulmonary lesions of oxygen toxicity in monkeys. II Ultrastructural and morphometric studies. Lab Invest 1969; 20:101–118.

173. Popovsky MA, Abel MD, Moore SB. Transfusion-related acute lung injury associated with passive transfer of antileukocyte antibodies. Am Rev Respir Dis 1983; 128:185–189.

174. Divertie MB. Diffuse alveolar damage, respiratory failure and blood transfusion. Mayo Clin Proc 1984; 59:643–644.

175. Dry SM, Bechard KM, Milford EL, Churchill WH, Benjamin RJ. The pathology of transfusion-related acute lung injury. Am J Clin Pathol 1999; 112:216–221.

176. Ratliff NB, Youg WG, Hackol DB, Mikat E, Wilson JW. Pulmonary injury - secondary to extracorporeal circulation. J Thorac Cardiovasc Surg 1973; 65:425–432.

177. Asada S, Yamaguchi M. Fine structural changes in the lungs following cardiopulmonary bypass. Chest 1971; 59:478–483.

178. Westaby S. Complement and the damaging effects of cardiopulmonary bypass. Thorax 1983; 38:321–325.

179. Tonz M, Mihaljevic T, Vonsegesser LK, et al. Acute lung injury during cardiopulmonary bypass: are the neutrophils responsible? Chest 1995; 108:1551–1556.

180. Wan S, LeClerc JL, Vincent JL. Inflammatory response to cardiopulmonary bypass: Mechanisms involved and possible therapeutic strategies. Chest 1997; 112:676–692.

181. Stauffer JL, Olson DE, Petty TL. Complications and consequences of endotracheal intubation and tracheotomy. A prospective study of 150 critically ill adult patients. Am J Med 1981; 70:65–75.

182. Vanheurn LWE, Theunissen PHMH, Ramsay G, Brink PRG. Pathologic changes of the trachea after percutaneous dilatational tracheotomy. Chest 1996; 109:1466–1469.

183. Phillips I. Pseudomonas aeruginosa respiratory tract infections in patients receiving mechanical ventilation. J Hyg 1967; 65:229–235.

184. Skim C. Cardiac arrhythmias resulting from tracheal suctioning. Ann Intern Med 1969; 71:1149–1153.

185. Deslee G, Brichet A, Lebuffe G, et al. Obstructive fibrinous tracheal pseudomembrane - A potentially fatal complication of tracheal intubation. Am J Respir Crit Care Med 2000; 162:1169–1171.

186. Jacobs IN, Wetmore RF, Tom LW, Handler SO, Potsic WP. Tracheobronchomalacia in children. Arch Otolaryngol Head Neck Surg 1994; 120:154–158.

187. Romagosa V, Bella MR, Truchero C, Moya J. Necrotizing sialometaplasia (adenometaplasia) of the trachea. Histopathology 1992; 21:280–282.

188. Rowley KM, Clubb BSS, Smith GJW, Cabin HS. Right sided infective endocarditis as a consequence of flow directed pulmonary artery catheterisation. N Engl J Med 1984; 311:1152–1156.

189. Connors AFJr. Castele RJ, Farhat NZ, Tomashefski JF. Complication of right heart catheterisation. Chest 1985; 88:567–572.

190. Stelzner TJ, King TE, Antony VB, Sahn SA. The pleuropulmonary manifestations of the postcardiac injury syndrome. Chest 1983; 84:383.

191. Weiser NJ, Kantor M, Russell HK, Murphy L. The postmyocardial infarction syndrome. The nonspecificity of the pulmonary manifestations. Circulation 1962; 25:643–650.

192. Khan AH. The postcardiac injury syndromes. Clin Cardiol 1992; 15:67–72.

193. Akl ES, Latif N, Dunn MJ, Rose ML, Yacoub MH. Antiheart antibodies following open heart surgery: incidence and correlation with postpericardiotomy syndrome. Eur J Cardiothorac Surg 1992; 6:503–507.

194. Kopec SE, Irwin RS. UmaliTorres CB, Balikian JP, Conlan AA. The postpneumonectomy state. Chest 1998; 114:1158–1184.

195. Biondetti PR, Fiore D, Sartori F, et al. Evaluation of post-pneumonectomy space by computed tomography. J Comput Assist Tomogr 1982; 6:238–242.

196. Suarez J, Clagett T, Brown AL. Jr. The postpneumonectomy space: factors influencing its obliteration. J Thorac Cardiovasc Surg 1969; 57:539–542.

197. Sakamaki Y, Matsumoto K, Mizuno S, et al. Hepatocyte growth factor stimulates proliferation of respiratory epithelial cells during postpneumonectomy compensatory lung growth in mice. Am J Respir Cell Molec Biol 2002; 26:525–533.

198. Williams EA, Quinlan GJ, Anning PB, Goldstraw P, Evans TW. Lung injury following pulmonary resection in the isolated, blood- perfused rat lung. Eur Resp J 1999; 14:745–750.

199. Jordan S, Mitchell JA, Quinlan GJ, Goldstraw P, Evans TW. The pathogenesis of lung injury following pulmonary resection. Eur Resp J 2000; 15:790–799.

200. Adams HD, Junod F, Aberdeen E, Johnson J. Severe airway obstruction caused by mediastinal displacement after right pneumonectomy in a child. A case report. J Thorac Cardiovasc Surg 1972; 63:534–539.

201. Grillo HC, Shepard JA, Mathisen DJ, Kanarek DJ. Postpneumonectomy syndrome: diagnosis, management, and results. Ann Thorac Surg 1992; 54:638–650.

202. Cordova FC, Travaline JM, O'Brien GM, Ball DS, Lippmann M. Treatment of left pneumonectomy syndrome with an expandable endobronchial prosthesis. Chest 1996; 109:567–570.

203. Boiselle PM, Shepard JA, McLoud TC, Grillo HC, Wright CD. Postpneumonectomy syndrome: another twist. J Thorac Imaging 1997; 12:209–211.

8

Vascular disease

8.1

Congestion and oedema; thrombosis, embolism and infarction; aneurysms

This section deals with several important pulmonary vascular diseases but others are dealt with elsewhere – congenital anomalies of pulmonary vessels in Chapter 2, shock in Chapter 4 and vascular tumours of the lung in Chapter 12.3.

PULMONARY CONGESTION AND OEDEMA

Congestion of the lungs may be active or passive, the former accompanying inflammation and the latter the result of an increase in pressure in the pulmonary veins, typically due to failure of the left ventricle or mitral stenosis. The active variety includes the congestive atelectasis that results from circulatory shock (see p. 132).

At necropsy the pulmonary vessels are engorged, the lungs are heavy and blood can be expressed from the cut surface. Histologically the capillaries are distended. Pulmonary congestion is often associated with pulmonary oedema and haemosiderosis.

Pulmonary oedema

Pathogenesis

In accordance with Starling's law, water moves between the vascular and interstitial compartments of the lung in response to net hydrostatic and osmotic forces acting across the vessel wall, modulated by the permeability of this membrane. The capillaries constitute the main site of microvascular fluid exchange, but small arteries and veins are also involved. Water movement chiefly takes place through the endothelial cell junctions;

beyond these the endothelial basement membrane offers no barrier to fluid transport.[1] Within the interstitium, water again flows along a hydrostatic gradient, in this case to the corners of the alveoli and thence to the connective tissue surrounding the arteries and bronchioles at the centres of the acini and the veins in the interlobular septa.[2,3] These are the sites where lymphatics commence.[3,4] There is considerable reserve in the clearance capacity of the pulmonary lymphatics, which may increase their load 10-fold when pulmonary oedema threatens,[5] but above this, spillover into the alveoli is inevitable. Before this the lungs sound dry on auscultation but the patient may nevertheless be breathless because the increased interstitial pressure triggers juxtacapillary nociceptors, which are represented by fine nerve terminals in the alveolar interstitium.[6,7]

In circumstances that involve only pressure changes, the oedema fluid is generally similar to normal interstitial fluid but in other circumstances the permeability of the vessels is increased and blood cells and high molecular weight plasma proteins, such as fibrinogen, escape into the tissues. Two main types of pulmonary oedema are therefore described, *haemodynamic* and *cytotoxic* (or *irritant*), characterised by the escape of low and high molecular weight blood substances respectively. Electron microscopy shows that in haemodynamic oedema there is widening of the interstitial spaces in the alveolar walls by fluid, with separation of the collagen and elastin fibres, but that this is confined to the thick side of the air/blood barrier. In contrast, in cytotoxic oedema fluid also accumulates in the thin part of the air/blood barrier so that the endothelial cells are detached from their basement membranes and are often stretched over large subendothelial blebs of fluid (Fig. 8.1.1),[8] changes that do not occur in uncomplicated haemodynamic pulmonary oedema.[9]

The separation of haemodynamic and cytotoxic oedema is not absolute: large haemodynamic forces alone can result in the escape of high molecular weight blood proteins.[10,11] Electron microscopy shows that when the alveolar capillary pressure is raised above 40 mmHg in anaesthetised rabbits, breaks develop in both the endothelium of the alveolar capillaries and the alveolar epithelium.[12–16] Such stress failure results in high permeability pulmonary oedema and even frank alveolar haemorrhage. This explains why the oedema fluid of mitral stenosis is often tinged with blood and why haemosiderosis is seen in other diseases characterised by raised pulmonary venous pressure, such as veno-occlusive disease (see p. 427) and lymphangioleiomyomatosis (see p. 297).

Stress failure of the alveoli also explains the occasional sudden demise of a thoroughbred racehorse from a 'burst blood vessel'.[17] These animals have been bred to such an extent that their cardiovascular systems develop very high pulmonary vascular pressures on exercise. Alveolar haemorrhage is common in these horses although it is seldom apparent to their attendants. Similar exercise-induced pulmonary haemorrhage has also been described in racing greyhounds and it is possible that the lungs of top athletes may also develop stress failure on occasion.[15,18] Stress failure is also seen when there is overinflation of the lung, such as that which occurs when there is a sudden drop

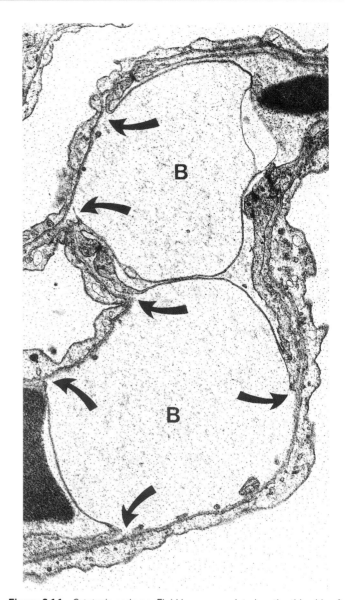

Figure 8.1.1 Cytotoxic oedema. Fluid has accumulated on the thin side of the air/blood barrier, raising the alveolar capillary endothelium off its basement membrane and producing two subendothelial blebs (B) which stretch right across the capillary. Arrows mark the points at which the endothelium is lifted off its basement membrane. Transmission electron micrograph of the lung of a rat that had been subjected to very high doses of the antidepressant drug iprindole. (Electron micrograph provided by Dr GS Balasubramaniam, Melbourne, Australia.)

in atmospheric pressure (see 'burst lung', p. 370) or when alveolar gas pressures are raised unduly by mechanical respiratory assistance devices in intensive care units.

Specific causes of pulmonary oedema
Pulmonary venous hypertension

This is the common factor by which conditions such as left ventricular failure, mitral stenosis and pulmonary veno-occlusive disease contribute to haemodynamic pulmonary oedema. A rise in pressure at the venous end of the pulmonary capillaries causes increased amounts of fluid to leave these vessels, with fluid that cannot be reabsorbed by the capillaries or drained by lymphatics accumulating as oedema. In left ventricular failure the accumulation of fluid is compounded by sodium retention, which is an important consequence of 'forward heart failure' through its effects on adrenocortical perfusion and aldosterone secretion.

Hypoproteinaemia

This is a potential cause of haemodynamic pulmonary oedema and underlies that occasionally observed in cirrhosis.

Intravenous fluid overload

Intravenous fluid overload may lead to pulmonary oedema by causing both left ventricular overload and dilution of the plasma proteins.

Re-expansion of the lungs

Rapid drainage of a pleural effusion or the removal of a large pleural tumour occasionally alters pulmonary haemodynamics to such an extent that pulmonary oedema results.[19] The oedema fluid is rich in protein suggesting that vascular permeability is increased and that there is stress failure of the alveolar walls.

Airway obstruction

Suggested mechanisms involved in the pulmonary oedema that occasionally accompanies airway obstruction include negative intrathoracic pressure causing transiently low interstitial pressure in the lungs, impaired left ventricular function and hypoxic postcapillary vasoconstriction.[20]

Inhalation of irritant gases

The accidental inhalation of gases such as ammonia, sulphur dioxide, chlorine, ozone and the oxides of nitrogen may cause widespread cytotoxic injury to the pulmonary capillaries as well as the alveolar epithelium, resulting in high permeability pulmonary oedema.[21]

Oxygen

Oxygen in high concentration, necessarily administered in some cases of severe lung injury, may further damage the lung and lead to cytotoxic pulmonary oedema.[22–24]

Acute pulmonary infection

Oedema is a common feature of most pulmonary infections. It is attributable to the direct or indirect effects on the capillary endothelium and alveolar epithelium of toxins produced by the infective agent.

Chemotherapy

Treatment with drugs such as busulphan is occasionally complicated by pulmonary oedema because of their cytotoxicity to alveolar endothelial and epithelial cells.

Shock lung

This condition is characterised by severe cytotoxic pulmonary oedema. The endothelial damage is attributable to several factors, notably nitric oxide, which is released in large amounts by activated macrophages and oxygen and hydroxyl radicals, which are released by activated polymorphs sequestered in the pulmonary capillaries. The detailed pathology of shock lung is described on p. 138.

Renal failure

Several mechanisms contribute to the development of pulmonary oedema in renal failure. They include fluid retention, hypertensive cardiac failure and hypoproteinaemia. The fluid is rich in protein suggesting that cytotoxic factors or stress failure may also operate.[25,26]

High altitude

The pulmonary oedema of acute mountain sickness (see p. 371) has a complex pathogenesis but the possibility that haemodynamic factors are involved is suggested by the undue susceptibility to the condition of persons with aplasia or hypoplasia of one pulmonary artery.[27,28] The lung lavage fluid is rich in protein[29] and electron microscopy shows subendothelial blebs characteristic of cytotoxic injury (Fig. 8.1.1) or even disruption of the alveolar walls,[30] indicating that there is haemodynamic stress failure.[12,31] The oedema can be prevented or treated successfully with vasodilators such as calcium channel blocking agents taken orally[32,33] or inhaled nitric oxide,[34] suggesting that hypoxic vasoconstriction plays an important pathogenetic role. Hypoxia is a powerful stimulus to pulmonary vasoconstriction but it mainly affects pre-capillary vessels and would therefore seem to protect the capillary bed. This apparent anomaly may be explained by the patchy nature of the oedema. If the hypoxic vasoconstriction affected some pulmonary arteries more than others some capillaries would be protected and the remainder subjected to abnormally high pressures: patchy vasoconstriction would lead to patchy stress failure. Hypoxic venous constriction may also be involved[35] (relevant to which is evidence that flow through the valveless pulmonary veins is controlled by sphincters).[36]

Cerebral injury

Neurogenic pulmonary oedema is a well recognised feature of cerebral damage, especially that caused by trauma or subarachnoid haemorrhage. Its pathogenesis appears to involve massive adrenergic release mediated by the hypothalamus.[37–39] This results in widespread vasoconstriction with marked systemic hypertension. Fluid then shifts from the systemic circulation to the relatively more compliant pulmonary circulation, with a resultant outpouring of fluid into the lung. Stress failure is invoked to explain the high permeability nature of the oedema fluid.[12]

Heroin overdosage

This is a well recognised cause of pulmonary oedema. Its pathogenesis is not well understood but high protein levels in the oedema fluid suggest increased pulmonary capillary permeability.[40] Adrenergic hyperactivity similar to that envisaged in neurogenic injury may be involved.

Prostacyclin therapy

Prostacyclin has been used to dilate the pulmonary arteries in patients with pulmonary hypertension but its continuous intravenous administration has been complicated by pulmonary oedema when the hypertension has been due to post-capillary obstruction, as in pulmonary veno-occlusive disease and pulmonary capillary haemangiomatosis.[41]

Pathological findings

At necropsy, an oedematous lung may weigh as much as 1 kg, nearly three times its normal weight. It feels firm and fails to collapse when the thorax is opened, so that the pleural surface remains smooth. Pleural effusion is often also present. Frothy fluid fills the airways when the lung is cut and watery fluid escapes from the exposed surface. The fibrin-containing fluid of 'toxic' oedema does not run from the cut surface as freely as the watery fluid of haemodynamic oedema due to its high fibrin content. The appearances may simulate haemorrhage if red cells have escaped in large numbers into the fluid. Interstitial oedema is seen to distend the loose connective tissue of the interlobular septa and that around the airways and arteries. The subpleural lymphatics may be visibly distended and often the hilar lymph nodes are considerably enlarged, soft and moist.

Microscopically, the interlobular septa and the periarterial connective tissue sheaths are swollen and lymphatics within them are dilated (see Fig. 2.8, p. 43). Alveolar oedema is seen as a homogenous, eosinophilic proteinaceous material filling the airspaces (Fig. 8.1.2). Entrapped air bubbles are represented by rounded spaces within the proteinaceous contents of the alveoli. Only scanty threads of fibrin are generally found, but in severe cases, especially of the toxic variety, much fibrin is present in the fluid. The lungs are then particularly firm and have been described as showing 'congestive consolidation'. There may also be many red blood cells in the air spaces. Iron-containing macrophages may be found in chronic cases.

Organisation of the fibrinous material may occur, leading to fibrosis in the alveoli.[42] This takes the form of intra-alveolar plugs of oedematous granulation tissue known as 'bourgeons conjonctifs' or Masson bodies.[43] Similar bodies develop in the bronchioles and the appearances closely mimic those found in healing bacterial pneumonia and in cryptogenic organising pneumonia (see p. 307). The connective tissue plugs may be incorporated into the alveolar walls, causing interstitial fibrosis by an accretive process.[44,45] Interstitial fibrosis may also arise as a direct consequence of interstitial oedema, so-called 'gefässlose' (vessel-less) organisation.[46] The combination of haemosiderosis and fibrosis spawned the term 'brown induration of the lungs' for the changes that develop in long-standing mitral stenosis (Fig. 8.1.3).[47]

The vascular changes resulting from pulmonary venous hypertension are described in Chapter 8.2.

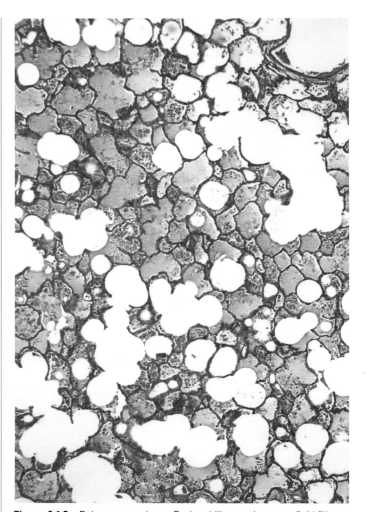

Figure 8.1.2 Pulmonary oedema. Eosinophilic proteinaceous fluid fills many alveoli.

Radiological findings[42,48,49]

Interstitial oedema is recognisable in radiographs of the chest by a combination of hilar enlargement, caused by peribronchial and periarterial cuffing, and peripheral linear opacities resulting from oedema of the interlobular septa. There is a greater concentration of perivascular and peribronchial connective tissue at the hila and consequently the hilar opacities are enlarged, denser and less well defined. Septal thickening is visualised radiologically as a series of non-branching, horizontal lines, 1–3 cm long, extending to the pleura at the lung bases. They are popularly known as 'Kerley B lines'.

Alveolar oedema exaggerates the hilar prominence of the interstitial oedema that precedes it to produce a 'bat's wing' or 'butterfly' shadow. This picture was first described in cases of uraemia but is now known to occur with other causes of pulmonary oedema. The opacification is particularly marked in severe oedema, such as occurs in shock, when there may be a total 'white-out' of the lung fields except for patent bronchi which are seen as if forming a 'negative bronchogram'.

In addition to the features of oedema, the chest radiograph often shows enlargement of the heart and widening of vessels

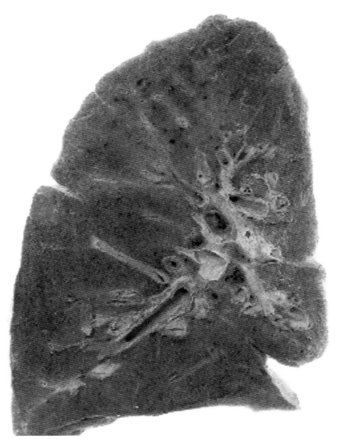

Figure 8.1.3 'Brown induration' representing a combination of haemosiderosis and interstitial fibrosis due to chronic pulmonary congestion and oedema in a patient with long-standing left-sided cardiac failure. Paper-mounted whole lung section. (Illustration provided by WGJ Edwards, London, UK.)

to upper zones of the lungs. The latter may be a direct effect of raised venous pressure on vessels that are normally at lower than alveolar pressure and therefore collapsed, or it may be a consequence of the vascular remodelling seen at the lung bases in pulmonary venous hypertension (described on p. 427).

Clinical features
Breathlessness is an early feature of pulmonary oedema, encountered when the process is still interstitial because of stimulation of the juxtacapillary nociceptors.[6,7] With the onset of alveolar oedema crepitations are heard on auscultation and in severe cases watery sputum is produced, sometimes tinged by blood and the patient is cyanosed and hypoxaemic. It is often essential to maintain cerebral oxygenation by augmenting the concentration of inspired oxygen despite the deleterious effect this may have on an already injured lung. Patients in left ventricular failure are prone to attacks of severe breathlessness when recumbent, typically at night. This is aptly termed paroxysmal nocturnal dyspnoea but is often still referred to by the older term cardiac asthma. The distinction from bronchial asthma (see p. 106) may be blurred by oedematous swelling of the bronchial wall causing the patient to wheeze.

PULMONARY THROMBOSIS AND THROMBOEMBOLISM

Pulmonary *thrombosis*, as distinct from thromboembolism, is seldom symptomatic in the absence of other pulmonary vascular disease. It is most commonly encountered as a complication of pulmonary hypertension of any cause and then confounds the histological distinction of thromboembolic pulmonary hypertension from that due to other causes, in particular the primary variety. It is necessary therefore to search for the specific histological features of the other varieties of pulmonary hypertension (dealt with in Chapter 8.2) whenever pulmonary thrombosis is recognised. Although atheroma is a feature of pulmonary hypertension (see Fig. 8.2.17),[50] it is generally confined to the large elastic pulmonary arteries and seldom attains the advanced, ulcerated degree that predisposes to aortic thrombosis. Thrombosis complicating pulmonary hypertension probably commences in the smaller muscular pulmonary arteries, which narrow in this condition.

As well as complicating pulmonary hypertension, pulmonary thrombosis and infarction also develop in systemic lupus erythematosus,[51] sickle cell disease,[52–56] spherocytosis,[57] thallasaemia,[58,59] paroxysmal nocturnal haemoglobinuria,[60] the antiphospholipid antibody syndrome,[51,61] the hypereosinophilic syndrome,[62,63] rare varieties of pulmonary vasculitis that affect the large elastic arteries,[64,65] and unusual varieties of vascular infection.[66] Pulmonary thrombosis is also predisposed to by low blood flow, as in congenital anomalies such as pulmonary stenosis and in pulmonary aneurysms.

Thromboembolism

Aetiology
Pulmonary thromboembolism is rare in the Third World but common in developed countries.[67] Economic development in Hong Kong has been accompanied by an increasing incidence of the disease[68,69] and in the USA, the incidence of pulmonary thromboembolism among non-whites is much the same as in whites.[70]

In western countries, thrombotic pulmonary emboli, often unsuspected in life, are commonly encountered at necropsy, especially in elderly and obese people who have been confined to bed with congestive cardiac failure and in adults of any age who have undergone major surgery, suffer from cancer or have been the victims of major trauma.[71–76] They develop in people who sleep in chairs that hinder venous return from the legs (e.g. deck chairs) and especially in air-travellers who are immobile for a long time. Nearly half prove fatal.[77] Pulmonary embolism is also prone to occur after childbirth. Contributing factors are listed in Box 8.1.1.[73,77–80] They operate in three ways, as described by Virchow in his well-known triad:

- by promoting blood stasis
- by damaging vascular endothelium
- by activating coagulation factors.

Table 8.1.1   Deaths from pulmonary embolism per million population by age and sex: England and Wales, 1988[82]

Age (years)	All ages	<45	45–54	55–64	65–74	75–84	>84
Men	20	0	5	16	67	210	461
Women	33	1	4	12	61	218	497

Box 8.1.1 Factors contributing to pulmonary thromboembolism[61,73,76–79]

Advancing age
Female sex
Obesity
Immobility
Congestive cardiac failure
Malignant disease
Trauma
Surgery
Childbirth
Haemoconcentration
Polycythaemia
Disseminated intravascular coagulation
Antiphospholipid antibody syndrome
High oestrogen contraceptive pills
Central venous cannulation
Cold weather

Table 8.1.2   Deaths from pulmonary embolism by season[a]

Season	Deaths (n)
January–March	2898
April–June	2651
July–September	2646
October–December	2893

[a]11 088 cases assembled from 23 reports from the Northern hemisphere.[85]

Table 8.1.3   Incidence of pulmonary embolism[a] according to the site of leg vein thrombosis[b,87]

Site	Pulmonary embolism
Calf vein thrombosis	0/21 patients
Calf and thigh vein thrombosis	8/15 patients

[a]Detected by lung perfusion and ventilation scans.
[b]Detected by venography, impedance plethysmography and radiofibrinogen leg scanning.

Thrombosis after operations and childbirth is promoted by the increased numbers of platelets that accompany any form of trauma. It often occurs in tributaries of the main veins of the legs and thighs, where the vascular stasis that follows immobilisation is known to be most pronounced. Puerperal thromboembolism is more frequent in women whose lactation has been suppressed by the administration of oestrogens than among those who breastfeed and in line with this it is known that the older high-oestrogen contraceptive pill carried a small risk of promoting thromboembolism by affecting the clotting factors VII and X and platelet aggregation. This risk is believed to be almost non-existent with the present low-oestrogen contraceptive pills. However, hypercoagulability is fairly prevalent in the general population and presumably augments the other factors contributing to thrombosis listed in Box 8.1.1. It can be recognised in 25% of patients with venous thromboembolism and in an even higher number of patients whose thrombosis is otherwise unexplained. High levels of factors VIII and XI are fairly common in the general population (each have a prevalence of about 10%) but abnormalities in the levels of many other clotting factors are also recognised.[81]

Despite the dangers of childbirth and oral contraception, the standardised mortality rate from thromboembolism is roughly the same for men and women, the increased risk of major trauma in young male adults balancing the risks special to women. However, the crude death rate from thromboembolism is much greater in women than in men[82] because of the marked effect of advancing age on the incidence of thromboembolism and the greater number of elderly women in the population (Table 8.1.1). There is also a significant but relatively minor seasonal variation in the incidence of pulmonary thromboembolism, the risk being greater in the colder months (Table 8.1.2).[83–86]

It is when calf vein thrombi propagate proximally to reach the main veins of the thigh that they are most likely to break off and reach the lungs as emboli (Table 8.1.3).[87] Proximal propagation is encountered in approximately 20% of patients with calf vein thrombosis and approximately 50% of those with proximal leg vein thrombosis develop pulmonary embolism.[88] Residual deep vein thrombosis can be demonstrated in most patients who have recently suffered pulmonary embolism.[89] The danger of leg vein thrombosis and embolism is lessened by the use of prophylactic massage and exercise. Treatment is mainly based on anticoagulation but may involve venous ligation proximal to the thrombus and thromboembolectomy. Leg vein thrombosis is nearly always bilateral and this should be kept in mind when ligation is being considered. Approximately 11% of patients with pulmonary thromboembolism die within one hour and only 29% of the remainder are correctly diagnosed and treated appropriately, which is unfortunate as there are ten times as many deaths in the undiagnosed and untreated majority (Fig. 8.1.4).[72]

The periprostatic venous plexus is another source of pulmonary emboli, particularly multiple small emboli. Thrombosis here is promoted by local inflammation as well as by sluggish venous flow as in heart failure. Less often, thrombotic emboli originate in the veins of the arms or in the chambers on

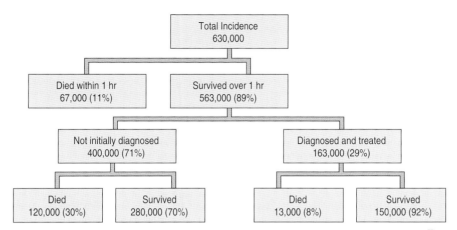

Figure 8.1.4 Annual incidence and survival in pulmonary thromboembolism in the USA.[72]

the right side of the heart. Other sources include intravenous cannulae and endocarditis affecting the valves on the right side of the heart. In one study 86% of thrombotic emboli reached the lungs via the inferior vena cava, 3% came via the superior vena cava, 3% originated in the heart and in 8% of cases the thrombosis was widespread.[80]

Clinical features

Sometimes the embolus is a massive one and its lodgement in the pulmonary trunk or main pulmonary artery is immediately fatal because it obstructs the pulmonary circulation. In only 28% of such cases is a diagnosis of pulmonary thromboembolism made before death.[80] More frequently, the embolus is small and without significant effect. Multiple microemboli as a cause of pulmonary hypertension is considered on p. 426.

The high prevalence of unsuspected pulmonary thromboembolism evident at autopsy has been demonstrated in life with perfusion scans, emphasising that once a diagnosis of peripheral venous thrombosis has been established, anticoagulant therapy should be instituted without delay.[90] Thromboendarterectomy is being increasingly undertaken.[91] Infarction is indicated clinically by an attack of localised pleural pain, dyspnoea and haemoptysis. Often there is more than one embolic episode and at necropsy infarcts of different ages are found.

Distribution of the emboli

When clots are introduced into a rabbit's systemic vein, both the size of the clots and the anatomy of the pulmonary arterial tree affect their subsequent distribution in the lungs.[92] While large emboli lodge in any of the main arteries, those of medium size are carried disproportionately often into the vessels of the posterior basal segments. In man, pulmonary infarcts are commoner in the posterior basal segments of the lower lobes[80] and solitary metastatic tumours are more frequently basal than apical. The explanation lies in the anatomy of the pulmonary arteries: they have a large axial trunk that gives off its branches at an angle and terminates in the posterior basal segment.

Pathological findings

The sudden impaction of a large embolus in the main pulmonary artery brings the circulation virtually to a halt. The small volume of blood that can percolate past the thrombotic mass is quite insufficient to fill the left side of the heart and maintain normal systemic arterial pressure and an adequate circulation through the cerebral and coronary arteries. In such cases, the embolus is found at necropsy to be coiled on itself, straddling the bifurcation of the pulmonary trunk (Fig. 8.1.5). The chambers of the right side of the heart and the venae cavae are distended, the left atrium and ventricle contracted and the lungs pale. The coiling distinguishes embolic thrombi from thrombi that have formed in the pulmonary arteries. When the

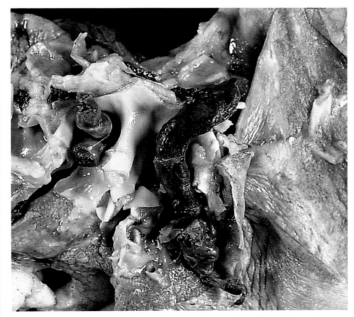

Figure 8.1.5 Massive pulmonary thromboembolism. Coiled thrombus occludes the pulmonary trunk and the main pulmonary arteries. (Illustration provided by Dr GA Russell, Tunbridge Wells, UK.)

embolus is removed from its site of impaction and is uncoiled it is seen to be of a diameter that corresponds to the calibre of the vessels in which it formed. Its surface is marked in correspondence with the venous valves: the broken ends of the thrombotic cast of the tributary veins can also be recognised and it may be possible to match these with the thrombus remaining in the veins.

Both thrombi formed *in situ* and thrombotic emboli are firm but friable and show striae of Zahn, which are evident naked-eye and indicative of their development during life (Fig. 8.1.6): these features distinguish them from clots, which are formed post mortem. Clots are shiny, soft and elastic: when pulled carefully from the vessels they show a characteristic 'horse's tail' appearance, their end being a cast of blood from the smaller branches of the pulmonary artery. Clots may show a transition from red to yellow, due to post mortem sedimentation of the cellular constituents of the stagnant blood, leaving a paler zone of serum in the eventual coagulum. This demarcation lacks the

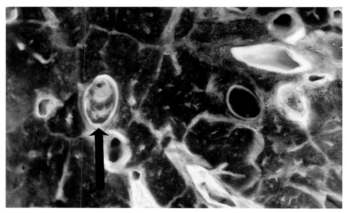

(a)

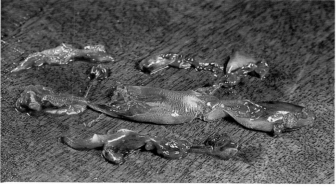

(b)

Figure 8.1.6 Thrombotic emboli showing the striae of Zahn. The striae represent successive layers of platelets and fibrin-enmeshed blood cells, indicating that the material was formed in life and therefore represents thrombus rather than clot. (a) Thrombus showing the striae is seen in pulmonary arteries on the cut surface of the lung (note that the post-mortem clot to the right lacks the striae). (b) Thrombus removed from the lung again shows the striae (centre).

alternate white and red layers formed respectively of platelets and fibrin-enmeshed blood cells that characterise the striae of Zahn in a thrombus.

Fresh thrombus may fragment and disperse into smaller pulmonary arteries, of which there is a great reserve, but within a few days thrombotic emboli undergo organisation and become firmly adherent to the vessel wall. In four to six weeks they are converted into fibrous tissue, often with recanalisation. Some emboli seem to disappear and it is presumed that they are destroyed by fibrinolysin. Thin fibrous bands stretching across the lumen of major pulmonary arteries are sometimes the only evidence of previous thromboembolism (Fig. 8.1.7a).[93] More often, the lumen of smaller arteries is divided up into multiple channels by the usual process of recanalisation (Fig. 8.1.7b).[94]

Pulmonary infarction

Like other infarcts, those in the lungs are generally wedge-shaped. An occluded pulmonary artery is found at the apex of the infarct; the base of the infarct is on the pleura. Often the edge of a lobe is involved, in which case the lesion is diamond-shaped rather than wedge-shaped (Fig. 8.1.8). Any part of the lung may be affected but infarction is commonest at the bases for the reasons explained above. Pulmonary infarcts are commonly multiple.

Partial and complete infarction

Completely infarcted tissue is beyond recovery and healing is only possible by repair (rather than by resolution), culminating in a fibrous scar. This is the situation in only a minority of pulmonary infarcts: most resolve completely, indicating that the lung tissue is not damaged irretrievably. The infarction is only partial. Frequently the lung escapes even this state of partial devitalization, despite complete obstruction of a pulmonary artery. The explanation for this is the dual blood supply to the lung and the lung's independence of the bloodstream for oxygen. True infarction is therefore rare and to produce even a partial infarct some factor other than failure of the pulmonary arterial supply is required. This factor is frequently a cardiac condition compromising the bronchial arterial supply. Although bronchial arteries normally supply little blood to peripheral lung tissue, they are capable of supplying more should the pulmonary artery supply fail. A common clinical setting for pulmonary infarction is the patient confined to bed with heart failure. This promotes thromboembolism and at the same time compromises the bronchial arterial supply. Pulmonary infarction is very rare in the absence of passive pulmonary venous congestion.

Partial infarcts are initially characterised by oedema but within 48 h, capillaries rupture and the resultant lesions are intensely haemorrhagic, swollen, firm and dark red (Fig. 8.1.8). The edge is sharply demarcated. Acute inflammation develops where infarcts border healthy lung and fibrin is found on the

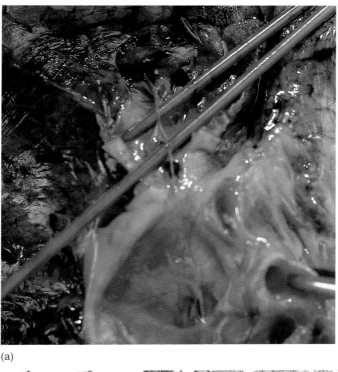

(a)

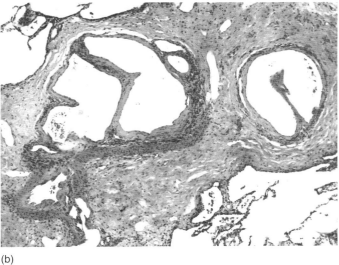

(b)

Figure 8.1.7 (a) Thin fibrous bands stretching across the lumen of pulmonary arteries may be the only remains of organised thrombotic emboli. (b) These are seen as intraluminal fibrous strands on microscopy.

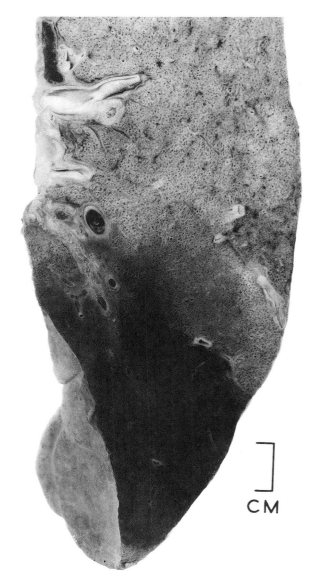

Figure 8.1.8 Recent infarct of lung. The dark area is infarcted lung in which the airspaces have become filled with blood. Just above the lesion can be seen the supplying pulmonary artery occluded by thrombus. (Reproduced with permission of the Curator of the Gordon Museum, Guy's Hospital, London, UK; photograph by Miss P Turnbull, Charing Cross Hospital and Medical School, London.)

pleural surface of the involved area. Microscopically, the alveoli are filled with blood. Their walls are intact however and the basic architecture of the tissue is unaltered. Complete and rapid resolution is frequently observed radiologically and should the patient then die, perhaps of a further massive embolism, no abnormality other than haemosiderin-laden macrophages can be detected in the recently infarcted area. Less often, necrosis is found, signifying true infarction. Healing is then by organisation, which is marked by slow paling and shrinkage,

until eventually only a barely detectable scar remains. As with most scars in organs that are subject to constant movement, such as the lung and the heart, they are rich in elastin.[95]

If the embolus is infected, as may happen with abdominal sepsis, infected venous cannulae or bacterial endocarditis affecting the valves on the right side of the heart, septic infarction is likely. Suppuration soon causes this to resemble any other lung abscess. A few initially sterile lung infarcts become abscesses by colonisation of the devitalised tissue by airborne bacteria.

Pulmonary venous infarction

In contrast to the infarcts caused by pulmonary artery occlusion, pulmonary venous infarction is very rare. This is attributable to the rich network of venous collateral vessels that drain the lung. Most of the few reported cases have been due to sclerosing mediastinitis. Other recorded causes include left atrial myxoma, left atrial thrombosis complicating mitral stenosis, venous thrombosis following pulmonary resection and carcinoma of the lung.[96,97] The infarcts are similar to those caused by arterial occlusion. Chronic venous obstruction, as seen in pulmonary veno-occlusive disease (see p. 427) may result in interstitial fibrosis. These areas of scarring are rich in haemosiderin and possibly represent healed venous infarcts.

NON-THROMBOTIC PULMONARY EMBOLI

Pulmonary embolism may result from various kinds of material forming in, or gaining access to, the systemic veins. Apart from thrombi, these include fat droplets, various types of tissue, clumps of tumour cells, gas bubbles and a variety of foreign substances. In some parts of the world parasitic emboli are important: these include the eggs of schistosomes (p. 252) and the adult form of the canine heart worm *Dirofilaria immitis* (p. 257).

Fat embolism

Fat embolism is usually the result of bone or soft tissue trauma,[98,99] but occasionally liposuction[100] or bone marrow infarction complicating haemoglobinopathy is the cause.[101] Under these circumstances, fat globules from the bone marrow or soft tissues enter the systemic veins and reach the lungs. Small fat globules can almost always be demonstrated in pulmonary capillaries after any fracture if frozen sections are stained appropriately and only a small proportion of patients develop symptoms referable to the embolism.

The classic fat embolism syndrome consists of hypoxaemia, cerebral disturbance, tachycardia and a petechial rash, which is typically maximal over the front of the chest. The hypoxaemia is attributed to the emboli blocking pulmonary capillaries and causing pulmonary arteriovenous anastomoses to open so that venous blood bypasses the lungs. The extrapulmonary symptoms are attributed to emboli that have similarly bypassed the pulmonary capillaries to occlude small systemic arteries. The presence or absence of lesions is determined by the extent of vascular anastomoses in the organ concerned and the relative susceptibility of the tissue to oxygen lack. For these reasons, the brain is particularly affected, showing petechial haemorrhages in the white matter. However, the kidney is the best organ in which to identify systemic fat embolism microscopically because it filters the blood and the fat accumulates in the glomeruli.

Some patients with fat embolism develop severe respiratory failure. This is seldom due to extensive occlusion of the pulmonary circulation. More often it is caused by traumatic shock, which has its own profound effects on the lungs (see p. 138). It has been suggested that release of irritant fatty acids in the course of lysis of neutral fat is responsible for the changes in the lungs[102,103] but the lack of an inflammatory reaction to the fat and experimental evidence[104–106] provide no support for lysis of neutral fat playing an important role in the development of the pulmonary changes.

Microembolism of agglutinated fat emulsions[99,107,108] or of crystals derived from infusions during the course of total parenteral nutrition[109] is described on p. 391.

Amniotic fluid embolism

Occasionally, during childbirth, amniotic fluid with its content of particulate debris, mostly epidermal squames and meconium, is forced by strong uterine contractions into the maternal circulation through small incomplete lower uterine tears. These particles may lead to fatal microembolism of the mother's small pulmonary arteries.[110] Recognition of their content of meconium mucus and epidermal squames is facilitated by the use of the combined Alcian blue/phloxine tartrazine stain.[111] Globules of vernix caseosa may also be demonstrated in frozen sections with fat stains. More sophisticated methods of confirming the diagnosis include the immunohistochemical identification of amniotic mucins[112] and of fetal isoantigen A in maternal tissues of B blood type.[113] Amniotic fluid embolism may be accompanied by disseminated intravascular coagulation, so that fibrin may also be demonstrable in the pulmonary capillaries. The emboli may be so sparse, even in fatal cases, that death is possibly due to shock rather than pulmonary vascular occlusion.

Trophoblastic embolism

Fragments of trophoblastic tissue may be found in the lungs in a large proportion of women who die during pregnancy or the puerperium.[114] The incidence is particularly high in cases of eclampsia, probably due to mechanical rather than metabolic factors. The trophoblastic tissue is recognisable as isolated multinucleated syncytiotrophoblastic cells within pulmonary blood vessels (Fig. 8.1.9). Chorionic villi are rarely observed. Immunocytochemical demonstration of human chorionic gonadotrophin helps in the identification of the trophoblast. It is believed that uterine contractions during pregnancy and especially those accompanying labour, dislodge the trophoblastic tissue and enable it to enter the bloodstream. The trophoblastic emboli cause no structural changes in the lung and appear to be immunologically inert, in spite of their fetal origin; they do not predispose to thrombosis and usually undergo early lysis.[114]

In exceptional cases of benign hydatidiform mole, it has been noted radiologically that masses within the lungs may persist for up to a year, but regress and totally disappear thereafter;[115] they presumably represent trophoblastic emboli that have gained a temporary foothold in the lungs.

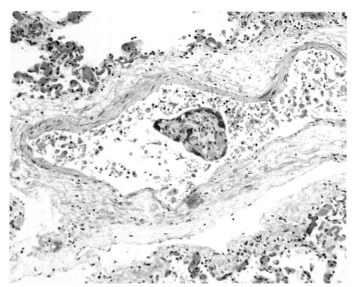

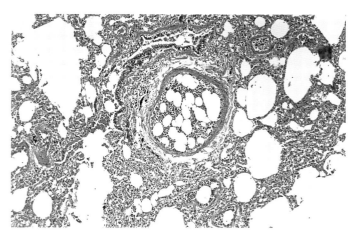

Figure 8.1.10   Bone marrow embolism incurred as a terminal event during unsuccessful attempts at cardiac massage in which ribs were fractured.

Figure 8.1.9   Trophoblast embolism. The trophoblast is recognisable as a clump of multinucleated syncytiotrophoblastic cells within a pulmonary artery.

Decidual embolism

Small foci of decidua are occasionally observed in the lungs in pregnancy. Such foci located immediately beneath the pleura[116] may represent focal metaplasia of the overlying serosa but deep in the lung an embolic aetiology is generally assumed although the decidual tissue is usually extravascular. The nature of pulmonary decidua is discussed further under the subject of pleuro-pulmonary endometriosis (see p. 494).

Tumour embolism

Tumour emboli are common in the lungs. A few survive to form metastatic deposits but most die very soon after arriving in the lungs; the embolus then becomes enclosed by platelets and finally undergoes organisation.[117] Vascular occlusion by tumour emboli is sometimes so widespread that it leads to right-sided heart failure,[118–124] while massive tumour emboli have sometimes proved fatal[125–127] or necessitated emergency embolectomy.[128] In other patients they have caused flitting radiographic opacities, which presumably represent infarcts.[129] Occlusion of the pulmonary arteries may be due to tumour alone or the tumour may promote thrombosis, organisation of which results in fibrocellular intimal thickening, so-called microscopic tumour angiopathy, carcinomatous arteriopathy or carcinomatous endarteritis (see p. 671).[130–133]

Other tissue embolism

Bone marrow is frequently seen plugging small pulmonary arteries post mortem when ribs have been broken during unsuccessful attempts at cardiac resuscitation or following trauma to other bones (Fig. 8.1.10). Other traumatic emboli may consist of brain tissue,[134,135] liver tissue,[136] bile,[137] bone fragments (Fig.

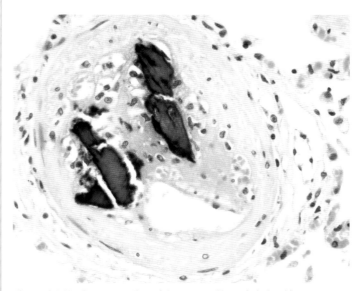

Figure 8.1.11   Bone embolism. A fragment of bone is lodged in a pulmonary artery after failed resuscitation.

8.1.11) or very rarely atheromatous cholesterol crystals.[138] Haemorrhage has been ascribed to the last of these but none of the others is of clinical consequence; they merely represent incidental necropsy findings.

Foreign body embolism

Some drug addicts break up preparations of drugs intended for oral use and inject an aqueous suspension intravenously. Substances used as fillers in the manufacture of tablets include starch, cellulose and talc. When injected intravenously, these lodge in pulmonary vessels and induce thrombosis and a local foreign body granulomatous reaction (Fig. 8.1.12).[139–146] Pulmonary hypertension may result if the injury to the vessels is extensive.[139] Widespread pulmonary fibrosis may also develop,

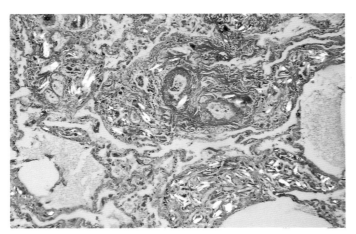

Figure 8.1.12 Drug addict's lung viewed with partially polarised light showing a granulomatous response to numerous birefringent plate-like talc crystals. Although reaching the lungs by the pulmonary arteries, the crystals work their way through the vessel walls and eventually become widely distributed in the lungs.

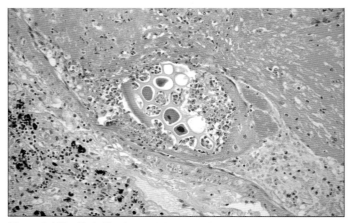

Figure 8.1.13 Embolised vegetable matter is present within a pulmonary artery in a patient who died of a ruptured oesophagus. (Case of Dr CA Seldenrijk, Nieuwegein, The Netherlands.)

occasionally mimicking pneumoconiotic progressive massive fibrosis.[147] Starch particles can be identified by their characteristic Maltese cross appearance on polarising microscopy and talc by its platy form on polarising microscopy and by elemental electron microprobe analysis.[147] Cellulose fibres can be distinguished from platy crystals such as talc by their reaction with periodic acid Schiff, silver methenamine and Congo red stains.[144,148] The particles leave the blood vessels and may be found in the interstitial tissues and even airspaces. Talc particles in the lung exceeding 5 μm in length should arouse suspicion of intravenous drug abuse,[149] but cellulose fibres up to 120 μm in length may reach the lungs and cause granulomatosis in addicts who inhale their illicit drugs.[148,150]

Other embolic foreign bodies described in pulmonary arteries include air gun pellets,[151] shrapnel, whole bullets,[152] masonry and stone fragments, food particles (Fig. 8.1.13), the broken-off ends of intravenous catheters and cannulas, plastic particles from dialysis tubing,[153] therapeutic injections or prosthetic implants of substances such as Teflon and silicone,[154–158] lymphangiography contrast medium,[159–162] various materials injected to occlude abnormal blood vessels,[163] and mercury, this last generally introduced into the circulation with suicidal intent.[164] Patients with psychiatric problems have also injected themselves with various other substances, such as olive oil, this resulting in pulmonary lipogranulomatosis.[165]

Bronchial, as opposed to pulmonary artery embolisation is sometimes carried out therapeutically in an attempt to stem intractable haemorrhage from lesions that are difficult to resect, such as an aspergilloma.[166] The same technique is used on occasion to induce infarction of neoplasms. It involves the cannulation of bronchial arteries via a femoral artery and the aorta. Bronchial arteries are chosen because aspergillomas and tumours derive their blood supply from these systemic vessels, as is the case with most pulmonary disease. If the procedure fails to stem the haemorrhage and surgery is resorted to, or the patient dies, the pathologist may be asked to confirm that the bronchial arteries do contain the injected material. This is usually a synthetic foam and is easily recognised as such (Fig. 8.1.14), but Verhoeff–van Gieson staining is recommended as a means of facilitating its recognition.[167]

Air embolism

Venous air embolism may occur whenever a vein above the level of the heart is opened and exposed to the atmosphere, for example during operations on the head and neck or pelvic operations in which the patient is put in the Trendelenburg position.

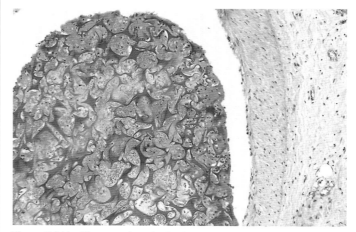

Figure 8.1.14 Therapeutic embolisation with foam introduced by percutaneous cannulation of the bronchial arteries in an unsuccessful attempt to stem haemorrhage into an aspergilloma cavity.

Air may also enter veins during peritoneal insufflation at laparoscopy or be inadvertently injected under pressure during urgent transfusions. Central venous cannulation carries a high risk of air embolism. Air embolism also occurs when the lungs burst due to dramatic changes in atmospheric pressure (see p. 370) or there is severe chest trauma. Systemic air embolism occurs most frequently during open heart surgery but may also develop after chest trauma or as a sequel to venous air embolism in patients with an arteriovenous shunt (paradoxical air embolism). It is also recorded in an aeroplane passenger who had a large intrapulmonary cyst.[168]

Following venous air embolism, the fine bubbles into which the air is churned during its passage through the heart are carried into the pulmonary arteries. The cause of death is generally acute heart failure and the embolism is recognised by a frothy mixture of air and blood filling the chambers of the right side of the heart and pulmonary trunk. The volume of air needed to produce fatal air embolism in this way may be 100–200 ml or more, but a few millilitres may prove fatal through obstruction of small vessels in the brain stem. More rarely, air embolism results in pulmonary oedema.[169]

PULMONARY ANEURYSMS

An aneurysm is defined as a localised vascular dilatation but the term is usually confined to arterial dilatations. Localised venous dilatations are generally termed varices. Both are rare in the pulmonary circulation. Either may be saccular or fusiform.

Historically, most pulmonary aneurysms have been syphilitic or tuberculous but these causes are now very rare. Today, various other causes are recognised but sometimes no cause can be identified (Table 8.1.4, Fig. 8.1.15).[170–172] The basic fault in all aneurysms is a localised defect in the arterial media.

Table 8.1.4   Causes of pulmonary artery aneurysms[170]
Congenital
with arteriovenous communication
Isolated
As part of hereditary haemorrhagic telangiectasia
Without arteriovenous communication
Vasculitic
Infective
Syphilitic
Tuberculous
'Mycotic' (from septic emboli)
Non-infective
Behçet's syndrome
Hughes–Stovin syndrome
Hypertensive
Traumatic
Idiopathic[171,172]

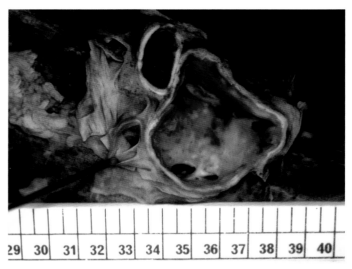

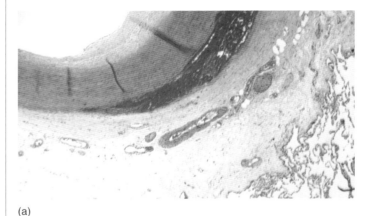

Figure 8.1.15   Idiopathic aneurysm of the pulmonary artery. The patient died of respiratory failure secondary to scoliosis, which was also idiopathic.

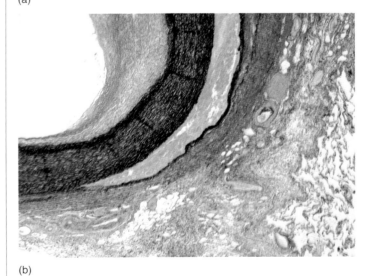

(a)

(b)

Figure 8.1.16   Dissection of a systemic artery supplying a pulmonary sequestration. (a) Haematoxylin and eosin stain, (b) elastin van Gieson stain.

Most are dealt with elsewhere: arteriovenous on p. 74; infective on p. 437; Behçet's syndrome and Hughes-Stovin syndromes on pp. 448, 479 and hypertensive on p. 431. Traumatic aneurysms may be true or false, the latter representing a haematoma alongside and communicating with the parent artery through a complete defect in the vessel wall but walled off externally by a fibrous capsule. Dissecting aneurysms have also been reported in pulmonary arteries, usually complicating pulmonary hypertension.[173,174] They may also be encountered in a systemic vessel supplying an extralobar sequestration (Fig. 8.1.16).

Pulmonary varix

A pulmonary varix is a localised dilatation of a pulmonary vein (Fig. 8.1.17).[175] Apart from rare examples that bleed, sometimes with fatal results, the condition is discovered incidentally at autopsy or by radiography.[176] In many cases the varix is assumed to represent a congenital anomaly or to develop postnatally because of a congenital defect in the vein wall. A substantial number of pulmonary varices, perhaps half, are secondary to mitral valve regurgitation.[177] Rarely, they are found in association with end-stage liver disease.[176]

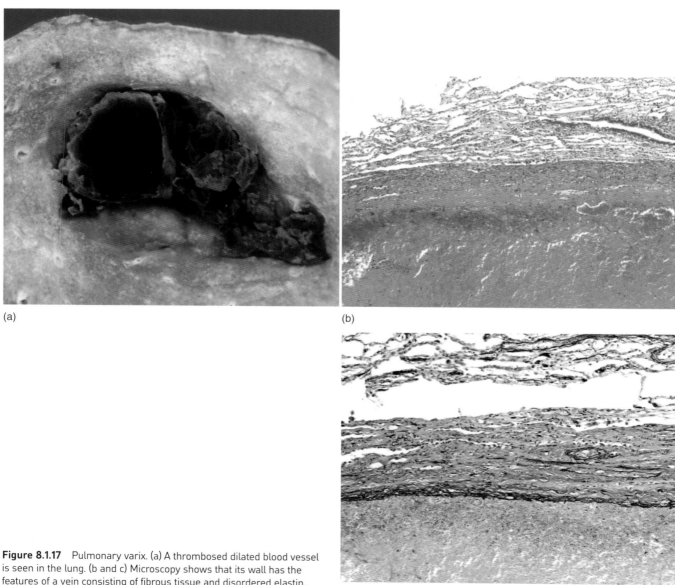

(a)

(b)

(c)

Figure 8.1.17 Pulmonary varix. (a) A thrombosed dilated blood vessel is seen in the lung. (b and c) Microscopy shows that its wall has the features of a vein consisting of fibrous tissue and disordered elastin. (c) Elastin van Gieson stain.

REFERENCES

Pulmonary congestion and oedema

1. Schneeberger-Keeley EE, Karnovsky MJ. The ultrastructural basis of alveolar-capillary membrane permeability to peroxidase used as a tracer. J Cell Biol 1968; 37:781–793.

2. Weibel ER, Bachofen H. Structural design of the alveolar septum and fluid exchange. In: Fishman ARE, ed. Pulmonary Edema. Baltimore: Williams and Wilkins; 1979:1–20.

3. Michel RP, Meterissian S, Poulsen RS. Morphometry of the distribution of hydrostatic pulmonary oedema in dogs. Br J Exp Pathol 1986; 67:865–877.

4. Staub NC, Nagano H, Pearce ML. Pulmonary edema in dogs, especially the sequence of fluid accumulation in lungs. J Appl Physiol 1967; 22:227–240.

5. Staub NC. The pathophysiology of pulmonary edema. Hum Pathol 1970; 1:419–432.

6. Spencer H, Leof D. The innervation of the human lung. J Anat 1964; 98:599–609.

7. Fox B, Bull TB, Guz A. Innervation of alveolar walls in the human lung: an electron microscopical study. J Anat 1980; 131:683–692.

8. Vijeyaratnam GS, Corrin B. Fine structural alterations in the lungs of iprindole-treated rats. J Pathol 1974; 114:233–239.

9. Kay JM, Edwards FR. Ultrastructure of the alveolar-capillary wall in mitral stenosis. J Pathol 1973; 111:239–245.

10. Pietra GG, Szidon JP, Leventhal MM, Fishman AP. Hemoglobin as a tracer in hemodynamic pulmonary edema. Science 1969; 166:1643–1646.

11. Schneeberger EE, Karnovsky MJ. The influence of intravascular fluid volume on the permeability of newborn and adult mouse lungs to ultrastructural protein tracers. J Cell Biol 1971; 49:319–334.

12. West JB, Mathieu-Costello O. Stress failure of pulmonary capillaries - role in lung and heart disease. Lancet 1992; 340:762–767.

13. Bachofen H, Schurch S, Michel RP, Weibel ER. Experimental hydrostatic pulmonary edema in rabbit lungs – morphology. Am Rev Respir Dis 1993; 147:989–996.

14. Bachofen H, Schurch S, Weibel ER. Experimental hydrostatic pulmonary edema in rabbit lungs – barrier lesions. Am Rev Respir Dis 1993; 147:997–1004.

15. Mathieu-Costello OA, West JB. Are pulmonary capillaries susceptible to mechanical stress? Chest 1994; 105;S102–S107.

16. Wu DXY, Weibel ER, Bachofen H, Schurch S. Lung lesions in experimental hydrostatic pulmonary edema: an electron microscopic and morphometric study. Exp Lung Res 1995; 21:711–730.

17. O'Callaghan MW, Pascoe JR, Tyler WS, Mason DK. Exercise-induced pulmonary haemorrhage in the horse: results of a detailed clinical, post mortem and imaging study. VIII. Conclusions and implications. Equine Vet J 1987; 19:428–434.

18. Weiler-Ravell D, Shupak A, Goldenberg I, et al. Pulmonary oedema and haemoptysis induced by strenuous swimming. BMJ 1995; 311:361–362.

19. Waller DA, Saunders NR. Unilateral pulmonary oedema following the removal of a giant pleural tumour. Thorax 1989; 44:682–683.

20. Boykett M. Pulmonary oedema after acute asphyxia in a child. BMJ 1989; 298:928.

21. Plopper CG, Dungworth DL, Tyler WS. Pulmonary lesions in rats exposed to ozone. Am J Pathol 1973; 71:375–394.

22. Kapanci Y, Weibel ER, Kaplan HP, Robinson FR. Pathogenesis and reversibility of the pulmonary lesions of oxygen toxicity in monkeys. II Ultrastructural and morphometric studies. Lab Invest 1969; 20:101–118.

23. Gould VE, Tosco R, Wheelis RF, Gould NF, Kapanci Y. Oxygen pneumonitis in man. Ultrastructural observations on the development of the alveolar lesions. Lab Invest 1972; 26:499–508.

24. Pratt PC. Pathology of pulmonary oxygen toxicity. Am Rev Respir Dis 1974; 110(suppl):51–57.

25. Rocker GM, Morgan AG, Pearson D, Basran GS, Shale DJ. Pulmonary vascular permeability to transferrin in the pulmonary oedema of renal failure. Thorax 1987; 42:620–623.

26. Crosbie WA, Snowden S, Parsons V. Changes in lung capillary permeability in renal failure. BMJ 1972; 4:388–390.

27. Hackett PH, Creagh CE, Grover RF, et al. High altitude pulmonary edema in persons without the right pulmonary artery. N Engl J Med 1980; 302:1070–1073.

28. Fiorenzano G, Rastelli V, Greco V, Distefano A, Dottorini M. Unilateral high-altitude pulmonary edema in a subject with right pulmonary artery hypoplasia. Respiration 1994; 61:51–54.

29. Schoene RB, Hackett PH, Henderson WR, et al. High altitude pulmonary oedema; characteristics of lung lavage fluid. JAMA 1986; 256:63–69.

30. Heath D, Moosavi H, Smith P. Ultrastructure of high altitude pulmonary oedema. Thorax 1973; 28:694–700.

31. West JB, Colice GL, Lee YJ, et al. Pathogenesis of high-altitude pulmonary oedema: direct evidence of stress failure of pulmonary capillaries. Eur Respir J 1995; 8:523–529.

32. Bartsch P, Maggiorini M, Ritter M, Noti C, Vock P, Oelz O. Prevention of high-altitude pulmonary edema by nifedipine. N Engl J Med 1991; 325:1284–1289.

33. Reeves JT, Schoene RB. When lungs on mountains leak - studying pulmonary edema at high altitudes. N Engl J Med 1991; 325:1306–1307.

34. Scherrer U, Vollenweider L, Delabays A, et al. Inhaled nitric oxide for high-altitude pulmonary edema. N Engl J Med 1996; 334:624–629.

35. Wagenvoort CA, Wagenvoort N. Pulmonary veins in high-altitude residents: a morphometric study. Thorax 1982; 37:931–935.

36. Schraufnagel DE, Patel KR. Sphincters in pulmonary veins. An anatomic study in rats. Am Rev Respir Dis 1990; 141:721–726.

37. Editorial. Neurogenic pulmonary oedema. Lancet 1985; 1:1430–1431.

38. Wray NP, Nicotra MB. Pathogenesis of neurogenic pulmonary oedema. Am Rev Respir Dis 1978; 118:783–786.

39. Carlson RW, Schaeffer RC, Michaels SG, Weil MH. Pulmonary oedema following intracranial haemorrhage. Chest 1979; 75:731–734.

40. Katz S, Aberman A, Frand UI, Stein IM, Fulop M. Heroin pulmonary edema. Evidence for increased pulmonary capillary permeability. Am Rev Respir Dis 1972; 106; 472–474.

41. Humbert M, Maitre S, Capron F, Rain B, Musset D, Simonneau G. Pulmonary edema complicating continuous intravenous prostacyclin in pulmonary capillary hemangiomatosis. Am J Respir Crit Care Med 1998; 157:1681–1685.

42. Heard BE, Steiner RE, Herdan A, Gleason D. Oedema and fibrosis of the lungs in left ventricular failure. Br J Radiol 1968; 41:161–171.

43. Masson P, Riopelle JL, Martin P. Poumon rheumatismal. Ann Anat Path 1937; 14:359–382.

44. Spencer H. Interstitial pneumonia. Ann Rev Med 1967; 18:423–442.

45. Spencer H. Chronic interstitial pneumonia. In: Liebow AA, ed. The Lung International Academy of Pathology, Monograph No 8. Baltimore: Williams & Wilkins; 1967:134–150.

46. Eppinger H. Die Permeabilitatspathologie als die Lehre vom Krankheitsbeginn. Vienna: Springer; 1949.

47. Goyette EM, Farinacci CJ, Forsee JH, Blake HA. The clinicopathologic correlation of lung biopsies in mitral stenosis. Am Heart J 1954; 47:645–652.

48. Herrnheiser G, Hinson KFW. An anatomical explanation of the formation of butterfly shadows. Thorax 1954; 9:198–210.

49. Grainger RG. Interstitial pulmonary oedema and its radiological diagnosis. A sign of pulmonary venous and capillary hypertension. Br J Radiol 1958; 31:201–217.

Pulmonary thrombosis and thromboembolism

50. Moore GW, Smith RRL, Hutchins GM. Pulmonary artery atherosclerosis. Correlation with systemic atherosclerosis and hypertensive pulmonary vascular disease. Arch Pathol Lab Med 1982; 106:378–380.

51. Boey ML, Colaco CB, Gharavi AE, Elkon KB, Loizou S, Hughes GRV. Thrombosis in systemic lupus erythematosus: striking association with the presence of circulating lupus anticoagulant. BMJ 1983; 287:1021–1023.

52. Oppenehimer EH, Esterly JR. Pulmonary changes in sickle cell disease. Am Rev Respir Dis 1971; 103:858–859.

53. Collins FS, Orringer EP. Pulmonary hypertension and cor pulmonale in the sickle hemoglobinopathies. Am J Med 1982; 73:814–821.

54. Athanasou NA, Hatton C, McGee JO, Weatherall DJ. Vascular occlusion and infarction in sickle cell crisis and the sickle chest syndrome. J Clin Pathol 1985; 38:659–664.

55. Gray A, Anionwu EN, Davies SC, Brozovic M. Patterns of mortality in sickle cell disease in the United Kingdom. J Clin Pathol 1991; 44:459–463.

56. Weil JV, Castro O, Malik AB, Rodgers G, Bonds DR, Jacobs TP. Pathogenesis of lung disease in sickle hemoglobinopathies. Am Rev Respir Dis 1993; 148:249–256.

57. Verresen D, Debacker W, Vanmeerbeeck J, Neetens I, Vanmarck E, Vermeire P. Spherocytosis and pulmonary hypertension: coincidental occurrence or causal relationship? Eur Respir J 1991; 4:629–631.

58. Landing BH, Nadorra R, Hyman CB, Ortega JA. Pulmonary lesions of thalassemia major. Perspect Pediatr Pathol 1987; 11:82–96.

59. Landing BH, Nadorra R, Hyman CB, Ortega JA. Pulmonary lesions of thalassemia major. In: Rosenberg HS, Bernstein J, eds. Respiratory and Alimentary Tract Diseases, Vol. 11: Perspectives in Pediatric Pathology. Basel: Karger; 1987:82–96.

60. Heller PG, Grinberg AR, Lencioni M, Molina MM, Roncoroni AJ. Pulmonary hypertension in paroxysmal nocturnal hemoglobinuria. Chest 1992; 102:642–643.

61. Pilling J, Cutaia M. The antiphospholipid antibody syndrome – A vascular disease with pulmonary manifestations. Chest 1997; 112:1451–1453.

62. Chusid MJ, Dale DC, West BC, Wolff SM. The hypereosinophilic syndrome: analysis of fourteen cases with review of the literature. Medicine 1975; 54:1–27.

63. Weller PF, Bubley GJ. The idiopathic hypereosinophilic syndrome. Blood 1994; 83:2759–2779.

64. Wagenaar SS, Westermann CJJ, Corrin B. Giant cell arteritis limited to large elastic pulmonary arteries. Thorax 1981; 36:876–877.

65. Wagenaar SS, van den Bosch JMM, Westermann CJJ, Brechot JM, Bosman HG, Lie JT. Isolated granulomatous giant cell vasculitis of the pulmonary elastic arteries. Arch Pathol Lab Med 1986; 110:962–964.

66. Stermer E, Bassan H, Oliven A, Grishkan A, Boss Y. Massive thrombosis as a result of triple infestation of the pulmonary arterial circulation by ascaris, candida and mucor. Hum Pathol 1984; 15:996–1001.

67. Thomas WA, Davies JNP, O'Neal RM, Dimakulangan AA. Incidence of myocardial infarction correlated with venous and pulmonary thrombosis and embolism. A geographic study based on autopsies in Uganda, East Africa and St Louis, USA. Am J Cardiol 1960; 5:41–47.

68. Chau KY, Yuen ST, Ng THK, Ng WF. An autopsy study of pulmonary thromboembolism in Hong-Kong Chinese. Pathology 1991; 23:181–184.

69. Chan CW. Pulmonary thromboembolism in Hong-Kong Chinese. Pathology 1993; 25:99–100.

70. Lilienfeld DE, Chan E, Ehland J, Godbold JH, Landrigan PJ, Marsh G. Mortality from pulmonary embolism in the United States: 1962 to 1984. Chest 1990; 98:1067–1072.

71. Fleming HA, Bailey SM. Massive pulmonary embolism in healthy people. BMJ 1966; 1:1322–1326.

72. Dalen JE, Alpert JS. Natural history of pulmonary embolism. Prog Cardiovasc Dis 1975; 17:259–270.

73. Saeger W, Genzkow M. Venous thromboses and pulmonary embolisms in post-mortem series - probable causes by correlations of clinical data and basic diseases. Pathol Res Pract 1994; 190:394–399.

74. Geerts WH, Code KI, Jay RM, Chen EL, Szalai JP. A prospective study of venous thromboembolism after major trauma. N Engl J Med 1994; 331:1601–1606.

75. Baglin TP, White K, Charles A. Fatal pulmonary embolism in hospitalised medical patients. J Clin Pathol 1997; 50:609–610.

76. Alikhan R, Peters F, Wilmott R, Cohen AT. Fatal pulmonary embolism in hospitalised patients: a necropsy review. J Clin Pathol 2004; 57:1254–1257.

77. Diebold J, Lohrs U. Venous thrombosis and pulmonary embolism – a study of 5039 autopsies. Pathol Res Pract 1991; 187:260–266.

78. Connors AF Jr, Castele RJ, Farhat NZ, Tomashefski JF. Complication of right heart catherisation. Chest 1985; 88:567–572.

79. Katsumura Y, Ohtsubo KI. Incidence of pulmonary thromboembolism, infarction and haemorrhage in disseminated intravascular coagulation: a necroscopic analysis. Thorax 1995; 50:160–164.

80. Morpurgo M, Schmid C. The spectrum of pulmonary embolism. Chest 1995; 107:18S–20S.

81. Dalen JE. Pulmonary embolism: What have we learned since Virchow? Natural history, pathophysiology and diagnosis. Chest 2002; 122:1440–1456.

82. Office of Population Censuses and Surveys. Mortality Statistics: Cause 1988. London: HMSO; 1990.

83. Chau KY, Yuen ST, Wong MP. Seasonal variation in the necropsy incidence of pulmonary thromboembolism in Hong Kong. J Clin Pathol 1995; 48:578–579.

84. Chau KY, Yuen ST, Wong MP. Seasonal variation in the necropsy incidence of pulmonary thromboembolism – comment. J Clin Pathol 1995; 48:883.

85. Allan TM, Douglas AS. Seasonal variation in deep vein thrombosis. Fatal pulmonary embolism is increased in both autumn and winter. BMJ 1996; 312:1227.

86. Boulay F, Berthier F, Schoukroun G, Raybaut C, Gendreike Y, Blaive B. Seasonal variations in hospital admission for deep vein thrombosis and pulmonary embolism: analysis of discharge data.

87. Moser KM, LeMoine JR. Is embolic risk conditioned by location of deep venous thrombosis? Ann Intern Med 1981; 94:439–444.

88. Hull RD, Raskob GE, Hirsh J. Prophylaxis of venous thromboembolism: an overview. Chest 1986; 89:374S–383S.

89. Girard P, Musset D, Parent F, Maitre S, Phlippoteau C, Simonneau G. High prevalence of detectable deep venous thrombosis in patients with acute pulmonary embolism. Chest 1999; 116:903–908.

90. Huisman MV, Buller HR, ten Cate JW, et al. Unexpected high prevalence of silent pulmonary embolism in patients with deep venous thrombosis. Chest 1989; 95:498–502.

91. Blauwet LA, Edwards WD, Tazelaar HD, Mcgregor CGA. Surgical pathology of pulmonary thromboendarterectomy: A study of 54 cases from 1990 to 2001. Hum Pathol 2003; 34:1290–1298.

92. Pryce DM, Heard BE. The distribution of experimental pulmonary emboli in the rabbit. J Pathol Bacteriol 1956; 71:15–25.

93. Morrell MT, Dunnill MS. Fibrous bands in conducting pulmonary arteries. J Clin Pathol 1967; 20:139–144.

94. Wagenvoort CA. Pathology of pulmonary thromboembolism. Chest 1995; 107;S10–S17.

95. Castleman B. Healed pulmonary infarcts. Arch Pathol 1940; 30:130–142.

96. Williamson WA, Tronic BS, Levitan N, Webb-Johnson DC, Shahian DM, Ellis FH. Pulmonary venous infarction. Chest 1992; 102:937–940.

97. Williamson WA, Tronic BS, Levitan N, Webb-Johnson DC, Shahian DM, Ellis FH. Pulmonary venous infarction secondary to squamous cell carcinoma. Chest 1992; 102:950–952.

Non-thrombotic pulmonary emboli

98. Sevitt S. The role of fat embolism in causation and of oxygen toxicity in the lung pathology. In: Williams WG, Smith RE, eds. Trauma of the Chest. Bristol: John Wright; 1977:164–175.

99. Hulman G. The pathogenesis of fat embolism. J Pathol 1995; 176:3–9.

100. Laub DR, Jr, Laub DR. Fat embolism syndrome after liposuction: a case report and review of the literature. Ann Plast Surg 1990; 25:48–52.

101. Zaidi Y, Sivakumaran M, Graham C, Hutchinson RM. Fatal bone marrow embolism in a patient with sickle cell beta⁺ thalassaemia. J Clin Pathol 1996; 49:774–775.

102. Moylan JA, Birnbaum M, Katz A, Ederson MA. Fat emboli syndrome. J Trauma 1976; 16:341–347.

103. Asnis DS, Saltzman HP, Melchert A. Shark oil pneumonia – an overlooked entity. Chest 1993; 103:976–977.

104. Reidbord HE. Pulmonary fat embolism. An ultrastructural study. Arch Pathol 1974; 98:122–125.

105. Derks CM, Derks DJ. Embolic pneumopathy induced by oleic acid. Am J Pathol 1977; 87:143–158.

106. Jacobovitz-Derks D, Derks CM. Pulmonary neutral fat embolism in dogs. Am J Pathol 1979; 95:29–42.

107. Hulman G, Levene M. Intralipid microemboli. Arch Dis Child 1986; 61:702–703.

108. Kitchell CC, Balogh K. Pulmonary lipid emboli in association with long-term hyperalimentation. Hum Pathol 1986; 17:83–85.

109. Reedy JS, Kuhlman JE, Voytovich M. Microvascular pulmonary emboli secondary to precipitated crystals in a patient receiving total parenteral nutrition – A case report and description of the high-resolution CT findings. Chest 1999; 115:892–895.

110. Attwood HD. Amniotic fluid embolism. Pathol Annu 1972; 7:145–172.

111. Attwood HD. The histological diagnosis of amniotic-fluid embolism. J Pathol Bacteriol 1958; 76:211–215.

112. Kobayashi H, Ooi H, Hayakawa H, et al. Histological diagnosis of amniotic fluid embolism by monoclonal antibody TKH-2 that recognises NeuAc alpha 2–6GalNAc epitope. Hum Pathol 1997; 28:428–433.

113. Ishiyama I, Mukaida M, Komuro E, Keil W. Analysis of a case of generalized amniotic fluid embolism by demonstrating the fetal isoantigen (A blood type) in maternal tissues of B blood type, using immunoperoxidase staining. Am J Clin Pathol 1986; 85:239–241.

114. Attwood HD, Park WW. Embolism to the lungs by trophoblast. J Opt Soc Am 1961; 68:611–617.

115. Savage MB. Trophoblastic lesions of the lungs following benign hydatidiform mole. Am J Obst Gyn 1951; 62:346–352.

116. Park WW. The occurrence of decidual tissue within the lung: report of a case. J Pathol Bacteriol 1954; 67:563–570.

117. Willis RA. The Spread of Tumours in the Human Body. London: Butterworths; 1973:47–48.

118. Morgan AD. The pathology of subacute cor pulmonale in diffuse carcinomatosis of the lungs. J Pathol Bacteriol 1949; 61:75–84.

119. Bagshawe KD, Brooks WDW. Subacute pulmonary hypertension due to chorionepithelioma. Lancet 1959; 1:653–658.

120. He XW, Tang YH, Luo ZQ, Cheng TO. Subacute cor pulmonale due to tumor embolization to the lungs. Angiology 1989; 40:11–17.

121. Seckl MJ, Rustin GJS, Newlands ES, Gwyther SJ, Bomanji J. Pulmonary embolism, pulmonary hypertension and choriocarcinoma. Lancet 1991; 338:1313–1315.

122. Veinot JP, Ford SE, Price RG. Subacute cor pulmonale due to tumor embolization. Arch Pathol Lab Med 1992; 116:131–134.

123. Soares FA, Landell GAM, Deoliveira JAM. Pulmonary tumor embolism to alveolar septal capillaries – an unusual cause of sudden cor pulmonale. Arch Pathol Lab Med 1992; 116:187–188.

124. Hibbert M, Braude S. Tumour microembolism presenting as 'primary pulmonary hypertension'. Thorax 1997; 52:1016–1017.

125. Storey PD, Goldstein W. Pulmonary embolization from primary hepatic carcinoma. Arch Intern Med 1962; 110:262–269.

126. Wakasa K, Sakurai M, Uchida A, Yoshikawa H, Maeda A. Massive pulmonary tumor emboli in osteosarcoma: occult and fatal complication. Cancer 1990; 66:583–586.

127. Ahmed AA, Heller DS. Fatal pulmonary tumor embolism caused by chondroblastic osteosarcoma. Report of a case and review of the literature. Arch Pathol Lab Med 1999; 123:437–440.

128. Watanabe S, Shimokawa S, Sakasegawa K, Masuda H, Sakata R, Higashi M. Choriocarcinoma in the pulmonary artery treated with emergency pulmonary embolectomy. Chest 2002; 121:654–656.

129. Edmondstone WM. Flitting radiographic shadows: an unusual presentation of cancer in the lungs. Thorax 1998; 53:906–908.

130. von Herbay A, Illes A, Waldherr R, Otto HF. Pulmonary tumor thrombotic microangiopathy with pulmonary hypertension. Cancer 1990; 66:587–592.

131. Systrom DM, Mark EJ, Bhalla M, Demirjian ZN, Kazemi H. A 55-year-old woman with acute respiratory failure and radiographically clear lungs – pulmonary embolic and lymphangitic carcinomatosis of breast origin. N Engl J Med 1995; 332:1700–1707.

132. Sato Y, Marutsuka K, Asada Y, Yamada M, Setoguchi T, Sumiyoshi A. Pulmonary tumor thrombotic microangiopathy. Pathol Int 1995; 45:436–440.

133. Kobayashi H, Tamashima S, Shigeyama J, Shimizu S, Suchi T. Vascular intimal carcinomatosis: An autopsy case of unusual form of pulmonary metastasis of transitional cell carcinoma. Pathol Int 1997; 47:655–657.

134. Levine SB. Embolism of cerebral tissue to lungs. Arch Pathol 1973; 96:183–185.

135. Bohm N, Keller KM, Kloke WD. Pulmonary and systemic cerebellar tissue embolism due to birth injury. Virchows Arch A Pathol Anat Histopathol 1982; 398:229–235.

136. Dunnill MS. The pathology of pulmonary embolism. Br J Surg 1968; 55:790794.

137. Balogh K. Pulmonary bile emboli. Sequelae of iatrogenic trauma. Arch Pathol Lab Med 1984; 108:814–816.

138. Sabatine MS, Oelberg DA, Mark EJ, Kanarek D. Pulmonary cholesterol crystal embolization. Chest 1997; 112:1687–1692.

139. Arnett EN, Battle WE, Russo JV, Roberts WC. Intravenous injection of talc-containing drugs intended for oral use. A cause of pulmonary granulomatosis and pulmonary hypertension. Am J Med 1976; 60:711–718.

140. Gross EM. Autopsy findings in drug addicts. Pathol Annu 1978; 13(part 2):35–67.

141. Pare JAP, Fraser RG, Hogg JC, Howlett JG, Murphy SB. Pulmonary 'mainline' granulomatosis: talcosis of intravenous methadone abuse. Medicine (Baltimore) 1979; 58:229–239.

142. Waller BF, Brownlee WJ, Roberts WC. Self induced pulmonary granulomatosis. A consequence of intravenous injection of drugs intended for oral use. Chest 1980; 78:90–94.

143. Tomashefski JF Jr, Hirsch CS. The pulmonary vascular lesions of intravenous drug abuse. Hum Pathol 1980; 11:133–145.

144. Tomashefski JF Jr, Hirsch CS, Jolly PN. Microcrystalline cellulose pulmonary embolism and granulomatosis. Arch Pathol Lab Med 1981; 105:89–93.

145. Farber HW, Fairman RP, Glauser FL. Talc granulomatosis: laboratory findings similar to sarcoidosis. Am Rev Respir Dis 1982; 125:258–261.

146. Rajs J, Harm T, Ormstad K. Postmortem findings of pulmonary lesions of older datum in intravenous drug addicts. A forensic–pathologic study. Virchows Arch A Pathol Anat Histopathol 1984; 402:405–414.

147. Crouch E, Churg A. Progressive massive fibrosis of the lung secondary to intravenous injection of talc. A pathologic and mineralogic analysis. Am J Clin Pathol 1983; 80:520–526.

148. Cooper CB, Bai TR, Heyderman E, Corrin B. Cellulose granulomas in the lungs of a cocaine sniffer. BMJ 1983; 286:2021–2022.

149. Abraham JL, Brambilla C. Particle size for differentiation between inhalation and injection pulmonary talcosis. Environ Res 1980; 21:94–96.

150. Buchanan DR, Lamb D, Seaton A. Punk rocker's lung: pulmonary fibrosis in a drug snorting fire-eater. BMJ 1981; 283:1661.

151. Lamb RK, Pawade A, Prior AL. Intravascular missile: apparent retrograde course from the left ventricle. Thorax 1988; 43:499–500.

152. Nehme AE. Intracranial bullet migrating to pulmonary artery. J Trauma 1980; 20:344–346.

153. Leong AS-Y, Disney APS, Gove DW. Spallation and migration of silicone from blood-pump tubing in patients on hemodialysis. N Engl J Med 1982; 306:135–140.

154. Chastre J, Basset F, Viau F, et al. Acute pneumonitis after subcutaneous injections of silicone in transsexual men. N Engl J Med 1983; 308:764–767.

155. Robinson MJ, Nestor M, Rywlin AM. Pulmonary granulomas secondary to embolic prosthetic valve material. Hum Pathol 1981; 12:759–762.

156. Mittleman RE, Marraccini JV. Pulmonary Teflon granulomas following periurethral Teflon injection for urinary incontinence. Arch Pathol Lab Med 1983; 107:611–612.

157. Vilde F, Arkwright S, Galliot M, Galle P, Labrousse J, Lissac J. Pneumopathie mortelle liee a l'injection sous-cutanee de silicone liquide dans les parties molles. Ann Pathol 1983; 3:307–312.

158. Lai YF, Chao TY, Wong SL. Acute pneumonitis after subcutaneous injections of silicone for augmentation mammaplasty. Chest 1994; 106:1152–1155.

159. Gough JH, Gough MH, Thomas ML. Pulmonary complications following lymphangiography with a note on technique. Br J Radiol 1964; 37:416–421.

160. Fraimow W, Wallace S, Lewis P, Greening RR, Cathcart RT. Changes in pulmonary function due to lymphangiography. Radiology 1965; 85:231–241.

161. Davidson JW. Pulmonary complications of lymphangiography. N Engl J Med 1971; 285:237.

162. Silvestri RC, Hyseby JS, Rughani I, Thorning D, Culver BH. Respiratory distress syndrome from lymphangiography contrast medium. Am Rev Respir Dis 1980; 122:543–549.

163. Coard K, Silver MD, Perkins G, Fox AJ, Vinuela EV. Isobutyl-2-cyanoacrylate pulmonary emboli associated with occlusive embolotherapy of cerebral arteriovenous malformations. Histopathology 1984; 8:917–926.

164. Oliver RM, Thomas MR, Cornaby AJ, Neville E. Mercury pulmonary emboli following intravenous self-injection. Br J Dis Chest 1987; 81:76–79.

165. Bhagat R, Holmes IH, Kulaga A, Murphy F, Cockcroft DW. Self-injection with olive oil: a cause of lipoid pneumonia. Chest 1995; 107:875–876.

166. Fairfax AJ, Ball J, Batten JC, Heard BE. A pathological study following bronchial artery embolization for haemoptysis in cystic fibrosis. Br J Dis Chest 1980; 74:345–352.

167. Kepes JJ, Yarde WL. Visualization of injected embolic material (polyvinyl alcohol) in paraffin sections with Verhoeff-van Gieson elastica stain. Am J Surg Pathol 1995; 19:709–711.

168. Zaugg M, Kaplan V, Widmer U, Baumann PC, Russi EW. Fatal air embolism in an airplane passenger with a giant intrapulmonary bronchogenic cyst. Am J Respir Crit Care Med 1998; 157:1686–1689.

169. Fitchet A, Fitzpatrick AP. Central venous air embolism causing pulmonary oedema mimicking left ventricular failure. BMJ 1998; 316:604–606.

Pulmonary aneurysms

170. Bartter T, Irwin RS, Nash G. Aneurysms of the pulmonary arteries. Chest 1988; 94:1065–1075.

171. Chiu B, Magil A. Idiopathic pulmonary arterial trunk aneurysm presenting as cor pulmonale: report of a case. Hum Pathol 1985; 16:947–949.

172. Onorato E, Festa P, Bourlon F, Yves L, Ballerini L. Idiopathic right pulmonary artery aneurysm with pulmonary valve insufficiency. Cathet Cardiovasc Diagn 1996; 37:162–165.

173. Shanks JH, Coup A, Howat AJ. Dissecting aneurysm of the pulmonary artery associated with a large facial cavernous haemangioma. Histopathology 1997; 30:390–392.

174. Inayama Y, Nakatani Y, Kitamura H. Pulmonary artery dissection in patients without underlying pulmonary hypertension. Histopathology 2001; 38:435–442.

175. Bartram C, Strickland B. Pulmonary varices. Br J Radiol 1971; 44:927–935.

176. Man KM, Keeffe EB, Brown CR, Egawa H, Esquivel CO. Pulmonary varices presenting as a solitary lung mass in a patient with end-stage liver disease. Chest 1994; 106:294–296.

177. Shida T, Ohashi H, Nakamura K, Morimoto M. Pulmonary varices associated with mitral valve disease: a case report and survey of the literature. Ann Thorac Surg 1982; 34:452–456.

8

Vascular disease

8.2

Pulmonary hypertension

Normally the pressure in the pulmonary artery seldom exceeds 30/15 mmHg, but in a variety of cardiopulmonary diseases this figure can increase up to 4-fold. In the great majority of cases the hypertension is secondary to a recognisable lesion in the heart or lungs but in a small minority, said to have primary pulmonary hypertension, no cause is apparent. The causes of pulmonary hypertension are listed in Box 8.2.1.[1] Occasional cases are familial.[2–6]

In diffuse pulmonary fibrosis, the pathology is dominated by the parenchymal disease, but with the other causes the vascular changes preponderate. These fall into distinct categories that largely correspond to the cause of the hypertension, the principal ones being plexogenic, hypoxic, thromboembolic and venous, as indicated in Box 8.2.1 and Fig. 8.2.1. Thus, to a large extent, the pathological changes indicate the cause of the hypertension, as well as its presence and severity.[7,8] However, certain common features are shared by all categories and these will be described first. An elastin stain is invaluable in appreciating the vascular changes.

The earliest vascular changes are not specific and are present irrespective of the cause. In mild pulmonary hypertension histological diagnosis will be entirely dependent on the recognition of these early changes. They consist of medial hypertrophy, which is followed by subendothelial intimal fibrosis (Fig. 8.2.2). Isolated intimal fibrosis is an age change encountered in the absence of pulmonary hypertension. Medial thickening is not an age change but is due to prolonged contraction of its smooth muscle and represents a form of work hypertrophy, probably stimulated by mediators released by the endothelium, notably endothelin, which counters the action of the endothelium-derived vasodilatory agent nitric oxide.[9] The cellular component of the intimal fibrosis is smooth muscle derived from the media.[10]

Medial thickening is conveniently quantitated if required by tracing the internal and external elastic laminae on a digitising tablet and using a microcomputer to express the media as a proportion of the whole vessel in terms of either its diameter or area. The vessel is often collapsed and the elastic laminae consequently wrinkled but the computer can be programmed to

Box 8.2.1 Causes of pulmonary hypertension and their principal pathological features

Cause	Pathology
Precapillary: constrictive[a]	Plexogenic arteriopathy
Unknown (primary pulmonary hypertension)	
Hyperkinetic congenital heart disease	
Chronic liver disease with portosystemic venous shunting	
HIV infection	
Appetite-suppressing drugs (aminorex, fenfluramine)	
Hereditary haemorrhagic telangiectasia	
Connective tissue disease	
Precapillary: hypoxic	
Prolonged residence at high altitude	Peripheral extension of medial muscle and the development of longitudinal muscle within the intima
Chronic obstructive lung disease	
Sleep apnoea obesity syndrome	
Precapillary: embolic	
Thromboembolic	Recanalisation
Parasitic (schistosomal)	
Tumour emboli	
Capillary	
Widespread pulmonary fibrosis	
Capillary haemangiomatosis	
Diffuse smooth muscle proliferation	
Postcapillary	
Left-sided heart disease	Venous muscular hypertrophy
Veno-occlusive disease	Venous luminal obliteration

[a]Termed pulmonary arterial hypertension in an international classification drawn up at Evian in 1998 (http://www.who.int/ncd/cvd/pph.html) and revised at Venice in 2003[1] despite hypoxic and embolic causes also directly affecting the pulmonary arteries.

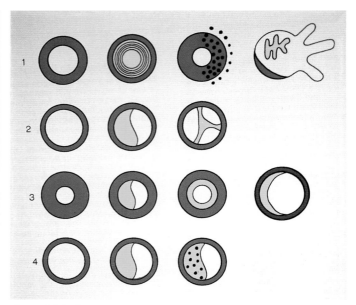

Figure 8.2.1 Patterns of vasculopathy in pulmonary hypertension. (1) Plexogenic arteriopathy characterised by medial hypertrophy, concentric intimal fibrosis, necrotising arteritis and a variety of dilatation lesions. (2) Thromboembolic, characterised by eccentric intimal thickening and duplication of the lumen by intimal bands. (3) Venous hypertension characterised by medial hypertrophy and either eccentric or concentric thickening of the arterial media coupled with intimal sclerosis of the post-capillary vessels. (4) Hypoxic characterised by mild medial hypertrophy and the development of longitudinal bundles of smooth muscle in the intima. (Reproduced from Wagenvoort CA. Classifying pulmonary vascular disease. Chest 1973; 64:503–504.[7] With permission from American College of Chest Physicians.)

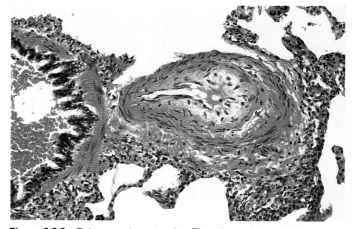

Figure 8.2.2 Pulmonary hypertension. There is marked medial hypertrophy and cellular intimal thickening. Pulmonary arteries normally have an extremely thin media and the thickening here represents marked hypertrophy. Its proximity to an airway indicates that this blood vessel is an artery rather than a vein.

express the diameter of the vessel as if it had been fixed in the filled state and the elastic laminae were smooth.[11] Normal values are best obtained by the same operator but the medial thickness of a normal muscular pulmonary artery has been given as 3–5% of its external diameter (compared with 15–20% in systemic arteries).[12]

Non-specific changes are also found in the smaller precapillary vessels. Below 100 μm diameter, the medial muscle normally spirals out and none at all is normally seen in vessels below about 30 μm in diameter: between 100 and 30 μm diameter, muscle is normally limited to one side of the vessel (see Fig. 1.35, p. 21). Fully muscularised vessels below 100 μm diameter and partially muscularised vessels below 30 μm diameter therefore indicate medial hypertrophy (Fig. 8.2.3).

Siderophages, cholesterol granulomas and focal fibrosis represent secondary changes consequent upon pulmonary haemorrhage, which may complicate severe or longstanding cases

of pulmonary hypertension.[13] Pulmonary arterial thrombosis, identical in appearance to thrombotic embolism, is generally a further secondary change[13] but in primary pulmonary hypertension it may be an inherent component of the pathogenetic process, as discussed below.[14]

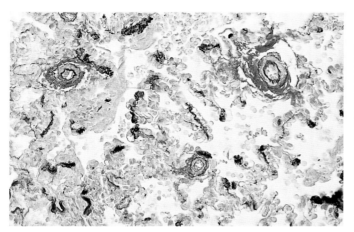

Figure 8.2.3 Intralobular arteries smaller than 30 μm diameter with a well-developed medial coat indicative of pulmonary hypertension. (Elastin van Gieson stain.)

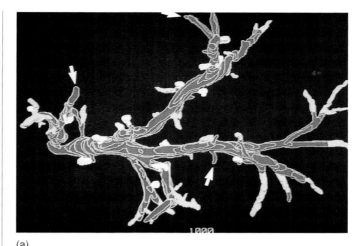

(a)

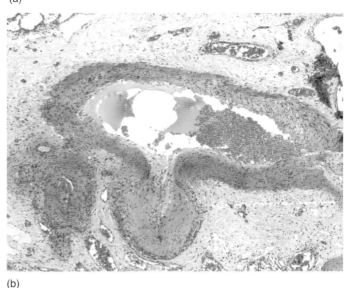

(b)

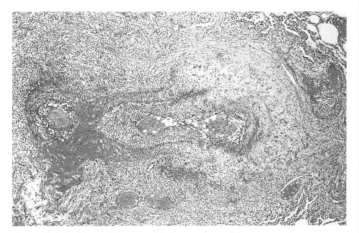

Figure 8.2.4 Necrotising arteritis in a patient with severe pulmonary hypertension secondary to a ventricular septal defect. Focal necrosis such as this leads to a variety of dilatation lesions.

Figure 8.2.5 (a) A computer-aided reconstruction of the distal pulmonary arteries in plexogenic pulmonary hypertension. Plexiform lesions (white) occur in supernumerary arteries just proximal to a point where the larger axial arteries are obliterated by intimal proliferation (yellow). Only a few patent vessels remain (arrows). (Reproduced from Yaginuma et al. Distribution of arterial lesions and collateral pathways in the pulmonary hypertension on congenital heart disease: a computer aided reconstruction study. Thorax 1990; 45:586–590.[18] With permission from British Medical Association.) (b) Histology shows a plexogenic lesion arising at the origin of a supernumerary artery.

PLEXOGENIC PULMONARY ARTERIOPATHY

In some conditions, which are listed in Box 8.2.1, further changes take place in the pulmonary arteries, notably a necrotising fibrinoid arteriopathy (Fig. 8.2.4) and the subsequent development of characteristic dilatation lesions, some of which are plexiform.[13,15–17] The necrotising arteriopathy is very similar morphologically to the auto-immune arteritides dealt with in Chapter 8.3 but is to be regarded as a consequence of severe medial contraction rather than an immune process. Because plexiform lesions occur only in the final stages of the disease the word 'plexogenic' (indicating a potential to develop plexiform lesions rather than their presence) was chosen to identify the disease as a whole, including the early stages.[17] It is notable that

plexiform lesions are not encountered in chronic pulmonary venous hypertension, chronic hypoxic pulmonary hypertension, or pulmonary hypertension due to chronic thromboembolic disease. They are limited to forms of pulmonary hypertension characterised by intense vasoconstriction.

Dilatation lesions are thin-walled vascular structures that come off a greatly thickened muscular artery. Beyond their point of origin, the parent artery is usually obliterated by intimal fibrosis (Fig. 8.2.5).[18] They are thought to represent 'blow-out lesions' at points of necrotising arteritis in the wall of the parent vessel.[16,18] It is therefore justifiable to condense into one, the last three grades of the traditional Heath and Edwards

Table 8.2.1   Heath and Edwards'[19] grading system of hypertensive pulmonary vascular disease

Grade	Histological criteria
1	Medial hypertrophy
2	Grade 1 plus cellular intimal thickening
3	Grade 1 plus fibrous intimal thickening
4	Grades 2 or 3 plus dilatation lesions
5	Grade 4 plus haemosiderosis
6	Grade 5 plus necrotising arteritis

This system was designed for use in connection with congenital heart disease. It is applicable to other causes of plexogenic pulmonary arteriopathy but not to other causes of pulmonary hypertension. Because dilatation lesions are now thought to be due to fibrinoid necrosis,[16] grades 4 to 6 could well be condensed into one. The critical area regarding reversibility lies in the region of grades 2 and 3 and there is a case for dividing these according to the degree of luminal narrowing.[20]

(Reprinted from Heath D, Edwards JE. The pathology of hypertensive pulmonary vascular disease. A description of six grades of structural changes in the pulmonary arteries with special reference to congenital cardiac septal defects. Circulation 1958; 18:533–547. With permission from Lippincott. www.lww.com)

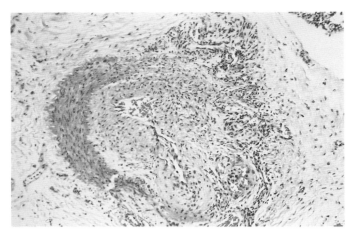

Figure 8.2.6   A plexiform lesion. The media of this pulmonary artery is deficient on one side and here the lumen communicates with a plexus of fine channels. On the other side of the artery the media is greatly hypertrophied.

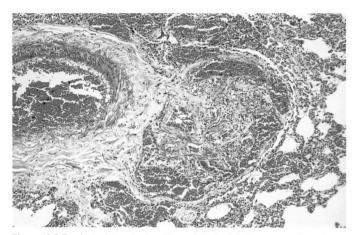

Figure 8.2.7   A plexiform lesion. The point of origin from the adjacent artery is not evident in this section but the plexiform lesion and its surrounding collection of wide thin-walled vessels are well represented.

grading system (Table 8.2.1),[16,19,20] which was devised specifically for patients with hyperkinetic pulmonary hypertension secondary to congenital heart disease but can be equally applied to plexogenic arteriopathy of whatever cause. Dilatation lesions involve the supernumerary arteries where these vessels leave the axial arteries.[18,21] Supernumerary arteries differ from axial arteries in that they do not accompany bronchioles or branch at a narrow angle: they leave the axial vessel at an obtuse angle and feed alveolar capillaries soon after their origin.[22] Thus, they rapidly narrow and there is considerable reduction in pressure over a short distance. When the arterial pressure is raised there is significant physical stress on these arteries and it is likely that this is involved in the development of the necrotising arteritis and subsequent dilatation lesions.

Dilatation lesions are described as being simple, plexiform or angiomatoid. Simple dilatation lesions are saccular aneurysms, whereas plexiform lesions represent such aneurysms filled by connective tissue that is rich in myofibroblasts and is intersected by a complex of fine endothelium-lined spaces (Fig. 8.2.6).[23,24] It is reported that the endothelial cell proliferation is monoclonal in primary but not secondary pulmonary hypertension.[25,26] Plexiform lesions often lead to wide thin-walled vessels which in turn feed into capillaries (Fig. 8.2.7).[18] They occasionally reach a diameter of 1 mm. The multiple fine channels probably represent organised and re-canalised thrombi within an otherwise simple dilatation lesion. The narrow channels of a plexiform lesion are probably responsible for the microangiopathic haemolytic anaemia that occasionally complicates plexogenic pulmonary arteriopathy.[27] The angiomatoid lesion consists of several thin-walled cavernous spaces linking a muscular pulmonary artery to its capillary bed and resembling a haemangioma (Fig. 8.2.8). They were once thought to represent congenital malformations but are now recognised to be acquired.

Plexiform lesions need to be distinguished from organised re-canalised thrombus with florid endothelial cell proliferation. The essential difference is that plexiform lesions lie alongside the parent artery whereas organised thrombus is within. Elastin stains are helpful in that pulmonary arteries containing re-canalised thrombus usually have intact internal and external elastic laminae whereas these structures are destroyed at the site of plexiform lesions.[28]

Congenital heart disease

Congenital cardiovascular anomalies characterised by left-to-right shunting, such as patent ductus arteriosus and septal defects, result in a hyperkinetic form of pulmonary hypertension in which the blood enters the pulmonary arteries in greater volume or at a higher pressure than usual. In cases of atrial septal defect, blood passes from the left to the right atrium, and so adds to the quantity of blood entering the pulmonary artery. This can usually be accommodated because of the marked dis-

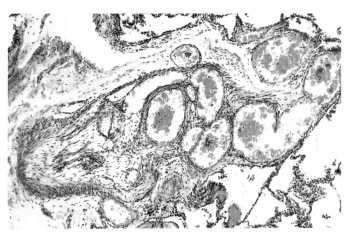

Figure 8.2.8   An angiomatoid lesion. A convoluted, wide, thin-walled vessel simulating a haemangioma leads directly off a hypertrophied pulmonary artery; the narrow sinusoids of a plexiform lesion are not apparent in this type of dilatation lesion.

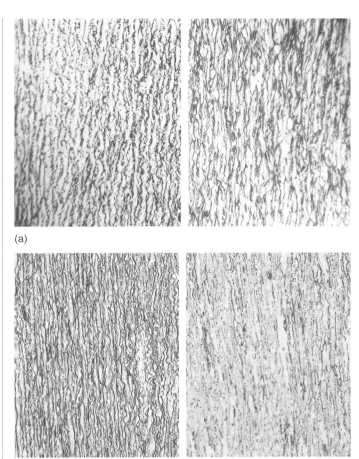

(a)

(b)

Figure 8.2.9   Aorta (left) and pulmonary trunk (right) in congenital pulmonary hypertension secondary to a ventricular septal defect (a), and in acquired pulmonary hypertension secondary to bronchopulmonary disease that developed in adult life (b). The fragmented elastin pattern of the normal adult pulmonary trunk is maintained in acquired pulmonary hypertension but in patients in whom the pulmonary hypertension has been present from birth the fetal pattern (which is identical to that in the aorta) is maintained. Elastin van Gieson stain.

tensibility of the pulmonary vasculature and hypertension seldom develops before middle age. However, when there is a ventricular septal defect or patent ductus arteriosus, the increase in the volume of the blood in the pulmonary circulation is accompanied by a substantial increase in pressure. The changes in the walls of the pulmonary arteries are consequently more severe and develop early in life. There is severe constriction of small muscular arteries, which undergo medial hypertrophy and raise the pulmonary resistance through their hypertonicity. At this stage, they are still capable of relaxation and there is enough circulatory reserve to meet the needs of exercise, but when severe hypertension persists the lumen of the small muscular arteries becomes further narrowed by thickening of the intima. Initially this is due to concentric laminar cellular proliferation but later intimal fibrosis supervenes. The vessels are then less capable of adaptive dilatation, the hypertension becomes irreversible, and the patient enters a perpetual state of high pulmonary resistance and low circulatory reserve. Further vascular changes are those described above under plexogenic arteriopathy. There may also be secondary pulmonary artery thrombosis, organisation of which leads to eccentric plaques of intimal fibrosis. The practical point is that the underlying congenital anomalies should be corrected before the pulmonary arteries are permanently narrowed by intimal fibrosis.

Lung biopsy can be useful in assessing the reversibility or otherwise of hyperkinetic pulmonary hypertension although most cases are now assessed by catheterisation.[29–31] Features that are compatible with a successful corrective operation include medial hypertrophy, cellular concentric intimal thickening of moderate degree, and eccentric intimal fibrosis consequent upon thrombosis. Conversely, severe intimal fibrosis, fibrinoid necrosis and dilatation lesions suggest that the pulmonary hypertension will progress despite corrective surgery. However, potential reversibility probably differs from safe operability.

Medial hypertrophy is potentially reversible but may be associated with fatal pulmonary hypertensive crises at operation.[32] The pathological criteria for operability have yet to be defined.

The major pulmonary arteries are elastic vessels and at birth the pattern of their elastic laminae closely resembles that of the aorta. However, within the first few months of life there is fragmentation of the elastic fibres and an irreversible 'adult pattern' is reached by about the age of 6 months. This 'adult pattern' is maintained even if pulmonary hypertension develops in later life, whereas in congenital pulmonary hypertension the 'aortic pattern' found at birth persists (Fig. 8.2.9).

In conditions leading to low pulmonary flow rates or diminished pulmonary artery pulse pressure, such as congenital pulmonary stenosis, perhaps as part of Fallot's tetrad, the pulmonary arteries show changes the reverse of those described above, namely medial atrophy, so that they are extremely thin-walled. A media is sometimes not apparent. The low blood flow and the almost invariably raised haematocrit promote thrombosis and evidence of this in the form of eccentric intimal plaques or subdivision of the lumen is often apparent. However, this is seldom so extensive that it causes pulmonary hypertension, but corrective procedures entailing shunts may lead to plexogenic arteriopathy.

Primary pulmonary hypertension

The microscopic features of primary pulmonary hypertension are those of plexogenic pulmonary arteriopathy, as described above. They are indistinguishable from those seen in plexogenic pulmonary hypertension due to any of the other causes listed in Box 8.2.1. A diagnosis of primary pulmonary hypertension can therefore only be made when all other possible causes of plexogenic pulmonary arteriopathy have been excluded by full clinical and radiological examination, cardiac catheterisation and, if necessary, surgical lung biopsy. Despite this, the term primary pulmonary hypertension has been used by clinicians when the condition remains unexplained after investigations that fall short of histological assessment. Pathological examination in 156 such cases showed that 70% were plexogenic, 20% were thrombotic and 6% showed venous obliteration.[15] Similar heterogeneity has been reported in other series.[33] Although plexogenic, thromboembolic and veno-occlusive pulmonary hypertension cannot be distinguished without histological assessment, their histological distinction is often blurred by plexogenic arteriopathy being complicated by thrombosis,[14] by the changes of veno-occlusive disease extending proximally to involve arteries, and by venous abnormalities being identified in plexogenic arteriopathy.[13] Some workers therefore regard primary plexogenic arteriopathy, thrombotic pulmonary vascular disease and veno-occlusion as facets of one condition and term this primary pulmonary hypertension on the basis that the cause is unknown whatever the predominant histological pattern.[3,33,34] Thus, the term primary pulmonary hypertension is currently used in three different ways, of which we prefer the first:

1 for primary plexogenic pulmonary hypertension
2 for pulmonary hypertension that cannot be explained despite full clinical investigation (but falling short of histological assessment)
3 for pulmonary hypertension due to intrinsic pulmonary vascular disease regardless of whether histology shows this to be thrombotic, plexogenic or veno-occlusive.

Primary plexogenic pulmonary hypertension can occur at any age but most commonly affects young adults, with women outnumbering men by about 2 to 1.[15,35] A family history is evident in approximately 6% of patients[35] but the identification first of the responsible gene on chromosome 2 (2q32-34),[36,37] and then its expression in seemingly sporadic cases of primary pulmonary hypertension[38] suggests that the true prevalence of familial cases is considerably higher. The gene concerned encodes for bone morphogenetic receptor protein-II, which controls the action of transforming growth factor-β on the vessel wall.[39–42] It is therefore relevant that the genes for hereditary haemorrhagic telangiectasia (Osler–Weber–Rendu disease – see pp. 75, 483), of which plexogenic pulmonary hypertension is a rare feature, also control the vascular transforming growth factor-β pathway.[43,44] Endothelial factors such as angiotensin-converting enzyme, endothelin and (deficiency of) nitric oxide are further likely mediators.[45–47] Female sex hormones may also play a role.[48] A reported increase in airway neuroendocrine cells[49–51] and the detection of *Chlamydia pneumoniae* in the hypertrophied pulmonary arteries of a patient dying of pulmonary hypertension[52] are of uncertain significance. Raynaud's phenomenon is found in 10% and a positive antinuclear antibody test in about 30% of patients with primary pulmonary hypertension.[35] There is also a high prevalence of autoimmune thyroid disease.[53] Pulmonary hypertension associated with more pronounced connective tissue disease is considered below.

Hepatic disease

The prevalence of plexogenic pulmonary hypertension in cirrhosis is in the order of 0.7%[54] and the fact that it takes this form of arteriopathy[55,56] suggests that it is vasoconstrictive, perhaps the result of metabolites that are normally inactivated in the liver. Paradoxically, some patients with cirrhosis of the liver develop pulmonary arterial dilatation and arteriovenous communications in the lungs,[57–59] while in one series pulmonary venous intimal thickening was identified in 65% of cirrhotic patients.[60]

Dietary pulmonary hypertension

A notable increase in the incidence of 'primary' pulmonary hypertension occurred in Switzerland, Austria and Germany during the period 1966–1968 when the anorectic drug aminorex was marketed.[61] It was not possible to reproduce the disease experimentally, but the epidemiological evidence that aminorex fumarate was responsible for the pulmonary hypertension is strong. The drug had been on sale only in these three countries and the increase in the frequency of pulmonary hypertension closely followed the rise in its sale, while following its withdrawal there was a corresponding fall in the number of cases of pulmonary hypertension. Another anorectic drug, fenfluramine, has also been linked to the development of pulmonary hypertension.[62–65] Plexiform lesions have been described with both these drugs.[66]

Pulmonary hypertension formed part of the Spanish toxic oil episode and the L-tryptophan-induced eosinophilia-myalgia syndrome. The changes wrought by these 'dietary' supplements include a pulmonary vasculitis and differ from those of plexogenic arteriopathy. They are described on pp. 376, 389.

Pyrollizidine alkaloids derived from various species of *Senecio* (ragworts and groundsels) cause intense vasoconstrictive pulmonary hypertension in laboratory animals but there is no evidence that ingestion of these plants causes pulmonary hypertension in man. Nevertheless, observations such as these support the histopathological evidence that primary plexogenic pulmonary hypertension is vasoconstrictive in nature due to an as yet unidentified neural or humoral agent.

HIV infection

An association of pulmonary hypertension with human immunodeficiency virus infection has been established but is as yet unexplained.[67–70] The virus cannot be identified in the pulmonary vessels but tubulo-reticular structures suggestive of cytokine accumulation have been identified there by electron microscopy in HIV positive individuals.[71] The incidence of pulmonary hypertension in HIV positive patients is 1 in 200, the male to female ratio is 1.6:1 and the age range is 3–56 years with a mean of 32 years.[72] The arteriopathy is generally plexogenic but thrombotic or veno-occlusive changes are described in 15% of cases.[72] Suggestions that Kaposi sarcoma-associated herpes virus is similarly associated with pulmonary hypertension have not been substantiated.[72a]

HYPOXIC PULMONARY HYPERTENSION

The pulmonary circulation differs from the systemic circulation in that it reacts to hypoxia by vasoconstriction rather than vasodilatation. Hypoxia, whether due to high altitude or a ventilatory lung defect, causes the muscular pulmonary arteries to constrict and although the consequent pulmonary hypertension may be life-threatening, the intense spasm that leads to the necrotising arteriopathy and dilatation lesions of plexogenic arteriopathy is not a feature. The mechanism by which hypoxia leads to pulmonary artery constriction is unclear but it operates at the local level, affecting only those vessels in the immediate vicinity of airways with low oxygen tensions.[73,74] It is likely that it involves changes in the levels of vasoactive factors synthesised and released by the arterial endothelium, in particular nitric oxide, which has vasodilatory properties, and endothelin, which is a vasoconstrictor (see p. 22).[45,46,75–77] The arteries involved are principally small precapillary vessels[73,74] but small pulmonary veins are also affected.[78] However, the earliest morphological response to hypoxia is found in the carotid bodies, which undergo hyperplasia before any structural changes are detectable in the lungs.[79]

Ventilatory disorders causing pulmonary hypertension include chronic bronchitis and emphysema, bronchiectasis and extrapulmonary causes of poor ventilation such as kyphoscoliosis and obesity. In emphysema, there is no correlation between the extent of capillary loss and right ventricular weight:[80,81] vasoconstriction is held to be responsible, as in other forms of hypoxic pulmonary hypertension. It is also possible that cigarette smoke components may augment the hypoxia by acting directly on the artery wall.[82] In bronchiectasis, both hypoxia and left-to-right shunts consequent upon bronchopulmonary arterial anastomoses contribute to the pulmonary hypertension.

Morphological changes characteristic of hypoxic pulmonary hypertension include mild medial hypertrophy and the extension of a complete muscular media into pre-capillary vessels

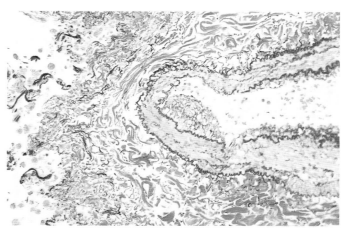

Figure 8.2.10   Hypoxic pulmonary hypertension. The arterial media is hypertrophied and longitudinal bundles of smooth muscle have developed in the intima.

below 80 μm in diameter (Fig. 8.2.3). A further feature is the occasional development of longitudinal bundles of smooth muscle in the intima of small pulmonary arteries (down to 80 μm diameter) and veins (Fig. 8.2.10).[83–86] It is suggested that the development of longitudinal smooth muscle in the intima is caused by repeated stretching of the small pulmonary vessels as a consequence of wide respiratory excursions: in some experimental models, stretching of vessels results in such laying down of longitudinal muscle,[87] but this is not confirmed by others, who regard the process as a component of normal repair.[88] Longitudinal smooth muscle is found in pulmonary arteries in other forms of pulmonary hypertension,[13,89] but not so noticeably as in the hypoxic forms. The arterial changes found in hypoxic pulmonary hypertension are reversible, but irreversible airway disease or prolonged residence at high altitude may result in death due to right-sided heart failure that is directly attributable to the hypoxic pulmonary hypertension.

In Rocky Mountain cattle, the dependent oedema of right-sided cardiac failure caused by hypoxic pulmonary hypertension affects the breast (brisket) particularly and such cattle are said to have 'brisket disease'.[90] A human counterpart of this has been described in children of Chinese ancestry who have been taken to reside in Tibet and who have developed a fatal form of subacute infantile mountain sickness.[91]

Only lowland cattle are affected by high altitude, the natural stock of the Himalayas and Ethiopian highlands apparently being immune. So too are other species long established at high altitude such as the llama and yak. These species are said to have adapted to their climate, that is, the forces of natural selection have bred out the pulmonary vasoconstrictive response to hypoxia. Cattle of European origin and man acclimatise to high altitude by processes such as increasing their red cell mass but generally they are not adapted like native species and suffer hypoxic pulmonary hypertension at altitudes in excess of 3000 m. Certain Himalayan highlanders may be an exception to this in that their small pulmonary arteries are reported not to show the muscularisation that characterises hypoxic pulmonary hypertension.[92]

PULMONARY HYPERTENSION IN DIFFUSE PARENCHYMAL LUNG DISEASE

Pulmonary hypertension develops when there is widespread pulmonary destruction, whatever the cause, but particularly pulmonary fibrosis. Thus, it is seen in advanced cryptogenic fibrosing alveolitis, sarcoidosis, pneumoconiosis and Langerhans cell histiocytosis. In the fibrotic parts of the lung, occlusive intimal fibro-elastosis akin to endarteritis obliterans is evident at a relatively early stage. With advancing disease there is widespread loss of capillaries and in less severely affected parts small precapillary vessels are fully muscularised. In sarcoidosis the granulomas may involve the media and even the intima of pulmonary blood vessels (see Fig. 6.1.33b, p. 289).

Two examples have been reported of middle-aged men with severe pulmonary hypertension and diffuse smooth muscle cell proliferation of the lungs.[93,94] The smooth muscle cell proliferation involved bronchioles, alveoli and small pulmonary arteries and veins, the vascular involvement accounting for the severe pulmonary hypertension, which resulted in cor pulmonale. The changes differ from those of pulmonary lymphangioleiomyomatosis (see p. 295) but are nevertheless also considered to be hamartomatous.[94]

EMBOLIC PULMONARY HYPERTENSION

Pulmonary hypertension may result from progressive diminution of the pulmonary vascular bed by multiple emboli. Thrombotic emboli may be very numerous but small and clinically silent. In these circumstances lung biopsy may show occlusion of small pulmonary arteries by thrombi in various stages of organisation. Totally organised emboli appear as eccentric fibrotic intimal plaques or show the multiple new lumina that indicate re-canalisation (Fig. 8.2.11).[95] Occasionally the organisation of the thrombus takes the form of multiple fine channels and the appearances mimic those of a plexiform lesion. However, the latter develops in a thrombosed dilatation lesion and is situated alongside the parent artery whereas organisation of thrombotic emboli is confined to the obliterated arterial lumen. The elastic laminae are intact in re-canalised arteries but destroyed at the site of a plexiform lesion.[28] We do not support the view that thromboembolic pulmonary hypertension is characterised by plexiform lesions, as proposed by some workers.[96] As well as re-canalisation by conventional thin-walled vessels, channels having a thick muscle coat and believed to be bronchial arteries are described within the fibrosed intima of affected pulmonary arteries (so-called vessel-within-vessel or double media lesion).[97,98] However, although many pulmonary arteries may be occluded, the lesions are focal and beyond them distal branches appear quite normal yet are non-functioning.

Changes such as these are generally taken to indicate thromboembolism[99] but could equally represent primary pulmonary thrombosis. Indeed, there are those who believe that

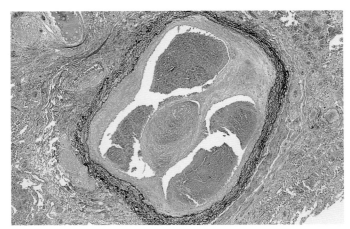

Figure 8.2.11 Thromboembolic pulmonary hypertension. The artery has a double lumen separated by a collagenous band that represents organised thrombus. (Elastin van Gieson stain.)

thromboembolism is seldom the cause of pulmonary hypertension; evidence adduced in favour of this includes the observation that it is very difficult to induce pulmonary hypertension experimentally by repeated embolisation of thrombi.[100] This is in line with the third use of the term primary pulmonary hypertension described above, namely it being applied irrespective of whether the changes are predominantly plexogenic, thrombotic or veno-occlusive.[3,33,34]

Pulmonary thrombosis occasionally causes pulmonary hypertension in conditions such as sickle cell disease[101–104] and paroxysmal nocturnal haematuria;[105] the morphological changes are then identical to those of multiple small thromboemboli but with plexiform lesions also described in some patients.[102,103] Secondary thrombosis is common in all forms of pulmonary hypertension and may make it difficult to distinguish thromboembolic pulmonary hypertension from other types complicated by thrombosis. If thromboembolic or thrombotic pulmonary hypertension can be recognised early enough, some mitigation of their progress can be achieved with anticoagulant drugs.

On rare occasions, emboli from malignant tumours obstruct the pulmonary circulation and cause pulmonary hypertension,[106–109] or excite a fibrocellular intimal proliferation that occludes small pulmonary arteries.[110] While in some countries severe schistosomiasis (see p. 252) is an important cause of embolic pulmonary hypertension. Schistosomal eggs block the lumen of the small pulmonary arteries, damage the wall to cause thrombosis, and work their way through into the surrounding tissues where they excite a severe foreign body inflammatory reaction. Proximal to the obstruction, changes indicative of severe pulmonary hypertension are found, including angiomatoid and possibly plexiform lesions.[55] The intravenous injection of drugs formulated for oral use is another embolic cause of pulmonary hypertension (see p. 379).

VENOUS PULMONARY HYPERTENSION

An increase of pressure in the pulmonary veins may result from mitral stenosis, prolonged left ventricular failure, fibrosing mediastinitis, or rarely, pulmonary veno-occlusive disease.[111]

Mitral stenosis

In mitral stenosis, the medial muscle of the pulmonary veins is hypertrophied, especially in the lower lobes, and there is a similar hypertrophy of the media on the arterial side of the capillaries.[112] In both arteries and veins there is also intimal sclerosis and again the changes are worse in the lower lobes. This is due to the added hydrostatic forces which result from our upright posture (Fig. 8.2.12).[112] In very severe cases there may be necrotising arteriopathy but this is unusual and plexiform lesions are not a feature of such passive pulmonary hypertension. The distinctive feature of passive pulmonary hypertension is the venous hypertrophy and sclerosis. However, in mitral stenosis the arterial changes do not merely reflect transmission of the raised left atrial pressure across the pulmonary capillary bed: pulmonary artery pressure rises disproportionately to the left atrial pressure, indicating that there is arterial constriction.[113] Pulmonary venous hypertension is also characterised by pulmonary oedema,[114,115] interstitial fibrosis[116] and haemosiderosis which together characterise the condition long known as 'brown induration of the lungs'.

Pulmonary veno-occlusive disease[117–123]

Pulmonary veno-occlusive disease is a rare disorder of unknown aetiology that is seldom diagnosed in life, and then usually by lung biopsy. However, the presence of Kerley B lines in the absence of any evidence of left atrial enlargement provides a valuable clue to the diagnosis in life.[119] As in true primary pulmonary hypertension, children and young adults are mainly affected but unlike primary pulmonary hypertension there is no female predominance: in children no predilection for either sex has been observed but in adults men are affected twice as often as women.[120] Familial cases are described.[2,124]

Aetiology

Pulmonary veno-occlusive disease is to be distinguished from pulmonary vein stenosis, which represents congenital atresia of the extrapulmonary veins (see p. 74). In pulmonary veno-occlusive disease the intra- or extra-pulmonary veins are narrowed or obliterated by fibrous thickening of the intima. This is presumed to be post-thrombotic but thrombosis is seldom seen. The cause of the fibrosis is unknown except in a few cases where factors such as chemotherapy,[125,126] radiotherapy,[127] bone marrow transplantation,[128] renal transplantation,[129] HIV infection,[130,131] Felty's syndrome[132] and systemic sclerosis[117,133] have been incriminated (Box 8.2.2[117,125–134]). There is no

Box 8.2.2 Causes of pulmonary veno-occlusive disease

Idiopathic – the great majority of cases
Chemotherapy[125,126]
Radiotherapy[127]
Bone marrow transplantation[a,128]
Renal transplantation[129]
HIV infection[b,130,131]
Felty's syndrome[132]
Systemic sclerosis[c,117,133]
Anti-phospholipid syndrome[134]
Sickle cell disease[102,103]
[a]Generally preceded by whole body radiation [b]Also associated with plexogenic arteriopathy [c]More often associated with arteriopathy

recognised connection with the bush teas that cause hepatic veno-occlusive disease, despite the observation that related pyrollizidine alkaloids cause an arterio-constrictive form of pulmonary hypertension in experimental animals.[55] Very rarely, immune complexes are identified in the pulmonary vessels,[135] or there is a granulomatous pulmonary phlebitis[136] or the disease is seen in the setting of a generalised venulopathy.[137] An onset characterised by fever may suggest a viral aetiology but could equally reflect pulmonary infarction attributable to the disease. However, in a case believed to have been contracted in utero, the baby also had myocarditis and the mother was thought to have had a viral infection when pregnant.[138]

Pathology

The condition is characterised by obliterative sclerosis of pulmonary veins. This venous obliteration causes venous hypertension, which in turn results in venous medial hypertrophy. This may be so extreme that the veins resemble arteries in structure, with internal and external elastic laminae, but the true nature of the affected vessel can still be recognised from its anatomical location in an interlobular septum, contrasting with the centriacinar position of the arteries alongside the airways (Fig. 8.2.13). The venous obstruction also results in marked pulmonary congestion and haemosiderosis. It also leads to the development of leashes of fine anastomotic vessels both around and within the occluded veins,[139] the appearances of pulmonary capillary haemangiomatosis (see below). The venous obstruction also results in prolonged severe interstitial oedema, which in turn causes interstitial fibrosis (Fig. 8.2.14).[140] Attention to the veins will help the pathologist avoid the error of diagnosing idiopathic pulmonary fibrosis in such cases.

Sometimes it is the small intralobular veins that are diseased. These are difficult to recognise without elastin stains but there are often clues that they are occluded. First there may be focal areas of intense capillary congestion within the affected lobules (Fig. 8.2.15),[117] a change that is practically pathognomonic of venular obstruction. Second, there may be so-called 'endogenous pneumoconiosis'. This oddly-termed process may be

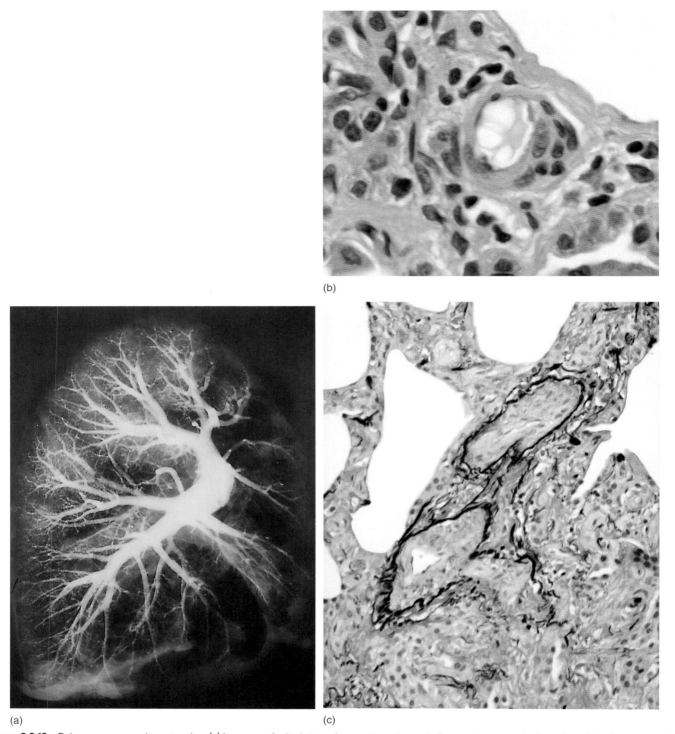

(b)

(a)

(c)

Figure 8.2.12 Pulmonary venous hypertension. (a) In a case of mitral stenosis, a post mortem arteriogram shows marked pruning of the finer vessels in the lower lobe, the lobar difference being due to the venous hypertension being added to the hydrostatic forces entailed in our upright posture. (b) In a patient with cardiomyopathy, small blood vessels show medial hypertrophy while in the same patient (c) pulmonary veins show intimal fibrosis. (Elastin van Gieson stain.)

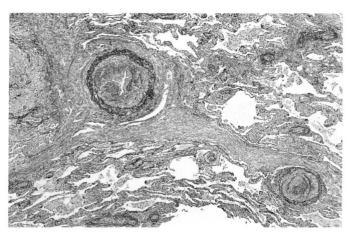

Figure 8.2.13 Pulmonary veno-occlusive disease. Two blood vessels are greatly narrowed by intimal fibrosis. The larger has distinct internal and external elastic laminae, as seen in pulmonary arteries, but the position of these blood vessels within an interlobular septum indicates that they are 'arterialised' pulmonary veins.

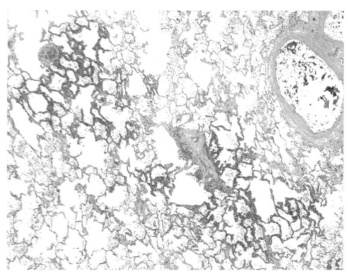

Figure 8.2.15 Pulmonary veno-occlusive disease affecting small interlobular vessels leading to focal areas of intense capillary engorgement. Venous occlusion is also evident (centre).

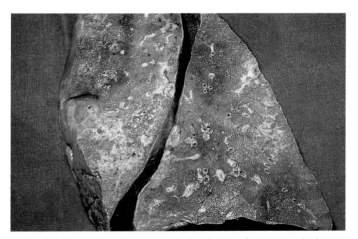

Figure 8.2.14 Pulmonary veno-occlusive disease. At necropsy the lungs show alternating areas of intense congestion and pallor, the latter due to interstitial fibrosis consequent upon severe interstitial oedema.

found whenever there is pulmonary haemosiderosis but is especially common in veno-occlusive disease. The haemosiderosis not only takes the form of iron-laden alveolar macrophages but encrusts the capillary basement membranes and venular elastic laminae, often with calcium being deposited there as well as iron. The heavily mineralised laminae are unduly rigid and break up to attract foreign body giant cells (see Figs 8.3.22, 8.3.23). Not realising the significance of this unusual change, earlier workers referred to it as 'endogenous pneumoconiosis'.[141] More recently it has been termed mineralising pulmonary elastosis.[142] It is not confined to veno-occlusive disease but is very suggestive of this condition. It is also seen, but less frequently, with other causes of pulmonary haemosiderosis.

Muscular pulmonary arteries show medial hypertrophy, and thrombosis may cause eccentric intimal thickening similar to

that seen in thrombo-embolic pulmonary hypertension or on rare occasions be the presenting feature.[143] It is debatable whether the arterial changes are entirely secondary, as implied by the name veno-occlusive disease, or represent a primary component of a wider process, in which case the name vaso-occlusive disease would be more appropriate.[122] Widespread small vessel occlusion justifying the term vaso-occlusive disease is seen in the pulmonary hypertension associated with sickle cell disease (see p. 484) and the anti-phospholipid syndrome[134] where the occlusion is due respectively to sludging of deformed red cells and platelets.

Pulmonary capillary haemangiomatosis

Pulmonary capillary haemangiomatosis is a very rare condition that represents one of the more unusual causes of pulmonary hypertension.[4,144–152] Its supposed neoplastic nature is questionable and it possibly represents an unusual manifestation of pulmonary veno-occlusive disease.[146]

Clinical features

Most patients are young adults (age range 14–71 years, mean 35 years) who present with dyspnoea and are found to be in cardiac failure. They may also complain of haemoptysis. Chest radiographs and computed tomography usually show pulmonary infiltrates or nodules, or pleural effusion. Radiological and hemodynamic findings are similar to those found in pulmonary veno-occlusive disease but differ from those identified with other causes of pulmonary hypertension.[153] The patient usually dies of right-sided heart failure within a few years, the median survival from the first clinical manifestation being 3 years. The diagnosis is rarely established before death[147] although focal lesions have been identified incidentally post mortem.[154] However, one patient diagnosed on biopsy went into complete remission when treated with doxycycline, an angiogenesis inhibitor.[155] In another patient, pulmonary capillary haemangiomatosis was associated with multiple pulmonary vascular malformations that formed part of hereditary haemorrhagic telangiectasia.[156]

Pathology

At autopsy, the lungs appear firm and haemorrhagic. They may be affected diffusely or there may be well circumscribed nodules, with the most severely affected areas found in the periphery of the lower lobes.[157] The characteristic histological finding is alveolar wall thickening by a proliferation of small, thin-walled, capillary-sized vessels (Fig. 8.2.16), although in one case the vessels were much larger, measuring up to 180μm in diameter.[158] The proliferating vessels also infiltrate the walls of larger blood vessels, particularly veins, and there is marked involvement of the interlobular septa. The veins are often obliterated, whereas arteries are usually less severely involved. In the most severely affected areas nodules of new capillaries replace the lung parenchyma. Where the pulmonary architecture is better preserved, alveolar walls, which at low magnification appear congested, can be seen on close examination to consist of a double layer of capillaries.[146] The process may extend to involve the pleura. It may also invade the walls of bronchi to form intraluminal tufts of capillaries (Fig. 8.2.16c). Haemorrhage and congestion lead to haemosiderosis, with accumulation of haemosiderin-laden macrophages. Secondary hypertensive changes in the arteries include medial hypertrophy and intimal fibrosis.

Aetiology and differential diagnosis

In the first reported case, the endothelial cells of the proliferating vessels were atypical and the authors regarded the process as being neoplastic.[144] However, atypia has not been seen in other examples and the disease remains confined to the lungs and pleura. Its age distribution (14–71 years) renders hamartomatous growth unlikely but its development in three siblings suggests that it might have a genetic basis, possibly involving the release of as yet unidentified angiogenic factors.[4] Rarely, the condition appears to complicate severe passive pulmonary congestion.[159]

The distinction between pulmonary capillary haemangiomatosis and pulmonary veno-occlusive disease is a fine one, if it exists at all. The histological similarities are close and described differences are debatable. The distinction is said to depend on the presence of infiltrating capillaries in the lung parenchyma and larger vessels, in contrast to fibroelastic obliteration of veins in veno-occlusive disease, but this may merely represent the establishment of more florid anastomoses bypassing occluded veins. Angiogenesis is a feature of pulmonary veno-occlusive disease[139] and pulmonary capillary haemangiomatosis may represent an exaggerated degree of such angiogenesis.

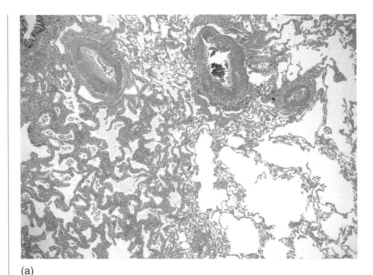

(a)

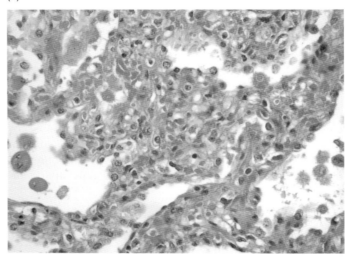

(b)

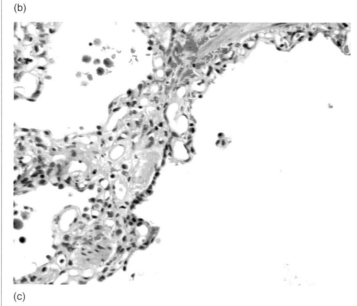

(c)

Figure 8.2.16 Pulmonary capillary haemangiomatosis. (a) At low power, an area of alveolar wall thickening is seen. (b) At high power, the thickening is seen to be due to an irregular proliferation of alveolar capillaries. (c) In a separate case, the proliferating capillaries infiltrate the bronchiolar epithelium.

Capillary haemangiomatosis should not be confused with the separate condition of diffuse pulmonary haemangiomatosis, which is a form of vascular malformation and is described on p. 621.

PULMONARY HYPERTENSION IN CONNECTIVE TISSUE DISEASE

Pulmonary disease of very varied type may develop in several connective tissue disorders (Table 10.1, p. 472). Pulmonary hypertension is one of the less common of these and when present may be secondary to another pulmonary manifestation of the connective tissue disorder, particularly fibrosing alveolitis. Pulmonary hypertension secondary to parenchymal lung disease is considered above and this section deals only with the pulmonary hypertension that develops in patients with connective tissue disorders who do not have parenchymal lung disease. Pathological studies are scanty,[6,69,132,133,160–170] possibly because lung biopsy carries a risk of haemorrhage in severe pulmonary hypertension. Furthermore, few accounts compare the changes in one connective tissue disease with those in another, or with those of primary pulmonary hypertension.

Although the changes in any one connective disease are often said to be distinctive, on comparing them they obviously have much in common, not only with each other but also with those of primary pulmonary hypertension, at least in the early stages of that disease. However, an important difference from primary pulmonary hypertension is a relative rarity of plexiform or angiomatoid lesions in the connective tissue diseases.

The characteristic changes in pulmonary hypertension associated with connective tissue diseases are to be found mainly in small intralobular pulmonary arteries and chiefly affect the intima, although such media as extends into these small vessels is often hypertrophied. The intima is thickened by a concentric spindle cell proliferation, which resembles the many skins of an onion, or by the deposition of acellular collagenous material, often resulting in gross reduction or obliteration of the lumen (Fig. 8.2.17). Although described in several connective tissue disorders, this pattern of disease is particularly seen in systemic sclerosis, in which condition such changes are well described in systemic arteries.[160] The form of systemic sclerosis most likely to be associated with pulmonary hypertension is that known as the CREST syndrome (Calcinosis, Raynaud's phenomenon, Esophageal dysfunction, Sclerodactyly and Telangiectasia).

Another change described in pulmonary hypertension associated with connective tissue disease is vasculitis. It is likely that this represents a true vasculitis, probably of an immune nature, rather than the necrotising arteritis of plexogenic arteriopathy, but this is disputed.[161]

A further association is seen in patients with the antiphospholipid syndrome, which may be idiopathic but is often associated with systemic lupus erythematosus or other connective tissue disorder.[134] In these patients lung biopsy shows platelet thrombi occluding small arteries and veins. The occlu-

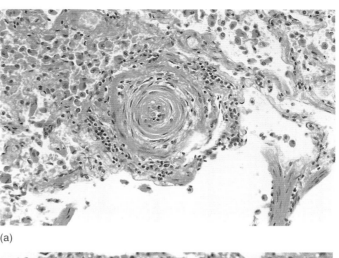

(a)

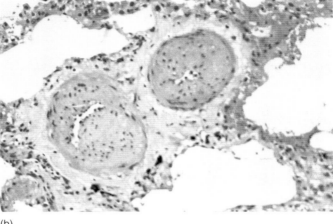

(b)

Figure 8.2.17 *Pulmonary arteries in two patients with the CREST variant of systemic sclerosis and severe pulmonary hypertension. In one (a) the pulmonary arteries show marked 'onion-skinning' (circumferential intimal cell proliferation) while in the other (b) there is hyaline intimal fibrosis. In both cases there is considerable narrowing of the lumen.*

sion of small intralobular veins leads to secondary changes such as the patchy capillary congestion and haemosiderosis described above under pulmonary veno-occlusive disease.

EFFECTS OF PULMONARY HYPERTENSION

In long-standing pulmonary hypertension, the larger pulmonary arteries may be dilated, and atheromatous plaques may be found in them at necropsy (Fig. 8.2.18).[171] Secondary thrombosis may supervene, occasionally resulting in pulmonary infarction. The dilatation may assume aneurysmal proportions and rupture is recorded, often in association with mucoid medial degeneration (cystic medial 'necrosis') and even dissection.[172–174] Some of the breathlessness associated with pulmonary hypertension may be due to aneurysmal dilatation of a major pulmonary artery pressing on the adjacent bronchus. Cholesterol granulomas have been described in the lungs of

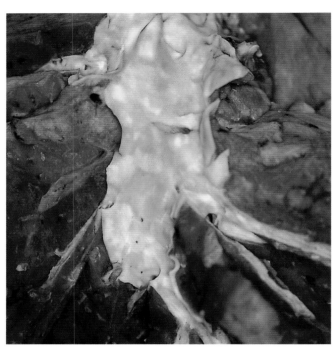

Figure 8.2.18 Atheroma of large pulmonary arteries, a change that is virtually confined to patients with pulmonary hypertension.

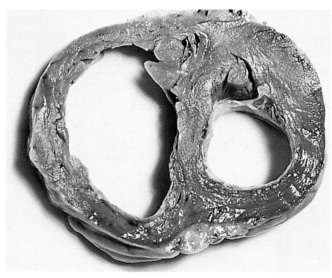

Figure 8.2.19 Cor pulmonale in a patient dying of pulmonary veno-occlusive disease. The dilated right ventricle is hypertrophied to such an extent that its thickness equals that of the left.

patients with pulmonary hypertension of varied aetiology,[175] but this is a rare finding.

Cor pulmonale

Irrespective of its pathogenesis, long-standing pulmonary hypertension leads to right heart strain and hypertrophy of the right ventricle (Fig. 8.2.19). For poorly understood reasons, the left ventricle also undergoes hypertrophy but not so markedly as the right.[176,177] Ultimately, the hypertrophied right ventricle fails and passive venous congestion develops in the systemic circulation. If the pulmonary hypertension is caused by disease within the lung, the term cor pulmonale may be used to denote the consequent right heart strain. Cor pulmonale is defined as *'hypertrophy of the right ventricle resulting from diseases affecting the function or structure of the lung, except when the pulmonary alterations are the result of diseases that primarily affect the left side of the heart or of congenital heart disease'*.[178] Hypertrophy of the right ventricle can only be assessed accurately from its weight; thickness of the ventricular muscle is affected by dilatation of the heart and is a poor index of hypertrophy.[177] To weigh the ventricles separately, the heart should be divided at the atrioventricular ring and the right ventricle trimmed away from the septum and left ventricle.[179] Normal values are right ventricle 65 g and left ventricle plus septum 185 g. Right ventricular hypertrophy is indicated by a right ventricular weight over 80 g or a ratio of the weights of the left ventricle plus septum to right ventricle of less than 2:1. This ratio normally lies between 2.3:1 and 3.3:1.

REFERENCES

1. Rubin LJ. Diagnosis and management of pulmonary arterial hypertension: ACCP evidence-based clinical practice guidelines. Chest 2004; 126:7S–10S.
2. Davies P, Reid L. Pulmonary veno-occlusive disease in siblings: case reports and morphometric study. Hum Pathol 1982; 13:922.
3. Loyd JE, Atkinson JB, Pietra GG, Virmani R, Newman JH. Heterogeneity of pathologic lesions in familial primary pulmonary hypertension. Am Rev Respir Dis 1988; 138:952–957.
4. Langleben D, Heneghan JM, Batten AP, et al. Familial pulmonary capillary hemangiomatosis resulting in primary pulmonary hypertension. Ann Intern Med 1988; 109:106–109.
5. Morse JH, Barst RJ, Fotino M. Familial pulmonary hypertension – immunogenetic findings in four Caucasian kindreds. Am Rev Respir Dis 1992; 145:787–792.
6. Wilson L, Tomita T, Braniecki M. Fatal pulmonary hypertension in identical twins with systemic lupus erythematosus. Hum Pathol 1991; 22:295–297.
7. Wagenvoort CA. Classifying pulmonary vascular disease. Chest 1973; 64:503–504.
8. Wagenvoort CA. Lung biopsy specimens in the evaluation of pulmonary vascular disease. Chest 1980; 77:614–625.
9. Giaid A. Nitric oxide and endothelin-1 in pulmonary hypertension. Chest 1998; 114:S208–S212.
10. Balk AG, Dingemans KP, Wagenvoort CA. The ultrastructure of the various forms of pulmonary arterial intimal fibrosis. Virchows Arch A Pathol Anat Histopathol 1979; 382:139–150.
11. Fernie JM, Lamb D. A new method for quantitating the medial component of pulmonary arteries. Arch Pathol Lab Med 1985; 109:156–162.
12. Hattano S., Strasser T. Primary Pulmonary Hypertension. Geneva: World Health Organisation; 1975.
13. Caslin AW, Heath D, Madden B, et al. The histopathology of 36 cases of plexogenic pulmonary arteriopathy. Histopathology 1990; 16:9–16.
14. Wagenvoort CA, Mulder PGH. Thrombotic lesions in primary plexogenic arteriopathy - similar pathogenesis or complication? Chest 1993; 103:844–849.

Plexogenic pulmonary hypertension

15. Wagenvoort CA, Wagenvoort N. Primary pulmonary hypertension. A pathologic study of the lung vessels in 156 clinically diagnosed cases. Circulation 1970; 42:1163–1184.

16. Yamaki S, Wagenvoort CA. Comparison of primary plexogenic arteriopathy in adults and children. A morphological study in 40 patients. Br Heart J 1985; 54:428–434.

17. Wagenvoort CA. Plexogenic arteriopathy. Thorax 1994; 49:S39–S45.

18. Yaginuma G, Mohri H, Takahashi T. Distribution of arterial lesions and collateral pathways in the pulmonary hypertension of congenital heart disease: a computer aided reconstruction study. Thorax 1990; 45:586–590.

19. Heath D, Edwards JE. The pathology of hypertensive pulmonary vascular disease. A description of six grades of structural changes in the pulmonary arteries with special reference to congenital cardiac septal defects. Circulation 1958; 18:533–547.

20. Wagenvoort CA. Grading of pulmonary vascular lesions – a reappraisal. Histopathology 1981; 5:595–598.

21. Jamison BM, Michel RP. Different distribution of plexiform lesions in primary and secondary pulmonary hypertension. Hum Pathol 1995; 26:987–993.

22. Elliott FM, Reid L. Some new facts about the pulmonary artery and its branching pattern. Clin Radiol 1965; 16:193–198.

23. Smith P, Heath D. Electron microscopy of the plexiform lesion. Thorax 1979; 34:177–186.

24. Tuder RM, Groves B, Badesch DB, Voelkel NF. Exuberant endothelial cell growth and elements of inflammation are present in plexiform lesions of pulmonary hypertension. Am J Pathol 1994; 144:275–285.

25. Lee SD, Shroyer KR, Markham NE, et al. Monoclonal endothelial cell proliferation is present in primary but not secondary pulmonary hypertension. J Clin Invest 1998; 101:927–934.

26. Tuder RM, Radisavljevic Z, Shroyer KR, Polak JM, Voelkel NF. Monoclonal endothelial cells in appetite suppressant-associated pulmonary hypertension. Am J Respir Crit Care Med 1998; 158:1999–2001.

27. Pare PD, Chan-Yan C, Wass H, Hooper R, Hogg JC. Portal and pulmonary hypertension with microangiopathic hemolytic anemia. Am J Med 1983; 74:1093–1096.

28. Kay JM. Pulmonary vascular lesions in chronic thromboembolic pulmonary hypertension. Chest 1994; 105:1619–1620.

29. Wagenvoort CA, Wagenvoort N, Draulans-Noe Y. Reversibility of plexogenic pulmonary arteriopathy following banding of the pulmonary artery. J Thorac Cardiovasc Surg 1984; 87:876–886.

30. Wagenvoort CA. Open lung biopsies in congenital heart disease for evaluation of pulmonary vascular disease. Predictive value with regard to corrective operability. Histopathology 1985; 9:417–436.

31. Gorenflo M, Vogel M, Hetzer R, et al. Morphometric techniques in the evaluation of pulmonary vascular changes due to congenital heart disease. Pathol Res Pr 1996; 192:107–116.

32. Haworth SG. Pulmonary vascular disease in ventricular septal defect: structural and functional correlations in lung biopsies from 85 patients, with outcome of intracardiac repair. J Pathol 1987; 152:157–168.

33. Pietra GG, Edwards WD, Kay JM, et al. Histopathology of primary pulmonary hypertension. A qualitative and quantitative study of pulmonary blood vessels from 59 patients in the National Heart, Lung, and Blood Institute primary pulmonary hypertension registry. Circulation 1989; 80:1198–1206.

34. Pietra GG. Histopathology of primary pulmonary hypertension. Chest 1994; 105:S2–S6.

35. Rich S, Dantzker DR, Ayres SM, et al. Primary pulmonary hypertension. Ann Intern Med 1987; 107:216–223.

36. Nichols WC, Koller DL, Slovis B, et al. Localisation of the gene for familial primary pulmonary hypertension to chromosome 2q31-32. Nat Genet 1997; 15:277–280.

37. Morse JH, Jones AC, Barst RJ, et al. Mapping of familial primary pulmonary hypertension locus (PPH1) to chromosome 2q31-q32. Circulation 1997; 95:2603–2606.

38. Newman JH, Wheeler L, Lane KB, et al. Mutation in the gene for bone morphogenetic protein receptor II as a cause of primary pulmonary hypertension in a large kindred. N Engl J Med 2001; 345:319–324.

39. Lane KB, Machado RD, Pauciulo MW, et al. Heterozygous germline mutations in BMPR2, encoding a TGF-beta receptor, cause familial primary pulmonary hypertension. Int PPH Consortium Nat Gen 2000; 26:81–84.

40. Rudarakanchana N, Trembath RC, Morrell NW. New insights into the pathogenesis and treatment of primary pulmonary hypertension. Thorax 2001; 56:888–890.

41. Loyd JE. Genetics and gene expression in pulmonary hypertension. Chest 2002; 121:46S–50S.

42. Eddahibi S, Morrell N. DOrtho MP, Naeije R, Adnot S. Pathobiology of pulmonary arterial hypertension. Eur Resp J 2002; 20:1559–1572.

43. Trembath RC, Thomson JR, Machado RD, et al. Clinical and molecular genetic features of pulmonary hypertension in patients with hereditary hemorrhagic telangiectasia. N Engl J Med 2001; 345:325–334.

44. Abdalla SA, Gallione CJ, Barst RJ, et al. Primary pulmonary hypertension in families with hereditary haemorrhagic telangiectasia. Eur Resp J 2004; 23:373–377.

45. Giaid A, Yanagisawa M, Langleben D, et al. Expression of endothelin-1 in the lungs of patients with pulmonary hypertension. N Engl J Med 1993; 328:1732–1739.

46. Giaid A, Saleh D. Reduced expression of endothelial nitric oxide synthase in the lungs of patients with pulmonary hypertension. N Engl J Med 1995; 333:214–221.

47. Orte C, Polak JM, Haworth SG, Yacoub MH, Morrell NW. Expression of pulmonary vascular angiotensin-converting enzyme in primary and secondary plexiform pulmonary hypertension. J Pathol 2000; 192:379–384.

48. Barberis MCP, Veronese S, Bauer D, Dejuli E, Harari S. Immunocytochemical detection of progesterone receptors: a study in a patient with pulmonary primary hypertension. Chest 1995; 107:869–872.

49. Heath D, Yacoub M, Gosney JR, et al. Pulmonary endocrine cells in hypertensive pulmonary vascular disease. Histopathology 1990; 16:21–28.

50. Madden BP, Gosney J, Coghlan JG, et al. Pretransplant clinicopathological correlation in end-stage primary pulmonary hypertension. Eur Respir J 1994; 7:672–678.

51. Gosney JR, Resl M. Pulmonary endocrine cells in plexogenic pulmonary arteriopathy associated with cirrhosis. Thorax 1995; 50:92–93.

52. Theegarten D, Anhenn O, Aretz S, Maass M, Mogilevski G. Detection of *Chlamydia pneumoniae* in unexplained pulmonary hypertension. Eur Resp J 2002; 19:192–194.

53. Chu JW, Kao PN, Faul JL, Doyle RL. High prevalence of autoimmune thyroid disease in pulmonary arterial hypertension. Chest 2002; 122:1668–1673.

54. McDonnell PJ, Toye PA, Hutchins GM. Primary pulmonary hypertension in cirrhosis: are they related? Am Rev Respir Dis 1983; 127:437–441.

55. Harris P, Heath D. The human pulmonary circulation. Its form and function in health and disease. Edinburgh, UK: Churchill Livingstone; 1986.

56. Budhiraja R, Hassoun PM. Portopulmonary hypertension – A tale of two circulations. Chest 2003; 123:562–576.

57. Rydell R, Hoffbauer FW. Multiple pulmonary arteriovenous fistulas in juvenile cirrhosis. Am J Med 1956; 21:450–460.

58. Berthelot P, Walker JG, Sherlock S, Reid L. Arterial changes in the lungs in cirrhosis of the liver – lung spider nevi. N Engl J Med 1966; 274:291–298.

59. Stanley NN, Williams AJ, Dewar CA, Blendis LM, Reid L. Hypoxia and hydrothoraces in a case of liver cirrhosis: correlation of physiological, radiographic, scintigraphic, and pathological findings. Thorax 1977; 32:457–471.

60. Lamps LW, Carson K, Bradley AL, et al. Pulmonary vascular morphological changes in cirrhotic patients undergoing liver transplantation. Liver Transpl Surg 1999; 5:57–64.

61. Kay JM, Smith P, Heath D. Aminorex and the pulmonary circulation. Thorax 1971; 26:262–270.

62. Douglas JG, Munro JF, Kitchin AH, Muir AL, Proudfoot AT. Pulmonary hypertension and fenfluramine. BMJ 1981; 283:881–883.

63. McMurray J, Bloomfield P, Miller HC. Irreversible pulmonary hypertension after treatment with fenfluramine. BMJ 1986; 292:239–240.

64. Abenhaim L, Moride Y, Brenot F, et al. Appetite-suppressant drugs and the risk of primary pulmonary hypertension. N Engl J Med 1996; 335:609–616.

65. Delcroix M, Kurz X, Walckiers D, Demedts M, Naeije R. High incidence of primary pulmonary hypertension associated with appetite suppressants in Belgium. Eur Resp J 1998; 12:271–276.

66. Kay JM. Dietary pulmonary hypertension. Thorax 1994; 49:S33–S38.

67. Speich R, Jenni R, Opravil M, Pfab M, Russi EW. Primary pulmonary hypertension in HIV infection. Chest 1991; 100:1268–1271.

68. Mette SA, Palevsky HI, Pietra GG, et al. Primary pulmonary hypertension in association with human immunodeficiency virus infection – a possible viral etiology for some forms of hypertensive pulmonary arteriopathy. Am Rev Respir Dis 1992; 145:1196–1200.

69. Cool CD, Kennedy D, Voelkel NF, Tuder RM. Pathogenesis and evolution of plexiform lesions in pulmonary hypertension associated with scleroderma and human immunodeficiency virus infection. Hum Pathol 1997; 28:434–442.

70. Mehta NJ, Khan IA, Mehta RN, Sepkowitz DA. HIV-Related pulmonary hypertension – Analytic review of 131 cases. Chest 2000; 118:1133–1141.

71. Orenstein JM, Preble OT, Kind P, Schulof R. The relationship of serum alpha-interferon and ultrastructural markers in HIV-seropositive individuals. Ultrastruct Pathol 1987; 11:673–679.

72. Mesa RA, Edell ES, Dunn WF, Edwards WD. Human immunodeficiency virus infection and pulmonary hypertension: two new cases and a review of 86 reported cases. Mayo Clin Proc 1998; 73:37–45.

72a. Laney AS, De Marco T, Peters JS, et al. Kaposi sarcoma-associated herpesvirus and primary and secondary pulmonary hypertension. Chest 2005; 127:762–767.

Hypoxic pulmonary hypertension

73. Kato M, Staub NC. Response of small pulmonary arteries to unilobar hypoxia and hypercapnia. Circ Res 1966; 19:426–439.

74. Nagasaka Y, Bhattacharya F, Nanjo S, Gropper MA, Staub NC. Micropuncture measurement of lung microvascular pressure profile during hypoxia in cats. Circ Res 1984; 54:90–95.

75. Kourembanas S, Bernfield M. Hypoxia and endothelial smooth muscle cell interactions in the lung. Am J Respir Cell Mol Biol 1994; 11:373–374.

76. Brij SO, Peacock AJ. Cellular responses to hypoxia in the pulmonary circulation. Thorax 1998; 53:1075–1079.

77. Nakanishi K, Tajima F, Nakata Y, et al. Expression of endothelin-1 in rats developing hypobaric hypoxia-induced pulmonary hypertension. Lab Invest 1999; 79:1347–1357.

78. Wagenvoort CA, Wagenvoort N. Pulmonary venous changes in chronic hypoxia. Virchows Arch A Pathol Anat Histopathol 1976; 372:51–56.

79. Smith P, Heath D, Williams D, et al. The earliest histopathological response to hypobaric hypoxia in rabbits in the Rifugio Torino (3370-m) on Monte Bianco. J Pathol 1993; 170:485–491.

80. Hicken P, Heath D, Brewer D. The relation between the weight of the right ventricle and the percentage of abnormal air space in the lung in emphysema. J Pathol Bacteriol 1966; 92:519–528.

81. Hicken P, Brewer D, Heath D. The relation between the weight of the right ventricle of the heart and the internal surface area and number of alveoli in the human lung in emphysema. J Pathol Bacteriol 1966; 92:529–546.

82. Barbera JA, Peinado VI, Santos S. Pulmonary hypertension in chronic obstructive pulmonary disease. Eur Resp J 2003; 21:892–905.

83. Hasleton PS, Heath D, Brewer DB. Hypertensive pulmonary vascular disease in states of chronic hypoxia. J Path Bact 1968; 95:431–440.

84. Wilkinson M, Langhorne CA, Heath D, Barer GR, Howard P. A pathophysiological study of 10 cases of hypoxic cor pulmonale. Q J Med 1988; 66:65–87.

85. Magee F, Wright JL, Wiggs BR, Pare PD, Hogg JC. Pulmonary vascular structure and function in chronic obstructive pulmonary disease. Thorax 1988; 43:183–189.

86. Ahmed Q, Chung-Park M, Tomashefski JF. Cardiopulmonary pathology in patients with sleep apnea/obesity hypoventilation syndrome. Hum Pathol 1997; 28:264–269.

87. Weibel E. Die Entstehung der Langsmuskulatur in den Asten der A.bronchialis. Z fur Zellforsch 1958; 47:440–468.

88. Wagenaar SJ, Wagenvoort CA. Experimental production of longitudinal smooth muscle cells in the intima of muscular arteries. Lab Invest 1978; 39:370–374.

89. Wagenvoort CA, Keutel J, Mooi WJ, Wagenvoort N. Longitudinal smooth muscle in pulmonary arteries. Occurrence in congenital heart disease. Virchows Arch A Pathol Anat Histopathol 1984; 404:265–274.

90. Harris P. Evolution, hypoxia and high altitude. In Heath D ed. Aspects of hypoxia. Liverpool, UK: Liverpool University Press; 1986:207–216.

91. Heath D, Harris P, Sui GJ, et al. Pulmonary blood vessels and endocrine cells in subacute infantile mountain sickness. Respir Med 1989; 83:77–81.

92. Gupta ML, Rao KS, Anand IS, Banerjee AK, Boparai MS. Lack of smooth muscle in the small pulmonary arteries of the native Ladakhi – is the Himalayan highlander adapted. Am Rev Respir Dis 1992; 145:1201–1204.

Pulmonary hypertension in diffuse parenchymal lung disease

93. Wagener OE, Roncoroni AJ, Barcat JA. Severe pulmonary hypertension with diffuse smooth muscle proliferation of the lungs. Pulmonary tuberous sclerosis? Chest 1989; 95:234–237.

94. Kay JM, Kahana LM, Rihal C. Diffuse smooth muscle proliferation of the lungs with severe pulmonary hypertension. Hum Pathol 1996; 27:969–974.

Embolic pulmonary hypertension

95. Wagenvoort CA. Pathology of pulmonary thromboembolism. Chest 1995; 107:S10–S17.

96. Moser KM, Bloor CM. Pulmonary vascular lesions in chronic thromboembolic pulmonary hypertension – reply. Chest 1994; 105:1620.

97. Wagenvoort CA, Mooi WJ. Biopsy pathology of the pulmonary vasculature. London: Chapman and Hall Medical; 1989.

98. Matsubara O, Yoshimura N, Tamura A, et al. Pathological features of the pulmonary artery in Takayasu arteritis. Heart Vessels 1992; Suppl 7:18–25.

99. Fedullo PF, Rubin LJ, Kerr KM, Auger WR, Channick RN. The natural history of acute and chronic thromboembolic disease: the search for the missing link. Eur Respir J 2000; 15:435–437.

100. Egermayer P, Peacock AJ. Is pulmonary embolism a common cause of chronic pulmonary hypertension? Limitations of the embolic hypothesis. Eur Respir J 2000; 15:440–448.

101. Collins FS, Orringer EP. Pulmonary hypertension and cor pulmonale in the sickle hemoglobinopathies. Am J Med 1982; 73:814–821.

102. Adedeji MO, Cespedes J, Allen K, Subramony C, Hughson MD. Pulmonary thrombotic arteriopathy in patients with sickle cell disease. Arch Pathol Lab Med 2001; 125:1436–1441.

103. Haque AK, Gokhale S, Rampy BA, et al. Pulmonary hypertension in sickle cell hemoglobinopathy: A clinicopathologic study of 20 cases. Hum Pathol 2002; 33:1037–1043.

104. Gladwin MT, Sachdev V, Jison ML, et al. Pulmonary hypertension as a risk factor for death in patients with sickle cell disease. N Engl J Med 2004; 350:886–895.

105. Heller PG, Grinberg AR, Lencioni M, Molina MM, Roncoroni AJ. Pulmonary hypertension in paroxysmal nocturnal hemoglobinuria. Chest 1992; 102:642–643.

106. Bagshawe KD, Brooks WDW. Subacute pulmonary hypertension due to chorionepithelioma. Lancet 1959; 1:653–658.

107. He XW, Tang YH, Luo ZQ, Cheng TO. Subacute cor pulmonale due to tumor embolisation to the lungs. Angiology 1989; 40:11–17.

108. Snyder LS, Harmon KR, Estensen RD. Intravascular lymphomatosis (malignant angioendotheliomatosis) presenting as pulmonary hypertension. Chest 1989; 96:1199–1200.

109. Hibbert M, Braude S. Tumour microembolism presenting as 'primary pulmonary hypertension'. Thorax 1997; 52:1016–1017.

110. Sato Y, Marutsuka K, Asada Y, et al. Pulmonary tumor thrombotic microangiopathy. Pathol Int 1995; 45:436–440.

Venous pulmonary hypertension

111. Chazova I, Robbins I, Loyd J, et al. Venous and arterial changes in pulmonary veno-occlusive disease, mitral stenosis and fibrosing mediastinitis. Eur Resp J 2000; 15:116–122.

112. Harrison CV. The pathology of the pulmonary vessels in pulmonary hypertension. Br J Radiol 1958; 31:217–226.

113. Goodwin JF. The nature of pulmonary hypertension. Br J Radiol 1958; 31:174–188.

114. Heard BE, Steiner RE, Herdan A, Gleason D. Oedema and fibrosis of the lungs in left ventricular failure. Br J Radiol 1968; 41:161–171.

115. Grainger RG. Interstitial pulmonary oedema and its radiological diagnosis. A sign of pulmonary venous and capillary hypertension. Br J Radiol 1958; 31:201–217.

116. Goyette EM, Farinacci CJ, Forsee JH, Blake HA. The clinicopathologic correlation of lung biopsies in mitral stenosis. Am Heart J 1954; 47:645–652.

117. Brewer DB, Humphreys DR. Primary pulmonary hypertension with obstructive venous lesions. Br Heart J 1960; 22:445–448.

118. Carrington CB, Liebow AA. Pulmonary veno-occlusive disease. Hum Pathol 1970; 1:322–324.

119. Liebow AA, Moser KM, Southgate MT. Clinical pathological conference; rapidly progressive dyspnoea in a teenage boy. JAMA 1973; 223:1243–1253.

120. Wagenvoort CA, Wagenvoort N. The pathology of pulmonary veno-occlusive disease. Virchows Arch A Pathol Anat Histopathol 1974; 364:69–79.

121. Thadani U, Burrow C, Whitaker W, Heath D. Pulmonary veno-occlusive disease. Q J Med 1975; 44:133–159.

122. Wagenvoort CA, Wagenvoort N, Takahashi T. Pulmonary veno-occlusive disease. Involvement of pulmonary arteries and review of the literature. Hum Pathol 1985; 16:1033–1041.

123. Mandel J, Mark EJ, Hales CA. Pulmonary veno-occlusive disease. Am J Respir Crit Care Med 2000; 162:1964–1973.

124. Voordes CG, Kuipers JRG, Elema JD. Familial pulmonary veno-occlusive disease: a case report. Thorax 1977; 32:763–766.

125. Lombard CM, Churg A, Winokur S. Pulmonary veno-occlusive disease following therapy for malignant neoplasms. Chest 1987; 92:871–876.

126. Swift GL, Gibbs A, Campbell IA, Wagenvoort CA, Tuthill D. Pulmonary veno-occlusive disease and Hodgkin's lymphoma. Eur Respir J 1993; 6:596–598.

127. Kramer MR, Estenne M, Berkman N, et al. Radiation-induced pulmonary veno-occlusive disease. Chest 1993; 104:1282–1284.

128. Williams LM, Fussell S, Veith RW, Nelson S, Mason CM. Pulmonary veno-occlusive disease in an adult following bone marrow transplantation: case report and review of the literature. Chest 1996; 109:1388–1391.

129. Canny GJ, Arbus GS, Wilson GJ, Newth CJ. Fatal pulmonary hypertension following renal transplantation. Br J Dis Chest 1985; 79:191–195.

130. Ruchelli ED, Nojadera G, Rutstein RM, Rudy B. Pulmonary veno-occlusive disease – another vascular disorder associated with human immunodeficiency virus infection? Arch Pathol Lab Med 1994; 118:664–666.

131. Escamilla R, Hermant C, Berjaud J, Mazerolles C, Daussy X. Pulmonary veno-occlusive disease in a HIV-infected intravenous drug abuser. Eur Respir J 1995; 8:1982–1984.

132. Devereux G, Evans MJ, Kerr KM, Legge JS. Pulmonary veno-occlusive disease complicating Felty's syndrome. Resp Med 1998; 92:1089–1091.

133. Morassut PA, Walley VM, Smith CD. Pulmonary veno-occlusive disease and the CREST variant of scleroderma. Can J Cardiol 1992; 8:1055–1058.

134. Levine JS, Branch DW, Rauch J. The antiphospholipid syndrome. N Engl J Med 2002; 346:752–763.

135. Corrin B, Spencer H, Turner-Warwick M, Beales SJ, Hamblin JJ. Pulmonary veno-occlusion – an immune complex disease? Virchows Arch A Pathol Anat Histopathol 1974; 364:81–91.

136. Crissman JD, Koss M, Carson RP. Pulmonary veno-occlusive disease secondary to granulomatous venulitis. Am J Surg Pathol 1980; 4:93–99.

137. Liang MH, Stern S, Fortin PR, et al. Fatal pulmonary veno-occlusive disease secondary to a generalized venulopathy: a new syndrome presenting with facial swelling and pericardial tamponade. Arthritis Rheum 1991; 34:228–233.

138. Wagenvoort CA, Losekoot G, Mulder E. Pulmonary veno-occlusive disease of presumably intrauterine origin. Thorax 1971; 26:429–434.

139. Schraufnagel DE, Sekosan M, McGee T, Thakkar MB. Human alveolar capillaries undergo angiogenesis in pulmonary veno-occlusive disease. Eur Respir J 1996; 9:346–350.

140. Eppinger H. Die Permeabilitatspathologie als die Lehre vom Krankheitsbeginn. Vienna: Springer; 1949.

141. Walford RI, Kaplan L. Pulmonary fibrosis and giant cell reaction to altered elastic tissue – endogenous pneumoconiosis. Arch Pathol Lab Med 1957; 63:75–90.

142. Pai UH, McMahon J, Tomashefski JF. Mineralizing pulmonary elastosis in chronic cardiac failure – endogenous pneumoconiosis revisited. Am J Clin Pathol 1994; 101:22–28.

143. Katz DS, Scalzetti EM, Katzenstein ALA, Kohman LJ. Pulmonary veno-occlusive disease presenting with thrombosis of pulmonary arteries. Thorax 1995; 50:699–700.

144. Wagenvoort CA, Beetstra A, Spijker J. Capillary haemangiomatosis of the lung. Histopathology 1978; 2:401–406.

145. Heath D, Reid R. Invasive pulmonary haemangiomatosis. Br J Dis Chest 1985; 79:284–294.

146. Tron V, Magee F, Wright JL, Colby T, Churg A. Pulmonary capillary hemangiomatosis. Hum Pathol 1986; 17:1144–1150.

147. SjSc W, Mulder JJS, Wagenvoort CA, Bosch JMM van den. Pulmonary capillary haemangiomatosis diagnosed during life. Histopathology 1989; 14:209–224.

148. Faber CN, Yousem SA, Dauber JH, et al. Pulmonary capillary hemangiomatosis. A report of three cases and a review of the literature. Am Rev Respir Dis 1989; 140:808–813.

149. Domingo C, Encabo B, Roig J, Lopez D, Morera J. Pulmonary capillary hemangiomatosis – report of a case and review of the literature. Respiration 1992; 59:178–180.

150. Masur Y, Remberger K, Hoefer M. Pulmonary capillary hemangiomatosis as a rare cause of pulmonary hypertension. Pathol Res Pr 1996; 192:290–295.

151. Ishii H, Iwabuchi K, Kameya T, Koshino H. Pulmonary capillary haemangiomatosis. Histopathology 1996; 29:275–278.

152. Unterborn J, Shepard JAO, Mark EJ, Kanarek DJ. A 45-year-old woman with exertional dyspnea, hemoptysis, and pulmonary nodules. Pulmonary-capillary hemangiomatosis. N Engl J Med 2000; 343:1788–1796.

153. Almagro P, Julia J, Sanjaume M, et al. Pulmonary capillary hemangiomatosis associated with primary pulmonary hypertension: report of 2 new cases and review of 35 cases from the literature. Medicine (Baltimore) 2002; 81:417–424.

154. Havlik DM, Massie LW, Williams WL, Crooks LA. Pulmonary capillary hemangiomatosis-like foci – An autopsy study of 8 cases. Am J Clin Pathol 2000; 113:655–662.

155. Ginns LC, Roberts DH, Mark EJ, Brusch JL, Marler JJ. Pulmonary capillary hemangiomatosis with atypical endotheliomatosis – Successful antiangiogenic therapy with doxycycline. Chest 2003; 124:2017–2022.

156. Varnholt H, Kradin R. Pulmonary capillary hemangiomatosis arising in hereditary hemorrhagic telangiectasia. Hum Pathol 2004; 35:266–268.

157. Erbersdobler A, Niendorf A. Multifocal distribution of pulmonary capillary haemangiomatosis. Histopathology 2002; 40:88–91.

158. Whittaker JS, Pickering CAC, Heath D, Smith P. Pulmonary capillary haemangiomatosis. Diag Histopathol 1983; 6:77–84.

159. Jing XF, Yokoi T, Nakamura Y, et al. Pulmonary capillary hemangiomatosis: A unique feature of congestive vasculopathy associated with hypertrophic cardiomyopathy. Arch Pathol Lab Med 1998; 122:94–96.

Pulmonary hypertension in connective tissue disease

160. Gardner DL, Duthie JJR, Macleod J, Allan WSA. Pulmonary hypertension in rheumatoid arthritis: report of a case with intimal sclerosis of the pulmonary and digital arteries. Scot Med J 1957; 2:183–188.

161. Kay JM, Banik S. Unexplained pulmonary hypertension with pulmonary arteritis in rheumatoid disease. Br J Dis Chest 1977; 71:53–59.

162. Young RH, Mark GJ. Pulmonary vascular changes in scleroderma. Am J Med 1978; 64:998–1004.

163. Kobayashi H, Sano T, Li K, et al. Mixed connective tissue disease with fatal pulmonary hypertension. Acta Pathol Jpn 1982; 32:1121–1129.

164. Asherson RA, Mackworth-Young CG, Boey ML, et al. Pulmonary hypertension in systemic lupus erythematosus. BMJ 1983; 287:1024–1025.

165. Wakaki K, Koizumi F, Fukase M. Vascular lesions in systemic lupus erythematosus [SLE] with pulmonary hypertension. Acta Pathol Jpn 1984; 34:593–604.

166. Sato T, Matsubara O, Tanaka Y, Kasuga T. Association of Sjogren's syndrome with pulmonary hypertension – report of two cases and review of the literature. Hum Pathol 1993; 24:199–205.

167. Kishida Y, Kanai Y, Kuramochi S, Hosoda Y. Pulmonary venoocclusive disease in a patient with systemic lupus erythematosus. J Rheumatol 1993; 20:2161–2162.

168. Ribadeau-Dumas S, Tillie-Leblond I, Rose C, et al. Pulmonary hypertension associated with POEMS syndrome. Eur Respir J 1996; 9:1760–1762.

169. Pronk LC, Swaak AJG. Pulmonary hypertension in connective tissue disease. Rheumatology 1991; 11:83–86.

170. Hoeper MM. Pulmonary hypertension in collagen vascular disease. Eur Resp J 2002; 19:571–576.

Effects of pulmonary hypertension

171. Moore GW, Smith RRL, Hutchins GM. Pulmonary artery atherosclerosis. Correlation with systemic atherosclerosis and hypertensive pulmonary vascular disease. Arch Pathol Lab Med 1982; 106:378–380.

172. Walley VM, Virmani R, Silver MD. Pulmonary arterial dissections and ruptures: to be considered in patients with pulmonary arterial hypertension presenting with cardiogenic shock or sudden death. Pathology 1990; 22:1–4.

173. Coard KCM, Martin MP. Ruptured saccular pulmonary artery aneurysm associated with persistent ductus arteriosus. Arch Pathol Lab Med 1992; 116:159–161.

174. Masuda S, Ishii T, Asuwa N, et al. Concurrent pulmonary arterial dissection and saccular aneurysm associated with primary pulmonary hypertension. Arch Pathol Lab Med 1996; 120:309–312.

175. Glancy DL, Frazier PD, Roberts WC. Pulmonary parenchymal cholesterol-ester granulomas in patients with pulmonary hypertension. Am J Med 1968; 45:198–210.

176. Kohama A, Tanouchi J, Hori M, Kitabatake A, Kamada T. Pathologic involvement of the left ventricle in chronic cor pulmonale. Chest 1990; 98:794–800.

177. Mitchell RS, Stanford RE, Silvers GW, Dart G. The right ventricle in chronic airway obstruction: a clinicopathologic study. Am Rev Respir Dis 1976; 114:147–154.

178. World Health Organisation. Chronic cor pulmonale: report of an expert committee. Circulation 1963; 27:594–615.

179. Fulton RM, Hutchinson EC, Jones AM. Ventricular weight in cardiac hypertrophy. Br Heart J 1952; 14:413–420.

8

Vascular disease

8.3

Vasculitis and granulomatosis, haemorrhage and haemosiderosis

This chapter deals with certain vasculitides in which the lungs are the sole or major site of involvement. In the Chapel Hill consensus classification, they largely come in the small vessel category (Box 8.3.1),[1] and are frequently combined with granulomatosis. Forms of vasculitis and granulomatosis dealt with elsewhere include bronchocentric granulomatosis on p. 463, allergic granulomatosis (Churg–Strauss syndrome) on p. 465, lymphomatoid granulomatosis on p. 653 and hypertensive arteritis on p. 421. Most of the diseases considered here have an immune basis and are treated by immunosuppressive therapy. However, they share many morphological features with the infective granulomas and it is very important that an infective aetiology is excluded before treatment is commenced. To emphasise the importance of this, infective vasculitis will be considered first.

INFECTIVE AND EMBOLIC VASCULITIS

Infective vasculitis may be due to bacterial, fungal or parasitic infection of the vessel wall. Haematogenous pseudomonas pneumonia is a good example as it is typically characterised by heavy bacterial colonisation of the arterial wall, which results in vasculitis, thrombosis and infarction (see Fig. 5.2.12). Such arterial involvement is also seen on occasion in pulmonary tuberculosis, with inflammatory weakening of the vessel wall resulting in aneurysm formation (Rasmussen aneurysms).[2] Aneurysms caused by infected emboli (so-called 'mycotic' aneurysms – a term used regardless of whether the infection is fungal of bacterial) are best known on the cerebral arteries but are occasionally encountered in the pulmonary circulation, the cause usually being infective endocarditis of the valves of the right side of the heart secondary to congenital disease or intravenous drug abuse.[3]

Drug addicts also develop granulomatous pulmonary arteritis because they inject substances intended for oral use. Many tablets include fillers such as talc, starch and cellulose, which impact in small pulmonary arteries causing foreign body granulomas within and around the vessel (see Fig. 7.2.9, p. 380). Subsequent thrombosis and re-canalisation may produce appearances similar to the plexiform lesions seen in some forms of pulmonary hypertension (see p. 421).[4–7a] A similar form of granulomatous arteritis is provoked by schistosome ova lodging in small pulmonary vessels but here, in addition to foreign body giant cells, there may also be a necrotising arteritis, which may represent an immune response to the ova (see p. 252).[8]

WEGENER'S GRANULOMATOSIS

A triad combining necrotising granulomatous inflammation and vasculitis of the upper and lower airways with glomerulonephritis was initially described by Klinger,[9] and only later by Wegener,[10,11] but it was the eponymous term Wegener's granulomatosis that was popularised by Godman and Churg.[12] These workers re-defined the triad as comprising:

Box 8.3.1 The Chapel Hill consensus classification of systemic vasculitis[1]

Large vessels
   Giant cell arteritis Typically involves the temporal arteries in patients older than 50. May involve the aorta. Pulmonary involvement rare.
   Takayasu's arteritis Typically involves the aorta in patients younger than 50. May involve the major pulmonary arteries.
Medium-sized vessels
   Polyarteritis nodosa Pulmonary involvement rare.
   Kawasaki disease Children. Pulmonary involvement not described.
Small vessels
   Wegener's granulomatosis Typically involves the respiratory tract.
   Churg–Strauss syndrome Typically involves the respiratory tract.
   Microscopic polyangiitis Typically involves the respiratory tract.
   Henoch–Schönlein purpura Respiratory involvement unusual.
   Essential cryoglobulinaemic vasculitis Respiratory involvement unusual.
   Cutaneous leukocytoclastic angiitis Limited to the skin.

- granulomatosis of the upper and lower respiratory tracts
- generalised vasculitis
- glomerulonephritis

thus recognising that the vasculitis has a wide distribution. So too does the granulomatosis but it is the respiratory tract that is most frequently affected (Table 8.3.1).[13] The glomerulonephritis was the major factor in the once high mortality of the disease but since cyclophosphamide became widely used in the 1960s the 5-year survival rate has improved from less than 10% to over 80%.[14] Limited forms of the disease, largely confined to the lungs, are dealt with below (p. 444).

Aetiology

The recognition of circulating anti-neutrophil cytoplasmic antibodies (ANCA) in Wegener's disease and related conditions provides considerable evidence that these diseases have an auto-immune basis.[15–17] Further evidence for this derives from the effectiveness of the immunosuppressive drugs cyclophosphamide and corticosteroids and a high titre of rheumatoid factor and raised levels of serum immunoglobulins. Studies of sputum and bronchoalveolar lavage fluid suggest that ANCA are produced in the lungs.[18] ANCA titres correlate with disease activity and *in vitro* it has been shown that ANCA cause cytokine-primed neutrophils to degranulate, releasing lysosomal enzymes and toxic oxygen radicals. This mechanism probably underlies the 'pathergic' process envisaged by Fienberg, which is characterised in its early stages by granulomas centred on small collections of neutrophils.[19,20] ANCA binding causes primed neutrophils to adhere to endothelial surfaces, with neutrophil degranulation at this site accounting for the vasculitis.[17] Immune deposits are not readily identifiable in the ANCA-associated diseases and they are therefore termed pauci-immune.

Clinical features[21]

Wegener's granulomatosis is a rare disease with a prevalence of about 3 per 100 000.[22] It affects men more than women and occurs at all ages. It generally presents with systemic features such as fever, weight loss, anaemia and arthralgia, combined with respiratory complaints such as nasal discharge and crusting, otitis media, cough, haemoptysis and chest pain. Rarer forms of presentation include acute pulmonary haemorrhage[23–25] and

---

Table 8.3.1 Frequency of organ involvement in Wegener's granulomatosis, microscopic polyangiitis and Churg–Strauss syndrome[13]

	Wegener's granulomatosis (%)	Microscopic polyangiitis (%)	Churg–Strauss syndrome (%)
Lung	90	50	70
Upper respiratory tract	90	35	50
Kidney	80	90	45
Musculoskeletal	60	60	50
Skin	40	40	60
Neurological	50	30	70
Gastrointestinal	50	50	50

glomerulonephritis: the latter usually follows the extra-renal manifestations of the disease.[14,26] Saddle deformity of the nose may occur and nasal destruction may be so great as to suggest lethal midline granuloma. All patients have involvement of the lungs or upper respiratory tract but virtually any organ may be affected. Radiological examination shows multiple lung masses resembling metastases or, if cavitating, abscesses. Eosinophilia is not a feature of the disease and if present should alert one to the possibility of Churg–Strauss granulomatosis (see p. 465). Fibroptic and aspiration biopsies are of limited use in the diagnosis of Wegener's granulomatosis but the identification of any one of the characteristic pathological features may suggest the diagnosis, provided that other processes such as infection have been ruled out. Serological tests, which are dealt with next, may also be helpful, but in many cases a surgical biopsy is required to establish the diagnosis.

Antineutrophil cytoplasmic antibodies

The recognition of circulating anti-neutrophil cytoplasmic antibodies (ANCA) in Wegener's disease and related conditions represents a major advance in diagnosis.[15,16,27–29] There are at least two such antibodies, both of which are of IgG type. Under indirect immunofluorescent microscopy, one antibody gives centrally accentuated granular staining in the cytoplasm of neutrophils: the antigen here is a 29 kD serine proteinase 3 and the antibody is known as cytoplasmic, c- or PR3-ANCA. The second antibody is recognised by perinuclear staining. It is directed principally against myeloperoxidase and is known as perinuclear, p- or MPO-ANCA (Fig. 8.3.1). However, atypical immunofluorescent patterns are sometimes encountered and more specific, solid phase enzyme-linked immunoabsorbent assays (ELISAs) are preferred.[30]

There is considerable overlap in the histological features associated with c- and p-ANCAs,[28,31] but Wegener's granulomatosis shows a strong association with c-ANCA, the Churg–Strauss syndrome with p-ANCA and microscopic polyangiitis with either c- or p-ANCA (Table 8.3.2).[32] The specificity of c-ANCA for Wegener's granulomatosis is high, about 95% in the classic form of the disease and about 65% in the limited form. The rare false positives are encountered with diseases of the lung such as tuberculosis, lymphoma, HIV infection and thromboembolism. The sensitivity varies with disease activity and this provides a useful means of monitoring treatment.[27,30,33]

Pathological features of the lung lesions[34–36]

At necropsy, multiple irregular but well-circumscribed masses of various size are seen in the lungs. They consist of grey indurated tissue surrounding a soft, friable, grey or haemorrhagic necrotic centre, which may cavitate (Fig. 8.3.2). There is

Table 8.3.2 Frequency of ANCA types in pauci-immune vasculitis[32]

ANCA type	Wegener's granulomatosis (%)	Microscopic polyangiitis (%)	Churg–Strauss syndrome (%)
Cytoplasmic (PR-3)	75	40	10
Perinuclear (MPO)	20	50	60

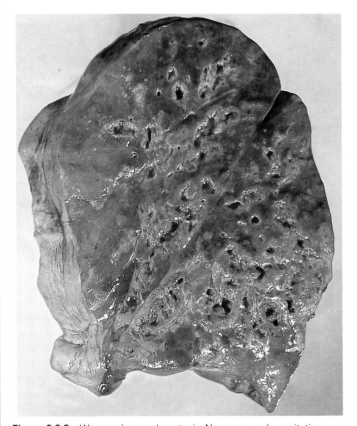

Figure 8.3.2 Wegener's granulomatosis. Numerous pale, cavitating masses replace the lung tissue, which elsewhere is haemorrhagic.

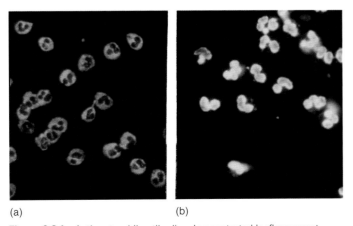

(a)   (b)

Figure 8.3.1 Antineutrophil antibodies demonstrated by fluorescent microscopy following the application of the patient's serum to test smears. (a) cytoplasmic antibodies (c-ANCA), (b) perinuclear antibodies (p-ANCA). (Illustration provided by Dr G Valesini, Rome, Italy.)

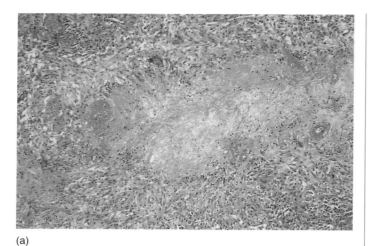

(a)

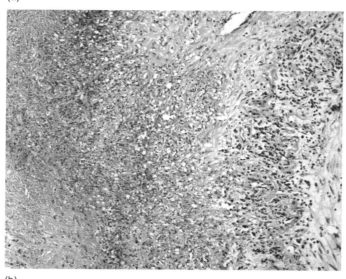

(b)

Figure 8.3.3 Wegener's granulomatosis. (a) A central area of necrosis is bordered by granulation tissue that is infiltrated by numerous lymphocytes and plasma cells and an occasional multinucleate giant cell. (b) The necrosis is often notably haematoxyphilic due to neutrophilic debris.

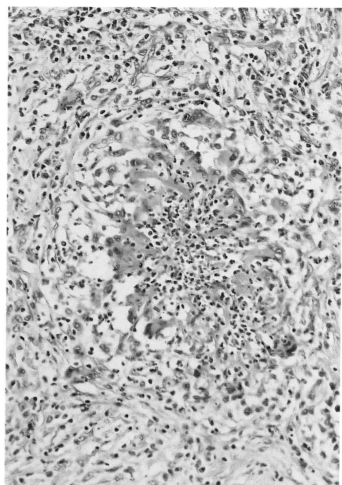

Figure 8.3.4 Wegener's granulomatosis. Neutrophilic microabscesses bordered by a granulomatous reaction probably represent an early stage in the development of the larger irregular areas of necrotising granulomatosis.

often a fibrinous pleurisy or effusion. The large airways may be ulcerated, thickened by nodules of granulation tissue, or stenotic.[37,38]

Microscopically, the nodules show irregular areas of necrosis surrounded by inflammatory granulation tissue (Fig. 8.3.3). The outlines of necrotic vessels or other structures may be evident centrally and there is often extensive karyorrhexis resulting in the accumulation of fine haematoxyphilic nuclear dust (Fig. 8.3.3). The inflammatory infiltrate of the surrounding granulation tissue includes lymphocytes, which are predominantly T-cells,[39] plasma cells, neutrophils and macrophages, the last often arranged in a palisade about the necrosis. Variable numbers of multinucleate giant cells may be seen, scattered individually or forming loose clusters, but seldom forming cohesive sarcoid-like granulomas. Neutrophilic microabscesses

form a further pattern of tissue necrosis and probably represent an early change (Fig. 8.3.4).[19,20] Eosinophils are seldom conspicuous, except in a rare eosinophilic variant of Wegener's granulomatosis[40] in which there is intense tissue eosinophilia within the inflammatory granulomatosis but not the eosinophilic pneumonia or the blood eosinophilia and asthma of the Churg–Strauss syndrome. The granulomatosis is fairly characteristic but the possibility of infection should always be kept in mind and stains for mycobacteria and fungi undertaken.

The necrotising granulomatosis is accompanied by focal vasculitis that involves medium-sized or small arteries or veins, or capillaries (Fig. 8.3.5). Its primary nature is best appreciated in areas not involved in the granulomatosis but this is seldom possible. Involved arteries and veins show transmural infiltration by neutrophils, lymphocytes, plasma cells and giant cells in varying proportions, and there is often fibrinoid necrosis. The vasculitis is sometimes granulomatous. Elastin stains are useful

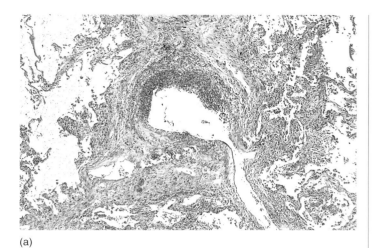

(a)

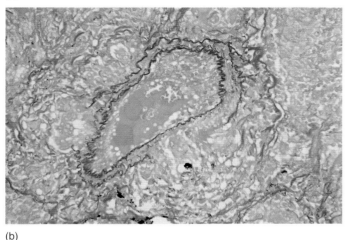

(b)

Figure 8.3.5 Wegener's granulomatosis. (a) A pulmonary artery is involved by necrotising vasculitis. (b) Deficiencies in the external elastic lamina of this pulmonary artery indicate that it has been previously affected by necrotising vasculitis (Elastin-van Gieson stain).

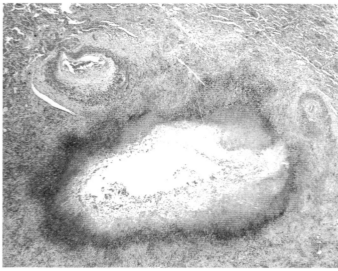

(a)

(b)

Figure 8.3.6 Bronchocentric injury in Wegener's granulomatosis. (a) A focus of necrosis is centred on a bronchiole. However, the necrosis is notably haematoxyphilic, raising the possibility of Wegener's granulomatosis. (b) An elastin stain shows destruction of a vessel wall adjacent to the necrotic area. Vasculitis was also evident elsewhere in the biopsy. (Sections provided by Dr D Rassl, Papworth, UK.)

for demonstrating the partial loss of elastic laminae indicative of a previous necrotising vasculitis (Fig. 8.3.5b). The process is usually focal, involving only a segment of the vessel wall.

Occasionally, the necrosis is strikingly bronchocentric (Fig. 8.3.6),[37] but vasculitis can also be identified. Capillaritis is manifest as a heavy neutrophil infiltrate of the alveolar septa (Fig. 8.3.7).[25] It may be leukocytoclastic and often leads to alveolar haemorrhage, which may obscure the inflammation (Fig. 8.3.8). Previous haemorrhagic episodes are characterised by haemosiderosis.

Immunofluorescence microscopy for immunoglobulins and complement is either negative or very weakly positive, the latter giving rise to the term pauci-immune.

The vasculitis causes thrombosis and wedge-shaped areas of haemorrhagic infarction but it is unlikely that the extensive necrosis is ischaemic as small foci are seen in the earliest form of the disease[20] and larger necrotising lesions are seen away from foci of vasculitis.[41] Fienberg referred to the necrosis as a pathergic process and introduced the term pathergic granulomatosis,[19,20] but the eponymous title remains in popular use.

Today, the pathologist is confronted with very small biopsy specimens from which the vasculitic lesions, formerly thought essential to the diagnosis, are often absent. However, foci of necrosis bordered by inflammatory granulation tissue with palisaded histiocytes at the interface are by themselves strongly suggestive – some would say diagnostic – of Wegener's granulomatosis.[20,42]

The lung between the lesions may show non-specific changes, including organising pneumonia, obstructive lipid

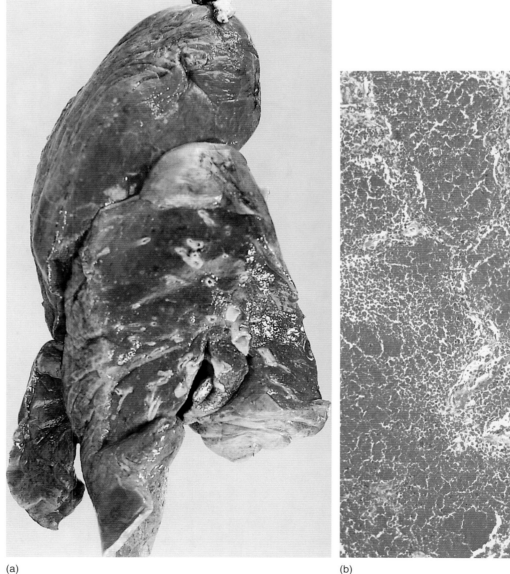

Figure 8.3.7 Wegener's granulomatosis. The vasculitis is sometimes manifest as a capillaritis, which is evident as a neutrophilic infiltrate of the alveolar walls.

pneumonia, haemorrhage and haemosiderosis, any of which may mask the characteristic lesions.[35,43] Also, the classic histological features may be considerably diminished if the biopsy is taken after the instigation of treatment.[44]

Extrapulmonary lesions

The same combination of necrotising granulomatous inflammation and vasculitis is seen in the upper respiratory tract[45–47] and skin[48,49] but biopsies may not show the full spectrum of changes. It is claimed that cutaneous biopsies characterised by leukocytoclastic vasculitis indicate a worse prognosis than those showing granulomatous inflammation.[49] The vascular lesions may be indistinguishable from those of classic polyarteritis nodosa. Such lesions may be present in the kidneys as well as the focal and segmental necrotising glomerulonephritis

(a)

(b)

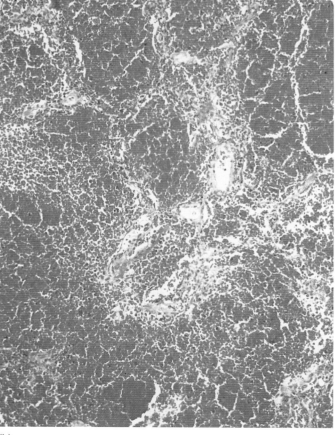

Figure 8.3.8 Wegener's granulomatosis resulting in diffuse pulmonary haemorrhage. (a) gross appearances, (b) microscopy.

that forms part of the classic triad of lesions (Fig. 8.3.9). The glomerulonephritis is characterised by fibrinoid necrosis of capillary loops and epithelial crescent formation.[50]

Differential diagnosis (Table 8.3.3)

Granulomatous fungal and mycobacterial infection must always be considered in the differential diagnosis of Wegener's

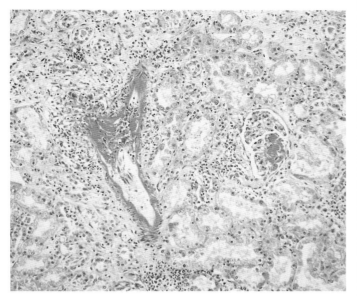

Figure 8.3.9 Wegener's granulomatosis. Kidney showing the classic focal necrotising glomerulonephritis and also necrotising arteritis.

granulomatosis. Well-formed granulomas favour infection (or sarcoidosis) but the histopathological appearances can be very similar and special stains, culture, serology or even molecular techniques may be necessary to identify infection. However, Wegener's granulomatosis entails a risk of opportunistic infection and both processes may be present. Tests for anti-neutrophil cytoplasmic antibodies (ANCA) are helpful as these are negative in patients with infection (apart from very occasional patients with tuberculosis) or sarcoidosis.

Churg–Strauss granulomatosis shares some histopathological features with Wegener's granulomatosis but there is also marked tissue eosinophilia. The p-ANCA test is positive and c-ANCA negative, and there is usually asthma and blood eosinophilia. The pattern of organ involvement also differs (see p. 465).

Wegener's granulomatosis that is predominantly bronchocentric[37,38,51] has to be distinguished from bronchocentric granulomatosis (see p. 463), which is characterised by necrotising granulomatous inflammation centred on airways but lacks the vasculitis of Wegener's disease.

Wegener's granulomatosis that is centred on the pulmonary capillaries has to be distinguished from microscopic polyangiitis (see p. 446), a condition that lacks the distinctive necrotising granulomatosis and is characterized by either p- or c-ANCA.

Other entities that enter the differential diagnosis of Wegener's granulomatosis include lymphomatoid granulomatosis (see p. 653), which is distinguished by the presence of atypical lymphoid cells of B-cell phenotype within the infiltrate and a relative absence of destructive vasculitis, and rheumatoid

Table 8.3.3   The differential diagnosis of pulmonary vasculitis and granulomatosis

	Vessels involved	ANCA type	Necrotising vasculitis	Parenchymal necrosis	Sarcoid granulomas	Palisaded granulomas	Blood eosinophilia	Asthma	Atypical cells
Polyarteritis nodosa	Small to medium systemic arteries	−	+	− (except infarction)	−	−	−	−	−
Microscopic polyangiitis	Capillaries	c = p	+	−	−	−	−	−	−
Wegener's granulomatosis	Small arteries, veins and capillaries	c > p	+	+	−	+	−	−	−
Necrotising sarcoid granulomatosis	Small arteries and veins	−	+	+	+	−	−	−	−
Churg–Strauss syndrome	Small arteries and veins	p > c	+	+	−	+	+	+	−
Lymphomatoid granulomatosis	Small arteries and veins	−	− (infiltration)	+	−	−	−	−	+
Bronchocentric granulomatosis	None	−	−	+	±	+	+	+	−
Sarcoidosis	Veins and small arteries	−	−	−	+	−	−	−	−
Infective granuloma	Any involved in the inflammation	−	+−	+	+	+	−	−	−
Rheumatoid nodule	Any near the granuloma	−	−	+	−	+	−	−	−

nodules (see p. 473), which also lack a vasculitic component and show even more prominent palisading.

Limited forms of Wegener's granulomatosis

Wegener's granulomatosis does not always show the widespread distribution described above. Limited forms of the disease have been described.[19,52,53] These lack the upper respiratory and glomerular components but show the typical pulmonary lesions, which are sometimes solitary.[54] Alternatively, there may be only capillaritis with diffuse pulmonary haemorrhage.[55,56] One biopsy series of Wegener's granulomatosis comprised 48 cases of classic disease and 19 of the limited form.[35]

Limited Wegener's granulomatosis affects women more than men and has a much better prognosis than the classic disease.[53] About 30% of patients with limited Wegener's granulomatosis lack anti-neutrophil cytoplasmic antibodies. As with the classic form of the disease, granulomatous infection figures prominently in the differential diagnosis. At one hospital, the application of simple stains for mycobacteria and fungi to 86 archival cases that had been filed as 'solitary necrotising granulomas' of the lung revealed an infectious aetiology in 75, presumably representing patients who had not received the appropriate treatment.[57]

CONDITIONS LINKING WEGENER'S GRANULOMATOSIS WITH SARCOIDOSIS AND OTHER DISORDERS

Vascular involvement is common in sarcoidosis (see Fig. 6.1.33, p. 289) but is usually no more than an incidental histological finding rather than a component of a systemic vasculitic syndrome. However, the two conditions that are about to be described indicate that there is a spectrum of conditions between sarcoidosis and Wegener's granulomatosis. In their classic forms sarcoidosis and Wegener's granulomatosis are very different but these intermediate conditions demonstrate that there can be considerable overlap. Other unusual combinations are pulmonary vascular lesions in the so-called 'non-infectious granulomatous angiitis with a predilection for the nervous system'[58] and temporal arteritis associated with Wegener's granulomatosis.[59,60] There are also occasional reports of Wegener's granulomatosis being associated with alpha-1 antitrypsin deficiency and bullous emphysema, all these conditions perhaps reflecting proteinase/antiproteinase imbalance in the lung.[61-63]

Necrotising sarcoid angiitis and granulomatosis

Necrotising sarcoid angiitis and granulomatosis combines the vasculitis and necrotising granulomatosis of Wegener's granulomatosis with numerous non-necrotising sarcoid granulomas.[64] Women are affected more than men and the age range is

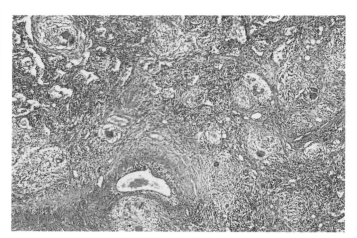

Figure 8.3.10 Necrotising sarcoid granulomatosis. The lung contains numerous non-necrotising epithelioid and giant cell granulomas and shows necrotising arteritis.

wide.[65-69] Some patients are asymptomatic but most have non-specific respiratory symptoms accompanied by malaise.

Chest radiographs usually show multiple nodules or masses measuring up to several centimetres in diameter, most numerous in the lower zones. Occasionally the lesions are unilateral or even single.[65,70] Cavitation is rare.

Evidence of extrapulmonary involvement is uncommon but hilar lymph node enlargement was a feature of more than half the patients in one series[66] and granulomas may be found in these nodes. Ocular and central nervous system involvement have also been reported[66,71-73] and in some patients the disease has been associated with ulcerative colitis[74] or cutaneous involvement.[75] Generally however, the disease is confined to the lungs and the prognosis is good, resolution occurring either spontaneously or following corticosteroid therapy.[69]

Pathological features

The lesions form irregular areas of induration, which microscopically consist of confluent aggregates of epithelioid and giant cell granulomas with surrounding fibrosis and chronic inflammation (Fig. 8.3.10). The granulomas are identical to those seen in sarcoidosis and, as in sarcoidosis, they tend to follow lymphatic pathways in the bronchovascular bundles, the interlobular septa and the pleura, and may show a small central area of necrosis. However, there are also larger areas of coagulative necrosis (Fig. 8.3.11). Regression of the inflammation may leave the necrotic areas surrounded only by hyaline connective tissue. Various patterns of vasculitis may be seen, all involving both arteries or veins, and destroying the vessel wall to a varying extent. The vessels may show discrete granulomas, a more diffuse proliferation of giant cells and epithelioid macrophages, or merely lymphocyte and plasma cell infiltration (Figs 8.3.11, 8.3.12). There may also be bronchial involvement, as in Wegener's granulomatosis.

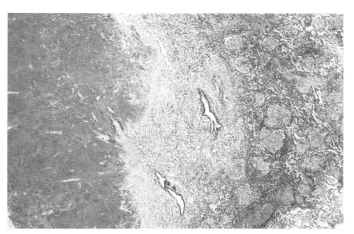

Figure 8.3.11 Necrotising sarcoid granulomatosis. This low power view shows non-necrotising sarcoid-like granulomas (right) in conjunction with a large area of necrosis (left).

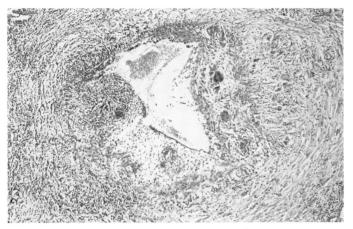

Figure 8.3.12 Necrotising sarcoid granulomatosis. A pulmonary artery shows a granulomatous vasculitis.

Aetiology

It has been suggested that necrotising sarcoid granulomatosis merely represents a variant of sarcoidosis in which mass lesions form, so-called nodular sarcoidosis.[66] This is supported by reports of raised levels of serum angiotensin-converting enzyme and selective migration of T-helper lymphocytes to the lung.[76] Furthermore, a granulomatous vasculitis is frequently seen in sarcoidosis.[77] However, the broad areas of necrosis seen in necrotising sarcoid granulomatosis are not a feature of classic sarcoidosis. In one case onset coincided with *Chlamydia pneumoniae* infection.[78]

Sarcoidosis combined with disseminated visceral giant cell angiitis

In contrast to necrotising sarcoid angiitis and granulomatosis, which, with the rare exceptions noted above, is confined to the

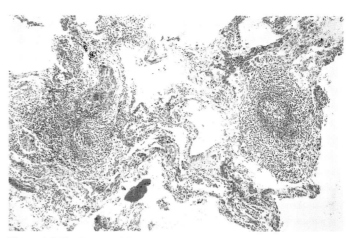

Figure 8.3.13 Polyarteritis nodosa affecting pulmonary arteries, an unusual feature of this disease.

lungs, occasional patients combine the features of sarcoidosis with those of disseminated visceral giant cell angiitis.[79–82] Such patients have disseminated necrotising granulomatosis, glomerulonephritis and systemic angiitis (the full spectrum of classic Wegener's granulomatosis) combined with typical sarcoid granulomas.

PULMONARY INVOLVEMENT IN OTHER FORMS OF SYSTEMIC VASCULITIS

Polyarteritis nodosa

When polyarteritis nodosa was first described in the nineteenth century it was stressed that it was a disease of the systemic circulation and that pulmonary involvement was unusual.[83] This has subsequently been borne out[84] but when a national survey of 'biopsy-proven' cases was conducted in 1957, roughly half were classified as being of 'respiratory type'.[85] However, the clinical details of these cases include features such as nasal granulomatosis or eosinophilia and it is evident that they represent Wegener's granulomatosis or Churg–Strauss granulomatosis rather than polyarteritis nodosa. This demonstrates that the same vasculitis is seen in these three conditions. The term 'polyangiitis overlap syndrome' has accordingly been applied to any systemic vasculitis that shows features of two or more of the well-defined vasculitic syndromes: polyarteritis nodosa, Churg–Strauss syndrome, Wegener's granulomatosis, temporal arteritis, Takayasu's arteritis and Henoch–Schonlein purpura.[86,87]

On the occasions when polyarteritis nodosa does affect the lungs it is generally limited to the bronchial vessels but it occasionally involves the pulmonary circulation in the absence of features such as granulomatosis or eosinophilia or the presence of anti-neutrophil cytoplasmic antibodies that place it in one of the other categories of vasculitis (i.e. Wegener's and Churg–Strauss granulomatosis), resulting in necrotising inflammation of medium sized muscular pulmonary arteries (Fig. 8.3.13).[88,89] So-called microscopic polyarteritis nodosa affects capillaries, arterioles and venules and is accordingly better known as microscopic polyangiitis, which is dealt with next.

Microscopic polyangiitis

Microscopic polyangiitis affects only the smallest blood vessels – arterioles, capillaries and venules – as opposed to the medium-sized arteries affected in polyarteritis nodosa. Most patients have glomerulonephritis and antineutrophil cytoplasmic antibodies, which may be of either cytoplasmic or perinuclear type (Table 8.3.2). About 50% of patients have pulmonary involvement and in about a third the upper respiratory tract is involved. Pulmonary involvement is generally characterised by lung haemorrhage; the granulomatosis of Wegener's disease is not a feature. Microscopic polyangiitis is the commonest cause of combined pulmonary and renal haemorrhagic failure (the pulmonary-renal syndrome). In the lungs, it is manifest as a haemorrhagic capillaritis characterised by neutrophil infiltration of the alveolar walls, sometimes with diffuse alveolar damage.[13,55,56,90–94] Cases in which the changes are limited to the lungs have been referred to as isolated pauci-immune pulmonary capillaritis.[95] Microscopic polyangiitis is touched upon again under diffuse pulmonary haemorrhage (see p. 452).

Hypersensitivity vasculitis

The term hypersensitivity vasculitis covers a variety of clinical conditions that are characterised pathologically by leukocytoclastic small vessel disease. They include such clinical syndromes as Henoch–Schonlein purpura[96,97] and essential mixed cryoglobulinaemia.[98] These conditions typically involve sites such as the skin or the bowel and pulmonary manifestations are unusual.[86,99] They are thought to be due to deposition of immune complexes in vessel walls. The antigen may be exogenous, such as a drug or infective agent, or endogenous, as in some connective tissue diseases. Haemoptysis is the principal complaint in all the hypersensitivity vasculitides that involve the lungs and the pathology is assumed to be a capillaritis, as described above. The hypocomplementaemic urticarial vasculitis syndrome is sometimes associated with progressive airflow obstruction due to emphysema, possibly related to the release of proteolytic enzymes from the disrupted leukocytes (Fig. 8.3.14).[100]

Vasculitis in the connective tissue diseases

Capillaritis has been identified in some patients with systemic lupus erythematosus complicated by alveolar haemorrhage,[101–106] and necrotising pulmonary vasculitis in rare rheumatoid patients (Figs 8.3.15, 8.3.16)[107–109] seen as either an autoimmune phenomenon or a component of plexogenic pulmonary hypertension.[110] Vasculitis is rare in the other connective diseases, but is recorded as an apparently isolated phenomenon in a patient with anti-Jo-1 antibodies, which are usually associated with myositis.[29]

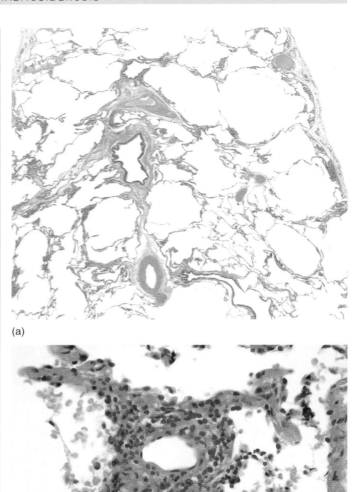

(a)

(b)

Figure 8.3.14 Hypocomplementaemic urticarial vasculitis syndrome associated with emphysema. (a) At low power, the main feature is panacinar emphysema. (b) At high power, capillaritis and focal small vessel vasculitis are evident.

Giant cell arteritis

Giant cell arteritis of the lung principally occurs in three clinical settings, Takayasu's disease,[111–113] temporal arteritis[114,115] and disseminated visceral giant cell arteritis.[116,117] These conditions differ in the distribution of the lesions, the size of the arteries involved and the type of patient they affect rather than the pathological changes within the affected vessels.

Takayasu's disease is a giant cell arteritis that typically affects the arch of the aorta and its branches, leading to so-called pulseless disease. It occurs predominantly in young women and is commonest in Japan whereas temporal arteritis typically affects elderly men and the racial distribution is wide. Only 10% of patients with temporal arteritis have extracranial involvement and pulmonary involvement is very rare, whereas evidence of pulmonary artery involvement is present in up to 70% of patients with Takayasu's disease.[111,112] Disseminated

visceral giant cell arteritis is very rare and involvement of the pulmonary arteries is usually overshadowed by disease of systemic arteries such as those supplying the myocardium. The age range is wide (infancy to old age) and the arteries affected are small muscular vessels whereas Takayasu's disease and temporal typically involve the large elastic arteries (Table 8.3.4).

Takayasu's disease is characterised by chronic giant cell inflammation of the affected arteries resulting in elastic tissue defects, eccentric intimal fibrosis or complete occlusion and re-canalisation (Fig. 8.3.17).[118–120] Some of the stenosis is caused by

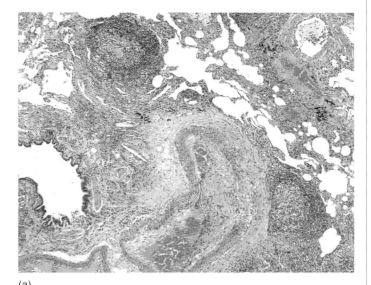

(a)

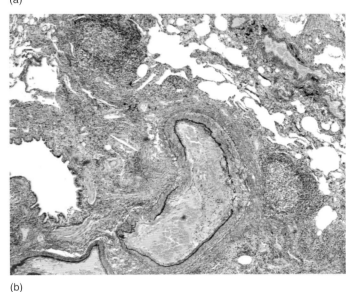

(b)

Figure 8.3.15 Vasculitis in systemic lupus erythematosus. The lung shows both follicular bronchiolitis and a small vessel vasculitis. Mixed patterns of lung disease are often seen in connective tissue disorders. (b, Elastin van Gieson stain.)

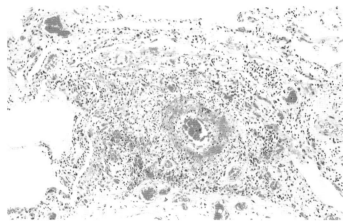

Figure 8.3.16 Pulmonary arteritis as a manifestation of rheumatoid disease.

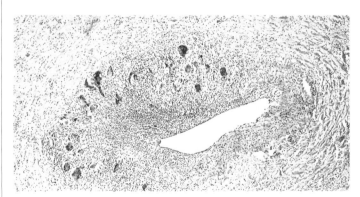

Figure 8.3.17 Takayasu's disease. This involvement of a medium sized pulmonary artery represents peripheral extension of disease that principally affected a lobar artery and led to infarction of that lobe. Giant cells are very prominent among the inflammatory infiltrate. (Case of Dr Sj Sc Wagenaar, Utrecht, Netherlands.)

Table 8.3.4   Giant cell arteritis involving the lungs

	Takayasu's disease	Temporal arteritis	Disseminated visceral giant cell arteritis
Age	Below 50 years	Over 50 years	Any age
Symptoms	Pulmonary infarction	Pulmonary infarction, headache, polymyalgia rheumatica	Sudden death, e.g. from myocardial infarction
Extrapulmonary distribution	Aorta and its major branches	Temporal artery	Coronary, renal, hepatic, pancreatic, gastric and mesenteric arteries
Pulmonary distribution	Large elastic arteries	Large elastic arteries	Small muscular arteries

cicatricial contracture, as indicated by the greatly reduced external diameter of the affected arteries.[120] Angiomatoid lesions (see p. 422) are also described, evidence that Takayasu's disease may cause pulmonary hypertension.[120] This is partly attributable to pulmonary artery obstruction and partly to re-canalisation by bronchial arteries establishing bronchopulmonary shunts.[120] More often, pulmonary Takayasu's disease is asymptomatic or mimics thromboembolic disease, sometimes resulting in infarction of a whole lung or lung lobe.[121–124]

Very rarely, giant cell arteritis is limited to the lesser circulation and categorisation then depends solely upon the age and sex of the patient, which is imprecise. Because pulmonary involvement is much commoner in Takayasu's disease than in temporal arteritis and because the pulmonary vessels affected are large elastic arteries it would be reasonable to regard isolated pulmonary disease as a manifestation of the Takayasu's disease, but if the patient was an elderly man, this would be a counter-argument. Few such patients have been reported.[121,122,124–128] Of five available for review by one author, three were women aged 25, 34 and 42 years, and two were men aged 33 and 66 years: only one was Japanese.[124]

Behçet's disease

Behçet's disease is a form of systemic vasculitis associated with immune-complex deposition.[129–131] It is particularly common in Japan and eastern Mediterranean countries and predominantly affects young men of HLA-B51 phenotype; the average age is 36 years and the male:female ratio 11.[132] The diagnostic criteria are oral ulceration and any two of genital ulceration, typical eye lesions (most commonly uveitis), pustular skin lesions and a positive pathergy test, the latter consisting of a sterile pustule that develops 24–48 h after a needle prick to the skin.[133]

Pulmonary lesions are rare and usually take the form of a vasculitis involving small arteries, veins and capillaries[134] but inflammation of segmental or lobar vessels may also occur. The lesions may be single or multiple. Small vessels usually show a leukocytoclastic vasculitis associated with deposition of IgA and complement, while larger vessels generally show a transmural, predominantly mononuclear, inflammatory infiltrate. Adventitial fibrosis may result in prominent perivascular cuffing while inflammatory destruction of the media leads to aneurysm formation (Fig. 8.3.18).[135,136] Computerised tomography shows aneurysms, irregularities or sharp cut-offs of the pulmonary arteries.[132,137] Repeated haemoptysis is common and may be fatal.[138,139]

Pulmonary artery aneurysms are also a feature of the Hughes–Stovin syndrome, which probably represents a variant of Behçet's disease.[137] It affects young males, in whom the aneurysms develop in association with recurrent episodes of peripheral venous thrombosis and a pyrexial illness. Blood cultures are negative and, although the oral and genital ulcers of Behçet's disease are lacking, pustular skin lesions may be present.[140–142] Occasionally, the bronchial arteries may be affected.[143]

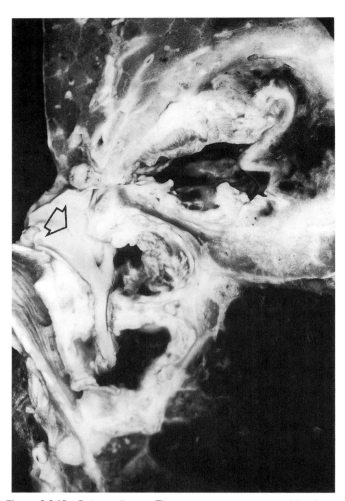

Figure 8.3.18 Behçets disease. Three aneurysms are seen arising from segmental branches of the lobar pulmonary artery. Rupture of one of these (arrow) resulted in fatal haemorrhage. (Case of Dr B J Addis, Brompton, UK.)

PULMONARY HAEMORRHAGE AND HAEMOSIDEROSIS

This section will concentrate on diseases that result in widespread alveolar haemorrhage. However, it should be remembered that haemorrhage from localised lesions such as neoplasms and tuberculosis may be disseminated widely through the lower respiratory tract by aspiration.

Aetiology (Box 8.3.2)

Widespread leakage of blood into alveolar spaces may be caused by:

- A bleeding diathesis
- Increased capillary pressure
- Capillary damage.

Box 8.3.2 Causes of pulmonary haemorrhage and haemosiderosis

Localised
  Tuberculosis, carcinoma, infarction, Wegener's granulomatosis
Diffuse
  Generalised bleeding disorders
  Capillary hypertension
    Mitral stenosis, atrial myxoma, mediastinal fibrosis
    Pulmonary veno-occlusive disease
    Pulmonary lymphangioleiomyomatosis
    Stress failure
  Chemical injury
    Silicone implants
    Lymphography
  Asphyxia
  Auto-immune vascular disease
    ANCA-associated capillaritis
      Microscopic polyangiitis
      Wegener's granulomatosis (capillaritis variety)
    Anti-basement membrane disease (Goodpasture's syndrome)
    Immune complex-mediated vasculitis
      Systemic lupus erythematosus
      Rheumatoid disease
      Behçet's disease
      Henoch–Schonlein purpura
      Coeliac disease
      Dermatitis herpetiformis
      Haemolytic anaemia
      Cows' milk hypersensitivity
      Trimellitic anhydride-induced
      Naphthylene-1,5-diisocyanate-induced
      Penicillamine-induced
Idiopathic pulmonary haemosiderosis

Table 8.3.5 Immunohistochemical and ultrastructural abnormalities in the lung in various immune disorders and idiopathic pulmonary haemosiderosis

	Immunofluorescent pattern	Electron dense deposits
Immune complex-mediated disease	Granular	Present
Goodpasture's (anti-basement membrane) disease	Diffuse	Absent
Neutrophil cytoplasmic antibody-mediated disease	Little or none (pauci-immune)	Absent
Idiopathic pulmonary haemorrhage	None	Absent

---

cent or electron microscopy (Table 8.3.5) and it may therefore be worth ensuring that some biopsy material is appropriately preserved if diffuse pulmonary haemorrhage is suspected clinically or on frozen section.

Clinical features

The clinical features of diffuse pulmonary haemorrhage vary from massive life-threatening haemoptysis to recurrent or continuous slow leakage leading to tiredness from iron deficiency anaemia. There is often concomitant haematuria and renal failure, forming a pulmonary-renal syndrome.[144] Chest radiographs show widespread, ill-defined, transient opacities. Carbon monoxide transfer may appear to be increased but the gas is being taken up by blood sequestered in the air spaces rather than transferred to the circulation. Serological tests for anti-neutrophil cytoplasmic antibodies, rheumatoid factor and antinuclear factor may give clues to the aetiology and help diagnostically.[55,56] Further diagnostic support is provided by the identification of haemosiderin-laden macrophages in sputum or lavage material,[145,146] but it should be noted that stains for iron may be positive in healthy smokers, foundry workers and patients with conditions as diverse as fibrosing alveolitis, chronic bronchitis and carcinoma of the lung.[147] Haemosiderin-laden macrophages are not a normal feature of the lung in infancy and if at autopsy the cause of an infant's death is not readily identified haemosiderin-laden macrophages should alert the pathologist to the possibility of an asphyxial death from overlying or smothering rather than the case being an example of the sudden infant death syndrome.[148,149]

Pathological features

Whatever the aetiology, biopsy shows a combination of alveolar haemorrhage and haemosiderosis (Fig. 8.3.19). The cause of the haemorrhage is often not evident histologically but there may be intense neutrophil infiltration of the alveolar walls representing capillaritis and rare cases show diffuse alveolar damage (see p. 131).[25,150]

Increased pulmonary capillary pressure generally reflects pulmonary venous hypertension or occlusion of pulmonary veins, the principal causes of which are mitral stenosis, left atrial myxoma, mediastinal fibrosis, pulmonary veno-occlusive disease (see p. 427), lymphangioleiomyomatosis (see p. 295) and capillary haemangiomatosis (see p. 429). Arterial constriction tends to protect the pulmonary capillary bed from pressure surges but if patchy the capillaries in those areas of the lung in which there is little upstream constriction are subjected to inordinately high pressures and may suffer stress failure. This is probably the mechanism underlying the haemorrhagic oedema seen in acute mountain sickness (see p. 371 and p. 402)

Diffuse capillary damage may be due to extraneous chemicals but is mainly auto-immune, representing small vessel vasculitis,[13,55,56,90–95] or idiopathic. Immune mechanisms fall into three categories: anti-basement membrane disease (Goodpasture's disease), immune complex-mediated injury and conditions characterised by antineutrophil cytoplasmic antibodies (pauci-immune vasculitis). These are considered separately below but together with idiopathic pulmonary haemosiderosis they share many clinical and pathological features and these aspects will be dealt with collectively. However, differences between these categories may be apparent on immunofluores-

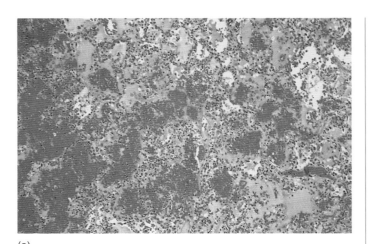

(a)

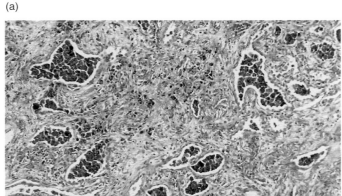

(b)

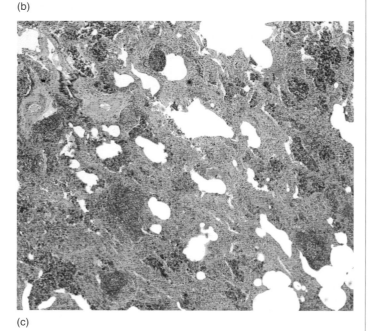

(c)

Figure 8.3.19 Pulmonary haemorrhage (a), haemosiderosis (b) and follicular lymphoid hyperplasia (c) in immune complex disease. In biopsy material haemorrhage is of uncertain significance as it could be operative but haemosiderosis provides firm evidence of previous bleeding.

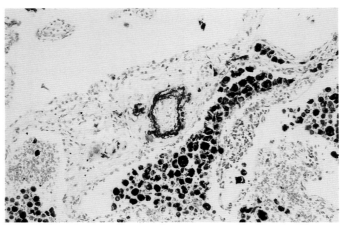

Figure 8.3.20 Pulmonary haemosiderosis giving a strongly positive Prussian blue reaction. The haemosiderin is largely contained within alveolar macrophages but also impregnates elastin in the walls of small pulmonary blood vessels. Perl's stain.

The haemosiderin is largely contained within alveolar macrophages, which generally congregate in the centres of the acini. It is a brown, coarsely granular pigment that gives a strongly positive Prussian blue reaction with Perl's stain (Figs 8.3.19b, 8.3.20), in contrast to smokers' pigment which is finely dispersed and gives a weaker Prussian blue reaction. Haemosiderin takes 2–3 days to develop after haemorrhage has occurred. It has been identified in tracheal macrophages 50 h after acute pulmonary haemorrhage and in cultured macrophages 72 h after the uptake of red blood cells.[151] A similar time course is reported in rats whose airways were injected with blood.[152,153]

In severe haemosiderosis, there is also encrustation of the elastic laminae of small blood vessels and alveolar walls (Figs 8.3.20, 8.3.21).[154] Calcium is often added to the iron (Fig. 8.3.22), as in the Gamna-Gandy nodules that develop in haemorrhagic splenic infarcts. The mineralised elastic fibres tend to fragment and attract giant cells of foreign body type, a process that has been termed 'endogenous pneumoconiosis' (Fig. 8.3.23).[155,156] Mild interstitial fibrosis and type II alveolar epithelial cell proliferation may also be seen.

Goodpasture's syndrome

The term Goodpasture's syndrome was first applied to the association of pulmonary haemorrhage and glomerulonephritis in 1958,[157] nearly 40 years after Goodpasture's original report, which was written in the wake of the 1918–1919 influenza pandemic with the primary object of discussing the aetiology of influenza.[158] The eponym is now reserved for those cases in which antibodies to glomerular or alveolar basement membrane can be demonstrated. Of 40 cases in one series in which lung haemorrhage was associated with glomerulonephritis only seven had basement membrane antibodies; of the others, 22 had systemic vasculitis and 11 had neither basement membrane antibodies nor systemic vasculitis.[159]

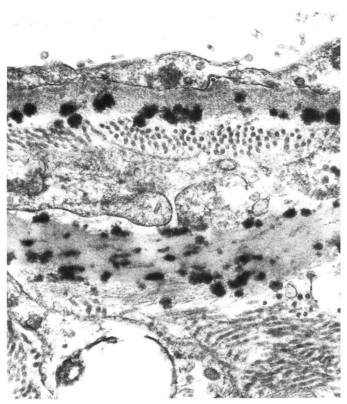

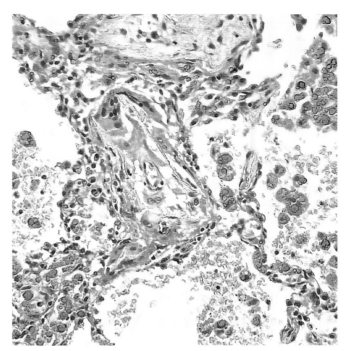

Figure 8.3.23 Pulmonary haemosiderosis. The heavily mineralised elastin fibres tend to fragment and attract foreign body giant cells giving an appearance that has been likened to pneumoconiosis although here the minerals are endogenous.

Figure 8.3.21 Electron microscopy shows that haemosiderin is preferentially deposited in the basement membrane and interstitial elastin tissue of the alveolar walls, sparing the collagen. Electron micrograph ×34 000. (Reproduced from Corrin et al. Fine structural changes in idiopathic pulmonary haemosiderosis. Journal of Pathology 1987; 153:249–256.[154] Copyright Pathological Society of Great Britain and Ireland. Reproduced with permission. Permission granted by John Wiley & Sons Ltd on behalf of PathSoc.)

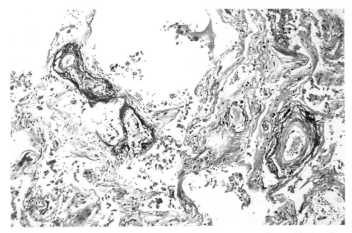

Figure 8.3.22 Pulmonary haemosiderosis. Calcium is often added to the haemosiderin deposits and being basophilic is evident without special stains.

Most patients with Goodpasture's syndrome are male. The mean age is about 20 years but the age range is wide and the disease has been reported in children.[160,161] Family clustering and associations with the major histocompatibility antigens HLA-DR2 and HLA-DQ have been reported.[162] Almost invariably, respiratory symptoms precede evidence of renal disease, sometimes by weeks or months.[163] Most patients have episodes of haemoptysis, although some develop anaemia, radiographic abnormalities and hypoxaemia without haemoptysis. Proteinuria, haematuria and renal failure indicate glomerular disease, which takes the form of a focal segmental glomerulonephritis with crescent formation. Therapy involves immunosuppression and removal of antibodies by plasma exchange.[93,164]

Immunofluorescence microscopy shows that antibodies are deposited along basement membranes in both glomeruli and alveolar walls (Fig. 8.3.24 and Table 8.3.5).[165] In 90% of cases they can also be demonstrated in the serum[166] and the disease can be passively transferred to animals.[167] The severity of the disease is proportional to the antibody titre. Cross-reactivity between pulmonary and renal basement membranes has been demonstrated.[168] The anti-glomerular basement membrane antibodies consist of a mixture of IgG subtypes[169] that react with a non-collagenous domain of the α_3 chain of type IV collagen.[170,171] The α_3 chain is restricted to sites such as the glomerular and alveolar basement membranes, in contrast to the ubiquitous α_1 and α_2 type IV chains. Antibody is deposited in a linear fashion along glomerular basement membranes, outlining the capillary loops, and similar linear fluorescence is seen in alveolar walls. In about two-thirds of cases immunoglobulin deposition is

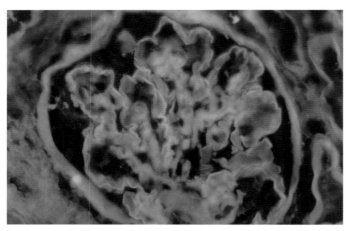

(a)

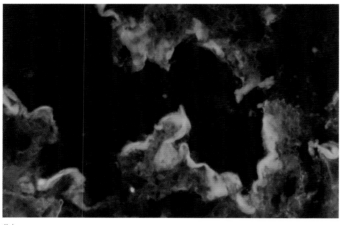

(b)

Figure 8.3.24 Goodpasture's syndrome. Immunofluorescent microscopy showing linear deposition of immunoglobulin in the glomerular (a) and alveolar (b) basement membranes. (Illustration provided by Dr A Paiva-Correia, Oporto, Portugal.)

accompanied by complement deposition with a similar pattern.[172]

Electron microscopy (Table 8.3.5) shows fragmentation of the basement membranes but not the dense deposits evident in immune complex-mediated disease.[173,174] It is not clear what initiates the disease but it has been suggested that damage to basement membrane by external agents, such as viruses or chemicals, alters its antigenicity.[175] Some patients have both anti-basement membrane and antineutrophil cytoplasmic antibodies and here it is possible that the former arise because of immune complex-mediated damage to the basement membrane.[176]

Antineutrophil cytoplasmic antibody-associated pulmonary haemorrhage

Antineutrophil cytoplasmic antibodies are associated with pulmonary haemorrhage in conditions such as microscopic polyangiitis (including cases limited the lungs known as isolated pauci-immune pulmonary capillaritis, see p. 446),[56,90–92,94,95]

Wegener's granulomatosis (including cases in which the vasculitic component is limited to the capillaries, see p. 438),[23–25,55,56,90,177,178] Churg–Strauss syndrome (see p. 465)[179] and systemic vasculitis.[104] In all these conditions, immunofluorescence microscopy shows only a weak or negative ('pauci-immune') reaction and electron microscopy fails to demonstrate electrondense deposits (Table 8.3.5). Wegener's granulomatosis and the Churg–Strauss syndrome usually show necrotising granulomatosis and inflammation of medium-sized vessels, but microscopic polyangiitis is limited to the smallest blood vessels and in the lung haemorrhage is the predominant lesion. Microscopic polyangiitis is the commonest cause of the pulmonary-renal syndrome.

Immune complex-mediated pulmonary haemorrhage

Immune complex deposition is the probable pathogenetic mechanism of diffuse pulmonary haemorrhage associated with conditions such as systemic lupus erythematosus,[102–106,180] Henoch–Schonlein purpura,[96,97] Behçet's disease,[134,181,182] rheumatoid disease,[108] cystic fibrosis[183] and various pulmonary-renal syndromes, as well as instances of isolated pulmonary haemorrhage.[95] Immune complex disease also appears to underlie occasional cases of pulmonary haemorrhage associated with penicillamine therapy[184] or exposure to epoxy resin paint powder containing the curing agent mellitic anhydride.[185,186] Diffuse pulmonary haemorrhage is also described in patients undergoing lymphangiography,[187,188] receiving silicone implants[189,190] or smoking cocaine[191] but the pathogenesis here is not well understood.

The haemorrhage is usually due to pulmonary capillaritis, which may develop in isolation, together with larger pulmonary vessel disease or as part of a systemic vasculitis. Capillaritis may be difficult to recognise but periodic acid-silver methenamine staining helps in the identification of basement membrane abnormalities.[94] In well established disease, neutrophils, nuclear debris, fibrin thrombi, fibrinoid necrosis, disruption of alveolar walls and fibrin lining alveoli may be seen.[25,104,105]

The association of immune complex-mediated glomerulonephritis and diffuse pulmonary haemorrhage is indistinguishable clinically from Goodpasture's syndrome. However, in contrast to Goodpasture's disease and idiopathic haemosiderosis, granular deposits of IgG may be demonstrated along alveolar walls[192] and electron-dense deposits in the capillary basement membrane (Table 8.3.5).[192] Sometimes there is evidence of immune complex deposition in the kidney but not in the lung,[193–195] or immunostaining may be negative in both organs[194] despite the presence of circulating complexes[196] or vasculitis.[84]

Idiopathic pulmonary haemosiderosis

Pulmonary haemorrhage and haemosiderosis may occur without evidence of vasculitis, immune complex deposition, anti-glomerular basement membrane antibodies or associated renal disease. If the other causes of pulmonary haemorrhage listed in Box 8.3.2 can be excluded the condition falls into the category of idiopathic pulmonary haemosiderosis.[197,198]

Epidemiology and clinical features

Idiopathic pulmonary haemosiderosis is predominantly a disease of children and young adults, usually occurring in the first three decades of life. The sex incidence is equal in children, whereas in adults there is 2 : 1 male predominance.[199] Familial cases have been described.[200–202] The disease tends to be more severe in children: they develop severe iron deficiency and have episodes of massive pulmonary haemorrhage, which may prove fatal. A more prolonged course is seen in adults and overt haemorrhage is not an invariable feature in this age group.[145] Treatment with steroids and azathioprine is empirical and because of the varying course of the disease, difficult to assess,[203] but immunosuppressive treatment has been successful in several cases.[204,205]

Aetiology

The cause of the disease is unknown but exposure to as yet unrecognised inhaled agents may play a role. Certain associations suggest that the disease has an immunological basis: these include coeliac disease, or at least a flattened jejunal mucosa,[206–209] dermatitis herpetiformis, autoimmune haemolytic anaemia,[210] thyrotoxicosis[211] and sensitivity to cow's milk, this last being seen in young children who have a positive skin test and serum precipitins to cows' milk, and who improve when cows' milk is removed from the diet.[212,213] An elevated serum IgA has also been noted in children with idiopathic pulmonary haemosiderosis.[214]

Pathological features

Bronchoalveolar lavage is the method of choice to confirm the alveolar bleeding, especially if this is occult.[215] The lavage fluid shows free red blood cells and phagocytosed erythrocytes within macrophages if there has been recent bleeding, and numerous haemosiderin-laden macrophages if the bleeding is old. Transbronchial biopsy can also show haemosiderosis.

The microscopic features are not specific, consisting merely of centriacinar collections of haemosiderin-laden macrophages, as described above (see Fig. 8.3.19). Interstitial fibrosis is sometimes regarded as being more characteristic of idiopathic pulmonary haemosiderosis than of other diseases which cause alveolar haemorrhage[216] but this is more likely to reflect the long duration of the disease than a specific process.

Immunostaining of the lung shows no evidence of immunoglobulin or complement deposition (Table 8.3.5). Various ultrastructural features have been described but no consistent pattern has emerged and it is uncertain whether the changes represent a primary manifestation of the disease or are secondary to the haemorrhage.[154,217] The abnormalities described include focal defects in the vascular endothelium and its basement membrane, and are more severe in children than adults. The capillary basement membrane may show focal thickening, splitting with the accumulation of fibrillar material and duplication.[154] Non-specific abnormalities include damage to type I epithelial cells and regeneration of type II epithelial cells.

REFERENCES

1. Jennette JC, Falk RJ, Andrassy K, et al. Nomenclature of systemic vasculitides. Proposal of an international consensus conference. Arthritis Rheum 1994; 37:187–192.

Infective and embolic vasculitis

2. Auerbach O. Pathology and pathogenesis of pulmonary arterial aneurysm in tuberculous cavities. Am Rev Tuberc 1939; 39:99–115.
3. Morgan JM, Morgan AD, Addis BJ, Bradley GW, Spiro SG. Fatal haemorrhage from mycotic aneurysms of the pulmonary artery. Thorax 1985; 41:70–71.
4. Gross EM. Autopsy findings in drug addicts. Pathol Annu 1978; 13(Part 2):35–67.
5. Tomashefski JFJr. Hirsch CS. The pulmonary vascular lesions of intravenous drug abuse. Hum Pathol 1980; 11:133–145.
6. Tomashefski JF, Hirsch CS, Jolly PN. Microcrystalline cellulose pulmonary embolism and granulomatosis. Arch Pathol Lab Med 1981; 105:89–93.
7. Rajs J, Harm T, Ormstad K. Postmortem findings of pulmonary lesions of older datum in intravenous drug addicts. A forensic-pathologic study. Virchows Arch A Pathol Anat Histopathol 1984; 402:405–414.
7a. Tomashefski JF Jr, Felo JA. The pulmonary pathology of illicit drug and substance abuse. Curr Diagn Pathol 2004; 10:413–426.
8. Chaves E. The pathology of the arterial pulmonary vasculature in Manson's schistosomiasis. Dis Chest 1966; 50:72–77.

Wegener's granulomatosis

9. Klinger H. Grenzformen der periarteritis nodosa. Frankf Z Pathol 1931; 42:455–480.
10. Wegener F. Uber generaliserte, septische Gefasserkrankungen. Verh Dtsch Ges Pathol 1936; 29:202–210.
11. Wegener F. Uber eine eigenartiger rhinogene Granulomatose mit besonderer Beteiligung des Arterien Systems und der Nieren. Beitr Pathol Anat 1939; 102:36–68.
12. Godman GC, Churg J. Wegener's granulomatosis. Arch Pathol Lab Med 1954; 58:533–553.
13. Jennette JC, Falk RJ. Small-vessel vasculitis. N Engl J Med 1997; 337:1512–1523.
14. Fauci AS, Haynes BF, Katz P, Wolff SM. Wegener's granulomatosis: prospective clinical and therapeutic experience with 85 patients for 21 years. Ann Intern Med 1983; 98:76–85.
15. Woude FJ van der, Rasmussen N, Lobatto S, et al. Autoantibodies against neutrophils and monocytes: tool for diagnosis and marker for disease activity in Wegener's granulomatosis. Lancet 1985; i:425–429.
16. Ramirez G, Khamashta MA, Hughes GRV. The ANCA test: its clinical relevance. Ann Rheum Dis 1990; 49:741–742.
17. Jennette JC, Falk RJ. Pathogenesis of the vascular and glomerular damage in ANCA- positive vasculitis. Nephrol Dial Transplant 1998; 13(Suppl 1):16–20.
18. Baltaro RJ, Hoffman GS, Sechler JMG, et al. Immunoglobulin G antineutrophil cytoplasmic antibodies are produced in the respiratory tracts of patients with Wegener's granulomatosis. Am Rev Respir Dis 1991; 143:275–278.
19. Fienberg R. Pathergic granulomatosis. Am J Med 1955; 19:829–831.
20. Mark EJ, Matsubara O, Tan-Liu N, Fienberg R. The pulmonary biopsy in the early diagnosis of Wegener's (pathergic) granulomatosis: a study based on 35 open lung biopsies from 67 patients. Hum Pathol 1988; 19:1065–1071.

21. Hoffman GS, Kerr GS, Levitt RY, et al. Wegener's granulomatosis. An analysis of 158 patients. Ann Intern Med 1992; 116:488–498.

22. Duna GF, Galperin C, Hoffman GS. Wegener's granulomatosis. Rheum Dis Clin North Am 1995; 21:949–986.

23. Travis WD, Carpenter HA, Lie JT. Diffuse pulmonary hemorrhage. An uncommon manifestation of Wegener's granulomatosis. Am J Surg Pathol 1987; 11:702–708.

24. Myers JL, Katzenstein A-LA. Wegener's granulomatosis presenting with massive pulmonary hemorrhage and capillaritis. Am J Surg Pathol 1987; 11:895–898.

25. Yoshimura N, Matsubara O, Tamura A, Kasuga T, Mark EJ. Wegener's granulomatosis-associated with diffuse pulmonary hemorrhage. Acta Pathol Jpn 1992; 42:657–661.

26. Fauci AS, Wolff SM. Wegener's granulomatosis: studies in eighteen patients and a review of the literature. Medicine (Baltimore) 1973; 52:535–561.

27. Nolle B, Specks U, Ludemann J, et al. Anticytoplasmic autoantibodies: their immunodiagnostic value in Wegener's granulomatosis. Ann Intern Med 1989; 111:28–40.

28. Gal AA, Salinas FF, Staton GW. The clinical and pathological spectrum of antineutrophil cytoplasmic autoantibody-related pulmonary disease: a comparison between perinuclear and cytoplasmic antineutrophil cytoplasmic autoantibodies. Arch Pathol Lab Med 1994; 118:1209–1214.

29. Brown I, Joyce C, Hogan PG, et al. Pulmonary vasculitis associated with anti-Jo-1 antibodies. Resp Med 1998; 92:986–988.

30. Higgs CMB. Anti-neutrophil cytoplasmic antibodies. Respir Med 1992; 86:367–369.

31. Gaudin PB, Askin FB, Falk RJ, Jennette JC. The pathologic spectrum of pulmonary lesions in patients with anti-neutrophil cytoplasmic autoantibodies specific for anti-proteinase 3 and anti-myeloperoxidase. Am J Clin Pathol 1995; 104:7–16.

32. Jennette JC, Thomas DB, Falk RJ. Microscopic polyangiitis (microscopic polyarteritis). Semin Diagn Pathol 2001; 18:3–13.

33. Specks U, Wheatley CL, McDonald TJ, Rohrbach MS, DeRemee RA. Anticytoplasmic antibodies in the diagnosis and follow-up of Wegener's granulomatosis. Mayo Clin Proc 1989; 64:28–38.

34. Yoskikawa Y, Watanabe T. Pulmonary lesions in Wegener's granulomatosis: a clinicopathologic study of 22 autopsy cases. Hum Pathol 1986; 17:401–410.

35. Travis WD, Hoffman GS, Leavitt RY, Pass HI, Fauci AS. Surgical pathology of the lung in Wegener's granulomatosis – review of 87 open lung biopsies from 67 Patients. Am J Surg Pathol 1991; 15:315–333.

36. Colby TV, Specks U. Wegener's granulomatosis in the 1990s – A pulmonary pathologist's perspective. In: Churg A, Katzenstein ALA, ed. The Lung. Current Concepts. Baltimore, MD: Williams & Wilkins; 1993:195–218.

37. Yousem SA. Bronchocentric injury in Wegener's granulomatosis – a report of five cases. Hum Pathol 1991; 22:535–540.

38. Daum TE, Specks U, Colby TV, et al. Tracheobronchial involvement in Wegener's granulomatosis. Am J Respir Crit Care Med 1995; 151: 522–526.

39. Gephardt GN, Ahmed M, Tubbs RR. Pulmonary vasculitis (Wegener's granulomatosis). Study of T and B cell markers. Am J Med 1983; 74:700–704.

40. Yousem SA, Lombard CM. The eosinophilic variant of Wegener's granulomatosis. Hum Pathol 1988; 19:682–688.

41. Goulart RA, Mark EJ, Rosen S. Tumefactions as an extravascular manifestation of Wegener's granulomatosis. Am J Surg Pathol 1995; 19:145–153.

42. Lombard CM, Duncan SR, Rizk NW, Colby TV. The diagnosis of Wegener's granulomatosis from transbronchial biopsy specimens. Hum Pathol 1990; 21:838–842.

43. Uner AH, Rozumslota B, Katzenstein ALA. Bronchiolitis obliterans-organizing pneumonia (BOOP)-like variant of Wegener's granulomatosis: a clinicopathologic study of 16 cases. Am J Surg Pathol 1996; 20:794–801.

44. Mark EJ, Flieder DB, Matsubara O. Treated Wegener's granulomatosis: Distinctive pathological findings in the lungs of 20 patients and what they tell us about the natural history of the disease. Hum Pathol 1997; 28:450–458.

45. Devaney KO, Travis WD, Hoffman GS, et al. Interpretation of head and neck biopsies in Wegener's granulomatosis. A pathologic study of 126 biopsies in 70 patients. Am J Surg Pathol 1990; 14:555–564.

46. Buono EA del, Flint A. Diagnostic usefulness of nasal biopsy in Wegener's granulomatosis. Hum Pathol 1991; 22:107–110.

47. Matsubara O, Yoshimura N, Doi Y, Tamura A, Mark EJ. Nasal biopsy in the early diagnosis of Wegener's (pathergic) granulomatosis – significance of palisading granuloma and leukocytoclastic vasculitis. Virchows Arch 1996; 428:13–19.

48. Hu CH, O'Loughlin S, Winkelmann RK. Cutaneous manifestations of Wegener's granulomatosis. Arch Derm 1977; 113:175–182.

49. Barksdale SK, Hallahan CW, Kerr GS, et al. Cutaneous pathology in Wegener's granulomatosis: a clinicopathologic study of 75 biopsies in 46 patients. Am J Surg Pathol 1995; 19:161–172.

50. Weiss MA, Crissman JD. Renal biopsy findings in Wegener's granulomatosis: segmental necrotising glomerulonephritis with glomerular thrombosis. Hum Pathol 1984; 15:943–956.

51. Cordier J-F, Valeyre D, Guillevin L, Loire R, Brechot J-M. Pulmonary Wegener's granulomatosis: a clinical and imaging study of 77 cases. Chest 1990; 97:906–912.

52. Carrington CB, Liebow AA. Limited forms of angiitis and granulomatosis of Wegener's type. Am J Med 1966; 41:497–527.

53. Cassan SM, Coles DT, Harrison EG. The concept of limited forms of Wegener's granulomatosis. Am J Med 1970; 49:366–379.

54. Katzenstein ALA, Locke WK. Solitary lung lesions in Wegener's granulomatosis: pathologic findings and clinical significance in 25 cases. Am J Surg Pathol 1995; 19:545–552.

55. Bosch X, Lopez-Soto A, Mirapeix E, et al. Antineutrophil cytoplasmic autoantibody-associated alveolar capillaritis in patients presenting with pulmonary hemorrhage. Arch Pathol Lab Med 1994; 118:517–522.

56. Schwarz MI, Brown KK. Small vessel vasculitis of the lung. Thorax 2000; 55:502–510.

57. Ulbright TM, Katzenstein A-LA. Solitary necrotising granulomas of the lung. Am J Surg Pathol 1980; 4:13–28.

Conditions linking Wegener's granulomatosis with sarcoidosis and other disorders

58. Cravioto H, Feigin I. Noninfectious granulomatous angiitis with a predilection for the nervous system. Neurology 1959; 9:599–609.

59. Nishino H, DeRemee RA, Rubino FA, Parisi JE. Wegener's granulomatosis associated with vasculitis of the temporal artery - report of five cases. Mayo Clin Proc 1993; 68:115–121.

60. Zenone T, Souquet PJ, Bohas C, Durand DV, Bernard JP. Unusual manifestations of giant cell arteritis: pulmonary nodules, cough, conjunctivitis and otitis with deafness. Eur Respir J 1994; 7:2252–2254.

61. Barnett VT, Sekosan M, Khurshid A. Wegener's granulomatosis and alpha1-antitrypsin-deficiency emphysema: proteinase-related diseases. Chest 1999; 116:253–255.

62. Mazodier P, Elzouki AN, Segelmark M, Eriksson S. Systemic necrotising vasculitides in severe alpha1-antitrypsin deficiency. QJM 1996; 89:599–611.

63. Mouly S, Brillet G, Stern M, Lesavre P, Guillevin L. Pulmonary giant bulla in Wegener's granulomatosis. Scand J Rheumatol 2000; 29:333–335.

64. Liebow AA. Pulmonary angiitis and granulomatosis. Am Rev Respir Dis 1973; 108:1–18.

65. Saldana MJ. Necrotising sarcoid granulomatosis: clinicopathologic observations in 24 patients. Lab Invest 1978; 38:364.

66. Churg A, Carrington CB, Gupta R. Necrotising sarcoid granulomatosis. Chest 1979; 76:406–413.

67. Koss MN, Hochholzer L, Feigin DS, Garancis JC, Ward PA. Necrotising sarcoid-like granulomatosis: clinical, pathologic and immunopathologic findings. Hum Pathol 1980; 11(Suppl):510–519.

68. Churg A. Pulmonary angiitis and granulomatosis revisited. Hum Pathol 1983; 14:868–883.

69. Chittock DR, Joseph MG, Paterson NAM, McFadden RG. Necrotising sarcoid granulomatosis with pleural involvement. Chest 1994; 106:672–676.

70. Stephen JG, Braimbridge MV, Corrin B, et al. Necrotising 'sarcoidal' angiitis and granulomatosis of the lung. Thorax 1976; 31:356–360.

71. Beach RC, Corrin B, Scopes JW, Graham E. Necrotising sarcoid granulomatosis with neurologic lesions in a child. J Pediatr 1980; 97:950–953.

72. Dykhuizen RS, Smith CC, Kennedy MM, et al. Necrotising sarcoid granulomatosis with extrapulmonary involvement. Eur Respir J 1997; 10:245–247.

73. Strickland-Marmol LB. Fessler RG, Rojiani AM. Necrotising sarcoid granulomatosis mimicking an intracranial neoplasm: Clinicopathologic features and review of the literature. Mod Pathol 2000; 13:909–913.

74. Legall F, Loeuillet L, Delaval P, et al. Necrotising sarcoid granulomatosis with and without extrapulmonary involvement. Pathol Res Pr 1996; 192:306–313.

75. Shirodaria CC, Nicholson AG, Hansell DM, Wells AU, Wilson R. Lesson of the month – Necrotising sarcoid granulomatosis with skin involvement. Histopathology 2003; 43:91–93.

76. Spiteri MA, Gledhill A, Campbell D, Clarke SW. Necrotising sarcoid granulomatosis. Br J Dis Chest 1987; 81:70–75.

77. Rosen Y, Moon S, Huang C-T, Lyons HA. Granulomatous pulmonary angiitis in sarcoidosis. Arch Pathol Lab Med 1977; 101:170–174.

78. Tauber E, Wojnarowski C, Horcher E, Dekan G, Fischer T. Necrotising sarcoid granulomatosis in a 14-yr-old female. Eur Resp J 1999; 13:703–705.

79. Gartside IB. Granulomatous arteritis in a lesion resembling sarcoidosis. J Pathol Bacteriol 1944; 56:61–66.

80. Marcussen N, Lund C. Combined sarcoidosis and disseminated visceral giant cell vasculitis. Pathol Res Pr 1989; 184:325–330.

81. Shintaku M, Mase K, Ohtsuki H, et al. Generalized sarcoid-like granulomas with systemic angiitis, crescentic glomerulonephritis, and pulmonary hemorrhage. Arch Pathol Lab Med 1989; 113:1295–1298.

82. Lie JT. Combined sarcoidosis and disseminated visceral giant cell angiitis – a third opinion. Arch Pathol Lab Med 1991; 115:210–211.

Pulmonary involvement in other forms of systemic vasculitis

83. Kussmaul A, Maier M. Ueber eine bisher nicht besdriebane eigenthumleche arteriomerkrankung (periarteritis nodosa) die mit morbus Briqhtii und rapid fortschreitender allgemeiner, Muskallahmung einherght. Deutches Arch Klin Med 1866; 1:484–518.

84. Thomashaw BM, Felton CP, Navarro C. Diffuse intrapulmonary haemorrhage, renal failure and a systemic vasculitis. Am J Med 1980; 68:299–304.

85. Rose GA, Spencer H. Polyarteritis nodosa. Q J Med 1957; 26:43–81.

86. Fauci AS, Haynes BF, Katz P. The spectrum of vasculitis: clinical, pathologic, immunologic and therapeutic considerations. Ann Intern Med 1978; 89:660–676.

87. Leavitt RY, Fauci AS. Polyangiitis overlap syndrome. Classification and prospective clinical experience. Am J Med 1986; 81:79–85.

88. Matsumoto T, Homma S, Okada M, et al. The lung in polyarteritis nodosa – a pathologic study of ten cases. Hum Pathol 1993; 24:717–724.

89. Nick J, Tuder R, May R, Fisher J. Polyarteritis nodosa with pulmonary vasculitis. Am J Respir Crit Care Med 1996; 153:450–453.

90. Haworth SJ, Savage CD, Carr D, Hughes JM, Rees AJ. Pulmonary haemorrhage complicating Wegener's granulomatosis and microscopic polyarteritis. BMJ 1985; 290:1775–1778.

91. Bosch X, Font J, Mirapeix E, et al. Antimyeloperoxidase autoantibody-associated necrotising alveolar capillaritis. Am Rev Respir Dis 1992; 146:1326–1329.

92. Akikusa B, Kondo Y, Irabu N, Yamamoto S, Saiki S. Six cases of microscopic polyarteritis exhibiting acute interstitial pneumonia. Pathol Int 1995; 45:580–588.

93. Green RJ, Ruoss SJ, Kraft SA, Berry GJ, Raffin TA. Pulmonary capillaritis and alveolar hemorrhage: update on diagnosis and management. Chest 1996; 110:1305–1316.

94. Akikusa B, Sato T, Ogawa M, Ueda S, Kondo Y. Necrotising alveolar capillaritis in autopsy cases of microscopic polyangiitis: incidence, histopathogenesis, and relationship with systemic vasculitis. Arch Pathol Lab Med 1997; 121:144–149.

95. Jennings CA, King TE, Tuder R, Cherniack RM, Schwarz MI. Diffuse alveolar hemorrhage with underlying isolated, pauciimmune pulmonary capillaritis. Am J Respir Crit Care Med 1997; 155:1101–1109.

96. Kathuria S, Chejfec G. Fatal pulmonary Henoch-Schonlein syndrome. Chest 1982; 82:654–656.

97. Markus HS, Clark JV. Pulmonary haemorrhage in Henoch-Schonlein purpura. Thorax 1989; 44:525–526.

98. Bombardieri S, Paoletti P, Ferro C, et al. Lung involvement in essential mixed cryoglobulinaemia. Am J Med 1979; 66:749–756.

99. Dreisen RB. Pulmonary vasculitis. Clin Chest Med 1982; 3:607–618.

100. Schwarz MI, Mortenson RL, Colby TV, et al. Pulmonary capillaritis. The association with progressive irreversible airflow limitation and hyperinflation. Am Rev Respir Dis 1993; 148:507–511.

101. Kuhn C. Systemic lupus erythematosus in a patient with ultrastructural lesions of the pulmonary capillaries previously reported in the review as due to idiopathic pulmonary hemosiderosis. Am Rev Respir Dis 1972; 106:931–932.

102. Churg A, Franklin W, Chan KL, Kopp E, Carrington CB. Pulmonary hemorrhage and immune-complex deposition in the lung. Complications in a patient with systemic lupus erythematosus. Arch Pathol Lab Med 1980; 104:388–391.

103. Marino CT, Pertschuk LP. Pulmonary haemorrhage in systemic lupus erythematosus. Arch Intern Med 1981; 141:201–203.

104. Mark EJ, Ramirez JF. Pulmonary capillaritis and hemorrhage in patients with systemic vasculitis. Arch Pathol Lab Med 1985; 109: 413–418.

105. Myers JL, Katzenstein AL. Microangiitis in lupus-induced pulmonary haemorrhage. Am J Clin Pathol 1986; 85:552–556.

106. Santos Ocampo AS, Mandell BF, Fessler BJ. Alveolar hemorrhage in systemic lupus erythematosus - Presentation and management. Chest 2000; 118:1083–1090.

107. Price TML, Skelton MO. Rheumatoid arthritis with lung lesions. Thorax 1956; 11:234–240.

108. Lemley PE, Katz P. Rheumatoid-like arthritis presenting as idiopathic pulmonary hemosiderosis: a report and review of the literature. J Rheumatol 1986; 13:954–957.

109. Baydur A, Mongan ES, Slager UT. Acute respiratory failure and pulmonary arteritis without parenchymal involvement. Demonstration in a patient with rheumatoid arthritis. Chest 1979; 75:518–520.

110. Kay JM, Banik S. Unexplained pulmonary hypertension with pulmonary arteritis in rheumatoid disease. Br J Dis Chest 1977; 71:53–59.

111. Kawai C, Ishikawa K, Kato M, Ishii Y, Nakao K. Pulmonary pulseless disease: pulmonary involvement in so-called Takayasu's disease. Chest 1978; 73:651–657.

112. Yamada I, Shibuya H, Matsubara O, et al. Takayasu arteritis: angiographic findings with special reference to pulmonary arterial change. Am J Radiol 1992; 159:263–269.

113. Johnston SL, Lock RJ, Gompels MM. Takayasu arteritis: a review. J Clin Pathol 2002; 55:481–486.

114. Bradley JD, Pinals RS, Poston WM. Giant cell arteritis with pulmonary nodules. Am J Med 1984; 77:135–140.

115. Doyle L, McWilliam L, Hasleton PS. Giant cell arteritis with pulmonary involvement. Br J Dis Chest 1988; 82:88–92.

116. Lie JT. Disseminated visceral giant cell arteritis. Am J Clin Pathol 1978; 69:299–305.

117. Kagata Y, Matsubara O, Ogata S, Lie JT, Mark EJ. Infantile disseminated visceral giant cell arteritis presenting as sudden infant death. Pathol Int 1999; 49:226–230.

118. Rose AG, Halper J, Factor SM. Primary arteriopathy in Takayasu's disease. Arch Pathol Lab Med 1984; 108:644–648.

119. Ladanyi M, Fraser RS. Pulmonary involvement in giant cell arteritis. Arch Pathol Lab Med 1987; 111:1178–1180.

120. Matsubara O, Yoshimura N, Tamura A, et al. Pathological features of the pulmonary artery in Takayasu arteritis. Heart Vessels 1992; Suppl 7:18–25.

121. Wagenaar SS, Westermann CJJ, Corrin B. Giant cell arteritis limited to large elastic pulmonary arteries. Thorax 1981; 36:876–877.

122. Wagenaar SS, Bosch JMM van den, Westermann CJJ, et al. Isolated granulomatous giant cell vasculitis of the pulmonary elastic arteries. Arch Pathol Lab Med 1986; 110:962–964.

123. Kerr KM, Auger WR, Fedullo PF, et al. Large vessel pulmonary arteritis mimicking chronic thromboembolic disease. Am J Respir Crit Care Med 1995; 152:367–373.

124. Lie JT. Isolated pulmonary Takayasu arteritis: clinicopathologic characteristics. Mod Pathol 1996; 9:469–474.

125. Okubo S, Kunieda T, Ando M, Nakajima N, Yutani C. Idiopathic isolated pulmonary arteritis with chronic cor pulmonale. Chest 1988; 94:665–666.

126. Masuda S, Ishii T, Asuwa N, Ishikawa Y, Kiguchi H. Isolated pulmonary giant cell vasculitis. Pathol Res Pr 1994; 190:1095–1100.

127. Lie JT. Pulmonary granulomatous (giant cell) vasculitides – commentary. Pathol Res Pr 1994; 190:1101–1102.

128. Brugiere O, Mal H, Sleiman C, et al. Isolated pulmonary arteries involvement in a patient with Takayasu's arteritis. Eur Resp J 1998; 11:767–770.

129. Chajek T, Fainaru M. Behçet's disease. Report of 41 cases and a review of the literature. Medicine (Baltimore) 1975; 54:179–196.

130. Witt C, John M, Martin H, et al. Behçet's syndrome with pulmonary involvement – combined therapy for endobronchial stenosis using neodym-YAG laser, balloon dilation and immunosuppression. Respiration 1996; 63:195–198.

131. Abadoglu O, Osma E, Ucan ES, et al. Behçet's disease with pulmonary involvement, superior vena cava syndrome, chyloptysis and chylous ascites. Respir Med 1996; 90:429–431.

132. Erkan F, Cavdar T. Pulmonary vasculitis in Behçet's disease. Am Rev Respir Dis 1992; 146:232–239.

133. International Study Group for Behçet's disease. Criteria for diagnosis of Behçet's disease. Lancet 1990; 335:1078–1080.

134. Gamble CN, Wiesner KB, Shapiro RF, Boyer WJ. The immune complex pathogenesis of glomerulonephritis and pulmonary vasculitis in Behçet's disease. Am J Med 1979; 66:1031–1039.

135. Lie JT. Cardiac and pulmonary manifestations of Behçet syndrome. Pathol Res Pr 1988; 183:347–352.

136. Aktogu S, Erer OF, Urpek G, Soy O, Tibet G. Multiple pulmonary arterial aneurysms in Behçet's disease: Clinical and radiologic remission after cyclophosphamide and corticosteroid therapy. Respiration 2002; 69:178–181.

137. Jerray M, Benzarti M, Rouatbi N. Possible Behçet's disease revealed by pulmonary aneurysms. Chest 1991; 99:1282–1284.

138. Raz I, Okon E, Chajek-Shaul T. Pulmonary manifestations in Behçet's syndrome. Chest 1989; 95:585–589.

139. Demontpreville VT, Macchiarini P, Dartevelle PG, Dulmet EM. Large bilateral pulmonary artery aneurysms in Behçet's disease: rupture of the contralateral lesion after aneurysmorrhaphy. Respiration 1996; 63:49–51.

140. Hughes JP, Stovin PGI. Segmental pulmonary artery aneurysms with peripheral venous thrombosis. Br J Dis Chest 1959; 53:19–27.

141. Kopp WL, Green RA. Pulmonary artery aneurysms with recurrent thrombophlebitis. The Hughes-Stovin syndrome. Ann Intern Med 1962; 56:105–114.

142. Frater R, Beck W, Shire V. The syndrome of pulmonary vascular aneurysms, pulmonary artery thrombi and peripheral venous thrombi. J Thorac Cardiovasc Surg 1965; 49:330–338.

143. Herb S, Hetzel M, Hetzel J, Friedrich J, Weber J. An unusual case of Hughes–Stovin syndrome. Eur Resp J 1998; 11:1191–1193.

Pulmonary haemorrhage and haemosiderosis

144. Young KR. Jr. Pulmonary-renal syndromes. Clin Chest Med 1989; 10:655–675.

145. Morgan PGM, Turner-Warwick M. Pulmonary haemosiderosis and pulmonary haemorrhage. Br J Dis Chest 1981; 75:225–242.

146. Delassence A, Fleury-Feith J, Escudier E, et al. Alveolar hemorrhage – diagnostic criteria and results in 194 immunocompromised hosts. Am J Respir Crit Care Med 1995; 151:157–163.

147. Corhay JL, Weber G, Bury T, et al. Iron content in human alveolar macrophages. Eur Respir J 1992; 5:804–809.

148. Becroft DMO, Lockett BK. Intra-alveolar pulmonary siderophages in sudden infant death: A marker for previous imposed suffocation. Pathology 1997; 29:60–63.

149. Yukawa N, Carter N, Rutty G, Green MA. Intra-alveolar haemorrhage in sudden infant death syndrome: a cause for concern? J Clin Pathol 1999; 52:581–587.

150. Lombard CM, Colby TV, Elliott CG. Surgical pathology of the lung in anti-basement membrane antibody-associated Goodpasture's syndrome. Hum Pathol 1989; 20:445–451.

151. Sherman JM, Winnie G, Thomassen MJ, Abdul-Karim FW, Boat TF. Time course of hemosiderin production and clearance by human pulmonary macrophages. Chest 1984; 86:409–411.

152. Magarey FR. Experimental pulmonary haemosiderosis. J Pathol Bacteriol 1951; 63:729–734.

153. Epstein CE, Elidemir O, Colasurdo GN, Fan LL. Time course of hemosiderin production by alveolar macrophages in a murine model. Chest 2001; 120:2013–2020.

154. Corrin B, Jagusch M, Dewar A, et al. Fine structural changes in idiopathic pulmonary haemosiderosis. J Pathol 1987; 153:249–256.

155. Walford RI, Kaplan L. Pulmonary fibrosis and giant cell reaction to altered elastic tissue - endogenous pneumoconiosis. Arch Pathol Lab Med 1957; 63:75–90.

156. Pai UH, McMahon J, Tomashefski JF. Mineralizing pulmonary elastosis in chronic cardiac failure – endogenous pneumoconiosis revisited. Am J Clin Pathol 1994; 101:22–28.

157. Stanton MC, Tange JD. Goodpasture's syndrome. Aust Ann Med 1958; 7:132–149.

158. Goodpasture EW. The significance of certain pulmonary lesions in relation to the aetiology of influenza. Am J Med Sci 1919; 158: 863–870.

159. Holdsworth S, Boyce N, Thomson NM, Atkins RC. The clinical spectrum of acute glomerulonephritis and lung haemorrhage (Goodpasture's syndrome). Q J Med 1985; 55:75–86.

160. Ozsoylu S, Hisconmex G, Berkel I, Say B, Tinaztepe B. Goodpasture's syndrome. Pulmonary haemosiderosis with nephritis. Clin Pediatr (Philadelphia) 1976; 15:358–360.

161. Briggs WA, Johnson JP, Teichman S, Yeager HC, Wilson CB. Antiglomerular basement membrane antibody mediated glomerulonephritis and Goodpasture's syndrome. Medicine (Baltimore) 1979; 58:348–361.

162. Huey B, McCormick K, Capper J, et al. Associations of HLA-DR and HLA-DQ types with anti-GBM nephritis by sequence-specific oligonucleotide probe hybridization. Kidney Int 1993; 44:307–312.

163. Tobler A, Schurch E, Altermatt HJ, Hof VI. Anti-basement membrane antibody disease with severe pulmonary haemorrhage and normal renal function. Thorax 1991; 46:68–69.

164. Peters DK, Rees AJ, Lockwood CM, Pusey CD. Treatment and prognosis in antibasement membrane antibody mediated nephritis. Transplant Proc 1982; 14:513–521.

165. Beechler CR, Enquist RW, Hunt KK, Ward GW, Knieser MR. Immunofluorescence of transbronchial biopsies in Goodpasture's syndrome. Am Rev Respir Dis 1980; 121:869–872.

166. Wilson CB, Dixon FJ. Anti-glomerular basement membrane induced glomerulonephritis. Kidney Int 1973; 3:74–89.

167. Lerner RA, Dixon FJ. The induction of acute glomerulonephritis in rabbits with soluble antigens isolated from normal homologous and autologous urine. J Immunol 1968; 100:1277.

168. Koffler D, Sandson J, Carr R. Immunologic studies concerning the pulmonary lesions in Goodpasture's syndrome. Am J Pathol 1969; 54:293–305.

169. Poskitt TR. Immunologic and electron microscopic studies in Goodpasture's syndrome. Am J Med 1970; 49:250–257.

170. Wieslander J, Heinegard D. The involvement of type IV collagen in Goodpasture's syndrome. Ann N Y Acad Sci 1985; 460:363–374.

171. Gunwar S, Bejarano PA, Kalluri R, et al. Alveolar basement membrane – molecular properties of the noncollagenous domain (hexamer) of collagen-IV and its reactivity with Goodpasture autoantibodies. Am J Respir Cell Mol Biol 1991; 5:107–112.

172. Thomas HM, Irwin RS. Classification of diffuse intrapulmonary haemorrhage. Chest 1975; 68:483–484.

173. Botting AJ, Brown AL Jr, Divertie MB. The pulmonary lesion in a patient with Goodpasture's syndrome, as studied with the electron microscope. Am J Clin Pathol 1964; 42:387–394.

174. Donald KJ, Edwards RL, McEvoy JDS. Alveolar capillary basement membrane lesions in Goodpasture's syndrome and idiopathic pulmonary haemosiderosis. Am J Med 1975; 59:642–649.

175. Markowitz AS, Battifora HA, Schwartz F, Aseron C. Immunological aspects of Goodpasture's syndrome. Clin Exp Immunol 1968; 3:585–591.

176. Fanburg BL, McLoud TC, Niles JL, et al. A 17-year-old girl with massive hemoptysis and acute oliguric renal failure – Goodpasture's syndrome, with ANCA and anti-GBM antibodies – Wegener's granulomatosis, involving lungs, kidneys, and spleen. N Engl J Med 1993; 329:2019–2026.

177. Stokes TC, McCann BG, Rees RT, Sims EH, Harrison BDW. Acute fulminating intrapulmonary haemorrhage in Wegener's granulomatosis. Thorax 1982; 37:315–316.

178. Travis WD, Colby TV, Lombard C, Carpenter HA. A clinicopathologic study of 34 cases of diffuse pulmonary hemorrhage with lung biopsy confirmation. Am J Surg Pathol 1990; 14:1112–1125.

179. Clutterbuck EJ, Pusey CD. Severe alveolar haemorrhage in Churg–Strauss syndrome. Eur J Respir Dis 1987; 71:158–163.

180. Hughson MD, He Z, Henegar J, McMurray R. Alveolar hemorrhage and renal microangiopathy in systemic lupus erythematosus – Immune complex small vascular injury with apoptosis. Arch Pathol Lab Med 2001; 125:475–483.

181. Davies JD. Behçet's syndrome with haemoptysis and pulmonary lesions. J Pathol 1973; 109:351–356.

182. Efthimiou J, Johnston C, Spiro SG, Turner-Warwick M. Pulmonary disease in Behçet's syndrome. Q J Med 1986; 58:259–280.

183. Finnegan MJ, Hinchcliffe J, Russell-Jones D, et al. Vasculitis complicating cystic fibrosis. Q J Med 1989; 72:609–622.

184. Sternlieb I, Bennett B, Scheinberg IH. D-penicillamine induced Goodpasture's syndrome in Wilson's disease. Ann Intern Med 1975; 82:673–676.

185. Ahmad D, Petterson R, Morgan WKC, Williams T, Zeiss CR. Pulmonary haemorrhage and haemolytic anaemia due to trimellitic anhydride. Lancet 1979; 2:328–330.

186. Kaplan V, Baur X, Czuppon A, et al. Pulmonary hemorrhage due to inhalation of vapor containing pyromellitic dianhydride. Chest 1993; 104:644–645.

187. Wiertz LM, Gagnon JH, Anthonisen NR. Intrapulmonary hemorrhage with anemia after lymphangiography. N Engl J Med 1971; 285:1364–1365.

188. Marglin SI, Castellino RA. Severe pulmonary haemorrhage following lymphography. Cancer 1979; 43:482–483.

189. Chastre J, Brun P, Soler P, et al. Acute and latent pneumonitis after subcutaneous injections of silicone in transsexual men. Am Rev Respir Dis 1987; 135:236–240.

190. Lai YF, Chao TY, Wong SL. Acute pneumonitis after subcutaneous injections of silicone for augmentation mammaplasty. Chest 1994; 106:1152–1155.

191. Murray RJ, Smialek JE, Golle M, Albin RJ. Pulmonary artery medial hypertrophy in cocaine users without foreign particle microembolization. Chest 1989; 96:1050–1053.

192. Eagen JW, Memoli VA, Roberts JL, et al. Pulmonary haemorrhage in systemic lupus erythematosus. Medicine (Baltimore) 1978; 57:545–560.

193. Loughlin GM, Taussig LM, Murphy SA, Strunk RC, Kohnen PW. Immune complex-mediated glomerulonephritis and pulmonary haemorrhage simulating Goodpasture's syndrome. J Pediatr 1978; 93:181–184.

194. Leatherman JW, Sibley RK, Davies SF. Diffuse intrapulmonary haemorrhage and glomerulonephritis unrelated to anti-glomerular basement antibody. Am J Med 1982; 72:401–410.

195. Goldstein J, Weil J, Liel Y. Intrapulmonary haemorrhages and immune complex glomerulonephritis masquerading as Goodpasture's syndrome. Hum Pathol 1986; 17:754–757.

196. Martinez JS, Kohler PF. Variant 'Goodpasture's Syndrome'? Ann Intern Med 1971; 75:67–76.

197. Turner-Warwick M, Dewar A. Pulmonary haemorrhage and pulmonary haemosiderosis. Clin Radiol 1982; 33:361–370.

198. Milman N, Pedersen FM. Idiopathic pulmonary haemosiderosis. Epidemiology, pathogenic aspects and diagnosis. Respir Med 1998; 92:902–907.

199. Soergel KH, Sommers SC. Idiopathic pulmonary hemosiderosis and related syndromes. Am J Med 1962; 32:499–511.

200. Thaell JF, Greipp PR, Stubbs SE, Siegal GP. Idiopathic pulmonary hemosiderosis. Two cases in a family. Mayo Clin Proc 1978; 53:113–118.

201. Breckenbridge RL, Ross JS. Idiopathic pulmonary haemosiderosis: a report of familial occurrence. Chest 1979; 75:636–639.

202. Beckerman RC, Taussig LM, Pinnas JL. Familial pulmonary hemosiderosis. Am J Dis Child 1979; 133:609–611.

203. Saeed MM, Woo MS, MacLaughlin EF, Margetis MF, Keens TG. Prognosis in pediatric idiopathic pulmonary hemosiderosis. Chest 1999; 116:721–725.

204. Byrd RB, Gracey DR. Immunosuppressive treatment of idiopathic pulmonary hemosiderosis. JAMA 1973; 226:458–459.

205. Yeager H, Powell D, Weinberg RM, et al. Idiopathic pulmonary hemosiderosis. Ultrastructural studies and response to azathioprine. Arch Intern Med 1976; 136:1145–1149.

206. Wright PH, Menzies IS, Pounder RE, Keeling PWN. Adult idiopathic pulmonary haemosiderosis and coeliac disease. Q J Med 1981; 197:95–102.

207. Wright PH, Buxton-Thomas M, Keeling PWN, Kreel L. Adult idiopathic pulmonary haemosiderosis: a comparison of lung function changes and the distribution of pulmonary disease in patients with and without coeliac disease. Br J Dis Chest 1983; 77:282–292.

208. Bouros D, Panagou P, Rokkas T, Siafakas NM. Bronchoalveolar lavage findings in a young adult with idiopathic pulmonary hemosiderosis and coeliac disease. Eur Respir J 1994; 7:1009–1012.

209. Hay JG, Turner-Warwick M. Pulmonary hemosiderosis, hemorrhagic syndromes and other rare infiltrative disorders. In: Murray JF, Nadel JA, eds. Textbook of Respiratory Medicine. Philadelphia, PA: WB Saunders; 1988:1501–1514.

210. Rafferty JR, Cook MK. Idiopathic pulmonary haemosiderosis with autoimmune haemolytic anaemia. Br J Dis Chest 1984; 78:282–285.

211. Bain SC, Bryan RL, Hawkins JB. Idiopathic pulmonary haemosiderosis and autoimmune thyrotoxicosis. Respir Med 1989; 83:447–450.

212. Stafford HA, Polmar SHJ, Boat TF. Immunologic studies in cow's milk-induced pulmonary haemosiderosis. Pediatr Res 1977; 11:898–903.

213. Cohen GA, Berman BA. Pulmonary hemosiderosis. Cutis 1985; 35:106–109.

214. Valassy-Adam H, Rouska A, Karpouzas J, Matsaniotis N. Raised IgA in idiopathic pulmonary hemosiderosis. Arch Dis Child 1975; 50:320–322.

215. Danel C, Israel-Biet D, Costabel U, Wallaert B, Klech H. The clinical role of BAL in rare pulmonary diseases. Eur Respir Rev 1992; 2:83–88.

216. Bradley JD. The pulmonary haemorrhage syndromes. Clin Chest Med 1982; 3:593–605.

217. Irwin RS, Cottrell TS, Hsu KC, Griswold WR. Thomas HM3. Idiopathic pulmonary hemosiderosis: an electron microscopic and immunofluorescent study. Chest 1974; 65:41–45.

9

Pulmonary eosinophilia

Pulmonary eosinophilia is a clinical term used to describe the association of radiographic lung opacities and blood eosinophilia.[1] Synonyms of pulmonary eosinophilia include 'pulmonary infiltrates with eosinophilia' and 'PIE syndrome'.[2] Some lung diseases that are characterised by an eosinophilic lung infiltrate are not associated with blood eosinophilia and are therefore dealt with elsewhere – eosinophilic granuloma on p. 290 and reactive eosinophilic pleurisy on p. 695. Other eosinophilic infiltrates are associated with blood eosinophilia but not with radiographic opacities, e.g. asthma. The eosinophilia-myalgia syndrome seen with the ingestion of certain tryptophan preparations may well have been considered in this chapter but is dealt with more fully under drug reactions (see p. 389).

Pulmonary eosinophilia may be classified clinically, aetiologically or pathologically. Here, the emphasis will be on pathology, but first the aetiology, pathogenesis and clinical types will be outlined.

Aetiology

Aetiologically, pulmonary eosinophilia may be classified as cryptogenic or of known cause, the latter including allergy to fungi, parasites or drugs (Box 9.1). Subsets of the cryptogenic category include the Churg–Strauss syndrome of allergic angiitis and granulomatosis and the hypereosinophilic syndrome, which are dealt with below.

In Britain, allergic aspergillosis is a common cause of pulmonary eosinophilia, whereas infestation by metazoan parasites is commoner in communities in which these parasites are prevalent (Box 9.2). In some parts of the world filariasis is the cause: this is *tropical pulmonary eosinophilia*, which can be readily diagnosed from the patient's history of residence in the tropics, by the presence of extraordinarily high levels of both serum IgE and antifilarial antibodies and by the dramatic therapeutic response to filaricides.[3–5] Pulmonary eosinophilia is also caused

---

Box 9.1 Aetiology of pulmonary eosinophilia

1	Allergic bronchopulmonary mycosis (usually aspergillosis)
2	Parasitic infestation (see Box 9.2)
3	Drug sensitivity (see Box 9.3)
4	Cryptogenic

Box 9.2 Parasites causing eosinophilic lung disease

Ancylostoma sp.	*Paragonimus westermani*
Ascaris sp.	Schistosoma sp.
Brugia malayi	*Strongyloides stercoralis*
Clonorchis sinensis	Toxocara sp.
Dirofilaria immitis	*Trichinella spiralis*
Echinococcus sp.	*Trichomonas tenax*
Opisthorchiasis sp.	Wuchereria bancrofti

Box 9.3 Drugs causing eosinophilic lung disease

Ampicillin	Methotrexate
Beclometasone dipropionate (inhaled)	Methylphenidate (Ritalin)
Bleomycin	Minocycline
Carbamazepine	Naproxen
Chlorpromazine	Nickel
Clofibrate	Nitrofurantoin
Cocaine (inhaled)	Para-aminosalicylic acid
Cromolyn (inhaled)	Penicillin
Desipramine	Pentamidine (inhaled)
Diclofenac	Phenytoin
Febarbamate	Pyrimethamine
Fenbufen	Rapeseed oil
Glafenine	Sulfadimethoxine
GM-CSF	Sulfadoxine
Ibuprofen	Sulfasalazine
Interleukin-2	Sulindac
Interleukin-3	Tamoxifen
Iodinated contrast dye	Tetracycline
L-tryptophan	Tolazamide
Mephenesin carbamate	Tolfenamic acid
	Vaginal sulfonamide cream

Leukotriene antagonists are not included as it is suspected that their association with Churg–Strauss syndrome represents an unmasking of this condition when these drugs are substituted for corticosteroids.[7]

---

by a number of drugs, notably nitrofurantoin but occasionally sulphonamides and aspirin, amongst others (Box 9.3). Pulmonary eosinophilia may also be a manifestation of rheumatoid disease.[6]

In other patients, the cause of the pulmonary eosinophilia is not recognised. Such cases are categorised as suffering from cryptogenic pulmonary eosinophilia.[8] A majority of these patients are atopic, giving a history of rhinitis or asthma.[9] There is a high level of activated helper T lymphocytes in their bronchoalveolar lavage fluid.[10] They also show a transient increase in circulating immune complexes.[11]

Pathogenesis

The eosinophil leukocyte is central to the pathogenesis of all the diseases in this chapter. Eosinophil leukocytes are produced in the bone marrow under the control of cytokines secreted by type 2 helper lymphocytes, notably interleukin-5. Once released into the blood they normally remain there for 12–18 h,

maintaining a count of 50–250/μl. An absolute count is more meaningful than the percentage in a differential white blood cell count. Tissue eosinophilia does not necessarily correlate with blood eosinophilia even though the two usually go together: blood counts may dip as eosinophils flood the lung and then rise as the infiltrate resolves due to a lag in bone marrow response.

Sputum and bronchoalveolar lavage counts reflect tissue eosinophilia better than blood counts but like neutrophils, eosinophils appear to be washed out of the lung more easily than macrophages so that raised lavage counts are encountered in diseases such as cryptogenic fibrosing alveolitis that are seldom characterised by any appreciable degree of tissue eosinophilia. Bronchoalveolar lavage eosinophils are usually expressed as a percentage of total cells recovered from the lungs, the normal being less than 3%. Eosinophils in sputum are generally expressed only in broad qualitative terms (e.g. 'small, moderate or large numbers'). When there is eosinophilic pneumonia, eosinophils are the predominant cell in both sputum and bronchoalveolar lavage fluid. They are represented at levels greatly in excess of those found in diseases such as cryptogenic fibrosing alveolitis.

Biopsy is the only way to establish tissue eosinophilia with certainty but in practice a tissue diagnosis is often inferred from the clinical features coupled with sputum, blood and bronchoalveolar lavage findings. If a tissue diagnosis is deemed essential a transbronchial biopsy will generally suffice because most of the conditions causing pulmonary eosinophilia affect sufficiently large areas of the lung to be targeted successfully by the bronchoscopist. However, some forms of tissue eosinophilia are characterised by an associated vasculitis and it is unlikely that a transbronchial biopsy will identify this. Vasculitis is more likely to be revealed by thoracoscopic biopsy. Alternatively, it may be identified in more accessible tissue, such as skin or muscle.

Eosinophils enter the tissues under the influence of chemotactic agents produced by a variety of cells, notably interleukins 5, 6 and 10 derived from type 2 helper lymphocytes and eosinophil chemotactic factor from mast cells.[12,13] Activated by these cytokines, eosinophils secrete a number of products, some of which counter the action of substances secreted by mast cells. Histaminase and aryl sulfatase for example respectively destroy histamine and the leukotriene complex formerly known as slow reacting substance of anaphylaxis. Eosinophils also phagocytose immune complexes and mast cell granules and tend to dampen reaginic hypersensitivity reactions. However, they also secrete substances such as reactive oxygen radicals, major basic protein and eosinophil cationic protein which, whilst helping to eliminate parasites, are also toxic to host cells (Fig. 9.1 and see Fig. 3.31, p. 113).[14–17] These eosinophil products are thought to be responsible for much of the tissue damage in the eosinophilic disorders about to be described. Activation of the cells involved in cryptogenic eosinophilic pneumonia is suggested by the demonstration that they express intercellular adhesion molecules, probably under the influence of the activated T lymphocytes referred to above.[18] Electron microscopy shows that released eosinophil granules are closely associated with degenerate and necrotic alveolar tissue.[19]

Corticosteroids act on eosinophils in a variety of ways.[20] They cause rapid eosinophil sequestration in peripheral blood vessels and inhibit their production in the bone marrow. They also reduce eosinophil survival by blocking lymphokines that inhibit eosinophil apoptosis. Eosinophil adherence and chemotaxis are also diminished by corticosteroids. In view of these many actions it is not surprising that corticosteroids are effective in treating many diseases characterised by eosinophilia.

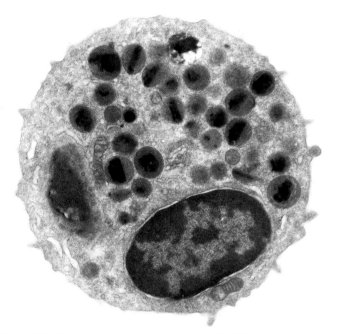

Figure 9.1   Electron micrograph of an eosinophil. A bilobed nucleus is surrounded by granules, many of which have a bar-shaped electron-dense core. The granule core consists of a basic protein, while the surrounding matrix contains cationic protein, both of which are highly toxic.[14] (Illustration provided by Miss A Dewar, Brompton, UK.)

Clinical patterns of pulmonary eosinophilia

The Swiss physician Löffler described two conditions that were characterised by blood eosinophilia. One is the hypereosinophilic syndrome (see below). The other is one that later came to be known as simple pulmonary eosinophilia.[21] Rarely, a patient may display features of both conditions.[22] The term Löffler's syndrome is confusingly applied to both. Crofton and colleagues recognised four further clinical patterns of pulmonary eosinophilia, dividing the condition into five groups: simple, prolonged, tropical, with asthma and with polyarteritis nodosa.[1] Table 9.1 correlates these categories with their usual aetiology and probable pathological basis.

Simple pulmonary eosinophilia is characterised by migratory pulmonary opacities accompanied by blood eosinophilia and minimal or no pulmonary symptoms. Ascariasis was prevalent in Switzerland in Löffler's day and was probably the cause of the eosinophilia in his cases. Löffler emphasised the benign transient nature of this condition. Corticosteroids are highly effective but are rarely required because the condition is usually idiopathic and self-limiting. However, an underlying cause such as parasitic infestation should be considered. The lung is seldom biopsied but it may be presumed to show changes similar to those seen in chronic eosinophilic pneumonia.

Subsequent to the classification outlined in Table 9.1 the terms chronic and acute eosinophilic pneumonia were introduced, the former synonymous with prolonged pulmonary eosinophilia and the latter for a newly recognised variety of eosinophilic lung disease. Modern pathological and imaging studies have tended to use these terms and this practice is followed here. As with the interstitial pneumonias, classical HRCT features correlated with appropriate clinical data often render biopsy unnecessary.[23]

CHRONIC EOSINOPHILIC PNEUMONIA[9,20,24–27]

Chronic eosinophilic pneumonia is a serious condition, which generally requires treatment with corticosteroids. These usually

Table 9.1   Traditional[1] classification of pulmonary eosinophilia with usual aetiological and probable pathological basis

		Probable pathological basis	Aetiology
1	Simple (Löffler's syndrome)	Eosinophilic pneumonia	Allergic aspergillosis Metazoa Drugs Cryptogenic
2	Prolonged	Eosinophilic pneumonia	Cryptogenic Allergic aspergillosis
		Mucoid impaction, bronchocentric granulomatosis	Allergic aspergillosis
		Hypereosinophilic syndrome	Leukoproliferative disorder
3	Tropical	Eosinophilic pneumonia	Filariasis
4	With asthma	Eosinophilic pneumonia	Cryptogenic Drugs
		Mucoid impaction, bronchocentric granulomatosis	Allergic aspergillosis
		Allergic granulomatosis	Allergy (cryptogenic)
5	With polyarteritis nodosa (Churg–Strauss syndrome)	Allergic granulomatosis	Allergy (cryptogenic)

prove efficacious but may have to be continued for many months, or even indefinitely, to prevent relapse. The disease is occasionally life-threatening. The peak incidence is in the fifth decade and females preponderate 2:1. There is often a history of atopic illnesses such as rhinitis or asthma. Any of the aetiological agents outlined above may be responsible.

Clinical features

The onset is insidious, with gradually worsening cough, dyspnoea, fever and weight loss. There is blood and sputum eosinophilia. However, blood and tissue eosinophil levels are not always elevated contemporaneously, the raised blood counts often having abated while eosinophils are still evident in the tissues. Bronchoalveolar lavage cell counts correlate better with the tissue findings, eosinophils being the predominant cell in lavage fluid from an involved segment.[13] The chest radiograph is distinctive, showing bilateral opacification that is peripheral and apical. It has been likened to the plume of a volcano or the photographic negative of the perihilar shadowing of pulmonary oedema. This is mirrored by subpleural consolidation on HRCT.

Pathology

In the occasional case that comes to autopsy the lungs are found to be heavy and firm with irregular areas of pale consolidation (Fig. 9.2). Microscopically, eosinophils fill the alveoli and infiltrate the interstitium (Fig. 9.3).[9,24,28] The alveoli also contain a variable number of macrophages, some of which may be multinucleate. The macrophages may outnumber the eosinophils to mimic the appearances of desquamative interstitial pneumonia (Fig. 9.4). Focal collections of eosinophils may undergo necrosis to form so-called eosinophil abscesses,[9] which are sometimes attended by foreign body type giant cells engulfing eosinophilic debris (Fig. 9.5). Sparse sarcoid-like granulomas are occasion-

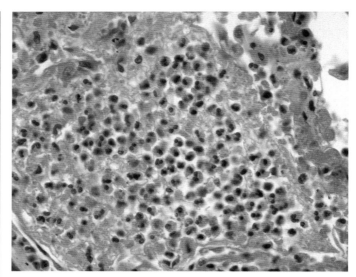

Figure 9.3 Eosinophilic pneumonia. The alveoli contain many eosinophil polymorphonuclear leukocytes.

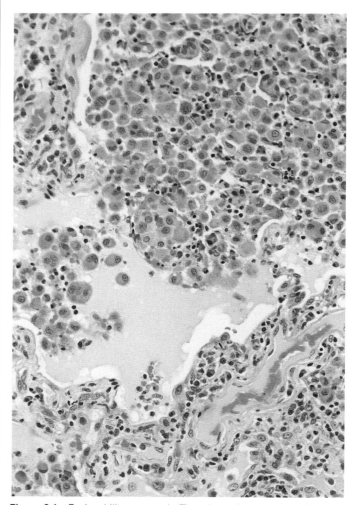

Figure 9.4 Eosinophilic pneumonia. There is moderate eosinophil exudation but these cells are outnumbered by alveolar macrophages.

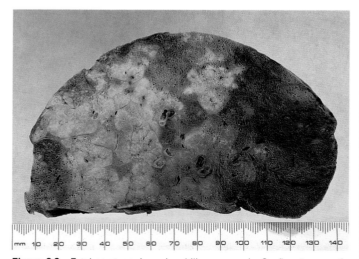

Figure 9.2 Fatal cryptogenic eosinophilic pneumonia. Confluent areas of consolidation represent alveoli filled with eosinophils.

ally seen and in rare cases are unduly prominent.[29] The eosinophil infiltrate may involve small blood vessels but necrotising vasculitis is not encountered: its presence would suggest Churg–Strauss allergic granulomatosis, which is dealt with below. Knowledge of treatment is important as eosinophils diminish with corticosteroid administration. Healing, whether occurring spontaneously or in response to treatment with steroids, usually results in complete resolution but may be by repair, this resulting in alveolar fibrosis that is indistinguishable from any other organising pneumonia.[11,30]

Differential diagnosis

The location of the eosinophils in air spaces as well as in the interstitium helps to distinguish eosinophilic pneumonia from eosinophilic granuloma of the lung, as does the presence of eosinophils in the blood, sputum and bronchoalveolar lavage fluid. Pneumothorax may provoke a reactive eosinophilic infiltrate but this is limited to the alveoli immediately beneath the

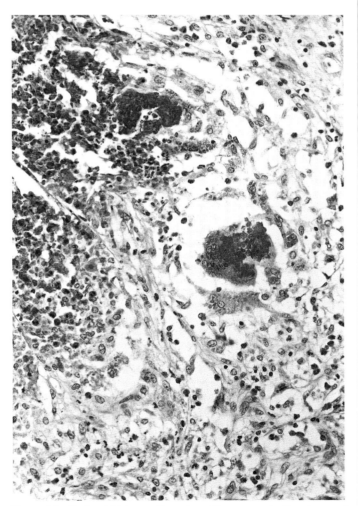

Figure 9.5 Eosinophil 'abscess' in eosinophilic pneumonia. Two clumps of amorphous eosinophilic material are seen, representing agglutinated dead eosinophils. There is a foreign body giant cell reaction to the lower clump.

pleura. In cases with abundant macrophages, desquamative interstitial pneumonia can be distinguished from eosinophilic pneumonia by HRCT review and a lack of blood eosinophilia.

ACUTE EOSINOPHILIC PNEUMONIA

Clinical features

The term acute eosinophilic pneumonia was introduced in 1989[31,32] for a condition characterised by the sudden onset of a febrile illness accompanied by myalgia, pleuritic pain and hypoxaemia. Patients may be of any age and either sex.[33] Chest radiographs show extensive bilateral opacification and effusions. Blood eosinophil counts are often normal but many eosinophils are found on bronchoalveolar lavage and pleural aspirates. A history of asthma is unusual but there may be one of allergic rhinitis.[34] Apart from the lavage and aspirate findings, the clinical features suggest severe infection or the acute respiratory distress syndrome. Most cases reported to date have been cryptogenic but a few appear to have represented drug reactions. An association with the commencement of cigarette smoking has also been reported in young Japanese patients.[35]

Pathology

Acute eosinophilic pneumonia shows the features of diffuse alveolar damage in its exudative or organising phases, coupled with a heavy interstitial infiltrate and a lesser alveolar exudate of eosinophils.[36] In its exudative phase diffuse alveolar damage is characterised by hyaline membranes and in its organising phase by interstitial fibroblast proliferation, prominent alveolar epithelial regeneration and organising alveolar exudates (Fig. 9.6).

Differential diagnosis

Acute eosinophilic pneumonia is more likely to be mistaken for diffuse alveolar damage than chronic eosinophilic pneumonia: therefore, whenever diffuse alveolar damage is being considered it is advisable to search for eosinophils, which may be focal in acute eosinophilic pneumonia. Chronic eosinophilic pneumonia lacks the features of diffuse alveolar damage seen in the acute condition and usually shows more eosinophils, which are often mixed with alveolar macrophages. The Churg–Strauss syndrome, which is described below, is also characterised by vasculitis, necrotising granulomatosis and asthma, features which are not seen in acute eosinophilic pneumonia.

BRONCHOCENTRIC GRANULOMATOSIS

Bronchocentric granulomatosis was first described by Liebow in 1973 as a necrotising granulomatous inflammation of the airway walls and surrounding lung tissue.[37] It may be associated with asthma but this is not always present.[38,39] In the patients with asthma, the disease appears to be a hypersensitivity reaction to inhaled antigens.[40–42] In the non-asthmatic

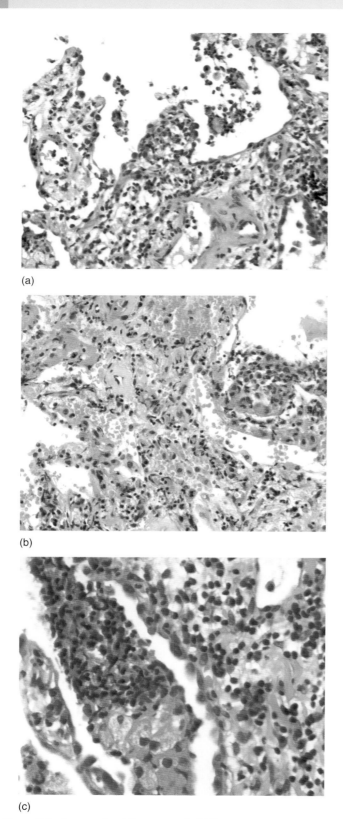

(a)

(b)

(c)

Figure 9.6 Acute eosinophilic pneumonia. (a) The alveolar walls are expanded by oedema and a mixed inflammatory cell infiltrate, which includes eosinophils. The alveolar epithelium shows focal desquamation and there is type II pneumocyte hyperplasia. (b) Hyaline membranes are evident. (c) Eosinophils are clumped together within an airspace and also infiltrate the interstitium. There is also atypical alveolar epithelial hyperplasia.

patients it most commonly represents a granulomatous response to airway infection.

Clinical features and prognosis

In one series of 23 patients, the mean age was 22 years in the ten asthmatic patients and 50 years in the 13 non-asthmatics. The sex distribution was almost equal in both groups.[38] Asthmatics with bronchocentric granulomatosis complain of increased wheezing, cough, fever and occasionally haemoptysis. Blood eosinophilia and positive sputum culture for Aspergillus are commonly seen.[38] The non-asthmatic patients are a more heterogeneous group. They may be asymptomatic or present with an acute febrile illness and cough. Blood eosinophilia is uncommon in this group. Chest radiographic abnormalities are similar in the two groups and include solitary or multiple infiltrates or tumour-like masses and areas of atelectasis, usually involving the upper lobes.[38,43] Apart from fever and blood eosinophilia the condition is confined to the lungs. The prognosis is good. Corticosteroids generally result in rapid clinical and radiological resolution. Some patients recover without treatment.

Aetiology and pathological findings

Bronchocentric granulomatosis usually represents a type of allergic bronchopulmonary aspergillosis that affects more distal airways than mucoid impaction. Medium or small bronchi, or even bronchioles, are affected rather than large central airways.[37,38,44,45] The condition is characterised by a necrotising granulomatous inflammation (Figs 9.7, 9.8). This destroys much of the airway wall and results in necrotic debris occluding the lumen (see Fig. 5.4.16 on p. 227 and Figs 9.7 and 9.8). The inflammation usually includes many eosinophils, together with lymphocytes, plasma cells and prominent epithelioid cells, which often border the necrotic debris in a palisade pattern. That the process is bronchocentric may sometimes be recognisable only from its location alongside unaffected pulmonary arteries or by tracing its distribution in step sections. Often, just a remnant of respiratory epithelium indicates that the disease is centred on the airways. Sparse hyphae are generally to be found within mucus plugs occluding larger airways. Rarely, bronchocentric granulomatosis may complicate an aspergilloma.[46]

In other cases, no allergen is ever identified: these cases differ from those caused by aspergilli in that there is no blood eosinophilia or history of asthma and eosinophils are sparse in the affected tissues, where plasma cells are predominant.[44] In other patients, bronchocentric granulomatosis is associated with other pathogens, such as echinococcus, mycobacteria, blastomyces, histoplasma or mucor.[47–50] Tuberculosis, histoplasmosis, blastomycosis and coccidioidomycosis may all show a histological process indistinguishable from bronchocentric granulomatosis and many cases of bronchocentric granulomatosis in non-asthmatic patients may represent unrecognised infections.[48] Atopy does not appear to be important in these cases but sometimes the patient is immunosuppressed.[49] A bronchocentric form of Wegener's granulomatosis is distin-

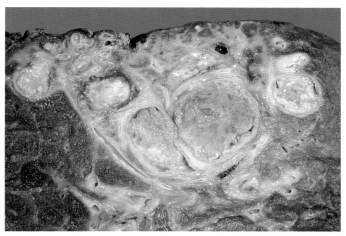

Figure 9.7 Bronchocentric granulomatosis as a manifestation of allergic bronchopulmonary aspergillosis. It formed a mass lesion that was thought to be neoplastic but this resection specimen shows dilated airways impacted with mucopurulent debris containing numerous eosinophils.

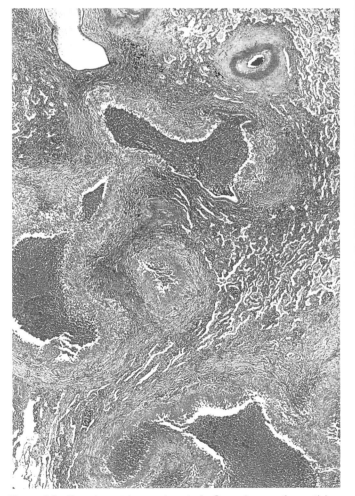

Figure 9.8 Bronchocentric granulomatosis. Several areas of necrotising granulomatous inflammation are seen. They are situated alongside arteries, which are themselves largely spared and an occasional remnant of respiratory epithelium confirms that they are centred on airways. In the absence of recognisable bronchial remnants the bronchocentricity of the lesion has to be inferred from its location next to a pulmonary artery.

guished from bronchocentric granulomatosis by its characteristic necrotising vasculitis.[51] Bronchocentric granulomatosis has also been reported in association with rheumatoid arthritis,[52–54] ankylosing spondylitis,[55] glomerulonephritis[56] and red cell aplasia.[57] It is also described beyond an obstructing bronchial carcinoma, the mechanism here being sustained non-allergic inflammation.[58,59]

ALLERGIC ANGIITIS AND GRANULOMATOSIS (CHURG–STRAUSS SYNDROME)

Allergic angiitis and granulomatosis is a clinico-pathological syndrome consisting of asthma, eosinophilia, vasculitis and necrotising granulomas, that was first described in 1951 by Churg and Strauss.[60] Since then, several additional series have appeared.[61–63] Among the cases of pulmonary polyarteritis nodosa reported by Rose and Spencer,[64] many had eosinophilia and were probably further examples of allergic angiitis. The cause is unknown but the predominant clinical features implicate the respiratory tract as the portal of entry of an as yet unidentified antigen. There are rare reports of allergic angiitis and granulomatosis developing in patients with allergic bronchopulmonary mycoses[65,66] or diffuse panbronchiolitis.[67]

Clinical features

The majority of patients are atopic. They initially suffer from allergic rhinitis and then asthma. They next develop pulmonary eosinophilia, as described above and finally enter a vasculitic phase.[61,63] In the eosinophilic stage blood eosinophil counts often exceed $5 \times 10^9/1$.[60] Serum IgE levels may be increased during the vasculitic phase.[63] Many patients have systemic symptoms, such as fever, weight loss and pulmonary infiltrates that may be diffuse and transient or massive and nodular and are generally non-cavitating. There may be eosinophilic pleural effusions. Myocardial or pericardial lesions are evident in about 50% of patients. Most deaths are associated with complications of cardiac involvement. Many patients also have involvement of the skin, gastrointestinal tract, joints, muscles, nervous system or lower urinary tract;[61] thymic lesions have also been described.[68] Renal disease is usually mild and renal failure is rare. Anti-myeloperoxidase antibodies (p-ANCA) are found in the majority of cases.[69,70] Unlike Wegener's granulomatosis, cytotoxic therapy is rarely indicated and corticosteroids usually provide effective treatment. The substitution of leukotriene antagonists for corticosteroids in the treatment of asthma appears to be unmasking previously unsuspected cases of Churg–Strauss syndrome[7,71]; the syndrome has also been recognised in asthmatic patients who have had their corticosteroid dosage reduced or who have been transferred from systemic to inhaled corticosteroids.[72]

In 1990, the American College of Rheumatology proposed six criteria, of which four were considered sufficient for a diagnosis of Churg–Strauss syndrome (Box 9.4). This yielded a sensitivity of 85% and a specificity of 99.7%. Alternatively, three particular criteria (asthma, blood eosinophilia greater than 10% and a history of allergy other than asthma or drug sensitivity) carried a sensitivity of 95% and a specificity of 99.2%.[73]

Pathology

Three histological features accompany the asthma and blood eosinophilia: tissue eosinophilia, vasculitis and necrotising granulomatosis. These features are not necessarily seen together and in practice the diagnosis is usually made on clinical grounds with histological verification of perhaps just one of them. The likelihood of all three features being identified increases with the size and number of the biopsies and is greatest in autopsy material.

At autopsy or in an adequate biopsy soft yellow nodules may be seen on the cut surface of the lung (Fig. 9.9). These represent foci of eosinophilic pneumonia within which irregular areas of necrosis containing the debris of dead eosinophils and Charcot–Leyden crystals are often seen.

Granulomas may be numerous but more usually are infrequent and may not be readily identifiable in biopsy material. Early granulomas consist of small irregular clusters of giant cells and histiocytes, usually with a small central focus of densely eosinophilic necrosis. Epithelioid cells are not a feature and the granulomas lack the cohesion and lymphocytic rim

typical of those seen in sarcoidosis. In larger granulomas the central necrotic area is surrounded by radially arranged palisading histiocytes and multinucleate cells (Fig. 9.10).

The vasculitis, which involves arteries, veins and even capillaries,[74] may be eosinophilic, neutrophilic or granulomatous[75] but usually takes the form of focal necrosis of vessel walls associated with perivascular and transmural infiltration by eosinophils (Fig. 9.11). Capillary involvement may cause alveolar haemorrhage.[76] If the vasculitis is neutrophilic the appearances are similar to those of polyarteritis nodosa[64] and the diagnosis of allergic granulomatosis has to depend upon extravascular features. Affected vessels may be obliterated by fibrous tissue. Electron dense deposits,[74] IgE[61] and IgM[63] have all been reported in the vascular basement membrane.

Other changes in the lungs include those of asthma (Figs 9.9 and 9.12). Extrapulmonary lesions show vasculitis

Box 9.4 American College of Rheumatology criteria for the diagnosis of Churg–Strauss syndrome[73]	
1	Asthma
2	Eosinophils >10% of the white cell differential count
3	Mononeuropathy or polyneuropathy
4	Non-fixed pulmonary infiltrates
5	Paranasal sinus abnormalities
6	Tissue eosinophils on biopsy

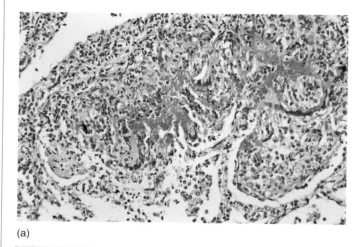

(a)

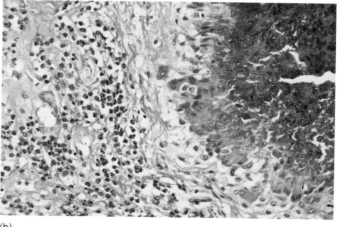

(b)

Figure 9.10 Allergic angiitis and granulomatosis (Churg–Strauss syndrome). (a) An eosinophilic 'abscess' has developed in an area of eosinophilic pneumonia. It consists of agglutinated necrotic eosinophils about which there is a granulomatous reaction. (b) Necrotising granulomatosis with prominent eosinophil accumulation in the pericardium of the same patient.

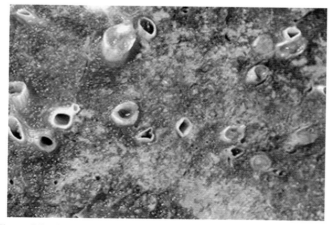

Figure 9.9 Allergic angiitis and granulomatosis (Churg–Strauss syndrome). Confluent yellow nodules representing foci of eosinophilic consolidation are seen while several airways show mucus plugging indicating underlying asthma.

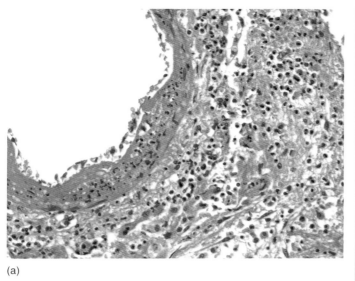

(a)

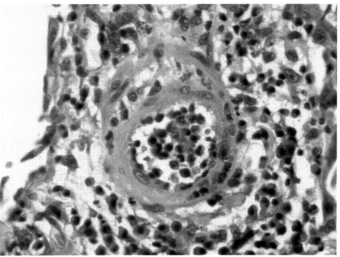

(b)

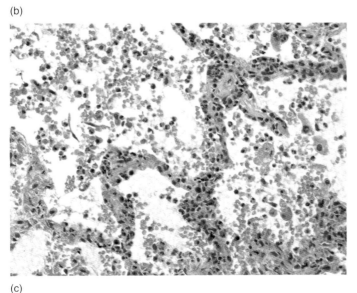

(c)

Figure 9.11 Allergic angiitis and granulomatosis (Churg–Strauss syndrome). The eosinophilic vasculitis predominantly involves medium-sized and small pulmonary arteries (a, b), but may also involve pulmonary capillaries (c).

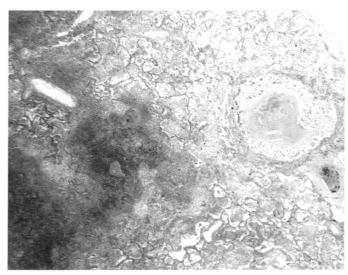

Figure 9.12 Allergic angiitis and granulomatosis (Churg–Strauss syndrome). An irregular area of eosinophilic necrosis, within which there is vasculitis. Note the small bronchus plugged by mucus (right).

and necrotising granulomatosis with prominent tissue eosinophilia, as in the lungs (Fig. 9.13).

Differential diagnosis

The relationship of the Churg–Strauss syndrome to other forms of vasculitis, hypereosinophilia and granulomatosis has been the subject of much debate.[63,77–79] Strictly speaking, the eponym should be reserved for cases in which all the criteria are present: asthma, eosinophilia, vasculitis and necrotising granulomatosis, but Churg and Strauss[60] considered the combination of marked tissue eosinophilia and granulomatosis to be pathognomonic. All their patients were asthmatic. Patients with the histological features of the Churg–Strauss syndrome but lacking a history of asthma and blood eosinophilia have been variously regarded as suffering from an eosinophilic variant of Wegener's granulomatosis[79] or atypical forms of the Churg–Strauss syndrome.[68,80] At various stages in the course of the Churg–Strauss syndrome, patients may fulfil the criteria for the hypereosinophilic syndrome (see below) or Löffler's syndrome (transient pulmonary infiltrates accompanied by peripheral blood eosinophilia, see above).

The differences between Churg–Strauss syndrome and Wegener's granulomatosis are both clinical and pathological. Asthma and blood eosinophilia are not features of Wegener's granulomatosis, while the destructive upper respiratory tract lesions of this condition are not present in the Churg–Strauss syndrome. The pulmonary lesions are generally less extensively necrotic in the Churg–Strauss syndrome than in Wegener's granulomatosis. Tissue eosinophilia is found in an eosinophilic variant of Wegener's granulomatosis[79] but is usually limited to the chronic inflammatory granulation tissue that surrounds areas of necrosis rather than flooding airspaces as in the eosinophilic pneumonia of the Churg–Strauss syndrome. The pathological changes in the kidney may be similar in the two

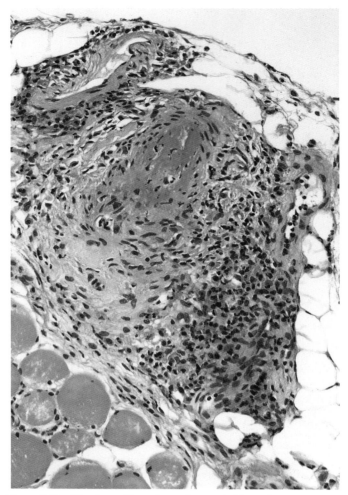

Figure 9.13 Allergic angiitis and granulomatosis (Churg-Strauss syndrome). A muscle biopsy shows necrotising vasculitis and eosinophilia.

Box 9.5 Systemic involvement by hypereosinophilic syndrome[85]	
Cardiovascular	58%
Cutaneous	56%
Neurological	54%
Pulmonary	49%
Splenic	43%
Hepatic	30%
Ocular	23%
Gastrointestinal	23%

(Box 9.5) and patients with cardiac or central nervous system involvement have a particularly poor prognosis. Vascular involvement is generally described as being thrombotic or haemorrhagic rather than vasculitic. Cases with fibrous endocarditis are often said to have Löffler's rather than the hypereosinophilic syndrome.

Aetiology

The proposed leukoproliferative basis of the hypereosinophilic syndrome is supported by the identification of monoclonal cell populations. Conventional cytogenetic analysis is often normal but a cryptic interstitial deletion of chromosome 4 resulting in the formation of an *FIP1L1-PDGFRA* fusion gene has led to the recognition that many patients who would previously have been regarded as having the hypereosinophilic syndrome actually have chronic eosinophilic leukaemia.[86,87] In other patients with hypereosinophilia there is a clonal proliferation of type 2 helper lymphocytes (Th2, CD4 cells).[82,88] Th2 cells produce cytokines implicated in eosinophil proliferation and activation, notably interleukin-5. The consequent eosinophil activation results in the release of cytotoxic factors such as major basic protein and eosinophil cationic protein that are probably responsible for much of the tissue damage encountered in the syndrome. In rare cases, lymphoma or leukaemia cells overproduce interleukin-5 and consequently hypereosinophilia.

Clinical features

The clinical picture is generally dominated by cardiovascular or neurological features. Vascular disease is characterised by an early thrombotic phase followed by fibrosis and cardiac involvement by dysrhythmia, valvular incompetence and ultimately heart failure. Neurological disease is characterised by intellectual impairment, a variety of localising signs and peripheral neuropathy. The commonest respiratory symptom is a nonproductive cough: asthma is rare. Pleural effusions are common but are generally transudates attributable to cardiac failure; they rarely contain eosinophils. Interstitial pulmonary infiltrates are detected in about a quarter of cases and these may progress to the acute respiratory distress syndrome.[89] The CT findings include small pulmonary nodules with or without a halo of ground-glass attenuation and focal areas of ground-glass attenuation which are mainly peripheral.[90] Many patients with pulmonary involvement respond to steroids but cytotoxic drugs have been deemed necessary in severe cases.[89]

diseases but they are rarely progressive in the Churg–Strauss syndrome and cause only mild impairment of function. Lastly, the p-ANCA test tends to be positive in the Churg–Strauss syndrome and c-ANCA negative, the reverse of that found in Wegener's granulomatosis. The Churg–Strauss syndrome, Wegener's granulomatosis and microscopic polyangiitis are compared in Tables 8.3.1 and 8.3.3 (see pp. 438, 443).

HYPEREOSINOPHILIC SYNDROME

The term hypereosinophilic syndrome was introduced in 1968.[81] It represents a rare and often fatal systemic disease of uncertain aetiology that is regarded by many as representing a leukoproliferative disorder.[82] The disease is marked by sustained overproduction of eosinophils (blood eosinophils in excess of $1.5 \times 10^9/l$, for longer than 6 months) and widespread organ damage.[83] It affects adults in the third and fourth decades and men outnumber women by 7 to 1.[84] Many organs are involved

Pathology

Pulmonary involvement is characterised by a heavy infiltrate of mature eosinophils and consolidation of the airspaces by the same cells, often with small foci of necrosis. There may be many Charcot–Leyden crystals, as with any heavy eosinophil infiltrate. Thus, in the lungs the pathological features of the hypereosinophilic syndrome are identical to those of eosinophilic pneumonia (see above). Secondary changes include widespread thrombosis and infarction.

REFERENCES

1. Crofton JW, Livingstone JL, Oswald NC, Roberts ATM. Pulmonary eosinophilia. Thorax 1952; 7:1–35.
2. Reeder WH, Goodrich BE. Pulmonary infiltration with eosinophilia (PIE syndrome). Ann Intern Med 1952; 36:1217–1240.
3. Danaraj TJ, Pacheco G, Shanmugaratnam K, Beaver PC. The etiology and pathology of eosinophilic lung (tropical eosinophilia). Am J Trop Med Hyg 1966; 15:183–189.
4. Udwadia FE. Tropical eosinophilia – a review. Respir Med 1993; 87:17–21.
5. Ong RKC, Doyle RL. Tropical pulmonary eosinophilia. Chest 1998; 113:1673–1679.
6. Norman D, Piecyk M, Roberts DH. Eosinophilic pneumonia as an initial manifestation of rheumatoid arthritis. Chest 2004; 126; 993–995.
7. Solans R, Bosch JA, Selva A, Orriols R, Vilardell M. Montelukast and Churg–Strauss syndrome. Thorax 2002; 57:183–185.
8. McCarthy DS, Pepys J. Cryptogenic pulmonary eosinophilias. Clin Allergy 1973; 3:339–351.
9. Liebow AA, Carrington CB. The eosinophilic pneumonias. Medicine (Baltimore) 1969; 48:251–285.
10. Albera C, Ghio P, Solidoro P, Mabritto I, Marchetti L, Pozzi E. Activated and memory alveolar T-lymphocytes in idiopathic eosinophilic pneumonia. Eur Respir J 1995; 8:1281–1285.
11. Miyagawa Y, Nagata N, Shigematsu N. Clinicopathological study of migratory lung infiltrates. Thorax 1991; 46:233–238.
12. Mukae H, Kadota J, Kohno S, Matsukura S, Hara K. Increase of activated T-cells in BAL fluid of Japanese patients with bronchiolitis obliterans organising pneumonia and chronic eosinophilic pneumonia. Chest 1995; 108:123–128.
13. Kita H, Sur S, Hunt LW, et al. Cytokine production at the site of disease in chronic eosinophilic pneumonitis. Am J Respir Crit Care Med 1996; 153:1437–1441.
14. Peters MS, Rodriguez M, Gleich GJ. Localization of human eosinophil granule major basic protein, eosinophil cationic protein and eosinophil-derived neurotoxin by immunoelectron microscopy. Lab Invest 1986; 54:656–662.
15. Plager DA, Loegering DA, Tang J, Kephart GM, Gleich GJ. Eosinophil proteins: Human eosinophil granule major basic protein homolog: biochemical, genetic and immunochemical aspects. Resp Med 2000; 94:1011–1012.
16. Ackerman SJ, Swaminathan GJ, Leonidas DD, et al. Eosinophil proteins: Structural biology of Charcot-Leyden crystal protein (Galectin-10): new insights into an old protein. Resp Med 2000; 94:1014–1016.
17. Venge P. Eosinophil Proteins: Eosinophil granule proteins as markers of eosinophil activity in vivo. Resp Med 2000; 94:1016–1017.
18. Azuma M, Nakamura Y, Sano T, Okano Y, Sone S. Adhesion molecule expression on eosinophils in idiopathic eosinophilic pneumonia. Eur Respir J 1996; 9:2494–2500.
19. Saitoh K, Shindo N, Toh Y, Yoshizawa A, Kudo K. Electron microscopic study of chronic eosinophilic pneumonia. Pathol Int 1996; 46:855–861.
20. Allen JN, Davis WB. Eosinophilic lung diseases. Am J Respir Crit Care Med 1994; 150:1423–1438.
21. Löffler W. Zur Differential-Diagnose der Lungeninfiltrierungen II. Uber fluchtige Succedan-Infiltrate (mit Eosinophilie). Beitr Z Klin D Tuberk 1932; 79:368–392.
22. Brink AJ, Weber HW. Fibroplastic parietal endocarditis with eosinophilia. Loffler's endocarditis. Am J Med 1963; 34:52–70.
23. Johkoh T, Muller NL, Akira M, et al. Eosinophilic lung diseases: diagnostic accuracy of thin-section CT in 111 patients. Radiology 2000; 216:773–780.

Chronic eosinophilic pneumonia
24. Carrington CB, Addington WW, Goff AM, et al. Chronic eosinophilic pneumonia. N Engl J Med 1969; 280:788–798.
25. Jederlinic PJ, Sicilian L, Gaensler EA. Chronic eosinophilic pneumonia: a report of 19 cases and a review of the literature. Medicine (Baltimore) 1988; 67:154–162.
26. Naughton M, Fahy J, FitzGerald MX. Chronic eosinophilic pneumonia – a long-term follow-up of 12 patients. Chest 1993; 103:162–165.
27. Hayakawa H, Sato A, Toyoshima M, Imokawa S, Taniguchi M. A clinical study of idiopathic eosinophilic pneumonia. Chest 1994; 105:1462–1466.
28. Baggenstoss AH, Bayley EC, Lindberg DON. Loffler's syndrome. Report of a case with pathologic examination of lungs. Proc Mayo Clin 1946; 21:457–465.
29. Shijubo N, Fujishima T, Morita S, et al. Idiopathic chronic eosinophilic pneumonia associated with noncaseating epithelioid granulomas. Eur Respir J 1995; 8:327–330.

Acute eosinophilic pneumonia
30. Yoshida K, Shijubo N, Koba H, et al. Chronic eosinophilic pneumonia progressing to lung fibrosis. Eur Respir J 1994; 7:1541–1544.
31. Allen JN, Pacht ER, Gadek JE, Davis WB. Acute eosinophilic pneumonia as a reversible cause of noninfectious respiratory failure. N Engl J Med 1989; 321:569–574.
32. Badesch DB, King TE, Schwarz MI. Acute eosinophilic pneumonia: a hypersensitivity pneumonia? Am Rev Respir Dis 1989; 139:249–252.
33. Alp H, Daum RS, Abrahams C, Wylam ME. Acute eosinophilic pneumonia: a cause of reversible, severe, noninfectious respiratory failure. J Pediatr 1998; 132:540–543.
34. King MA, Pope-Harman AL, Allen JN, Christoforidis GA, Christoforidis AJ. Acute eosinophilic pneumonia: radiologic and clinical features. Radiology 1997; 203:715–719.
35. Shintani H, Fujimura M, Yasui M, et al. Acute eosinophilic pneumonia caused by cigarette smoking. Intern Med 2000; 39:66–68.
36. Tazelaar HD, Linz LJ, Colby TV, Myers JL, Limper AH. Acute eosinophilic pneumonia: histopathologic findings in nine patients. Am J Respir Crit Care Med 1997; 155:296–302.

Bronchocentric granulomatosis
37. Liebow AA. Pulmonary angiitis and granulomatosis. Am Rev Respir Dis 1973; 108: 1–18.
38. Katzenstein ALA, Liebow AA, Friedman PJ. Bronchocentric granulomatosis, mucoid impaction and hypersensitivity reaction to fungi. Am Rev Respir Dis 1975; 111:497–537.
39. Koss MN, Robinson RG, Hochholzer L. Bronchocentric granulomatosis. Hum Pathol 1981; 12:632–638.
40. Hanson G, Flod N, Wells I, Novey H, Galant S. Bronchocentric granulomatosis: A complication of allergic bronchopulmonary aspergillosis. J Allergy Clin Immunol 1977; 59:83–90.
41. Bosken CH, Myers JL, Greenberger PA, Katzenstein A-LA. Pathologic features of allergic bronchopulmonary aspergillosis. Am J Surg Pathol 1988; 12:216–222.
42. Sulavik SB. Bronchocentric granulomatosis and allergic bronchopulmonary aspergillosis. Clin Chest Med 1988; 9:609–621.
43. Robinson RB, Wehunt WD, Tsou E, Koss MN, Hochholzer L. Bronchocentric granulomatosis: roentgenographic manifestations. Am Rev Respir Dis 1982; 125:751–756.
44. Koss MN, Robinson RG, Hochholzer L. Bronchocentric granulomatosis. Hum Pathol 1981; 12:632–638.

45. Saldana MJ. Bronchocentric granulomatosis: clinicopathologic observations in 17 patients. Lab Invest 1979; 40:281–282.

46. Makker H, McConnochie K, Gibbs AR. Postirradiation pulmonary fibrosis complicated by aspergilloma and bronchocentric granulomatosis. Thorax 1989; 44:676–677.

47. Den Hertog RW, Wagenaar SjSc, Westermann CJJ. Bronchocentric granulomatosis and pulmonary echinococcosis. Am Rev Respir Dis 1982; 126:344–347.

48. Myers JL, Katzenstein A-LA. Granulomatous infection mimicking bronchocentric granulomatosis. Am J Surg Pathol 1986; 10:317–322.

49. Tazelaar HD, Baird AM, Mill M, Grimes MM, Schulman LL, Smith CR. Bronchocentric mycosis occurring in transplant recipients. Chest 1989; 96:92–95.

50. Maguire GP, Lee M, Rosen Y, Lyons HA. Pulmonary tuberculosis and bronchocentric granulomatosis. Chest 1986; 89:606–608.

51. Yousem SA. Bronchocentric injury in Wegener's granulomatosis – a report of five cases. Hum Pathol 1991; 22:535–540.

52. Berendsen HH, Hofstee N, Kapsenberg PD, van Reesema DRS, Klein JJ. Bronchocentric granulomatosis associated with rheumatoid arthritis. Chest 1983; 5:831–832.

53. Bonafede RP, Benatar SR. Bronchocentric granulomatosis and rheumatoid arthritis. Br J Dis Chest 1987; 81:197–201.

54. Hellems SO, Kanner RE, Renzetti AD. Bronchocentric granulomatosis associated with rheumatoid arthritis. Chest 1983; 5:831–832.

55. Rohatgi PK, Turrisi BC. Bronchocentric granulomatosis and ankylosing spondylitis. Thorax 1984; 39:317–318.

56. Warren J, Pitchenik AE, Saldana MJ. Bronchocentric granulomatosis with glomerulonephritis. Chest 1985; 125:751–756.

57. Martinez-Lopez MA, Pena JM, Quiralte J, et al. Bronchocentric granulomatosis associated with pure red cell aplasia and lymphadenopathy. Thorax 1992; 47:131–133.

58. Clee MD, Lamb D, Clark RA. Bronchocentric granulomatosis: a review and thoughts on pathogenesis. Br J Dis Chest 1983; 77:227–234.

59. Houser SL, Mark EJ. Bronchocentric granulomatosis with mucus impaction due to bronchogenic carcinoma. An association with clinical relevance. Arch Pathol Lab Med 2000; 124:1168–1171.

Allergic angitis and granulomatosis (Churg–Strauss syndrome)

60. Churg J, Strauss L. Allergic granulomatosis, allergic angiitis and periarteritis nodosa. Am J Pathol 1951; 27:277–301.

61. Chumbley LC, Harrison EG, DeRemee RA. Allergic granulomatosis and angiitis (Churg–Strauss syndrome). Mayo Clin Proc 1977; 52:477–484.

62. Koss MN, Antonovych T, Hochholzer L. Allergic granulomatosis (Churg–Strauss syndrome): pulmonary and renal morphological findings. Am J Surg Pathol 1981; 5:21–28.

63. Lanham JC, Elkon KB, Pusey CD, Hughes GR. Systemic vasculitis with asthma and eosinophilia; a clinical approach to the Churg–Strauss syndrome. Medicine (Baltimore) 1984; 63:65–81.

64. Rose GA, Spencer H. Polyarteritis nodosa. Q J Med 1957; 26:43–81.

65. Stephens M, Reynolds S, Gibbs AR, Davies B. Allergic bronchopulmonary aspergillosis progressing to allergic granulomatosis and angiitis (Churg–Strauss syndrome). Am Rev Respir Dis 1988; 137:1226–1228.

66. Matsumoto H, Niimi A, Suzuki K, Kawai M, Matsui Y, Amitani R. Allergic granulomatous angiitis (Churg–Strauss syndrome) associated with allergic bronchopulmonary candidiasis. Respiration 2000; 67:577–579.

67. Sasaki A, Hasegawa M, Nakazato Y, Ishida Y, Saitoh S. Allergic granulomatosis and angiitis (Churg–Strauss syndrome). Report of an autopsy case in a nonasthmatic patient. Acta Pathol Jpn 1988; 38:781–788.

68. Jessurun J, Azevedo M, Saldana M. Allergic angiitis and granulomatosis (Churg–Strauss syndrome): report of a case with massive thymic involvement in a non-asthmatic patient. Hum Pathol 1986; 17:637–639.

69. Gaskin G, Ryan JJ, Rees AJ, Pusey CD. Anti-myeloperoxidase antibodies in vasculitis: relationship to ANCA and clinical diagnosis. APMIS 1990; 98(Suppl. 19):33.

70. Tervaert JWC, Elema JD, Kallenberg CGM. Clinical and histopathological association of 29kD-ANCA and MPO-ANCA. APMIS 1990; 98(Suppl. 19):35.

71. Wechsler ME, Finn D, Gunawardena D, et al. Churg–Strauss syndrome in patients receiving montelukast as treatment for asthma. Chest 2000; 117:708–713.

72. LeGall C, Pham S, Vignes S, et al. Inhaled corticosteroids and Churg–Strauss syndrome: a report of five cases. Eur Resp J 2000; 15(5):978–981.

73. Masi AT, Hunder GG, Lie JT, et al. The American College of Rheumatology 1990 criteria for the classification of Churg–Strauss syndrome (allergic granulomatosis and angiitis). Arthritis Rheum 1990; 33:1094–1100.

74. Lichtig C, Ludatscher R, Eisenberg E, Bental E. Small blood vessel disease in allergic granulomatous angiitis (Churg–Strauss syndrome). J Clin Pathol 1989; 42:1001–1002.

75. Clausen KP, Bronstein H. Granulomatous pulmonary arteritis. A hypereosinophilic syndrome. Am J Clin Pathol 1974; 62:82–87.

76. Clutterbuck EJ, Pusey CD. Severe alveolar haemorrhage in Churg–Strauss syndrome. Eur J Respir Dis 1987; 71:158–163.

77. Katzenstein ALA. Diagnostic features and differential diagnosis of Churg–Strauss syndrome in the lung – A review. Amer J Clin Pathol 2000; 114:767–772.

78. Dreisen RB. Pulmonary vasculitis. Clin Chest Med 1982; 3:607–618.

79. Yousem SA, Lombard CM. The eosinophilic variant of Wegener's granulomatosis. Hum Pathol 1988; 19:682–688.

80. Lipworth BJ, Slater DN, Corrin B, Kesseller ME, Haste AR. Allergic granulomatosis without asthma: a rare 'forme fruste' of the Churg–Strauss syndrome. Respir Med 1989; 83:249–250.

Hypereosinophilic syndrome

81. Hardy WR, Anderson RE. The hypereosinophilic syndrome. Ann Intern Med 1968; 68:1220–1229.

82. Schwartz RS. The hypereosinophilic syndrome and the biology of cancer. N Engl J Med 2003; 348:1199–1200.

83. Chusid MJ, Dale DC, West BC, Wolff SM. The hypereosinophilic syndrome: analysis of fourteen cases with review of the literature. Medicine 1975; 54:1–27.

84. Spry CJF, Davies J, Tai PC, Olsen EGJ, Oakley CM, Goodwin JF. Clinical features of fifteen patients with the hypereosinophilic syndrome. Q J Med 1983; 205:1–22.

85. Weller PF, Bubley GJ. The idiopathic hypereosinophilic syndrome. Blood 1994; 83:2759–2779.

86. Cools J, DeAngelo DJ, Gotlib J, et al. A tyrosine kinase created by fusion of the PDGFRA and FIP1L1 genes as a therapeutic target of imatinib in idiopathic hypereosinophilic syndrome. N Engl J Med 2003; 348:1201–1214.

87. Bain BJ. Relationship between idiopathic hypereosinophilic syndrome, eosinophilic leukemia and systemic mastocytosis. Am J Hematol 2004; 77:82–85.

88. Cogan E, Schandené L, Crusiaux A, Cochaux P, Velu T, Goldman M. Brief report: clonal proliferation of type 2 helper T-cells in a man with the hypereosinophilic syndrome. N Engl J Med 1994; 330:535–538.

89. Winn RE, Kollef MH, Meyer JI. Pulmonary involvement in the hypereosinophilic syndrome. Chest 1994; 105:656–660.

90. Kang EY, Shim JJ, Kim JS, Kim KI. Pulmonary involvement of idiopathic hypereosinophilic syndrome: CT findings in five patients. J Comput Assist Tomogr 1997; 21:612–615.

10

Pulmonary manifestations of systemic disease

Some systemic diseases particularly affect the lungs but are dealt with exclusively in other chapters: examples of these include sarcoidosis (p. 285), vasculitis and granulomatosis (p. 437) and Langerhans cell histiocytosis (p. 290). Other diseases often affect the lungs in isolation and are described in full elsewhere but as, on occasion, they also form part of systemic illnesses they also have to be referred to here: examples of these include cryptogenic fibrosing alveolitis, which is associated with many of the systemic connective tissue disorders. Drug reactions are usually systemic, but are dealt with separately on pp. 383–392.

CONNECTIVE TISSUE DISEASES

The connective tissue diseases form a heterogeneous group of immunologically mediated disorders that share certain characteristics, notably inflammation of synovial and serosal membranes, connective tissue and blood vessels in various tissues. The lung is often involved in this group of diseases, probably because of its abundant connective tissue and vasculature. Pulmonary associations of connective tissue diseases include abnormalities of airways, alveoli, pulmonary blood vessels, pleura and chest wall, any of which may precede, accompany or follow the onset of the systemic disease (Table 10.1). Many of the pulmonary associations of connective tissue diseases also occur in isolation (although often accompanied by serological markers), leading to terms such as 'lone' and 'systemic' cryptogenic fibrosing alveolitis. Pathologically, the systemic form of fibrosing alveolitis differs from that seen in 'lone' cryptogenic fibrosing alveolitis in that the histological pattern is more often that of NSIP than UIP.[1–4a] Also, its progression is often slower and its prognosis correspondingly better.[5–7] The few patients with connective tissue diseases who show a UIP pattern have fewer fibroblastic foci than patients with idiopathic interstitial pneumonia and UIP.[8]

The histological features of connective tissue diseases need to be separated from the effects of therapy, including drug reactions and opportunistic infections, as well as any co-existent disease processes not directly associated with the connective tissue diseases. This may be difficult as, in most cases, the

Table 10.1 Respiratory associations of acquired connective tissue disorders

	Airways	Alveoli	Pulmonary vessels	Pleura	Diaphragm and chest wall
Rheumatoid arthritis (see Box 10.1)	Bronchitis Bronchiectasis Follicular bronchiolitis Constrictive bronchiolitis	Pneumonia Interstitial pneumonia (NSIP or rarely UIP or LIP) Rheumatoid nodules	Hypertension Vasculitis	Pleurisy Empyema	
Systemic lupus erythematosus		Interstitial pneumonia (DAD or rarely NSIP, UIP or OP)	Hypertension Thrombosis Vasculitis Haemorrhage	Pleurisy	'Shrinking lungs' with high diaphragm
Systemic sclerosis		Interstitial pneumonia (NSIP or rarely UIP, OP, DAD or LIP) Aspiration pneumonia	Haemorrhage		'Hidebound' chest
Sjögren's syndrome	'Sicca' features	Interstitial pneumonia (NSIP or LIP, rarely UIP, OP or DAD) Lymphoma		Pleurisy	
Dermatomyositis and polymyositis		Aspiration pneumonia Interstitial pneumonia (NSIP or OP, rarely UIP, DAD)			Myositis
Ankylosing spondylitis		Upper lobe fibrosis			Costovertebral restriction
Behçet's syndrome	Stenosis Ulceration		Arteritis Aneurysms		
Relapsing polychondritis	Stenosis				
Rheumatic fever		DAD	Vasculitis		Pleurisy Diaphragmatic paralysis

NSIP, non-specific interstitial pneumonia; UIP, usual interstitial pneumonia; LIP, lymphoid interstitial pneumonia; OP, organising pneumonia; DAD, diffuse alveolar damage.

histological patterns found in the lung are rarely specific for a particular connective tissue disease and are indistinguishable from those in patients without an underlying systemic disorder. Detailed clinicopathological correlation is therefore essential.[6]

A further association of lung disease and various connective tissue disorders is seen with the pneumoconioses, particularly silicosis. There is a well recognised association between silicosis and disorders such as systemic sclerosis and rheumatoid disease.[9–11] It is doubtful whether the relationship is causal but the one seems to aggravate the other and may lead to its earlier development. For example, the presence of dust results in rheumatoid lesions in the lungs being particularly florid (see p. 337 'immunology and silicosis' and p. 344 'Caplan's syndrome').

Rheumatoid disease

It was the association of pulmonary fibrosis with rheumatoid arthritis that first drew attention to the fact that this disease is not confined to the joints, and led to the use of the term rheumatoid disease (rather than arthritis) to indicate the generalised nature of the disorder.[12] It is now recognised that rheumatoid disease has many pleuropulmonary manifestations (see Table 10.1 and Box 10.1).

Box 10.1 Respiratory abnormalities in rheumatoid disease

Cricoarytenoid arthritis
Pleurisy
Empyema
Necrobiotic nodules
Non-specific interstitial pneumonia
Usual interstitial pneumonia
Organising pneumonia
Lymphoid interstitial pneumonia
Diffuse alveolar damage
Apical fibrosis
Bronchitis
Bronchiectasis
Bronchocentric granulomatosis
Follicular bronchiolitis
Constrictive obliterative bronchiolitis
Diffuse panbronchiolitis
Pulmonary hypertension
Pulmonary vasculitis
Pulmonary drug toxicity
Carcinoma of the lung
Lymphoma of the lung
Pulmonary involvement in systemic amyloidosis

Although rheumatoid disease is more common in women, pulmonary complications are more frequent in men, possibly reflecting the prevalence of smoking, which may increase pulmonary vascular permeability and aggravate the inflammatory process in the lung. As with many connective tissue disorders, the pulmonary manifestations of rheumatoid disease may precede other clinical or serological evidence of the disease, although in most cases there are other features, such as arthritis, subcutaneous nodules, digital vasculitis and positive serology.

Pleurisy[13–16]

Pleural effusion is the most common respiratory manifestation of rheumatoid disease. The effusion is often small and asymptomatic but it may be large and bilateral and cause pleuritic pain, fever and breathlessness. It is an exudate rather than a transudate (see p. 698). Most rheumatoid pleural effusions resolve spontaneously. Biopsy usually shows non-specific chronic inflammation of the pleura but multiple rheumatoid nodules[13] or a linear granulomatous process showing prominent palisading of histiocytes may replace the mesothelium (see Fig. 13.7, p. 698), in which case epithelioid histiocytes recognisable in the pleural aspirate may permit a cytological diagnosis.[17]

Empyema

Patients with rheumatoid disease are prone to infections[18] and sometimes a pleural effusion in a rheumatoid patient is found to be purulent. Occasionally there is pyopneumothorax,[19,20] probably due to rupture into the pleural cavity of a pleural or subpleural rheumatoid nodule.

Rheumatoid nodules

Nodules identical to those found in the subcutis of patients with rheumatoid disease occasionally develop in the substance of the lung or the trachea.[21–24] They may be the only manifestation of rheumatoid disease, developing before there is any arthritis or seroconversion.[21] Thus, they may herald generalised disease. As they may develop in any part of the body, the occasional involvement of the major airways should occasion no surprise.[23]

The nodules in the lungs may be recurrent or appear first in one lung and then the other. They may be solitary or multiple and may enlarge, remain static or shrink to an insignificant scar. Resolution is usually by absorption but occasionally a nodule cavitates and discharges its necrotic contents through an airway. Erosion of both an airway and the pleura establishes a bronchopleural fistula, and perhaps pyopneumothorax.[19,20] Direct involvement of the pleura by rheumatoid nodules is considered on p. 698.

Patients with rheumatoid nodules may present with haemoptysis, or chest pain if there is pleural involvement, or they may have no symptoms. The radiographic findings may be suspected of representing malignant disease. Rheumatoid nodules have a tendency to develop in the subpleural regions of the upper and mid zones.[22] They are round and typically measure up to 3 cm across but larger nodules are sometimes found, particularly when synergistic factors such as mine dust are also present (see 'Caplan's syndrome', p. 344).[25] As elsewhere, the nodules have a necrotic centre of finely granular eosinophilic debris surrounded by a capsule of chronic inflammatory granulation tissue (Fig. 10.1). The boundary between dead and viable tissue is marked by a characteristic palisade of radially oriented macrophages (Fig. 10.2). The inflammatory cells include a small number of giant cells as well as plentiful lymphocytes and plasma cells. Fungal colonisation is a rare complication of rheumatoid nodules.[26]

The differential diagnosis is principally from infection and Wegener's granulomatosis (see Table 8.3.3, p. 443). The satellite granulomas seen in tuberculosis are not a feature of rheumatoid nodules, and special stains for mycobacteria and fungi give negative results. However, staining for these organisms should always be undertaken if there is any doubt about the diagnosis. Less common infective granulomas that enter the differential

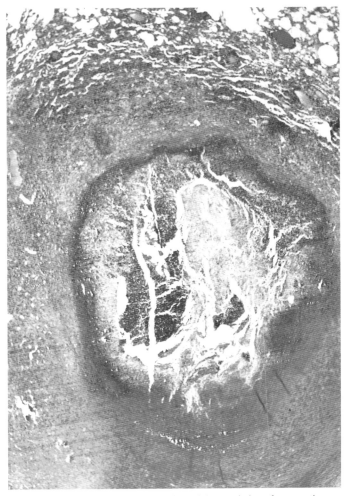

Figure 10.1 A pulmonary rheumatoid nodule consisting of a necrotic centre surrounded by a thick fibrous capsule and an intervening inflammatory zone.

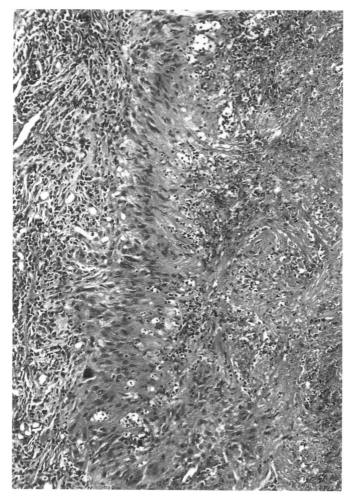

Figure 10.2 A pulmonary rheumatoid nodule. As in the subcutaneous nodules of rheumatoid disease, a palisade of radially oriented macrophages borders the central necrosis.

diagnosis include syphilis and dirofilariasis, the former requiring serological investigation and the latter step sections to identify fragments of the worm (see pp. 214 and p. 257, respectively). In Wegener's granulomatosis (see p. 438) there is also vasculitis whereas blood vessels near rheumatoid nodules show intimal fibrosis and a cuff of lymphocytes, but not a true vasculitis.

Interstitial pneumonias

Clinically overt pulmonary parenchymal disease in the form of interstitial pneumonia is reported in approximately 5% of patients with rheumatoid arthritis. All seven patterns of interstitial pneumonias in the consensus classification (see p. 263) have been described in patients with rheumatoid arthritis, although the association of respiratory bronchiolitis and desquamative interstitial pneumonia with rheumatoid disease is questionable, given that all recorded cases were smokers.[27–30] In earlier studies, UIP and organising pneumonia were the patterns most frequently reported but more recent data using

current criteria suggest that an NSIP pattern is the most common, often with superimposed follicular bronchiolitis.[1–4,7,31] There are few data on the prognoses of these patterns of lung disease in rheumatoid disease but the prognosis appears to be close to that seen in idiopathic NSIP.[1,5–7]

Apical fibrosis

Occasional patients with rheumatoid disease develop cavitating upper lobe fibrosis similar to that described in ankylosing spondylitis (see below).[32–34]

Bronchial disease

Bronchitis and bronchiectasis are more common in patients with rheumatoid arthritis coming to autopsy than in matched controls[35,36] and occasional rheumatoid patients develop bronchocentric granulomatosis.[37] Computerised tomography has permitted the recognition of airway disease in a high proportion of patients with rheumatoid arthritis.[38]

Follicular bronchiolitis

Rheumatoid disease is characterised by widespread lymphoid hyperplasia. This is best seen in lymph nodes but the bronchopulmonary lymphoid tissue is also affected, resulting in the development of lymphoid follicles alongside the bronchioles, a process termed follicular bronchiolitis (see Fig. 12.4.3, p. 643).[39,40] Patients complain of breathlessness with cough, fever or recurrent pneumonia. They have bilateral reticulonodular radiographic opacities and lung function tests show an obstructive, restrictive or combined defect. When follicular bronchiolitis accompanies an interstitial pneumonia it suggests that the latter is part of a systemic connective tissue disorder.

Constrictive obliterative bronchiolitis

Rare patients with rheumatoid disease and other connective tissue disorders develop a bronchiolar disorder that is of considerably greater clinical consequence than follicular bronchiolitis, one that is characterised by a severe ventilatory disturbance that often proves fatal. This is the constrictive form of obliterative bronchiolitis (see Figs 3.39, 3.40, p. 120).[41,42] The primary lesion appears to involve continuing autoimmune damage to the respiratory epithelium. This is replaced by granulation tissue, which is laid down in a circumferential pattern and gradually narrows and finally obliterates the airway lumen. It has been suggested that the process is a consequence of penicillamine[43,44] or gold[45] anti-rheumatoid therapy rather than a direct result of the connective tissue disease but as rheumatoid patients who have not received these drugs have also developed constrictive obliterative bronchiolitis this appears unlikely. Furthermore, constrictive obliterative bronchiolitis has not been reported in patients treated with penicillamine for disorders such as Wilson's disease and primary biliary cirrhosis. Alternatively, it has been suggested that the bronchiolitis may have an infective basis. However, the obliterative process has the constrictive pattern seen when there is constant attrition of

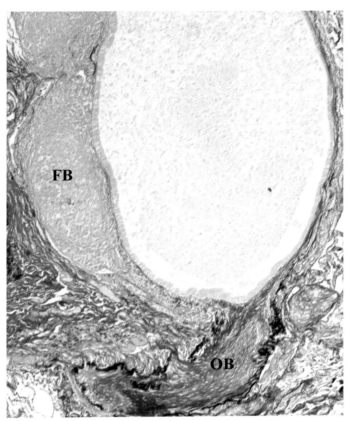

Figure 10.3 Follicular bronchiolitis (FB) and constrictive obliterative bronchiolitis (OB) in a patient with rheumatoid arthritis. (Elastin van Gieson stain.)

the respiratory epithelium rather than the classic intralumenal organising form of the disease seen after brief viral or chemical injury (see Fig. 3.38, p. 119). It is notable that a case of obliterative bronchiolitis attributed to the domestic inhalation of a common cleansing agent concerned a patient with rheumatoid disease and that the airway obliteration was of the constrictive variety,[46] suggesting that the process was the result of continuing injury rather than an isolated episode of fume inhalation. Constrictive obliterative bronchiolitis is characteristic of transplantation rejection and in the connective tissue disorders a primary autoimmune process appears to be the most likely mechanism. As with all patterns of lung disease in the connective tissue diseases, constrictive obliterative bronchiolitis may be seen in association with other patterns of rheumatoid lung disease (Fig. 10.3).

Diffuse panbronchiolitis

This disease, which is described on p. 122, is also recorded in association with rheumatoid arthritis.[47,48]

Pulmonary hypertension

Pulmonary hypertension is occasionally reported in rheumatoid disease. The vascular changes are described as showing

advanced fibroelastic intimal proliferation that obliterates the lumen of small arteries, either in isolation[49,50] or in combination with pulmonary arteritis.[51] The dilatation lesions of plexogenic arteriopathy are not observed.[49–51]

Pulmonary vasculitis

Digital vasculitis is a common manifestation of rheumatoid disease and identical changes are occasionally encountered in the pulmonary vasculature (see Fig. 8.3.16, p. 447).[51–53] It is likely that this represents a true vasculitis, probably of an immune nature, rather than the necrotising arteritis of plexogenic arteriopathy, although this is disputed.[51]

Pulmonary drug toxicity

Adverse pulmonary effects may be caused by drugs used in the treatment of rheumatoid disease. For example, aspirin and other non-steroidal anti-inflammatory drugs may cause asthma and eosinophilic pneumonia while gold and penicillamine may exert a cytotoxic effect resulting in diffuse alveolar damage and pulmonary fibrosis. Similarly, methotrexate may result in varying patterns of interstitial pneumonias.[54]

Pulmonary eosinophilia

As well as representing a reaction to the drugs used to treat rheumatoid disease, eosinophilic pneumonia may be a manifestation of the rheumatoid process itself.[55]

Pulmonary malignancy

Carcinoma of the lung is a well recognised complication of cryptogenic fibrosing alveolitis, whether it is 'lone' or systemic,[56] and occasionally arises at the edge of a rheumatoid nodule.[56a] It would appear that pulmonary lymphoma is a further complication.[56,57]

Rheumatic fever

Rheumatic fever is now rare in developed countries but remains common in many parts of the world. It involves serosal surfaces and often results in pleurisy, which generally manifests as a sterile exudative effusion. Less commonly there is a fibrinous alveolar exudate, organisation of which results in Masson bodies, hyaline membrane formation, as in diffuse alveolar damage, chronic interstitial pneumonia or a focal necrotising process involving alveoli and pulmonary blood vessels.[58–61]

Systemic sclerosis

Pulmonary involvement in systemic sclerosis may take the form of interstitial pneumonia,[3,6,62] pulmonary hypertension[63] or diffuse alveolar haemorrhage,[64,65] while oesophageal involvement may result in aspiration pneumonia.

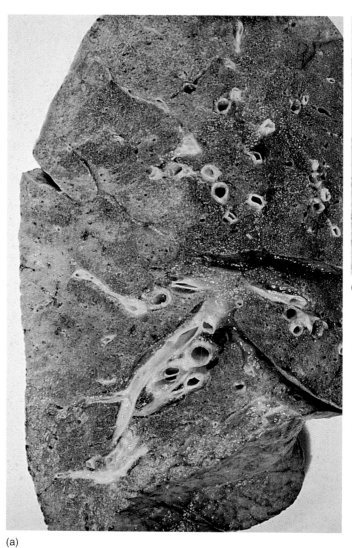

(a)

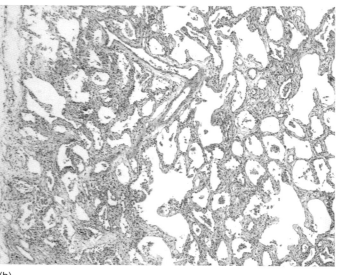

(b)

Figure 10.4 Pulmonary fibrosis as a manifestation of systemic sclerosis. (a) The fibrosis is seen as a subpleural band of pallor, chiefly affecting the base and posterior of the lung. (b) Microscopy shows a fibrotic pattern of non-specific interstitial pneumonia.

Interstitial pneumonia

Interstitial pneumonia is the most common pulmonary manifestation of systemic sclerosis (Fig. 10.4), the prevalence at autopsy being approximately 70%.[66,67] However, many of these cases have subclinical involvement[68] and the prognosis is better than in idiopathic interstitial pneumonia.[6,69–71] Non-specific interstitial pneumonia is the most common pattern, accounting for 55–77% of cases.[2–4] The second most common pattern is usual interstitial pneumonia but the adverse prognosis associated with this pattern in idiopathic disease is not seen in patients with systemic sclerosis.[3,4] This may be related to differences in neutrophil numbers and degranulation in the lung.[72] Other histological patterns seen in systemic sclerosis include desquamative interstitial pneumonia and respiratory bronchiolitis although, as discussed earlier, it is likely that these patterns are related to smoking more than systemic sclerosis.[29,30] Organising pneumonia has been reported in occasional patients,[73] as has diffuse alveolar damage,[65,74] Sarcoid granulo-

mas have also been noted but whether they relate to systemic sclerosis or are incidental is unknown.[3,75]

Pulmonary hypertension

In some patients with systemic sclerosis the lung parenchyma is unremarkable but there are marked vascular changes. These patients have severe pulmonary hypertension and are mainly those with the CREST variant of systemic sclerosis, i.e. those with Calcinosis cutis, Raynaud's phenomenon, Esophageal dysfunction, Sclerodactyly and Telangiectasia.[76] Pathologically, there is generally myxoid thickening of the wall of small pulmonary arteries, usually involving intimal fibroblasts arranged circumferentially in an 'onion skin' pattern (see Fig. 8.2.17, p. 431); the appearances are similar to those described in the kidney in systemic sclerosis.[77,78] Plexiform lesions are not seen.[77] In other patients with the CREST variant of systemic sclerosis pulmonary hypertension is caused by veno-occlusive disease.[79] Pulmonary hypertension is also recorded in the POEMS

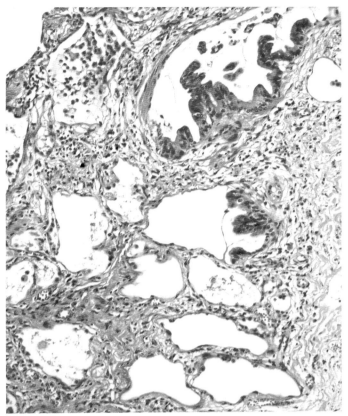

Figure 10.5 Malignant change in systemic sclerosis. There is both non-specific interstitial pneumonia and bronchioloalveolar carcinoma.

syndrome,[80,81] a rare variant of plasma cell dyscrasia with multisystem features. The name POEMS is an acronym for its principal features, Polyneuropathy, Organomegaly, Endocrinopathy, M protein and Skin changes, the last of which resemble scleroderma. It is noteworthy that in the POEMS syndrome, there is overproduction of the endothelial-cell-specific mitogen and the potent angiogenic peptide vascular endothelial growth factor,[81] which has also been reported in the plexiform lesions of other patients with pulmonary hypertension.[82]

Bronchial disease

Occasional patients have both systemic sclerosis and small airways disease.[29]

Malignant change

There is an increased risk of lung cancer in patients with systemic sclerosis, adenocarcinoma, often of bronchioloalveolar pattern, being the most common type (Fig. 10.5).[83,84]

Systemic lupus erythematosus

Pleuropulmonary involvement is more common in systemic lupus erythematosus[85] (SLE) than in any other connective tissue disease but the prognosis is more dependent upon renal than pleuropulmonary involvement.

Pleural disease

Pleuritis, seen either as a dry fibrinous exudate or an exudative effusion, is the most common respiratory manifestation of SLE. The effusion contains neutrophils, lymphocytes, LE cells and antinuclear factor in high titre, and shows positive nuclear immunofluorescence.

Parenchymal disease

Although parenchymal disease is less common than pleural involvement it is more serious. Acute lupus pneumonitis is characterised by diffuse alveolar damage or less commonly by cryptogenic organising pneumonia.[86–89] In either case infection needs to be excluded.[90] In survivors, healing may be by resolution but more commonly leaves the lungs permanently scarred. Chronic pulmonary injury is rarer in SLE than in rheumatoid disease and systemic sclerosis but both UIP and NSIP have been reported,[86,91] and more rarely organising pneumonia,[88,89] amyloidosis[92] and LIP.[93] Renal disease is also common in SLE and may lead to uraemic pulmonary oedema. Some patients with SLE are severely breathless and radiologically appear to have small lungs. The term 'shrinking lungs' is often applied to these cases but this is misleading as the fault lies in the respiratory muscles, which show myopathic changes, rather than the lungs.[94] Dyspnoea has been attributed to the tight skin about the chest but the cutaneous changes rarely affect respiratory function.

Pulmonary vascular disease

Pulmonary vascular disease in SLE may be secondary to systemic venous thrombosis (pulmonary thromboembolism), or widespread thrombosis may affect the pulmonary as well as the systemic circulation.[87] Pulmonary thrombosis, infarction and haemorrhage have been linked to the presence of circulating phospholipid antibody (also known as cardiolipin or lupus anticoagulant; see blood disorders, below) in SLE.[95] Thrombosis may underlie the pulmonary hypertension that has been reported in association with SLE,[95–100] or the pathogenesis of the hypertension may involve vasospasm, which is suggested by the frequent association of Raynaud's phenomenon with pulmonary hypertension in SLE.[96] As in systemic sclerosis, the dilatation lesions of plexogenic arteriopathy are seldom observed.[97,98,100] Pulmonary veno-occlusive disease has also been described in SLE.[101]

Other patients with SLE have pulmonary vasculitis or capillaritis with evidence of immune-complex deposition.[86,102–106] The vasculitis may be complicated by massive pulmonary haemorrhage[107–110] or haemosiderosis.[111] Tubuloreticular endothelial cell inclusions once thought to be specific for SLE but later identified in AIDS and other conditions are probably non-specific indicators of cell damage, possibly mediated by interferon.[112]

Malignant change

Rare examples of pulmonary lymphoma are recorded in SLE.[113,114]

Polymyositis and dermatomyositis

The most common pleuropulmonary complication of these diseases is aspiration pneumonia due to a depressed cough reflex and weakness of pharyngeal and intercostals muscles and the diaphragm.[115]

Interstitial pneumonia

Patients with myositis may develop interstitial pneumonia, the incidence of this complication being less than 10% in patients with polymyositis[116] but in the region of 41–67% in dermatomyositis.[115,117,118] Patients with polymyositis and the anti-Jo-1 antibody also have a high incidence of interstitial lung disease.[119,120] The most common histological pattern is NSIP,[1,121] which is often mixed with a component of organising pneumonia.[7,122,123] Other patterns of interstitial lung disease that have been associated with myositis include DAD, UIP and rarely alveolar proteinosis.

Pulmonary vascular disease

Pulmonary vasculitis has also been reported in association with the anti-Jo-1 syndrome.[122–124] Antibodies against endothelial cells may underlie the capillaritis and resultant pulmonary haemorrhage that has been described in a few patients with dermatomyositis.[124,125]

Pulmonary malignancy

Dermatomyositis is often a complication of malignant disease and so may be secondary to bronchopulmonary carcinoma. Pulmonary lymphoma has also been described in association with dermatomyositis.[126]

Mixed connective tissue disease

Mixed connective tissue disease is characterised by overlapping features of other connective tissue disorders, notably systemic lupus erythematosus, systemic sclerosis and polymyositis, in association with high titres of an antinuclear antibody that gives a speckled pattern of immunofluorescence.[127] The frequency of pulmonary involvement has ranged from 25 to 85%, the most common form being interstitial disease, followed by pleuritis, pulmonary hypertension and vasculitis.[128–132] The interstitial disease may take the form of diffuse alveolar damage or fibrosing alveolitis.[130,132] Pulmonary hypertension is especially seen when features of systemic sclerosis are prominent but the pathological features are those of plexogenic arteriopathy rather than the myxoid intimal thickening seen in systemic sclerosis.[133]

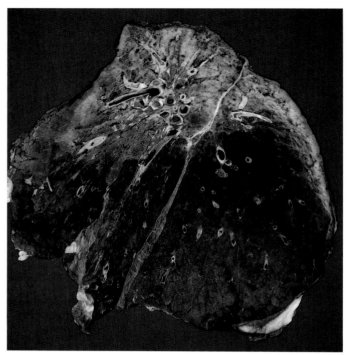

Figure 10.6   Gross apical fibrosis in a patient with ankylosing spondylitis.

Ankylosing spondylitis

Ankylosing spondylitis typically affects the spine of young men with an HLA-B27 haplotype. Pulmonary associations include apical fibrosis. This develops in 1–2% of patients with ankylosing spondylitis, typically many years after the onset of the joint disease.[134,135] Whereas the spinal lesions typically appear early in adult life, it is not until the fifth decade or so that pulmonary disease develops, often being discovered incidentally on chest radiographs. Initially, the changes may be unilateral but they have often become bilateral if cough or dyspnoea first draw attention to pulmonary involvement. As the disease progresses, cystic changes develop and the appearances resemble those of tuberculosis, but mycobacteria do not appear to play a causal role. However, like all cavities in the lungs, those of ankylosing spondylitis are liable to secondary saprophytic infection by aspergillus species or colonisation by opportunistic mycobacteria.[136]

At necropsy, there is bilateral apical fibrosis (Fig. 10.6), which may be associated with bronchiectasis and bulla formation. Secondary infection may be found but generally microscopy shows only fibrosis and lymphocytic infiltration. The process is not granulomatous and the aetiology is unknown. The changes cannot be attributed to the irradiation that was formerly used to treat ankylosing spondylitis as this was confined to the spine and the pulmonary changes may develop without such therapy. Occasionally, identical changes are found in association with rheumatoid disease[32] or with psoriatic spondylitis.[137]

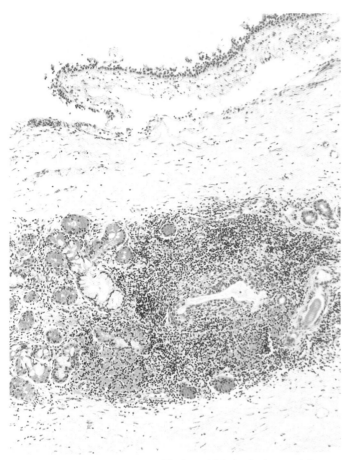

Figure 10.7 Sjögren's syndrome. The bronchial glands show an intense lymphoid infiltrate.

Sicca syndrome and Sjögren's syndrome

Bronchial disease

The sicca syndrome of dry eyes and dry mouth, due respectively to keratoconjunctivitis sicca and xerostomia, may be combined with one of the connective tissue disorders, usually rheumatoid disease, to form Sjögren's syndrome. The dryness of the eyes and mouth is due to inflammatory destruction of the lachrymal and salivary glands. The same process may extend into the lower respiratory tract to destroy the tracheobronchial glands and lead to dryness of the trachea and bronchi.[138–141] Airway clearance is impaired and bronchitis, bronchiectasis, bronchiolitis and pneumonia may develop. The destruction of the glands is of unknown cause in some patients and in both these and those with the full Sjögren's syndrome, the glands show a heavy lymphoid infiltrate with destruction of the secretory acini (Fig. 10.7).[142] Further extensions of the sicca syndrome are encapsulated in the term TASS syndrome (Thyroiditis, Addison's disease, Sjögren's and Sarcoidosis).[143] The association with rheumatoid disease, thyroiditis and Addison's disease

suggests an auto-immune aetiology. The immunoparesis associated with HIV infection is also reported in the sicca syndrome.[144]

Parenchymal disease

Parenchymal disease occurs in both primary and secondary Sjögren's disease but is more common in the latter where it often reflects the pulmonary manifestations of the associated connective tissue disease. Parenchymal disease includes amyloidosis and the formation of bullae (Fig. 10.8).[145–149] Interstitial pneumonia is uncommon and when present, usually takes the form of NSIP.[150] Less commonly there is pulmonary hypertension, LIP, UIP or organising pneumonia.[150–155]

Pulmonary malignancy

Primary pulmonary lymphoma has been reported in Sjögren's syndrome, usually marginal zone non-Hodgkin's lymphomas of mucosa-associated lymphoid tissue.[156–158]

Relapsing polychondritis

Relapsing polychondritis is a rare systemic disorder affecting connective tissues with a high content of glycosaminoglycans, notably cartilage, the aorta, the sclera and cornea.[159–163] It is associated with rheumatoid arthritis in about 20% of cases. Auto-antibodies to cartilage and type III collagen are sometimes found[164] and there may be vasculitis, glomerulonephritis, rheumatoid disease, Sjögren's syndrome, SLE or other auto-immune disease.[163,165,166]

Constitutional symptoms are common while involvement of the pinnae and nasal cartilage leads to crumpled ears and a saddle nose deformity.[161,162] Involvement of the lower respiratory tract is uncommon, especially in isolation, but may result in life-threatening tracheobronchial narrowing (see p. 91).[167–169]

Histologically, there is erosion of the edges of the affected cartilages by a dense lymphocytic, plasma cell and giant cell infiltrate (see Fig. 3.4, p. 91). Immunoglobulins and complement components have been demonstrated at the chondrofibrous junction.[170] Resolution of the inflammation, which may be spontaneous, may leave a deformed cartilage showing fibrosis and metachromasia of its ground substance.[169]

Behçet's syndrome and Hughes–Stovin syndrome

Behçet's syndrome combines recurrent orogenital ulceration with a variety of systemic disorders. A family history is sometimes obtained and the disease is associated with HLA-B51, suggesting that it has a genetic basis. Pulmonary involvement occurs in up to 8% of cases, most commonly as multiple pulmonary artery aneurysms due to a necrotising arteritis (see Fig. 8.3.18, p. 448). Leakage or rupture of the aneurysms causes pulmonary haemorrhage, which may be fatal. Other respiratory manifestations include pleurisy, pulmonary fibrosis, bronchial

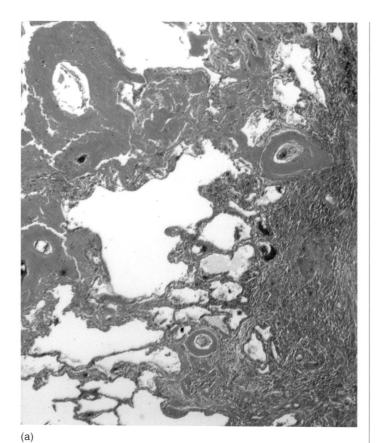

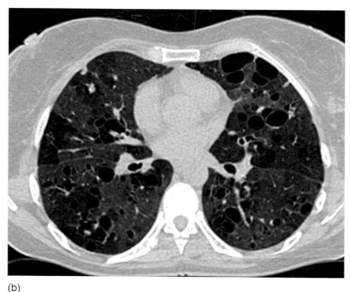

Figure 10.8   Sjögren's syndrome. (a) The lung shows amyloidosis, lymphoid hyperplasia and air-space destruction. (b) HRCT shows cystic destruction and peripheral nodules, the latter probably reflecting the focal amyloid deposition.

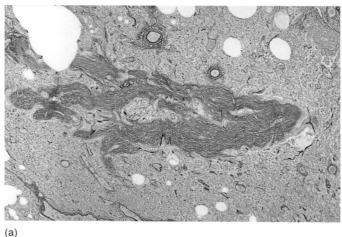

(a)

(b)

Figure 10.9   Ehlers–Danlos syndrome. (a) Fibrous scars, shown red in this van Gieson stain are probably the result of spontaneous tearing of the lung and (b) Fibrous pseudotumours may represent a development of the same process.

Cutis laxa

Cutis laxa is a rare hereditary disease of connective tissue in which the skin lacks its normal elasticity and hangs in folds like the dewlaps of a bloodhound. It may be associated with dissection of the aorta and pulmonary emphysema.[181]

Ehlers–Danlos syndrome

Ehlers–Danlos syndrome is another hereditary defect of connective tissue. There are ten recognised subtypes, with corresponding clinical heterogeneity. The syndrome is generally characterised by soft, hyperextensible skin and hyperextensibility of the joints. Visceral abnormalities include fragility of blood vessels with consequent haemorrhage, hernias, visceral rupture, mitral valve prolapse and premature rupture of the membranes in pregnancy. Pulmonary complications include haemorrhage, tracheobronchomegaly, cystic change, recurrent pneumothoraces and fibrous pseudotumours (Fig. 10.9)[182,183] and occasionally some of these are seen in isolation.[184]

ulceration and stenosis, and chyloptysis.[171–178] The Hughes–Stovin syndrome of haemoptysis due to pulmonary artery aneurysms probably represents a limited form of Behçet's syndrome.[179,180]

Ehlers–Danlos syndrome and cutis laxa have both been associated with Mounier–Kuhn's (see p. 63) and Klippel–Trenauny syndromes (see p. 483).

Pseudoxanthoma elasticum

Pseudoxanthoma elasticum is a further generalised connective tissue disorder that has its principal manifestations in the skin but may involve the lung. As in other tissues the pulmonary elastic tissue is damaged and the site of dystrophic calcification.[185]

Marfan's syndrome

Marfan's syndrome is a further hereditary disorder of connective tissue. Patients with this disorder are of a tall thin build and have arachnodactyly, a high arched palate, pectus excavatum, scoliosis, flat feet, dislocation of the lens, aortic incompetence, dissection of the aorta and mitral valve prolapse. Pulmonary complications of the connective tissue fragility include recurrent pneumothoraces and emphysema.[186–188]

VASCULAR DISEASE

Cardiovascular disease often leads to cardiac hypertrophy and if this is severe it may affect the lungs. For example, the enlarged heart may come to occupy a significant proportion of the thoracic space, restricting lung volume, or a very enlarged left atrium may compress the oesophagus, causing swallowing difficulties and so promoting aspiration pneumonia. The narrow, pliable bronchi of infants are liable to be compressed at certain points, with consequent absorption collapse, if the pulmonary arteries are distended, as in acyanotic congenital cardiac disease (Fig. 10.10).[189] Congenital heart disease may have profound effects upon the pulmonary circulation, as may failure of the left ventricle and mitral stenosis but these conditions are considered in Chapters 2 and 8.1, respectively. Pulmonary hypertension secondary to disorders of the heart and systemic vasculature is dealt with in Chapter 8.2 and vasculitis in Chapter 8.3.

Congenital anomalies characterised by direct communication between the two circulations

Some of the more severe pulmonary effects of cardiovascular disease are caused by congenital abnormalities that establish a direct communication between the systemic and pulmonary circulations – anomalies such as septal defects, patent ductus arteriosus, transposition of the great arteries, and variants of the tetrad of Fallot in which there is little obstruction to right ventricular outflow. These all lead to shunting of oxygenated blood back into the lesser circulation.

With atrial septal defects, the principal effect is that the output of the right ventricle is greater than that of the left. In many cases, the increased flow is accommodated by under-perfused vessels being recruited. This lowers pulmonary artery resistance so that there is no rise in pressure. However, with large defects, hyperkinetic pulmonary hypertension eventually develops, a complication that occurs much earlier with communications at the ventricular or aortic level than with atrial septal defects. Hyperkinetic pulmonary hypertension is characterised by plexogenic arteriopathy (see p. 421). The major pulmonary arteries are distended and where they are in close proximity to bronchi, the latter may be compressed, particularly in young infants in whom the bronchial cartilages are still soft and pliable (Fig. 10.10).[189] The result is pulmonary collapse, or if the obstruction is partial, infantile lobar emphysema. Eventually, the right ventricle becomes dominant and the left-to-right shunt is reversed, causing cyanosis, a process known as Eisenmenger's reaction or syndrome. Eisenmenger's own case combined a ventricular septal defect with an overriding aorta, an arrangement that is termed Eisenmenger's complex. Eisenmenger attributed the cyanosis to the biventricular origin of the aorta but cardiac catheter studies have subsequently shown that acquired pulmonary hypertension is the responsible factor.

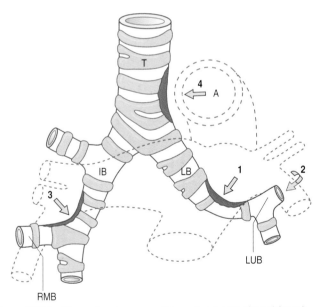

Figure 10.10 The major airways and thoracic arteries viewed from in front with the latter in dotted outline demonstrating the sites where the bronchi and arteries are in particularly close proximity and the narrow, pliable bronchi of infants are liable to be compressed if the pulmonary arteries are distended. (1) The superior aspect of the left bronchus (LB) is compressed where it is crossed by a distended left pulmonary artery. (2) The posterior aspect of the left upper lobe bronchus (LUB) is compressed as the left pulmonary artery hooks around it. (3) The lateral side of the junction of the intermediate (IB) and right middle lobe bronchi (RMB) is compressed by the right lower lobe artery. (4) A distended left pulmonary artery pushes the aorta (A) medially and upwards against the left lateral aspect of the trachea (T) to accentuate the normal indentation of the trachea by the aorta. (Redrawn from Stanger et al.[189])

Tetrad of Fallot and congenital pulmonary stenosis

The tetrad of Fallot consists of a ventricular septal defect, an over-riding aorta, pulmonary stenosis and right ventricular hypertrophy. The dominant factor is usually the pulmonary stenosis, which leads to a right-to-left ventricular shunt, the clinical features of which, cyanosis, polycythaemia and clubbing, develop in infancy, in contrast to Eisenmenger's syndrome in which cyanosis develops later. In all patients with cyanotic congenital heart disease, but particularly those with Fallot's tetrad, a sudden reduction in systemic resistance or increase in pulmonary resistance leads to episodes of more profound cyanosis and hypoxaemia, which can be fatal. With pulmonary stenosis, the attenuation of the pulmonary artery walls that normally takes place after birth proceeds apace so that the normal medial thinning is greatly exaggerated, in contrast to Eisenmenger's syndrome in which the pulmonary arteries are hypertrophied.

Anomalies of the great vessels compressing the trachea

Four vascular anomalies are liable to compress the trachea. These are the left pulmonary artery sling syndrome and three varieties of vascular ring.

The left pulmonary artery sling syndrome

In this syndrome,[190] the left pulmonary artery crosses to the right in front of the trachea, curls around it above the origin of the right main bronchus and runs to the left between the trachea and the oesophagus (Fig. 10.11). The lower trachea is liable to be compressed, causing stridor or wheeze.

Vascular rings

Certain congenital anomalies of the great vessels result in a ring of arteries surrounding and possibly compressing the trachea. Three conditions are liable to do this:

1 A double aortic arch in which the ring is formed by the heart to the front, the twin arches to either side and the common descending aorta behind.
2 An anomalous right subclavian artery. Here the ring consists of the heart to the front, the aortic arch to the left, an anomalous right subclavian artery behind and a ductus (or ligamentum) arteriosus connecting the anomalous right subclavian artery to the right pulmonary artery to the right.
3 A right-sided aortic arch with an anomalous left subclavian artery. This is the mirror image of the above and here the vascular ring is formed by the heart in front, the aortic arch to the right, an anomalous left subclavian artery behind and a ductus (or ligamentum) arteriosus connecting the left subclavian artery to the left pulmonary artery to the left (Fig. 10.12).[191]

It will be noted that in two of these conditions there is a right-sided aortic arch. This can be identified radiologically and in a child thought to have steroid-resistant asthma is a valuable indication that the true cause of the child's wheezing is a vascular ring compressing the trachea.[192]

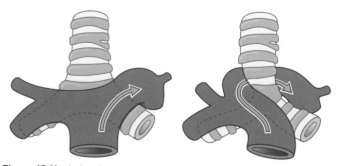

Figure 10.11 Left pulmonary artery sling syndrome. In comparison with the normal arrangement shown on the left, the left pulmonary artery passes to the right and then backwards over the origin of the right main bronchus before crossing to the left side behind the trachea just above its bifurcation and in front of the oesophagus. The arrows indicate the course of the left pulmonary artery. (Redrawn from Brewis RAL, Corrin B, Geddes DM, Gibson GJ, eds. Respiratory Medicine, 2nd edn. London: Saunders; 1995. With permission from Elsevier Ltd.)

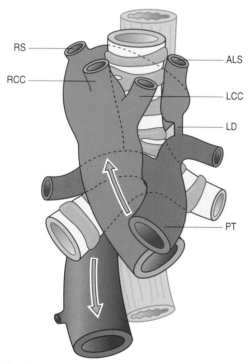

Figure 10.12 Right-sided aortic arch with anomalous left subclavian artery. In this condition a vascular ring is formed by a right-sided aortic arch, an anomalous left subclavian artery, the ductus arteriosus, the left pulmonary artery, the pulmonary trunk and the heart. Arrows indicate aortic flow. PT, pulmonary trunk; RCC, right common carotid artery; LCC, left common carotid artery; LD, left ductus; RS, right subclavian artery; ALS, aberrant left subclavian artery. (Redrawn from Stewart et al.[191])

Hereditary haemorrhagic telangiectasia (Osler–Weber–Rendu disease)

Hereditary haemorrhagic telangiectasia is an autosomal dominant condition characterised by multiple telangiectases in the skin and mucous membranes, often resulting in distressing and sometimes life-threatening haemorrhage.[193–195] Epistaxis and gastrointestinal haemorrhage are common manifestations. There may also be haemoptysis, haematuria and iron deficiency anaemia. Viscera such as the lungs, liver and brain may be involved. The telangiectases connect arteries and veins, bypassing the normal resistance vessels so that they are subject to arterial pressure.[196] They act as arteriovenous fistulae and increase cardiac output. They also permit paradoxical embolisation or form a nidus for thrombosis and infection with the danger of subsequent systemic embolisation. About 15% of patients have large pulmonary arteriovenous fistulae (see p. 74).[197] Genetic mutations have been identified at three loci involving cell surface receptors for transforming growth factor-β. Two, which are located at 9q33-34 and 3p22 and respectively encode for endoglin and ALK1, are found in families in whom pulmonary arteriovenous fistulae are common.[198,199] The third mutation, which is less common, has been mapped to the long arm of chromosome 12.[200] This mutation is associated with primary pulmonary hypertension rather than pulmonary arteriovenous fistulae.[200–202]

Klippel–Trenaunay syndrome

This is a congenital disorder characterised by a triad of cutaneous vascular lesions, venous abnormalities of the extremities and soft tissue or bony hypertrophy. Venous thromboembolism is a common complication, sometimes leading to pulmonary hypertension and right heart failure.[203–205] Occasionally, there are also pulmonary angiomas.

Idiopathic arterial calcification of infancy

In this condition, there is calcification of the arterial internal elastic laminae, generally involving systemic vessels but also pulmonary arteries on occasion.[206] Affected babies usually die in infancy and the diagnosis is often made at autopsy. Medium-sized arteries are rigid and as well as showing calcification of the internal elastic lamina they are often obliterated by secondary thrombosis and fibrosis.

Blue rubber bleb disease

Blue rubber bleb disease is characterised by cavernous haemangiomas involving the skin and gastrointestinal tract. Rarely the lesions extend into the trachea and bronchi where they are seen as discrete bluish mucosal nodules.[207]

RENAL DISEASE

A combination of haematuria and pulmonary haemorrhage (or haemosiderosis) is seen in a variety of pulmonary–renal syndromes (Box 10.2). Those associated with systemic connective

---

> **Box 10.2 Renal disease associated with pulmonary haemorrhage**
>
> With anti-glomerular basement membrane antibody
>   Goodpasture's syndrome
> Without anti-glomerular basement membrane antibody
>   Without systemic disease
>   Glomerulonephritis
>   Penicillamine-associated disease
>   With connective tissue disorders
>   Systemic lupus erythematosus
>   Systemic sclerosis
>   Rheumatoid disease
>   Mixed connective tissue disease
>   With systemic vasculitis
>   Wegener's granulomatosis
>   Polyangiitis overlap syndrome
>   Henoch–Schönlein purpura
>   Behçet's disease

tissue disorders are considered above and the remainder on pp. 448–453.

Renal failure

The most common respiratory conditions encountered in renal failure are infection and pulmonary oedema. The latter is often described as 'uraemic lung' but is indistinguishable from pulmonary oedema of other cause, described in full on p. 401. Several mechanisms may contribute to the development of pulmonary oedema in renal failure. They include fluid retention; hypertensive left ventricular failure secondary to chronic glomerulonephritis, chronic pyelonephritis and polycystic renal disease; and hypoproteinaemia, which is a prominent feature of the nephrotic syndrome.[208] Cytotoxic factors may also operate.[209] Pleural effusion may develop for the same reasons.

Renal failure may be complicated by secondary hyperparathyroidism, leading to absorption of bone and a secondary rise in serum calcium levels. This may be followed by metastatic calcification, in which the lungs are amongst the most commonly affected organs (see below). Pulmonary hypertension is also reported in chronic renal failure, affecting 29% of such patients in one study; its aetiology is poorly understood but it appears to be unrelated to secondary hyperparathyroidism or pulmonary vascular calcification.[210]

The treatment of renal failure introduces further respiratory hazards. The immunosuppression involved in renal transplantation is associated with azathioprine-associated interstitial pneumonitis, opportunistic infection and post-transplantation lymphoproliferative disease, while dialysis has its own detrimental effects on lung function. Peritoneal dialysis entails a reduction in diaphragmatic excursions so that a low vital capacity and hypoxaemia are regularly seen with this form of dialysis. Haemodialysis may be accompanied by hypoxaemia, probably because the filters employed activate complement and lead to the sequestration of neutrophils in the pulmonary capillaries, as in shock (see p. 139 and Figs 4.19 and 4.20, p. 140).

BLOOD DISORDERS

Attention here will be concentrated on the respiratory associations of diseases that are essentially haematological, although it may be noted that any lung disease liable to impair oxygenation of the blood may give rise to secondary polycythaemia while the paraneoplastic syndromes associated with lung tumours include conditions such as red cell aplasia (see Box 12.1.8, p. 539).[211] Lymphoproliferative disease is dealt with in Chapter 12.4.

Anaemia

Anaemia from any cause is liable to give rise to breathlessness because of impaired oxygen transport, even when cardiorespiratory function is normal. More specific, is an association of autoimmune haemolytic anaemia with cryptogenic fibrosing alveolitis.[212]

Hypercoaguability

Hypercoaguability of the blood gives rise to pulmonary thromboembolism, pulmonary thrombosis and pulmonary infarction, conditions that are accordingly seen in association with polycythaemia, thrombocythaemia, myelomatosis, macroglobulinaemia,[213] cryoglobulinaemia,[214] cryofibrinogenaemia,[215] the anti-phospholipid syndrome,[216–219] the hypereosinophilic syndrome (see p. 468) and haemoglobinopathies such as sickle cell disease,[220–225] spherocytosis,[226] thallasaemia[227–229] and paroxysmal nocturnal haemoglobinuria.[230] The thrombosis and subsequent organisation may be widespread and lead to pulmonary hypertension of the pattern seen in thromboembolic disease (see p. 426).[230]

Sickle cell disease

Sickle cell disease is a serious haemolytic disorder caused by homozygosity for haemoglobin S. The sickle cell trait is its milder heterozygous counterpart in which there is both haemoglobin S and A. The gene is found in Africa and Mediterranean countries. Whenever oxygen tension drops, haemoglobin S is liable to alter its molecular shape and deform the red blood cell, causing haemolysis and thrombosis. Infarction is widespread and may involve the lungs. Two major clinical forms of pulmonary involvement are recognised: an acute chest syndrome and sickle cell chronic lung disease. Acute chest syndrome is characterised by fever, chest pain, and the appearance of new radiographic opacities. It represents an acute pulmonary vaso-occlusive crisis leading to acute right ventricular failure and sometimes death. Histologically, this may mimic veno-occlusive disease by causing patchy congestion through capillary sludging of the abnormal red blood cells (Fig. 10.13). Exchange transfusion has been shown to be effective.[231] Chronic lung disease on the other hand is manifest as radiographic infiltrates, impaired pulmonary function, and, in its most severe form, pulmonary hypertension.[232,232a] The pulmonary hyperten-

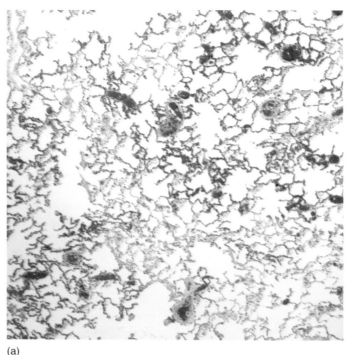

(a)

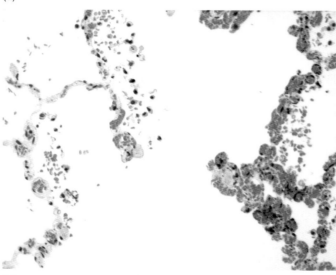

(b)

Figure 10.13 Sickle cell disease. (a) In a patient who died of an acute vaso-occlusive crisis, the lungs show differential congestion similar to that seen in veno-occlusive disease but here due to sludging of the abnormal red blood cells rather than post-capillary obstruction. (b) High power contrasting normal alveolar capillaries on the left with those showing congestion on the right.

sion is due to pulmonary thrombosis (Fig. 10.14).[220–225] In severe cases there is plexogenic arteriopathy.[233,234] Veins as well as arteries thrombose and when the venous thrombus organises the appearances are similar to those seen in veno-occlusive disease. Pneumococcal septicaemia is also seen in sickle cell disease, possibly because of the splenic infarction that occurs in this condition. Fatal bone marrow embolism is a further occasional complication of sickle cell disease.[229,235]

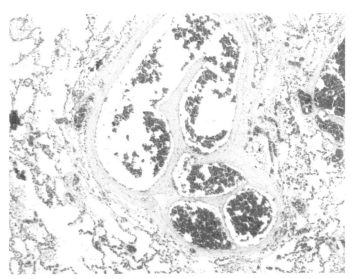

Figure 10.14   Sickle cell disease. A pulmonary artery shows recanalisation, following thrombosis.

Thalassaemia

Thalassaemia is another serious haemoglobinopathy, in this case caused by persistence of fetal haemoglobin because of a genetic inability to form adult haemoglobin A. Again there is haemolysis coupled with hypercoaguability of the blood, leading to thrombosis and infarction. Pulmonary hypertension may develop but is not as common as in sickle cell disease.[227] Haemosiderin deposition is a prominent pulmonary change and may lead to interstitial fibrosis.[228,229,236,237] Hypoxaemia is often noted in thalassaemia; this is possibly due to arterio-venous anastomoses in the form of 'spider naevi' that have been demonstrated in the periphery of the lung by postmortem injection techniques in thalassaemia patients that also have cirrhosis, which is a further complication of this disease.[228] Such anastomoses are recorded in the lungs of other patients with liver disease (see below). Mixed sickle cell thalassaemia has led to fatal bone marrow embolism.[229]

Myeloproliferative disease

Myeloproliferative disease may extend from the bone marrow to the interstitium of the lung. Pulmonary involvement in myelofibrosis is seen as interstitial pulmonary fibrosis accompanied by foci of extramedullary haemopoiesis.[238–240] Leukaemic processes also infiltrate the interstitial compartment of the lung, but generally as a terminal event:[241] before the lungs are directly involved they are liable to be the seat of opportunistic infection. Alveolar lipoproteinosis is also described (see p. 317). Pulmonary fibrosis is recorded in occasional patients with human T-cell lymphotropic virus type I associated myelopathy[242] and leukaemia.[243] The pulmonary effects of treating leukaemia with cytotoxic drugs and by bone marrow transplantation are discussed on pp. 385, 658.

Chronic granulomatous disease

Chronic granulomatous disease is characterised by opportunistic infections, both bacterial and fungal.[244,245] It is due to a genetic disorder that impairs the production of oxygen metabolites by neutrophils, eosinophils and macrophages. The phagocytic cells lack nicotinamide adenine dinucleotide phosphate oxidase and ingested microbes are therefore not killed following phagocytosis. Abscesses develop throughout the body in the first year of life, the lung being only one of many organs affected (Fig. 10.15). Often a balance is arrived at whereby viable microbes survive within granulomas composed of lymphocytes and yellow-brown, foamy macrophages centred on collections of neutrophils and eosinophils. The granulomatosis may affect the lung parenchyma or be centred on the airways.[246]

Sea-blue histiocytosis

Sea-blue histiocytosis takes its name from the appearance of macrophages laden with cytoplasmic granules of this colour in Giemsa stained preparations. In haematoxylin and eosin stained sections the macrophages have an abundant pale, granular cytoplasm. Such cells are seen in Niemann–Pick disease (see below) and occasionally within the pulmonary interstitium and air spaces in a variety of acquired haematological disorders, including myelofibrosis.[247]

Mastocytosis

Mastocytosis is a rare disease of uncertain aetiology, characterised by infiltration and proliferation of mast cells in the skin (urticaria pigmentosa), bone marrow, gastrointestinal tract and lymph nodes. Pulmonary mast cell infiltration is particularly rare.[248]

ALIMENTARY TRACT DISORDERS

Disorders of the upper alimentary tract

A variety of upper alimentary tract disorders may be associated with pulmonary disease, chiefly the consequence of aspiration of ingested material or of alimentary tract secretions (Box 10.3). Gastro-oesophageal reflux that is otherwise asymptomatic has been associated with several respiratory disorders.[249] Complications of aspiration include chronic cough, asthma, recurrent

---

Box 10.3 Disorders of the upper alimentary tract associated with aspiration syndromes

Dental sepsis
Neuromuscular disease
Congenital oesophageal atresia
Congenital tracheo-oesophageal fistula
Pharyngeal diverticulum
Aplasia of the oesophagus
Oesophageal stricture
Hiatus hernia with gastro-oesophageal reflux

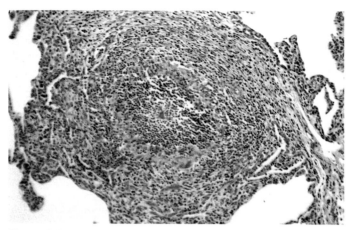

Figure 10.15 Chronic granulomatous disease. A collection of neutrophils is surrounded by epithelioid and giant cells and beyond that chronic inflammatory granulation tissue. Eosinophils are prominent throughout. (Case of Dr K Dhaene, Ghent, Belgium.)

infections, aspiration pneumonia, abscess, empyema, bronchiectasis, exogenous lipid pneumonia, Mendelson's syndrome (see p. 141) and chronic interstitial pneumonia and fibrosis.

Coeliac disease

In coeliac disease there is villous atrophy in the small intestine because of allergy to dietary gluten. Some patients with coeliac disease experience respiratory problems and it is likely that these are also based on hypersensitivity.

Allergy to avian protein

When it was discovered that some patients with coeliac disease and respiratory symptoms had serum antibodies against avian antigens,[250] it was naturally assumed that they also had bird fanciers' lung, a form of extrinsic allergic alveolitis. However, further investigations showed that the antigen concerned was a globulin and that this was not found in bird droppings, unlike the avian albumin responsible for bird fanciers' lung.[251] The source of the allergen is believed to be egg yolk and the allergy probably stems from the ingestion of hens' eggs rather than the inhalation of bird droppings. Attempts to establish a link between coeliac disease and other forms of extrinsic allergic alveolitis such as farmers' lung[252] have proved inconclusive. The relationship of the antibodies against avian globulin to the patients' respiratory disease is unclear. Increased lung permeability and reduced gas transfer suggest that there is an alveolitis, but most histological investigations have been limited to transbronchial biopsies. These are reported to show peribronchiolar fibrosis and chronic inflammation.[253] Radiology has occasionally identified bronchiectasis in coeliac patients.[254]

Pulmonary haemosiderosis

Some patients diagnosed as having idiopathic pulmonary haemosiderosis are found to be suffering from malabsorption associated with jejunal villous atrophy, and some of them improve on removing gluten from the diet.[255-257] The association appears to be more than coincidental but its basis is unclear.

Inflammatory bowel disease

Pulmonary abnormalities are much more common with ulcerative colitis than with Crohn's disease but are nevertheless among the rarest extraintestinal features of both these diseases.[258,259] However, although rare, a wide variety of pulmonary associations has now been described (Table 10.2).[259-283] Furthermore, it is possible that some patients have subclinical lung involvement as bronchoalveolar lavage has shown lymphocytosis in Crohn's disease patients who are free of pulmonary symptoms.[284,285] Similarly, lung function studies have shown that about 20% of patients with active bowel disease have a reduced diffusing capacity.[286] In a minority of cases the lung disease precedes that in the bowel.[259] Lung disease has also developed many years after the colon has been totally removed.

The most common respiratory association of inflammatory bowel disease is inflammation of the airways.[259-268] There is a productive cough yet the patient is usually a non-smoker.[262] Biopsy shows either severe non-specific chronic inflammation[263] or non-necrotising tuberculoid granulomas.[266,282,283] The appearances have been likened to those in the bowel and it is possible that the gut and the lung are both affected because they share common antigens. Progression of the bronchitis to bronchiectasis[260,262,263,267,268,281] and tracheobronchial stenosis[264] has been reported, and occasionally the airway disease causes acute respiratory failure.[287]

Other respiratory associations include follicular bronchiolitis,[271] constrictive bronchiolitis, organising pneumonia,[272] fibrosing alveolitis,[271,273-275] pulmonary eosinophilia,[282] sterile suppurative nodules resembling pyoderma gangrenosa,[259] focal lymphoid infiltrates,[288] involvement in systemic amyloidosis,[276] apical fibrosis similar to that seen with ankylosing spondy-

Table 10.2 Respiratory associations of inflammatory bowel disease

	Ulcerative colitis	Crohn's disease
Bronchitis[259-267]	+	+
Granulomatous bronchitis/bronchiolitis[266,280]	–	+
Bronchiectasis[260,262,263,267-269,281]	+	+
Bronchial stenosis[264]	+	+
Bronchiolitis[271]	+	+
Organising pneumonia[272]	+	+
Pulmonary fibrosis[271,273-275]	+	+
Pulmonary eosinophilia (drug related)[282]	+	+
Pyogenic nodules[259]	+	–
Amyloidosis[276]	–	+
Apical fibrosis[277]	+	–
Thromboembolism	+	+
Hypoproteinaemic oedema[278]	–	+
Pleurisy	+	+
Antineutrophil cytoplasmic antibody[279]	+	+

litis,[277] hypoproteinaemic pulmonary oedema caused by malabsorption,[278] vasculitis[289] and the development of antineutrophil cytoplasmic antibody.[279] Many of these associations have been reported in patients under treatment with salazine type drugs but except for pulmonary eosinophilia they are all recorded in patients who were not under treatment. However, drug effects need to be excluded before attributing pulmonary symptoms to the inflammatory bowel disease.

Whipple's disease

Whipple's disease[290] is a rare disorder that was for long considered to be a storage disorder of uncertain aetiology but is now known to represent infection by the bacilliform bacterium *Tropheryma whippelii*.[291–293] Patients usually give a long history of polyarthritis and insidious weight loss due to malabsorption, which later results in anaemia and diarrhoea.[294] Diagnosis is usually by jejunal biopsy, which shows heavy mucosal infiltration by macrophages distended by diastase-resistant periodic acid-Schiff-positive material. Electron microscopy shows large numbers of bacilli within the macrophages.[293] Few other inflammatory cells are seen. Plasma cells are reduced in number and it is postulated that a cytopathic effect of *T. whippelii* to plasma cells contributes to the bacilli evading the local immune response.[293] The condition usually responds to antibiotic treatment.[295–297]

The changes may extend to lymph nodes and other viscera, including the lungs.[295–299] Respiratory symptoms such as breathlessness, cough and pleuritic pain may precede the diarrhoea, and rarely pulmonary disease may be detected in the absence of intestinal features.[296] Radiographs show pleural thickening and effusion and patchy pulmonary opacification. Some patients suffer from pulmonary hypertension.[297]

Lung biopsy shows nodular collections of foam cells surrounding the centriacinar bronchioles and arteries and thickening the interlobular septa and pleura. As in the intestine, the foam cells stain strongly with diastase-controlled periodic acid-Schiff reagents and electron microscopy shows that they contain numerous bacilli.[295]

Pneumatosis coli

In this condition, there are numerous gas-filled cysts beneath the mucosa of the colon. It has been associated with emphysema and was once thought to be due to interstitial emphysema tracking through the mediastinal and retroperitoneal tissues. However, it is now considered that the gas is produced locally by intestinal bacteria and that the association with emphysema is not a causal one.

Hepatic disease

Pulmonary vascular disease

A number of abnormalities of the pulmonary blood vessels may be found in association with cirrhosis.[300] It is suspected that

vasoactive substances that are normally metabolised in the liver and thereby prevented from reaching the lungs do so through the portosystemic anastomoses that develop in cirrhosis. Pulmonary hypertension of the plexogenic variety (see p. 421) is a particularly serious but rare complication of cirrhosis associated with portal hypertension.[301–305] Hypoxaemia is a more common finding, often referred to as the hepatopulmonary syndrome.[305,306] Although pulmonary arteriovenous anastomoses ('spider naevi') have been demonstrated in such patients[228,307–309] they are uncommon and a more likely explanation of the syndrome is that the normal vasoconstrictive response of the lungs to hypoxia is inhibited, with consequent ventilation/perfusion mismatching.[310–312]

Ascites and pleural effusion

Ascites is common in cirrhosis because of portal hypertension and hypoproteinaemia. If the effusion is large, lung volumes are reduced resulting in breathlessness. In many patients this is aggravated by a concomitant right-sided pleural effusion, which is attributed to the pressure difference between the pleural and peritoneal cavities drawing fluid into the thorax through diaphragmatic defects.[313]

Primary biliary cirrhosis

The pathological basis of this liver disease is a granulomatous destruction of intrahepatic bile ducts and it is therefore noteworthy that there are reports of pulmonary or multiorgan granulomas similar to those of sarcoidosis in association with the condition.[314–316] Other biopsy studies have demonstrated a nongranulomatous lymphocytic infiltrate of either the alveoli[317,318] or the airways.[319] Sjögren's syndrome, the pulmonary manifestations of which are described earlier in this chapter, has also been reported in association with primary biliary cirrhosis.[320] Fibrosing alveolitis is largely confined to those patients with primary biliary cirrhosis who also have another autoimmune disease, such as systemic sclerosis.[318,321] It is possible that many patients with primary biliary cirrhosis have subclinical lung disease as they have been shown to have a pulmonary lymphocytosis by bronchoalveolar lavage.[322]

Hepatitis

The incidence of hepatitis C virus infection appears to be raised in idiopathic pulmonary fibrosis, leading to speculation that the association is causal, although not necessarily direct.[323] Autoimmune factors are prominent in several forms of hepatitis and some patients with chronic active hepatitis and non-organ specific autoantibodies also develop cryptogenic fibrosing alveolitis.[212,324] Bronchiectasis,[325] lymphoid interstitial pneumonia[326] and pulmonary haemorrhage[327] have also been reported in association with autoimmune hepatitis on occasion.

α₁-Antitrypsin deficiency

This genetic disorder may cause panacinar emphysema or cirrhosis. The coexistence of the two conditions in affected patients is recorded, but is rare.[328]

Liver abscess

Pyogenic or amoebic abscesses in the liver are prone to spread through the diaphragm to cause right-sided pleurisy, pneumonia, lung abscess or hepatobronchial fistula.

Pancreatic disease

The inflammation involved in acute pancreatitis may spread through the diaphragm to cause left-sided, or rarely bilateral, pleurisy. Acute pancreatitis of severe degree causes shock and the clinical and pathological features of this condition may develop, namely the acute respiratory distress syndrome and diffuse alveolar damage.[329]

NEUROMUSCULAR DISEASE

Neuromuscular diseases secondary to non-metastatic bronchopulmonary neoplasia (the paraneoplastic neuromuscular syndromes) are considered on p. 539 and this section will be limited to the pulmonary manifestations of neuromuscular disease.

'Neurogenic' pulmonary oedema

'Neurogenic' pulmonary oedema is a well recognised feature of cerebral damage, especially that due to trauma and subarachnoid haemorrhage. Its pathogenesis is thought to involve widespread adrenergic vasoconstriction resulting in marked systemic hypertension.[330–332] Fluid then shifts from the systemic circulation to the relatively more compliant pulmonary circulation, with a resultant outpouring of fluid into the lung.

Tuberous sclerosis

Tuberous sclerosis is an autosomal dominant hereditary disease characterised by hamartomas in multiple tissues, notably the brain, skin and kidney. Pulmonary involvement generally takes the form of lymphangioleiomyomatosis, which is described on p. 295. This is clinically evident in only 2.3% of tuberous sclerosis patients[333] but accounts for 10% of their deaths.[334] Radiological scans show lung cysts suggestive of lymphangioleiomyomatosis in 34–39% of women with tuberous sclerosis.[335,336]

An even rarer pulmonary manifestation of tuberous sclerosis is the multifocal micronodular type II pneumocyte hyperplasia described on p. 689. This lesion may be seen alone or in association with pulmonary lymphangioleiomyomatosis but has not been described in patients who do not have tuberous

sclerosis. Aneurysms of systemic arteries are a rare feature of tuberous sclerosis and occasionally affect a pulmonary artery.[337]

The benign clear cell tumour of the lung described on p. 613 may also develop in patients with tuberous sclerosis,[338] and it is notable that the multifocal micronodular type II pneumocyte hyperplasia referred to above is occasionally composed of cells that have an unusually clear cytoplasm.[339] It is also notable that the benign clear cell tumour expresses HMB45, a feature that it shares with two other lesions found in tuberous sclerosis, pulmonary lymphangioleiomyomatosis and angiomyolipoma.

Angiomyolipomas of the kidney, retroperitoneum and liver are a further feature of tuberous sclerosis and are found in about half the women with lymphangioleiomyomatosis.[340] A few examples have been reported in the lungs (see p. 619), one in a patient with tuberous sclerosis but not lymphangioleiomyomatosis.[341] It is reported that patients with tuberous sclerosis have a higher than expected incidence of renal carcinoma but re-evaluation of these tumours has shown that most of them represent atypical epithelioid angiomyolipomas that manifest unusually malignant behaviour.[342] Renal angiomyolipomas are more common in women and those associated with tuberous sclerosis often have progesterone receptors, suggesting that hormonal factors are important in their pathogenesis, as in lymphangioleiomyomatosis.[343] It is now thought that both angiomyolipomas and benign clear cell tumours of the lung derive from certain 'perivascular epithelioid cells' and may therefore be collectively termed PEComas.[344]

Neurofibromatosis

Neurofibromatosis is occasionally associated with interstitial lung disease described as fibrosing alveolitis indistinguishable pathologically from the cryptogenic variety.[345–348] However, these reports antedate current concepts of disease patterns in interstitial pneumonia and although they describe fibrocystic disease the appearances are not those of usual interstitial pneumonia. Occasional scar cancers are encountered,[348,349] as in other fibrosing lung conditions. The thoracic neurofibromas of von Recklinghausen's disease and their obstructive complications are dealt with on p. 629.

Neuromuscular disease

Neuromuscular disease of varying aetiology may promote pulmonary infection by impairing the cough reflex and weakening respiration. Also, there is a danger of aspiration if swallowing is affected.

METABOLIC AND ENDOCRINE DISORDERS

Obesity

Obesity restricts ventilation by the fat splinting the chest wall and buttressing the underside of the diaphragm. This increases the work of breathing and contributes to the common symptom of breathlessness, which may be present at rest but is accentuated by the effort of moving an overweight body.

A few grossly obese patients have a severely disturbed sleep pattern due to repeated episodes of nocturnal apnoea, attributable to neck fat compressing the pharyngeal airway. The resultant daytime somnolence is well illustrated by the fat messenger boy Joe described by Charles Dickens in his Pickwick Papers, hence the term Pickwickian syndrome (see obstructive sleep apnoea, p. 89).

Hypercalcaemia and metastatic calcification

The causes of hypercalcaemia include hyperparathyroidism, skeletal metastases, tumours secreting a parathormone-like peptide, sarcoidosis and hypervitaminosis D (Box 10.4). In sarcoidosis the epithelioid cells of the granulomas participate in a number of metabolic activities, including the final hydroxylation and hence activation of vitamin D,[350] thereby accounting for the hypercalcaemia that is so frequently found in this condition.[351–353] Activation of vitamin D normally takes place in the kidneys and renal failure may be complicated by secondary hyperparathyroidism, again leading to hypercalcaemia and metastatic calcification. Metastatic calcification involving viscera takes the form of whitlockite ($(CaMg)_3(PO_4)_2$) whereas in the soft tissues it is deposited as hydroxyapatite ($(Ca_{10}(PO_4)_6(OH)_2$).

The lungs, kidneys and stomach are particularly likely to be involved in metastatic calcification. Virchow suggested that this was because all these organs excrete acid and are therefore slightly alkaline.[354] In line with this is the observation that metastatic calcification may be localised to lung tissue beyond an obstructed pulmonary artery, the increased ventilation-perfusion ratio there raising the pH.[355] Basement membranes and elastic fibres are favoured sites of calcium deposition and the walls of blood vessels and alveoli are therefore particularly affected by metastatic calcification.[354,356–358] In severe cases, every alveolar wall is delicately impregnated. The calcium is recognisable in routine sections due to its affinity for haematoxylin (Fig. 10.16) but if little is present the diagnosis may be confirmed with von Kossa's stain. Not surprisingly, the permeability of the alveolar walls may be increased. Some patients with severe pulmonary involvement have died of massive pulmonary oedema.[359] Organisation of such protein-rich oedema fluid may explain the alveolar fibrosis that sometimes accompanies metastatic calcification. In rare cases the calcification is confined to the airway mucosa.[360]

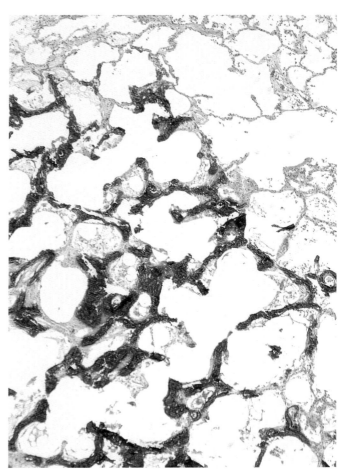

Figure 10.16   Metastatic calcification in a patient with hypercalcaemia. Heavy deposition of calcium salts renders the alveolar walls basophilic.

Systemic amyloidosis and systemic light chain deposition

Pathological evidence of pulmonary involvement is common in all forms of systemic amyloidosis, including the rare familial and senile (cardiac) forms[361–367] and the β_2-microglobulin-derived amyloidosis that sometimes complicates long-term haemodialysis.[364,368] Despite this multiplicity of amyloid types evident pathologically, most patients with respiratory symptoms attributable to systemic amyloidosis have primary or myeloma-associated disease. The amyloid is therefore of the light chain (AL) type. This is also true of amyloidosis confined to the lungs (which is dealt with under tumour-like conditions on p. 684). The distinction of localised from systemic amyloidosis is clinically important. The two forms are distinguished by organ distribution, as revealed by cardiac echocardiography and serum amyloid protein (SAP) scintigraphy, screening for plasma cell dyscrasias and biopsy.

In primary systemic amyloidosis there is usually a fine diffuse interstitial deposition. Multifocal nodules may develop but the mass lesions of localised amyloid are not seen. Microscopy shows a widespread delicate thickening of the

---

Box 10.4 The causes of hypercalcaemia

Hyperparathyroidism
Skeletal metastases
Neoplastic parathormone-like activity
Sarcoidosis
Hypervitaminosis D

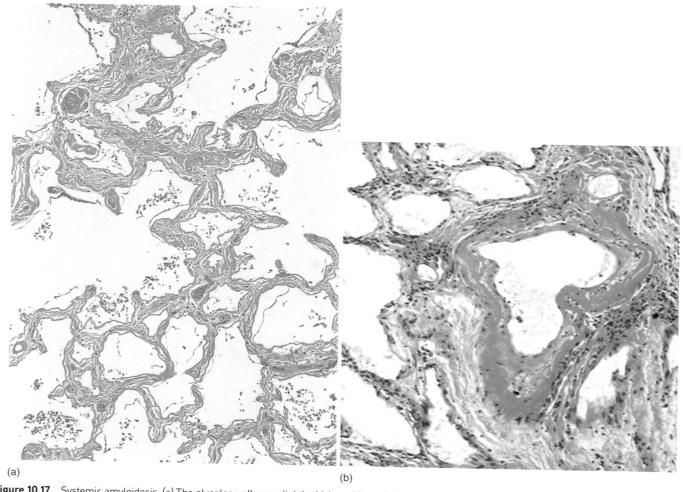

(a)　　　　　　　　　　　　　　　　　　　　　　　　　　　　(b)

Figure 10.17 Systemic amyloidosis. (a) The alveolar walls are slightly thickened by a diffuse interstitial deposition of amyloid. (b) The media of a pulmonary artery shows deposition of amyloid.

alveolar and vascular walls by an eosinophilic, amorphous deposit (Fig. 10.17). Larger pulmonary vessels are also involved, in similar fashion to systemic vessels. Electron microscopy shows that the amyloid is preferentially deposited in the alveolar epithelial and endothelial basement membranes.[366] On occasion there may be prominent pleural involvement.[369] The alveolar wall thickening is liable to be mistaken for interstitial fibrosis but the inflammatory component that usually accompanies such scarring is not a feature and a Congo red stain should quickly lead to the correct diagnosis. The potassium permanganate/Congo red reaction conforms to the amyloid being of the AL type (derived from immunoglobulin).[362] and this is supported by immunohistochemistry.[370,371] If what appears to be amyloid fails to stain as such, it might represent pulmonary involvement in systemic light chain deposition disease.[372] Multifocal nodules of amyloid may stimulate the foreign body giant cell reaction that is more characteristic of localised bronchopulmonary amyloidosis (see p. 684).

The severity of the pulmonary involvement generally parallels that in the heart.[362] It is often an incidental post-mortem finding in patients known to have amyloid elsewhere but it may impair gas transfer and only be discovered when lung biopsy is undertaken to investigate the cause of abnormal blood gases or, rarely, dyspnoea. Pulmonary blood vessels are particularly involved and rarely this may be so severe as to cause pulmonary hypertension.[373,374]

In secondary (AA type) amyloidosis, pulmonary involvement is generally limited to blood vessels and bronchial glands: alveolar walls are not affected and there is seldom any clinical evidence of lung disease.[361]

Storage disorders

The storage disorders comprise a wide variety of rare congenital defects involving specific lysosomal enzymes. They are generally manifest by the accumulation of the enzyme's substrate and deficiency of its reaction product. They are best known by the chemical character of the substrate and are often grouped under terms such as lipidoses, mucopolysaccharidoses and glycogenoses. The excess substrate is stored in the reticuloendothelial system and hepatosplenomegaly is a common feature of many storage diseases. The lungs contain many cells of the histiocyte series and pulmonary involvement is therefore commonly found post-mortem. It is seldom troublesome in life but may cause significant morbidity, for example in adults with Niemann–Pick disease type B, in which case whole lung lavage may be successful.[375]

In the lungs there is an increase in both alveolar and interstitial macrophages, the cytoplasm of which is swollen by the indigestible lysosomal substrate (Figs 10.18, 10.19). In *Gaucher's*

disease (glucosylceramide lipidosis)[376–381] the macrophage cytoplasm may be foamy or finely granular and eosinophilic and the appearances may mimic those of desquamative interstitial pneumonia (Fig. 10.18). In *Niemann–Pick's disease* (sphingomyelin-cholesterol lipidosis)[375,382–384] the macrophage cytoplasm is more foamy and the features are those of endogenous lipid pneumonia. The process also involves the ciliated epithelium but relatively spares the pneumocytes (Fig. 10.20). In the *mucopolysaccharidoses* the macrophage cytoplasm is weakly haematoxyphil, and in *cystine storage disease* free crystals can be identified if an alcoholic fixative and polarisers are used. The lungs may also be involved in *Fabry's disease*, when PAS-

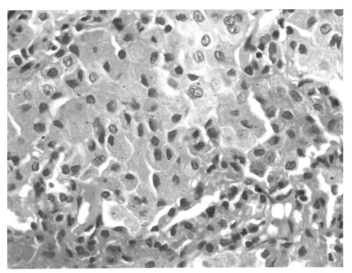

Figure 10.18   Macrophages with eosinophilic cytoplasm fill the alveoli.

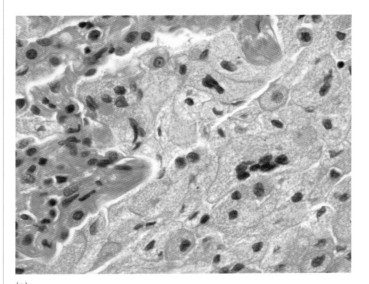

(a)

(b)

Figure 10.20   Niemann–Pick disease. (a) There is a florid endogenous lipoid pneumonia with Touton-type giant cell formation. (b) Bronchiolar epithelial cells have a foamy cytoplasm but the type 2 pneumocytes seen in (a) do not.

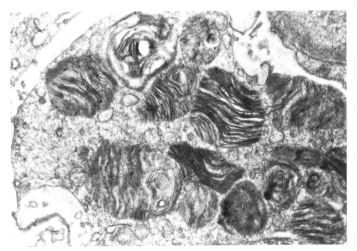

Figure 10.19   Fabry's disease. Electron microscopy shows osmiophilic lamellar inclusions of α-galactoside within the cytoplasm of epithelial cells.

positive inclusion bodies of α-galactoside are found in endothelial cells, alveolar epithelial cells and bronchial muscle,[385] sometimes narrowing the airways.[386]

The lungs are seldom affected in isolation but very occasionally conspicuous pulmonary lipidosis is associated with insignificant systemic involvement,[387] particularly in patients with malignant cachexia who develop *ceroidosis*.[388] In these cases the swollen macrophages contain much brown ceroid pigment. The histological appearances simulate those of haemosiderosis but stains for iron and ceroid readily distinguish these two conditions.

Generalised ceroid storage, albinism and platelet dysfunction resulting in a bleeding diathesis characterise the *Hermansky–Pudlak syndrome*.[389,390] This familial condition, largely confined to Dutch and Puerto Rican patients, is of particular interest to pulmonologists because it is sometimes associated with chronic interstitial pneumonitis and fibrosis with honeycombing (Fig. 10.21). The changes are widespread and lack the basal and subpleural predilection seen in idiopathic pulmonary fibrosis. Lung biopsy shows that the fibrosis is maximal around respiratory bronchioles and is accompanied by florid foamy swelling of type II pneumocytes.[390–397] The foamy pneumocytes contain giant lamellar bodies but stain only weakly for surfactant apoprotein, suggesting that there is a fundamental abnormality in surfactant production (which involves lysosomal activity, see p. 16). The ceroid accumulation is thought to reflect lipid peroxidation, with oxygen radical release during this process being responsible for the pulmonary fibrosis. Identification of the ceroid from its autofluorescent properties in urinary sediment or buccal scrapings aids the diagnosis.

Morquio's disease is a further storage disorder that is occasionally responsible for respiratory disability. It represents a deficiency of galactosamine-6-sulphatase, which leads to a build-up of keratin sulphate. Deposits of this substance may obstruct the upper airways or impair movement of the chest wall.[398]

Xanthogranulomatosis

This condition is characterised by focal collections of foamy macrophages rich in cholesterol and other lipids. Such deposits are found in the lung in diabetes mellitus and generalised xanthomatosis.[399] Cholesterol pneumonitis is considered further on p. 320.

Alkane lipogranulomatosis

Certain indigestible waxes found in the skin of apples and other foodstuffs are absorbed unaltered. The amounts are usually trivial and of no importance but persons consuming inordinate amounts of such foodstuffs are liable to have these alkane waxes deposited in their tissues. One French farmer for example was estimated to have consumed 5 tons of apples. He was found to have lipogranulomatous nodules throughout his lungs while being investigated for angina, and after he died of coronary disease similar deposits were identified in many other organs, including the liver, spleen, adrenal glands and lymph nodes.[400] Mass spectrometry showed the lipid to consist of straight-line saturated aliphatic hydrocarbons (n-alkanes) with the formula $C_{29}H_{60}$ or $C_{31}H_{64}$. Histologically the deposits resemble cholesterol granulomas as they take the form of acicular crystals being engulfed by macrophages and foreign body giant cells (Fig. 10.22).

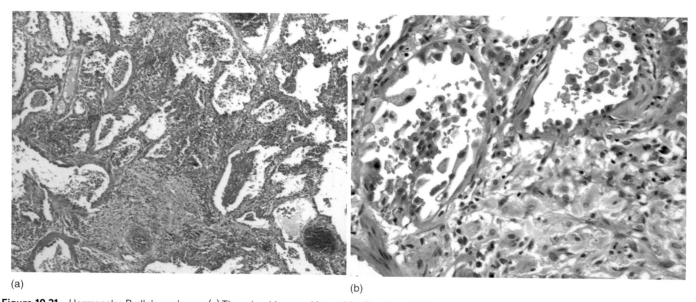

(a)

(b)

Figure 10.21 Hermansky–Pudlak syndrome. (a) There is widespread interstitial fibrosis and inflammation resembling non-specific interstitial pneumonia. (b) Higher magnification shows vacuolation of the type II pneumocytes (top left) and an interstitial accumulation of pale histiocytes, occasionally containing golden brown pigment.

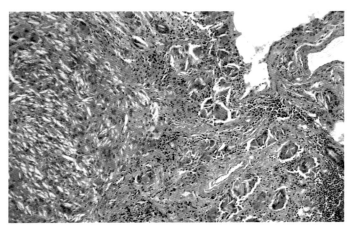

Figure 10.22 Alkane lipogranulomatosis. The granulomas consist of macrophages and foreign body giant cells surrounding alkane crystals, which are acicular and resemble those of cholesterol. (Case of Dr Duboucher, Paris, France.)

Erdheim–Chester disease

Erdheim–Chester disease is a rare form of generalised xanthomatosis that is chiefly characterised by fibrosis and foam cell infiltration of the bone marrow resulting in osteosclerosis, particularly of the long bones.[401,402] Clonality has been reported.[403] A fibrosing, non-lipidic macrophage infiltrate may affect the lungs where it is variously reported as causing marked thickening of the interlobular septa and bronchovascular bundles, sparing the alveolar tissue (Fig. 10.23),[404–406a] or as causing granulomatous disease.[407] Diabetes insipidus and pulmonary fibrosis are features that Erdheim–Chester disease shares with Langerhans cell histiocytosis,[408,409] and occasionally the two diseases are associated.[404] However, in Erdheim–Chester disease the infiltrate fails to react for the Langerhans cell marker CD1a. The osteosclerotic lesions of Erdheim–Chester disease also differ from the osteolysis seen in Langerhans cell histiocytosis. Pulmonary involvement generally augers a poor prognosis,[405,406] although one case showed a response to immunosuppressive therapy.[410]

Acromegaly

The lungs share in the general visceromegaly seen in acromegaly. Being a disease of adult life, they are affected after development is complete and for this reason the lung enlargement represents an increase in alveolar size rather than number. Acromegalic enlargement of the tongue and laryngeal tissues may cause upper airway obstruction, and pulmonary venous hypertension may stem from acromegalic cardiomyopathy.

Thyroid disease

A retrosternal goitre may compress the trachea, thyrotoxicosis may result in pulmonary hypertension secondary to high output cardiac failure[411] and myxoedema may be associated with pericardial and pleural transudates[412] related to the

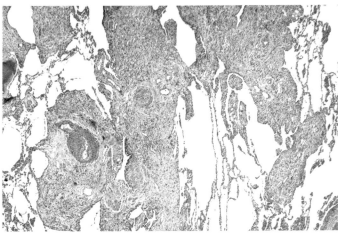

(a)

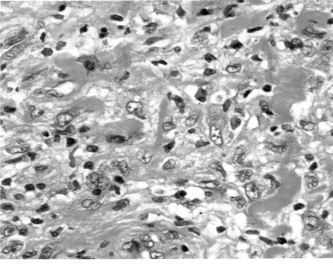

(b)

Figure 10.23 Erdheim–Chester disease. (a) There is prominent fibrous thickening of the interlobular septa. (b) At high power, histiocytes and eosinophils are seen. The histiocytes are S-100 positive but unlike Langerhans cells they fail to stain for CD1a. (Illustration (a) from a case of Dr M Kambouchner, Paris, France; (b) from a case of Dr T Ashcroft, Newcastle-upon-Tyne, UK.)

perivascular deposits of amorphous, eosinophilic material that have been described in this disease.[413]

Diabetes mellitus

Lung function is impaired in diabetes mellitus because of autonomic neuropathy and pulmonary microangiopathy. The former is probably responsible for diminished ventilatory responses to hypoxaemia and hypercapnia, and the latter for a mild reduction in diffusing capacity and pulmonary capillary blood volume.[414,415] Changes within the lungs develop independently of those attributable to diabetes in other organs.

No dramatic morphological changes are evident in the lungs in diabetes but microangiopathy similar to that observed elsewhere in the body has been reported – principally thickening of the alveolar capillary and epithelial basement membranes.[416–420] Micronodular fibrosis of alveolar walls is a rarely reported phenomenon.[421] Occasional perivascular xanthogranulomatous deposits have also been identified.[399] Similar basement membrane and connective tissue alterations have been described in laboratory animals rendered diabetic with alloxan or streptozotocin,[422–426] together with impairment of lung growth in young animals:[424] insulin treatment prevented all these changes.

Diabetes mellitus predisposes to infection and confers an increased risk of bronchitis, bronchiectasis, pneumonia, pulmonary tuberculosis and fungal lung disease.

Hypovitaminosis A

Vitamin A is essential to the integrity of the respiratory mucosa. Deficiency leads to squamous metaplasia.[427] This has led to proposals that hypovitaminosis A is a co-factor promoting the development of lung cancer. Extensive trials of vitamin A and carotene supplementation have consequently been conducted, but these have failed to show that these dietary measures have any effect on the incidence of lung cancer.[428,429]

SKIN DISEASE

Cutaneous manifestations of malignant lung disease

Apart from skin metastases and infections of the skin secondary to impaired host defence consequent upon disseminated cancer, there are several skin conditions that although not malignant themselves, are sometimes associated with systemic cancer, including bronchopulmonary carcinoma. They include the cutaneous consequences of *thrombophlebitis migrans* (one of Trousseau's signs), *dermatomyositis, acanthosis nigricans, arsenical keratoses* and several *non-metastatic endocrinopathies* that elicit changes in the skin, for example ectopic adrenocorticotrophic hormone secretion and acromegaly. Lastly, nicotine staining of the fingers should alert the physician to the increased danger of cancer and other lung diseases caused by smoking.

Skin disease associated with non-malignant lung disease

Psoriasis may be associated with spondylitis, including that of the ankylosing variety, which is sometimes associated with apical lung fibrosis.[137] *Pemphigoid* of the sclerosing variety, also known as benign mucous membrane pemphigoid, rarely extends below the larynx but has caused fatal tracheobronchial obstruction.[430] Necrotising tracheobronchitis has also complicated paraneoplastic *pemphigus*,[431] and pustules similar to those seen in the skin in *acute febrile neutrophilic dermatosis (Sweet's syndrome)* have been described in the bronchial mucosa and lung in patients with this disease.[432–434] Pulmonary manifestations of *pyoderma gangrenosa* are rare but multiple nodules showing aseptic necrosis are recorded,[435] similar to those occasionally

seen in the lungs in inflammatory bowel disease (see above).[259] *Cutis laxa* and *Ehlers–Danlos syndrome* sometimes involve the lungs, as described on p. 480. Other diseases manifest in both the skin and lungs, which are also described elsewhere include *tuberous sclerosis* (p. 488), various *vasculitides* (p. 437), *systemic sclerosis* (p. 475), *rheumatoid disease* (p. 472), *Langerhans cell histiocytosis* (p. 290) and *sarcoidosis* (p. 285). *Erythema multiforme* may be a manifestation of sarcoidosis or changing immunity to tuberculosis and a variety of *infections* may be common to the skin and lungs. Lastly, *drug reactions* developing during the treatment of many lung diseases may be first evident in the skin.

GYNAECOLOGICAL AND OBSTETRIC CONDITIONS

Meigs' syndrome

Meigs' syndrome consists of a pleural effusion associated with ascites and a pelvic neoplasm, removal of which results in resolution of both effusions.[436,437] The ascitic fluid is thought to spread to the pleural space through small apertures in the diaphragm. The effusion is right-sided in 70% of cases, bilateral in 20% and left-sided in 10%. The pelvic tumour is usually an ovarian fibroma but ovarian cysts and uterine fibroids have also been responsible.[438]

Pregnancy

Increased levels of progesterone result in an increased respiratory drive from the early weeks of pregnancy while in the third trimester the mechanical effects of the enlarging uterus may cause breathlessness. Successful deliveries have been achieved despite severe lung disease but pulmonary hypertension may deteriorate during pregnancy. Accelerated lung transplant rejection is also recorded during pregnancy.[439] Complications of pregnancy that may have an adverse affect on the lungs include uterine haemorrhage and infection, either of which may result in 'shock lung' (see p. 138), and eclampsia, which is sometimes associated with pulmonary oedema.[440,441] The incidence of thromboembolism is also increased in pregnancy. Embolism of amniotic fluid, trophoblast and decidua is considered on pp. 410 and 411.

Thoracic endometriosis

Thoracic endometriosis generally affects the pleura and subpleural lung tissue but occasionally the process appears to be entirely intrapulmonary.[442] The mechanisms underlying pleural and pulmonary endometriosis appear to be quite different but proffered explanations are not entirely satisfactory. Pleural deposits may represent serosal metaplasia or be due to transdiaphragmatic spread of pelvic endometriosis, whereas embolism is the probable explanation of the parenchymal lesions. The clinical effects of pleural and pulmonary endometriosis also differ, except that either may first be identified coincidentally as an asymptomatic tumour.

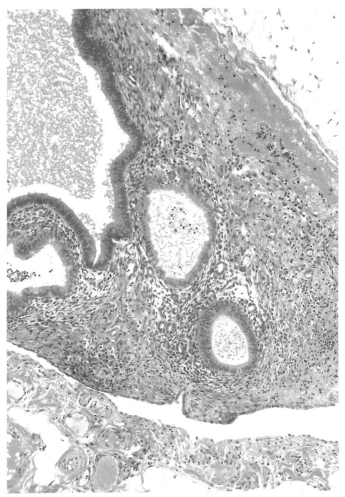

Figure 10.24 Pleural endometriosis comprising both endometrial glands and endometrial stroma. (Case of Dr M Neyra, Lyons, France.)

Pleural endometriosis is usually characterised by catamenial pneumothorax,[443–445] and occasionally by catamenial haemothorax,[446] both of which are almost always limited to the right side. Although serosal metaplasia is a possible explanation, many cases have pelvic endometriosis, congenital diaphragmatic perforations and multiple endometriotic implants on both the visceral and the parietal pleura and in these, transdiaphragmatic spread of pelvic endometriosis seems likely. The almost universal limitation of the disease to the right side is attributed to diaphragmatic fenestrations preponderating on that side.[447] Pneumothorax secondary to pneumoperitoneum, and haemothorax secondary to haemoperitoneum are also largely limited to the right, as is the pleural effusion of Meigs' syndrome (see above).[447] Many small diaphragmatic fenestrae must go unnoticed but a complicating factor is that some diaphragmatic perforations may be secondary to endometriotic implants.[447]

Intrapulmonary endometriosis is even rarer than the pleural variety.[448–450] It is typically characterised by catamenial haemoptysis, affects either or both lungs and is seldom associated with pelvic endometriosis.[450] On the other hand, there is a strong association with gynaecological surgery,[450] suggesting that blood-borne endometrial seeding of the lung following uterine instrumentation or parturition is responsible. This is supported by animal experiments in which intravenously injected endometrial tissue migrated from pulmonary blood vessels into the lung substance where it remained viable and underwent cyclic change.[451]

Whatever its pathogenesis, thoracic endometriosis is similar in its age distribution (23–45 years) and pathological appearance to that encountered more commonly elsewhere. CT findings include irregular opacities, nodular lesions, cystic change and bulla formation.[452,453] Magnetic resonance imaging is also useful in as it highlights changes related to bleeding.[454] Grossly, lesions may be single or multifocal, well-circumscribed or infiltrative, nodular, cystic, or nodulo-cystic. Rarely the disease may be predominantly endobronchial.[454,455] The heterotopic tissue consists of both stroma and glands and reproduces the appearances of normal endometrium in every way (Fig. 10.24). Decidual change takes place in pregnancy[456,457] and cyclic haemorrhagic disruption, with consequent haemosiderosis, may obscure the nature of the tissue. The ectopic tissue also responds to steroid derivatives that suppress gonadotrophin release[450] and this has proved successful therapeutically.[442,458] Others prefer local surgical resection to avoid the side-effects of hormonal therapy.[459] Pleural abrasion is superior to hormonal treatment in the management of pneumothorax.[458]

REFERENCES

Connective tissue disease

1. Douglas WW, Tazelaar HD, Hartman TE, et al. Polymyositis-dermatomyositis-associated interstitial lung disease. Am J Respir Crit Care Med 2001; 164:1182–1185.
2. Fujita J, Yoshinouchi T, Ohtsuki Y, et al. Non-specific interstitial pneumonia as pulmonary involvement of systemic sclerosis. Ann Rheum Dis 2001; 60:281–283.
3. Bouros D, Wells AU, Nicholson AG, et al. Histopathologic subsets of fibrosing alveolitis in patients with systemic sclerosis and their relationship to outcome. Am J Respir Crit Care Med 2002; 165:1581–1586.
4. Kim DS, Yoo B, Lee JS, et al. The major histopathologic pattern of pulmonary fibrosis in scleroderma is nonspecific interstitial pneumonia. Sarcoidosis Vasc Diffuse Lung Dis 2002; 19:121–127.
4a. Kitaichi M, Nagai S, Ito I, Yanagi S. Pulmonary pathology in association with connective tissue disorders. Curr Diagnost Pathol 2004; 10:291–303.
5. Agusti C, Xaubet A, Roca J, Agusti AGN, Rodriguez-Roisin R. Interstitial pulmonary fibrosis with and without associated collagen vascular disease – results of a two year follow up. Thorax 1992; 47:1035–1040.
6. Homma Y, Ohtsuka Y, Tanimura K, et al. Can interstitial pneumonia as the sole presentation of collagen vascular diseases be differentiated from idiopathic interstitial pneumonia? Respiration 1995; 62:248–251.
7. Tansey D, Wells AU, Colby TV, et al. Variations in histological patterns of interstitial pneumonia between connective tissue disorders and their relationship to prognosis. Histopathology 2004; 44:585–596.
8. Flaherty KR, Colby TV, Travis WD, et al. Fibroblastic foci in usual interstitial pneumonia. Idiopathic versus collagen vascular disease. Am J Respir Crit Care Med 2003; 167:1410–1415.
9. Erasmus LD. Scleroderma in gold-miners on the Witwatersrand with particular reference to pulmonary manifestations. S Afr J Lab Clin Med 1957; 3:209–231.

10. Scheule RK, Holian A. Mini-review – immunologic aspects of pneumoconiosis. Exp Lung Res 1991; 17:661–685.

11. Beckett W, Abraham J, Becklake M, et al. Adverse effects of crystalline silica exposure. Am J Respir Crit Care Med 1997; 155:761–768.

12. Ellman P, Ball RE. 'Rheumatoid disease' with joint and pulmonary manifestations. BMJ 1948; 2:816.

13. Ellman P, Cudkowicz L, Elwood JS. Widespread serous membrane involvement by rheumatoid nodules. J Clin Pathol 1954; 7:239–244.

14. MacFarlane JD, Dieppe PA, Rigden BG, Clark TJH. Pulmonary and pleural disease in rheumatoid disease. Br J Dis Chest 1978; 72:288–300.

15. Engel U, Aru A, Francis D. Rheumatoid pleurisy. Acta Path Microbiol Immunol 1986; 94:53–56.

16. Anderson RJ, Hansen KK, Kuzo RS, et al. A 38-year-old woman with chronic rheumatoid arthritis and a new pleural effusion – rheumatoid pleuritis. N Engl J Med 1994; 331:1642–1647.

17. Nosanchuk JS, Naylor B. A unique cytologic picture in pleural fluid from patients with rheumatoid arthritis. Am J Clin Pathol 1968; 50:330–335.

18. Walker WC. Pulmonary infections and rheumatoid arthritis. Q J Med 1967; 36:239–251.

19. Hindle W, Yates DAH. Pyopneumothorax complicating rheumatoid lung disease. Ann Rheum Dis 1965; 24:57–60.

20. Davies D. Pyopneumothorax in rheumatoid lung disease. Thorax 1966; 21:230–235.

21. Eraut D, Evans J, Caplin M. Pulmonary necrobiotic nodules without rheumatoid arthritis. Br J Dis Chest 1978; 72:301–306.

22. Walters MN-I, Ojeda VJ. Pleuropulmonary necrobiotic rheumatoid nodules. A review and clinicopathological study of six patients. Med J Aust 1986; 144:648–651.

23. Ip MSM, Wong MP, Wong KL. Rheumatoid nodules in the trachea. Chest 1993; 103:301–303.

24. White DA, Mark EJ, Kradin RL, Bloch KJ. A 53-year-old woman with arthritis and pulmonary nodules. Rheumatoid lung disease with rheumatoid nodules, pleuritis, and interstitial fibrosis. N Engl J Med 2001; 344:997–1004.

25. Gough J, Rivers D, Seal RME. Pathological studies of modified pneumoconiosis in coal-miners with rheumatoid arthritis (Caplan's syndrome). Thorax 1955; 10:9–18.

26. Cavazza A, Paci M, Turrini E, Dallari R, Rossi G. Fungus colonisation of pulmonary rheumatoid nodule. J Clin Pathol 2003; 56:636–637.

27. Carrington CB, Gaensler EA, Coutu RE, FitzGerald MX, Gupta RG. Natural history and treated course of usual and desquamative interstitial pneumonia. N Engl J Med 1978; 298:801–809.

28. Yousem SA, Colby TV, Gaensler EA. Respiratory bronchiolitis-associated interstitial lung disease and its relationship to desquamative interstitial pneumonia. Mayo Clin Proc 1989; 64:1373–1380.

29. Yousem SA. The pulmonary pathologic manifestations of the CREST syndrome. Human Pathology 1990; 21:467.

30. Moon J, Dubois RM, Colby TV, Hansell DM, Nicholson AG. Clinical significance of respiratory bronchiolitis on open lung biopsy and its relationship to smoking related interstitial lung disease. Thorax 1999; 54:1009–1014.

31. Dixon AStJ, Ball J. Honeycomb lung and chronic rheumatoid arthritis. Ann Rheum Dis 1957; 16:241–245.

32. Petrie GR, Bloomfield P, Grant IWB, Crompton GK. Upper lobe fibrosis and cavitation in rheumatoid disease. Br J Dis Chest 1980; 74:263–267.

33. MacFarlane JD, Francken CK, Van Leeuwen AW. Progressive cavitating pulmonary changes in rheumatoid arthritis. Ann Rheum Dis 1984; 43:98–101.

34. Cheung CY, Chan HP, Kurshner I. Apical fibrocavitary lesions of the lung in rheumatoid arthritis. Am J Med 1986; 81:741–746.

35. Takanami I, Imamuma T, Yamamoto Y, Yamamoto T, Kodaira S. Bronchiectasis complicating rheumatoid arthritis. Respir Med 1995; 89:453–454.

36. Despaux J, Manzoni P, Toussirot E, Auge B, Cedoz JP, Wendling D. Prospective study of the prevalence of bronchiectasis in rheumatoid arthritis using high-resolution computed tomography. Rev Rhum Engl Ed 1998; 65:453–461.

37. Bonafede RP, Benatar SR. Bronchocentric granulomatosis and rheumatoid arthritis. Br J Dis Chest 1987; 81:197–201.

38. Perez T, Remy Jardin M, Cortet B. Airways involvement in rheumatoid arthritis: Clinical, functional, and HRCT findings. Am J Respir Crit Care Med 1998; 157:1658–1665.

39. Yousem SA, Colby TV, Carrington CB. Follicular bronchitis/bronchiolitis. Hum Pathol 1985; 16:700–706.

40. Fortoul TI, Cano Valle F, Oliva E, Barrios R. Follicular bronchiolitis in association with connective tissue diseases. Lung 1985; 163:305–314.

41. Geddes DM, Corrin B, Brewerton DA, Davies RJ, Turner-Warwick M. Progressive airway obliteration in adults and its association with rheumatoid disease. Q J Med 1977; 46:427–444.

42. Hakala M, Paakko P, Sutinen S, Huhti E, Koivisto O, Tarkka M. Association of bronchiolitis with connective tissue disorders. Ann Rheum Dis 1986; 45:656–662.

43. Epler GR, Snider GL, Gaensler EA, Cathcart ES, FitzGerald MX, Carrington CB. Bronchiolitis and bronchitis in connective tissue disease. A possible relationship to the use of penicillamine. JAMA 1979; 242:528–532.

44. Boehler A, Vogt P, Speich R, Weder W, Russi EW. Bronchiolitis obliterans in a patient with localized scleroderma treated with D-penicillamine. Eur Respir J 1996; 9:1317–1319.

45. Schwartzman KJ, Bowie DM, Yeadon C, Fraser R, Sutton ED, Levy RD. Constrictive bronchiolitis obliterans following gold therapy for psoriatic arthritis. Eur Respir J 1995; 8:2191–2193.

46. Murphy DMF, Fairman RP, Lapp NL, Morgan WKC. Severe airway disease due to inhalation of fumes from cleansing agents. Chest 1976; 69:372–376.

47. Sugiyama Y, Saitoh K, Kano S, Kitamura S. An autopsy case of diffuse panbronchiolitis accompanying rheumatoid arthritis. Respir Med 1996; 90:175–177.

48. Homma S, Kawabata M, Kishi K, et al. Diffuse panbronchiolitis in rheumatoid arthritis. Eur Resp J 1998; 12:444–452.

49. Gardner DL, Duthie JJR, Macleod J, Allan WSA. Pulmonary hypertension in rheumatoid arthritis: report of a case with intimal sclerosis of the pulmonary and digital arteries. Scot Med J 1957; 2:183–188.

50. Balagopal VP, DaCosta P, Greenstone MA. Fatal pulmonary hypertension and rheumatoid vasculitis. Eur Respir J 1995; 8:331–333.

51. Kay JM, Banik S. Unexplained pulmonary hypertension with pulmonary arteritis in rheumatoid disease. Br J Dis Chest 1977; 71:53–59.

52. Price TML, Skelton MO. Rheumatoid arthritis with lung lesions. Thorax 1956; 11:234–240.

53. Baydur A, Mongan ES, Slager UT. Acute respiratory failure and pulmonary arteritis without parenchymal involvement. Demonstration in a patient with rheumatoid arthritis. Chest 1979; 75:518–520.

54. Imokawa S, Colby TV, Leslie KO, Helmers RA. Methotrexate pneumonitis: review of the literature and histopathological findings in nine patients. Eur Resp J 2000; 15(2):373–381.

55. Norman D, Piecyk M, Roberts DH. Eosinophilic pneumonia as an initial manifestation of rheumatoid arthritis. Chest 2004; 126:993–995.

56. Mellemkjaer L, Linet MS, Gridley G, Frisch M, Moller H, Olsen JH. Rheumatoid arthritis and cancer risk. Eur J Cancer 1996; 32A:1753–1757.

56a. Baruch AC, Steinbronn K, Sobonya R. Pulmonary adenocarcinomas associated with rheumatoid nodules: a case report and review of the literature. Arch Pathol Lab Med 2005; 129:104–106.

57. Nicholson AG, Wotherspoon AC, Jones AL, Sheppard MN, Isaacson PG, Corrin B. Pulmonary B-cell non-Hodgkin's lymphoma associated with autoimmune disorders: a clinicopathological review of six cases. Eur Respir J 1996; 9:2022–2025.

58. Paul JR. Pleural and pulmonary lesions in rheumatic fever. Medicine (Baltimore) 1928; 7:383–410.

59. Masson P, Riopelle JL, Martin P. Poumon rheumatismal. Ann Anat Path 1937; 14:359–382.

60. Neuberger KT, Geever EF, Rutledge EK. Rheumatic pneumonia. Arch Pathol 1944; 37:1–15.

61. Grunow WA, Esterly JR. Rheumatic pneumonitis. Chest 1972; 61:298–301.

62. Harrison NK, Myers AR, Corrin B, et al. Structural features of interstitial lung disease in systemic sclerosis. Am Rev Respir Dis 1991; 144:706–713.

63. Hoeper MM. Pulmonary hypertension in collagen vascular disease. Eur Resp J 2002; 19:571–576.

64. Griffin MT, Robb JD, Martin JR. Diffuse alveolar haemorrhage associated with progressive systemic sclerosis. Thorax 1990; 45:903–904.

65. Nishi K, Myou S, Ooka T, Fujimura M, Matsuda T. Diffuse cutaneous systemic sclerosis associated with pan- serositis, disseminated intravascular coagulation, and diffuse alveolar haemorrhage. Respir Med 1994; 88:471–473.

66. D'Angelo WA, Fries JF, Masi AT, Shulman LE. Pathologic observations in systemic sclerosis scleroderma: a study of fifty-eight autopsy cases and fifty-eight matched controls. Am J Med 1969; 46:428–440.

67. Wiedemann HP, Matthay RA. Pulmonary manifestations of the collagen vascular diseases. Clin Chest Med 1989; 10:677–722.

68. Harrison NK, Glanville AR, Strickland B, et al. Pulmonary involvement in systemic sclerosis: the detection of early changes by thin section CT scan, bronchoalveolar lavage and 99mTc-DTPA clearance. Respir Med 1989; 83: 403–414.

69. Chan TYK, Hansell DM, Rubens MB, Dubois RM, Wells AU. Cryptogenic fibrosing alveolitis and the fibrosing alveolitis of systemic sclerosis: morphological differences on computed tomographic scans. Thorax 1997; 52:265–270.

70. Wells AU, Cullinan P, Hansell DM, et al. Fibrosing alveolitis associated with systemic sclerosis has a better prognosis than lone cryptogenic fibrosing alveolitis. Am J Respir Crit Care Med 1994; 149:1583–1590.

71. Wells AU, Hansell DM, Rubens MB, et al. Fibrosing alveolitis in systemic sclerosis: indices of lung function in relation to extent of disease on computed tomography. Arthritis Rheum 1997; 40:1229–1236.

72. Cailes JB, O'Connor C, Pantelidis P, et al. Neutrophil activation in fibrosing alveolitis: a comparison of lone cryptogenic fibrosing alveolitis and systemic sclerosis. Eur Respir J 1996; 9:992–999.

73. Bridges AJ, Hsu KC, Dias-Arias AA, Chechani V. Bronchiolitis obliterans organizing pneumonia and scleroderma. J Rheumatol 1992; 19:1136–1140.

74. Muir TE, Tazelaar HD, Colby TV, Myers JL. Organizing diffuse alveolar damage associated with progressive systemic sclerosis. Mayo Clin Proc 1997; 72:639–642.

75. Biasi D, Caramaschi P, Carletto A, Bambara LM. Localized scleroderma associated with sarcoidosis. Clin Exp Rheumatol 1998; 16:761–762.

76. Stupi AM, Steen VD, Owens GR, Barnes EL, Rodnan GP, Medsger TA Jr. Pulmonary hypertension in the CREST syndrome variant of systemic sclerosis. Arthritis Rheum 1986; 29:515–524.

77. Young RH, Mark GJ. Pulmonary vascular changes in scleroderma. Am J Med 1978; 64:998–1004.

78. Landzberg MJ, Ko J, King ME, Roberts DJ, Castro MA. A 38-year-old woman with increasing pulmonary hypertension after delivery - Scleroderma overlap syndrome with pulmonary vasculopathy and malignant pulmonary hypertension accelerated during puerperium. N Engl J Med 1999; 340:455–464.

79. Morassut PA, Walley VM, Smith CD. Pulmonary veno-occlusive disease and the CREST variant of scleroderma. Can J Cardiol 1992; 8:1055–1058.

80. Ribadeau-Dumas S, Tillie-Leblond I, Rose C, et al. Pulmonary hypertension associated with POEMS syndrome. Eur Respir J 1996; 9:1760–1762.

81. Lesprit P, Godeau B, Authier FJ, et al. Pulmonary hypertension in POEMS syndrome: A new feature mediated by cytokines. Am J Respir Crit Care Med 1998; 157:907–911.

82. Hirose S, Hosoda Y, Furuya S, Otsuki T, Ikeda E. Expression of vascular endothelial growth factor and its receptors correlates closely with formation of the plexiform lesion in human pulmonary hypertension. Pathol Int 2000; 50:472–479.

83. Rosenthal AK, McLaughlin JK, Linet MS, Persson I. Scleroderma and malignancy: an epidemiological study. Ann Rheum Dis 1993; 52:531–533.

84. Yang Y, Fujita J, Tokuda M, Bandoh S, Ishida T. Lung cancer associated with several connective tissue diseases: with a review of literature. Rheumatol Int 2001; 21:106–111.

85. Keane MP, Lynch JP. Pleuropulmonary manifestations of systemic lupus erythematosus. Thorax 2000; 55(2):159–166.

86. Miller LR, Greenberg SD, McLarty JW. Lupus lung. Chest 1985; 88:265–269.

87. Matthay RA, Schwarz MI, Petty TL, et al. Pulmonary manifestations of systemic lupus erythematosus: review of twelve cases of acute lupus pneumonitis. Medicine (Baltimore) 1974; 54:397–408.

88. Gammon RB, Bridges TA, Alnezir H, Alexander CB, Kennedy JI. Bronchiolitis obliterans organizing pneumonia associated with systemic lupus erythematosus. Chest 1992; 102:1171–1174.

89. Mana F, Mets T, Vincken W, Sennesael J, Vanwaeyenbergh J, Goossens A. The association of bronchiolitis obliterans organizing pneumonia, systemic lupus erythematosus, and Hunner's cystitis. Chest 1993; 104:642–644.

90. Kim WU, Kim SI, Yoo WH, et al. Adult respiratory distress syndrome in systemic lupus erythematosus: causes and prognostic factors: a single center, retrospective study. Lupus 1999; 8:552–557.

91. Kim JS, Lee KS, Koh EM, Kim SY, Chung MP, Han J. Thoracic involvement of systemic lupus erythematosus: clinical, pathologic, and radiologic findings. J Comput Assist Tomogr 2000; 24:9–18.

92. Marenco JL, Sanchez-Burson J, Ruiz CJ, Jimenez MD, Garcia-Bragado F. Pulmonary amyloidosis and unusual lung involvement in SLE. Clin Rheumatol 1994; 13:525–527.

93. Yood RA, Steigman DM, Gill LR. Lymphocytic interstitial pneumonitis in a patient with systemic lupus erythematosus. Lupus 1995; 4:161–163.

94. Gibson GJ, Edmonds JP, Hughes GRV. Diaphragm function and lung involvement in systemic lupus erythematosus. Am J Med 1977; 63:926–932.

95. Boey ML, Colaco CB, Gharavi AE, Elkon KB, Loizou S, Hughes GRV. Thrombosis in systemic lupus erythematosus: striking association with the presence of circulating lupus anticoagulant. BMJ 1983; 287:1021–1023.

96. Asherson RA, Mackworth-Young CG, Boey ML, et al. Pulmonary hypertension in systemic lupus erythematosus. BMJ 1983; 287:1024–1025.

97. Wakaki K, Koizumi F, Fukase M. Vascular lesions in systemic lupus erythematosus [SLE] with pulmonary hypertension. Acta Pathol Jpn 1984; 34:593–604.

98. Wilson L, Tomita T, Braniecki M. Fatal pulmonary hypertension in identical twins with systemic lupus erythematosus. Hum Pathol 1991; 22:295–297.

99. Nair SS, Askari AD, Popelka CG, Kleinerman JF. Pulmonary hypertension and systemic lupus erythematosus. Arch Intern Med 1980; 140:109–111.

100. Yokoi T, Tomita Y, Fukaya M, Ichihara S, Kakudo K, Takahashi Y. Pulmonary hypertension associated with systemic lupus erythematosus: Predominantly thrombotic arteriopathy accompanied by plexiform lesions. Arch Pathol Lab Med 1998; 122:467–470.

101. Kishida Y, Kanai Y, Kuramochi S, Hosoda Y. Pulmonary venoocclusive disease in a patient with systemic lupus erythematosus. J Rheumatol 1993; 20:2161–2162.

102. Olsen EGJ, Lever JV. Pulmonary changes in systemic lupus erythematosus. Br J Dis Chest 1972; 66:71–77.

103. Fayemi AO. Pulmonary vascular disease in systemic lupus erythematosus. Am J Clin Pathol 1976; 65:284–290.

104. Churg A, Franklin W, Chan KL, Kopp E, Carrington CB. Pulmonary hemorrhage and immune-complex deposition in the lung. Complications in a patient with systemic lupus erythematosus. Arch Pathol Lab Med 1980; 104:388–391.

105. Gross M, Esterly JR, Earle RH. Pulmonary alterations in systemic lupus erythematosus. Am Rev Respir Dis 1972; 105:572–577.

106. Brown JH, Doherty CC, Allen DC, Morton P. Fatal cardiac failure due to myocardial microthrombi in systemic lupus erythematosus. BMJ 1988; 296:1505.

107. Marino CT, Pertschuk LP. Pulmonary haemorrhage in systemic lupus erythematosus. Arch Intern Med 1981; 141:201–203.

108. Myers JL, Katzenstein AL. Microangiitis in lupus-induced pulmonary haemorrhage. Am J Clin Pathol 1986; 85:552–556.

109. Santos Ocampo AS, Mandell BF, Fessler BJ. Alveolar hemorrhage in systemic lupus erythematosus – presentation and management. Chest 2000; 118:1083–1090.

110. Hughson MD, He Z, Henegar J, McMurray R. Alveolar hemorrhage and renal microangiopathy in systemic lupus erythematosus. Immune complex small vascular injury with apoptosis. Arch Pathol Lab Med 2001; 125:475–483.

111. Kuhn C. Systemic lupus erythematosus in a patient with ultrastructural lesions of the pulmonary capillaries previously reported in the review as due to idiopathic pulmonary hemosiderosis. Am Rev Respir Dis 1972; 106:931–932.

112. Hammar SP, Winterbauer RH, Bockus D, Remington F, Sale GE, Meyers JD. Endothelial cell damage and tubuloreticular structures in interstitial lung disease associated with collagen vascular disease and viral pneumonia. Am Rev Respir Dis 1983; 127:77–84.

113. Yum M, Ziegler J, Walker P, et al. Pseudolymphoma of the lung in a patient with systemic lupus erythematosus. Am J Med 1979; 66:172.

114. Dux S, Pitlik S, Rosenfeld JB, Pick J, Ben-Bassat M. Localised visceral immunocytoma associated with serological findings suggesting systemic lupus erythematosus. BMJ 1984; 288:898–899.

115. Lakhanpal S, Lie JT, Conn DL, Martin WJ. Pulmonary disease in polymyositis and dermatomyositis: a clinico-pathological analysis of 65 autopsy cases. Ann Rheum Dis 1987; 46:23–29.

116. Salmeron G, Greenberg SD, Lidsky MD. Polymyositis and diffuse interstitial lung disease. A review of the pulmonary histopathologic findings. Arch Intern Med 1981; 141:1005–1010.

117. Takizawa H, Shiga J, Moroi Y, Miyachi S, Nishiwaki M, Miyamoto T. Interstitial lung disease in dermatomyositis: clinicopathological study. J Rheumatol 1987; 14:102–107.

118. Fathi M, Dastmalchi M, Rasmussen E, Lundberg IE, Tornling G. Interstitial lung disease, a common manifestation of newly diagnosed polymyositis and dermatomyositis. Ann Rheum Dis 2004; 63:297–301.

119. Bernstein RM, Morgan SH, Chapman J, et al. Anti-Jo-1 antibody: a marker for myositis with interstitial lung disease. BMJ 1984; 289:151–152.

120. Kiely JL, Donohoe P, Bresnihan B, McNicholas WT. Pulmonary fibrosis in polymyositis with the Jo-1 syndrome: an unusual mode of presentation. Resp Med 1998; 92:1167–1169.

121. Cottin V, Thivolet-Bejui F, Reynaud-Gaubert M, et al. Interstitial lung disease in amyopathic dermatomyositis, dermatomyositis and polymyositis. Eur Resp J. 2003; 22: 245–250.

122. Chan WM, Ip M, Lau CS, Wang E, Peh WCG. Anti-Jo-1 syndrome presenting as cryptogenic organizing pneumonia. Respir Med 1995; 89:639–641.

123. Brown I, Joyce C, Hogan PG, Armstrong J, Steele R, Bansal AS. Pulmonary vasculitis associated with anti-Jo-1 antibodies. Resp Med 1998; 92:986–988.

124. Schwarz MI, Sutarik JM, Nick JA, Leff JA, Emlen JW, Tuder RM. Pulmonary capillaritis and diffuse alveolar hemorrhage - a primary manifestation of polymyositis. Am J Respir Crit Care Med 1995; 151:2037–2040.

125. Cervera R, Ramirez G, Fernandez-Sola J, et al. Antibodies to endothelial cells in dermatomyositis: association with interstitial lung disease. BMJ 1991; 302:880–881.

126. Kamel OW, van de Rijn M, Lebrun DP, Weiss LM, Warnke RA, Dorfman RF. Lymphoid neoplasms in patients with rheumatoid arthritis and dermatomyositis: frequency of Epstein–Barr virus and other features associated with immunosuppression. Hum Pathol 1994; 25:638–643.

127. Sharp GS, Irvin WS, Tan EM, Gould RG, Holman HR. Mixed connective tissue disease: an apparently distinct rheumatic disease syndrome associated with a specific antibody to an extractable nuclear antigen (ENA). Am J Med 1972; 52:148–159.

128. Bennett RM, O'Connell DJ. Mixed connective tissue disease: a clinicopathologic study of 20 cases. Sem Arthritis Rheum 1980; 10:25–51.

129. Kobayashi H, Sano T, Li K, Hizawa K, Yamanoi A, Otsuka T. Mixed connective tissue disease with fatal pulmonary hypertension. Acta Pathol Jpn 1982; 32:1121–1129.

130. Sullivan WD, Hurst DJ, Harmon CE, et al. A prospective evaluation emphasizing pulmonary involvement in patients with mixed connective tissue disease. Medicine (Baltimore) 1984; 63:92–102.

131. Prakash UBS, Luthra HS, Divertie MB. Intrathoracic manifestations in mixed connective tissue disease. Mayo Clin Proc 1985; 60:813–821.

132. Lazarus DS, Mark EJ, McLoud TC. A 46-year old woman with dermatomyositis, increasing pulmonary insufficiency, and terminal right ventricular failure – mixed connective-tissue disease, with diffuse alveolar damage, interstitial pneumonitis, pulmonary hypertension, epicarditis, esophageal fibrosis, and sclerodactyly. N Engl J Med 1995; 333:369–377.

133. Wiener-Kronish JP, Solinger AM, Warnock ML, Churg A, Ordonez N, Golden JA. Severe pulmonary involvement in mixed connective tissue disease. Am Rev Respir Dis 1981; 124:499–503.

134. Rosenow EC, Strimlan CV, Muhm JR, Ferguson RH. Pleuropulmonary manifestations of ankylosing spondylitis. Mayo Clin Proc 1977; 52:641–649.

135. Davies D. Ankylosing spondylitis and lung fibrosis. Q J Med 1972; 41:395–417.

136. Levy H, Hurwitz MD, Strimling M, Zwi S. Ankylosing spondylitis lung disease and Mycobacterium scrofulaceum. Br J Dis Chest 1988; 82:84–87.

137. Guzman LR, Gall EP, Pitt M, Lull G. Psoriatic spondylitis. Association with advanced nongranulomatous upper lobe pulmonary fibrosis. JAMA 1978; 239:1416–1417.

138. Ellman P, Weber FP, Goodier TEW. A contribution to the pathology of Sjogren's disease. Q J Med 1951; 20:33–42.

139. Bucher UG, Reid L. Sjogren's syndrome - report of a fatal case with pulmonary and renal lesions. Br J Dis Chest 1959; 53:237–252.

140. Bloch KJ, Buchanan WW, Wohl MJ, Bunim JJ. Sjogren's syndrome. A clinical, pathological, and serological study of sixty-two cases. Medicine (Baltimore) 1965; 44:187–231.

141. Constantopoulos SH, Papdimitrious CS, Moutsopoulos HM. Respiratory manifestations in primary Sjogren's syndrome. Chest 1985; 88:226–229.

142. Amin K, Ludviksdottir D, Janson C, et al. Inflammation and structural changes in the airways of patients with primary Sjogren's syndrome. Resp Med 2001; 95:904–910.

143. Deheinzelin D, de Carvalho CR, Tomazini ME, Barbas Filho JV, Saldiva PH. Association of Sjogren's syndrome and sarcoidosis. Report of a case. Sarcoidosis 1988; 5:68–70.

144. Itescu S, Brancato LJ, Winchester R. A sicca syndrome in HIV infection: association with HLA-DR5 and CD8 lymphocytosis. Lancet 1989; ii:466–468.

145. Inase N, Usui Y, Tachi H, et al. Sjogren's syndrome with bronchial gland involvement and multiple bullae. Respiration 1990; 57:286–288.

146. Bonner H, Ennis RS, Geelhoed GW, Tarpley TM. Lymphoid infiltration and amyloidosis of lung in Sjogren's syndrome. Arch Pathol Lab Med 1973; 95:42–44.

147. Kobayashi H, Matsuoka R, Kitamura S, Tsunoda N, Saito K. Sjogren's syndrome with multiple bullae and pulmonary nodular amyloidosis. Chest 1988; 94:438–440.

148. Desai SR, Nicholson AG, Stewart S, Twentyman OM, Flower CD, Hansell DM. Benign pulmonary lymphocytic infiltration and amyloidosis: computed tomographic and pathologic features in three cases. J Thorac Imaging 1997; 12:215–220.

149. Harris RS, Mark EJ. A 42-year-old man with multiple pulmonary cysts and recurrent respiratory infections. Sjogren's syndrome involving the lungs, with follicular bronchiolitis, air trapping with cyst formation, and deposition of amyloid-like material. N Engl J Med. 2001; 344, 1701–1708.

150. Yamadori I, Fujita J, Bandoh S, et al. Nonspecific interstitial pneumonia as pulmonary involvement of primary Sjogren's syndrome. Rheumatol Int 2002; 22:89–92.

151. Sato T, Matsubara O, Tanaka Y, Kasuga T. Association of Sjogren's syndrome with pulmonary hypertension – report of two cases and review of the literature. Hum Pathol 1993; 24:199–205.

152. Sowa JM. The association of Sjogrens syndrome and primary pulmonary hypertension. Hum Pathol 1993; 24:1035.

153. Kadota J, Kusano S, Kawakami K, Morikawa T, Kohno S. Usual interstitial pneumonia associated with primary Sjogren's syndrome. Chest 1995; 108:1756–1758.

154. Deheinzelin D, Capelozzi VL, Kairalla RA, Barbas JV, Saldiva PHN, Decarvalho CRR. Interstitial lung disease in primary Sjogren's syndrome – clinical-pathological evaluation and response to treatment. Am J Respir Crit Care Med 1996; 154:794–799.

155. Gardiner P, Ward C, Allison A, et al. Pleuropulmonary abnormalities in primary Sjogren's syndrome. J Rheumatol 1993; 20:831–837.

156. Schuurman H-J, Gooszen HCh, Tan IWN, Kluin PM, Wagenaar SjSc, Van Unnik JAM. Low-grade lymphoma of immature T-cell phenotype in a case of lymphocytic interstitial pneumonia and Sjogren's syndrome. Histopathology 1987; 11:1193–1204.

157. Mariette X. Lymphomas in patients with Sjogren's syndrome: review of the literature and physiopathologic hypothesis. Leuk Lymphoma 1999; 33:93–99.

158. Kojima M, Nakamura S, Ban S, et al. Primary pulmonary low-grade marginal zone B-cell lymphoma of mucosa-associated lymphoid tissue type with prominent hyalinosis. A case report. Pathol Res Pract 2002; 198:685–688.

159. Pearson CM, Cline HM, Newcomer VD. Relapsing polychondritis. N Engl J Med 1960; 263:51–58.

160. Verity MA, Larson WM, Madden SC. Relapsing polychondritis. Report of two necropsied cases with histochemical investigation of the cartilage lesion. Am J Pathol 1963; 42:251–269.

161. Kaye RL, Sones DA. Relapsing polychondritis. Clinical and pathological features in 14 cases. Ann Intern Med 1964; 60:653–664.

162. Hughes RAC, Berry CL, Seifert M, Lessof MH. Relapsing polychondritis. Three cases with a clinico-pathological study and literature review. Q J Med 1972; 41:363–380.

163. McAdam LP, O'Hanlan MA, Bluestone R, Pearson CM. Relapsing polychondritis: prospective study of 23 patients and a review of the literature. Medicine (Baltimore) 1976; 55:193–215.

164. Ebringer R, Rook G, Swana GT, Botazzo GF, Doniach D. Autoantibodies to cartilage and type II collagen in relapsing polychondritis and other rheumatic diseases. Ann Rheum Dis 1979; 40:473–479.

165. Somers G, Potvliege P. Relapsing polychondritis: relation to periarteritis nodosa. BMJ 1978; 2:603–604.

166. Neild GH, Cameron JS, Lessof MH, Ogg CS, Turner DR. Relapsing polychondritis with crescentic glomerulonephritis. BMJ 1978; 1:743–745.

167. Higgenbottam T, Dixon J. Chondritis associated with fatal intramural bronchial fibrosis. Thorax 1979; 34:563–564.

168. Rogerson ME, Higgins EM, Godfrey RC. Tracheal stenosis due to relapsing polychondritis in rheumatoid arthritis. Thorax 1987; 42:905–906.

169. Sheffield E, Corrin B. Fatal bronchial stenosis due to isolated relapsing chondritis. Histopathology 1992; 20:442–443.

170. Valenzuela R, Cooperrider PA, Gogate P, Deodhar SD, Bergfeld WF. Relapsing polychondritis. Immunomicroscopic findings in cartilage of ear biopsy specimens. Hum Pathol 1980; 11:19–22.

171. Chajek T, Fainaru M. Behcet's disease. Report of 41 cases and a review of the literature. Medicine (Baltimore) 1975; 54:179–196.

172. Slavin RF, de Groot WJ. Pathology of the lung in Behcet's disease: case report and review of the literature. Am J Surg Pathol 1981; 5:779–788.

173. Efthimiou J, Johnston C, Spiro SG, Turner-Warwick M. Pulmonary disease in Behcet's syndrome. Q J Med 1986; 58:259–280.

174. Lie JT. Cardiac and pulmonary manifestations of Behcet syndrome. Pathol Res Pract 1988; 183:347–352.

175. Demontpreville VT, Macchiarini P, Dartevelle PG, Dulmet EM. Large bilateral pulmonary artery aneurysms in Behcet's disease: rupture of the contralateral lesion after aneurysmorrhaphy. Respiration 1996; 63:49–51.

176. Witt C, John M, Martin H, et al. Behcet's syndrome with pulmonary involvement - combined therapy for endobronchial stenosis using neodym-YAG laser, balloon dilation and immunosuppression. Respiration 1996; 63:195–198.

177. Erkan F, Gul A, Tasali E. Pulmonary manifestations of Behcet's disease. Thorax 2001; 56:572–578.

178. Aktogu S, Erer OF, Urpek G, Soy O, Tibet G. Multiple pulmonary arterial aneurysms in Behcet's disease: Clinical and radiologic remission after cyclophosphamide and corticosteroid therapy. Respiration 2002; 69:178–181.

179. Kopp WL, Green RA. Pulmonary artery aneurysms with recurrent thrombophlebitis. The Hughes-Stovin syndrome. Ann Intern Med 1962; 56:105–114.

180. Jerray M, Benzarti M, Rouatbi N. Possible Behcet's disease revealed by pulmonary aneurysms. Chest 1991; 99:1282–1284.

181. Corbett E, Glaisyer H, Chan C, Madden B, Khaghani A, Yacoub M. Congenital cutis laxa with a dominant inheritance and early onset emphysema. Thorax 1994; 49:836–837.

182. Ayres JG, Pope FM, Reidy JF, Clark TJH. Abnormalities of the lungs and thoracic cage in the Ehlers-Danlos syndrome. Thorax 1985; 40:300–305.

183. Corrin B, Simpson CGB, Fisher C. Fibrous pseudotumours and cyst formation in the lungs in Ehlers-Danlos syndrome. Histopathology 1990; 17:478–479.

184. Watanabe A, Kawabata Y, Okada O, et al. Ehlers–Danlos syndrome type IV with few extrathoracic findings: a newly recognised point mutation in the COL3A1 gene. Eur Resp J 2002; 19:195–198.

185. Jackson A, Loh C-L. Pulmonary calcification and elastic tissue damage in pseudoxanthoma elasticum. Histopathology 1980; 4:607–611.

186. Sharma BK, Talukdar B, Kapoor R. Cystic lung in Marfan's syndrome. Thorax 1989; 44:978–979.

187. Yellin A, Shiner RJ, Lieberman Y. Familial multiple bilateral pneumothorax associated with Marfan syndrome. Chest 1991; 100:577–578.

188. Rigante D, Segni G, Bush A. Persistent spontaneous pneumothorax in an adolescent with Marfan's syndrome and pulmonary bullous dysplasia. Respiration 2001; 68:621–624.

Vascular diseases

189. Stanger P, Lucas RV, Jr, Edwards JE. Anatomic factors causing respiratory distress in acyanotic congenital cardiac disease. Special reference to bronchial obstruction. Pediatrics 1969; 43:760–769.

190. Cohen SR, Landing BH. Tracheostenosis and bronchial anomalies associated with pulmonary artery sling. Ann Otol Rhinol Laryngol 1976; 85:1.

191. Stewart JR, Kincaid OW, Titus JL. Right aortic arch: plain film diagnosis and significance. Am J Roentgen 97, 377–389. 1966.

192. Stoica SC, Lockowandt U, Coulden R, Ward R, Bilton D, Dunning J. Double aortic arch masquerading as asthma for thirty years. Respiration 2002; 69:92–95.

193. Dines DE, Arms RA, Bernatz PE, Gomes MR. Pulmonary arteriovenous fistulas. Mayo Clin Proc 1974; 49:460–465.

194. Hughes JMB. Intrapulmonary shunts: coils to transplantation. J R Coll Physicians Lond 1994; 28:247–253.

195. Shovlin CL, Letarte M. Hereditary haemorrhagic telangiectasia and pulmonary arteriovenous malformations: issues in clinical management and review of pathogenic mechanisms. Thorax 1999; 54:714–729.

196. Braverman IM, Keh A, Jacobson BS. Ultrastructure and three-dimensional organisation of the telangiectases of hereditary hemorrhagic telangiectasia. J Invest Dermatol 1990; 95:422–427.

197. Hodgson CH, Burchell HB, Good CA, Clagett OT. Hereditary hemorrhagic telagiectasia and pulmonary arteriovenous fistula. Survey of a large family. N Engl J Med 1959; 261:625–636.

198. McAllister KA, Lennon F, Bowles-Biesecker B, et al. Genetic heterogeneity in hereditary haemorrhagic telangiectasia: possible correlation with clinical phenotype. J Med Genet 1994; 31:927–932.

199. McAllister KA, Grogg KM, Johnson DW, et al. Endoglin, a TGF-beta binding protein of endothelial cells, is the gene for hereditary haemorrhagic telangiectasia type 1. Nat Genet 1994; 8:345–351.

200. Vincent P, Plauchu H, Hazan J, Faure S, Weissenbach J, Godet J. A third locus for hereditary haemorrhagic telangiectasia maps to chromosome 12q. Hum Mol Genet 1995; 4:945–949.

201. Trell E, Johansson BW, Linell F, Ripa J. Familial pulmonary hypertension and multiple abnormalities of large systemic arteries in Osler's disease. Am J Med 1972; 53:50–63.

202. Trembath RC, Thomson JR, Machado RD, et al. Clinical and molecular genetic features of pulmonary hypertension in patients with hereditary hemorrhagic telangiectasia. N Engl J Med 2001; 345:325–334.

203. Joshi M, Cole S, Knibbs D, Diana D. Pulmonary abnormalities in Klippel–Trenaunay syndrome – a histologic, ultrastructural, and immunocytochemical study. Chest 1992; 102:1274–1277.

204. Gianlupi A, Harper RW, Dwyre DM, Marelich GP. Recurrent pulmonary embolism associated with Klippel–Trenaunay–Weber syndrome. Chest 1999; 115:1199–1201.

205. Walder B, Kapelanski DP, Auger WR, Fedullo PF. Successful pulmonary thromboendarterectomy in a patient with Klippel–Trenaunay syndrome. Chest 2000; 117:1520–1522.

206. Morton R. Idiopathic arterial calcification in infancy. Histopathology 1978; 2:423–432.

207. Gilbey LK, Girod CE. Blue rubber bleb nevus syndrome – Endobronchial involvement presenting as chronic cough. Chest 2003; 124; 760–763.

Renal disease

208. Rocker GM, Morgan AG, Pearson D, Basran GS, Shale DJ. Pulmonary vascular permeability to transferrin in the pulmonary oedema of renal failure. Thorax 1987; 42:620–623.

209. Crosbie WA, Snowden S, Parsons V. Changes in lung capillary permeability in renal failure. BMJ 1972; 4:388–390.

210. Amin M, Fawzy A, Hamid MA, Elhendy A. Pulmonary hypertension in patients with chronic renal failure - Role of parathyroid hormone and pulmonary artery calcifications. Chest 2003; 124; 2093–2097.

Blood disorders

211. Entwistle CC, Fentem PH, Jacobs A. Red-cell aplasia with carcinoma of the bronchus. BMJ 1964; 2:1504–1506.

212. Williams AJ, Marsh J, Stableforth DE. Cryptogenic fibrosing alveolitis, chronic active hepatitis and autoimmune haemolytic anaemia in the same patient. Br J Dis Chest 1985; 79:200–203.

213. Rausch PG, Herion JC. Pulmonary manifestations of Waldenstroms's macroglobulinaemia. Am J Hematol 1980; 9:201–209.

214. Bombardieri S, Paoletti P, Ferri C, et al. Lung involvement in mixed cryoglobulinaemia. Am J Med 1979; 66:748–756.

215. Nash JW, Ross P, Crowson AN, et al. The histopathologic spectrum of cryofibrinogenemia in four anatomic sites – Skin, lung, muscle, and kidney. Am J Clin Pathol 2003; 119:114–122.

216. Lai YP, Kuo PH, Wu HD, Yang PC. A patient with haemoptysis, rapidly changing pulmonary infiltrates and left flank pain – primary antiphospholipid syndrome with pulmonary infarction, pulmonary haemorrhage and left adrenal haemorrhage. Eur Respir J 1996; 9:2184–2187.

217. Pilling J, Cutaia M. The antiphospholipid antibody syndrome – A vascular disease with pulmonary manifestations. Chest 1997; 112:1451–1453.

218. Kerr JE, Poe R, Kramer Z. Antiphospholipid antibody syndrome presenting as a refractory noninflammatory pulmonary vasculopathy. Chest 1997; 112:1707–1710.

219. Greaves M. Antiphospholipid syndrome. J Clin Pathol 1997; 50:973–974.

220. Heath D, Thompson IM. Bronchopulmonary anastomoses in sickle cell anaemia. Thorax 1969; 24:232–238.

221. Oppenehimer EH, Esterly JR. Pulmonary changes in sickle cell disease. Am Rev Respir Dis 1971; 103:858–859.

222. Collins FS, Orringer EP. Pulmonary hypertension and cor pulmonale in the sickle hemoglobinopathies. Am J Med 1982; 73:814–821.

223. Athanasou NA, Hatton C, McGee JO, Weatherall DJ. Vascular occlusion and infarction in sickle cell crisis and the sickle chest syndrome. J Clin Pathol 1985; 38:659–664.

224. Gray A, Anionwu EN, Davies SC, Brozovic M. Patterns of mortality in sickle cell disease in the United Kingdom. J Clin Pathol 1991; 44:459–463.

225. Weil JV, Castro O, Malik AB, Rodgers G, Bonds DR, Jacobs TP. Pathogenesis of lung disease in sickle hemoglobinopathies. Am Rev Respir Dis 1993; 148:249–256.

226. Verresen D, Debacker W, Vanmeerbeeck J, Neetens I, Vanmarck E, Vermeire P. Spherocytosis and pulmonary hypertension: coincidental occurrence or causal relationship? Eur Respir J 1991; 4:629–631.

227. Landing BH, Nadorra R, Hyman CB, Ortega JA. Pulmonary lesions of thalassemia major. Perspect Pediatr Pathol 1987; 11:82–96.

228. Landing BH, Nadorra R, Hyman CB, Ortega JA. Pulmonary lesions of thalassemia major. In: Rosenberg HS, Bernstein J, eds. Respiratory and Alimentary Tract Diseases, Vol. 11 Perspectives in Pediatric Pathology. Basel: Karger; 1987:82–96.

229. Zaidi Y, Sivakumaran M, Graham C, Hutchinson RM. Fatal bone marrow embolism in a patient with sickle cell beta⁺ thalassaemia. J Clin Pathol 1996; 49:774–775.

230. Heller PG, Grinberg AR, Lencioni M, Molina MM, Roncoroni AJ. Pulmonary hypertension in paroxysmal nocturnal hemoglobinuria. Chest 1992; 102:642–643.

231. Adedeji MO, Cespedes J, Allen K, Subramony C, Hughson MD. Pulmonary thrombotic arteriopathy in patients with sickle cell disease. Arch Pathol Lab Med 2001; 125:1436–1441.

232. Haque AK, Gokhale S, Rampy BA, Adegboyega P, Duarte A, Saldana MJ. Pulmonary hypertension in sickle cell hemoglobinopathy: A clinicopathologic study of 20 cases. Hum Pathol 2002; 33:1037–1043.

232a. Gladwin MT, Sachdev V, Jison ML, et al. Pulmonary hypertension as a risk factor for death in patients with sickle cell disease. N Engl J Med 2004; 350:886–895.

233. Emre U, Miller ST, Gutierez M, Steiner P, Rao SP, Rao M. Effect of transfusion in acute chest syndrome of sickle cell disease. J Pediatr 1995; 127:901–904.

234. Siddiqui AK, Ahmed S. Pulmonary manifestations of sickle cell disease. Postgrad Med J 2003; 79:384–390.

235. McMahon LEC, Mark EJ, Shepard JAO. A 22-year-old man with a sickle cell crisis and sudden death – Sickle cell anemia. N Engl J Med 1997; 337:1293–1301.

236. Aessopos A, Stamatelos G, Skoumas V, Vassilopoulos G, Mantzourani M, Loukopoulos D. Pulmonary hypertension and right heart failure in patients with beta-thalassemia intermedia. Chest 1995; 107:50–53.

237. Tai DYH, Wang YT, Lou J, Wang WY, Mak KH, Cheng HK. Lungs in thalassaemia major patients receiving regular transfusion. Eur Respir J 1996; 9:1389–1394.

238. Asakura S, Colby TV. Agnogenic myeloid metaplasia with extramedullary hematopoiesis and fibrosis in the lung - report of two cases. Chest 1994; 105:1866–1868.

239. Yusen RD, Kollef MH. Acute respiratory failure due to extramedullary hematopoiesis. Chest 1995; 108:1170–1172.

240. Coyne JD, Burton IE. Interstitial pneumonitis due to extramedullary haematopoiesis (EMH) in agnogenic myeloid metaplasia. Histopathology 1999; 34:275–276.

241. Doran HM, Sheppard MN, Collins PW, Jones L, Newland AC, Vanderwalt JD. Pathology of the lung in leukaemia and lymphoma – a study of 87 autopsies. Histopathology 1991; 18:211–219.

242. Couderc LJ, Rain B, Desgranges C. Pulmonary fibrosis in association with human T cell lymphotropic virus type 1 (HTLV-1) infection. Respir Med 2000; 94:1010.

243. Yoshioka R, Yamaguchi K, Yoshinaga T, Takatsuki K. Pulmonary complications in patients with adult T-cell leukemia. Cancer 1985; 55:2491–2494.

244. Moskaluk CA, Pogrebniak HW, Pass HI, Gallin JI, Travis WD. Surgical pathology of the lung in chronic granulomatous disease. Am J Clin Pathol 1994; 102:684–691.

245. Del G, I, Iori AP, Mengarelli A, et al. Allogeneic stem cell transplant from HLA-identical sibling for chronic granulomatous disease and review of the literature. Ann Hematol 2003; 82:189–192.

246. Moltyaner Y, Geerts WH, Chamberlain DW, et al. Underlying chronic granulomatous disease in a patient with bronchocentric granulomatosis. Thorax 2003; 58: 1096–1098.

247. Yamauchi K, Shimamura K. Pulmonary fibrosis and sea-blue histiocyte infiltration in a patient with primary myelofibrosis. Eur Respir J 1995; 8:1620–1623.

248. Schmidt M, Dercken C, Loke O, et al. Pulmonary manifestation of systemic mast cell disease. Eur Resp J 2000; 15:623–625.

Alimentary tract disorders

249. Allen CJ, Newhouse MT. Gastroesophageal reflux and chronic respiratory disease. Am Rev Respir Dis 1984; 129:645–647.

250. Berrill WT, Fitzpatrick PF, Macleod WM, Eade OE, Hyde I, Wright R. Bird-fancier's lung and jejunal villous atrophy. Lancet 1975; 2:1006–1008.

251. Faux JA, Hendrick DJ, Amand B. Precipitins to different avian serum antigens in bird fanciers' lung and coeliac disease. Clin Allergy 1978; 8:101–108.

252. Robinson TJ. Coeliac disease with farmers' lung. BMJ 1976; 1:745–746.

253. Edwards C, Williams A, Asquith P. Bronchopulmonary disease in coeliac patients. J Clin Pathol 1985; 38:361–367.

254. Mahadeva R, Flower C, Shneerson J. Bronchiectasis in association with coeliac disease. Thorax 1998; 53:527–529.

255. Wright PH, Menzies IS, Pounder RE, Keeling PWN. Adult idiopathic pulmonary haemosiderosis and coeliac disease. Q J Med 1981; 197:95–102.

256. Wright PH, Buxton-Thomas M, Keeling PWN, Kreel L. Adult idiopathic pulmonary hemosiderosis: a comparison of lung function changes and the distribution of pulmonary disease in patients with and without coeliac disease. Br J Dis Chest 1983; 77:282–292.

257. Bouros D, Panagou P, Rokkas T, Siafakas NM. Bronchoalveolar lavage findings in a young adult with idiopathic pulmonary haemosiderosis and coeliac disease. Eur Respir J 1994; 7:1009–1012.

258. Shapiro MS, Dobbins JW, Matthay RA. Pulmonary manifestations of gastrointestinal disease. Clin Chest Med 1989; 10:617–643.

259. Camus P, Piard F, Ashcroft T, Gal AA, Colby TV. The lung in inflammatory bowel disease. Medicine 1993; 72:151–183.

260. Butland RJA, Cole P, Citron KM, Turner-Warwick M. Chronic bronchial suppuration and inflammatory bowel disease. Q J Med 1981; 50:63–75.

261. Wilcox P, Miller R, Miller G, et al. Airway involvement in ulcerative colitis. Chest 1987; 92:18–21.

262. Moles KW, Varghese G, Hayes JR. Pulmonary involvement in ulcerative colitis. Br J Dis Chest 1988; 82:79–83.

263. Kraft SC, Earle RH, Roesler M, Esterly JR. Unexplained bronchopulmonary disease with inflammatory bowel disease. Arch Intern Med 1976; 136:454–459.

264. Rickli H, Fretz C, Hoffman M, Walser A, Knoblauch A. Severe inflammatory upper airway stenosis in ulcerative colitis. Eur Respir J 1994; 7:1899–1902.

265. Vasishta S, Wood JB, McGinty F. Ulcerative tracheobronchitis years after colectomy for ulcerative colitis. Chest 1994; 106:1279–1281.

266. Lemann M, Messing B, D'Agay F, Modigliani R. Crohn's disease with respiratory tract involvement. Gut 1987; 28:1669–1672.

267. Gibb WRG, Dhillon DP, Zilkha KJ, Cole PJ. Bronchiectasis with ulcerative colitis and myelopathy. Thorax 1987; 42:155–156.

268. Higenbottam T, Cochrane GM, Clark TJH, Turner O, Millis R, Seymour W. Bronchial disease in ulcerative colitis. Thorax 1980; 35:581–585.

269. Eaton TE, Lambie N, Wells AU. Bronchiectasis following colectomy for Crohn's disease. Thorax 1998; 53:529–531.

270. Spira A, Grossman R, Balter M. Large airway disease associated with inflammatory bowel disease. Chest 1998; 113:1723–1726.

271. Kayser K, Probst F, Gabius HJ, Muller KM. Are there characteristic alterations of lung tissue associated with Crohn's disease? Pathol Res Pract 1990; 186:485–490.

272. Swinburne CR, Jackson GJ, Cobden I, Ashcroft T, Morritt GN, Corris PA. Bronchiolitis obliterans organising pneumonia in a patient with ulcerative colitis. Thorax 1988; 43:735–736.

273. Shneerson JM. Steroid-responsive alveolitis associated with ulcerative colitis. Chest 1992; 101:585–586.

274. Dawson A, Gibbs AR, Anderson G. An unusual perilobular pattern of pulmonary interstitial fibrosis associated with Crohn's disease. Histopathology 1993; 23:553–556.

275. Hotermans G, Benard A, Guenanen H, Demarcqdelerue G, Malart T, Wallaert B. Nongranulomatous interstitial lung disease in Crohn's disease. Eur Respir J 1996; 9:380–382.

276. Beer TW, Edwards CW. Pulmonary nodules due to reactive systemic amyloidosis (AA) in Crohn's disease. Thorax 1993; 48:1287–1288.

277. Meadway J, Hills EA. Ulcerative colitis, colitic spondylitis and associated apical pulmonary fibrosis. Proc R Soc Med 1974; 67:324–325.

278. Bradshaw MJ, Harvey RF, Burns-Cox CJ. Crohn's disease presenting as recurrent pulmonary edema. BMJ 1981; ii:1437–1438.

279. Hardarson S, Labrecque DR, Mitros FA, Neil GA, Goeken JA. Antineutrophil cytoplasmic antibody in inflammatory bowel and hepatobiliary diseases – high prevalence in ulcerative colitis, primary sclerosing cholangitis, and autoimmune hepatitis. Am J Clin Pathol 1993; 99:277–281.

280. Vandenplas O, Casel S, Delos M, Trigaux JP, Melange M, Marchand E. Granulomatous bronchiolitis associated with Crohn's disease. Am J Respir Crit Care Med 1998; 158:1676–1679.

281. Cohen M, Sahn SA. Bronchiectasis in systemic diseases. Chest 1999; 116:1063–1074.

282. Faller M, Gasser B, Massard G, Pauli G, Quoix E. Pulmonary migratory infiltrates and pachypleuritis in a patient with Crohn's disease. Respiration 2000; 67:459–463.

283. Casey MB, Tazelaar HD, Myers JL, et al. Noninfectious lung pathology in patients with Crohn's disease. Am J Surg Pathol 2003; 27:213–219.

284. Wallert B, Colombel JF, Tonnel AB, et al. Evidence of lymphocyte alveolitis in Crohn's disease. Chest 1985; 87:363–367.

285. Bonniere P, Wallaert B, Cortot A, et al. Latent pulmonary involvement in Crohn's disease: biological, functional, bronchoalveolar lavage and scintigraphic studies. Gut 1986; 27:919–925.

286. Tzanakis N, Bouros D, Samiou M, et al. Lung function in patients with inflammatory bowel disease. Respir Med 1998; 92:516–522.

287. Lamblin C, Copin MC, Billaut C, et al. Acute respiratory failure due to tracheobronchial involvement in Crohn's disease. Eur Respir J 1996; 9:2176–2178.

288. Golpe R, Mateos A, PerezValcarcel J, Lapena JA, GarciaFigueiras R, Blanco J. Multiple pulmonary nodules in a patient with Crohn's disease. Respiration 2003; 70; 306–309.

289. Isenberg JI, Goldstein H, Korn AS, Ozeran RS, Rosen V. Pulmonary vasculitis – an uncommon complication of ulcerative colitis. N Engl J Med 1968; 279:1376–1377.

290. Whipple GH. A hitherto undescribed disease characterised anatomically by deposits of fat and fatty acids in the intestinal and mesenteric lymphatic tissues. Bull Johns Hopkins Hospital 1907; 18:382.

291. Bayless TM, Knox DL. Whipple's disease: a multisystemic infection. N Engl J Med 1979; 300:920–921.

292. Relman DA, Schmidt TM, MacDermott RP, Falkow S. Identification of the uncultured bacillus of Whipple's disease. N Engl J Med 1992; 327:293–301.

293. Eck M, Kreipe H, Harmsen D, Muller-Hermelink HK. Invasion and destruction of mucosal plasma cells by Tropheryma whippelii. Hum Pathol 1997; 28:1424–1428.

294. Fleming JL, Weisner RH, Shorter RG. Whipple's disease: clinical, biochemical, and histopathologic features and assessment of treatment in 29 patients. Mayo Clin Proc 1988; 63:539–551.

295. Winberg CD, Rose ME, Rappaport H. Whipple's disease of the lung. Am J Med 1978; 65:873–880.

296. Kelly CA, Egan M, Rawlinson J. Whipple's disease presenting with lung involvement. Thorax 1996; 51:343–344.

297. Riemer H, Hainz R, Stain C, et al. Severe pulmonary hypertension reversed by antibiotics in a patient with Whipple's disease. Thorax 1997; 52:1014–1015.

298. Symmons DPM, Shepherd AN, Boardman PL, Bacon PA. Pulmonary manifestations of Whipple's disease. Q J Med 1985; 56:497–504.

299. MacDermott RP, Shepard JAO, GraemeCook FM, Bloch KJ. A 59-year-old man with anorexia, weight loss, and a mediastinal mass – Whipple's disease involving the small intestine and mesenteric and mediastinal lymph nodes. N Engl J Med 1997; 337:1612–1619.

300. Herve P, Lebrec D, Brenot F, et al. Pulmonary vascular disorders in portal hypertension. Eur Resp J 1998; 11:1153–1166.

301. Mantz FA, Craige E. Portal axis thrombosis with spontaneous portacaval shunt and resultant cor pulmonale. Arch Pathol 1951; 52:91–97.

302. McDonnell PJ, Toye PA, Hutchins GM. Primary pulmonary hypertension in cirrhosis: are they related? Am Rev Respir Dis 1983; 127:437–441.

303. Lockhart A. Pulmonary arterial hypertension in portal hypertension. Clin Gastroenterol 1985; 14:123–138.

304. Robalina BD, Moodie DS. Association between primary pulmonary hypertension and portal hypertension: analysis of its pathophysiology and clinical laboratory and hemodynamic manifestations. J Am Coll Cardiol 1991; 17II:492–498.

305. Rodriguez-Roisin R, Krowka MJ, Herve P, Fallon MB, on behalf of the ERS Task Force Pulmonary-Hepatic Vascular Disorders Scientific Committee ERS Task Force PHD Scientific Committee. Pulmonary-Hepatic vascular Disorders (PHD). Eur Respir J 2004; 24:861–880.

306. Stratakos G, Malagari K, Broutzos E, Zakynthinos E, Roussos C, Papiris S. Dyspnoea and cyanosis in a cirrhotic patient – Diagnosis: Hepatopulmonary syndrome with diffuse (Type I) intrapulmonary vascular dilatations. Eur Resp J 2002; 19:780–783.

307. Rydell R, Hoffbauer FW. Multiple pulmonary arteriovenous fistulas in juvenile cirrhosis. Am J Med 1956; 21:450–460.

308. Berthelot P, Walker JG, Sherlock S, Reid L. Arterial changes in the lungs in cirrhosis of the liver - lung spider nevi. N Engl J Med 1966; 274:291–298.

309. Stanley NN, Williams AJ, Dewar CA, Blendis LM, Reid L. Hypoxia and hydrothoraces in a case of liver cirrhosis: correlation of physiological, radiographic, scintigraphic, and pathological findings. Thorax 1977; 32:457–471.

310. Andrivet P, Cadranel J, Housset B, Herigault R, Harf A, Adnot S. Mechanism of impaired arterial oxygenation in patients with liver cirrhosis and severe respiratory insufficiency. Chest 1993; 103:500–507.

311. Rodriguez-Roisin R, Roca J, Agusti AG, Mastai R, Wagner PD, Bosch J. Gas exchange and pulmonary vascular reactivity in patients with liver cirrhosis. Am Rev Respir Dis 1987; 135:1085–1092.

312. Krowka MJ, Cortese DA. Hepatopulmonary syndrome – current concepts in diagnostic and therapeutic considerations. Chest 1994; 105:1528–1537.

313. Lazaridis KN, Frank JW, Krowka MJ, Kamath PS. Hepatic hydrothorax: pathogenesis, diagnosis, and management.

314. Stanley NN, Fox RA, Whimster WF, Sherlock S, James DG. Primary biliary cirrhosis or sarcoidosis – or both. N Engl J Med 1972; 287:1282–1284.

315. Fagan EA, Moore-Gillon JC, Turner-Warwick M. Multiorgan granulomas and mitochondrial antibodies. N Engl J Med 1983; 308:572–575.

316. Hughes P, McGavin CR. Sarcoidosis and primary biliary cirrhosis with co-existing myositis. Thorax 1997; 52:201–202.

317. Weissman E, Becker N. Interstitial lung disease in primary biliary cirrhosis. Am J Med Sci 1983; 285:21–27.

318. Wallace JG, Tong MJ, Ueki BH, Quismorio FP. Pulmonary involvement in primary biliary cirrhosis. J Clin Gastroenterol 1987; 9:431–435.

319. Chatte G, Streichenberger N, Boillot O, Gille D, Loire R, Cordier JF. Lymphocytic bronchitis/bronchiolitis in a patient with primary biliary cirrhosis. Eur Respir J 1995; 8:176–179.

320. Tsianos EV, Hoofnagle JH, Fox PC, et al. Sjogren's syndrome in patients with primary biliary cirrhosis. Hepatology 1990; 11:730–734.

321. Golding PL, Smith M, Williams R. Multisystem involvement in chronic liver disease: studies on the incidence and pathogenesis. Am J Med 1973; 55:772–782.

322. Johnson MA, Spiteri MA, Epstein U, et al. Subclinical alveolitis in patients with primary biliary cirrhosis. Eur Respir J 1988; 1:246.

323. Meliconi R, Andreone P, Fasano L, et al. Incidence of hepatitis C virus infection in Italian patients with idiopathic pulmonary fibrosis. Thorax 1996; 51:315–317.

324. Turner-Warwick M. Fibrosing alveolitis and chronic liver disease. Q J Med 1968; 37:133.

325. Kayser K, Paul K, Feist D, Hofmann W, Wille L, Gabius HJ. Alteration of the lung parenchyma associated with autoimmune hepatitis. Virchows Arch A Pathol Anat Histopathol 1991; 419:153–157.

326. Helman CA, Keeton GR, Benatar SR. Lymphoid interstitial pneumonia with associated chronic active hepatitis and renal tubular acidosis. Am Rev Respir Dis 1977; 115:161–164.

327. Kagalwalla AF, Rahman A, Taleb A, Kagalwalla YA, Ali MM, Yaish H. Pulmonary hemorrhage in association with autoimmune chronic active hepatitis. Chest 1993; 103:634–636.

328. Glasgow JFG, Lynch MJ, Herez A, et al. Alpha-1 antitrypsin deficiency in association with both cirrhosis and chronic obstructive lung disease in two sibs. Am J Med 1973; 54:181.

329. Bachofen M, Weibel ER. Basic pattern of tissue repair in human lungs following unspecific injury. Chest 1974; 65(Suppl):14s–19s.

Neuromuscular diseases

330. Editorial. Neurogenic pulmonary oedema. Lancet 1985; 1:1430–1431.

331. Wray NP, Nicotra MB. Pathogenesis of neurogenic pulmonary oedema. Am Rev Respir Dis 1978; 118:783–786.

332. Carlson RW, Schaeffer RC, Michaels SG, Weil MH. Pulmonary oedema following intracranial haemorrhage. Chest 1979; 75:731–734.

333. Castro M, Shepherd CW, Gomez MR, Lie JT, Ryu JH. Pulmonary tuberous sclerosis. Chest 1995; 107:189–195.

334. Shepherd CW, Gomez MR, Lie JT, Crowson CS. Causes of death in patients with tuberous sclerosis. Mayo Clin Proc 1991; 66:792–796.

335. Franz DN, Brody A, Meyer C, et al. Mutational and radiographic analysis of pulmonary disease consistent with lymphangioleiomyomatosis and micronodular pneumocyte hyperplasia in women with tuberous sclerosis. Am J Respir Crit Care Med 2001; 164:661–668.

336. Moss J, Avila NA, Barnes PM, et al. Prevalence and clinical characteristics of lymphangioleiomyomatosis (LAM) in patients with tuberous sclerosis complex. Am J Respir Crit Care Med 2001; 164:669–671.

337. Burrows NJ, Johnson SR. Pulmonary artery aneurysm and tuberous sclerosis. Thorax 2004; 59: 86.

338. Flieder DB, Travis WD. Clear cell 'Sugar' tumor of the lung: Association with lymphangioleiomyomatosis and multifocal micronodular pneumocyte hyperplasia in a patient with tuberous sclerosis. Am J Surg Pathol 1997; 21:1242–1247.

339. Chuah KL, Tan PH. Multifocal micronodular pneumocyte hyperplasia, lymphangiomyomatosis and clear cell micronodules of the lung in a Chinese female patient with tuberous sclerosis. Pathology 1998; 30:242–246.

340. Chu SC, Horiba K, Usuki J, et al. Comprehensive evaluation of 35 patients with lymphangioleiomyomatosis. Chest 1999; 115:1041–1052.

341. Wu K, Tazelaar HD. Pulmonary angiomyolipoma and multifocal micronodular pneumocyte hyperplasia associated with tuberous sclerosis. Hum Pathol 1999; 30:1266–1268.

342. Pea M, Bonetti F, Martignoni G, et al. Apparent renal cell carcinomas in tuberous sclerosis are heterogeneous: The identification of malignant epithelioid angiomyolipoma. Am J Surg Pathol 1998; 22:180–187.

343. Henske EP, Ao X, Short MP, et al. Frequent progesterone receptor immunoreactivity in tuberous sclerosis-associated renal angiomyolipomas. Modern Pathol 1998; 11:665–668.

344. Bonetti F, Pea M, Martignoni G, et al. Clear cell ('sugar') tumor of the lung is a lesion strictly related to angiomyolipoma - the concept of a family of lesions characterised by the presence of the perivascular epithelioid cells (PEC). Pathology 1995; 26:230–236.

345. Davies PDB. Diffuse pulmonary involvement in von Recklinghausen's disease: a new syndrome. Thorax 1963; 18:198.

346. Israel-Asselain R, Chebat J, Sors C, Basset F, Le Rolland A. Diffuse interstitial pulmonary fibrosis in a mother and son with von Recklinghausen's disease. Thorax 1965; 20:153–157.

347. Massaro D, Katz S. Fibrosing alveolitis: its occurrence, roentgenographic, and pathologic features in von Recklinghausen's neurofibromatosis. Am Rev Respir Dis 1966; 93:934–942.

348. Webb WR, Goodman PC. Fibrosing alveolitis in patients with neurofibromatosis. Radiology 1977; 122:289–293.

349. De Scheerder I, Elinck W, Van Renterghem D, Cuvelier C, Tasson J, Van der Straeten M. Desquamative interstitial pneumonia and scar cancer of the lung complicating generalised neurofibromatosis. Eur J Respir Dis 1984; 65:623–626.

Metabolic and endocrine disorders

350. Adams JS, Sharma OP, Glacad MA, Singer FR. Metabolism of 25-hydroxyvitamin D3 by cultured pulmonary alveolar macrophages in sarcoidosis. J Clin Invest 1983; 72:1856–1860.

351. Bell NH, Stern PH, Pantzer E, Sinha TK, DeLuca HF. Evidence that increased circulating 1-alpha, 25-dihydroxyvitamin D is the probable cause of abnormal calcium metabolism in sarcoidosis. J Clin Invest 1979; 64:218–225.

352. Papapoulos SE, Frahjer LJ, Sandler LM, Clemens TL, Lewin IG, O'Riordan JLH. 1,25-dihydroxycholecalciferol in the pathogenesis of the hypercalcemia of sarcoidosis. Lancet 1979; ii:627–630.

353. Sharma OP. Vitamin D, calcium, and sarcoidosis. Chest 1996; 109:535–539.

354. Virchow R. Kalk-Metastasen. Virchows Arch A Pathol Anat Histopathol 1855; 8:103–113.

355. Bloodworth J, Tomashefski JF. Localised pulmonary metastatic calcification associated with pulmonary artery obstruction. Thorax 1992; 47:174–178.

356. Mulligan RM. Metastatic calcification. Arch Pathol 1947; 43:177–230.

357. Kaltreider HB, Baum GL, Bogaty G, McCoy MD, Tucker M. So-called 'metastatic' calcification of the lung. Am J Med 1969; 46:189–196.

358. Hartman TE, Muller NL, Primack SL, et al. Metastatic pulmonary calcification in patients with hypercalcaemia. Am J Roentol 1994; 162:799–802.

359. Holmes F, Harlan J, Felt S, Ruhlen J, Murphy B. Pulmonary oedema in hypercalcaemic crisis. Lancet 1974; 1:311–312.

360. Wright J, Jones E. Diffuse calcification of the airways. Modern Pathol 2001; 14:717–719.

361. Celli BR, Rubinow A, Cohen AS, Brody JS. Patterns of pulmonary involvement in systemic amyloidosis. Chest 1978; 74:543–547.

362. Smith RRL, Hutchins GM, Moore GW, Humphrey RL. Type and distribution of pulmonary parenchymal and vascular amyloid: correlation with cardiac amyloidosis. Am J Med 1979; 66:96–104.

363. Ishi T, Hosoda Y, Ikegami N, Shimada H. Senile amyloid deposition. J Pathol 1983; 139:1–22.

364. Theaker JM, Raine AEG, Rainey AJ, Heryet A, Clark A, Oliver DO. Systemic amyloidosis of B2-microglobulin type: a complication of long term haemodialysis. J Clin Pathol 1987; 40:1247–1251.

365. Planes C, Kleinknecht D, Brauner M, Battesti JP, Kemeny JL, Valeyre D. Diffuse interstitial lung disease due to AA amyloidosis. Thorax 1992; 47:323–324.

366. Cordier JF, Loire R, Brune J. Amyloidosis of the lower respiratory tract. Chest 1986; 90:827–831.

367. Utz JP, Swensen SJ, Gertz MA. Pulmonary amyloidosis. The Mayo Clinic experience from 1980 to 1993. Ann Intern Med 1996; 124:407–413.

368. Gal R, Korzets A, Schwartz A, Rathwolfson L, Gafter U. Systemic distribution of beta2microglobulin-derived amyloidosis in patients who undergo long-term hemodialysis - report of seven cases and review of the literature. Arch Pathol Lab Med 1994; 118:718–721.

369. Kavuru MS, Adamo JP, Ahmad M, Mehta AC, Gephardt GN. Amyloidosis and pleural disease. Chest 1990; 98:20–23.

370. Gillmore JD, Hawkins PN. Amyloidosis and the respiratory tract. Thorax 1999; 54:444–451.

371. Shah PL, Gillmore JD, Copley SJ, et al. The importance of complete screening for amyloid fibril type and systemic disease in patients with amyloidosis in the respiratory tract. Sarcoidosis Vasc Diffuse Lung Dis 2002; 19:134–142.

372. Kijner CH, Yousem SA. Systemic light chain deposition disease presenting as multiple pulmonary nodules. A case report and review of the literature. Am J Surg Pathol 1988; 12:405–413.

373. Shiue S-T, McNally DP. Pulmonary hypertension from prominent vascular involvement in diffuse amyloidosis. Arch Intern Med 1988; 148:687–689.

374. Johnson WJ, Lie JT. Pulmonary hypertension and familial Mediterranean fever – a previously unrecognised association. Mayo Clin Proc 1991; 66:919–925.

375. Nicholson AG, Wells AU, Hooper J, Hansell DM, Kelleher A, Morgan C. Successful treatment of endogenous lipoid pneumonia due to Niemann–Pick type B disease with whole-lung lavage. Am J Respir Crit Care Med 2002; 165:128–131.

376. Wolsen AH. Pulmonary findings in Gaucher's disease. Am J Roentol 1975; 123:712–715.

377. Schneider EL, Epstein CJ, Kaback MJ, Brandes D. Severe pulmonary involvement in adult Gaucher's disease: report of three cases and review of the literature. Am J Med 1977; 63:475–480.

378. Smith RRL, Hutchins GM, Sack GH, Ridolfi RL. Unusual cardiac, renal and pulmonary involvement in Gaucher's disease. Interstitial glucocerebroside accumulation, pulmonary hypertension and fatal bone marrow embolisation. Am J Med 1978; 65:352–359.

379. Morimura Y, Hojo H, Abe M, Wakasa H. Gaucher's disease, type i (adult type), with massive involvement of the kidneys and lungs. Virchows Arch 1994; 425:537–540.

380. Santamaria F, Parenti G, Guidi G, et al. Pulmonary manifestations of Gaucher disease: an increased risk for L444P homozygotes? Am J Respir Crit Care Med 1998; 157:985–989.

381. Amir G, Ron N. Pulmonary pathology in Gaucher's disease. Hum Pathol 1999; 30:666–670.

382. Minai OA, Sullivan EJ, Stoller JK. Pulmonary involvement in Niemann–Pick disease: Case report and literature review. Resp Med 2000; 94:1241–1251.

383. Elleder M, Houstkova H, Zeman J, Ledvinova J, Poupetova H. Pulmonary storage with emphysema as a sign of Niemann–Pick type C2 disease (second complementation group). Report of a case. Virchows Archiv 2001; 439:206–211.

384. Niggemann B, Rebien W, Rahn W, Wahn U. Asymptomatic pulmonary involvement in two children with Niemann–Pick disease type B. Respiration 1994; 61:55–57.

385. Smith P, Heath D, Rodgers B, Helliwell T. Pulmonary vasculature in Fabry's disease. Histopathology 1991; 19:567–569.

386. Brown LK, Miller A, Bhuptani A, et al. Pulmonary involvement in Fabry disease. Amer J Respir Crit Care Med 1997; 155:1004–1010.

387. Sastre J, Renedo G, Mangado NG, Cabrera P, Lahoz F. Pulmonary ceroidosis. Chest 1987; 91:281–283.

388. Takahashi K, Hakozaki H, Kojima M. Idiopathic pulmonary ceroidosis. Acta Pathol Jpn 1978; 28:301–311.

389. Hermansky F, Pudlak P. Albinism associated with hemorrhagic diathesis and unusual pigmented cells in the bone marrow: report of two cases with histochemical studies. Blood 1959; 14:162–169.

390. Gahl WA, Brantly M, Kaiser Kupfer MI, et al. Genetic defects and clinical characteristics of patients with a form of oculocutaneous albinism (Hermansky-Pudlak syndrome). N Engl J Med 1998; 338:1258–1264.

391. Garay SM, Gardella JE, Fazzini EP, Goldring RM. Hermansky-Pudlak syndrome. Pulmonary manifestations of a ceroid storage disorder. Am J Med 1979; 66:737–747.

392. Luisetti M, Fiocca R, Pozzi E, De Rose V, Magrini U, Grassi C. The Hermansky-Pudlak syndrome. A case with macrophage-neutrophil alveolitis. Eur J Respir Dis 1986; 68:301–305.

393. Shinella RA, Greco MA, Garay SM. Hermansky-Pudlak syndrome: a clinicopathologic study. Hum Pathol 1985; 16:366–376.

394. White DA, Walker Smith GJ, Cooper JAD, et al. Hermansky–Pudlak syndrome and interstitial lung disease: a report of a case with lavage findings. Am Rev Respir Dis 1984; 130:138–141.

395. Reynolds SP, Davies BH, Gibbs AR. Diffuse pulmonary fibrosis and the Hermansky–Pudlak syndrome: clinical course and postmortem findings. Thorax 1994; 49:617–618.

396. Wockel W, Sultz J. Diffuse pulmonary fibrosis and Hermansky–Pudlak syndrome. Thorax 1995; 50:591.

397. Nakatani Y, Nakamura N, Sano J, et al. Interstitial pneumonia in Hermansky–Pudlak syndrome: significance of florid foamy swelling/degeneration (Giant lamellar body degeneration) of type-2 pneumocytes. Virchows Archiv 2000; 437:304–313.

398. Walker PP, Rose E, Williams JG. Upper airways abnormalities and tracheal problems in Morquio's disease. Thorax 2003; 58:458–459.

399. Reinila A. Perivascular xanthogranulomatosis in the lungs of diabetic patients. Arch Pathol Lab Med 1976; 100:542–543.

400. Duboucher C, Escamilla R, Rocchiccioli F, Negre A, Lageron A, Migueres J. Pulmonary lipogranulomatosis due to excessive consumption of apples. Chest 1986; 90:611–612.

401. Rosier RN, Rosenberg AE, Hornicek FJ. A 41-year-old man with multiple bony lesions and adjacent soft-tissue masses – Erdheim–Chester disease involving multiple bones, with pathologic fractures and soft-tissue masses. N Engl J Med 2000; 342:875–883.

402. AlQuran S, Reith J, Bradley J, Rimsza L. Erdheim–Chester disease: Case report, PCR-based analysis of clonality, and review of literature. Modern Pathol 2002; 15:666–672.

403. Chetritt J, Paradis V, Dargere D, et al. Chester–Erdheim disease: A neoplastic disorder. Hum Pathol 1999; 30:1093–1096.

404. Kambouchner M, Colby TV, Domenge C, Battesti JP, Soler P, Tazi A. Erdheim–Chester disease with prominent pulmonary involvement

associated with eosinophilic granuloma of mandibular bone. Histopathology 1997; 30:353–358.

405. Egan AJM, Boardman LA, Tazelaar HD, et al. Erdheim–Chester disease – Clinical, radiologic, and histopathologic findings in five patients with interstitial lung disease. Am J Surg Pathol 1999; 23: 17–26.

406. Rush WL, Andriko JAW, GalateauSalle F, et al. Pulmonary pathology of Erdheim–Chester disease. Modern Pathol 2000; 13:747–754.

406a. Allen TC, Chevez-Barrios P, Shetlar DJ, Cagle PT. Pulmonary and ophthalmic involvement with Erdheim-Chester disease: a case report and review of the literature. Arch Pathol Lab Med 2004; 128:1428–1431.

407. Devouassoux G, Lantuejoul S, Chatelain P, Brambilla E, Brambilla C. Erdheim–Chester disease: A primary macrophage cell disorder. Am J Respir Crit Care Med 1998; 157:650–653.

408. Brower AC, Worsham GF, Dudley AH. Erdheim–Chester disease: a distinct lipoidosis or part of the spectrum of histiocytosis? Radiology 1984; 151:35–38.

409. Athanasou NA, Barbatis C. Erdheim–Chester disease with epiphyseal and systemic disease. J Clin Pathol 1993; 46:481–482.

410. Bourke SC, Nicholson AG, Gibson GJ. Erdheim–Chester disease: pulmonary infiltration responding to cyclophosphamide and prednisolone. Thorax 2003; 58:1004–1005.

411. Marvisi M, Brianti M, Marani G, DelBorello P, Bortesi ML, Guariglia A. Hyperthyroidism and pulmonary hypertension. Resp Med 2002; 96:215–220.

412. Gottehrer A, Roa J, Stanford GG, Chernow B, Sahn SA. Hypothyroidism and pleural effusion. Chest 1990; 98:1130–1132.

413. Naeye RL. Capillary and venous lesions in myxedema. Lab Invest 1963; 12:465–470.

414. Sandler M, Bunn AE, Stewart RI. Cross-section study of pulmonary function in patients with insulin-dependent diabetes mellitus. Am Rev Respir Dis 1987; 135:223–229.

415. Guazzi M, Brambilla R, DeVita S, Guazzi MD. Diabetes worsens pulmonary diffusion in heart failure, and insulin counteracts this effect. Am J Respir Crit Care Med 2002; 166:978–982.

416. Vracko R, Thorning D, Huang TW. Basal lamina of alveolar epithelium and capillaries: quantitative changes with aging and diabetes mellitus. Am Rev Respir Dis 1979; 120:973–983.

417. Sandler M. Is the lung a target organ in diabetes mellitus? Arch Intern Med 1990; 150:1385–1388.

418. Watanabe K, Senju S, Toyoshima H, Yoshida M. Thickness of the basement membrane of bronchial epithelial cells in lung diseases as determined by transbronchial biopsy. Resp Med 1997; 91:406–410.

419. Weynand B, Jonckheere A, Frans A, Rahier J. Diabetes mellitus induces a thickening of the pulmonary basal lamina. Respiration 1999; 66:14–19.

420. Minette P, Buysschaert M, Rahier J, Veriter C, Frans A. Pulmonary gas exchange in life-long nonsmoking patients with diabetes mellitus. Respiration 1999; 66:20–24.

421. Farina J, Furio V, Fernandezacenero MJ, Muzas MA. Nodular fibrosis of the lung in diabetes mellitus. Virchows Arch 1995; 427:61–63.

422. Sugahara K, Ushijima K, Morioka T, Usuku G. Studies of the lung in diabetes mellitus. I. Ultrastructural studies of the lungs in alloxan-induced diabetic rats. Virchows Arch A Pathol Anat Histopathol 1981; 390:313–324.

423. Kida K, Utsuyama M, Thurlbeck WM. Changes in lung morphologic features and elasticity caused by streptozotocin-induced diabetes mellitus in growing rats. Am Rev Respir Dis 1983; 128:125–131.

424. Ofulue AF, Kida K, Thurlbeck WM. Experimental diabetes and the lung. I. Changes in growth, morphometry, and biochemistry. Am Rev Respir Dis 1988; 137:162–166.

425. Ofulue AF, Thurlbeck WM. Experimental diabetes and the lung. II. In vivo connective tissue metabolism. Am Rev Respir Dis 1988; 138:284–289.

426. Popov D, Simionescu M. Alterations of lung structure in experimental diabetes, and diabetes associated with hyperlipidaemia in hamsters. Eur Resp J 1997; 10:1850–1858.

427. Shields PA, Jeffery PK. The combined effects of vitamin A-deficiency and cigarette smoke on rat tracheal epithelium. Br J Exp Pathol 1987; 68:705–717.

428. Hennekens CH, Buring JE, Manson JE, et al. Lack of effect of long-term supplementation with beta carotene on the incidence of malignant neoplasms and cardiovascular disease. N Engl J Med 1996; 334:1145–1149.

429. Omenn GS, Goodman GE, Thornquist MD, et al. Effects of a combination of beta carotene and vitamin A on lung cancer and cardiovascular disease. N Engl J Med 1996; 334:1150–1155.

Skin diseases

430. de Carvalho CRR, Amato MBP, da Silva LMMF, Barbas CSV, Kairalla RA, Saldiva PHN. Obstructive respiratory failure in cicatricial pemphigoid. Thorax 1989; 44:601–602.

431. Osmanski JP, Fraire AE, Schaefer OP. Necrotising tracheobronchitis with progressive airflow obstruction associated with paraneoplastic pemphigus. Chest 1997; 112:1704–1707.

432. Takimoto CH, Warnock M, Golden JA. Sweet's syndrome with lung involvement. Am Rev Respir Dis 1991; 143:177–179.

433. Lazarus AA, McMillan M, Miramadi A. Pulmonary involvement in Sweet's syndrome (acute febrile neutrophilic dermatosis). Preleukemic and leukemic phases of acute myelogenous leukemia. Chest 1986; 90:922–924.

434. Thurnheer R, Stammberger U, Hailemariam S, Russi EW. Bronchial manifestation of acute febrile neutrophilic dermatosis (Sweet's syndrome). Eur Resp J 1998; 11:978–980.

435. Kruger S, Piroth W, Takyi BA, Brener C, Schwarz ER. Multiple aseptic pulmonary nodules with central necrosis in association with pyoderma gangrenosum. Chest 2001; 119: 977–978.

Gynaecological and obstetric conditions

436. Meigs JV, Cass JW. Fibroma of the ovary with ascites and hydrothorax. Am J Obstet Gynecol 1937; 33:249–267.

437. Meigs JV. Fibroma of the ovary with ascites and hydrothorax – Meigs' syndrome. Am J Obstet Gynecol 1954; 67:962.

438. Meigs JV. Pelvic tumours other than fibromas of the ovary with ascites and hydrothorax. Obstet Gynecol 1954; 3:471.

439. Parry D, Hextall A, Robinson VP, Banner NR, Yacoub MH. Pregnancy following a single lung transplant. Thorax 1996; 51:1162–1164.

440. Phelan JP. Pulmonary edema in obstetrics. Obstet Gynecol Clin North Am 1991; 18:319–331.

441. Sibai BM, Mabie WC. Hemodynamics of preeclampsia. Clin Perinatol 1991; 18:727–747.

442. Flieder DB, Moran CA, Travis WD, Koss MN, Mark EJ. Pleuro-pulmonary endometriosis and pulmonary ectopic deciduosis: A clinicopathologic and immunohistochemical study of 10 cases with emphasis on diagnostic pitfalls. Hum Pathol 1998; 29:1495–1503.

443. Maurer RR, Schall JA, Mendex FLJ. Chronic recurring spontaneous pneumothorax due to endometriosis of the diaphragm. JAMA 1972; 168:2012–2014.

444. Stern H, Toole A, Merino M. Catamenial pneumothorax. Chest 1980; 78:480–482.

445. Alifano M, Roth T, Broet SC, Schussler O, Magdeleinat P, Regnard JF. Catamenial pneumothorax – A prospective study. Chest 2003; 124; 1004–1008.

446. Wilkins SB, Bell-Thompson J, Tyras DH. Hemothorax associated with endometriosis. J Thorac Cardiovasc Surg 1985; 89:636–638.

447. Slasky BS, Siewers RD, Lecky JW, Zajko A, Burkholder JA. Catamenial pneumothorax: the roles of diaphragmatic defects and endometriosis. Am J Roentol 1982; 138:639–643.

448. Jelihovsky T, Grant AF. Endometriosis of the lung. A case report and brief review of the literature. Thorax 1968; 23:434–437.

449. Di Palo S, Mari G, Castoldi R, Staudacher C, Taccagni G, Di Carlo V. Endometriosis of the lung. Respir Med 1989; 83:255–258.

450. Bateman ED, Morrison SC. Catamenial haemoptysis from endobronchial endometriosis - a case report and review of previously reported cases. Respir Med 1990; 84:157–161.

451. Hobbs JE, Bortnick R. Endometriosis of the lung: an experimental and clinical study. Am J Obstet Gynecol 1940; 40:832–843.

452. Kiyan E, Kilicaslan Z, Caglar E, Yilmazbayhan D, Tabak L, Gurgan M. An unusual radiographic finding in pulmonary parenchymal endometriosis. Acta Radiol 2002; 43:164–166.

453. Orriols R, Munoz X, Alvarez A, Sampol G. Chest CT scanning: utility in lung endometriosis. Respir Med 1998; 92:876–877.

454. Cassina PC, Hauser M, Kacl G, Imthurn B, Schroder S, Weder W. Catamenial hemoptysis. Diagnosis with MRI. Chest 1997; 111:1447–1450.

455. Kuo PH, Wang HC, Liaw YS, Kuo SH. Bronchoscopic and angiographic findings in tracheobronchial endometriosis. Thorax 1996; 51:1060–1061.

456. Park WW. The occurrence of decidual tissue within the lung: report of a case. J Pathol Bacteriol 1954; 67:563–570.

457. Cameron HM, Park WW. Decidual tissue within the lung. J Obstet Gynaec Brit Commonw 1965; 72:748–752.

458. Joseph J, Sahn SA. Thoracic endometriosis syndrome: new observations from an analysis of 110 cases. Am J Med 1996; 100:164–170.

459. Inoue T, Kurokawa Y, Kaiwa Y, et al. Video-assisted thoracoscopic surgery for catamenial hemoptysis. Chest 2001; 120:655–658.

11

Lung transplantation

Revised by Margaret Burke

Human lung transplantation was first performed in 1963 but few patients survived and the operation was largely abandoned until the advent of cyclosporin and the development of combined heart and lung transplantation nearly 20 years later. Today over 20 000 lung transplants have been performed and the procedure is firmly established among the therapeutic options available for patients with severe lung disease.[1] Donor shortage is the main factor limiting its application. This has caused the number of lung transplants to plateau at about 1700 procedures per year worldwide and has led to the occasional use of live donors.[2] About 2% of lung transplants are repeat operations, performed because of graft failure. Patients receiving lung transplants have ranged from infants to the elderly, with the peak age being about 50 years. The principal conditions treated by lung transplantation in adults have been chronic obstructive pulmonary disease/emphysema (48%), pulmonary fibrosis (17%), cystic fibrosis (16%) and primary pulmonary hypertension (4%).[1] The most common indication for lung transplantation in adolescents is cystic fibrosis and in children congenital heart disease.[3]

TYPES OF LUNG TRANSPLANT

Combined heart and lung transportation, which was first performed in 1981, was followed by single lung transplantation, then double lung transplantation and lastly sequential bilateral lung transplantation. The combined operation requires total cardiopulmonary bypass and if successful carries a risk of accelerated coronary atheroma and problems resulting from cardiac denervation. However, it is relatively simple technically, maintains coronary-tracheobronchial arterial anastomoses that help the tracheal anastomosis to heal, and is particularly suitable when both heart and lungs are damaged, as in pulmonary hypertension. In cystic fibrosis, it is necessary to replace both lungs to avoid the risk of spillover infection. Double lung transplantation is a complex procedure but was initially used in emphysema because it was feared that with single lung transplantation the native diseased lung would be preferentially ventilated. This proved not to be the case and single lung transplantation is now widely used for both severe emphysema and pulmonary fibrosis. It is the most common procedure, the simplest to perform, is associated with the fewest postoperative complications, requires the least amount of donor tissue and enables the greatest number of recipients to benefit from a single donor.

Except for bronchial artery re-vascularisation, which is undertaken in only a few centres,[4,5] no attempt is made to re-anastomose the severed tracheal or bronchial blood vessels and nerves in any of these operations, or the lymphatics, which are also severed if the heart is not included. Loss of these structures promotes postoperative haemorrhage, breakdown of the tracheal or bronchial anastomosis, a reduction in the cough reflex and pulmonary oedema. A further aspect of lung transplantation is that some lymphatic tissue is inevitably included in the allograft, entailing a risk of graft-versus-host disease. This is greatest when the whole mediastinum is transferred, as in combined heart and lung transplantation.

The mortality associated with lung transplantation is constantly diminishing, as techniques and immunosuppression improve. In 2004 the International Society of Heart-Lung Transplantation (*www.ishlt.org*) reported survival rates of 74%, 47% and 24% at 1, 5 and 10 years, respectively for lung transplantation and 62%, 41% and 26% at the same periods for combined heart-lung transplantation (Fig. 11.1).[1,6] In the first postoperative month, mortality is chiefly due to sepsis, haemorrhage and poor lung preservation. After the first month the principal causes of death are infection and rejection in the form of obliterative bronchiolitis.

RECIPIENT SELECTION

Lung transplantation is an operation of last resort. There are insufficient donors and patients are unlikely to be considered unless other measures have failed and their short-term prognosis is otherwise poor. The presence of uncontrolled systemic disease precludes consideration and good renal and hepatic function is essential, particularly in view of immunosuppres-

sant drug toxicity.[7] This is particularly important in α-1 antitrypsin deficiency and cystic fibrosis, both of which may affect the liver directly. Any infection that cannot be eliminated, either before or by the operation, is likely to disseminate postoperatively because of the immunosuppression and therefore militates against successful transplantation. An aspergilloma is a contraindication to any form of lung transplantation as its attempted removal inevitably leads to seeding of the pleural cavity and mediastinum. Previous thoracic surgery may make it difficult to operate and the possibility of a future lung transplant should therefore be borne in mind when considering the best treatment for conditions such as pneumothorax. Left ventricular function should be normal or near normal although treatable coronary artery disease is not an absolute contraindication. Ventilator support prior to transplantation is a significant risk factor at 1 and 5 years.[1] Pulmonary neoplasia is generally regarded as a contraindication because of its early dissemination but bronchioloalveolar carcinoma is often limited to the lungs and double lung transplantation has been employed to treat this form of lung cancer.[8–10]

DONOR MATCHING

The selection and management of donors and preservation of the harvested lung are crucial to reducing the impact of brain stem death on the lung and minimising re-implantation injury. Brain stem death leads to adrenergic systemic hypertension, which results in fluid shifting to the lesser circulation and neurogenic pulmonary oedema. Such injury is part of a generalised release of cytokines and other inflammatory mediators that damage many organs, including the lungs, where it may compound the other causes of injury so that only about 20% of donated cadaver lungs can be used.[11]

Current donor selection criteria include age less than 65 years, ABO compatibility, a clear chest X-ray, no airway mucosal

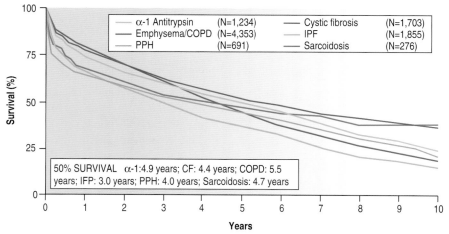

Figure 11.1 Adult lung transplantation: actuarial survival by diagnosis. COPD, chronic obstructive pulmonary disease; IPF, idiopathic pulmonary fibrosis; PPH, primary pulmonary hypertension. (Adapted from Hertz *et al.* The registry of the International Society for Heart and Lung Transplantation introduction to the Twentieth Annual Reports – 2003. Journal of Heart Lung Transplant 2003; 22:610–615,[6] with permission from the International Society for Heart and Lung Transplantation.)

inflammation at bronchoscopy and no history of lung contusion, severe chest trauma, previous cardiopulmonary surgery or aspiration.[12] Donor seropositivity for cytomegalovirus is dangerous in a seronegative recipient.[1] Persistent hepatitis B antigenaemia and HIV infection are further contraindications. Physiotherapy, bronchial toilet, prophylactic antibiotics (if required) and monitoring of blood gases and pulmonary wedge pressure are all important in managing a potential donor. Harvested lungs are best stored inflated, cooled and flushed through the pulmonary artery with Euro-Collins solution. Ischaemia is tolerated for up to 8 h.[12] Donor-recipient matching includes an approximate similarity in chest size. One lobe of an adult's lung may be used to replace a whole lung of a child. Tissue transplanted into a child grows at a normal rate.[13]

Potential recipients are screened for donor-specific lymphocytic antibodies ('panel-reactive antibodies') against a wide range of HLA-A, -B and -DR antigens. The result is considered positive if the recipient's serum reacts to more than 10% of the HLA antigens in the panel, in which case donor-specific T- and B-lymphocytotoxic antibody cross-matching is required, a positive result here contraindicating transplantation from that donor as it promotes accelerated graft rejection.[14,15]

IMMUNOSUPPRESSION

The recipient's immunity is suppressed with a combination of cyclosporin, azathioprine and prednisolone with backup provided by drugs such as tacrolimus, mycophenolate mofetil, everolimus and sirolimus. All these drugs have side-effects, notably renal, hepatic and bone marrow toxicity, and an increased risk of neoplasia. Antithymocyte globulin is now seldom used and cyclophosphamide and plasmapheresis are reserved for use in antibody-mediated rejection. Low-dose septrin is administered prophylactically against pneumocystis infection.

RECIPIENT MONITORING

Frequent monitoring of the lung transplant recipient is essential in the first 6 months after transplantation when the risk of the main complications, acute rejection and infection, is greatest. Recipients undergo frequent clinical review and bronchoscopy is undertaken in response to symptoms, radiographic changes, unexplained fever or a sudden deterioration in lung function. Both bronchoalveolar lavage and transbronchial biopsy are generally performed.[16] Lavage is particularly useful for detecting infection while transbronchial lung biopsy, despite a false-negative rate of about 20% is the mainstay in the diagnosis of allograft rejection.[17] Rejection of the heart in combined heart and lung transplant recipients is rare and endomyocardial biopsies provide an unreliable guide to pulmonary rejection.[18]

Production of *de novo* donor-specific HLA antibodies and of non-HLA antibodies such as anti-endothelial antibodies may predict the development of chronic rejection,[19,20] and testing for these is now common.

Recent advances in genetic research have led to the development of DNA microarrays, or gene chips, capable of identifying genes specific to cellular immunity.[21] Preliminary results suggest that their identification may predict acute cellular rejection and hence assist in defining treatment strategies specific to the individual recipient.[22]

ROLE OF THE HISTOPATHOLOGIST

Histopathology plays a major role in assessing the postoperative complications of transplantation, but can contribute more than this to the management of transplant recipients, both before and after the operation (Box 11.1).[23,24] An accurate preoperative diagnosis is important because histopathological reassessment of the potential recipient may affect the choice of transplantation procedure and identify conditions treatable by other means or that need to be eradicated before transplantation is undertaken. It may also predict the presence of systemic disease and the likelihood of the original disease recurring in the allograft, or detect malignant disease, which apart from bronchioloalveolar carcinoma is an absolute contraindication to transplantation. Explanted lungs should also be examined, and without delay, in case they show unsuspected diseases such as tuberculosis, sarcoidosis or malignancy that may be active elsewhere in the recipient.[25] Similarly, if only one donor lung is used, the other should be examined, as this may identify unsuspected infection or other disease that is likely also to be present in the graft. Thus, histopathologists should not be concerned solely in assessing complications, but this is undoubtedly their major role and the rest of this chapter will be largely confined to this aspect of transplantation.

COMPLICATIONS (Box 11.2)

To assess complications, at least five pieces of alveolated lung should be examined at a minimum of three levels each, using connective tissue and fungal stains in addition to haematoxylin and eosin. Because sequential sampling is common, the possibility of observed abnormalities being due to previous biopsies always has to be considered. It is also important to remember that some patterns of lung injury are non-specific.

Box 11.1 The role of the histopathologist in lung transplantation

Diagnosis of the underlying disease before transplantation
Examination of the explanted lung to verify the diagnosis and identify any other diseases that may be present
Examination of any unused donor tissue
Biopsy assessment of post-transplant complications
Post mortem examination

As well as contributing to the outcome of the transplantation, the histopathologist is well-placed to undertake collaborative research.

Box 11.2 Complications of lung transplantation

Postoperative
   Haemorrhage and other surgical complications
   Reimplantation syndrome
   Diffuse alveolar damage
Early and late airway complications
   Anastomotic dehiscence, granulation tissue overgrowth
   Bronchial stenosis, chondromalacia, ectasia
Rejection
Infection
Neoplasia
Post-transplantation lymphoproliferative disorders
Graft-versus-host disease
Recurrence of the underlying disease
Drug effects

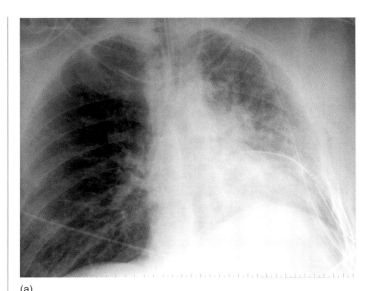

(a)

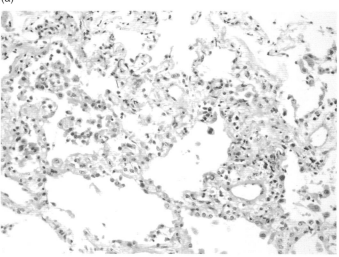

(b)

Figure 11.2 Reimplantation injury presenting as (a) hazy shadowing of left donor lung 3 days after single lung transplantation for emphysema; (b) biopsy shows focal interstitial oedema, subacute inflammation, pneumocyte hyperplasia and aggregates of alveolar macrophages.

For example, diffuse alveolar damage may reflect severe re-perfusion injury, infection or acute rejection. It may require special stains for infective agents and a consideration of the timing of events to distinguish these causes. There may be both rejection and infection and as their histological features overlap the biopsy findings should always be interpreted in the light of the clinical and radiological features, previous biopsy findings and results of current microbiological and serological investigations.

Perioperative allograft injury

Even if the operation goes well and there are no surgical complications, the early postoperative period is often marked by a temporary period of dyspnoea. Chest radiographs at this time often show hilar opacification and if biopsy is undertaken this generally shows pulmonary oedema accompanied by a mild neutrophil exudate (Fig. 11.2).[26] These changes, termed reimplantation injury, are variously attributed to deterioration of the graft, surgical trauma, ischaemia, severance of the pulmonary lymphatics and the release of free radicals and chemokines from neutrophils interacting with the graft endothelium damaged by ischaemia.[27] They settle as lymphatics regenerate and lung drainage is re-established but may be complicated by airway infection promoted by slow recovery of mucociliary clearance.[28,29]

More severe changes include those of diffuse alveolar damage, to which the term primary graft failure has been applied.[30] It may represent a reimplantation response, rejection, infection or occur for no obvious cause. It may progress to parenchymal fibrosis. It is associated with reduced survival at 1 year.[31]

Alveolar proteinosis and an unusual neutrophil-rich pattern of mixed interstitial pneumonitis have also been described in the perioperative period.[32,33]

Complications involving the airway anastomosis

Apart from the combined heart-lung procedure, lung transplantation inevitably involves severance of the tracheobronchial blood supply so that the donor airway receives only retrograde pulmonary arterial blood until new bronchial arterial anastomoses develop. It is not surprising therefore that poor healing at the airway anastomosis has been a serious complication, although improved surgical techniques such as bronchial artery revascularisation, performed at the time of transplantation, have rendered it less common.[4,5] The anastomosis is also subject to infection until the surface epithelium heals and mucociliary clearance recovers.[29] Denervation contributes to the risk of infection by eliminating the cough reflex and promoting aspiration.[34] Dehiscence of the airway anastomosis is a devastating early complication, but one that is fortunately now rare. More common is the development of exuberant granulation tissue. This may seriously narrow the airway and require endoscopic removal or cryotherapy.[35] Late airway complications include

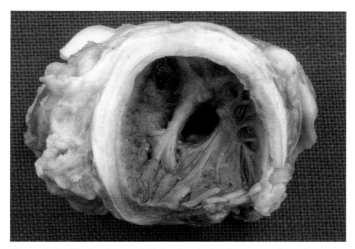

Figure 11.3 Tracheal stenosis following double lung transplantation.

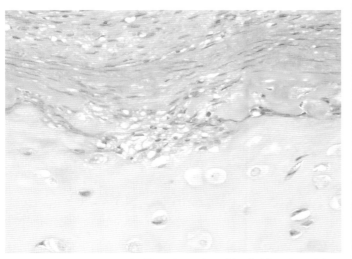

Figure 11.4 Bronchomalacia. There is erosion of the limiting plate of the bronchial cartilage.

stenosis and bronchomalacia (Figs 11.3, 11.4), requiring the insertion of stents.[36]

Rejection

The mechanisms underlying lung allograft rejection are not fully understood but the process is probably initiated by T-cell recognition of histocompatibility antigens on the surface of donor cells.[37] The brunt of the rejection damage is on the blood vessels and airways, this presumably reflecting the increased expression of histocompatibility antigens by the pulmonary vascular endothelium and airway epithelium that has been shown to follow transplantation.[37] Incompatibility is followed by the activation and sequestration of platelets, neutrophils and macrophages within the pulmonary capillaries, the release of reactive oxygen species and inflammatory cytokines, and increased expression of endothelin and inducible nitric oxide synthase.[38–40] The rejection process probably involves both antibody and cell-mediated immune mechanisms but the extent to which these each contribute varies: hyperacute rejection is generally regarded as being antibody-mediated whereas acute and chronic rejection are thought to be predominantly cell-mediated.

Hyperacute allograft rejection

Hyperacute rejection occurs within 48 h of transplantation. It is characterised by marked congestion and oedema, resulting in the production of copious frothy bloodstained fluid from the bronchial orifice of the allograft. Risk factors include multiple blood transfusions, pregnancy, surgery and previous transplantation, any of which necessitates donor-specific pre-transplant T- and B-lymphocytotoxic antibody cross-matching (see above).

Microscopy shows marked pulmonary congestion and oedema, alveolar haemorrhage, vascular thrombosis, neutrophil infiltration, endothelial and epithelial damage, and ultimately diffuse alveolar damage (Fig. 11.5). The diagnosis is confirmed by the detection by immunofluorescence of IgG deposition on endothelium, along vessel walls and in alveolar spaces, and by a strongly positive IgG-mediated lymphocytotoxic reaction to donor T and/or B-lymphocytes.[41–43]

Acute allograft rejection

Acute rejection is characterised clinically by dyspnoea, fever, hypoxaemia and pleuropulmonary opacification (Fig. 11.6). It is most frequent in the first postoperative year, typically developing within a few months of the operation but sometimes within a few weeks or several years later.

Acute and chronic rejection are classified and graded according to internationally agreed histological criteria (Box 11.3).[44,45] Acute rejection may be centred on the blood vessels or the airways but predominantly affects the former and the surrounding lung parenchyma. The vascular changes (Class A) are treated separately from those involving the airways (Class B) because the latter may also reflect chronic infection, ischaemia, aspiration or chronic rejection.[28,34,46,47]

Histologically, the vascular changes are characterised by an infiltrate of variable intensity comprising small lymphocytes, plasma cells, histiocytes and occasional neutrophils surrounding small blood vessels and infiltrating the adjacent alveolar interstitium. They are graded as minimal (grade A1) if they can hardly be discerned without high magnification and mild (grade A2) if they are just evident at low magnification and consist of an infiltrate that includes large activated lymphocytes with pyroninophilic cytoplasm and angulated nuclei. Neutrophils and eosinophils are also seen and there is infiltration of the vascular intima (lymphocytic intimitis or endothelialitis). Endothelial cells show hyperplasia. Moderate acute rejection (grade A3) is characterised by extension of the infiltrate into the alveolar interstitium, while in severe (grade A4) acute rejection, which is usually fatal, the infiltrate is widespread and accompanied by haemorrhagic oedema, increased numbers of alveolar macrophages, fibrinous exudates, hyaline membranes and

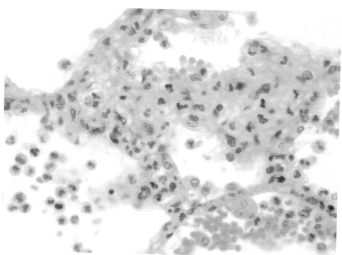

Figure 11.5 Hyperacute rejection. Neutrophils engorge the blood vessels and have passed into the alveolar interstitium and lumen. The patient died during the operation. Panel reactive antibodies were positive and a donor-specific lymphocytotoxic cross-match was strongly positive for T- and B-lymphocytes.

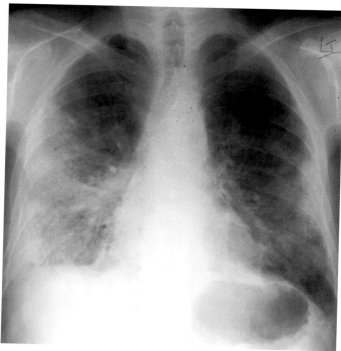

Figure 11.6 Chest radiograph in acute rejection showing opacification of the lower zone of the right lung, which was transplanted because of emphysema.

destructive changes typical of diffuse alveolar damage (Fig. 11.7). With successful suppression of the rejection, follow-up biopsies show a reduction in the infiltrate (termed resolving rejection/lower grade) and a change in its make-up to a mixture of small lymphocytes and haemosiderin-laden macrophages (termed resolved rejection or grade A0).[48]

Immunohistochemistry shows that the majority of the lymphoid cells are CD8-suppressor lymphocytes (Fig. 11.8).[49] They are often pyroninophilic and may express the lymphocyte activation antigen CD30 and the proliferation antigen Ki-67. B-lymphocytes are usually sparse; larger numbers may reflect rejection based on humoral rather than cellular mechanisms and therefore predict a poor response to the usual cell-based immunosuppressive regimes.[50] However, their presence should also prompt consideration of other entities such as eosinophilic pneumonia, fungal infection and lymphoproliferative disease.[51,52] The vascular endothelium and alveolar epithelium both show upregulation of class II HLA (HLA-DR) antigens.[37]

Although perivascular lymphoid cell infiltration is the hallmark of acute rejection, similar infiltrates may be seen in patients with infections and other conditions for which augmented immunosuppression is inappropriate. For this reason, acute rejection should only be diagnosed and graded in the absence of infection.[45] The opportunistic infections may be viral, particularly herpes simplex and cytomegalovirus. The distinctive inclusions of the latter may be modified by prior antiviral treatment and therefore difficult to identify (Fig. 11.9).[53] However, the infiltrates of a viral infection are generally more extensive and the pattern is predominantly that of an interstitial pneumonitis with secondary involvement of vessels.[53] Perivascular lymphoid infiltrates may also be seen in *P. jerovici* pneumonia.[54] and in other fungal and bacterial infections,

---

Box 11.3 Revised working formulation for the classification and grading of pulmonary rejection[45]

A	Acute rejection		
	Grade	0	None
		1	Minimal
		2	Mild
		3	Moderate
		4	Severe
B	Airway inflammation – lymphocytic bronchitis/bronchiolitis[a]		
	Grade	0	None
		1	Minimal
		2	Mild
		3	Moderate
		4	Severe
		BX	Ungradeable (sampling problems, infection, tangential sectioning)
C	Chronic airway rejection – obliterative bronchiolitis		
	a	Active	
	b	Inactive	
D	Chronic vascular rejection – accelerated graft vascular sclerosis		

A and B may coexist, as may C and D
[a]The grading of airway inflammation is frequently impractical and may be omitted

---

necessitating special stains, and in difficult cases immunocytochemistry and *in situ* hybridization.[55,56] Eosinophilic pneumonia is an uncommon manifestation of graft rejection and before accepting it as such, infection by organisms such as aspergillus should be excluded.[57,58] A predominantly neutrophilic infiltrate,

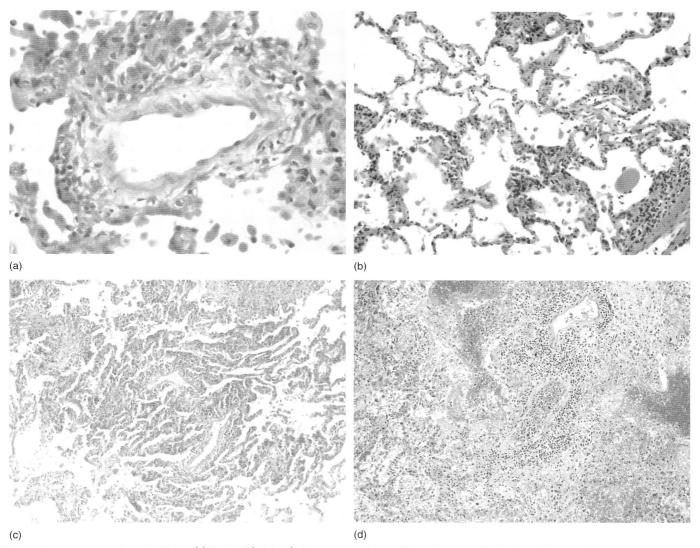

(a)

(b)

(c)

(d)

Figure 11.7   Acute parenchymal rejection. (a) Grade A1 (minimal) changes are not discernible at low magnification but high power shows a sparse perivascular lymphoid infiltrate. (b) Grade A2 (mild) shows a more marked infiltrate but this is still restricted to the vessels and the alveolar septa are spared. (c) Grade A3 (moderate) acute rejection showing spread of the infiltrate into surrounding alveolar septa. (d) Grade A4 (severe) acute rejection is characterised by diffuse alveolar damage and a dense perivascular lymphoid infiltrate.

necrosis and granuloma formation all favour infection rather than rejection.

Acute rejection should also be distinguished from the ischaemia-reperfusion injury described above and from the lymphoproliferative disorders described below.[52] Ischaemia-reperfusion injury lacks the perivascular and interstitial infiltration of rejection while a polymorphous, perivascular infiltrate of B- and T-lymphocytes with a predominance of the latter favours rejection rather than lymphoproliferative disease, which is characterised by a monomorphous infiltrate of large B-lymphocytes.[51] Mass lesions also favour lymphoproliferative disease or infection rather than rejection. Recurrence in the allograft of diseases such as sarcoidosis and Langerhans cell histiocytosis may also be misinterpreted as acute rejection if their characteristic features are not well represented.

Airway inflammation is the other major pattern of acute rejection. Evidence for it representing rejection is its progression to chronic rejection (obliterative bronchiolitis) and frequent response to augmented immunosuppression.[59] It may accompany or succeed the perivascular infiltrates described above or be seen alone, but most frequently follows the vascular changes.[28,28,47] The changes range from sparse airway cuffing by small lymphoid cells to diffuse infiltration of the lamina propria and epithelium by medium and large lymphoid cells and epithelial apoptosis (Fig. 11.10). In severe cases, the lymphoid cell infiltrate is particularly dense and there is ulceration and fibrinopurulent exudation. Airway inflammation may be graded in the same way as the perivascular infiltration but in practice the small size of the biopsies generally precludes the precision required for this.

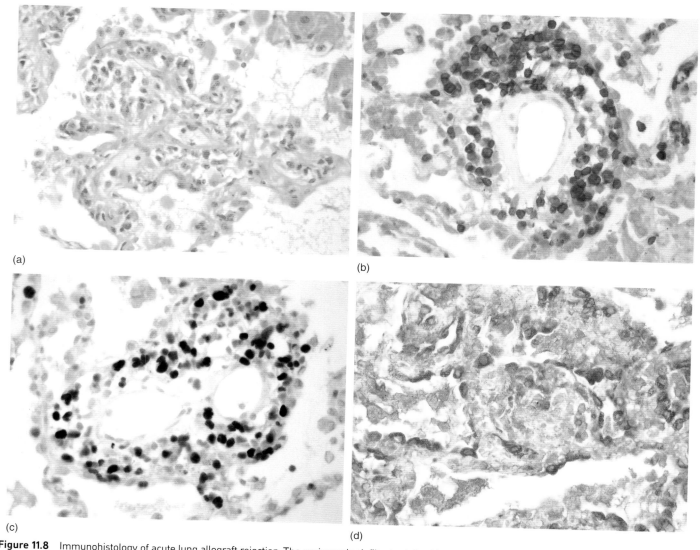

(a)

(b)

(c)

(d)

Figure 11.8 Immunohistology of acute lung allograft rejection. The perivascular infiltrate stained by haematoxylin and eosin in (a) expresses the T cell marker CD3 (b) and the proliferation marker Kiel-67 (c), while class II HLA-DR antigens are strongly expressed by alveolar epithelium and macrophages (d).

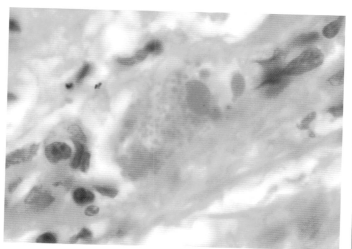

Figure 11.9 Fragmented cytomegalovirus inclusions after treatment with ganciclovir.

The differential diagnosis of airway inflammation includes the presence of bronchus-associated lymphoid tissue of donor origin, low-grade infection and the consequences of aspiration. Airway or parenchymal infection, notably by cytomegalovirus, may accompany rejection.[60]

Chronic allograft rejection

Chronic rejection of the transplanted lung is marked by progressive breathlessness, cough, which is often productive, fever and a decline in lung function.[61] The changes, which can be monitored by spirometry and imaging (Fig. 11.11), are centred on the bronchioles (Class C) and blood vessels (Class D). The former show constrictive obliterative bronchiolitis in which there is concentric or eccentric hyaline fibrous thickening of the bronchiolar submucosa, encroaching on the airway lumen and eventually resulting in total occlusion (Fig. 11.12).[62–65] The

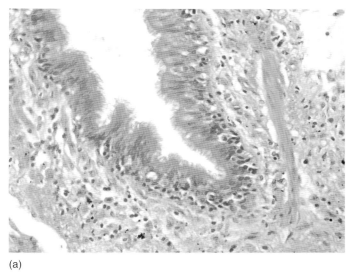

(a)

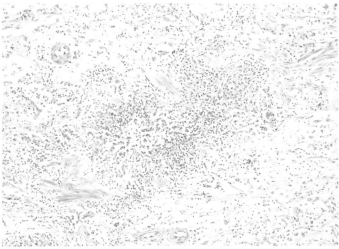

(b)

Figure 11.10 Acute airway rejection (lymphocytic bronchiolitis). (a) Grade B1 acute rejection is characterised by occasional small lymphocytes infiltrating the bronchiolar epithelium and lamina propria. (b) Grade B3 acute airway rejection shows extensive infiltration and obliteration of bronchiolar epithelium by lymphocytes.

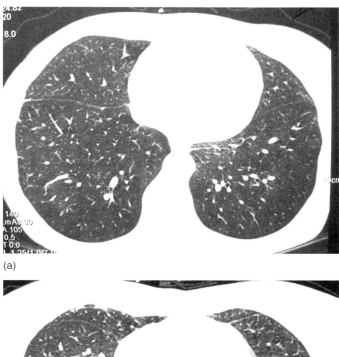

(a)

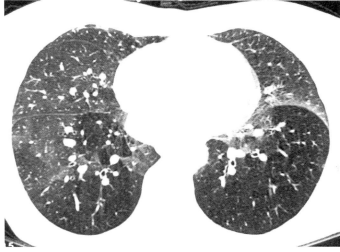

(b)

Figure 11.11 CT scan appearances in bronchiolitis obliterans syndrome: (a) the inspiratory image shows mild generalised hyperinflation with bronchial dilatation and wall thickening while (b) the expiratory image shows irregular dark areas of focal air-trapping.

recognition of obliterative bronchiolitis is the key discriminator between acute and chronic rejection. Residual bronchiolar epithelium may show squamous metaplasia and there is usually disruption of the muscle coat. The process may be active (i.e. associated with lymphocytic bronchiolitis) or inactive (consisting of dense fibrous scarring with minimal or no inflammation). The infiltrating cells are T-lymphocytes.[66] The process is patchy and therefore not always evident in small biopsies,[67,68] but its presence may be suggested by obstructive features such as the accumulation of foamy macrophages in distal airspaces. The adjacent lung may also show evidence of concomitant acute rejection (Fig. 11.13). Most patients with obliterative bronchiolitis also have bronchiectasis (Fig. 11.14), which probably results

from a combination of factors, including rejection, infection and denervation. Concomitant acute airway inflammation suggests post-obstructive infection.

Unfortunately, sampling error renders the diagnosis of obliterative bronchiolitis unreliable on small biopsies and its identification generally depends upon recognition of a bronchiolitis obliterans syndrome (BOS), which is defined as 'graft deterioration due to progressive airways disease for which there is no other cause'.[69–71] The principal role of transbronchial lung biopsy is therefore to exclude treatable causes of deterioration in lung function.

Obliterative bronchiolitis is seldom seen within 6 months of the operation and while its incidence diminishes after 1–2 years it affects 50% of recipients by 5 years.[67] Risk factors

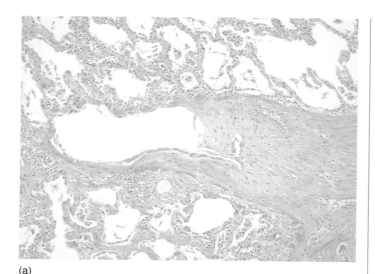

(a)

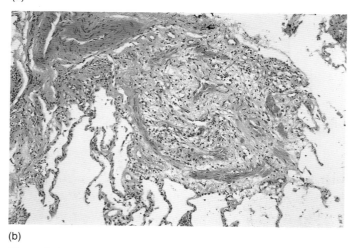

(b)

Figure 11.12 The histological spectrum of chronic airway rejection (obliterative bronchiolitis). (a) Partial occlusion of a bronchiole by plaque-like submucosal fibrous tissue with sparse chronic inflammation. (b) An incomplete ring of smooth muscle provides the only evidence that this focal pulmonary scar represents an obliterated bronchiole.

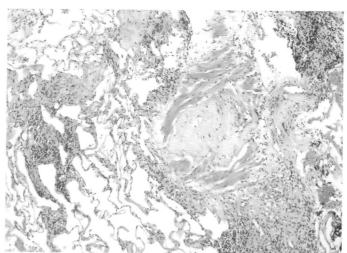

Figure 11.13 Concomitant acute and chronic rejection. Acute rejection is evidenced by a perivascular lymphoid infiltrate while a bronchiole totally obstructed by fibrous tissue is indicative of chronic rejection.

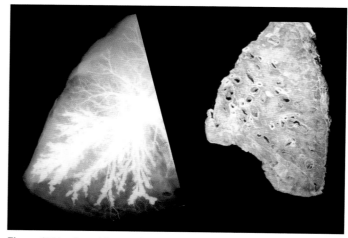

Figure 11.14 Bronchiographic and macroscopic appearances of chronic airway rejection complicated by bronchiectasis. (Illustration provided by Dr H. Tazelaar, Rochester, Minnesota, USA.)

include earlier rejection episodes and histocompatibility mismatch,[51,64,72,73] supporting the view that it represents a late manifestation of rejection,[47,74] with an immunological pathogenesis analogous to that occurring in rheumatoid and graft-versus-host disease.[75–78] The development of *de novo* anti-HLA antibodies following transplantation is also associated with an increased incidence of obliterative bronchiolitis.[19,20] Other causes include cytomegalovirus infection,[28,53,72,79,80] community acquired viral infection[81,82] and ischaemia.[83]

Chronic rejection may also involve the pulmonary vasculature, resulting in fibrointimal sclerosis of arteries and veins analogous to that occurring in the coronary arteries of heart and heart-lung allografts (Fig. 11.15).[84,85] It may be active or inactive and may be seen in association with obliterative bronchiolitis, which would then dominate the clinical picture. Its appearance

in biopsies is regarded as non-specific as it may also follow ischaemia, acute rejection, non-rejection related pulmonary inflammation and non-specific donor-related factors. It may be associated with similar coronary artery disease in combined heart-lung allografts.[62,86]

Infection

Infection[87] is a major hazard for the immunosuppressed recipient of a lung allograft. It is often multiple and may affect the native lung and other organs as well as the allograft. Its recognition in the lungs largely depends upon the microbiological examination of bronchoalveolar lavage fluid but the addition of

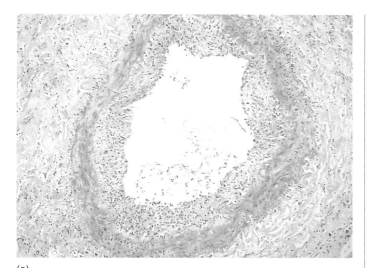

(a)

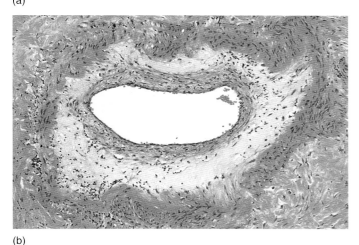

(b)

Figure 11.15 Chronic vascular rejection. (a) Active chronic rejection affecting a muscular artery. (b) A pulmonary artery shows severe intimal fibrosis.

Figure 11.16 Cytomegalovirus antigenaemia. Positive immunohistochemical staining of peripheral blood leukocytes for cytomegalovirus pp65 antigen.

transbronchial lung biopsy increases the detection rate.[16] Problems in biopsy interpretation include distinguishing rejection from infection, which is compounded by the atypical host response of the immunosuppressed patient. Distinguishing colonisation, subclinical infection and clinically-significant disease may also be difficult. The pathology of pulmonary infection is described in Chapter 5 but the special circumstances associated with transplantation warrant further comment on some infective agents here.

Viruses

Cytomegalovirus infection of a seronegative recipient, transmitted by blood transfusion or the graft, increases the incidence of rejection, probably by promoting the expression of the major histocompatibility antigens in the alveolar epithelium.[37,88,89] The recognition of clinically significant disease (as opposed to

mere carriage of the virus) is based upon identification of blood cytomegalovirus pp65 antigen (Fig. 11.16),[90,91] biopsy evidence of interstitial pneumonitis and bronchiolitis[92] and the detection of the virus. The latter often requires immunohistochemistry or molecular techniques such as the polymerase chain reaction because in the early stages of infection typical viral inclusions are often sparse (Fig. 11.17). Only in the later stages are there numerous intranuclear and cytoplasmic inclusions (Fig. 11.18). Other patterns of cytomegalovirus disease include poorly formed granulomas, diffuse alveolar damage and mass lesions simulating a tumour.[93] Viral prophylaxis may result in fragmented inclusions and an acute neutrophilic pneumonitis (Fig. 11.9).

Infection by *Herpes simplex* virus is infrequent in lung allograft recipients but may cause necrotizing tracheobronchitis and pneumonia in these patients.[94] Similarly, infection by influenza and respiratory syncytial viruses may cause significant morbidity and contribute to the development of bronchiolitis obliterans.[82,95] Other viral infections of note in transplant patients include pulmonary and systemic infection by varicella-zoster (Fig. 11.19).

Bacteria

Opportunistic mycobacteria originating in either the donor or recipient infect lung allograft recipients on rare occasions, or merely colonise the graft without causing disease.[96,97] Other bacterial infections of these patients include nocardiosis and legionella pneumonia.

Fungi

Pneumocystis jiroveci pneumonia is rare in lung transplantation because of chemoprophylaxis, the reported incidence being

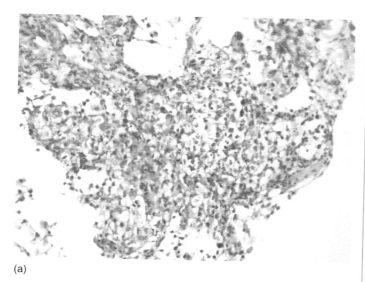

(a)

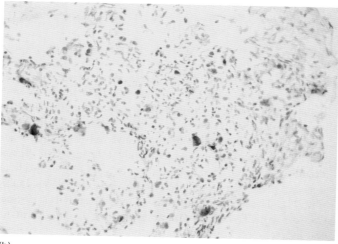

(b)

Figure 11.17 Early cytomegalovirus pneumonitis. (a) Focal acute interstitial pneumonitis with several possible cytomegaloviral inclusions, (b) confirmed by immunohistochemistry.

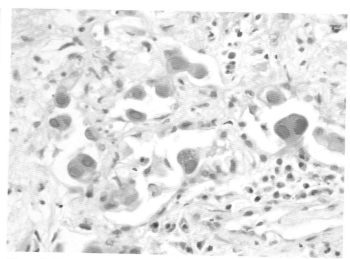

Figure 11.18 Severe cytomegalovirus pneumonitis in a cytomegalovirus-negative recipient of a cytomegalovirus-positive lung.

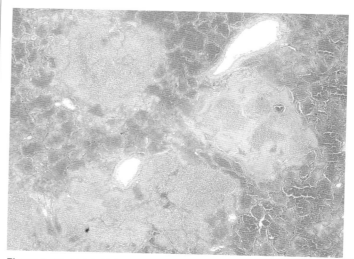

Figure 11.19 Fatal chickenpox pneumonitis. Foci of necrosis are surrounded by haemorrhage.

less than 1%.[24] It mostly follows the immunosuppression being increased because of acute rejection.[98] The histological patterns include a predominantly lymphoplasmacytic interstitial pneumonitis with scanty exudate, and a granulomatous pneumonitis. The fungal cysts are sparse and the classic foamy alveolar exudate is rarely encountered. The perivascular component of the lymphoplasmacytic pattern resembles that of acute rejection, hence the mandatory use of silver staining techniques for all transbronchial lung allograft biopsies and the routine screening of all bronchoalveolar lavage specimens using immunocytochemistry or the polymerase chain reaction.[99]

Other fungi that infect lung allograft patients include *Candida* and *Aspergillus*. These agents may merely colonise the airways[100] or cause ulcerative tracheobronchitis, dehiscence of the anastomosis, bronchocentric granulomatosis, cavitating pneumonia, mediastinitis and multiple haematogenous abscesses.[101–105]

Toxoplasmosis

Infection of the lung allograft by *Toxoplasma gondii* is rare, having been largely eliminated in seronegative solid organ transplant recipients given a positive organ by prophylaxis with pyrimethamine. It usually occurs as part of systemic infection following graft mismatch.[106] Identification of the organism in biopsy material may be difficult as the cysts of *T. gondii* are sparse and extracellular tachyzoites may be mistaken for haematoxyphil debris (see Fig. 5.5.2, p. 251). The diagnosis may be confirmed by immunohistochemistry or by the polymerase chain reaction applied to tissue, body fluids or peripheral blood.[107]

Neoplasia

After rejection, neoplasia is the most significant factor limiting long-term survival in solid organ transplantation.[1,108] It ranges in incidence from 6–11%.[109,110] The tumours may arise *de novo* or be inadvertently introduced within the allograft. They are often particularly aggressive. Predisposing factors in addition to immunosuppression include ultraviolet irradiation and activation of oncogenic viruses such as Epstein–Barr virus, papilloma virus and herpesvirus. Molecular techniques have shown that those arising *de novo* may be of donor rather than recipient origin.[111]

The most frequently encountered *de novo* tumours include the post-transplantation lymphoproliferative disorders (see below) and cutaneous tumours, notably squamous carcinoma and premalignant skin lesions, which are often multiple. The carcinomas frequently metastasise and may contain papilloma virus.[108,112] Intra-epithelial neoplasia and squamous carcinomas of the uterine cervix, vulva and perineum, also associated with papilloma virus infection, may occur. Other tumours reputed to occur with greater frequency than in the general population include carcinomas of the kidney, hepatobiliary tract and lung, the last of these often presenting at an advanced stage and being of donor origen.[87,113,114] Cytological specimens of the bronchi often show epithelial atypia but this is more often reactive than malignant.[115]

Other tumours seen more commonly in lung transplant recipients than the general population include Kaposi's sarcoma[116] and low-grade leiomyosarcoma,[117,118] which are described on pp. 624 and 619, respectively.

Post-transplantation lymphoproliferative disorders

A spectrum of lymphoproliferative disorders may complicate transplantation of many organs, including the lungs.[119–122] Immunosuppression would appear to underlie this escape from normal control as similar disease is seen in other persons suffering from profound immunosuppression – AIDS patients for example. Epstein–Barr virus is suspected of playing a part in the causation of these lesions, having been identified in many of them by immunostaining and the application of molecular probes.[123–125] The incidence of lymphoproliferative disease is higher in recipients who are sero-negative for Epstein–Barr virus before the operation,[126] suggesting that the viral infection is primary rather than representing re-infection or re-activation of latent disease.[123] The virus is detectable more often with early than late disease. A notable feature is that the lesions are potentially reversible once immunosuppression is reduced.[121,127]

Post-transplantation lymphoproliferative disorders have been described in association with virtually all currently used immunosuppressive agents and are thought to result from uncontrolled proliferation of Epstein–Barr virus-immortalised B-cells due to loss of cytotoxic T-cell control.[124,128] Risk factors include the type of transplant, young age, multiple rejection episodes, multi-agent immunosuppression, anti-T-cell therapy and pre-transplant Epstein–Barr virus sero-negativity.[126,129] The

interval between lung transplantation and the development of the lymphoproliferative process is generally short (median time 7 months), as is the median time to death following presentation (5 months).[125]

The incidence of post-transplantation lymphoproliferative disorders ranges from about 1% with bone marrow and kidney transplants to nearly 10% with lung and heart-lung and 17% with intestine.[130] With bone marrow transplants the disorders are usually of donor origin whereas with solid organ transplants they are generally of recipient origin.[130–132] Nevertheless, they often first present in the allograft itself.[123,125,130]

Post-transplantation lymphoproliferative disease may involve the lung in isolation or as part of disseminated disease.[122,123,125] The lungs may also be involved by post-transplantation lymphoproliferative disease in recipients of other solid organ transplants.[133,134] The disease may be asymptomatic or cause cough, fever and malaise. Radiographs may show diffuse infiltrates or single or multiple nodules. Tissue should be examined for Epstein–Barr virus by immunocytochemistry or *in situ* hybridisation, cell phenotype and immunoglobulin clonality, and the lesion classified according to the scheme advocated by the World Health Organisation (Box 11.4).[135] Synchronous and metachronous lesions should all be investigated as variations in clonality and morphology occur both within an individual lesion and between simultaneous or subsequent lesions. Difficulties encountered in diagnosis, especially on core biopsies, stem from the small size of the sample, crush artefact and extensive necrosis caused by angioinvasion. The differential diagnosis includes infections by agents such as cytomegalovirus and pneumocystis, inflammation caused by previous biopsies, the presence of bronchus-associated lymphoid tissue and, in the transplanted lung, acute allograft rejection and, rarely, graft-versus-host disease.

The chief pulmonary manifestations of post-transplantation lymphoproliferative disease are lymphoid hyperplasia, lym-

---

Box 11.4 WHO classification of post transplantation lymphoproliferative disorders (PTLD)[135]

1 Early lesions
      Reactive plasmacytic hyperplasia
      Infectious mononucleosis
2 PTLD – polymorphic
      Polyclonal (rare)
      Monoclonal
3 PTLD monomorphic (classify according to lymphoma classification)
      B-cell lymphomas
         Diffuse large B-cell lymphoma (immunoblastic, centroblastic, anaplastic)
         Burkitt/Burkitt-like
         Plasma cell myeloma
      T-cell lymphomas
         Peripheral T-cell lymphoma, not otherwise categorised
         Other types (hepatosplenic, gamma-delta, T/NK)
4 Other types (rare)
      Hodgkin's disease-like lesions
      Plasmacytoma-like lesions

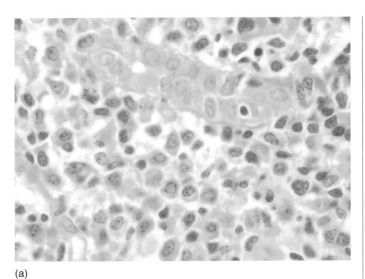

(a)

(b)

Figure 11.20 Pulmonary post-transplantation lymphoproliferative disorder (polymorphous, lymphoplasmacytoid). (a) Plasma cells, plasmacytoid cells and medium-sized lymphocytes surround an alveolar duct. (b) CD79a-positivity shows that the infiltrate is of B cell origin.

phoid interstitial pneumonia and the full spectrum of lymphomas,[123] all of which are described in Chapter 12.4. Lymphomas predominantly comprise B-lymphocytes whereas T-lymphocytes predominate in the infiltrates that characterise rejection.[122] Diffuse large cell lymphomas often show angio-invasion and extensive necrosis, thereby resembling lymphomatoid granulomatosis. Early lesions may be rich in mature plasma cells or show changes suggestive of infectious mononucleosis. Polymorphous infiltrates often include plasmacytoid cells (Fig. 11.20). Monomorphous infiltrates may consist of transformed blasts, centroblast-like, centrocyte-like cells or immunoblasts showing a high proliferation index (Fig. 11.21). Single cell necrosis is common. Histiocytes and T lymphocytes often cuff the lesion and infiltrate the bronchiolar epithelium while the uninvolved lung may show patchy organising pneu-

monia. Immunoglobulin clonality is variable. Early lesions tend to be polyclonal. Monomorphous lesions are usually monoclonal while polymorphous lesions may be either polyclonal or monoclonal.[130,136]

A reduction of immunosuppression and treatment with antiviral agents usually leads to rapid resolution[123] but relapse is frequent and may require radiation treatment or chemotherapy. Newer, less toxic, treatments such as cytotoxic T-lymphocyte infusions, interferon-α and antibodies to B cells (anti-CD20) are currently being evaluated.

Graft-versus-host disease

The transplanted heart-lung block contains a significant amount of lymphoid tissue and on rare occasions a rash, colitis, pancytopenia and liver dysfunction may suggest that graft-versus-host disease has developed.[137] The identification of donor lymphocytes in the blood and bronchoalveolar lavage fluid of such patients supports this possibility. Graft-versus-host disease tends to develop in the early postoperative period. It may be severe but is fortunately rare and usually responds to increased immunosuppression. The graft-versus-host disease of bone marrow transplantation may cause constrictive obliterative bronchiolitis that is indistinguishable from that seen in lung rejection[76,77,138,139] but of course in lung transplantation the donor lung is spared this complication.

Biopsy diagnosis is generally dependent upon the histological appearances in the skin rather than the lung. The diagnosis may be confirmed by demonstrating donor and recipient chimerism on HLA typing of peripheral blood lymphocytes and bronchoalveolar lavage fluid.

Recurrent disease in the allograft

The systemic effects of underlying diseases such as cystic fibrosis may impact significantly on recovery but only recurrence in the allograft will be considered here.

The aetiology of many diseases treated by lung transplantation is imperfectly understood but our knowledge of them has been broadened by their behaviour following transplantation. Some of these diseases are prone to recur in the new lungs whereas others are not. Of particular interest is the finding that lungs transplanted into patients with cystic fibrosis do not appear to develop the basic defect of membrane transport that underlies this disease[140,141] It is also notable that whereas asthma appears to be cured by lung transplantation, it may also be transferred by transplanting the lungs of asthmatic donors to non-atopic patients.[142] Sarcoidosis has recurred in the graft in up to 60% of cases[143–146] but is seldom of clinical significance.[146] Other diseases which have recurred in the graft include the giant cell pneumonia of hard metal workers,[147] desquamative interstitial pneumonia,[148,149] panbronchiolitis,[150] alveolar proteinosis,[151] Langerhans cell histiocytosis[152–154] and lymphangioleiomyomatosis.[155–157] This last disease is almost entirely confined to women and it is notable that the donors of some lungs affected by recurrent disease were men; the recur-

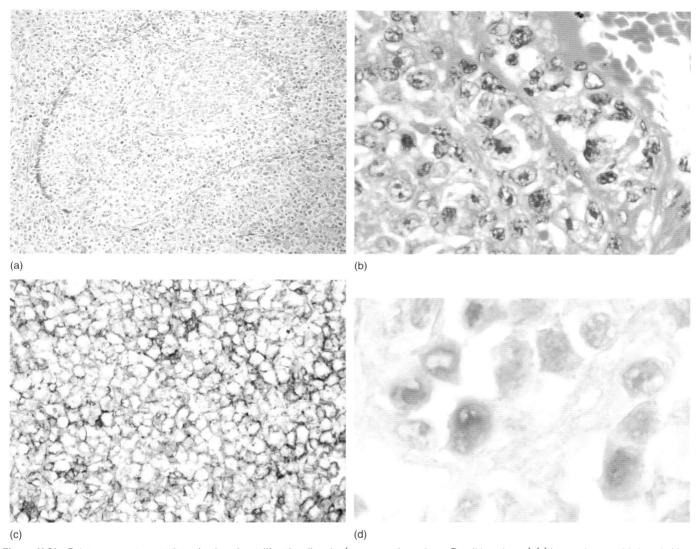

Figure 11.21 Pulmonary post-transplantation lymphoproliferative disorder (monomorphous, large B-cell lymphoma). (a) Large pleomorphic lymphoid cells, some with immunoblastic features, show angiocentricity. (b) Some of the lymphoid cells infiltrating the vessel wall show immunoblastic features. (c) CD20-positivity shows that the infiltrate is of B-cell origin. (d) *In situ* hybridisation for EBV-encoded RNA shows strong nuclear positivity. (Fig. (d) was kindly provided by Dr JA Thomas, London, UK.)

rent smooth muscle proliferation is reported to have been of donor origin in some patients[157] and recipient origin in others.[158] Recurrent bronchioloalveolar cell carcinoma has been shown to have originated in the recipient and the recurrence to have taken place despite both lungs having been replaced and there being no evidence of extrapulmonary involvement.[9] Diseases that have not yet been reported to recur in the new lungs include idiopathic pulmonary fibrosis and emphysema.

Drug injury

Some of the immunosuppressive drugs used to maintain an organ transplant may cause dysfunction in other organs. For example cyclosporine may be responsible for renal damage and rhabdomyolysis and azathioprine for hepatotoxicity and bone marrow failure. Recently several patterns of lung disease have been described in renal transplant patients treated with sirolimus: they include lymphocytic interstitial pneumonia, cryptogenic organising pneumonia and pulmonary haemorrhage.[159]

REFERENCES

1. Trulock EP, Edwards LB, Taylor DO, et al. The Registry of the International Society for Heart and Lung Transplantation: twenty-first official adult heart transplant report – 2004. J Heart Lung Transplant 2004; 23:804–815.

2. Starnes VA, Bowdish ME, Woo MS, et al. A decade of living lobar lung transplantation: recipient outcomes. J Thorac Cardiovasc Surg 2004; 127:114–122.

3. Boucek MM, Edwards LB, Keck BM, et al. Registry for the International Society for Heart and Lung Transplantation: seventh official pediatric report–2004. J Heart Lung Transplant 2004; 23:933–947.

Types of lung transplant

4. Kshettry VR, Kroshus TJ, Hertz MI, et al. Early and late complications after lung transplantation: incidence and management. Ann Thorac Surg 1997; 63:1576–1583.

5. Norgaard MA, Andersen CB, Pettersson G. Does bronchial artery revascularization influence results concerning bronchiolitis obliterans syndrome and/or obliterative bronchiolitis after lung transplantation? Eur J Cardiothorac Surg 1998; 14:311–318.

6. Hertz MI, Mohacsi PJ, Taylor DO, et al. The registry of the International Society for Heart and Lung Transplantation: introduction to the twentieth annual reports–2003. J Heart Lung Transplant 2003; 22:610–615.

Recipient selection

7. Tazelaar HD, Yousem SA. The pathology of combined heart-lung transplantation: an autopsy study. Hum Pathol 1988; 19:1403–1416.

8. Etienne B, Bertocchi M, Gamondes JP, et al. Successful double-lung transplantation for bronchioloalveolar carcinoma. Chest 1997; 112: 1423–1424.

9. Garver RI, Zorn GL, Wu X, et al. Recurrence of bronchioloalveolar carcinoma in transplanted lungs. N Engl J Med 1999; 340:1071–1074.

10. Zorn GL, McGiffin DC, Young KR, et al. Pulmonary transplantation for advanced bronchioloalveolar carcinoma. J Thorac Cardiovasc Surg 2003; 125:45–48.

Donor matching

11. Pratschke J, Wilhelm MJ, Kusaka M, et al. Brain death and its influence on donor organ quality and outcome after transplantation. Transplantation 1999; 67:343–348.

12. Dark J. Single and bilateral lung transplantation. In: Banner NR, Polak JM, Yacoub M, eds. Lung Transplantation. Cambridge: Cambridge University Press; 2003:132–140.

13. Cohen AH, Mallory GB, Ross K, et al. Growth of lungs after transplantation in infants and in children younger than 3 years of age. Am J Respir Crit Care Med 1999; 159:1747–1751.

14. Smith JD, Danskine AJ, Laylor RM, Rose ML, Yacoub MH. The effect of panel reactive antibodies and the donor specific crossmatch on graft survival after heart and heart-lung transplantation. Transpl Immunol 1993; 1:60–65.

15. Scornik JC, Zander DS, Baz MA, Donnelly WH, Staples ED. Susceptibility of lung transplants to preformed donor-specific HLA antibodies as detected by flow cytometry. Transplantation 1999; 68:1542–1546.

Recipient monitoring

16. Guilinger RA, Paradis IL, Dauber JH, et al. The importance of bronchoscopy with transbronchial biopsy and bronchoalveolar lavage in the management of lung transplant recipients. Am J Respir Crit Care Med 1995; 152:2037–2043.

17. Higenbottam T, Stewart S, Penketh A, Wallwork J. Transbronchial lung biopsy for the diagnosis of rejection in heart-lung transplant patients. Transplantation 1988; 46:532–539.

18. Novitzy D, Cooper DKC, Rose AG, Reichart B. Acute isolated pulmonary rejection following transplantation of the heart and both lungs: experimental and clinical observations. Ann Thorac Surg 1986; 42: 180–184.

19. Palmer SM, Davis RD, Hadjiliadis D, et al. Development of an antibody specific to major histocompatibility antigens detectable by flow cytometry after lung transplant is associated with bronchiolitis obliterans syndrome. Transplantation 2002; 74:799–804.

20. Rose ML. De novo production of antibodies after heart or lung transplantation should be regarded as an early warning system. J Heart Lung Transplant 2004; 23:385–395.

21. Mansfield ES, Sarwal MM. Arraying the orchestration of allograft pathology. Am J Transplant 2004; 4:853–862.

22. Mehra MR, Kobashigawa JA. Advances in heart and lung transplantation 2004: Report from the 24th International Society for Heart and Lung Transplantation Annual Meeting, San Francisco. J Heart Lung Transplant 2004; 2004; 23:925–930.

Role of the histopathologist

23. Wallace WAH, Bellamy COC, Rassl DM, Harrison DJ. Transplant histopathology for the general histopathologist. Histopathology 2003; 43:313–322.

24. Burke M. Transplant pathology. In: Banner NR, Polak JM, Yacoub M, eds. Lung Transplantation. Cambridge: Cambridge University Press; 2005: 294–325.

25. Stewart S, McNeil K, Nashef SA, et al. Audit of referral and explant diagnoses in lung transplantation: a pathologic study of lungs removed for parenchymal disease. J Heart Lung Transplant 1995; 14: 1173–1186.

Complications

26. Khan SU, Salloum J, Odonovan PB, et al. Acute pulmonary edema after lung transplantation – The pulmonary reimplantation response. Chest 1999; 116:187–194.

27. Ng CSH, Wan S, Yim APC. Pulmonary ischaemia-reperfusion injury: role of apoptosis. Eur Respir J 2005; 25:356–363.

28. Ohori NP, Iacono AT, Grgurich WF, Yousem SA. Significance of acute bronchitis/bronchiolitis in the lung transplant recipient. Am J Surg Pathol 1994; 18:1192–1204.

29. Rivero DHRF, Lorenzi G, Pazetti R, Jatene FB, Saldiva PHN. Effects of bronchial transection and reanastomosis on mucociliary system. Chest 2001; 119:1510–1515.

30. Zenati M, Yousem SA, Dowling RD. Primary graft failure following pulmonary transplantation. Transplantation 1990; 50:165–167.

31. Gammie JS, Stukus DR, Pham SM, et al. Effect of ischemic time on survival in clinical lung transplantation. Ann Thorac Surg 1999; 68: 2015–2019.

32. Yousem SA. Alveolar lipoproteinosis in lung allograft recipients. Hum Pathol 1997; 28:1383–1386.

33. McDonald JW, Keller CA, Ramos RR, Brunt EM. Mixed (neutrophil-rich) interstitial pneumonitis in biopsy specimens of lung allografts: a clinicopathologic evaluation. Chest 1998; 113:117–123.

34. Yousem SA, Paradis IL, Dauber JA, et al. Large airway inflammation in heart-lung transplant recipients–its significance and prognostic implications. Transplantation 1990; 49:654–656.

35. Maiwand MO, Zehr KJ, Dyke CM, et al. The role of cryotherapy for airway complications after lung and heart-lung transplantation. Eur J Cardiothorac Surg 1997; 12:549–554.

36. Yousem SA, Dauber JH, Griffith BP. Bronchial cartilage alterations in lung transplantation. Chest 1990; 98:1121–1124.

37. Taylor PM, Rose M, Yacoub MH. Expression of class I and class II MHC antigens in normal and transplanted human lung. Transplant Proc 1989; 21:451–452.

38. Karamsetty MR, Klinger JRNO. More than just a vasodilator in lung transplantation. Am J Respir Cell Molec Biol 2002; 26:1–5.

39. Mason NA, Springall DR, Pomerance A, et al. Expression of inducible nitric oxide synthase and formation of peroxynitrite in posttransplant obliterative bronchiolitis. J Heart Lung Transplant 1998; 17:710–714.

40. Gabbay E, Haydn WE, Orsida B, et al. In stable lung transplant recipients, exhaled nitric oxide levels positively correlate with airway neutrophilia and bronchial epithelial iNOS. Am J Respir Crit Care Med 1999; 160: 2093–2099.

41. Roberts F, Harper CM, Downie I, Burnett RA. Immunohistochemical analysis still has a limited role in the diagnosis of malignant mesothelioma – A study of thirteen antibodies. Am J Clin Pathol 2001; 116:253–262.

42. Choi JK, Kearns J, Palevsky HI, et al. Hyperacute rejection of a pulmonary allograft. Immediate clinical and pathologic findings. Am J Respir Crit Care Med 1999; 160:1015–1018.

43. Bittner HB, Dunitz J, Hertz M, Bolman MR, III, Park SJ. Hyperacute rejection in single lung transplantation–case report of successful management by means of plasmapheresis and antithymocyte globulin treatment. Transplantation 2001; 71:649–651.

44. Yousem SA, Berry GJ, Brunt EM, et al. A working formulation for the standardisation of nomenclature in the diagnosis of the heart and lung rejection: lung rejection study group. J Heart Transplant 1990; 9:593–601.

45. Yousem SA, Berry GR, Cagle PT, et al. Revision of the 1990 working formulation for the classification of pulmonary allograft rejection: lung rejection study group. J Heart Lung Transplant 1996; 15:11–15.

46. Yousem SA, Duncan SR, Griffith BP. Interstitial and airspace granulation tissue reactions in lung transplant recipients. Am J Surg Pathol 1992; 16: 877–884.

47. Yousem SA. Lymphocytic bronchitis/bronchiolitis in lung allograft recipients. Am J Surg Pathol 1993; 17:491–496.

48. Clelland CA, Higenbottam TW, Stewart S, Scott JP, Wallwork J. The histological changes in transbronchial biopsy after treatment of acute lung rejection in heart-lung transplants. J Pathol 1990; 161:105–112.

49. Blic J de, Peuchmaur M, Carnot F, et al. Rejection in lung transplantation–an immunohistochemical study of transbronchial biopsies. Transplantation 1992; 54:639–644.

50. Yousem SA, Martin T, Paradis IL, Keenan R, Griffith BP. Can immunohistological analysis of transbronchial biopsy specimens predict responder status in early acute rejection of lung allografts? Hum Pathol 1994; 25:525–529.

51. Rosendale B, Yousem SA. Discrimination of Epstein-Barr virus-related posttransplant lymphoproliferations from acute rejection in lung allograft recipients. Arch Pathol Lab Med 1995; 119:418–423.

52. Longchampt E, Achkar A, Tissier F, et al. Coexistence of acute cellular rejection and lymphoproliferative disorder in a lung transplant patient. Arch Pathol Lab Med 2001; 125:1500–1502.

53. Nakhleh RE, Bolman RM. III, Henke CA, Hertz MI. Lung transplant pathology. A comparative study of pulmonary acute rejection and cytomegaloviral infection. Am J Surg Pathol 1991; 15:1197–1201.

54. Tazelaar HD. Perivascular inflammation in pulmonary infections: implications for the diagnosis of lung rejection. J Heart Lung Transplant 1991; 10:437–441.

55. Niedobitek G, Finn T, Herbst H, et al. Detection of cytomegalovirus by in-situ hybridisation and histochemistry using a monoclonal antibody CCH2: a comparison of methods. J Clin Pathol 1988; 41:1005–1009.

56. Weiss LM, Movahed LA, Berry GJ, Billingham ME. In situ hybridization studies for viral nucleic acids in heart and lung allograft biopsies. Am J Clin Pathol 1990; 93:675–679.

57. Yousem SA. Graft eosinophilia in lung transplantation. Hum Pathol 1992; 23:1172–1177.

58. Gerhardt SG, Tuder RM, Girgis RE, et al. Pulmonary eosinophilia following lung transplantation for sarcoidosis in two patients. Chest 2003; 123: 629–632.

59. Husain AN, Siddiqui MT, Holmes EW, et al. Analysis of risk factors for the development of bronchiolitis obliterans syndrome. Am J Respir Crit Care Med 1999; 159:829–833.

60. Sibley RK, Berry GJ, Tazelaar HD, et al. The role of transbronchial biopsies in the management of lung transplant recipients. J Heart Lung Transplant 1993; 12:308–324.

61. Scott JP, Peters SG, McDougall JC, Beck KC, Midthun DE. Posttransplantation physiologic features of the lung and obliterative bronchiolitis. Mayo Clin Proc 1997; 72:170–174.

62. Burke CM, Theodore J, Dawkins KD, et al. Post-transplant obliterative bronchiolitis and other late lung sequelae in human heart-lung transplantation. Chest 1984; 86:824–829.

63. Yousem SA, Burke CM, Billingham ME. Pathologic pulmonary alterations in long-term human heart-lung transplantation. Hum Pathol 1985; 16: 911–923.

64. Kramer MR. Bronchiolitis obliterans following heart-lung and lung transplantation. Respir Med 1994; 88:9–15.

65. Cagle PT, Brown RW, Frost A, Kellar C, Yousem SA. Diagnosis of chronic lung transplant rejection by transbronchial biopsy. Mod Pathol 1995; 8: 137–142.

66. Milne DS, Gascoigne A, Wilkes J, et al. The immunohistopathology of obliterative bronchiolitis following lung transplantation. Transplantation 1992; 54:748–750.

67. Kramer MR, Stoehr C, Whang JL, et al. The diagnosis of obliterative bronchiolitis following heart-lung and lung transplantations: Low yield of transbronchial lung biopsy. J Heart Lung Transplant 1993; 12:675–681.

68. Pomerance A, Madden B, Burke MM, Yacoub MH. Transbronchial biopsy in heart and lung transplantation: clinicopathologic correlations. J Heart Lung Transplant 1995; 14:761–773.

69. Cooper JD, Billingham M, Egan T, et al. A working formulation for the standardization of nomenclature and for clinical staging of chronic dysfunction in lung allografts. International Society for Heart and Lung Transplantation. J Heart Lung Transplant 1993; 12:713–716.

70. Estenne M, Maurer JR, Boehler A, et al. Bronchiolitis obliterans syndrome 2001: an update of the diagnostic criteria. J Heart Lung Transplant 2002; 21:297–310.

71. Ramsey R, Hachem RR, Chakinala MM, et al. The Predictive Value of Bronchiolitis Obliterans Syndrome Stage 0-p. Am J Respir Crit Care Med 2004; 169:468–472.

72. Heng D, Sharples LD, McNeil K, et al. Bronchiolitis obliterans syndrome: incidence, natural history, prognosis, and risk factors. J Heart Lung Transplant 1998; 17:1255–1263.

73. Boehler A, Estenne M. Post-transplant bronchiolitis obliterans. Eur Resp J 2003; 22:1007–1018.

74. Clelland C, Higenbottam T, Otulana B, et al. Histologic prognostic indicators for the lung allografts of heart-lung transplants. J Heart Transplant 1990; 9:177–185.

75. Geddes DM, Corrin B, Brewerton DA, Davies RJ, Turner-Warwick M. Progressive airway obliteration in adults and its association with rheumatoid disease. Q J Med 1977; 46:427–444.

76. Urbanski SJ, Kossakowska AE, Curtis J, et al. Idiopathic small airways pathology in patients with graft-versus-host disease following allogeneic bone marrow transplantation. Am J Surg Pathol 1987; 11:965–971.

77. Epler GR. Bronchiolitis obliterans and airway obstruction associated with graft-versus-host disease. Clin Chest Med 1988; 9:551–556.

78. Yousem SA. The histological spectrum of pulmonary graft versus host disease in bone marrow transplant recipients. Hum Pathol 1995; 26: 668–675.

79. Kroshus TJ, Kshettry VR, Savik K, et al. III. Risk factors for the development of bronchiolitis obliterans syndrome after lung transplantation. J Thorac Cardiovasc Surg 1997; 114:195–202.

80. Koskinen PK, Kallio EA, Bruggeman CA, Lemstrom KB. Cytomegalovirus infection enhances experimental obliterative bronchiolitis in rat tracheal allografts. Am J Respir Crit Care Med 1997; 155:2078–2088.

81. Billings JL, Hertz MI, Savik K, Wendt CH. Respiratory viruses and chronic rejection in lung transplant recipients. J Heart Lung Transplant 2002; 21: 559–566.

82. Khalifah AP, Hachem RR, Chakinala MM, et al. Respiratory viral infections are a distinct risk for bronchiolitis obliterans syndrome and death. Am J Respir Crit Care Med 2004; 170:181–187.

83. Luckraz H, Goddard M, McNeil K, et al. Microvascular changes in small airways predispose to obliterative bronchiolitis after lung transplantation. J Heart Lung Transplant 2004; 23:527–531.

84. Yousem SA, Paradis IL, Dauber JH, et al. Pulmonary arteriosclerosis in long-term human heart-lung transplant recipients. Transplantation 1989; 47:564–569.

85. Hasleton PS, Brooks NH. Severe pulmonary vascular change in patients dying from right ventricular failure after heart transplantation. Thorax 1995; 50:210–212.

86. Pucci A, Forbes RD, Berry GJ, Rowan RA, Billingham ME. Accelerated posttransplant coronary arteriosclerosis in combined heart-lung transplantation. Transplant Proc 1991; 23:1228–1229.

87. Kotloff RM, Ahya VN. Medical complications of lung transplantation. Eur Resp J 2004; 23:334–342.

88. Arbustini E, Morbini P, Grasso M, et al. Human cytomegalovirus early infection, acute rejection, and major histocompatibility class II expression in transplanted lung. Molecular, immunocytochemical, and histopathologic investigations. Transplantation 1996; 61:418–427.

89. You XM, Steinmuller C, Wagner TO, et al. Enhancement of cytomegalovirus infection and acute rejection after allogeneic lung transplantation in the rat: virus-induced expression of major histocompatibility complex class II antigens. J Heart Lung Transplant 1996; 15:1108–1119.

90. Egan JJ, Barber L, Lomax J, et al. Detection of human cytomegalovirus antigenaemia: a rapid diagnostic technique for predicting cytomegalovirus infection/pneumonitis in lung and heart transplant recipients. Thorax 1995; 50:9–13.

91. Tikkanen J, Lemstrom K, Halme M, et al. Cytological monitoring of peripheral blood, bronchoalveolar lavage fluid, and transbronchial biopsy specimens during acute rejection and cytomegalovirus infection in lung and heart–lung allograft recipients. Clin Transplant 2001; 15: 77–88.

92. Fend F, Prior C, Margreiter R, Mikuz G. Cytomegalovirus pneumonitis in heart-lung transplant recipients: histopathology and clinicopathologic considerations. Hum Pathol 1990; 21:918–926.

93. Allen TC, Bag R, Zander DS, Cagle PT. Cytomegalovirus infection masquerading as carcinoma in a lung transplant patient. Arch Pathol Lab Med 2005; 129:e1–e3.

94. Smyth RL, Higenbottam TW, Scott JP, et al. Herpes simplex virus infection in heart-lung transplant recipients. Transplantation 1990; 49:735–739.

95. Vilchez R, McCurry K, Dauber J, et al. Influenza and parainfluenza respiratory viral infection requiring admission in adult lung transplant recipients. Transplantation 2002; 73:1075–1078.

96. Dromer C, Nashef SA, Velly JF, Martigne C, Couraud L. Tuberculosis in transplanted lungs. J Heart Lung Transplant 1993; 12:924–927.

97. Kesten S, Chaparro C. Mycobacterial infections in lung transplant recipients. Chest 1999; 115:741–745.

98. Gryzan S, Paradis IL, Zeevi A, et al. Unexpectedly high incidence of pneumocystis carinii infection after heart–lung transplantation. Implications for lung defense and allograft survival. Am Rev Respir Dis 1988; 137:1268–1274.

99. Wakefield AE, Miller RF, Guiver LA, Hopkin JM. Granulomatous Pneumocystis carinii pneumonia: DNA amplification studies on bronchoscopic alveolar lavage samples. J Clin Pathol 1994; 47:664–666.

100. Cahill BC, Hibbs JR, Savik K, et al. Aspergillus airway colonization and invasive disease after lung transplantation. Chest 1997; 112:1160–1164.

101. Tazelaar HD, Baird AM, Mill M, et al. Bronchocentric mycosis occurring in transplant recipients. Chest 1989; 96:92–95.

102. Skerrett SJ, Martin TR. Alveolar macrophage activation in experimental legionellosis. J Immunol 1991; 147:337–345.

103. Kramer MR, Denning DW, Marshall SE, et al. Ulcerative tracheobronchitis after lung transplantation – a new form of invasive aspergillosis. Am Rev Respir Dis 1991; 144:552–556.

104. Egan JJ, Yonan N, Carroll KB, et al. Allergic bronchopulmonary aspergillosis in lung allograft recipients. Eur Respir J 1996; 9:169–171.

105. Mehrad B, Paciocco G, Martinez FJ, et al. Spectrum of aspergillus infection in lung transplant recipients – Case series and review of the literature. Chest 2001; 119:169–175.

106. Wreghitt TG, Hakim M, Gray JJ, et al. Toxoplasmosis in heart and heart and lung transplant recipients. J Clin Pathol 1989; 42:194–199.

107. Holliman R, Johnson J, Savva D, Cary N, Wreghitt T. Diagnosis of toxoplasma infection in cardiac transplant recipients using the polymerase chain reaction. J Clin Pathol 1992; 45:931–932.

108. Penn I. Occurrence of cancers in immunosuppressed organ transplant recipients. Clin Transpl 1998; :147–158.

109. Mihalov ML, Gattuso P, Abraham K, Holmes EW, Reddy V. Incidence of post-transplant malignancy among 674 solid-organ-transplant recipients at a single center. Clin Transplant 1996; 10:248–255.

110. Rinaldi M, Pellegrini C, D'Armini AM, et al. Neoplastic disease after heart transplantation: single center experience. Eur J Cardiothorac Surg 2001; 19:696–701.

111. DeSoyza AG, Dark JH, Parums DV, Curtis A, Corris PA. Donor-acquired small cell lung cancer following pulmonary transplantation. Chest 2001; 120:1030–1031.

112. Harwood CA, Surentheran T, McGregor JM, et al. Human papillomavirus infection and non-melanoma skin cancer in immunosuppressed and immunocompetent individuals. J Med Virol 2000; 61:289–297.

113. Torbenson M, Wang J, Nichols L, Randhawa P, Nalesnik MA. Renal cortical neoplasms in long term survivors of solid organ transplantation. Transplantation 2000; 69:864–868.

114. Anyanwu AC, Townsend ER, Banner NR, et al. Primary lung carcinoma after heart or lung transplantation: management and outcome. J Thorac Cardiovasc Surg 2002; 124:1190–1197.

115. Ohori NP. Epithelial cell atypia in bronchoalveolar lavage specimens from lung transplant recipients. Am J Clin Pathol 1999; 112:204–210.

116. Sleiman C, Mal H, Roue C, et al. Bronchial Kaposi's sarcoma after single lung transplantation. Eur Respir J 1997; 10:1181–1183.

117. Flint A, Lynch JP, Martinez FJ, Whyte RI. Pulmonary smooth muscle proliferation occurring after lung transplantation. Chest 1997; 112: 283–284.

118. Somers CR, Tesoriero AA, Hartland E, et al. Multiple leiomyosarcomas of both donor and recipient origin arising in a heart-lung transplant patient. Am J Surg Pathol 1998; 22:1423–1428.

119. Swerdlow SH. Post-transplant lymphoproliferative disorders: a morphologic, phenotypic and genotypic spectrum of disease. Histopathology 1992; 20:373–385.

120. Craig FE, Gulley ML, Banks PM. Posttransplantation lymphoproliferative disorders. Am J Clin Pathol 1993; 99:265–276.

121. Swerdlow SH. Post-transplant lymphoproliferative disorders: a working classification. Curr Diagn Pathol 1997; 4:28–35.

122. Reams D, McAdams HP, Howell DN, et al. Posttransplant lymphoproliferative disorder – Incidence, presentation, and response to treatment in lung transplant recipients. Chest 2003; 124:1242–1249.

123. Yousem SA, Randhawa P, Locker J, et al. Posttransplant lymphoproliferative disorders in heart-lung transplant recipients: primary presentation in the allograft. Hum Pathol 1989; 20:361–369.

124. Delecluse HJ, Kremmer E, Rouault JP, et al. The expression of Epstein–Barr virus latent proteins is related to the pathological features of post-transplant lymphoproliferative disorders. Am J Pathol 1995; 146: 1113–1120.

125. Ramalingam P, Rybicki L, Smith MD, et al. Posttransplant lymphoproliferative disorders in lung transplant patients: The Cleveland Clinic experience. Mod Pathol 2002; 15:647–656.

126. Aris RM, Maia DM, Neuringer IP, et al. Post-transplantation lymphoproliferative disorder in the Epstein–Barr virus-naive lung transplant recipient. Am J Respir Crit Care Med 1996; 154:1712–1717.

127. Starzl TE, Nalesnik MA, Porter KA, et al. Reversibility of lymphomas and lymphoproliferative lesions developing under cyclosporin-steroid therapy. Lancet 1984; 1:583–587.

128. Thomas JA, Crawford DH, Burke M. Clinicopathologic implications of Epstein–Barr virus related B cell lymphoma in immunocompromised patients. J Clin Pathol 1995; 48:287–290.

129. Swerdlow AJ, Higgins CD, Hunt BJ, et al. Risk of lymphoid neoplasia after cardiothoracic transplantation. a cohort study of the relation to Epstein–Barr virus. Transplantation 2000; 69:897–904.

130. Nalesnik MA, Jaffe R, Starzl TE, et al. The pathology of posttransplant lymphoproliferative disorders occurring in the setting of cyclosporine A-prednisone immunosuppression. Am J Pathol 1988; 133:173–192.

131. Weissmann DJ, Ferry JA, Harris NL, et al. Posttransplantation lymphoproliferative disorders in solid organ recipients are predominantly aggressive tumors of host origin. Am J Clin Pathol 1995; 103:748–755.

132. Chadburn A, Suciufoca N, Cesarman E, et al. Post-transplantation lymphoproliferative disorders arising in solid organ transplant recipients are usually of recipient origin. Am J Pathol 1995; 147:1862–1870.

133. Ohori NP, Whisnant RE, Nalesnik MA, Swerdlow SH. Primary pleural effusion posttransplant lymphoproliferative disorder: Distinction from secondary involvement and effusion lymphoma. Diagn Cytopathol 2001; 25:50–53.

134. Halkos ME, Miller JI, Mann KP, Miller DL, Gal AA. Thoracic presentations of posttransplant lymphoproliferative disorders. Chest 2004; 126:2013–2020.

135. Immunodeficiency associated lymphoproliferative disorders. In: Jaffe ES, Harris NL, Stein H, Vardiman JW, eds. Tumours of Haemopoietic and Lymphoid Tissues. Lyon, France: IARC Press; 2001:264–269.

136. Knowles DM, Cesarman E, Chadburn A, et al. Correlative morphologic and molecular genetic analysis demonstrates three distinct categories of posttransplantation lymphoproliferative disorders. Blood 1995; 85:552–565.

137. Chau EM, Lee J, Yew WW, Chiu CS, Wang EP. Mediastinal irradiation for graft-versus-host disease in a heart-lung transplant recipient. J Heart Lung Transplant 1997; 16:974–979.

138. Roca J, Granena A, Rodriguez-Roisin R, et al. Fatal airway disease in an adult with chronic graft-versus-host disease. Thorax 1982; 37:77–78.

139. Ralph DD, Springmeyer SC, Sullivan KM, et al. Rapidly progressive air-flow obstruction in marrow transplant recipients. Possible association between obliterative bronchiolitis and chronic graft-versus-host disease. Am Rev Respir Dis 1984; 129:641–644.

140. Alton EWFW, Khagani A, Taylor RFH, et al. Effect of heart-lung transplantation on airway potential difference in patients with and without cystic fibrosis. Eur Respir J 1991; 4:5–9.

141. Tsang VT, Alton EWFW, Hodson ME, Yacoub M. In vitro bioelectric properties of bronchial epithelium from transplanted lungs in recipients with cystic fibrosis. Thorax 1993; 48:1006–1011.

142. Corris PA, Dark JH. Aetiology of asthma – lessons from lung transplantation. Lancet 1993; 341:1369–1371.

143. Johnson BA, Duncan SR, Ohori NP, et al. Recurrence of sarcoidosis in pulmonary allograft recipients. Am Rev Respir Dis 1993; 148:1373–1377.

144. Kazerooni EA, Jackson C. Cascade PN. Sarcoidosis: recurrence of primary disease in transplanted lungs. Radiology 1994; 192:461–464.

145. Martinez FJ, Orens JB, Deeb M, et al. Recurrence of sarcoidosis following bilateral allogeneic lung transplantation. Chest 1994; 106:1597–1599.

146. Walker S, Mikhail G, Banner N, et al. Medium term results of lung transplantation for end stage pulmonary sarcoidosis. Thorax 1998; 53:281–284.

147. Frost AE, Keller CA, Brown RW, et al. Giant cell interstitial pneumonitis - disease recurrence in the transplanted lung. Am Rev Respir Dis 1993; 148:1401–1404.

148. King MB, Jessurun J, Hertz MI. Recurrence of desquamative interstitial pneumonia after lung transplantation. Am J Respir Crit Care Med 1997; 156:2003–2005.

149. Verleden GM, Sels F, VanRaemdonck D, et al. Possible recurrence of desquamative interstitial pneumonitis in a single lung transplant recipient. Eur Resp J 1998; 11:971–974.

150. Baz MA, Kussin PS, Vantrigt P, et al. Recurrence of diffuse panbronchiolitis after lung transplantation. Am J Respir Crit Care Med 1995; 151:895–898.

151. Parker LA, Novotny DB. Recurrent alveolar proteinosis following double lung transplantation. Chest 1997; 111:1457–1458.

152. Etienne B, Bertocchi M, Gamondes JP, et al. Relapsing pulmonary Langerhans cell histiocytosis after lung transplantation. Am J Respir Crit Care Med 1998; 157:288–291.

153. Habib SB, Congleton J, Carr D, et al. Recipient Langerhans cell histiocytosis recurring following bilateral lung transplantation. Thorax 1998; 53:323–325.

154. Gabbay E, Dark JH, Ashcroft T, et al. Recurrence of Langerhans' cell granulomatosis following lung transplantation. Thorax 1998; 53:326–327.

155. Nine JS, Yousem SA, Paradis IL, Keenan R, Griffith BP. Lymphangioleiomyomatosis recurrence after lung transplantation. J Heart Lung Transplant 1994; 13:714–719.

156. O'Brien JD, Lium JH, Parosa JF, et al. Lymphangiomyomatosis recurrence in the allograft after single-lung transplantation. Am J Respir Crit Care Med 1995; 151:2033–2036.

157. Bittmann I, Dose TB, Muller C. Dienemann H. Lymphangioleiomyomatosis: Recurrence after single lung transplantation. Hum Pathol 1997; 28:1420–1423.

158. Carsillo T, Astrinidis A, Henske EP. Mutations in the tuberous sclerosis complex gene TSC2 are a cause of sporadic pulmonary lymphangioleiomyomatosis. Proc Natl Acad Sci USA 2000; 97:6085–6090.

159. Pham PT, Pham PC, Danovitch GM, et al. Sirolimus-associated pulmonary toxicity. Transplantation 2004; 77:1215–1220.

12

Tumours

12.1

Carcinoma of the lung

INCIDENCE AND MORTALITY

The last 100 years have seen the incidence of lung cancer transformed from it being an almost unknown disease to it far outstripping all other forms of cancer as a cause of death in many western countries. The death rate from lung cancer exceeds 60 per 100000 in the UK and is close to this in many developed countries. In British men, it is responsible for about 35% of cancer deaths, and about 8% of all deaths, while in women, it now rivals breast cancer as the major cause of cancer mortality. In many developed countries the incidence in men has levelled off and in some it has started to decline, but in women it is still rising,[1,2] the lag being almost totally due to women taking to smoking later than men. The male to female ratio was nearly equal in England and Wales at the end of the nineteenth century but climbed to six:one by 1951.[3] Now it is again verging on equality as deaths in men decline slightly and deaths in women rise at a rate comparable with that seen in men in the first half of the twentieth century. Furthermore, for a given level of smoking, women are at higher risk of developing lung cancer than men, the relative risk being 1.7.[4,5] A higher level of aromatic DNA adducts (indicating DNA damage) is reported in the lungs of female smokers.[6]

Many developing countries have a relatively low incidence of lung cancer but are beginning to see the rises already experienced elsewhere as the inhabitants take to smoking in increasing numbers. There are also substantial racial differences in susceptibility to the carcinogenic effect of cigarette smoke. For example, at any level of smoking, black Americans have a risk of lung cancer 1.8 times greater than that of their white compatriots.[4] It is likely that in the twenty-first century there will be a significant shift in the geographical distribution of lung cancer.

Lung cancer is largely a disease of later life. In patients younger than 40 years of age, there is a lower male to female ratio and a higher proportion of adenocarcinoma but as in the elderly, cigarette smoking is the most important cause.[7]

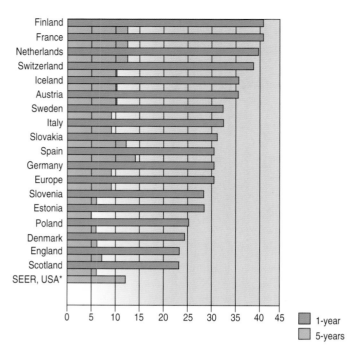

Figure 12.1.1 National 1-year and 5-year survival rates (%) from lung cancer in men. Rates in women are slightly better but broadly similar.[10,11] *5-year survival only.

The tumour is very rare in children but occasional cases are encountered.[8]

Lung cancer carries a very poor prognosis. Surgical survival figures may reach 50% (and over 70% for T1N0M0 tumours)[9] but they are based on a highly selected group of patients. Spread of the tumour often results in it being inoperable at presentation while many patients with lung cancer also have coexistent chronic obstructive lung disease that renders them unfit for surgery. Overall 5-year survival rates vary from 6–17%, mainly due to national differences in access to specialist care (Fig. 12.1.1).[10–12]

AETIOLOGY

There is convincing evidence that cigarette smoking is by far the most important cause of lung cancer. This is based mainly on sound epidemiological studies, supplemented by pathological findings. Other factors have been identified but these are considerably less important than cigarette smoking.

Smoking

The evidence linking cigarette smoking and lung cancer was first established in the early 1950s when the smoking habits of large groups of patients with lung cancer were compared with those of matched controls. These provided clear evidence that the majority of patients with carcinoma of the lung were heavy cigarette smokers and that the incidence of the disease in non-smokers was low.[13–15] Later, prospective studies in which the

incidence of lung cancer was determined over a long period of time in large groups of people with different smoking habits were even more conclusive. One of the best known of these studies was carried out in Britain on a group of 40 000 doctors. In 1951, each completed a questionnaire asking for details of their smoking habits. By 1964, there was ample evidence of a clear link between cigarette smoking and deaths from lung cancer.[16,17] Similar studies were carried out in the USA with identical conclusions.[18,19] These studies established that the risk of lung cancer is increased in smokers compared with non-smokers by a factor of 10. Pipe smokers and cigar smokers have a significantly lower incidence than cigarette smokers, probably due to them not inhaling their smoke to the same degree.[20] The risk increases with the number of cigarettes smoked and is proportional to the length of time a person has smoked, being greatest in those who commenced at an early age.[18] The term 'pack years' is often used to quantify this combination of risk factors, 'one pack year' equating to 20 cigarettes per day for 1 year or 40 per day for 6 months, etc. In those who stop smoking, the risk begins to decline immediately but it takes about 15 years for the risk in ex-smokers to approach that of non-smokers.[16] The incidence of lung cancer is increased in those with other smoking-related diseases, such as chronic bronchitis.[21]

The risk of lung cancer is reduced by switching to filter tip and low tar cigarettes,[22] and from cigarettes to cigars or pipes.[23] However, it is suggested that the switch to low tar cigarettes has led smokers to inhale more deeply and thereby contributed to the increased incidence of peripheral tumours, particularly adenocarcinomas. There is no clear evidence that French cigarettes, which contain air-cured tobacco, are any safer than those made of flue-cured tobacco, but the resultant smoke is more alkaline and the contained nicotine can be absorbed from the mouth. Consequently, fewer French than British cigarette smokers admit to inhaling their smoke and this may contribute to the observed lower incidence of lung cancer in France than Britain, but there are other differences between the two countries: dietary differences are mentioned below.

Passive smoking, which is exposure to the cigarette smoke exhaled by others and the smoke emitted by their smouldering cigarettes (referred to as mainstream and sidestream smoke respectively), carries a small risk of lung cancer.[24,25] Compared with a non-smoker, the increased risk of lung cancer is generally quoted as a percentage for a passive smoker but so-many-fold for an active smoker, the respective figures being in the order of 25% and 13-fold (which equate to 1.25-fold *vs* 13-fold). A comparison of nicotine metabolite levels suggests that passive smoking entails an exposure equivalent of up to one cigarette a day. It is estimated that passive smoking accounts for one extra death from lung cancer or heart disease for every 10 000.

Numerous carcinogens have been identified in cigarette smoke. The more important ones are listed in Table 12.1.1. Many of them are thought to act by binding to DNA. Of particular note are the polycyclic hydrocarbons found in the neutral fraction of the particulate phase and the nitrosamines of the basic fraction. The former has been linked to squamous cell

Table 12.1.1   Major carcinogens of tobacco smoke

Particulate phase

(a) Neutral fraction	Benzpyrene
	Dibenzanthracene
	Benzofluoranthenes
(b) Basic fraction	Nitrosamines
(c) Acidic fraction	Nickel
(d) Residual fraction	Cadmium
	Polonium–210

Vapour phase

Nickel carbonyl
Hydrazine
Vinyl chloride
Nitrogen oxides
Nitrosodiethylamine

carcinoma and the latter to adenocarcinoma.[26] There appears to be genetic susceptibility to the carcinogenic effects of these chemicals, which is possibly based on differences in the amounts of activating enzymes in the lung, many of which are P450 cytochromes.[27]

Direct evidence of the effects of cigarette smoke on bronchial epithelium is provided by pathological studies, which demonstrate a close association between metaplasia and atypia and the number of cigarettes smoked.[28,29] Long-term animal experiments have been difficult to institute but have provided further support evidence of the link between tobacco smoke and lung cancer.[30,31]

Cigarette smoking predisposes to pulmonary carcinoma of all the major histological types, but the link is strongest with squamous cell and small cell carcinoma, which generally arise in central airways, and weakest with adenocarcinoma, which is commoner in the periphery of the lung.[32,33]

Environmental carcinogens

As with constituents of cigarette smoke, many inhaled chemicals are not hazardous as such but are transformed to reactive intermediates within the lungs, often by enzymes of the P450 family. After allowing for differences in smoking habits it is found that the risk of lung cancer is higher in urban areas than in rural areas, suggesting a role for general atmospheric pollution.[34,35] Major atmospheric pollutants include polycyclic hydrocarbons from the combustion of fossil fuels. Domestic coal fires were formerly the prime source of polycyclic hydrocarbons in Britain and it was estimated that in the 1950s air pollution accounted for about 10% of lung cancer in men.[36] Since that time coal fires have been eliminated in most major conurbations and concentrations of benzpyrene have fallen dramatically, by a factor of 30 in London over a period of 30 years.[37] The main source in Britain, as in many countries, is now motor vehicle exhaust and particular attention is being paid to diesel smoke. Some epidemiological studies have identified an increased risk of lung cancer in occupational groups having heavy exposure to diesel exhaust, notably one that examined American mainte-

nance workers exposed to fumes from diesel locomotives.[38] A review by an international agency concluded that there was evidence that diesel engine exhaust was carcinogenic in experimental animals and that there was limited support for this in man.[39] There appears to be only a weak link between urban nitrogen oxide and sulphur dioxide pollution and lung cancer.[40]

Ionising radiation

One of the earliest examples of occupational lung cancer is provided by the miners of the Erzgebirge ('Ore Mountains'), which separate Saxony from the Czech Republic. For four centuries ore from these mountains has proved a rich source of many metals – silver, copper, lead, cobalt, bismuth, iron and, recently, uranium. For much of this time, miners in Schneeberg on the Saxony side and Joachimstal on the Czech side suffered from a fatal respiratory disease – Bergkrankheit – that was recognised as lung cancer in the late nineteenth century. It is estimated that as many as 50% of the miners died from this cause, the average time from starting work in the mines to the development of a tumour being about 17 years. The overall risk of developing lung cancer was about 30 times that of the general population and repeated widowhood was commonplace. The lung cancer is attributable to the miners being exposed to very high levels of ionising radiation in the form of radon gas that is emitted from the rock face and when inhaled subjects the respiratory epithelium to α-irradiation.

Similar increases in lung cancer incidence were seen in North American miners exposed to radon and its daughter products[41,42] and such exposure probably accounts for the increased incidence seen in English haematite miners.[43] The increase involves both squamous cell carcinoma and small cell carcinoma, but particularly the latter.[44,45] Cigarette smoking is an important co-factor in uranium miners. The increased risk is 67 times greater in heavy smokers exposed to heavy doses of irradiation than in non-smokers with comparable radiation exposure,[46,47] indicating a multiplicative effect, as seen with asbestos.

Radon levels may also reach dangerous levels within the home, the degree of danger depending upon the character of the underlying rock.[48,48a] It is difficult to prevent radon seeping into buildings and easier to instal beneath solid floors a radon sump, which can be exhausted to the exterior. In Britain new homes are now required to be built with preventive measures against radon exposure.

Irradiation also results in there being an increased incidence of lung carcinoma in patients given therapeutic irradiation to the spine for ankylosing spondylitis[49] or to the breast for mammary carcinoma.[50,51] Survivors of the Hiroshima and Nagasaki nuclear bombings were also at increased risk of lung cancer.[52,53]

Asbestos

An association between exposure to asbestos and carcinoma of the lung was first demonstrated conclusively in 1955.[54] As with mesothelioma, the association is stronger with amphibole asbestos than chrysotile, but much higher levels of exposure are required. There is some uncertainty whether asbestos causes lung cancer in the absence of asbestosis but compensation for lung carcinoma is more likely to be awarded to an asbestos worker if asbestosis is also present (see p. 352). Whereas lung cancer in the general population preferentially affects the upper lobes, with asbestos a higher proportion arises in the lower lobes, at the sites where asbestos fibres are most numerous and where asbestosis is most pronounced. All histological types are involved but the proportion of adenocarcinoma is increased.[55–57] Cigarette smoking is an important co-factor. In a study of 17 800 asbestos workers, the risk in smokers was 14 times that in non-smokers.[58] Table 7.1.4 (p. 352) provides further data on this, showing that the lung cancer risk for workers heavily exposed to asbestos is five times that of unexposed persons whatever their smoking status, while the risk for smokers is 11 times that of non-smokers whether they are exposed to asbestos or not. As a consequence, the lung cancer incidence among smokers exposed to asbestos is 53 times higher than that among unexposed non-smokers – a multiplicative rather than additive effect.[59] The risk diminishes in those who cease smoking. A practical preventive point arising from this is that most of the excess risk can be abolished by eliminating or decreasing exposure to either asbestos or cigarette smoke. Also, it suggests that asbestos acts as a promoting agent rather than a primary carcinogen.

Other industrial chemicals

Apart from asbestos and ionising radiation, six other agents encountered in industry are accepted pulmonary carcinogens: arsenic, chloromethyl ethers, chromium, nickel, polyaromatic hydrocarbons and vinyl chloride. Many others, including cadmium, formaldehyde and dioxin are suspected of having a similar effect (Table 12.1.2).[60] Cigarette smoking is often an additional factor.[61]

Workers in the coal gas industry exposed to polyaromatic hydrocarbons were found to have a lung cancer risk twice that of the general population,[62] and lung cancer has also been associated with a range of metal refining and smelting processes: nickel, chromium, arsenic and cadmium have all been incriminated.[63,64] In the 1930s a higher incidence was reported among workers at the Clydach nickel refinery in South Wales. Changes in the process later resulted in a reduction of the risk but the hazard remains in several other nickel refineries.[65] Exposure to both nickel and cadmium was related to lung cancer in workers in a battery plant.[66] Poorly soluble hexavalent chromium pigments cause lung cancer but very soluble chromium compounds are comparatively safe.[67,68] Arsenic and its compounds are associated with skin and lung carcinomas, an increased incidence being found in people administered arsenic therapeutically, in vineyard workers involved in spraying arsenical insecticides, and in copper smelters exposed to arsenic.[69] Arsenic may also be responsible for an increased risk of lung cancer identified in antimony workers.[70] It is also anticipated

Table 12.1.2 Occupational agents associated with lung cancer, categorized by the criteria of the International Agency for Research on Cancer[60]

Known carcinogens (Group 1)
Arsenic
Asbestos
Bis(chloromethyl)ether
Chromium, hexavalent
Nickel and nickel compounds
Polycyclic aromatic compounds
Radon
Vinyl chloride
Probable carcinogens (Group 2A)
Acrylonitrile
Beryllium
Cadmium
Formaldehyde
Possible carcinogens (Group 2B)
Acetaldehyde
Man-made fibres
Silica
Welding fumes

that the next decade will witness widespread arsenic-induced cancer in Bengal and Bangladesh following the provision of water free of bacterial contamination by extraction from shallow aquifers. Up to 10 million shallow tube wells have been dug and it is estimated that one million of these are heavily contaminated with naturally occurring arsenic released by anaerobic metal-reducing bacteria.[71] At least 100 000 cases of arsenic-induced skin growths have been identified and it seems inevitable that cancer of the skin and respiratory tract will follow.

Exposure to the alkylating agent chloromethyl methyl ether, which is used as a cross-linking agent in ion exchange resins and as an intermediate in the production of organic chemicals, carries an increased risk of lung cancer, particularly if there is contamination with bis (chloromethyl) ether.[72] Small cell carcinoma is particularly increased.[73]

Epidemiological studies have also incriminated silica exposure as a risk factor for lung cancer, and as with asbestos there is uncertainty as to whether the risk is due to high silica levels alone or to the fibrotic process.[74] Claims for compensation are therefore more likely to succeed if silicosis as well as carcinoma can be demonstrated.

Diet

Many of the differences in disease incidence seen between Mediterranean and northern European countries have been ascribed to diet, especially the differing intake of antioxidants. Dietary differences are probably important in regard to cardiovascular disease but may also affect cancer incidence. Many cigarette smokers have therefore gleefully increased their consumption of red wine on evidence that is to date at best equivocal.[75]

Vitamin A deficiency leads to squamous metaplasia of mucosal surfaces, dryness of the skin, eyes and mouth, and to an increased susceptibility to cancer.[76] Cigarette smoke augments the metaplastic action of vitamin A deficiency in rats,[77] while in man low vitamin A intake leads to an increased incidence of lung cancer in smokers.[78] Folate is another dietary component that protects against squamous metaplasia.[79] Diets high in carotenoid-rich fruits and vegetables are associated with a reduced risk of lung cancer, as are high serum levels of vitamin E and beta carotene, but long-term dietary supplementation with these substances either had no effect or resulted in a slightly higher incidence of lung cancer in male smokers.[80–82]

Pulmonary fibrosis

Idiopathic pulmonary fibrosis is associated with a 14-fold increased incidence of lung cancer,[83,84] similar to that noted above in asbestosis.[58] In both these diseases, the tumours are of all histological types and they arise more frequently in the periphery of the lower lobes where the fibrosis is most marked.[85,86] Although the original publications suggested that adenocarcinoma was the most common histological type, it is now believed that the cell type distribution is similar to that in the general population.[56] In contrast to these forms of diffuse pulmonary fibrosis, the role of localised scars in the development of lung cancer is now questioned (see p. 551). Sarcoidosis has been reported to convey an increased risk of lung cancer in some studies[87,88] but not others.[89]

Viruses

Viral oncogenes participate in carcinogenesis by the RNA of the viral genome being transcribed into the DNA genome of the host by the enzyme reverse transcriptase. The DNA sequences transcribed by viral oncogenes are virtually identical to sequences in the cellular DNA of most animal species and presumably have the same potential for affecting malignant growth as cellular oncogenes. Viruses have been suggested in the past as being related to the development of some lung cancers and the development of molecular probes has given some impetus to such investigations. Papilloma virus has been identified in a small proportion of squamous cell carcinomas of the bronchus (types 16,18,31,33,35), as well as papillomatosis (types 6 and 11),[90–93] and Epstein–Barr virus has been shown to be associated with bronchopulmonary as well as nasopharyngeal lymphoepithelial carcinomas (but with only occasional lung tumours of the more common histological types).[94,95] There is an increased incidence of lung cancer in AIDS but this is not thought to be directly attributable to the human immunodeficiency virus.[96]

Heredity

The great majority of smokers reaching old age do not die of lung cancer, suggesting that individuals differ greatly in the way they metabolise xenobiotic substances.[97] These differences are presumably inborn. Genetic differences could influence the risk of cancer in several ways.[98] For example, they could affect the enzymatic elimination or activation of carcinogens,[99,100] or the expression of oncogenes or tumour suppressor genes (see below). Epidemiological studies have shown an excess of lung cancer in close relatives,[101,102] despite there being confounding factors,[103] but a study of 15 924 pairs of male twins failed to identify any evidence of an inherited predisposition to lung cancer.[104]

PATHOGENESIS

Pre-malignant changes evident morphologically

Carcinoma of the lung largely arises from the epithelial cells lining the airspaces. The few carcinomas that develop in the bronchial glands are dealt with in the next chapter. The next chapter also considers diffuse neuroendocrine hyperplasia as a precursor of tumourlets and carcinoids (but not of neuroendocrine carcinomas). Bronchioloalveolar carcinoma is now defined as a pre-invasive condition but is nevertheless considered under adenocarcinoma. Attention here is confined to squamous metaplasia and atypical adenomatous hyperplasia. No precursor of small cell carcinoma has been identified.

Four main cell types make up the surface epithelium of the bronchi – basal, mucous, neuroendocrine and ciliated (see p. 7) – and only the last of these appear to be end cells. The others are all capable of division and thus have malignant potential. Clara cells and type II pneumocytes are the respective stem cells of the bronchioles and the alveoli and are found in some adenocarcinomas of the lung.

Squamous metaplasia and dysplasia

The regenerative capability of bronchial epithelial cells has been extensively studied. Hyperplasia of the surviving basal cells is an early regenerative event that is followed by the development of a stratified squamous epithelium.[105] Further differentiation into mucous cells and thence ciliated cells follows but mucous differentiation is dependent upon the availability of vitamin A.[77,106] The application of carcinogens such as benz-pyrene, asbestos or nitrosamines results in the proliferation of bronchial neuroendocrine cells, which may undergo squamous metaplasia.[107–109] It is clear therefore that basal, mucous, neuroendocrine and metaplastic squamous cells are closely related and readily transform one to another. This marked metaplastic potential of the bronchial epithelium provides no support for facile suppositions regarding the histogenesis of particular types of lung carcinoma from particular precursor cells.

The sequence of hyperplasia – metaplasia – dysplasia – carcinoma-*in-situ* – invasive carcinoma (Fig. 12.1.2) is well documented in human airways[110,111] and a grading system, which details the histological features evident in the surface epithelium, has been introduced (Table 12.1.3).[112] Changes are also found in the mucosal blood vessels. Several groups have

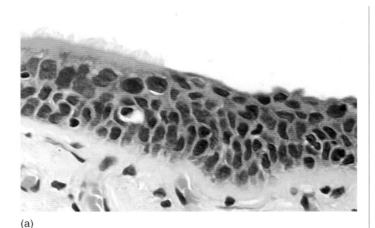

(a)

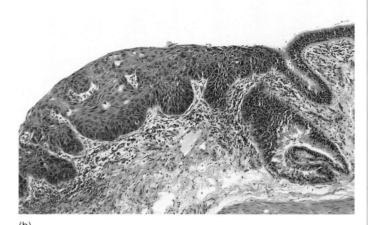

(b)

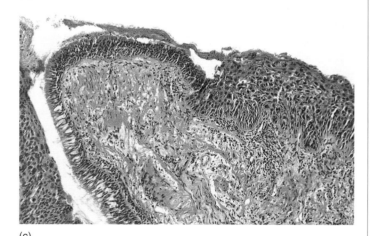

(c)

Figure 12.1.2 Smokers' bronchi showing (a) basal cell hyperplasia (left) and squamous metaplasia (right). (b) moderate squamous dysplasia and (c) carcinoma *in situ* (right).

described hyperplastic capillary loops in close apposition to dysplastic epithelium, giving rise to the term angiogenic squamous dysplasia.[113] The vascular changes can be detected by fluorescence bronchoscopy, suggesting that it may be possible to eradicate the lesions before they become invasive.[114]

Uranium miners in the USA provided cytopathologists with the opportunity of studying the gradual evolution of bronchial carcinoma. Periodic sputum examination showed squamous metaplasia followed by gradually increasing cellular atypia in those miners who later developed invasive carcinoma of either squamous or small cell type. Atypical cells could be identified in the sputum for many years prior to the development of invasive tumours: on average, dysplastic changes lasted 16 years and carcinoma-*in-situ* a further 2 years before there was invasion.[110] Isolated foci of *in-situ* squamous cell carcinomas amenable to limited surgical procedures are occasionally identified[115] but at presentation invasion has generally supervened.

Further evidence of dysplasia preceding carcinoma came from a large autopsy study in which the whole bronchial tree was examined in a series of patients dying of lung cancer.[28] This showed widespread premalignant changes involving mucosa that appeared macroscopically normal, including foci of carcinoma-*in-situ* and occasional microinvasive cancers distant from the main tumour.

Foci of hyperplasia, metaplasia and dysplasia are also frequently seen adjacent to invasive tumours in surgical specimens,[116] and similar changes have been described in experimental dogs exposed to cigarette smoke.[30] Full thickness squamous metaplasia is not necessary before atypical features are seen in the proliferating basal cells; dysplasia may be present beneath an intact surface layer of columnar cells.[28] The transition from normal bronchial epithelium to squamous epithelium is usually abrupt. Atypical epithelium may extend deeply into bronchial glands replacing duct and acinar lining cells. The appearances may mimic microinvasive carcinoma but the basement membrane as yet remains intact.

In view of the extent of these pre-malignant changes, it is not surprising that there is a high incidence of double or second primary lung cancers;[117] even triple primary tumours are described.[118] Using standard criteria of a double primary growth, namely involvement of different lobes, or different histological types, or a time interval over 3 years, it has been shown that 4% of lung cancer patients have more than one lung tumour at presentation and that a further 6% develop a second primary lung growth later.[117] The patients most at risk of developing lung cancer are therefore those who have had one in the past. These patients might therefore be worth following up particularly frequently.

Patients with squamous dysplasia or carcinoma-*in-situ* may be asymptomatic or present with cough and haemoptysis. However, it is often difficult to know how much their cough is due to the dysplastic change rather than other smoking related diseases such as chronic bronchitis. The epithelial changes are focal, usually developing at the bifurcations of segmental bronchi and subsequently extending proximally and distally. They are not always visible to the bronchoscopist but are sometimes evident as grey plaque. Treatment is problematic because the lesions are frequently multiple.[119] Patients are therefore liable to be followed up by serial bronchoscopy until inva-

Table 12.1.3   Morphology of squamous dysplasia and carcinoma-*in-situ*[112]

Abnormality	Thickness	Cell size	Maturation/Orientation	Nuclei
Mild dysplasia	Mildly increased	Mildly increased	Continuous progression of maturation	Mild variation of nuclear/cytoplasmic ratio
		Mild anisocytosis, pleomorphism	Basilar zone expanded with cellular crowding in lower-third	Finely granular chromatin
			Distinct intermediate (prickle cell) zone present	Minimal angulation
			Superficial flattening of epithelial cells	Nucleoli inconspicuous or absent
				Nuclei vertically oriented in lower third
				Mitoses absent or very rare
Moderate dysplasia	Moderately increased	Mild increase in cell size	Partial progression of maturation	Moderate variation of N/C ratio
		Moderate anisocytosis, pleomorphism	Basilar zone expanded; cellular crowding in lower two-thirds	Finely granular chromatin
			Intermediate zone confined to upper third of epithelium	Nuclear angulations, grooves, lobulations present
			Superficial flattening of epithelial cells	Nucleoli inconspicuous or absent
				Nuclei vertically oriented in lower two-thirds
				Mitotic figures present in lower third
Severe dysplasia	Markedly increased	Markedly increased	Little progression of maturation from base to luminal surface	Nuclear/cytoplasmic ratio often high and variable
		Marked anisocytosis, pleomorphism	Basilar zone expanded with cellular crowding well into upper third	Chromatin coarse and uneven
			Intermediate zone greatly attenuated	Nuclear angulations and folding prominent
			Superficial flattening of epithelial cells	Nucleoli frequently present and conspicuous
				Nuclei vertically oriented in lower two-thirds
				Mitotic figures present in lower two-thirds
Carcinoma *in situ*	May or may not be increased	May be markedly increased	No progression of maturation from base to luminal surface, epithelium could be inverted with little change in appearance	Nuclear/cytoplasmic ratio often high and variable
		Marked anisocytosis, pleomorphism	Basilar zone expanded with cellular crowding throughout epithelium	Chromatin coarse and uneven
			Intermediate zone absent	Nuclear angulations and folding prominent
			Surface flattening only of most superficial cells	Nucleoli frequently present and conspicuous
				No consistent orientation of nuclei in relation to epithelial surface
				Mitotic figures present through full thickness

sion is apparent when the lesion may be treated by local ablation or surgical resection.

Atypical adenomatous hyperplasia

The hyperplasia – dysplasia – neoplasia sequence is again encountered in the periphery of the lung,[120,121] particularly when there is diffuse pulmonary fibrosis.[83,84] Accompanying such fibrosis there is often hyperplasia of type II alveolar epithelial cells, sometimes accompanied by extension of bronchiolar epithelium into adjacent alveoli and occasionally by squamous metaplasia and dysplasia. The tumours that develop in pulmonary fibrosis may be of any histological type but there is a disproportionately large number of adenocarcinomas, especially bronchioloalveolar carcinomas.[122] However, the development of a carcinoma in relation to a solitary lung scar (so-called 'scar cancer') is less common than was once believed (see p. 551).

Atypical alveolar hyperplasia is also reported as a focal premalignant change accompanying carcinoma in lungs that are not affected by fibrosis (Fig. 12.1.3), when it is generally termed atypical adenomatous hyperplasia.[123–126] Remarkably, such foci are quite commonly found when sought in lungs resected for cancer yet they have evidently lain undiscovered by generations of pathologists dealing with such specimens. Admittedly, they are generally small and easily overlooked. Their identification is facilitated by immersion in Bouin's solution[127] or microscopically by the immunocytochemical demonstration of cytokeratin for they represent foci of hyperplastic type II alveolar epithelial cells or bronchiolar Clara cells. An autopsy study of 100 cases free of lung cancer identified focal adenomatous hyperplasia in six,[128] while in lungs resected for cancer atypical adenomatous hyperplasia has been reported in up to 23% of cases.[127,129,130] The tumour that atypical adenomatous hyperplasia most often accompanies is an adenocarcinoma, particularly a peripheral adenocarcinoma, but it is sometimes a large cell or

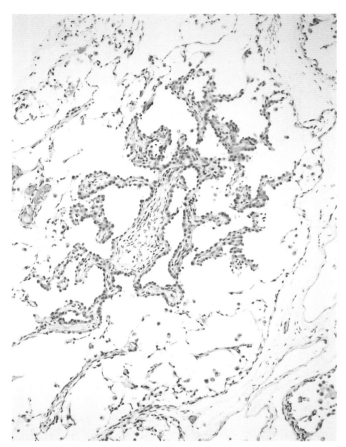

Figure 12.1.3 A focus of atypical adenomatous hyperplasia identified in a random section of lung excised because of carcinoma.

squamous cell carcinoma.[131] Multiple lesions may be found, particularly in association with multiple adenocarcinomas. Molecular studies show that individual lesions differ in their genetic make-up, establishing that they are independent of each other and of any accompanying carcinoma and do not represent micrometastases of the latter.[132]

Atypical adenomatous hyperplasia is a focal lesion, generally less than 5mm in diameter, in which the alveoli are lined by cuboidal to low columnar cells with dense chromatin, prominent nucleoli and sparse cytoplasm.[112,133] The interstitium may show some fibrosis but this is generally mild. Atypical adenomatous hyperplasia is distinguished from non-mucinous bronchioloalveolar carcinoma by its size (generally less than 5mm whereas most carcinomas exceed 10mm), gaps between the epithelial cells as opposed to a continuous cell line, and the cells being cuboidal rather than columnar. Mitoses are rarely evident but varying degrees of atypia are observed[125,134] and the familiar hyperplasia – dysplasia – neoplasia sequence is easily envisaged. Morphometry,[135,136] argyrophilic nucleolar-organiser counts,[137] DNA status,[136,137] loss of heterozygosity[138] and the identification of a range of oncogenes within the atypical lesions[124,135,139–141] provide further support for this form of hyperplasia being premalignant. The demonstration of monoclonality suggests that it is neoplastic[123,142] and it is now widely regarded as being the precursor of non-mucinous bronchio-

loalveolar carcinoma and subsequently most peripheral adenocarcinomas. Nevertheless, the presence of multiple foci of atypical adenomatous hyperplasia does not appear to be related to patient survival.[143,144] Patients without cancer who are found to have harboured this lesion should be kept under surveillance: further intervention is not warranted.

More recently, bronchiolar columnar cell dysplasia has been described as a further precursor of adenocarcinoma.[145] The micronodular hyperplasia of type II pneumocytes reported in tuberous sclerosis (see p. 689) is not recognised as being premalignant. Some congenital lung cysts have a low but appreciable malignant potential (see p. 61).

Molecular factors in the development of lung cancer

That the morphological changes described above are truly premalignant is supported by the demonstration of genetic abnormalities similar to those found in adjacent invasive cancer.[146–153] They reflect a multistep accumulation of genetic abnormalities, the number of which gradually increases as dysplasia progresses.[154–156] The earliest molecular changes may be detected before any abnormality is evident at the microscopic level. Mutations involving a single gene are generally insufficient to cause cancer. Successive mutations affecting 10–20 different oncogenes or anti-oncogenes are required before malignant change is eventually established.[156] Molecular techniques therefore enable the identification of premalignant change in tissues that may be normal histologically.[147,149–151,157] Some of the earliest genetic changes involve loci on chromosomes 3p and 9p.[158,159] Inactivation of the *p16* gene is also an early event whereas mutations involving the K-*ras* and *p53* genes occur late in the sequence of genetic alterations.

Many of the carcinogens discussed above act by inducing mutations in the genes that control cell growth, either by activating genes that enhance cell growth (proto-oncogenes) or inactivating tumour suppressor genes (anti-oncogenes).[160,161] The activity of growth factors is largely dependent on proto-oncogenes because these involve receptors on the cell surface concerned in signal transduction. These cellular oncogenes (c-*onco* genes) control normal cell growth and differentiation and have the potential to influence tumour behaviour. Other oncogenes (v-*onc* genes) have been identified in a large group of RNA viruses, the retroviruses, and the possible role of these viruses in pulmonary carcinogenesis is touched upon above. Proto-oncogenes are generally dominant and mutation of only one allele is therefore sufficient to promote undue cell growth. Tumour suppressor genes on the other hand are generally recessive and mutation of both alleles is therefore required for their inactivation. The first mutation usually results in a small alteration and the second a large one involving complete loss or translocation of the gene. The second mutation can be detected following suitable amplification, for example by the polymerase chain reaction, as a single band on gel electrophoresis, a change that is often termed 'loss of heterozygosity'. Molecular factors that have been implicated in lung cancer are listed in Table 12.1.4.

Table 12.1.4 Molecular markers associated with lung cancer

Gene mutation	Chromosome involved	Type of mutation
Proto-oncogene activation		
Ki-ras, Ha-ras, N-ras	12p	Point mutation
c-erb-B2 (Her-2/neu) (Epidermal growth factor receptor gene)	17q	Translocation
c-myc, L-myc, N-myc	8	Translocation
bcl-2	14-18	Translocation
Tumour suppressor gene inactivation		
FHIT, the fragile histidine triad gene	3p	Deletion
Retinoblastoma gene	13q	Point mutation
p53	17p	Deletion
Growth factors/receptors		
Epidermal growth factor receptor		
Transforming growth factor		
Vascular endothelium growth factor		
Gastrin-releasing peptide		
Transferrin		
Insulin-like growth factor		
Endothelin		

Proto-oncogenes involved in lung cancer include those belonging to the *ras* and *myc* families, especially K-*ras* and c-*myc*. Activating point mutations of *ras* genes result in an aberrant p21 membrane-associated protein that continuously transduces an inappropriate growth signal. K-*ras* is mutated in 30% of pulmonary adenocarcinomas,[162] and particularly in the mucinous type of bronchioloalveolar carcinoma.[163] It is recorded in the precursor lesion atypical alveolar hyperplasia that is described above. K-*ras* mutation is therefore a good candidate for the early detection of lung cancer as it should be detectable in bronchioloalveolar cells shed in sputum or recovered by lavage.

Myc genes encode for cell cycle specific nuclear phosphoproteins and thereby control cell growth and differentiation. Amplification of the *myc* group of oncogenes accounts for *myc* protein accumulation in 20% of small cell carcinomas and 10% of non-small cell carcinomas. It is found particularly in patients with recurrent tumour.[164-166] Conversely, *myc* genes are seldom amplified in carcinomas from patients who have not undergone treatment and thus appear to be associated with tumour progression rather than initiation. Some drug regimens result in *myc* amplification more than others.

Apoptosis is promoted by the Bax gene and blocked by the bcl-2 (B cell lymphoma-2) gene, the latter thereby preventing cell death. The bcl-2 gene is over-expressed in pre-invasive lesions, a variable number of non-small cell carcinomas of the lung,[167-169] most small cell carcinomas and a variety of other lung tumours showing neuroendocrine differentiation.[170,171] A high bcl-2:bax ratio generally accompanies mutation of the p53 tumour suppressor gene.[171]

Tumour suppressor genes (anti-oncogenes) are believed to play an important role in the pathogenesis of lung cancer because deletions or mutations of chromosomes 3p, 13q and 17p are frequently found.[172-174] 13q is the site of the retinoblastoma gene, 17p the p53 gene and 3p the FHIT (fragile histidine triad) anti-oncogene. 3p deletion is particularly common in small cell carcinoma and 13q and 17p deletion in non-small cell carcinoma.[175-177] FHIT deletion is one of the earliest mutations and p53 deletion one of the last in the lung cancer gene sequence. p53 mutation is the most common genetic alteration in human cancer and occurs in over half of lung cancers. p53 is normally responsible for apoptosis and abnormalities of this gene are thought to permit unchecked cell proliferation. The normal p53 protein product is generally undetectable due to a short half-life but mutations frequently extend this so that the protein accumulates and can be detected immunocytochemically. Accumulation of p53 protein product has been associated with an adverse prognosis in lung cancer and may provide a marker for early diagnosis or pre-malignant states.[178]

Recognition of a structural homology between certain growth factor receptors and oncogenes, and acceptance of the concept of autocrine activity by which tumour cells secrete substances that induce self-proliferation have stimulated much interest. Gastrin releasing peptide (human bombesin) is one of the best known autocrine factors and is particularly involved in the remarkably rapid growth of small cell carcinomas.[179] The gastrin releasing peptide receptor gene appears to be activated by cigarette smoke and being located on the X chromosome is more strongly expressed in women than men,[180] possibly contributing to the greater female susceptibility to tobacco-induced lung cancer noted above.[5] Other autocrine factors secreted by small cell carcinoma include transferrin, an insulin-like growth factor and endothelin,[181-183] while epidermal growth factor receptor gene (c-erbB-2 [HER2/neu] oncogene) is over-expressed in non-small cell carcinoma.[184]

Telomerase is a molecular marker that can be detected in most lung cancers and is frequently found in bronchial epithelium showing premalignant change. It is the enzyme that adds nucleotide repeats to the ends (telomeres) of chromosomes to compensate for the nucleotide losses that occur with each round of DNA replication.[185-187] Normal somatic cells show no telomerase activity and stop dividing when their telomers are sufficiently shortened. The indefinite proliferation of cancer cells probably owes much to their telomerase activity.

Oncogenes and growth factors are obviously important to the prognosis of lung cancer and are touched upon again under that heading on p. 567.

Screening for lung cancer

Lung cancer fulfils many of the criteria necessary for a successful screening programme: the condition is common, the population at risk is well known and pre-malignant changes can be detected cheaply (by sputum cytology). Unfortunately the premalignant changes cannot be easily eradicated: there is no bronchopulmonary equivalent of a uterine cone biopsy. Nor

Table 12.1.5	Natural history of lung cancer[190]		
Cell type	Volume doubling time (days)	Years from malignant change to the tumour reaching	
		1 cm (diagnosis)	10 cm (death)
Squamous cell carcinoma	88	8.4	9.6
Adenocarcinoma	161	15.4	17.6
Large cell carcinoma	86	8.2	9.4
Small cell carcinoma	29	2.8	3.2

does screening for early invasive growths by a combination of sputum cytology and radiography appear to reduce mortality.[188,189] The relative failure of surgery, radical radiotherapy and preventive screening programmes is partly explained by backward extrapolations of observed tumour size doubling times, which suggest that malignant change takes place years before a tumour is first detectable clinically (Table 12.1.5).[190] Nevertheless, sparked by the advances in molecular pathology described above and refinements in HRCT, there has been a renewal of interest in early detection.[188] For example, it appears that p53 immunohistochemistry may assist in the identification of preneoplastic lesions,[152] the detection of *p16(INK4a)* inactivation in sputum may identify smokers at increased risk of developing lung cancer[191,192] and low dose CT screening trials are proving more sensitive in detecting small peripheral tumours.[193–198] Wedge resection rather than lobectomy is undertaken for these small asymptomatic lesions, with good results, particularly for those showing ground-glass opacification, which is characteristic of bronchioloalveolar carcinoma.[199–202]

SITE OF ORIGIN AND SPREAD

As might be expected from the relative size of the two lungs, slightly more carcinomas arise on the right than the left. There is also a slight preponderance in the upper lobes. Most carcinomas arise in large central bronchi (Fig. 12.1.4), particularly at bifurcations where inhaled particles tend to impinge and mucociliary clearance is delayed (Fig. 12.1.5)[203–205] Primary carcinoma of the trachea is rare,[206] possibly because of its lack of branches, the mouths of which present a barrier to mucociliary clearance in the bronchi: the few tumours that arise in the trachea are generally of salivary gland type or carcinoids.[207]

Despite the large central bronchi being the most common site of origin, a substantial number of carcinomas are peripheral and the proportion of these tends to be underestimated because hilar lymph node metastases may grow into an adjacent bronchus and simulate a primary bronchial growth, the smaller but real primary in the periphery of the lung being overlooked or mistaken for a metastasis.[120,208,209] The ratio of central to peripheral growths is about 2:1[210–212] Historically, squamous cell and small cell carcinomas have preponderated in the main airways and

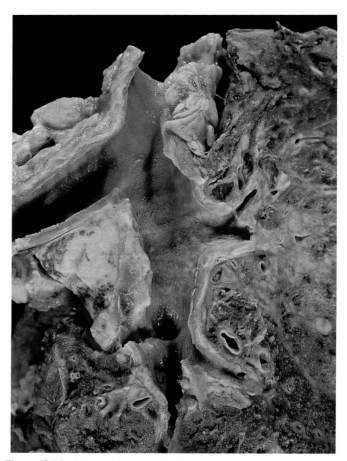

Figure 12.1.4 Most carcinomas arise in large central bronchi. Note the slight roughening of the bronchial mucosa and the invasion of adjacent hilar lymph nodes. (Illustration provided by Dr GA Russell, Tunbridge Wells, UK.)

adenocarcinoma in the periphery of the lung but with the current changes in the proportions of the various histological types (see p. 542) this difference is becoming less marked.[213]

Dissemination of the tumour is chiefly along lymphatic routes, at least initially. Blood spread usually follows. Metastases in hilar and mediastinal lymph nodes, and perhaps beyond, have often developed by the time symptoms first cause the patient to seek attention. Retrograde spread within the lung may lead to widespread lymphatic permeation, resulting in so-called 'lymphangitis carcinomatosa', which is described in the chapter on secondary tumours, as are extralymphatic routes of tumour spread within the lung (see p. 669). Further tumour growth and dissemination give rise to a variety of clinical effects, which will now be described.

CLINICAL EFFECTS

Most lung cancers are diagnosed because the patient presents with symptoms: less than 15% are discovered by chance, usually during the course of radiological investigations performed for other purposes, such as routine preoperative assess-

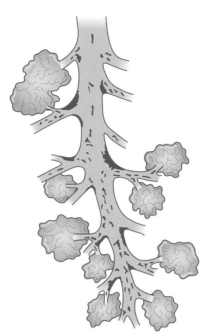

Figure 12.1.5 Mucociliary clearance is impaired at bronchial branching points, as shown in this drawing of a rat's airways following the experimental insufflation of carbon. (Reproduced from Iravani J, van As A. Mucous transport in the tracheobronchial tree of normal and bronchitic rats. Journal of Pathology 1972; 106:81–93.[203] Copyright Pathological Society of Great Britain and Ireland. Reproduced with permission. Permission granted by John Wiley & Sons on behalf of PathSoc.)

Table 12.1.6 Histological findings in two series of 'peripheral coin lesions' (%)

	A German series (n = 955)[214]	A New Zealand series (n = 114)[215]
Malignant neoplasm	49	71
Primary carcinoma	38	64
Other primary malignancy	2	7
Metastasis	9	
Benign lesion	51	29
Benign neoplasm	14	
'Hamartoma'	8	
Nerve tumour	2	
Adenoma	1	
Localised fibrous tumour	<1	
Others	2	
Non-neoplastic lesion	37	
Tuberculosis	24	
Pneumonia/abscess	2	
Echinococcal cyst	2	
Bronchogenic cyst	2	
Aspergilloma	1	
Others	5	

ment, the investigation of chest injuries, the detection of metastases of other tumours, or life insurance.

An asymptomatic solitary pulmonary nodule ('coin lesion')

The management of an asymptomatic patient in whom a solitary, well-circumscribed pulmonary opacity has been discovered has to be based on the supposition that the lesion is malignant until proved otherwise. Radiological evidence of central calcification and a slow growth rate suggest that the lesion is benign whereas fine linear strands radiating from the edge of the nodule favour the converse, but these features are not wholly reliable. Not infrequently all investigations short of thoracotomy fail to provide a diagnosis and the lesion is resected or submitted for frozen section. While it may well prove to be fungal in the USA, an echinococcal cyst in the Orient, and tuberculosis worldwide, a malignant tumour is often the cause. Details of two large series are provided in Table 12.1.6.[214,215]

Local effects

Central tumours are prone to obstruct the larger airways (Fig. 12.1.6), leading to pulmonary collapse, infection and endogenous lipid pneumonia (see p. 316). This results in cough, dyspnoea, pain and fever. Haemoptysis caused by ulceration of the tumour is another common symptom but is not usually severe. However, many peripheral tumours reach a substantial size and metastasise before causing any symptoms

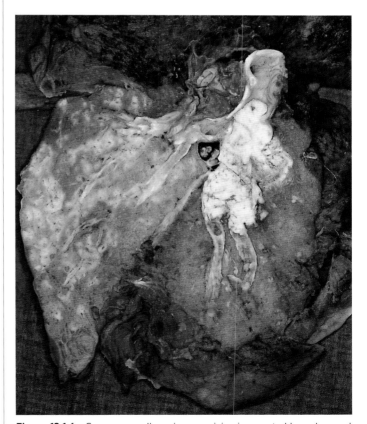

Figure 12.1.6 Squamous cell carcinoma arising in a central bronchus and growing in largely endobronchial manner within the intermediate and right lower lobe bronchi to obstruct the lumen and cause distal bronchiectasis (in the lower lobe) and obstructive pneumonia (in the middle lobe).

at all. Cavitation is often evident radiologically, particularly with squamous cell carcinomas, while the radiographic features of bronchioloalveolar carcinomas often simulate those of pneumonic consolidation.

Patients being treated for pneumonia should be observed until there is complete roentographic resolution. Any pneumonia that does not resolve within 4 weeks should be evaluated further to exclude carcinoma.

Intrathoracic spread

Direct spread may cause pleural or chest wall pain, while either pleural involvement or post-stenotic bronchopneumonia may cause pleural effusion, which if neoplastic is characteristically haemorrhagic.

Apical tumours are prone to invade the ribs, the brachial plexus and the cervical part of the sympathetic system (Fig. 12.1.7) causing pain in the shoulder and the ulnar side of the arm, atrophy of the hand muscles, Horner's syndrome (ptosis, constricted pupil, enophthalmos and decreased ipsilateral facial sweating), bone destruction and an apical radiographic opacity. This syndrome was first described by Hare in 1838,[216] but it is generally named after Pancoast who described it afresh a century later;[217] the term 'superior sulcus syndrome' is also used.[218] Most tumours that cause Pancoast's syndrome are squamous cell carcinomas.

Involvement of the left recurrent laryngeal nerve as it loops around the aorta to cause hoarseness is another characteristic neurological complication of bronchopulmonary carcinoma.

Superior vena caval obstruction may be caused by compression and infiltration of the vein by either the primary tumour or metastases in superior mediastinal lymph nodes (Fig. 12.1.8). Small cell carcinoma is particularly likely to present in this way, with massive mediastinal nodes and a small or even undetectable primary. Hilar lymph node metastases may also cause bronchial narrowing and its sequelae. Any lung tumour that

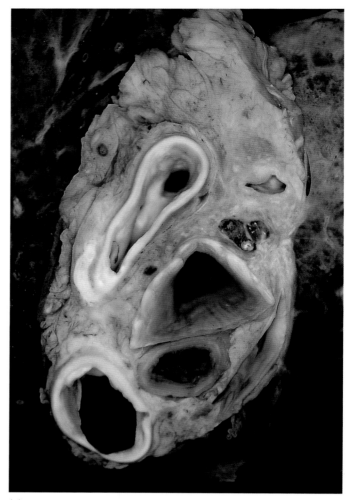

(a)

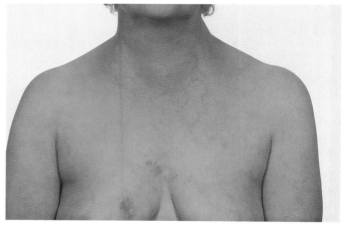

(b)

Figure 12.1.8 Superior vena caval compression by mediastinal tumour. (a) Cross-section of the mediastinum viewed from above at the level of the aortic arch showing compression of the superior vena cava by metastatic small cell carcinoma. The compressed vein is situated to the right of the ascending aorta and in front of the carbon-pigmented pretracheal lymph node. (b) In life, the patient had shown distension of veins over the front of the chest.

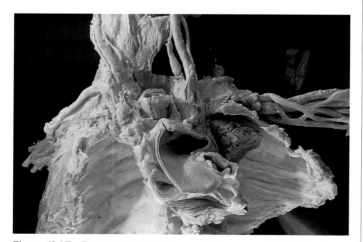

Figure 12.1.7 Pancoast tumour. A tumour in the apex of the left lung has invaded the ribs, the cervical sympathetic chain and the brachial plexus

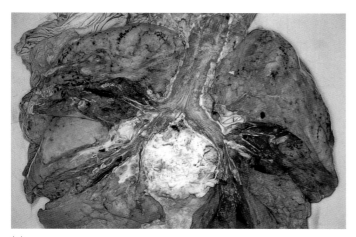

(a)

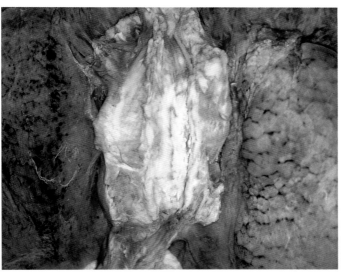

(b)

Figure 12.1.9 Anterior (a) and posterior (b) views of a squamous cell carcinoma of the left main bronchus that metastasised to subcarinal lymph nodes and thence invaded the oesophagus.

Table 12.1.7 Metastatic patterns of lung cancer at autopsy (%) in patients dying of lung cancer[219]

	Squamous cell	Adeno	Large cell	Small cell
Hilar/mediastinal nodes	77	80	84	96
Pleura	34	60	67	34
Chest wall	20	20	20	13
Limited to thorax	46	18	14	4
Liver	25	41	48	74
Adrenals	23	50	59	55
Bone	20	36	30	37
Abdominal nodes	10	23	30	52
CNS	NS	37	25	29

NS, incidence not stated.

Table 12.1.8 Paraneoplastic syndromes associated with lung cancer

Neuromuscular	**Musculoskeletal and cutaneous**
Polymyositis	Hypertrophic osteoarthropathy
Myasthenic syndrome	Clubbing
Sensory motor neuropathy	Dermatomyositis
Encephalopathy	Acanthosis nigricans
Myelopathy	Pruritus
Cerebellar degeneration	Urticaria
Psychosis	Erythema multiforme
Dementia	Hyperpigmentation
Endocrine	**Haematological**
Cushing's syndrome	Haemolytic anaemia
Inappropriate ADH secretion	Red cell aplasia
Hypercalcaemia	Polycythaemia
Carcinoid syndrome	Thrombocytopenic purpura
Gynaecomastia	Thrombocytosis
Hyperglycaemia	Dysproteinaemia
Hypoglycaemia	Eosinophilia
Galactorrhoea	Leukoerythroblastic reaction
Growth hormone excess	including thrombocytopenia
Secretion of TSH	
Calcitonin secretion	**Others**
	Nephrotic syndrome
Cardiovascular	Hyperuricaemia
Superficial thrombophlebitis	Amyloidosis
(Trousseau's syndrome)	Secretion of alkaline phosphatase
Thrombosis	Secretion of immunoglobulin A
Marantic endocarditis	

ADH, antidiuretic hormone; TSH, thyroid stimulating hormone.

extends into the pericardium or oesophagus (Fig. 12.1.9) is likely to cause cardiac tamponade or dysphagia, respectively, but invasion of the heart itself is unusual.

Extrathoracic spread

Many patients with carcinoma of the lung eventually develop cervical or abdominal lymph node involvement, while about a third present with distant metastases, which may obviously lead to a wide variety of symptoms, depending on the site involved. Blood-borne metastases of lung carcinoma occur most often in the liver, adrenal glands, brain, skeleton and kidneys: in many countries the most common cerebral tumour of adults is metastatic carcinoma of the lung. The pattern of metastases varies with the histological type (Table 12.1.7).[219]

Paraneoplastic manifestations

Paraneoplastic syndromes are non-metastatic disorders of distant organs. They develop in 10–20% of cases of lung cancer. Some of the better established paraneoplastic syndromes are listed in Table 12.1.8.

Neuromuscular paraneoplastic syndromes are quite varied. They include the carcinomatous neuromyopathies, a term that covers a variety of encephalopathies, myelopathies, peripheral neuropathies and myopathies.[220] Polymyositis and dermato-myositis come within the myopathies and up to 30% of patients with these diseases have an underlying neoplasm.[221] Carcinomatous neuropathy and the myasthenia gravis-like Eaton–Lambert syndrome are particularly associated with small cell lung cancer.[222] The Eaton–Lambert myasthenic syndrome is a disorder of acetylcholine production at neuromuscular junctions in which an autoantibody directed against determinants on the tumour cell membrane cross-reacts with components of the nerve terminal.[223] Autoantibodies directed against a neuronal or muscle cell antigen underlie many carcinomatous neuromyopathies.[224] These syndromes are not related to the size or duration of the tumour and may develop months before the tumour becomes apparent.

Inappropriate or ectopic hormone secretion is responsible for another important group of paraneoplastic syndromes. It is most often associated with small cell carcinoma; common examples include the secretion of adrenocorticotrophic hormone and antidiuretic hormone by the tumour.[225] Antidiuretic hormone is raised in the serum of 30–40% of patients with small cell carcinoma but the clinical syndrome of severe hyponatraemia, hypo-osmolality of the serum and continued urinary sodium excretion is recognised in only 5–10%.[226] Excess antidiuretic hormone is sometimes found with non-neoplastic lung disease but here it is pituitary in origin rather than ectopic.

Severe clinical symptoms due to adrenocorticotrophic hormone production are seen in 3–7% of patients with small cell carcinoma. They generally lack the classic features of Cushing's syndrome (Fig. 12.1.10) but glucose intolerance and hypokalaemic alkalosis are often severe and hyperpigmentation is usually pronounced.[227]

Less common is the production of atrial natriuretic peptide and vasopressin[228] or the kinins responsible for the carcinoid syndrome.[229] Rare peptide syndromes include hypoglycaemia, hyperpigmentation and hypercalcaemia. Cancer-associated hypercalcaemia is usually due to bone metastases but occasionally occurs without metastatic disease, when it is generally mediated by parathyroid-related protein which increases both bone resorption and renal tubular reabsorption of calcium: serum parathyroid hormone levels are characteristically low or unmeasurable in these cases. The lung tumour most commonly associated with such hypercalcaemia is squamous cell carcinoma.[230] Gynaecomastia and testicular atrophy are occasionally encountered, again with squamous cell carcinoma. Adenocarcinoma of the lung is occasionally responsible for elevated serum levels of amylase.[231] Elevated levels of human chorionic gonadotrophin, α-fetoprotein and other trophoblast markers are sometimes associated with a variety of non-small cell carcinomas of the lung,[232] but notably ones resembling hepatocellular carcinoma ('hepatoid carcinoma of the lung').[233]

Common haematological abnormalities include the anaemia of chronic disease and thrombocytosis. As with many other cancers, there may be activation of the coagulation cascade resulting in venous thrombosis or disseminated intravascular coagulation. Cardiovascular syndromes also include non-bacterial thrombotic (marantic) endocarditis, the vegetations of

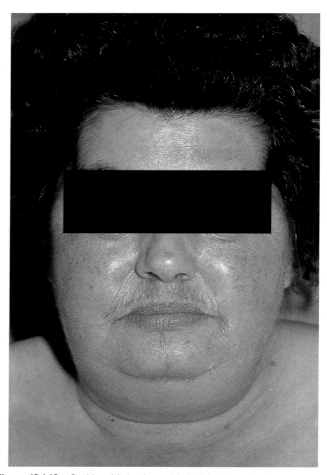

Figure 12.1.10 Cushingoid obesity and facial hirsutism due to inappropriate production of adrenocorticotrophic hormone in a patient with small cell carcinoma of the bronchus.

which may embolise and cause transient ischaemia. Less commonly, carcinoma of the lung releases haemopoietic growth or chemotactic factors, resulting in either blood or local tissue eosinophilia[234] or neutrophilia.[235–237]

Other associated disorders include pulmonary hypertrophic osteoarthropathy, acanthosis nigricans and scleroderma while lung tumour antigens may result in immune-complex glomerulonephritis and vasculitis.[238,239]

DIAGNOSTIC PROCEDURES FOR OBTAINING TUMOUR MATERIAL

The main methods of obtaining material for the pathological diagnosis of lung cancer are sputum collection, bronchoscopy and transthoracic needle aspiration, supplemented as required by tissue obtained at mediastinoscopy, mediastinotomy and thoracotomy, or on biopsies or aspirates of distant metastases. Thoracotomy is now generally video-assisted.

If necessary, sputum production can be induced by the inhalation of a saline spray. When cancer is present, the detection rate after four good specimens of sputum, obtained on waking and after cleaning the mouth, is about 85%.[240] Poor quality specimens result in this figure being considerably lower. A freshly fixed smear stained with Papanicolaou's stain, haematoxylin and eosin or other stain of choice may be examined, or sputum may be collected for several days in a container of alcohol, and the specimen then smeared or blocked for the preparation of paraffin sections. Alternatively, the sputum may first be homogenised.[241] Cytological typing of lung tumours is possible in most cases[242] and is often superior to histological typing.[243]

The flexible fibre-optic bronchoscope has greatly facilitated the collection of bronchopulmonary samples. The specimens are small but many can be taken. It is reported that four biopsies are sufficient to ensure the diagnosis of central tumours but that six may be required if the tumour is peripheral.[244]

Typing is relatively easy if the tumour is well-differentiated but it can be very difficult to type poorly-differentiated tumours in small fibroptic biopsies[245,246] and clinicians often fail to appreciate how a biopsy diagnosis of undifferentiated large cell carcinoma comes to be re-categorised when the resection specimen is examined. For this reason, it is better to use the term undifferentiated non-small cell carcinoma when specimens are small, and only diagnose large cell carcinoma when the tumour can be widely sampled and differentiation excluded.[245,247] The degree of differentiation varies greatly from one part of a tumour to another and adequate grading of lung tumours is never possible on biopsy specimens. Surface abnormalities may not reflect the cell type of an underlying tumour and caution is needed if the biopsy is unduly superficial. For instance, small cell carcinoma may be covered by atypical metaplastic epithelium or even squamous carcinoma-*in-situ* and if the invasive tumour is not sampled an erroneous report may be issued (Fig. 12.1.11).[248]

Cytological specimens may also be obtained at bronchoscopy, by washing, brushing or transbronchial fine needle aspiration[249,250] and the combination of cytology and biopsy has been shown to be cost-effective.[251] Brushing of many branches increases the detection rate and can identify the site of an occult carcinoma.[252] When the tumour is located peripherally and cannot be visualised by bronchoscopy, selective bronchial lavage can be useful.[253]

Fine needle aspiration is usually reserved for peripheral growths. It requires fluoroscopic control and the radiologist greatly appreciates the attendance of a laboratory worker in the radiology suite to attend to the rapid fixation of material for cytology and on the spot verification that the specimen is adequate. However, with the introduction of spring-loaded widebore (18 gauge) needles, excellent specimens sufficient for histology are now obtained (see p. 736). Transbronchial needle aspiration is also useful in staging, often obviating the need for mediastinoscopy. By this means, lymph node involvement suspected on imaging (usually by either CT, PET or a combined scan) can be confirmed at the same time as the diagnostic bronchial biopsy.[254,255]

HISTOLOGICAL TYPING

The histological typing of lung cancer has long been subject to debate. This is partly due to the heterogeneity many lung tumours display. Many are of mixed cell type[256–259] or their cell type changes on treatment,[257,260,261] thus supporting Willis's unitary view that all pulmonary carcinomas arise from a common stem cell that has the potential to differentiate along various pathways.[262] On the other hand, the different tumour types clearly differ in their clinical behaviour and response to treatment, so histological typing is of considerable clinical importance.[263–265] Unfortunately, the small size of fibroptic bronchoscopic biopsy specimens imposes considerable problems in the accurate typing of lung tumours.[266]

The classification adopted here is that advocated by the World Health Organization (Table 12.1.9).[112,267] It is based solely on light microscopy and consequently can be used by histopathologists everywhere, which is important in epidemiological studies of causation and response to treatment. However, electron microscopy and immunohistochemistry can undoubtedly sharpen the histological diagnosis on occasion.[268–271]

The relative frequency of the various histological types varies according to the type of material examined (Table 12.1.10)[55,211,219,240,272–280] and thus depends upon the site and metastatic potential of the tumour. Surgical series include more peripheral tumours than bronchoscopic studies while those tumours that disseminate early are more numerous in autopsy series. Figures derived from large surveys provide the most reliable information but even these vary with time as smoking patterns change. There are also geographical differences. Squamous cell carcinoma has been the most common type in many countries but adenocarcinoma is increasing in frequency and is now the most common type in many American and Japanese series.[281–284] Figures also vary according to the detail

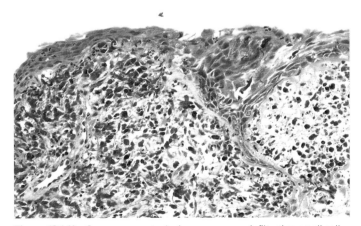

Figure 12.1.11 Squamous metaplasia seen over an infiltrating small cell carcinoma. Superficial sampling could lead to erroneous cell typing. The tumour has a classic 'oat cell' morphology, which is probably attributable to biopsy trauma.

put into the pathological examination. If mucus stains are neglected, many poorly-differentiated adenocarcinomas will be classified as undifferentiated large cell carcinoma, while if electron microscopy and immunocytochemistry are used the undifferentiated category is eliminated altogether and adenosquamous carcinoma becomes the most common. There may also be considerable interobserver variability: one group of

pathologists reached agreement on 72% of small cell carcinomas, 56% of adenocarcinomas, 48% of squamous cell carcinomas and only 5% of large cell carcinomas.[285] However, less interobserver variation is reported in other studies.[245,246,286]

Many pulmonary carcinogens are associated with particular histological types of lung cancer. The association with smoking has been stronger with centrally situated tumours such as squamous and small cell carcinomas than with tumours such as large cell and adenocarcinomas that are commoner in the periphery of the lung but this is changing with changes in cigarette manufacture.[211,287,288] Asbestos is particularly associated with adenocarcinoma[55–57,289] while irradiation and chloromethyl ether are both particularly associated with small cell carcinoma.[73] It has also been claimed that polyaromatic hydrocarbons, arsenic, chromates and nickel are all associated with squamous cell carcinoma but this is not well substantiated.[73]

In considering trends in the proportions of the various histological types, it should be borne in mind that the criteria for histological classification of lung carcinomas have changed.[290] Thus, the 1981 revision of the WHO classification is possibly relevant to some reports that adenocarcinoma is on the increase, because the revision recommended that solid tumours showing mucin secretion should be categorised as adenocarcinoma, rather than large cell carcinoma, as previously. However, quite apart from this, there appears to be a genuine increase in the proportion of adenocarcinomas.[211,282–284,291–293] This is seen in both men and women but is more marked among women.[283] It presumably reflects the increased popularity of low tar and filter-tipped cigarettes[288] and the increasing proportion of female smokers. This change in the proportions of the various histological types appears to be accompanied by a change in their distribution within the lung so that the historical predominance of adenocarcinomas in the periphery and squamous cell carcinomas in the central region is now less distinct.[213]

Table 12.1.9 World Health Organization histological classification of malignant epithelial tumours of lung[112]

Squamous cell carcinoma
  Variants:
    Papillary
    Clear cell
    Small cell
    Basaloid
Small cell carcinoma
  Variant:
    Combined
Adenocarcinoma
  Mixed adenocarcinoma
  Acinar adenocarcinoma
  Papillary adenocarcinoma
  Bronchioloalveolar carcinoma
  Solid adenocarcinoma with mucus formation
  Variants:
    Fetal adenocarcinoma
    Mucinous ('colloid') carcinoma
    Mucinous cystadenocarcinoma
    Signet ring adenocarcinoma
    Clear cell adenocarcinoma
Large cell carcinoma
  Variants:
    Large cell neuroendocrine carcinoma
    Basaloid carcinoma
    Lymphoepithelioma-like carcinoma
    Clear cell carcinoma
    Large cell carcinoma with rhabdoid phenotype
Adenosquamous carcinoma
Sarcomatoid carcinoma
  Pleomorphic carcinoma
  Spindle cell carcinoma
  Giant cell carcinoma
  Carcinosarcoma
  Pulmonary blastoma
Carcinoid tumour
  Typical carcinoid
  Atypical carcinoid
Salivary gland tumours
  Mucoepidermoid carcinoma
  Adenoid cystic carcinoma
  Epithelial-myoepithelial carcinoma

SQUAMOUS CELL CARCINOMA

Squamous cell carcinoma has classically been regarded as a tumour of the central bronchi (Figs 12.1.6, 12.1.9) but peripheral examples (Fig. 12.1.7) are now just as common.[294] The cut surface is often granular or friable and large tumours frequently cavitate because of central necrosis (Fig. 12.1.12). Hilar lymph nodes are often directly invaded. Metastasis occurs later than with the other histological types of bronchopulmonary carcinoma.

Table 12.1.10 Frequency (%) of histological subtypes of lung carcinoma by source of specimen[272–276]

	Biopsy/Cytology	Surgery[275,277]	Autopsy (hospital)[211,219,278]	All sources (community)[240]	All sources (asbestosis)[279,280]	All sources[55]
Squamous cell	44	56	34	47	52	19
Small cell	16	3	21	17	30	28
Adeno	22	28	26	16	13	38
Large cell	16	10	17	17	5	15

Histological appearances

Squamous cell carcinomas form irregular nests and strands of tumour cells separated by varying amounts of fibrous stroma. The tumour cells have large irregular nuclei, clumped chromatin and nucleoli of varying size. Stratification is often evident but by itself this is considered inadequate evidence of squamous differentiation as it is also seen in occasional poorly-differentiated adenocarcinomas. Categorisation of a pulmonary carcinoma as squamous cell requires evidence of either keratinisation or intercellular bridging.[112] Keratinisation may involve single tumour cells but is easier to recognise when it forms concentrically laminated squamous 'pearls' (Fig. 12.1.13). Individually keratinised cells are rounded and have slightly refractile eosinophilic cytoplasm. Their nuclei may be pyknotic or show karyolysis, but all these features are seen in any apoptotic tumour cell. To be confident that cytoplasmic eosinophilia represents keratinisation it is necessary to concentrate on cells with viable nuclei. Intercellular bridging is another marker of squamous differentiation. The bridges (or 'prickles') represent desmosomal cell junctions that are evident at the light microscopic level only because artefactual cell shrinkage results in them being stretched across intercellular spaces, where they are seen as regularly spaced thin cytoplasmic threads (Fig. 12.1.14).

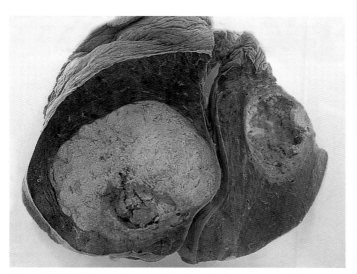

Figure 12.1.12   Two carcinomas of the lung, both squamous cell in type and both showing central cavitation. They are in different lobes, thereby fulfilling one of the criteria for double primary tumours.

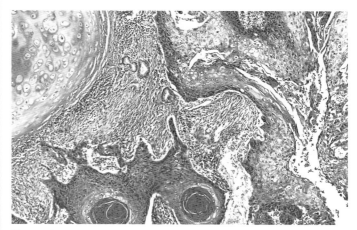

Figure 12.1.13   Well-differentiated squamous cell carcinoma of the bronchus showing stratification and two keratin 'pearls'.

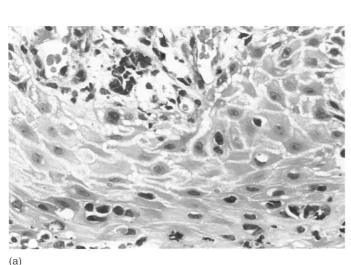

(a)

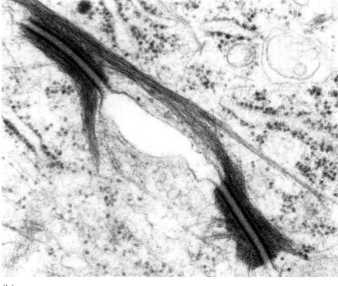

(b)

Figure 12.1.14   (a) Well-differentiated squamous cell carcinoma showing well-developed 'prickles' connecting the tumour cells and representing desmosomes highlighted by artefactual cell shrinkage. (b) Electron micrograph of the desmosomes, without shrinkage artefact. (Electron micrograph provided by Professor W. Mooi, Amsterdam, Netherlands.)

Central necrosis is often evident within groups of squamous carcinoma cells, often sharply demarcated from the viable tumour cells. Squamous debris may elicit a foreign body giant cell reaction. Alternatively, the necrotic debris may be absorbed, leaving a space that could be misinterpreted as evidence of glandular differentiation. Some squamous cell carcinomas show oncocytic change, due to large numbers of mitochondria within the cytoplasm. Osteocartilaginous stromal metaplasia is a further rare feature.[295] Rarely, squamous carcinomas of the lung have a distinctly adenoid structure and correspond to those more frequently encountered in the skin, where they are termed adenoacanthoma or adenoid or pseudovascular (pseudoangiosarcomatous) squamous cell carcinoma.[296] Pilomatricoma-like differentiation is particularly rare.[297]

Squamous cell carcinomas may be graded but this is best confined to resection specimens, as there is often considerable variation within a tumour: small biopsies are inadequate for tumour grading. Well-differentiated squamous cell carcinomas show prominent keratinisation throughout whereas poorly-differentiated tumours require careful scrutiny to identify keratinisation or intercellular bridging.

Histological variants

Four variants of squamous cell carcinoma are recognised – papillary, clear cell, small cell and basaloid.[112]

- *Papillary variant* (Fig. 12.1.15a): This variant has a papillary architecture and is very well-differentiated. Most examples are endobronchial. Often there is no evidence of stromal invasion, in which case they are better classified as carcinoma *in situ* with papillary architecture or even solitary squamous papilloma with dysplasia.[298] Most of these tumours are T1N0 and have a 5-year survival of over 60%.[299] Examples of the papillary variant developing in the periphery of the lung may show an alveolar filling pattern.[294]
- *Clear cell variant* (Fig. 12.1.15b): Small foci of clear cell change are commonly seen in squamous cell carcinomas but seldom predominate.[300] Pure clear cell carcinomas are classified as variant of large cell carcinoma and are described under that heading below. Focal clear cell change in a squamous cell carcinoma is of no prognostic significance.
- *Small cell variant:* (Fig. 12.1.15c): This a poorly-differentiated squamous cell carcinoma in which the cells are small but retain the nuclear characteristics of a non-small cell carcinoma and show focal squamous differentiation. Thus, it is composed of cells that bear a resemblance to small cell carcinoma in that they are small, but their nuclei are vesicular and contain evident nucleoli, lacking the 'salt and pepper' chromatin pattern of small cell carcinoma. It is to be distinguished from the combined variant of small cell carcinoma described below.[301] The prognosis is that of a poorly-differentiated squamous cell carcinoma.
- *Basaloid variant:* (Fig. 12.1.15d): This variant of squamous cell carcinoma is characterised by foci resembling basal cell carcinoma of the skin in that there is peripheral palisading

and the tumour cells are small and have hyperchromatic nuclei. Tumours with such features throughout are classified as a variant of large cell carcinoma and are described below under this heading. Some studies have shown that the basaloid variant of squamous cell carcinoma carries a worse prognosis than other poorly-differentiated squamous cell carcinomas in Stage I and II disease,[302,303] while others have failed to confirm this.[304]

Immunohistochemistry

Squamous cell carcinomas of the lung stain strongly for low molecular weight cytokeratins, and in the better differentiated tumours high molecular weight cytokeratins and carcinoembryonic antigen are also found.[305] There may also be focal staining for epithelial membrane antigen. Many squamous cell carcinomas stain for a variety of trophoblast markers.[232,306–308] Negative reactions are usually obtained for thyroid transcription factor-1 and the neuroendocrine marker CD56 (Table 12.1.11).

Electron microscopy

Electron microscopy generally shows a wealth of tonofibrils, many of which converge on desmosomes and extend into the intercellular bridges (Fig. 12.1.14). The cytoplasm otherwise contains relatively few organelles. Keratinisation is marked by increased numbers of tonofibrils, sometimes in a perinuclear arrangement. Thickening of the cell membrane by the deposition of small granules on its inner surface[309] appears to render the membrane impermeable and is followed by cytoplasmic shrinkage, pyknosis of the nucleus and ultimately cell death.

Differential diagnosis

There is seldom any difficulty in recognising squamous cell carcinoma but both histopathologists and cytopathologists need to beware of misinterpreting regenerative atypical squamous metaplasia. Quite alarming, but reversible changes may be seen

Table 12.1.11 Immunophenotypic characterisation of carcinoma of the lung. Immunohistochemistry may be used as an adjunct to histology, but not a substitute	
Cell type	*Usual immunophenotype*
Squamous cell carcinoma (including the basaloid variants of both squamous cell carcinoma and large cell carcinoma)	CK5 +ve, CK7 −ve > +ve, TTF1 −ve, CD56 −ve
Adenocarcinoma and some large cell carcinomas (including sarcomatoid carcinoma)	CK5 −ve, CK7 +ve, TTF1 +ve,[a] CD56 −ve
Small cell carcinoma and large cell neuroendocrine carcinoma	CK5 −ve, CK7 +ve, TTF1 +ve, CD56 +ve

CK, cytokeratin; TTF1, thyroid transcription factor 1.
[a]Mucinous bronchioloalveolar cell carcinomas are usually TTF1 −ve.

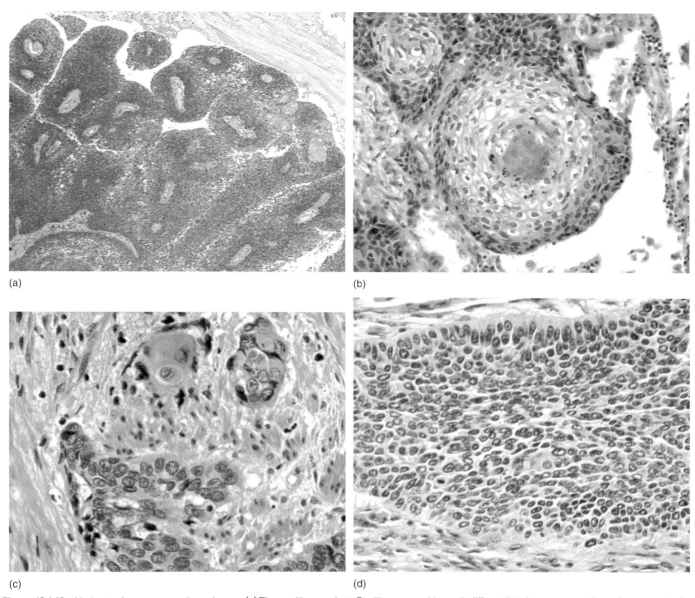

(a)

(b)

(c)

(d)

Figure 12.1.15 Variants of squamous cell carcinoma. (a) The papillary variant. Papillae covered by well-differentiated squamous cell carcinoma protrude into the bronchial lumen. (b) In the clear cell variant the tumour cell cytoplasm appears empty. (c) The small cell variant. Although the tumour cells are small (bottom) they lack the characteristic nuclear features of a small cell carcinoma and keratinisation is present in the upper half of the field. (d) The basaloid variant. Groups of tumour cells show peripheral palisading while the individual tumour cells are cuboidal or fusiform, have scanty cytoplasm and hyperchromatic nuclei devoid of prominent nucleoli. Squamoid elements were present elsewhere in the tumour.

bordering a necrotising process in the lung, such as a tuberculous cavity, an infarct or Wegener's granulomatosis, or in the bronchus if a recent biopsy site is again sampled.[105] Irradiation, cytotoxic therapy or even previous instrumentation may also give rise to false positive cytology results. Prolonged tracheal intubation may cause necrosis with extension of regenerative metaplasia into the submucosal glands, a process known as necrotising sialometaplasia, which also needs to be distinguished from invasive carcinoma.[310,311] The basaloid variant stains for high molecular weight cytokeratins but not for TTF-1 and neuroendocrine markers.[312] Small cell variants of squamous cell carcinoma also fail to stain for neuroendocrine markers.

ADENOCARCINOMA

In many parts of the world, adenocarcinoma of the lung shows an increase in its incidence that cannot be ascribed solely to changes in histological typing.[211,281,282,284,292] This may be connected with the increasing number of women who smoke, for women appear to have a propensity to develop carcinoma of this particular histological pattern,[291] but the major factor is probably the increasing popularity of filter-tipped cigarettes, the carcinogens of which are thought to penetrate more deeply into the lungs. Although most patients with pulmonary adeno-carcinoma are elderly cigarette smokers, there is a higher proportion of adenocarcinoma in non-smokers[313] and the young.[314]

Most adenocarcinomas of the lung arise in the periphery of the lung and it is usually difficult to determine whether they arise in a small bronchus, a bronchiole or the alveoli. In a Japanese study, less than 3% of adenocarcinomas arose in large central bronchi,[315] whereas this figure was over 13% in a British series.[316] It has been suggested that a simple division into central and peripheral would be better than histological subtyping, first because of histological heterogeneity and second because location has prognostic relevance, the central growths having the worse outlook.[316] Molecular studies demonstrating different mutations support the classification of pulmonary adenocarcinoma into bronchial and peripheral subtypes.[132]

Central adenocarcinomas often show polypoid endobronchial growth whereas peripheral adenocarcinomas often show central scarring with in-drawing of the overlying pleura (Fig. 12.1.16). Central cavitation is not so common as with squamous cell carcinomas. Occasionally peripheral adenocarcinomas spread out over the pleura, thereby mimicking mesothelioma (so-called pseudomesotheliomatous carcinoma of the lung).[317] The bronchioloalveolar pattern of adenocarcinoma has its own distinctive gross appearances and is dealt with separately.

Histological appearances

The WHO classification of lung tumours (Table 12.1.9) recognises five subtypes of adenocarcinoma and several rarer variants. However, adenocarcinomas of the lung form a heterogeneous group of tumours histologically, often showing variations in architecture, hence the *mixed* subtype (Fig. 12.1.17a), which makes up about 80% of cases. The periphery of the tumour frequently has a papillary, or bronchiovascular architecture, and the centre an acinar, papillary or solid pattern. For this reason, adenocarcinomas of the lung should not be subtyped or graded when dealing with small biopsies.

In the *acinar* pattern, there is a predominance of glandular structures, i.e. acini and tubules (Fig. 12.1.17b). The lining tumour cells are typically cuboidal or columnar with moderately abundant cytoplasm that may contain mucin. The tubules of an acinar adenocarcinoma have to be distinguished from the pseudoglandular structures that may develop in squamous cell carcinomas and large cell carcinomas as a result of central necrosis and absorption. Remnants of entrapped alveoli may also be mistaken for glandular differentiation.[318] Adenocarcinomas of acinar pattern mostly occur in the larger bronchi whereas predominantly papillary and bronchioloalveolar tumours constitute the commoner peripherally situated adenocarcinomas. In the *papillary* pattern (Fig. 12.1.17c) the tumour cells are again cuboidal or columnar and may again contain mucin but here they generally cover complex secondary and tertiary papillary

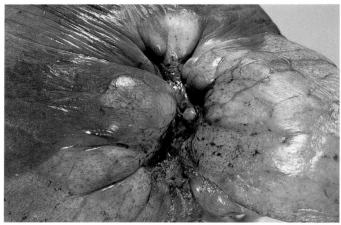

(a)

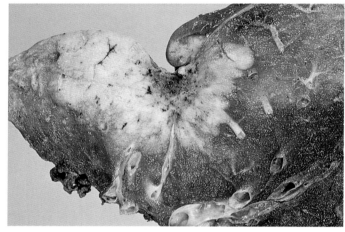

(b)

Figure 12.1.16 (a,b) A peripheral adenocarcinoma of the lung showing a central pigmented scar and indrawing of the overlying pleura.

structures with fibrovascular cores, as opposed to the simple papillary structures seen in the bronchioloalveolar carcinoma described below.[319] However, a *micropapillary* pattern of adenocarcinoma, in which the papillae lack stromal cores has also been described (Fig. 12.1.18).[320–322a] It is reputed to have a relatively poor prognosis. The *bronchioloalveolar* pattern of adenocarcinoma (Fig. 12.1.17d) is characterised by the tumour cells growing along the alveolar walls without destroying them. This is sometimes referred to as a lepidic growth pattern. It is commonly seen at the advancing edge of many adenocarcinomas that have a central acinar or papillary pattern. In the past, such mixed adenocarcinomas were often termed bronchioloalveolar but this category is now reserved for those that show a non-invasive, non-destructive pattern of mural growth throughout. The entire lesion is therefore required to determine whether a tumour grows exclusively in this fashion and bronchioloalveolar carcinoma is not a diagnosis that can be made on biopsy samples. It is considered separately below. The *solid* pattern of adenocarcinoma (Fig. 12.1.17e) is represented by sheets of polygonal cells devoid of intercellular bridges and neuroen-

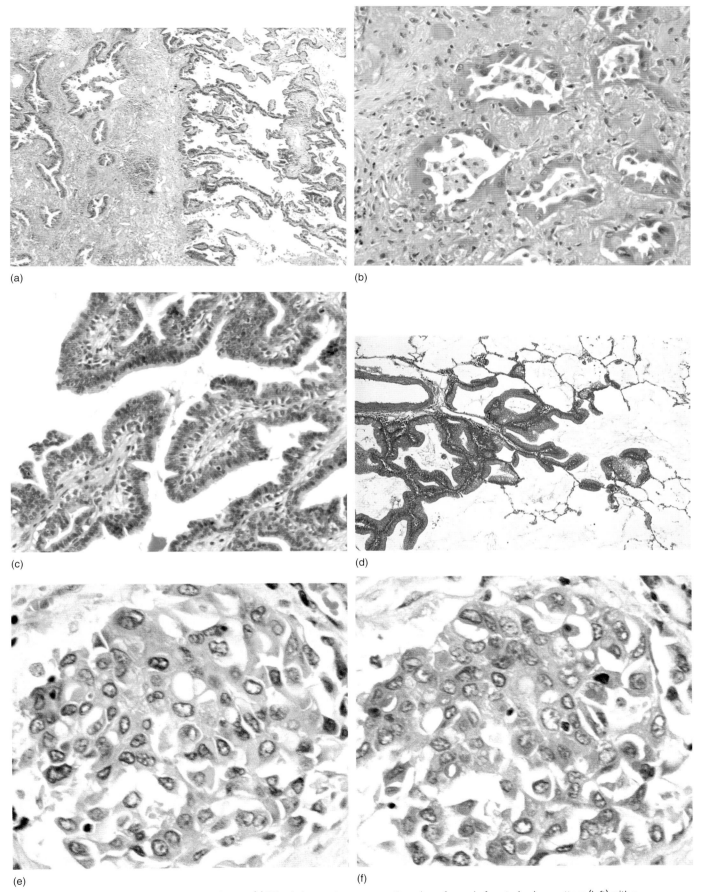

Figure 12.1.17 Common patterns of adenocarcinoma. (a) Mixed, the most common pattern, here formed of central acinar pattern (left) with a bronchioloalveolar pattern at the periphery (right), (b) Acinar, (c) Papillary, (d) Bronchioloalveolar, (e, f) Solid with mucus formation (f, D-PAS stain).

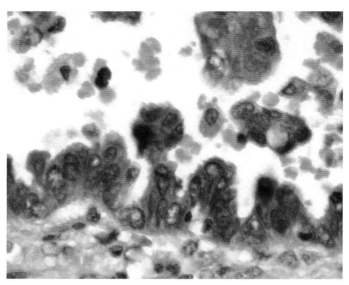

Figure 12.1.18 Micropapillary pattern of adenocarcinoma. Clusters of tumour cells form small papillary structures that lack stromal cores.

docrine features but containing histochemically demonstrable mucus vacuoles. A little mucin may be present in squamous cell carcinoma, carcinoid or small cell lung carcinoma and only when a tumour that would otherwise be classified as a large cell carcinoma contains substantial amounts of mucin (at least five mucin-positive cells in two high power fields) is it categorised as a poorly-differentiated adenocarcinoma of solid pattern (Fig. 12.1.17f).[112] With the exception of the rare mucinous cystadenocarcinomas considered below, mucin-forming adenocarcinomas generally carry a worse prognosis regardless of histological pattern.[323,324] This is possibly because of differences in host response, the non-mucous tumours showing more pronounced HLA expression and inflammatory reaction.[325,326] Whatever the histological pattern, individual tumour cells generally have large vesicular nuclei, prominent nucleoli and moderately abundant cytoplasm. Nuclear inclusion bodies are sometimes observed.

The pulmonary metastases of adenocarcinomas of other organs are usually indistinguishable from primary lung adenocarcinomas, so that in practice the diagnosis of primary adenocarcinoma of the lung should not be made before the patient has been screened for a primary tumour elsewhere and immunocytochemical markers have been sought, notably surfactant apoprotein and thyroid transcription factor-1 as markers of primary lung adenocarcinoma (see below), and markers that are available for an increasing range of other adenocarcinomas, e.g. thyroid and prostate. It is particularly important that the metastases of adenocarcinomas that are amenable to hormonal manipulation or chemotherapy are identified. Breast cancer generally carries oestrogen receptors, which are rare in primary adenocarcinoma of the lung.[327]

Immunohistochemistry

Adenocarcinomas of the lung express a wide range of cytokeratins, but not 5 and 6, which are characteristic of epithelioid mesotheliomas,[328] and 20, which is found more frequently in intestinal carcinomas. They also generally stain for carcinoembryonic antigen, BerEP4, AUA1, epithelial membrane antigen and vimentin. Surfactant apoprotein[329–333] and thyroid transcription factor-1[334,335] are sensitive and specific markers of pulmonary adenocarcinomas, thyroid transcription factor-1 being the more sensitive of the two. The neuroendocrine markers chromogranin and neuron-specific enolase can be demonstrated in some pulmonary adenocarcinomas and it is reported that this is associated with increased sensitivity to chemotherapy.[336] However, CD56 is generally negative. Trophoblastic markers can often be demonstrated adenocarcinomas, as well as in other non-small cell carcinomas of the lung.[232,308]

Electron microscopy

The heterogeneity of adenocarcinoma of the lung noted above is again evident when these tumours are examined by electron microscopy.[324,337] Some reflect the embryological derivation of the lower respiratory tract from the primitive foregut by showing the microvillous core rootlets and glycocalyceal bodies that are better known in intestinal carcinomas,[338–340] while many are composed of cells rich in cytoplasmic organelles that indicate active mucin synthesis and storage. The mucin granules vary in size and electron density and tend to coalesce into large vacuoles. Sometimes, the secretory product is amylase rather than mucin and the cytoplasm contains large zymogen-like granules.[231] Occasionally, neuroendocrine granules are seen, indicating dual differentiation.[231] Many adenocarcinomas are composed of cells resembling type II pneumocytes[341] or Clara cells,[342] while in some adenocarcinomas, type II pneumocytes may be seen alongside mucous or Clara cells, and occasionally overlying a basal layer of myoepithelial cells.[343] These mixed phenotypes make it difficult to classify pulmonary adenocarcinomas by cell type. A variety of nuclear inclusions are described, the most common being granular and staining for surfactant apoprotein,[344] while others consist of tubular structures derived from the nuclear envelope.[345]

Bronchioloalveolar carcinoma[346–347a]

These tumours arise in the periphery of the lung: a bronchial origin cannot be identified. They are characterised by the tumour cells growing along the alveolar walls without destroying them (Fig. 12.1.17d). As emphasised above, this category is now reserved for primary lung adenocarcinomas that show a non-invasive, non-destructive pattern of mural growth throughout, which requires step-sectioning. Bronchioloalveolar carcinomas may be mucinous, non-mucinous or, rarely, mixed (Fig. 12.1.19a–c). In the mucinous type, the tumour cells are relatively monomorphic, show little atypia, and produce large amounts of mucin, which may lead to bronchorrhoea. This

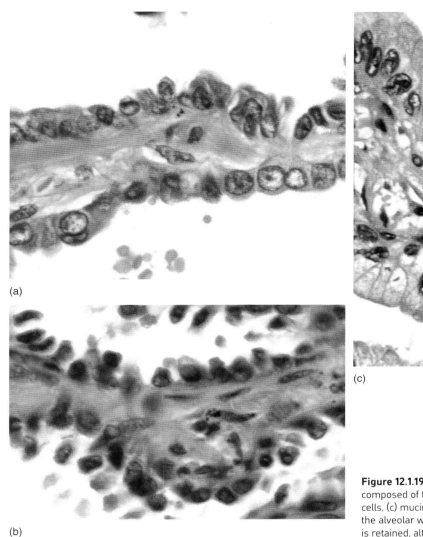

(a)

(b)

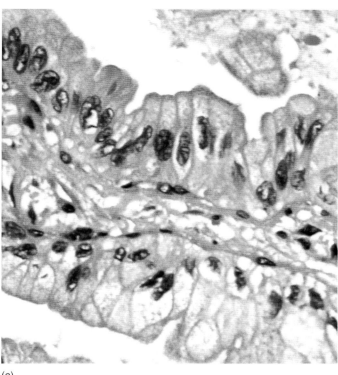

(c)

Figure 12.1.19 Bronchioloalveolar carcinoma. (a) nonmucinous composed of type II pneumocytes, (b) nonmucinous composed of Clara cells, (c) mucinous. Whatever the cell type, the tumour cells grow along the alveolar walls without destroying them and the alveolar architecture is retained, although there may be focal interstitial fibrosis.

type tends to involve a whole lobe or be multifocal and bilateral, and carries a worse prognosis than the non-mucinous type, which produces little mucin, shows more atypia and is often solitary.[348–350] The lung structure is maintained and when a whole lobe is involved the appearances may simulate those of lobar pneumonia, particularly the mucinous variety produced by Klebsiella species (Fig. 12.1.20). The non-mucinous type consists of Clara cells or type II pneumocytes, often in combination.[342,349] The Clara cells have a narrow base and a bulbous apex, resulting in a characteristic 'hobnail' pattern (Fig. 12.1.19b). Immunocytochemistry shows distinct differences: the non-mucinous variety expresses the pulmonary marker thyroid transcription factor (TTF-1) but fails to stain with the colonic marker cytokeratin 20 whereas the reverse is found with mucinous bronchioloalveolar carcinomas.[351–354] The latter also displays a specific pattern of mucin gene expression.[355]

Invasive activity excludes a diagnosis of bronchioloalveolar carcinoma but it can be difficult to recognise early invasion. The presence of intraluminal macrophages implies continuity between the malignant cells and surrounding alveolar spaces, favouring bronchioloalveolar carcinoma. Conversely, basement membrane stains, such as those recognising type IV collagen, facilitate the identification of invasion[356,357] and demonstrate that the epithelial basement membrane is destroyed when there is central fibrosis.[358] Not surprisingly therefore it has been shown that prominent central scarring as opposed to simple collapse is an adverse prognostic feature in small peripheral lung cancers.[359,360] Microinvasion, defined as invasion no greater than 5 mm, carries a prognosis intermediate between that of bronchioloalveolar carcinoma (i.e. no invasion) and adenocarcinoma containing invasive areas greater than 5 mm across.[361]

The multicentric nature of many bronchioloalveolar carcinomas could reflect either multifocal origin or metastasis. The mediastinal lymph nodes are generally free of growth, but this has only led to the view that the multicentricity represents aerogenous dissemination rather than multifocal origin. A sparsity of intercellular junctions that would minimise cellular cohesion and promote such aerial metastasis has been noted on

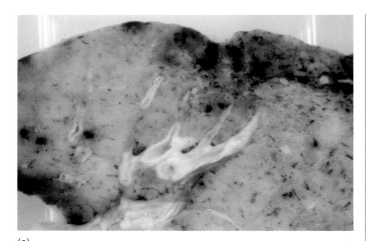

(a)

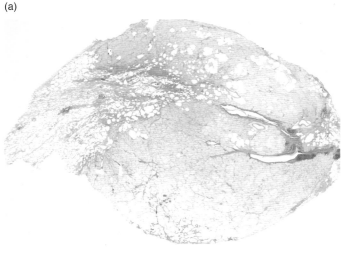

(b)

Figure 12.1.20 Bronchioloalveolar carcinoma. The lung is consolidated throughout by mucinous bronchioloalveolar carcinoma, the gross appearances (a) mimicking those of lobar pneumonia. (b) Consolidation is due to accumulation of mucus within alveoli. (Fig. (a) provided by Dr JW Seo, Seoul, Korea.)

electron microscopy.[362] Molecular studies of multifocal bronchioloalveolar carcinomas and multifocal atypical adenomatous hyperplasia, the putative precursor of peripheral pulmonary adenocarcinomas, have so far led to contrary views and at present do not allow a firm conclusion as to whether they represent independent lesions or metastases derived from a single source.[132,142,363,364]

On occasion it can be difficult to distinguish bronchioloalveolar carcinoma from reactive hyperplasia. Features favouring malignancy include a tall columnar cell shape, cellular crowding, cytological atypia and papillary infolding. Alternatively, morphometry may be applied to identify the significantly larger nuclei of a carcinoma.[365] The presence of cilia does not exclude malignancy,[366] but renders it unlikely.

The characteristic growth pattern of a bronchioloalveolar cell carcinoma is also seen on occasion in the pulmonary metastases of adenocarcinomas arising in other sites, especially the pan-

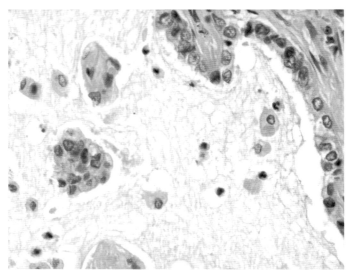

Figure 12.1.21 Colloid carcinoma. Small groups of tumour cells lie free within their abundant mucus secretion.

creas, stomach, colon, breast and ovary,[367,368] some of which can now be distinguished by their expression of specific markers, for example the colonic marker CDX2.[354,369,370]

An infectious disease of sheep known as jaagsiekte, droning sickness or pulmonary adenomatosis closely resembles human bronchioloalveolar carcinoma[371] but the two are considered to be separate diseases. A report of a protein immunologically related to the jaagsiekte sheep retrovirus in some human lung carcinomas[372] has not been supported by subsequent molecular investigations.[373]

Mucinous 'colloid' adenocarcinoma

'Colloid' carcinoma similar to the tumour of the same name in the gastrointestinal tract also develops in the lungs.[374] It affects the middle-aged or elderly of either sex. The mucoid nature of the tumour is evident upon macroscopic examination of the cut surface. Microscopically, tumour cells float free within copious amounts of mucin that fill and often distend alveoli; growth along the alveolar walls is often deficient (Fig. 12.1.21). Colloid carcinoma lacks the capsule of a mucinous cystadenocarcinoma and the pools of tumour-cell bearing mucin frequently spill over into neighbouring air spaces that are not themselves lined by neoplastic cells. One group reports the tumour cells as being of either goblet cell or 'signet ring' type, with the former having a better prognosis, but the numbers classified in this way have so far been small.[370] Variable reactions are reported for CK7 and CK20.[370]

'Signet ring cell' adenocarcinoma

On occasion 'signet ring cell carcinoma' similar to the tumour of the same name found in the stomach develops in the lung (Fig. 12.1.22).[375,376] One series comprised 12 men and 3 women

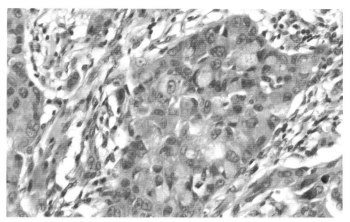

Figure 12.1.22 Signet ring cell carcinoma. A primary pulmonary adenocarcinoma of signet ring cell morphology, mimicking metastatic gastric carcinoma.

with a mean age of 53 years.[376] The tumours formed glands or diffuse sheets of cells with a prominent cytoplasmic globule of mucus indenting the nucleus. There was no evidence of a primary tumour elsewhere and reactions compatible with a pulmonary origin were obtained: thyroid transcription factor-1 and cytokeratin 7 positive, cytokeratin 20 negative.

Mucinous cystadenoma/cystadenocarcinoma

This is a particularly rare tumour. It occurs in patients who are middle-aged or elderly and of either sex. It shows a wide range of behaviour and is often of borderline malignancy. Some examples have shown no evidence of malignancy whatsoever and have been termed cystadenoma[377,378] while others have included only a few foci suspicious of adenocarcinoma.[379–381] Some have seeded out onto the pleura in a manner reminiscent of pseudomyxoma peritoneii produced by comparable tumours of the appendix or ovary.[382] Cytological atypia and microglandular solid areas may suggest malignancy but there is seldom any evidence of invasive activity. Most can be excised in their entirety and do not recur.

The tumour is typically peripheral, well-demarcated, cystic and either unilocular or multilocular. It is filled with mucus and microscopically is lined by stratified mucous cells, which are sometimes thrown into folds. The cyst wall is fibrous but the tumour displays no desmoplasia.

These tumours differ from bronchogenic cysts in the older age of the patient, the peripheral location of the tumour and an absence of bronchial glands and cartilage, and from congenital cystic adenomatoid malformations in the age of the patient again and the entirely mucous nature of the epithelial lining. They are distinguished from cystically degenerate adenocarcinomas, both primary and metastatic, by their lack of obvious malignancy and the presence of a cyst wall. They differ from mucous gland adenomas of bronchial gland origin (see p. 594) in that the latter are generally solid tumours that protrude into

the lumen of proximal bronchi; sometimes the term mucous gland cystadenoma is applied to the bronchial gland tumours but this is for varieties that have a cystic pattern microscopically, as opposed to the grossly cystic form of the tumour under consideration. A more difficult distinction is that from colloid carcinoma of the lung, which is similar microscopically but does not show gross cystic change and lacks the fibrous capsule of these mucinous cystic tumours.

Well-differentiated fetal adenocarcinoma (pulmonary endodermal tumour resembling fetal lung, pulmonary adenocarcinoma with endometrioid features)

Some well-differentiated adenocarcinomas of the lung show a distinct resemblance to the epithelial elements of fetal lung in the pseudoglandular stage of development.[383–387] It has been suggested that they represent one-sided development in pulmonary blastomas,[383,388,389] but that view is not followed here. The age range is wide but high-grade tumours tend to affect the elderly and low-grade ones the middle-aged.[389] They are generally parenchymal growths but may be endobronchial.[386,390] They vary in histological grade but are generally indolent growths.[388]

Histologically, these tumours form complex glandular structures lined by columnar cells with glycogen-rich clear cytoplasm (Fig. 12.1.23). The glands are separated by sparse fibromyxoid stroma. In places, the epithelial cells form solid squamoid collections that have been termed morulae. Immunocytochemistry shows focal neuroendocrine differentiation in the morulae.[386] Also in the morulae, the nuclei are often clear, the chromatin forming a thin peripheral rim due to the central accumulation of biotin.[387,391] Biotin is an essential co-factor for several enzymes but is normally found in the cytoplasm rather than the nucleus. However, biotin is stored in the nuclei of endometrial epithelial cells in pregnancy and in endometrioid ovarian carcinoma, supporting this tumour's alternative name of pulmonary endometrioid adenocarcinoma. Morular cells that express neuroendocrine markers and have optically clear, biotin-rich nuclei also show accumulation of β-catenin, a component of cell junctions that also acts as a transcriptional activator of the Wnt signalling pathway. Its accumulation reflects mutation of the β-catenin gene, a feature that well-differentiated fetal adenocarcinoma shares with pulmonary blastoma.[392]

Scar cancer

Pulmonary adenocarcinomas showing pronounced pleural puckering and central scarring (Fig. 12.1.16) are often assumed to represent 'scar cancers', meaning that the scar preceded and predisposed to the cancer. However, except in conditions such as fibrosing alveolitis, it is often impossible to tell whether a tumour has developed in a pre-existing scar, and can therefore be designated a true scar cancer, or whether the central scar is secondary to the tumour.[393] Nevertheless, there is considerable evidence, both radiological and pathological, supporting the view that the scar is the product of the tumour rather than

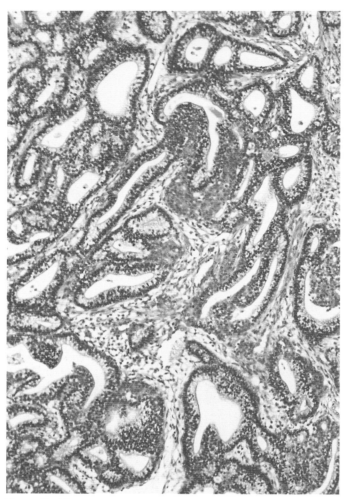

Figure 12.1.23 Well-differentiated adenocarcinoma resembling fetal lung.

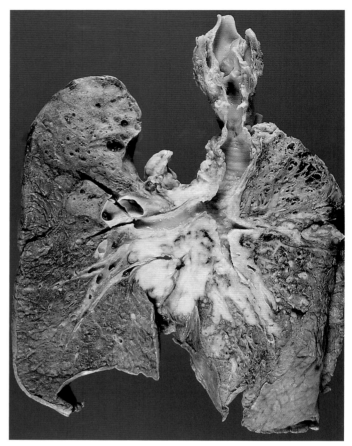

Figure 12.1.24 Small cell carcinoma that recurred after chemotherapy, extended within the thorax and metastasised widely.

the reverse. Relevant radiological observations[394] include the following:

- a scar is not usually evident in previous radiographs
- as peripheral tumours develop they may shrink in size despite involving a greater proportion of the affected lobe
- initially soft opacities often become more opaque centrally
- adjacent airways and blood vessels increasingly converge on the tumour.

Pathological observations[395–399] supporting the view that central scars are usually a product of the tumour rather than the reverse include the following:

- the size of the scar generally matches that of the tumour
- similar scars develop in extrapulmonary metastases
- similar scars are found in the pulmonary metastases of other adenocarcinomas
- psammoma bodies derived from the carcinoma may be found deep within the central scar

- the scars often show a predominance of myofibroblasts and type III collagen
- elastin stains often show that the central scar is formed on an area of collapse consequent upon airway or arterial obstruction by the tumour.

Despite all the evidence that the scar is the product of the cancer, the incidence of lung carcinoma is undoubtedly increased when pulmonary fibrosis is widespread, as in fibrosing alveolitis. The increased risk in this condition involves all cell types but there is a disproportionately large number of adenocarcinomas, especially bronchiolo-alveolar carcinomas.[393]

Irrespective of whether the scar or the tumour comes first, central scarring in a pulmonary adenocarcinoma is an adverse prognostic indicator, being associated with increased vascular and pleural invasion and lymph node metastasis.[395,400]

SMALL CELL CARCINOMA

Small cell carcinoma generally arises in major airways (Fig. 12.1.24), grows rapidly, metastasises early and initially at least is sensitive to chemotherapy. Oncologists classify small cell carcinoma only as 'limited' and 'extensive', believing that it has always disseminated by the time it is clinically manifest. Untreated patients survive on average less than three months. With treatment, the patient usually dies with widely disseminated disease within one to two years: long term disease-free survival is seen in only a minority of patients treated with chemotherapy.[401] Surgeons claim to be able to treat a few patients successfully[402–404] but these cases are highly selected and may have included atypical carcinoids. Although small cell carcinomas are generally central tumours, rare cases present as a peripheral nodule and it is these that have the best chances of successful surgical resection.

Histological subtypes

In the 1981 WHO classification,[405] small cell carcinoma was divided into oat cell, intermediate cell and combined subtypes but this has not proved to be of prognostic significance.[406–408] The combined subtype, which is reported to comprise between 3 and 28% of the total, is characterised by the presence of squamous cell carcinoma, adenocarcinoma or large cell carcinoma in addition to small cell carcinoma, combinations that are generally easy to recognise.[409,410] The differences between the oat cell and the intermediate cell types are imprecise and probably artefactual. Classic oat cell carcinoma is most often observed in traumatised biopsies or poorly-preserved autopsy material, whereas in well-preserved surgical material the intermediate cell type is seen almost exclusively. Accordingly, a recommendation that the terms oat cell and intermediate cell be abandoned[411] has been adopted in the 3rd and 4th editions of the WHO classification, only the combined variant being retained (Table 12.1.9).[112]

Histological appearances

Small cell carcinomas consist of closely packed small or medium-sized round or elongated cells, arranged in nests or strands or scattered singly within a scanty stroma.[412,413] The edge of the tumour is ill-defined and lacks a capsule. Extensive necrosis is commonly seen. Mitoses are numerous and the nuclei of adjacent tumour cells characteristically press on one another, a feature termed nuclear moulding, which is especially prominent in cytological specimens (Fig. 12.1.25).[414] Rosettes of radially arranged tumour cells may be formed and genuine lumina may also be present, sometimes containing a little mucin.

Classic oat cells, which as explained above are probably artefactual, have dense pyknotic nuclei and very sparse cytoplasm. Well preserved tumour cells are a little larger, have a discernible but still small amount of cytoplasm and a nucleus with a finely divided chromatin pattern (Fig. 12.1.26). Nucleoli are inconspicuous in paraffin sections but may be quite striking in plastic sections. These nuclear characteristics are more important than cell size in separating small cell carcinoma from large cell carcinoma.[414–416] Some small cell carcinomas show scattered tumour cells with hyperchromatic giant nuclei. This phenomenon can also be seen in other lung tumour types, and is especially common in tumours that have responded well to

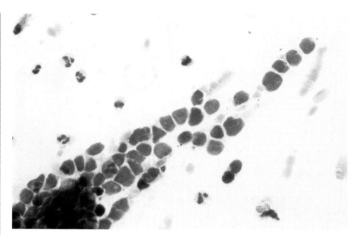

Figure 12.1.25 Small cell carcinoma. Nuclear moulding is clearly evident in this sputum sample.

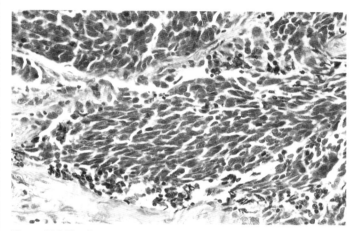

Figure 12.1.26 Small cell carcinoma. The tumour cells have little cytoplasm and finely dispersed nuclear chromatin. Nucleoli are not readily evident.

radiotherapy or chemotherapy.[417] A partial change to non-small cell histology during the course of the disease is encountered in about a fifth of patients.[418]

Haematoxyphil, Feulgen-positive nucleoprotein derived from degenerate tumour cells may be deposited in the walls of stromal blood vessels (so-called Azzopardi[412] effect, Fig. 12.1.27) but this feature is also found in other cellular tumours, such as lymphoma, seminoma and even other types of lung carcinoma. In biopsy specimens, the tumour cells are often crushed so that long strands and masses of haematoxyphil material are seen. This finding should prompt a careful search for viable, non-traumatised tumour cells. By itself, it does not justify a diagnosis of small cell lung carcinoma because other tumours, such as lymphomas, and also inflammatory infiltrates, may show the same crush artefact.

In bronchial biopsies, the tumour cells are often seen beneath an intact surface epithelium that shows atypical squamous metaplasia (Fig. 12.1.11), which is possibly due to the secretion

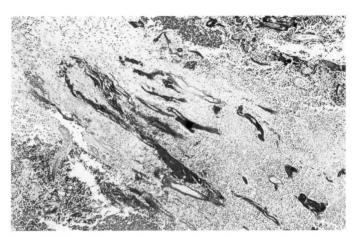

Figure 12.1.27 DNA deposition in vessel walls is seen in highly cellular necrotic tumours such as this small cell carcinoma.

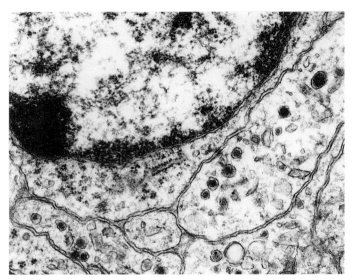

Figure 12.1.28 Small cell carcinoma. Electron microscopy demonstrates the presence of dense-core neuroendocrine granules. (Electron micrograph provided by Professor W. Mooi, Amsterdam, Netherlands.)

Table 12.1.12   Comparison of small cell carcinoma and large cell carcinoma, other than on cell size

	Small cell carcinoma	Large cell carcinoma
Cell shape	Fusiform	Polygonal
Nuclear/cytoplasmic ratio	High	Low
Chromatin	Fine	Coarse
Nucleoli	Indistinct	Prominent
DNA staining of vessels	Frequent	Rare

of growth factors by the tumour.[248] Superficial sampling limited to this surface change may lead to erroneous histological classification and hence the wrong treatment: it is essential that invasive tumour be examined. On the other hand, there may be infiltration of the overlying epithelium by small groups of tumour cells, similar to that seen in Paget's disease of the nipple.

Differential diagnosis

Small cell carcinoma is liable to be mistaken for large cell carcinoma if attention is concentrated on cell size and the presence of discernible amounts of cytoplasm, but these two tumours are generally separable on their nuclear characteristics: the finely divided, evenly dispersed chromatin of a small cell carcinoma contrasts greatly with the clumped chromatin and prominent nucleolus set in an otherwise vesicular nucleus of a large cell carcinoma (Table 12.1.12). Lymphocytes, either reactive or neoplastic, may also be mistaken for small cell carcinoma, especially if the tissue is traumatised: however, the carcinoma cells are larger than reactive lymphocytes and may be distinguished from lymphoma cells by immunocytochemistry, using antibodies against leukocytes (CD45) and cytokeratin. Some squamous cell and adenocarcinomas are composed of small tumour cells but these lack the nuclear features of small cell carcinoma and

show no immunohistochemical or ultrastructural evidence of neuroendocrine differentiation. Wider sampling generally reveals their true nature. If adequate, non-traumatised tissue is provided, small cell carcinomas are relatively easily distinguished from other histological types,[419] but problematical cases are certainly not rare,[420] particularly in small bronchial biopsies.[245] This is one of the areas where immunohistochemistry, electron microscopy[421] and image analysis[422] may prove to be important.

Electron microscopy

Ultrastructurally, small cell lung carcinomas usually show neuroendocrine differentiation, the hallmark of which is the presence of small cytoplasmic granules.[423,424] These granules are round and have a central homogeneously electron-dense core that is separated from an outer membrane by a thin electron-lucent halo (Fig. 12.1.28). They measure 50–200 nm and are often concentrated near the cell membrane. The granules may be difficult to find, there being far fewer than in carcinoid tumours. They have to be distinguished from bristle-coated vesicles, small lysosomes and small exocrine granules. Bristle-coated vesicles have a fuzzy surrounding membrane while lysosomes and exocrine granules lack the halo separating the central core from the outer membrane. Exocrine granules are also usually more pleomorphic, and are concentrated near intercellular lumina lined by microvilli.

A minority of carcinomas of apparent small cell morphology show undoubted ultrastructural evidence of squamous or mucous cell differentiation, alone or in combination with neuroendocrine features.[301,421,425–427] Of 46 such small cell carcinomas examined by electron microscopy, 22 proved to be neuroendocrine, 6 were squamous cell, 2 were mucous and 16 were not categorised.[428] However, these ultrastructural variations do not appear to be reflected in clinical behaviour or response to chemotherapy.[429] Conversely, a variety of non-small cell carcinomas are sometimes found to contain dense-core granules on electron microscopy.[430]

Immunocytochemistry

In line with their epithelial nature, a range of cytokeratins may be demonstrated in small cell lung carcinoma,[431] generally with a paranuclear dot-like distribution due to the formation of filament whorls.[432] Similarly most small cell carcinomas express TTF-1.

Immunohistochemistry has been widely used in attempts to distinguish small cell and non-small cell lung carcinoma but to date, no completely satisfactory marker of neuroendocrine differentiation is available. At present, chromogranin A, synaptophysin and CD56 probably represent the best compromise between specificity and sensitivity.[433–436] Chromogranin A is a fairly specific protein component of endocrine granules but is usually difficult to detect because small cell lung carcinomas are only sparsely granulated. *In situ* hybridisation may be useful here for it demonstrates high levels of chromogranin A mRNA in these tumours.[437] CD56 detects the neural cell adhesion molecule and is very sensitive but lacks specificity.[438,439] The enzyme neuron-specific enolase and the neural protein PGP 9.5 are not granule-associated, and are positive in many small cell carcinomas, but are of low specificity. Leu-7, a surface antigen present on human natural killer cells and neuroendocrine cells,[440] is also of low specificity. In contrast to these neuroendocrine markers, CD44 is reported to be expressed only by non-small cell carcinomas.[441]

LARGE CELL CARCINOMA

Large cell carcinomas of the lung are aggressive tumours[442] distinguished by an absence of differentiation when examined by light microscopy. The tumour cells are arranged in monotonous fields and individually are distinguished from small cell carcinoma by a variety of cytological features, of which size is one of the least and nuclear detail one of the most important (Table 12.1.12): they generally have a moderate amount of cytoplasm, chromatin that is clumped at the periphery of the nucleus and a prominent nucleolus (Fig. 12.1.29).[414–416]

Immunocytochemistry shows that these tumours often express both cytokeratin and vimentin and that over 50% express an adenocarcinoma immunophenotype (CK5–ve, CK7+ve, TTF1+ve).[271,443] Electron microscopy usually reveals evidence of squamous, glandular or neuroendocrine differentiation, or even a combination of these (Fig. 12.1.30).[444,445] Thus, large cell carcinoma is not a distinct entity, but rather a collection of very poorly-differentiated epithelial tumours. However, the clinical significance of subtyping large cell carcinoma by these special techniques is uncertain.[268,269]

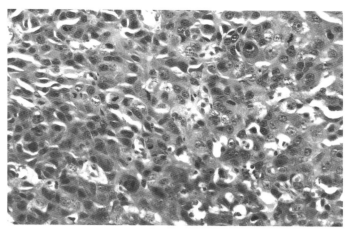

Figure 12.1.29 Large cell carcinoma. The tumour is undifferentiated and consists of cells with appreciable amounts of cytoplasm and nuclei that show coarse chromatin clumping and prominent nucleoli.

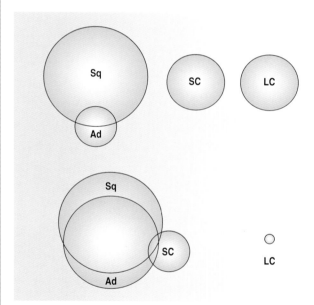

Figure 12.1.30 Types of lung carcinoma: frequency assessed by light microscopy (top) and electron microscopy (bottom). Sq, squamous cell carcinoma; Ad, adenocarcinoma; SC, small cell carcinoma; LC, large cell carcinoma. Adenosquamous carcinoma is represented by the overlapping Sq and Ad circles. For the electron microscopist adenosquamous carcinoma is the most common pattern, large cell carcinoma is very rare, small cell carcinoma is less distinct and rare tumours showing tripartite differentiation are recognised.

The diagnosis of large cell carcinoma should only be made on resection specimens: if the diagnosis is made on a biopsy, the subsequent resection specimen of the tumour often reveals focal differentiation, requiring the diagnosis to be amended. When a biopsy shows a non-small cell carcinoma without evidence of differentiation, the diagnosis 'undifferentiated carcinoma, non-small cell type' is appropriate.[245,247]

Clear cell carcinoma

Primary clear cell carcinoma of the lung forms a subgroup of large cell carcinoma in which most of the tumour cells have a pale, watery cytoplasm, usually due to the presence of glycogen (Fig. 12.1.31).[300,446] Early series[447] included those that owed their clear cytoplasm to mucus but today such tumours would be classified as adenocarcinomas, despite their lack of glandular differentiation. The term clear cell carcinoma is now restricted to tumours that give negative mucus stains. They show no evidence of squamous or glandular differentiation on light microscopy but either may be detected by electron microscopy.[446] Focal clear cell change is sometimes seen in squamous cell carcinomas and adenocarcinomas but this is considered insufficient to justify a diagnosis of clear cell carcinoma.

The nuclei may show little atypicality, in which case the distinction from benign clear cell tumour of the lung (see p. 613) may be difficult. However, the thin-walled sinusoidal blood vessels of a benign clear cell tumour are not evident in clear cell carcinoma. Metastatic renal carcinoma is perhaps a more likely

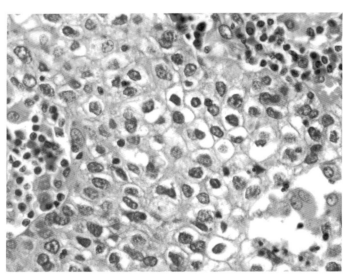

Figure 12.1.31 Clear cell variant of large cell carcinoma. The tumour is composed solely of undifferentiated large tumour cells with clear cytoplasm.

alternative, one that would be supported by the presence of sudanophilic fat within the cytoplasm of tumour cells; however, fat stains are not possible if the material has all been embedded in paraffin, and in these circumstances recourse to renal imaging is probably the best option.[448] If mucin stains are positive, metastatic renal carcinoma, primary clear cell carcinoma and benign clear cell tumour can all be excluded.

Large cell neuroendocrine carcinoma

Some large cell carcinomas display neuroendocrine features and are appropriately termed large cell neuroendocrine carcinomas. Their diagnosis is based on recognition of both neuroendocrine morphology and the immunohistochemical demonstration of at least one specific neuroendocrine marker. As in any large cell carcinoma the cells have moderate amounts of cytoplasm and nuclei that show peripheral clumping of chromatin and a prominent nucleolus. There is much mitotic activity and extensive necrosis. However, it is soon noticed that the tumour has an organoid pattern with its cells arranged in cords or well demarcated groups showing rosette formation or peripheral palisading (Fig. 12.1.32). Some of these features are also seen in carcinoid tumours and the relationship to carcinoid is strengthened by shared immunocytochemical, ultrastructural and molecular features of neuroendocrine differentiation, such as the presence of chromogranin, synaptophysin or CD56, or their gene expression, and scanty dense-core granules evident on electron microscopy.[434,449–452] Certain squamous cell carcinomas also show these neuroendocrine features: these have been termed non-small cell carcinoma with neuroendocrine features.[453] Neuroendocrine differentiation can be demonstrated by electron microscopy or immunohistochemistry in 10–15% of non-small cell carcinomas of the lung despite an absence of morphological neuroendocrine features.[451,453–456]

The differential diagnosis of large cell neuroendocrine carcinoma includes atypical carcinoid tumour (Table 12.1.13) but the organoid pattern of that tumour is not so well developed in large cell neuroendocrine carcinoma and the degree of atypia, mitotic activity and necrosis all far exceed those seen in an atypical carcinoid. A criterion recommended for distinguishing atypical carcinoid from large cell neuroendocrine carcinoma is mitotic number, atypical carcinoid having fewer than 10 mitoses

Table 12.1.13 Comparison of neuroendocrine large cell carcinoma and atypical carcinoid		
	Neuroendocrine large cell carcinoma	*Atypical carcinoid*
Histological pattern	Large well circumscribed cell groups with peripheral palisading	Small cell groups usually in a trabecular or mosaic pattern
Cell size	Large	Medium
Mitoses	10 or more/10 high power fields	More than 2/10 and up to 10/10 high per fields
Nuclear/cytoplasmic ratio	Low	Moderate
Chromatin	Coarse	Fine
Nucleoli	Prominent	Indistinct
Necrosis	Large areas	Usually confined to the centres of the cell groups
Atypia	Prominent	Moderate
Neuroendocrine stains	Necessary (positive)	Optional (positive)

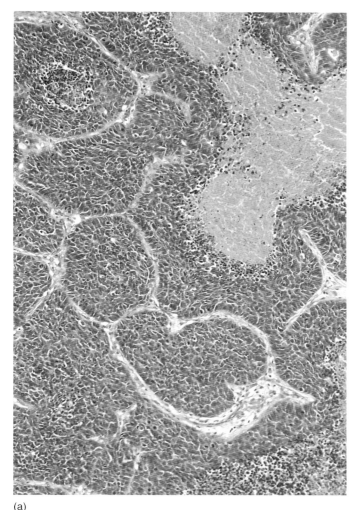

(a)

(b)

Figure 12.1.32 Large cell neuroendocrine carcinoma (a) There is peripheral palisading reminiscent of a carcinoid tumour but the tumour also exhibits much more extensive necrosis than is seen in an atypical carcinoid. (b) Immunoperoxidase staining for chromogranin is positive.

per 10 high power fields and large cell carcinoma 10 or more (if 1 high power field = an area of 0.2 mm²).[450] Most large cell neuroendocrine carcinomas show considerably more mitotic activity than this, the average number of mitoses per 10 high power fields being in the order of 75. Large 'geographic' areas of necrosis characterise large cell neuroendocrine carcinoma whereas in atypical carcinoid necrosis is generally confined to the centres of individual cell groups. Small cell carcinoma also enters into the differential diagnosis of large cell neuroendocrine carcinoma;[457] here reliance has to be placed upon the different nuclear characteristics, the fine granularity of the small cell carcinoma's chromatin differing from the clumped chromatin and prominent nucleoli of neuroendocrine large cell carcinoma.

In general, large cell neuroendocrine carcinomas are tumours of middle-aged or elderly cigarette smokers that arise in central bronchi. Despite the morphological evidence of neuroendocrine differentiation, ectopic hormone secretion is not a feature. The clinical significance of these tumours has yet to be fully evaluated but their recognition is of potential therapeutic significance for their undoubted neuroendocrine nature links them to classic small cell carcinoma and it would be important if their metastases were similarly sensitive to chemotherapy. Reports available to date regarding their chemosensitivity are contradictory.[336,430,458–462] Some advise that these tumours behave like small cell carcinoma,[463] others that they are more aggressive than ordinary large cell carcinomas,[452,456,464–466] and yet others that neuroendocrine expression in large cell carcinoma is of no prognostic significance,[467–470a] or even that it confers longer survival.[462,471] The presence of neuroendocrine markers in pulmonary adenocarcinoma is reported to be associated with increased sensitivity to chemotherapy,[336,455,458,461,469] and to be an independent favourable prognostic factor in chemotherapy-treated non-small cell lung carcinoma,[462] leading to suggestions that this treatment may be considered for those non-small cell carcinomas that express neuroendocrine features and are inoperable.[456,467] However, as yet there have been no large scale, prospective, controlled trials of small cell chemotherapy for this subgroup of large cell carcinomas or for other non-small cell carcinomas showing neuroendocrine differentiation. Furthermore, the clinical importance of neuroendocrine differentiation may diminish if a current trend towards treating all inoperable lung carcinomas with aggressive chemotherapy continues.

Basaloid carcinoma

Basaloid carcinoma of the lung[294,302–304,312,472–474] is relatively rare, forming only about 3% of non-small cell carcinomas of the lung. It often shows an exophytic, endobronchial pattern of growth and a well-defined edge (Fig. 12.1.33). Carcinoma-*in-situ* can often be recognised in the adjacent or distant bronchial epithelium.

Histologically, basaloid carcinoma displays a lobular or anastomosing trabecular pattern with peripheral palisading of radially arranged small cuboidal or fusiform cells with scanty cytoplasm and a hyperchromatic nucleus devoid of prominent

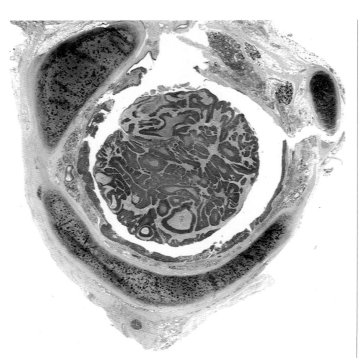

Figure 12.1.33 Basaloid carcinoma. The tumour shows an exophytic endobronchial pattern of growth. Carcinoma-*in-situ* is also present.

nucleoli (see Fig. 12.1.15d). Mitoses are frequent (over 25 per 10 high power fields) and there is often centrilobular comedo-like necrosis. Like other non-small cell carcinomas, a small proportion (<10%) of tumour cells may express neuroendocrine markers. Basaloid carcinoma also expresses high molecular weight cytokeratins typical of bronchial basal cells (cytokeratins 1, 5, 6 and 14)[312] but not the low molecular weight cytokeratins (4, 10 and 11) that are more typical of cornifying squamous epithelium or the TTF-1 expressed by most adenocarcinomas and small cell carcinomas of the lung. There may, however, be a substantial squamous cell, large cell or adenocarcinomatous component. Other features occasionally present include stromal cartilage or bone formation and hyaline change. Basaloid carcinoma is liable to be confused with small cell carcinoma, large cell neuroendocrine carcinoma and poorly-differentiated squamous cell carcinoma but none of these has the full constellation of features listed above.

In their pure form these tumours resemble basal cell carcinoma of the skin and anus but when there is a squamous component the WHO classifies these tumours as basaloid variants of squamous cell carcinoma (see p. 544),[112] akin to the basaloid-squamous cell carcinoma of the upper aerodigestive tract.[475]

Patients with basaloid carcinoma do not differ from those with other undifferentiated pulmonary carcinomas in age, clinical presentation or pattern of relapse.[302–304,472] The median survival rate is 22 months for Stage I and II disease, which is considerably worse than that of poorly-differentiated squamous cell carcinoma but better than that of small cell carcinoma, and not dissimilar to that of large cell carcinoma or the basaloid variant of squamous cell carcinoma.[302,303,472]

Lymphoepithelial carcinoma

Lymphoepithelial carcinoma is a term usually applied to a type of nasopharyngeal carcinoma that shows prominent lymphoid infiltration. Recently this tumour has been described in a number of other sites, including the lung.[94,476,476–480] As with the nasopharyngeal tumours, pulmonary lymphoepithelial carcinoma mainly affects Asians, in whom it is associated with the Epstein–Barr virus (Fig. 12.1.34). Most of the few lymphoepithelial carcinomas of the lung reported in non-Asian patients do not contain Epstein–Barr virus,[481,482] suggesting that the presence of this agent may be an epiphenomenon. However, Epstein–Barr virus was not found in any other form of lung cancer in a Hong Kong laboratory reporting pulmonary lymphoepithelial carcinomas associated with this virus.[477] Pulmonary lymphoepithelial carcinoma is also associated with the bcl-2 oncogene, chemosensitivity and a better survival rate than other large cell carcinomas of the lung.[478,479,483]

Pulmonary lymphoepithelial carcinoma affects adults of all ages and the sexes are affected equally. There is no strong association with cigarette smoking.[478] The tumour usually forms a solitary, discrete, subpleural nodule that is amenable to surgery. Major bronchi are not usually affected but the tumour may replace the lining of small bronchi. It generally has a soft fleshy appearance on its cut surface. Microscopy shows sheets of large cells with vesicular nuclei and prominent nucleoli, mixed with numerous lymphocytes and plasma cells, and occasionally, granulomas (Fig. 12.1.34). Thymoma of mixed cellularity may be suggested but the less mature lymphocytes of CD1a phenotype encountered in thymoma are not identified. The lymphoid infiltrate may be so prominent as to suggest lymphoma, from which it is distinguished by the immunocytochemical demonstration of sheets of cytokeratin-positive cells.

Rhabdoid carcinoma

This rare subtype of large cell carcinoma is characterised by the presence of a hyaline eosinophilic globule indenting the nucleus.[484] The globule represents a tangle of intermediate filaments, both vimentin and cytokeratin (Fig. 12.1.35).[485,486] Rhabdoid foci are also found in lung tumours showing varying lines of differentiation, where they are thought to represent areas of dedifferentiation.[487,488] Not surprisingly therefore, rhabdoid tumours appear to carry a poor prognosis, although numbers of analysed cases are small.[489,490]

ADENOSQUAMOUS CARCINOMA

Many non-small cell carcinomas of the lung show ultrastructural evidence of both squamous and glandular differentiation but the diagnosis of adenosquamous carcinoma is reserved for tumours that show both squamous and adenocarcinomatous differentiation on light microscopy (Fig. 12.1.36).[491–494] These are rare but the exact incidence is uncertain because until recently there were no agreed criteria as to how much of the minor com-

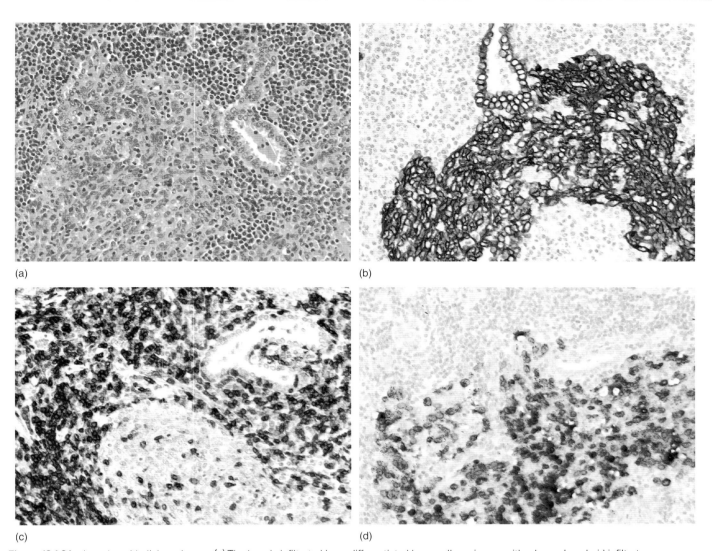

(a)

(b)

(c)

(d)

Figure 12.1.34 Lymphoepithelial carcinoma. (a) The lung is infiltrated by undifferentiated large cell carcinoma with a heavy lymphoid infiltrate. (b) Cytokeratin (MNF116) and (c) lymphocyte (CD3) staining distinguishes the two components of the tumour. (d) EBERS *in situ* hybridisation demonstrates Epstein–Barr virus.

ponent should be present: however, the current WHO classification[112] stipulates at least 10%. Alveoli entrapped within squamous carcinomas may be mistaken for tumour acini[318] but their lining cells are smaller and more uniform that those lining tumour acini.

Clinically and macroscopically, adenosquamous carcinomas resemble adenocarcinomas.[495] They are often peripheral tumours that metastasise widely, often showing the same intermingling of the two components in this metastasis as in the primary tumour. The prognosis is poor, worse than for either pure squamous cell carcinoma or pure adenocarcinoma.[493,494]

SARCOMATOID CARCINOMA

Occasional carcinomas show foci of malignant spindle or giant cells, suggesting that the tumour is composed of a mixture of carcinoma and sarcoma. Such tumours were formerly thought to result from the merging of separate carcinomas and sarcomas (so-called 'collision tumours'), or were considered to represent carcinomas merely exhibiting exuberant stromal growth. The current view is that they represent carcinomas showing connective tissue differentiation. This is an extension of the widely accepted concept of tumour heterogeneity used to explain tumours of mixed epithelial phenotype, such as adenosquamous carcinoma and the combined subgroup of small cell carcinoma. What appears to be a sarcomatous element may seem to stream from an obvious epithelial element (Fig. 12.1.37) and there is now considerable electron microscopic and immunohistochemical evidence that tumours that appear to be of mixed epithelial and connective tissue phenotype, or composed only of what appears histologically to be sarcoma, are entirely epithelial.[496–499] Molecular studies are in accord with this, showing identical mutations in the spindle cells and more obvi-

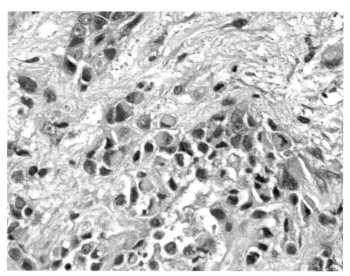

Figure 12.1.35 Rhabdoid variant of large cell carcinoma. Large cell carcinoma cells show indentation of nuclei by a hyaline eosinophilic globule.

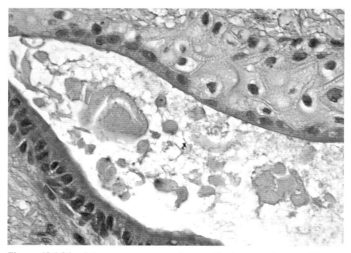

Figure 12.1.36 Adenosquamous carcinoma. The tumour shows evidence of both squamous and glandular differentiation, with each component making up more than 10% of the whole.

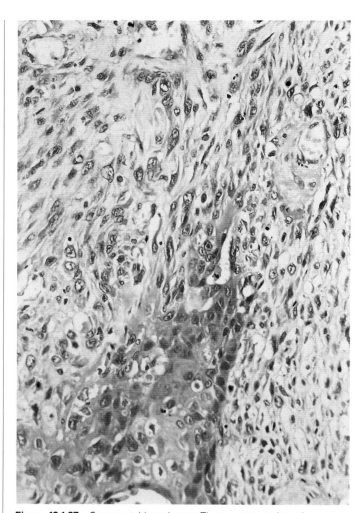

Figure 12.1.37 Sarcomatoid carcinoma. The tumour consists of squamous and spindle cells, the latter obviously derived from the adjacent squamous cell carcinoma. Both components gave a strongly positive immunoreaction for cytokeratin.

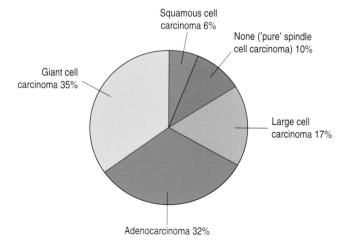

Figure 12.1.38 Frequency of patterns found to be associated with spindle cell carcinoma, illustrating the diversity that led to the introduction of the term pleomorphic cell carcinoma.[502]

ously epithelial components.[500,501] The term sarcomatoid carcinoma is therefore appropriate and could well supplant older terms such as carcinosarcoma and pulmonary blastoma. The latter are inaccurate but are retained in the WHO classification for historic reasons.

Some sarcomatoid carcinomas consist entirely of spindle or giant cells and for these the terms *spindle cell carcinoma* and *giant cell carcinoma* are appropriate. Spindle cell carcinoma was formerly classed as a variant of squamous cell carcinoma but it is now appreciated that spindle cell change may be found in any type of non-small cell carcinoma (Fig. 12.1.38), including giant cell carcinoma. This has led to the introduction of the term *pleo-*

morphic carcinoma for a tumour that combines spindle and/or giant cell carcinoma with any of the more usual patterns of non-small cell carcinoma.[502] Occasionally, there is an even greater degree of connective tissue differentiation so that bone, cartilage or muscle is formed. The WHO classification retains the inaccurate term *carcinosarcoma* for sarcomatoid carcinomas containing such heterologous elements although it recognises them to be basically epithelial in nature. In one form of carcinosarcoma, the neoplastic glands and stroma have an embryonic appearance so that the tumour bears a spurious resemblance to fetal lung in its canalicular phase of development: the traditional (but inaccurate) term pulmonary *blastoma* is retained for this pattern in the WHO classification.[112] In one of the largest series of sarcomatoid carcinomas, 58 cases were classified as pleomorphic carcinoma, 10 as spindle cell carcinoma, 3 as giant cell carcinoma, 3 as carcinosarcoma and 1 as pulmonary blastoma.[503]

An alternative classification to that advocated by WHO recognises only monophasic and biphasic sarcomatoid carcinomas, with the latter subdivided into homologous and heterologous varities.[504,505] In this classification a *monophasic sarcomatoid carcinoma* is one in which the epithelial nature of the tumour is only recognisable by the application of immunohistochemistry to demonstrate cytokeratin or other epithelial markers. It thus corresponds to both spindle cell and giant cell carcinoma. Biphasic sarcomatoid carcinoma combines an obvious epithelial component (e.g. glandular or squamous cell carcinoma) with a malignant stroma (spindle cell or giant cell), as in Fig. 12.1.37. If the stroma shows chondroid, osseous or myogenic differentiation the tumour is classified as a *heterologous biphasic sarcomatoid carcinoma* (corresponding to carcinosarcoma and blastoma); if not it is termed a *homologous biphasic sarcomatoid carcinoma* (corresponding to pleomorphic carcinoma). This classification has the merit of being understood by those unversed in the historic development of our understanding of lung tumours. It is also familiar to general histopathologists because it is applied to similar tumours that are encountered in the upper aerodigestive and genitourinary systems. The two classifications are compared in Table 12.1.14.

Sarcomatoid carcinomas are rare, accounting for about only 1% of all lung malignancies.[502,503] Patients are usually elderly and have been heavy smokers.[503] They typically give a short history, yet have bulky tumours. The prognosis is generally poor.[505] Tumours that are operable have a worse[503] or similar[506] prognosis to large cell carcinoma of the lung, which is itself

Table 12.1.14 Sarcomatoid carcinoma. Corresponding terminology used in different classifications

Wick[504,505]	*World Health Organization*[112]
Monophasic	Spindle cell
	Giant cell
Biphasic	
Homologous	Pleomorphic
Heterologous	Carcinosarcoma
	Blastoma

poor. Signs and symptoms are related to tumour localisation Haemoptysis, fever due to recurrent pneumonia, cough, and progressive dyspnoea are common with endobronchial lesions. Peripheral tumours may be asymptomatic and only discovered incidentally on chest radiography, but most eventually cause pleuritic pain.

Spindle cell carcinoma is a non-small cell carcinoma that consists only of spindle-shaped tumour cells. It is a rare tumour but is nevertheless the most common spindle cell malignancy encountered in the lung. When encountering a tumour of such pattern one should therefore think of spindle cell carcinoma before considering a diagnosis of primary pulmonary sarcoma. It is distinguished from sarcoma by its expression of epithelial markers such as cytokeratin, epithelial membrane antigen and carcinoembryonic antigen.[497,507] Difficulty may be encountered in distinguishing spindle cell carcinoma from synovial sarcoma because they both express epithelial markers but synovial sarcoma also expresses the bcl-2 oncogene and shows t(X;18)(p11.2;q11.2) translocation (see p. 620). When there is pleural involvement it is particularly difficult to distinguish monophasic sarcomatoid carcinoma from sarcomatoid mesothelioma. Pankeratin, calretinin and thrombomodulin are frequently expressed in both while neither commonly expresses cytokeratin 5/6 or WT1, but some difference is reported for smooth muscle actin (positive in 60% of sarcomatoid mesotheliomas compared with only 10% of sarcomatoid carcinomas).[499] *Inflammatory sarcomatoid carcinoma* is an unusual variant of spindle cell carcinoma that closely mimics an inflammatory myofibroblastic tumour. It shows a proliferation of cytologically bland neoplastic spindle cells in a myxoid background while lymphocytes and plasma cells surround or infiltrate the tumour. However, a dearth of neutrophils, eosinophils and foam cells together with small foci of necrosis and invasion of bronchi and blood vessels all favour sarcomatoid carcinoma.

Giant cell carcinoma is a non-small cell carcinoma composed of very large cells that are frequently multinucleate. The many nuclei are large, pleomorphic and often multilobed. The mitotic rate is high. The tumour cells are poorly cohesive and show a marked tendency to dissociate from each other (Fig. 12.1.39).[337] There is generally a rich inflammatory infiltrate, usually of neutrophils, which frequently invade the tumour cells.[235] This phenomenon was initially thought to represent phagocytosis by the tumour cells,[508] but more probably reflects emperipolesis[509] (active penetration of the leukocytes into the tumour cells, in contrast to passive engulfment). The inflammation is not necessarily associated with necrosis and is seen in metastases as well as the primary growth. Neutrophil sequestration within the tumour may be associated with peripheral granulocytosis and even a leukaemoid reaction. The granulocytosis is not dependent upon bone marrow metastases. An unidentified chemoattractant is presumably responsible for both the granulocytosis and the sequestration of neutrophils within the tumour.[235] The phenomenon is also seen in the inflammatory sarcomatoid carcinoma mentioned above.

The tumour cells often co-express cytokeratin, vimentin, carcinoembryonic antigen and thyroid transcription factor-1. By

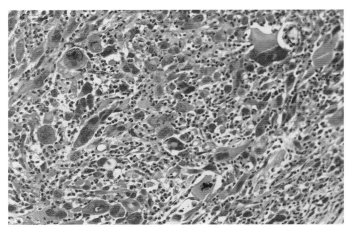

Figure 12.1.39 Giant cell carcinoma. The tumour cells are poorly cohesive and there is a rich polymorph infiltrate. Multinucleate tumour giant cells are evident.

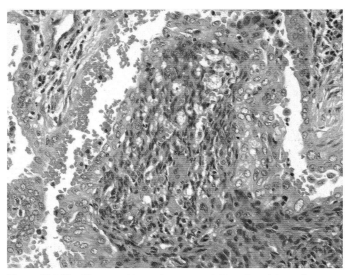

Figure 12.1.40 Pleomorphic carcinoma consisting of a mixture of glandular and spindle cell growth.

electron microscopy aggregates of paranuclear filaments may be seen but otherwise the tumour cells possess few tonofibrils and are very poorly-differentiated. Only very occasional desmosomes are identified, which is in accordance with the poor cohesiveness of the tumour cells.[510]

The differential diagnosis of giant cell carcinoma includes not only other types of lung carcinoma, but also primary and metastatic malignant fibrous histiocytoma, pleomorphic rhabdomyosarcoma, metastatic adrenocortical carcinoma and other pleomorphic malignant tumours, most of which can be distinguished by their own distinctive markers.

Pleomorphic carcinoma is a poorly-differentiated non-small cell carcinoma in which spindle cell carcinoma and/or giant cell carcinoma form at least 10% of what would otherwise be a pure squamous cell, adeno- or large cell carcinoma (Fig. 12.1.40), or a carcinoma consisting only of spindle and giant cells.

Immunostaining is only required if the tumour lacks an obvious epithelial component. *Pseudoangiosarcomatous carcinoma* is a variety of pleomorphic carcinoma in which squamous cell carcinoma is accompanied by an angiosarcomatoid component showing anastomosing channels lined by anaplastic cells focally aggregated in pseudopapillae. The channels contain erythrocytes and occasionally form 'blood lakes', thus simulating an angiosarcoma. However, the lining cells express epithelial rather than endothelial markers and represents the pulmonary counterpart of pseudovascular adenoid squamous cell carcinoma that one may see in other organs. Distinction from pleuropulmonary angiosarcoma is based on the carcinoma's lack of atypical endothelial cells, negative immunostaining for vascular markers, and the presence of at least focal areas of squamous cell carcinoma.

Carcinosarcoma (heterologous type of biphasic sarcomatoid carcinoma)

Carcinosarcomas of the lung are malignant tumours that contain both epithelial and connective tissue elements, with the latter showing heterologous differentiation into bone, cartilage or smooth muscle. They are similar to those described in the upper aero-digestive tract, the urogenital organs and other sites as carcinosarcomas, biphasic sarcomatoid carcinomas or malignant mixed Müllerian tumours. The first description of pulmonary carcinosarcoma is attributed to Kika in 1908.[511] Immunocytochemistry and electron microscopy (see below) support the view that carcinosarcoma is basically an epithelial tumour that shows varying degrees of mesenchymal differentiation. In line with this, molecular studies showing that the epithelial and sarcomatoid components have a common genome.[501,512] Further support derives from experiments involving the transplantation of human lung carcinomas into inbred mice, in which environment these epithelial neoplasms showed connective tissue differentiation.[513]

Clinical and gross features

Pulmonary carcinosarcomas occur in the same type of patient as the more common forms of lung cancer, namely elderly or middle-aged cigarette smokers, and carry a similarly poor prognosis.[514,515] The male:female ratio is about seven, with a mean and median age 65 years.[516] Two-thirds arise in the walls of large airways and form polypoid endobronchial lesions but some grow into large intrapulmonary masses that may invade the chest wall.[517] Central tumours cause cough, haemoptysis and recurrent chest infection whereas peripheral lesions may be asymptomatic until they reach the pleura and give rise to effusion or pleurisy.

Histological features

By definition, these tumours are biphasic, composed of an intimate mixture of epithelial and connective tissue.[268,317] The demarcation between the two may be sharp or poorly defined.

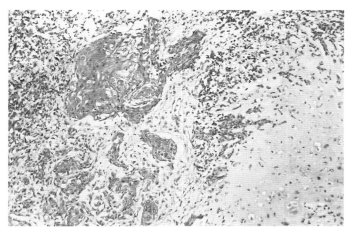

Figure 12.1.41 Carcinosarcoma (biphasic sarcomatoid carcinoma with heterologous elements) composed of squamous and spindle cell carcinoma, the latter showing chondroid differentiation.

Table 12.1.15 Pathological features of 46 cases of carcinosarcoma[517]

	Endobronchial (n = 32)	Peripheral (n = 14)
Epithelial component	Squamous 29 (91%) Glandular 3 (9%)	Squamous 6 (43%) Glandular 7 (50%) Other 1 (7%)
Mesenchymal component	Undifferentiated spindle cell 26 (81%) Differentiated 6 (19%)	Undifferentiated spindle cell 11 (79%) Differentiated 3 (21%)
Differentiated includes chondrosarcoma and rhabdomyosarcoma.		

The most frequent epithelial element is squamous cell carcinoma, followed by adenocarcinoma, large cell carcinoma, small cell carcinoma and carcinoid tumour but glandular differentiation is commoner in the rarer peripheral growths (Fig. 12.1.41 and Table 12.1.15).[517,518] The connective tissue component usually consists of undifferentiated spindle cells in which there are foci of malignant osteoid, cartilage or striated muscle.[497,514,515,519] These connective tissue elements are clearly malignant, in contrast to the osteocartilaginous stromal metaplasia that is recorded in occasional squamous cell carcinomas.[295] Such differentiation may be sparse, rendering the distinction from spindle cell carcinoma and undifferentiated sarcoma difficult. Furthermore, the relative proportions of carcinoma and sarcoma vary considerably: it should therefore be borne in mind that sarcomas of the lung are very rare and before making such a diagnosis the lesion should be sampled widely to exclude the possibility that the tumour is a carcinosarcoma of predominantly sarcomatous pattern, particularly if it has the characteristic endobronchial growth pattern of a central carcinosarcoma.

The malignant epithelial cells frequently express cytokeratin, epithelial membrane antigen, carcinoembryonic antigen and thyroid transcription factor-1, and the mesenchymal cells vimentin, but any of these markers may be found in either component.[497,498,520–522] Electron microscopy may also show epithelial features such as desmosomes in the spindle cell component, further emphasising the close relation between carcinosarcoma and spindle cell carcinoma.[497,498]

The metastases of a carcinosarcoma may consist of carcinoma or sarcoma or both.[520,523] If the epithelial component is glandular, pleural involvement may lead to confusion with a mesothelioma of mixed pattern but the identification of mucus and carcinoembryonic antigen excludes mesothelioma.[519]

Blastoma

The term pulmonary blastoma was coined by Spencer[524] in 1961, superseding Barnard's earlier one of embryoma of lung.[525,526] At that time it was thought that the peripheral part of the lung was of mesenchymal origin and Spencer considered pulmonary blastomas to be analogous to nephroblastomas in that both their epithelial and mesenchymal components were derived from a common mesodermal blastoma. The embryological basis for this concept is now known to be false (see p. 39). Occasional reports of tumours intermediate in structure between blastoma and carcinosarcoma,[523,527–529] suggest that blastomas are related to carcinosarcomas,[497] and hence to spindle cell carcinomas. It has been suggested that the well-differentiated fetal adenocarcinoma represents one-sided epithelial development of a pulmonary blastoma, but this is unconvincing and it is therefore considered with other adenocarcinomas on p. 551. Pleuropulmonary blastoma, a purely connective tissue tumour of the young that is described on p. 612 is now considered to represent the true blastoma of the lung.

Clinical features

Pulmonary blastoma is a rare tumour that affects males three times more commonly than females. It may occur at any age from childhood to the ninth decade with the mean age being about 40 years, earlier than that of carcinosarcoma but considerably later than blastomas of other organs. Blastomas may reach a considerable size before cough, haemoptysis or chest pain cause the patient to seek attention, or they may be discovered incidentally by radiography. Pulmonary blastomas vary greatly in their behaviour but the prognosis is generally unfavourable: the overall 5-year survival is only 16%.[530]

Pathological features

Pulmonary blastomas are generally peripheral growths and often form large well-demarcated masses with foci of cystic change and haemorrhage (Fig. 12.1.42). However, up to one-quarter are similar to carcinosarcomas in forming polypoid endobronchial tumours.[388,530] Microscopically, they are biphasic tumours composed of branching epithelial tubules or cords set in an undifferentiated stroma. The latter is formed of loosely arranged polygonal cells which have fairly uniform, small, dark, oval or spindle-shaped nuclei and scanty cytoplasm (Fig. 12.1.43): both components are malignant and either or both may be seen in the metastases. The mesenchymal cells tend to be

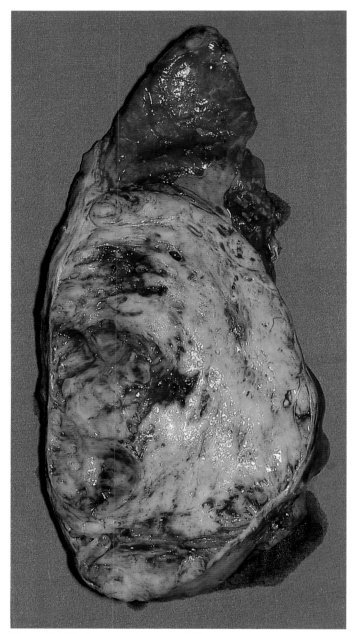

Figure 12.1.42 Pulmonary blastoma. A 20 cm partly necrotic and haemorrhagic tumour occupies much of the lower lobe. (Case of Dr PF Roberts, Norwich, UK.)

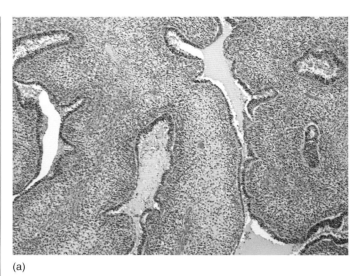

(a)

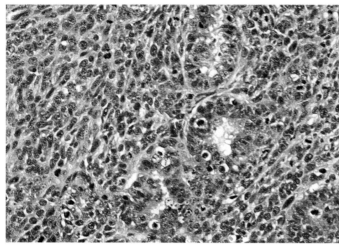

(b)

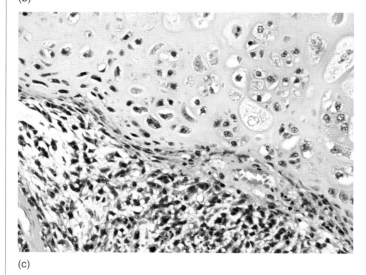

(c)

Figure 12.1.43 Pulmonary blastoma. (a) The tumour consists of malignant epithelial elements, resembling those seen in fetal lung, set in a sarcomatoid stroma. (b) High power shows compact epithelial tubules within a dense blastomatous stroma. (c) Elsewhere there is chondroid differentiation.

arranged more compactly around the epithelial tubules, which are lined by cuboidal or columnar cells with clear glycogen-rich cytoplasm; the appearances closely resemble first trimester fetal lung, hence the term blastoma.[524,531,532] The stromal component shows focal differentiation into cartilage, bone, fat and smooth or striated muscle in up to 25% of cases (Fig. 12.1.43c).[388,533] In some tumours, the epithelial element shows squamous differentiation. Occasional morules associated with β-catenin mutation are observed, as seen in well-differentiated adenocarcinomas of fetal type (see p. 551).[392] Other examples have had melanomatous,[534] small cell carcinoma[535] or yolk sac components.[536] Transition to carcinosarcoma is also described.[523,527–529] Immunohistochemistry and electron microscopy support the view that pulmonary blastomas are true mixed tumours: epithelial markers are confined to the epithelial elements and connective tissue markers to the stromal component.[497,531–533,537–540] However, the features they share with carcinosarcoma indicate that they represent a further type of sarcomatoid carcinoma.

PROGNOSTIC FACTORS[541]

Staging: the role of the pathologist

The appalling prognosis of carcinoma of the lung has already been touched upon, when it was noted that the best overall 5-year survival rates are no better than 17%. This poor outlook is due to a combination of late presentation, early metastasis and a poor sustained response to chemotherapy. Surgeons can achieve 5-year survival rates of 50%, but only by being extremely rigorous in assessing operability and thereby excluding many patients (up to 80%).[9] Staging is therefore extremely important in both treatment and prognosis. Some believe it to be the only significant predictor of survival.[542]

An early step in the spread of a carcinoma is the transition from *in situ* to invasive growth, recognition of which can sometimes be difficult, in which case staining for constituents of the epithelial basement membrane such as laminin and type IV collagen can be helpful.[543] Similarly the integrity of lymphatic and capillary endothelium can be investigated with antibodies to factor VIII-related antigen, *Ulec europeus*, CD31 and CD34.

The accurate assessment of metastasis requires histology and a variety of tissues suspected of harbouring metastatic tumour may be submitted to the laboratory for this purpose. Mediastinal lymph nodes are often sampled by mediastinoscopy or mediastinotomy, usually because they are enlarged although histology shows that the correlation between size and involvement by tumour is poor.[544,545] Alternatively, enlarged mediastinal lymph nodes may be sampled by transbronchial needle aspiration.[250] If the tumour is known to be a small cell carcinoma, bone marrow may be aspirated. The histological detection of micrometastases in these tissues may be helped by the use of epithelial or neuroendocrine markers.[546,547] Molecular techniques have also been used for this purpose.[548] However, the clinical impact of applying these special techniques is questionable.[549,550]

After surgery, pathological staging provides a useful adjunct to the clinical assessment of tumour size and lymph node involvement.[551,552] Protocols for the examination of specimens from patients with lung cancer have been drawn up,[553] one of which is outlined in Table A1 on p. 740. The resection specimen should be dissected and sampled in such a way that apart from ensuring adequate typing of the tumour, all questions pertaining to the pathological tumour stage can be answered. As a routine, the bronchial resection margin, the peribronchial and hilar lymph nodes, the resection margins of the large vessels

Table 12.1.16   Staging of a tumour according to its TNM features[554]

Primary tumour (T)	
TX	Tumour proven by the presence of malignant cells in bronchopulmonary secretions but not visualised roentgenographically or bronchoscopically, or any tumour that cannot be assessed.
T0	No evidence of primary tumour.
TIS	Carcinoma *in situ*
T1	A tumour that is 3.0 cm or less in greatest dimension, surrounded by lung or visceral pleura, and without evidence of invasion proximal to a lobar bronchus at bronchoscopy.
T2	A tumour more than 3.0 cm in greatest dimension, or a tumour of any size that either invades the visceral pleura or has associated atelectasis or obstructive pneumonitis extending to the hilar region. At bronchoscopy, the proximal extent of demonstrable tumour must be within a lobar bronchus or at least 2.0 cm distal to the carina. Any associated atelectasis or obstructive pneumonitis must involve less than an entire lung.
T3	A tumour of any size with direct extension into the chest wall (including 'superior sulcus' tumours), diaphragm, or the mediastinal pleura or pericardium without involving the heart, great vessels, trachea, oesophagus or a vertebra, or a tumour in the main bronchus within 2 cm of the carina without involving the carina.
T4	A tumour of any size with invasion of the mediastinum or involving heart, great vessels, trachea, oesophagus, a vertebra or carina, or in the presence of malignant pleural effusion.
Nodal involvement (N)	
N0	No demonstrable metastasis to regional lymph nodes.
N1	Metastasis to lymph nodes in the peribronchial or the ipsilateral hilar region, or both, including direct extension.
N2	Metastasis to ipsilateral mediastinal lymph nodes and subcarinal lymph nodes.
N3	Metastasis to contralateral mediastinal lymph nodes, contralateral hilar lymph nodes, or ipsilateral or contralateral scalene or supraclavicular lymph nodes.
Distant metastasis (M)	
M0	No (known) distant metastasis.
M1	Distant metastasis present – specify site(s).

and the pleura nearest to the tumour should be sampled. Lung tissue away from the tumour should also be sampled to detect occult spread and for the assessment of conditions such as asbestosis that might have led to the development of the tumour.

The full pathological TNM classification[554] is shown in Tables 12.1.16, 12.1.17 and the effect of stage in Figure 12.1.44.[555] Size greater than 3 cm or pleural involvement puts the tumour into the T2 category. If the tumour is close to, but not obviously through the pleura, an elastin stain is useful to delineate the deep margin of the pleura.[556] The pathologist should attempt to identify and sample lymph nodes at the hilum of the resection specimen, involvement of these taking the tumour stage to N1. The laboratory will usually receive several separate specimens of higher lymph node stations, all numbered according to an international classification.[557] The assessment of these will decide whether stage N2 has been reached. It is usually suffi-

Table 12.1.17 Stage grouping and survival of TNM subsets after pathological examination of the excised specimen (pTNM)

Stage grouping	pTNM subset	5-year survival (%)	Median survival (months)
Occult carcinoma	TX N0 M0		
Stage 0	TIS N0 M0		
Stage Ia	T1 N0 M0	69	60+
Stage Ib	T2 N0 M0	59	60+
Stage IIa	T1 N1 M0	54	60+
Stage IIb	T2 N1 M0	40	29
	T3 N0 M0	44	26
Stage IIIa	T3 N1 M0	18	16
	T1–3 N2 M0	29	22
Stage IIIb	Any T N3 M0		
	T4 Any N M0		
Stage IV	Any T Any N M1		

Stage IIIb and IV tumours are considered to be inoperable.

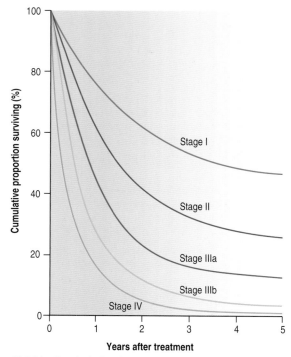

Figure 12.1.44 Survival of patients with carcinoma of the lung: cumulative proportion surviving up to 5 years after treatment. (Data from Mountain.[555])

cient for the pathologist to record the presence or absence of tumour in each of these. Some surgeons wish to know whether the lymph node capsule has been breached but the higher nodes are often received piecemeal. There is some evidence that direct spread to N1 nodes has a better prognosis than metastatic spread to these nodes[558] and similarly that intrapulmonary N1 lymph node involvement is better than extrapulmonary N1 disease.[559]

Histological type and grade

Bearing in mind that stage is far more important than any other prognostic factor,[542] histological type, subtype and grade cannot be considered to have a major impact, but all have some relevance to prognosis.[263,265,286,560–563] In regard to tumour typing, interobserver variability is reported to be small[245,246] but grading is more subjective. The worst histological type, small cell carcinoma, has a 5-year survival rate of only 4% (Fig. 12.1.45).[10] Many oncologists regard all small cell carcinomas as inoperable and only divide them according to whether spread is limited or extensive. Adenocarcinoma is recognised as having more metastatic potential than squamous cell carcinoma and with this cell type it is worth extending preoperative screening procedures for metastases to include the brain. Histological typing is also important in regard to treatment, small cell carcinoma

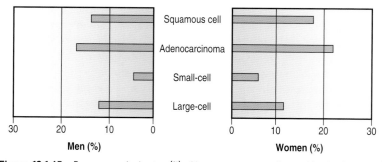

Figure 12.1.45 5-year survival rates (%) of lung cancer according to histological type.[10]

generally being considered the only type that responds to chemotherapy, if only temporarily. However, the introduction of neoadjuvant chemotherapy for non-small cell carcinoma implies that these tumours are also chemosensitive,[564] albeit to a lesser extent than small cell carcinoma. Considerable attention is being paid today to the implications of neuroendocrine differentiation in non-small cell carcinomas, in particular to the possibility that such differentiation may be associated with the chemosensitivity shown by small cell carcinoma: the limited evidence for this is discussed under large cell neuroendocrine carcinoma (see p. 557).

Other prognostic factors[565]

After tumour stage and histological type, factors such as DNA content,[566–568] ploidy,[569–571] nuclear/cytoplasmic ratio,[572] proliferation markers,[573–576] nucleolar organiser regions,[577–579] telomerase activity,[580] apoptosis,[581] tumour doubling time,[582] tumour specific markers,[336,583,584] oestrogen receptor,[585] inflammatory response,[326,586–588] fibrosis,[395] vascularity,[589–592] vascular invasion,[593,594] cell adhesion molecule expression,[595,596] the production of immunosuppressive oncogenes by the tumour,[597] widespread disruption of the epithelial basement membrane[598,599] and the secretion of metalloproteinases[600–602] are all reported to carry prognostic significance, albeit rather limited, but reports tend to be conflicting. Furthermore, this discordance is compounded by the heterogeneity of lung tumours, which is found to apply to the results of these more sophisticated investigations as much as to simple histological typing: therefore, if it were planned to introduce any of these techniques into routine laboratory practice quite extensive standardised sampling of the tumour would be required.[603,604]

Oncogene expression also appears to be linked to prognosis.[605–608] Not all groups have found a positive correlation,[609–611] but expression of the *ras* oncogene in lung tumours is widely reported to auger a poor prognosis[612–615] and mutations of genes that control cell growth and apoptosis, such as p53, RB and bcl-2 are found in many lung neoplasms,[576,614,616–621] with obvious implications for the growth of the tumour. Furthermore, genetic abnormalities enhancing tumour growth may be induced by the very chemotherapy aimed at eliminating the tumour. For example, amplification of c-*myc* is more often present in small cell carcinomas from patients who have relapsed after chemotherapy than in newly diagnosed patients; patients in relapse who showed amplification had shorter survivals than those who did not.[622]

Drug resistance is a major problem in chemotherapy, and one that is compounded by the observation that tumours that acquire resistance to one drug often simultaneously become resistant to a variety of other structurally unrelated drugs. This multidrug resistance is under genetic control. The genes responsible encode glycoproteins in the cell membrane that eliminate various drugs from the cell and can be detected immunocytochemically.[623–625]

One mechanism whereby aberrant gene expression may be linked to tumour aggressiveness is over-elaboration of growth factors. Endothelin for example is a growth factor that has been demonstrated in large amounts in squamous cell and adenocarcinoma of the lung,[183] and transforming growth factor β-1 is reported to be a prognostic factor for pulmonary adenocarcinoma.[626] Over 30 other growth factors are known to be synthesised by small cell lung cancer.[627] Some growth factors, notably gastrin releasing peptide (human bombesin), evince autocrine activity by stimulating the proliferation of the cancer cells that produce them.[628,629] A further mechanism by which faulty genetic regulation may influence tumour growth is in the production of receptors for specific growth factors. An example of this is the strong expression of epidermal growth factor receptor demonstrated in pulmonary squamous cell carcinoma.[184]

FUTURE DEVELOPMENTS IN TREATMENT

The traditional treatment of lung cancer is 3-fold: surgery for those patients whose tumours appear to be operable after extensive staging, aggressive chemotherapy for most small cell carcinomas, and palliative chemotherapy or radiotherapy for inoperable non-small carcinoma. Neoadjuvant chemotherapy extends this by reducing the extent of the tumour to operable proportions, so providing curative treatment to patients formerly offered only palliation.[564] New chemotherapeutic drugs are constantly being introduced and aggressive chemotherapy is being increasingly offered to patients with inoperable non-small cell carcinoma.[630]

Totally new anticancer treatments are also being introduced. Some of these involve the use of natural or recombinant cytokines such as the interferons, the interleukins and tumour necrosis factor, or inhibitors of matrix proteinases involved in neoplastic infiltration and metastasis.[97] Others involve modification of the signal transduction pathways important in the continued growth of lung cancer. Activation of tyrosine kinase receptors is an important growth signal for all histological types of lung cancer[631] and inhibitors of cyclin-dependent kinase have now reached the stage of being tested in clinical trials.[632–635] Epidermal growth factor receptor (Her-2) is over-expressed in some non-small carcinomas and drugs have been developed to block this receptor.[636] There is currently much interest in this area as it has been shown that those who respond to chemotherapy with gefitinib have somatic mutations in the tyrosine kinase domain of the EGFR gene, providing a possible avenue for targeted therapy.[637,638] Certain antagonists to gastrin releasing peptide (human bombesin) are also of potential clinical importance.[639,640]

Other new lines of cancer therapy now undergoing evaluation involve antibodies to tumour antigens. For example, vaccination with mutant *k-ras* peptides are in progress.[641] That immune mechanisms may provide an effective host response is suggested by reports of spontaneous regression of small cell lung carcinoma in patients with paraneoplastic neuronal antibodies.[642] Some of the antigens being targeted are not strictly specific to tumours but represent normal cell components that

85. Mizushima Y, Kobayashi M. Clinical characteristics of synchronous multiple lung cancer associated with idiopathic pulmonary fibrosis: a review of Japanese cases. Chest 1995; 108:1272–1277.

86. Hironaka M, Fukayama M. Pulmonary fibrosis and lung carcinoma: A comparative study of metaplastic epithelia in honeycombed areas of usual interstitial pneumonia with or without lung carcinoma. Pathol Int 1999; 49:1060–1066.

87. Askling J, Grunewald J, Eklund A, Hillerdal G, Ekbom A. Increased risk for cancer following sarcoidosis. Am J Respir Crit Care Med 1999; 160:1668–1672.

88. Bouros D, Hatzakis K, Labrakis H, Zeibecoglou K. Association of malignancy with diseases causing interstitial pulmonary changes. Chest 2002; 121:1278–1289.

89. Seersholm N, Vestbo J, Viskum K. Risk of malignant neoplasms in patients with pulmonary sarcoidosis. Thorax 1997; 52:892–894.

90. Nakazato I, Hirayasu T, Kamada Y, Tsuhako K, Iwamasa T. Carcinoma of the lung in Okinawa, Japan: With special reference to squamous cell carcinoma and squamous metaplasia. Pathol Int 1997; 47:659–672.

91. Bohlmeyer T, Le TN, Shroyer AL, Markham N, Shroyer KR. Detection of human papillomavirus in squamous cell carcinomas of the lung by polymerase chain reaction. Am J Respir Cell Molec Biol 1998; 18:265–269.

92. Iwamasa T, Miyagi J, Tsuhako K, et al. Prognostic implication of human papillomavirus infection in squamous cell carcinoma of the lung. Pathol Res Pr 2000; 196:209–218.

93. Syrjanen KJ. HPV infections and lung cancer. J Clin Pathol 2002; 55:885–891.

94. Chan JKC, Hui PK, Tsang WYW, et al. Primary lymphoepithelioma-like carcinoma of the lung – a clinicopathologic study of 11 cases. Cancer 1995; 76:413–422.

95. Conway EJ, Hudnall SD, Lazarides A, et al. Absence of evidence for an etiologic role for Epstein-Barr virus in neoplasms of the lung and pleura. Mod Pathol 1996; 9:491–495.

96. Chan TK, Aranda CP, Rom WN. Bronchogenic carcinoma in young patients at risk for acquired immunodeficiency syndrome. Chest 1993; 103:862–864.

97. Smyth JF. Cancer genetics and cell and molecular biology: is this the way forward? Chest 1996; 109:S125–S129.

98. Schwartz AG. Genetic predisposition to lung cancer. Chest 2004; 125:86S–89S.

99. Ayesh R, Idle JR, Ritchie JC, Crothers MJ, Hetzel MR. Metabolic oxidation phenotypes as markers for susceptibility to lung cancer. Nature 1984; 312:169–170.

100. Philpot RM. Modulation of the pulmonary cytochrome-p450 system as a factor in pulmonary-selective toxic responses – fact and fiction. Am J Respir Cell Mol Biol 1993; 9:347–349.

101. Shaw GL, Falk RT, Pickle LW, Mason TJ, Buffler PA. Lung cancer risk associated with cancer in relatives. J Clin Epidemiol 1991; 44:429–437.

102. Ambrosone CB, Rao U, Michalek AM, Cummings KM, Mettlin CJ. Lung cancer histologic types and family history of cancer – analysis of histologic subtypes of 872 patients with primary lung cancer. Cancer 1993; 72:1192–1198.

103. Lynch HT, Kimberling WJ, Markvicka SE, et al. Genetics and smoking-associated cancers. A study of 485 families. Cancer 1986; 57:1640–1646.

104. Braun MM, Caporaso NE, Page WF, Hoover RN. Genetic component of lung cancer: cohort study of twins. Lancet 1994; 344:440–443.

Pathogenesis

105. Chandraratnam EA, Henderson DW, Meredith DJ, Jain S. Regenerative atypical squamous metaplasia in fibreoptic bronchial biopsy sites – a lesion liable to misinterpretation as carcinoma on rebiopsy report of 5 cases. Pathology 1987; 19:419–424.

106. Ayers MM, Jeffery PK. Proliferation and differentiation in mammalian airway epithelium. Eur Respir J 1988; 1:58–80.

107. Chopra DP, Cooney RA. Histogenesis of benzo(a)pyrene-induced lesions in tracheal explants. Virchows Arch B Cell Pathol 1985; 48:299–315.

108. Johnson NF, Wagner JC, Wills HA. Endocrine cell proliferation in the rat lung following asbestos exposure. Lung 1980; 158:221–228.

109. Reznik-Schuller H. Sequential morphologic alterations in the bronchial epithelium of Syrian golden hamsters during N-nitrosomorpholine-induced pulmonary tumorigenesis. Am J Pathol 1977; 89:59–66.

110. Saccomanno G, Archer VE, Auerbach O, Saunders RP, Brennan LM. Development of carcinoma of the lung as reflected in exfoliated cells. Cancer 1974; 33:256–270.

111. Franklin WA. Premalignant Evolution of Lung Cancer: Gilles F. Filley Lecture. Chest 2004; 125:90S–994.

112. World Health Organization. Tumours of the lung, pleura, thymus and heart. Lyons, France: IARC Press; 2004.

113. Keith RL, Miller YE, Gemmill RM, et al. Angiogenic squamous dysplasia in bronchi of individuals at high risk for lung cancer. Clin Cancer Res 2000; 6:1616–1625.

114. Shibuya K, Hoshino H, Chiyo M, et al. Subepithelial vascular patterns in bronchial dysplasias using a high magnification bronchovideoscope. Thorax 2002; 57:902–907.

115. Nagamoto N, Saito Y, Sato M, et al. Clinicopathological analysis of 19 cases of isolated carcinoma insitu of the bronchus. Am J Surg Pathol 1993; 17:1234–1243.

116. Solomon MD, Greenberg SD, Spjut HJ. Morphology of bronchial epithelium adjacent to adenocarcinoma of the lung. Mod Pathol 1990; 3:684–687.

117. Bodegom PC, van Wagenaar SjSc, Corrin B, Baak JPA, Berkel J, Vanderschueren RGJRA. Second primary lung cancer: importance of long term follow up. Thorax 1989; 44:788–793.

118. Okada M, Tsubota N, Yoshimura M, Kubota M, Murotani A. Simultaneous occurrence of three primary lung cancers. Chest 1994; 105:631–632.

119. Banerjee AK, Rabbitts PH, George J. Lung cancer center dot 3: Fluorescence bronchoscopy: clinical dilemmas and research opportunities. Thorax 2003; 58:266–271.

120. Raeburn C, Spencer H. A study of the origin and development of lung cancer. Thorax 1953; 8:1–10.

121. Spencer H, Raeburn C. Atypical proliferation of bronchiolar epithelium. J Path Bact 1954; 67:187–193.

122. Weng SY, Tsuchiya E, Kasuga T, Sugano H. Incidence of atypical bronchioloalveolar cell hyperplasia of the lung – relation to histological subtypes of lung cancer. Virchows Arch A Pathol Anat Histopathol 1992; 420:463–471.

123. Nakayama H, Noguchi M, Tsuchiya R, Kodama T, Shimosato Y. Clonal growth of atypical adenomatous hyperplasia of the lung: cytofluorometric analysis of nuclear DNA content. Mod Pathol 1990; 3:314–320.

124. Kerr KM, Carey FA, King G, Lamb D. Atypical alveolar hyperplasia: relationship with pulmonary adenocarcinoma, p53, and c-erbB-2 expression. J Pathol 1994; 174:249–256.

125. Rao SK, Fraire AE. Alveolar cell hyperplasia in association with adenocarcinoma of lung. Mod Pathol 1995; 8:165–169.

126. Chapman AD, Kerr KM. The association between atypical adenomatous hyperplasia and primary lung cancer. Br J Cancer 2000; 83:632–636.

127. Miller RR, Nelems B, Evans KG, Muller NL, Ostrow DN. Glandular neoplasia of the lung. A proposed analogy to colonic tumors. Cancer 1988; 61:1009–1014.

128. Sterner DJ, Mori M, Roggli VL, Fraire AE. Prevalence of pulmonary atypical alveolar cell hyperplasia in an autopsy population: a study of 100 cases. Mod Pathol 1997; 10:469–473.

129. Miller RR. Bronchioloalveolar cell adenomas. Am J Surg Pathol 1990; 14:904–912.

130. Nakahara R, Yokose T, Nagai K, Nishiwaki Y, Ochiai A. Atypical adenomatous hyperplasia of the lung: a clinicopathological study of 118 cases including cases with multiple atypical adenomatous hyperplasia. Thorax 2001; 56:302–305.

131. Koga T, Hashimoto S, Sugio K, et al. Lung adenocarcinoma with bronchioloalveolar carcinoma component is frequently associated with foci of high-grade atypical adenomatous hyperplasia. Am J Clin Pathol 2002; 117:464–470.

132. Cooper CA, Carey FA, Bubb VJ, et al. The pattern of K-ras mutation in pulmonary adenocarcinoma defines a new pathway of tumour development in the human lung. J Pathol 1997; 181:401–404.

133. Mori M, Rao SK, Popper HH, Cagle PT, Fraire AE. Atypical adenomatous hyperplasia of the lung: A probable forerunner in the development of adenocarcinoma of the lung. Mod Pathol 2001; 14:72–84.

134. Mori M, Chiba R, Takahashi T. Atypical adenomatous hyperplasia of the lung and its differentiation from adenocarcinoma – characterization of atypical cells by morphometry and multivariate cluster analysis. Cancer 1993; 72:2331–2340.

135. Kitamura H, Kameda Y, Nakamura N, et al. Atypical adenomatous hyperplasia and bronchoalveolar lung carcinoma: analysis by morphometry and the expressions of p53 and carcinoembryonic antigen. Am J Surg Pathol 1996; 20:553–562.

136. Yokozaki M, Kodama T, Yokose T, Matsumoto T, Mukai K. Differentiation of atypical adenomatous hyperplasia and adenocarcinoma of the lung by use of DNA ploidy and morphometric analysis. Mod Pathol 1996; 9:1156–1164.

137. Nakanishi K, Hiroi S, Kawai T, Suzuki M, Torikata C. Argyrophilic nucleolar-organizer region counts and DNA status in bronchioloalveolar epithelial hyperplasia and adenocarcinoma of the lung. Hum Pathol 1998; 29:235–239.

138. Takamochi K, Ogura T, Suzuki K, et al. Loss of heterozygosity on chromosomes 9q and 16p in atypical adenomatous hyperplasia concomitant with adenocarcinoma of the lung. Am J Pathol 2001; 159:1941–1948.

139. Ohshima S, Shimizu Y, Takahama M. Detection of c-ki-ras gene mutation in paraffin sections of adenocarcinoma and atypical bronchioloalveolar cell hyperplasia of human lung. Virchows Arch 1994; 424:129–134.

140. Kurasono Y, Ito T, Kameda Y, Nakamura N, Kitamura H. Expression of cyclin D1, retinoblastoma gene protein, and p16 MTS1 protein in atypical adenomatous hyperplasia and adenocarcinoma of the lung – An immunohistochemical analysis. Virchows Arch 1998; 432:207–215.

141. Kitamura H, Kameda Y, Ito T, Hayashi H. Atypical adenomatous hyperplasia of the lung – Implications for the pathogenesis of peripheral lung adenocarcinoma. Am J Clin Pathol 1999; 111:610–622.

142. Niho S, Yokose T, Suzuki K, et al. Monoclonality of atypical adenomatous hyperplasia of the lung. Am J Pathol 1999; 154:249–254.

143. Logan PM, Miller RR, Evans K, Muller NL. Bronchogenic carcinoma and coexistent bronchioloalveolar cell adenomas: assessment of radiologic detection and follow-up in 28 patients. Chest 1996; 109:713–717.

144. Suzuki K, Nagai K, Yoshida J, et al. The prognosis of resected lung carcinoma associated with atypical adenomatous hyperplasia: A comparison of the prognosis of well-differentiated adenocarcinoma associated with atypical adenomatous hyperplasia and intrapulmonary metastasis. Cancer 1997; 79:1521–1526.

145. Ullmann R, Bongiovanni M, Halbwedl I, et al. Bronchiolar columnar cell dysplasia – genetic analysis of a novel preneoplastic lesion of peripheral lung. Virchows Arch 2003; 442:429–436.

146. Nuorva K, Soini Y, Kamel D, et al. Concurrent p53 expression in bronchial dysplasias and squamous cell lung carcinomas. Am J Pathol 1993; 142:725–732.

147. Hirano T, Franzen B, Kato H, Ebihara Y, Auer G. Genesis of squamous cell lung carcinoma – sequential changes of proliferation, DNA ploidy and p53 expression. Am J Pathol 1994; 144:296–302.

148. Dosakaakita H, Shindoh M, Fujino M, et al. Abnormal p53 expression in human lung cancer is associated with histologic subtypes and patient smoking history. Am J Clin Pathol 1994; 102:660–664.

149. Kitamura H, Kameda Y, Nakamura N, et al. Proliferative potential and p53 overexpression in precursor and early stage lesions of bronchioloalveolar lung carcinoma. Am J Pathol 1995; 146:876–887.

150. Walker C, Robertson LJ, Myskow MW, Pendleton N, Dixon GR. p53 expression in normal and dysplastic bronchial epithelium and in lung carcinomas. Br J Cancer 1994; 70:297–303.

151. Boers JE, Tenvelde GPM, Thunnissen FBJM. p53 in squamous metaplasia: a marker for risk of respiratory tract carcinoma. Am J Respir Crit Care Med 1996; 153:411–416.

152. Ponticiello A, Barra E, Giani U, Bocchino M, Sanduzzi A. p53 immunohistochemistry can identify bronchial dysplastic lesions proceeding to lung cancer: a prospective study. Eur Resp J 2000; 15:547–552.

153. Sanz-Ortega J. Saez MC, Sierra E et al. 3p21, 5q21, and 9p21 allelic deletions are frequently found in normal bronchial cells adjacent to non-small-cell lung cancer, while they are unusual in patients with no evidence of malignancy. J Pathol 2001; 195:429–434.

154. Sundaresan V, Ganly P, Hasleton P, et al. p53 and chromosome 3 abnormalities, characteristic of malignant lung tumours, are detectable in preinvasive lesions of the bronchus. Oncogene 1992; 7:1989–1 997.

155. Chung GT, Sundaresan V, Hasleton P, et al. Sequential molecular genetic changes in lung cancer development. Oncogene 1995; 11:2591–2598.

156. Park IW, Wistuba II, Maitra A, et al. Multiple clonal abnormalities in the bronchial epithelium of patients with lung cancer. J Natl Cancer Inst 1999; 91:1863–1868.

157. Hayashi H, Miyamoto H, Ito T, et al. Analysis of p21(Waf1/Cip1) expression in normal, premalignant, and malignant cells during the development of human lung adenocarcinoma. Am J Pathol 1997; 151:461–470.

158. Hung J, Kishimoto Y, Sugio K, et al. Allele-specific chromosome 3p deletions occur at an early stage in the pathogenesis of lung carcinoma [published erratum appears in JAMA 1995; 273:1908]. JAMA 1995; 273:558–563.

159. Kishimoto Y, Sugio K, Hung JY, et al. Allele-specific loss in chromosome 9p loci in preneoplastic lesions accompanying non-small-cell lung cancers. J Natl Cancer Inst 1995; 87:1224–1229.

160. Giaccone G. Oncogenes and antioncogenes in lung tumorigenesis. Chest 1996; 109:S130–S134.

161. Rom WN, Hay JG, Lee TC, Jiang YX, TchouWong KM. Molecular and genetic aspects of lung cancer. Am J Respir Crit Care Med 2000; 161:1355–1367.

162. Westra WH, Slebos RJC, Offerhaus GJA, et al. K-ras oncogene activation in lung adenocarcinomas from former smokers – evidence that k-ras mutations are an early and irreversible event in the development of adenocarcinoma of the lung. Cancer 1993; 72:432–438.

163. Marchetti A, Buttitta F, Pellegrini S, et al. Bronchioloalveolar lung carcinomas: k-ras mutations are constant events in the mucinous subtype. J Pathol 1996; 179:254–259.

164. Nau MM, Brooks BJ, Carney DN, et al. Human small-cell lung cancers show amplification and expression of the N-myc gene. Proc Natl Acad Sci USA 1986; 83:1092–1096.

165. Scott GM, Jones IG. A study of myc-related gene expression in small cell lung cancer by in situ hybridization. Am J Pathol 1988; 132:13–17.

166. Gazdar AF. Oncogenes, antioncogenes and growth factors in the pathogenesis of small cell lung cancer (SCLC). Proceedings Second International Conference on Small Cell Lung Cancer, 1990.

167. Pezzella F, Turley H, Kuzu I, et al. bcl-2 protein in non-small-cell lung carcinoma. N Engl J Med 1993; 329:690–694.

168. Walker C, Robertson L, Myskow M, Dixon G. Expression of the BCL-2 protein in normal and dysplastic bronchial epithelium and in lung carcinomas. Br J Cancer 1995; 72:164–169.

169. Rao SK, Krishna M, Woda BA, Savas L, Fraire AE. Immunohistochemical detection of bcl-2 protein in adenocarcinoma and non-neoplastic cellular compartments of the lung. Mod Pathol 1996; 9:555–559.

170. Jiang SX, Kameya T, Sato Y, et al. Bcl-2 protein expression in lung cancer and close correlation with neuroendocrine differentiation. Am J Pathol 1996; 148:837–846.

171. Brambilla E, Negoescu A, Gazzeri S, et al. Apoptosis-related factors p53, Bcl2 and Bax in neuroendocrine lung tumors. Am J Pathol 1996; 149:1941–1 952.

172. Kok K, Osinga J, Carritt B, et al. Deletion of a DNA sequence at the chromosomal region 3p21 in all major types of lung cancer. Nature 1987; 330:578–581.

173. Yokota J, Wada M, Shimosato Y, Terada M, Sugimura T. Loss of heterozygosity on chromosomes 3, 13, and 17 in small-cell carcinoma and on chromosome 3 in adenocarcinoma of the lung. Proc Natl Acad Sci USA 1987; 84:9252–9256.

174. Lehman TA, Bennett WP, Metcalf RA, et al. p53 mutations, ras mutations, and p53 – heat shock 70 protein complexes in human lung carcinoma cell lines. Cancer Res 1991; 51:4090–4096.

175. Whang-Peng J, Bunn PAJr, Kao-Shan CS et al. A nonrandom chromosomal abnormality, del 3p,[14–23] in human small cell lung cancer (SCLC). Cancer Genet Cytogenet 1982; 6:119–134.

176. Caamano J, Ruggeri B, Momiki S, et al. Detection of p53 in primary lung tumors and nonsmall cell lung carcinoma cell lines. Am J Pathol 1991; 139:839–845.

177. Barbareschi M, Girlando S, Mauri FA, et al. Tumour suppressor gene products, proliferation, and differentiation markers in lung neuroendocrine neoplasms. J Pathol 1992; 166:343–350.

178. Klein N, Vignaud JM, Sadmi M, et al. Squamous metaplasia expression of proto-oncogenes and p-53 in lung cancer patients. Lab Invest 1993; 68:26–32.

179. Hamid Q, Addis BJ, Springall DR, et al. Expression of the C-terminal peptide of human pro-bombesin in 361 lung endocrine tumours, a reliable marker and possible prognostic indicator for small cell carcinoma. Virchows Arch A Pathol Anat Histopathol 1987; 411:185–192.

180. Shriver SP, Bourdeau HA, Gubish CT, et al. Sex-specific expression of gastrin-releasing peptide receptor: relationship to smoking history and risk of lung cancer. J Natl Cancer Inst 2000; 92:24–33.

181. Nakashini Y, Mulshine JL, Kasprzyk PG, et al. Insulin-like growth factor-1 can mediate autocrine proliferation of human small cell lung cancer cell lines. J Clin Invest 1988; 82:354–359.

182. Vostrejs M, Moran PL, Seligman PA. Transferrin synthesis by small cell lung cancer acts as an autocrine regulator of cellular proliferation. J Clin Invest 1988; 82:331–339.

183. Giaid A, Hamid QA, Springall DR, et al. Detection of endothelin immunoreactivity and mRNA in pulmonary tumours. J Pathol 1990; 162:15–22.

184. Berger MS, Gullick WJ, Greenfield C, et al. Epidermal growth factor receptors in lung tumours. J Pathol 1987; 152:297–307.

185. Hiyama K, Hiyama E, Ishioka S, et al. Telomerase activity in small-cell and non-small-cell lung cancers. J Natl Cancer Inst 1995; 87:895–902.

186. Albanell J, Lonardo F, Rusch V, et al. High telomerase activity in primary lung cancers: association with increased cell proliferation rates and advanced pathologic stage. J Natl Cancer Inst 1997; 89:1609–1615.

187. Arinaga M, Shimizu S, Gotoh K, et al. Expression of human telomerase subunit genes in primary lung cancer and its clinical significance. Ann Thorac Surg 2000; 70:401–405.

188. Bach PB, Kelley MJ, Tate RC, McCrory DC. Screening for lung cancer – A review of the current literature. Chest 2003; 123:72S–82S.

189. Manser RL, Irving LB, Byrnes G, et al. Screening for lung cancer: a systematic review and meta-analysis of controlled trials. Thorax 2003; 58:784–789.

190. Geddes DM. The natural history of lung cancer: a review based on rates of tumour growth. Br J Dis Chest 1979; 73:1–17.

191. Belinsky SA, Palmisano WA, Gilliland FD, et al. Aberrant promoter methylation in bronchial epithelium and sputum from current and former smokers. Cancer Res 2002; 62:2370–2377.

192. Palmisano WA, Divine KK, Saccomanno G, et al. Predicting lung cancer by detecting aberrant promoter methylation in sputum. Cancer Res 2000; 60:5954–5958.

193. Simpson NK, Johnson CC, Ogden SL, et al. Recruitment strategies in the Prostate, Lung, Colorectal and Ovarian (PLCO) Cancer Screening Trial: the first six years. Control Clin Trials 2000; 21:356S–378S.

194. Henschke CI, Naidich DP, Yankelevitz DF, et al. Early lung cancer action project: initial findings on repeat screenings. Cancer 2001; 92: 153–159.

195. Henschke CI, Yankelevitz DF, Mirtcheva R, et al. CT screening for lung cancer: frequency and significance of part-solid and nonsolid nodules. AJR Am J Roentgenol 2002; 178:1053–1057.

196. Henschke CI, Yankelevitz DF, McCauley D, et al. CT screening for lung cancer. Cancer Chemother Biol Response Modif 2002; 20:665–676.

197. Sagawa M, Nakayama T, Tsukada H, et al. The efficacy of lung cancer screening conducted in 1990s: four case-control studies in Japan. Lung Cancer 2003; 41:29–36.

198. Bach PB, Niewoehner DE, Black WC. Screening for lung cancer: the guidelines. Chest 2003; 123:83S–88S.

199. Yamato Y, Tsuchida M, Watanabe T, et al. Early results of a prospective study of limited resection for bronchioloalveolar adenocarcinoma of the lung. Ann Thorac Surg 2001; 71:971–974.

200. Kodama K, Higashiyama M, Yokouchi H, et al. Prognostic value of ground-glass opacity found in small lung adenocarcinoma on high-resolution CT scanning. Lung Cancer 2001; 33:17–25.

201. Si W, Watanabe T, Arai K, et al. Results of wedge resection for focal bronchioloalveolar carcinoma showing pure ground-glass attenuation on computed tomography. Ann Thorac Surg 2002; 73:1071–1075.

202. Suzuki K, Asamura H, Kusumoto M, Kondo H. Tsuchiya R. 'Early' peripheral lung cancer: prognostic significance of ground glass opacity on thin-section computed tomographic scan. Ann Thorac Surg 2002; 74:1635–1639.

Site of origin and spread

203. Iravani J, As A van. Mucus transport in the tracheobronchial tree of normal and bronchitic rats. J Pathol 1972; 106:81–93.

204. Hilding AC. Ciliary streaming in the bronchial tree and the time element in carcinogenesis. N Engl J Med 1957; 256:634–640.

205. Churg A, Vedal S. Carinal and tubular airway particle concentrations in the large airways of non-smokers in the general population: evidence for high particle concentration at airway carinas. Occup Environ Med 1996; 53:553–558.

206. Salm R. Primary carcinoma of the trachea: a review. Br J Dis Chest 1964; 58:61–72.

207. Gelder CM, Hetzel MR. Primary tracheal tumours – a national survey. Thorax 1993; 48:688–692.

208. Rigler LG. A roentgen study of the evolution of carcinoma of the lung. J Thorac Surg 1957; 34:283–297.

209. Rigler LG, O'Loughlin BJ, Tucker RC. The duration of carcinoma of the lung. Dis Chest 1953; 23:50–57.

210. Kerr IH. Radiological assessment. Recent Results Cancer Res 1984; 92:30–42.

211. Auerbach O, Garfinkel L. The changing pattern of lung carcinoma. Cancer 1991; 68:1973–1977.

212. Walter JB, Pryce DM. The site of origin of lung cancer and its relation to histological type. Thorax 1955; 10:107–126.

213. Quinn D, Gianlupi A, Broste S. The changing radiographic presentation of bronchogenic carcinoma with reference to cell types. Chest 1996; 110:1474–1479.

Clinical effects

214. Toomes H, Delphendahl A, Manke H-G, Vogt-Moykopf I. The coin lesion of the lung. A review of 955 resected coin lesions. Cancer 1983; 51:534–537.

215. Baldwin DR, Eaton T, Kolbe J, et al. Management of solitary pulmonary nodules: how do thoracic computed tomography and guided fine needle biopsy influence clinical decisions? Thorax 2002; 57:817–822.

216. Hare ES. Tumour involving certain nerves. Lond Med Gaz 1838; 23:16.

217. Pancoast HK. Superior pulmonary sulcus tumor: tumor characterized by pain, Horner's syndrome, destruction of bone and atrophy of hand muscles. JAMA 1932; 99:1391–1396.

218. Arcasoy SM, Jett JR. Current concept: Superior pulmonary sulcus tumors and Pancoast's syndrome. N Engl J Med 1997; 337:1370–1376.

219. Matthews MJ. Problems in morphology and behavior of bronchopulmonary malignant disease. In: Israel L, Chahinain P, eds. Lung cancer natural history, prognosis and therapy. New York, NY: Academic Press; 1976:23–62.

220. Gomm SA, Thatcher N, Barber PV, Cumming WJK. A clinicopathological study of the paraneoplastic neuromuscular syndromes associated with lung cancer. Q J Med 1990; 75:577–595.

221. Bohan A, Peter JB. Polymyositis and dermatomyositis. N Engl J Med 1975; 293:344–347.

222. Newsom-David J. Lambert-Eaton myasthenic syndrome. Semin Immunopathol 1985; 8:129–140.

223. Kiers L, Altermatt HJ, Lennon VA. Paraneoplastic anti-neuronal nuclear IgG autoantibodies (type-I) localize antigen in small cell lung carcinoma. Mayo Clin Proc 1991; 66:1209–1216.

224. Grunwald GB, Klein R, Simmonds M, Kornguth SE. Autoimmune basis for visual paraneoplastic syndrome in patients with small cell lung cancer. Lancet 1985; i:658–661.

225. Levine RJ, Metz SA. A classification of ectopic hormone-producing tumors. Ann N Y Acad Sci 1974; 230:533–546.

226. Troyer A De, Demaner JC. Clinical, biological and pathogenic features of the syndrome of inappropriate secretion of ADH. Q J Med 1976; 45:521–531.

227. Imura H, Matsukura S, Yamamoto H. Studies on ectopic ACTH-producing tumors. Cancer 1975; 35:1430–1437.

228. Campling BG, Sarda IR, Baer KA, et al. Secretion of atrial natriuretic peptide and vasopressin by small cell lung cancer. Cancer 1995; 75:2442–2451.

229. Salyer DC, Eggleston JC. Oat cell carcinoma of the bronchus and the carcinoid syndrome. Arch Pathol 1975; 99:513–515.

230. Davidson LA, Black M, Carey FA, Logue F, McNicol AM. Lung tumours immunoreactive for parathyroid hormone related peptide: analysis of serum calcium levels and tumour type. J Pathol 1996; 178:398–401.

231. Yoshida Y, Mori M, Sonoda T, et al. Ultrastructural, immunohistochemical and biochemical studies on amylase and ACTH producing lung cancer. Virchows Arch A Pathol Anat Histopathol 1985; 408:163–172.

232. Boucher LD, Yoneda K. The expression of trophoblastic cell markers by lung carcinomas. Hum Pathol 1995; 26:1201–1206.

233. Hiroshima K, Iyoda A, Toyozaki T, et al. Alpha-fetoprotein-producing lung carcinoma: report of three cases. Pathol Int 2002; 52:46–53.

234. Sawyers CL, Golde DW, Quan S, Nimer SD. Production of granulocyte-macrophage colony-stimulating factor in two patients with lung cancer, leukocytosis, and eosinophilia. Cancer 1992; 69:1342–1346.

235. Johnson RL, Donnell RM. Diffuse granulocytic infiltration of giant cell carcinoma of the lung: a distinctive histologic finding with clinical significance. Lab Invest 1979; 40:262.

236. Ascensao JL, Oken MM, Ewing SL, Goldberg RJ, Kaplan ME. Leukocytosis and large cell lung cancer. A frequent association. Cancer 1987; 60:903–905.

237. Adachi N, Yamaguchi K, Morikawa T, et al. Constitutive production of multiple colony-stimulating factors in patients with lung cancer associated with neutrophilia. Br J Cancer 1994; 69:125–129.

238. Boon ES, Vrij AA, Nieuwhof C, Vannoord JA, Zeppenfeldt E. Small cell lung cancer with paraneoplastic nephrotic syndrome. Eur Respir J 1994; 7:1192–1193.

239. Ponge T, Boutoille D, Moreau A, et al. Systemic vasculitis in a patient with small-cell neuroendocrine bronchial cancer. Eur Resp J 1998; 12:1228–1229.

Diagnostic procedures for obtaining tumour material
240. Oswald NC, Hinson KFW, Canti G, Miller AB. The diagnosis of primary lung cancer with special reference to sputum cytology. Thorax 1971; 26:623–631.

241. Tang CS, Tang CMC, Lau YY, Kung ITM. Sensitivity of sputum cytology after homogenization with dithiothreitol in lung cancer detection – two years of experience. Acta Cytol 1995; 39:1137–1140.

242. Evans DMD, Shelley G. Respiratory cytodiagnosis: study in observer variation and its relation to quality of material. Thorax 1982; 37:259–263.

243. Mennemeyer R, Hammar SP, Bauermeister DE, et al. Cytologic, histologic and electron microscopic correlations in poorly-differentiated primary lung carcinoma. Study of 43 cases. Acta Cytol 1979; 23:297–302.

244. Popovich J, Kvale PA, Eichenhorn MS, et al. Diagnostic accuracy of multiple biopsies from flexible fiberoptic bronchoscopy. A comparison of central versus peripheral carcinoma. Am Rev Respir Dis 1982; 125:521–523.

245. Thomas JSJ, Lamb D, Ashcroft T, et al. How reliable is the diagnosis of lung cancer using small biopsy specimens? Report of a UKCCCR lung cancer working party. Thorax 1993; 48:1135–1139.

246. Burnett RA, Howatson SR, Lang S, et al. Observer variability in histopathological reporting of non-small cell lung carcinoma on bronchial biopsy specimens. J Clin Pathol 1996; 49:130–133.

247. Edwards SL, Roberts C, McKean ME, et al. Preoperative histological classification of primary lung cancer: accuracy of diagnosis and use of the non-small cell category. J Clin Pathol 2000; 53:537–540.

248. Yoneda K, Boucher LD. Bronchial epithelial changes associated with small cell carcinoma of the lung. Hum Pathol 1993; 24:1180–1183.

249. Reichenberger F, Weber J, Tamm M, et al. The value of transbronchial needle aspiration in the diagnosis of peripheral pulmonary lesions. Chest 1999; 116:704–708.

250. Hermens FHW, VanEngelenburg TCA, Visser FJ, et al. Diagnostic yield of transbronchial histology needle aspiration in patients with mediastinal lymph node enlargement. Respiration 2003; 70:631–635.

251. Govert JA, Kopita JM, Matchar D, Kussin PS, Samuelson WM. Cost-effectiveness of collecting routine cytologic specimens during fiberoptic bronchoscopy for endoscopically visible lung tumor. Chest 1996; 109:451–456.

252. Sato M, Saito Y, Nagamoto N, et al. Diagnostic value of differential brushing of all branches of the bronchi in patients with sputum positive or suspected positive for lung cancer. Acta Cytol 1993; 37:879–883.

253. Pirozynski M. Bronchoalveolar lavage in the diagnosis of peripheral, primary lung cancer. Chest 1992; 102:372–374.

254. Bilaceroglu S, Cagirici U, Gunel O, Bayol U, Perim K. Comparison of rigid and flexible transbronchial needle aspiration in the staging of bronchogenic carcinoma. Respiration 1998; 65:441–449.

255. Chin R, McCain TW, Lucia MA, et al. Transbronchial needle aspiration in diagnosing and staging lung cancer – How many aspirates are needed? Am J Respir Crit Care Med 2002; 166:377–381.

Histological typing
256. Walter JB, Pryce DM. The frequency of differentiation in oat-cell carcinoma of the lung. J Pathol Bacteriol 1960; 80:121–125.

257. Yesner R. The dynamic histopathologic spectrum of lung cancer. Yale J Biol Med 1981; 54:447–456.

258. Roggli VL, Vollmer RT, Greenberg SD, et al. Lung cancer heterogeneity: a blinded and randomized study of 100 consecutive cases. Hum Pathol 1985; 16:569–579.

259. Bombi JA, Martinez A, Ramirez J, et al. Ultrastructural and molecular heterogeneity in non-small cell lung carcinomas: Study of 110 cases and review of the literature. Ultrastruct Pathol 2002; 26:211–218.

260. Gray SR, Hahn IS, Cornog JL. Short-term effect of radiation on human neoplasms. Arch Pathol 1974; 97:74–78.

261. Begin P, Sahai S, Wang N-S. Giant cell formation in small cell carcinoma of the lung. Cancer 1983; 52:1875–1879.

262. Willis RA. Pathology of Tumours. London: Butterworths; 1967.

263. Shields TW, Yee J, Conn JH. Relationship of cell type and lymph node metastasis to survival after resection of bronchial carcinoma. Am J Thorac Surg 1975; 20:501–510.

264. Petrovitch Z, Stanley K, Cox JD, Paig C. Radiotherapy in the management of locally advanced lung cancer of all cell types: final report of randomized trial. Cancer 1981; 48:1335–1340.

265. Mayer JE, Ewing SL, Ophoren TJ, Sumner HW, Humphrey EW. Influence of histological type on survival after curative resection for undifferentiated lung cancer. J Thorac Cardiovasc Surg 1982; 84:641–648.

266. Chuang MT, Marchevsky A, Teirstein A, Kirschner PA, Kleinerman J. Diagnosis of lung cancer by fibreoptic bronchoscopy: problems in the histological classification of non-small carcinomas. Thorax 1984; 39:175–178.

267. World Health Organization. Histological typing of lung and pleural tumors. Geneva, Switzerland: World Health Organization; 1999.

268. Horie A, Ohta M. Ultrastructural features of large cell carcinoma of the lung with reference to the prognosis of patients. Hum Pathol 1981; 12:423–432.

269. Albain KS, True LD, Golomb HM, Hoffman PC, Little AG. Large cell carcinoma of the lung. Ultrastructural differentiation and clinicopathologic correlations. Cancer 1985; 56:1618–1623.

270. Mooi WJ, Zandwijk N van, Dingemans KP, Koolen MGJ, Wagenvoort CA. The 'grey area' between small cell and non-small cell lung carcinomas: light and electron microscopy versus clinical data in 14 cases. J Pathol 1986; 149:49–54.

271. Johansson L. Histopathologic classification of lung cancer: Relevance of cytokeratin and TTF-1 immunophenotyping. Ann Diagn Pathol 2004; 8:259–267.

272. Yesner R, Gerstl B, Auerbach O. Application of the World Health Organization classification of lung carcinoma to biopsy material. Ann Thorac Surg 1965; 1:33–45.

273. Mountain CF, Carr DT, Anderson WAD. A system for the clinical staging of lung cancer. AJR 1974; 120:130–138.

274. Feinstein AR, Gelfman NA, Yesner RA. The diverse effects of histopathology on manifestations and outcome of lung cancer. Chest 1974; 66:225–229.

275. Matthews MJ, Gordon PR. Morphology of pulmonary and pleural malignancies. In: Strauss MJ, ed. Lung cancer: clinical diagnosis and treatment. New York, NY: Grune & Stratton; 1977:49–69.

276. Johnston WW. Histologic and cytologic patterns of lung cancer in 2,580 men and women over a 15-year period. Acta Cytol 1987; 32:163–168.

277. Edinburgh Lung Cancer Group. Patients presenting with lung cancer in South East Scotland. Thorax 1987; 42:853–857.

278. Auerbach O, Garfinkel L, Parks VR. Histologic type of lung cancer in relation to smoking habits, year of diagnosis and sites of metastases. Chest 1975; 67:382–387.

279. Kannerstein M, Churg J. Pathology of carcinoma of the lung associated with asbestos exposure. Cancer 1972; 30:14–21.

280. Huhti E, Sutinen S, Reinila A, Poukkula A, Saloheimo M. Lung cancer in a defined geographical area: history and histological types. Thorax 1980; 35:660–667.

281. Valaitis J, Warren S, Gamble D. Increasing incidence of adenocarcinoma of the lung. Cancer 1981; 47:1042–1046.

282. Barsky SH, Cameron R, Osann KE, Tomita D, Holmes EC. Rising incidence of bronchioloalveolar lung carcinoma and its unique clinicopathologic features. Cancer 1994; 73:1163–1170.

283. Zheng TZ, Holford TR, Boyle P, et al. Time trend and the age-period-cohort effect on the incidence of histologic types of lung cancer in Connecticut, 1960–1 989. Cancer 1994; 74:1556–1567.

284. Travis WD, Travis LB, Devesa SS. Lung cancer. Cancer 1995; 75:191–202.

285. Keehn R, Auerbach O, Nambu S, et al. Reproducibility of major diagnoses in a binational study of lung cancer in uranium miners and atomic bomb survivors. Am J Clin Pathol 1994; 101:478–482.

286. Sorensen JB, Hirsch FR, Gazdar A, Olsen JE. Interobserver variability in histopathologic subtyping and grading of pulmonary adenocarcinoma. Cancer 1993; 71:2971–2976.

287. Barbone F, Bovenzi M, Cavallieri F, Stanta G. Cigarette smoking and histologic type of lung cancer in men. Chest 1997; 112:1474–1479.

288. Stellman SD, Muscat JE, Thompson S, Hoffmann D, Wynder EL. Risk of squamous cell carcinoma and adenocarcinoma of the lung in relation to lifetime filter cigarette smoking. Cancer 1997; 80:382–388.

289. Coutts II, Gilson JC, Kerr IH, Parkes WR, Turner-Warwick M. Mortality in cases of asbestosis diagnosed by a pneumoconiosis medical panel. Thorax 1987; 42:111–116.

290. Caldwell CJ, Berry CL. Is the incidence of primary adenocarcinoma of the lung increasing? Virchows Arch 1996; 429:359–363.

291. Vincent RG, Pickren JW, Lane WW. The changing histopathology of lung cancer: a review of 1682 cases. Cancer 1977; 39:1647–1655.

292. Lam KY, Fu KH, Wong MP, Wang EP. Significant changes in the distribution of histologic types of lung cancer in Hong-Kong. Pathology 1993; 25:103–105.

293. Levi F, Franceschi S, LaVecchia C, Randimbison L, Te VC. Lung carcinoma trends by histologic type in Vaud and Neuchatel, Switzerland, 1974–1 994. Cancer 1997; 79:906–914.

Squamous cell carcinoma

294. Funai K, Yokose T, Ishii G, et al. Clinicopathologic characteristics of peripheral squamous cell carcinoma of the lung. Am J Surg Pathol 2003; 27:978–984.

295. Flanagan P, McCracken AW, Cross RMP. Squamous carcinoma of the lung with osteocartilaginous stroma. J Clin Pathol 1965; 18:403–407.

296. Nappi O, Swanson PE, Wick MR. Pseudovascular adenoid squamous cell carcinoma of the lung: clinicopathologic study of three cases and comparison with true pleuropulmonary angiosarcoma. Hum Pathol 1994; 25:373–378.

297. GarciaEscudero A, NavarroBustos G, JuradoEscamez P, RiosMartin J, GonzalezCampora R. Primary squamous cell carcinoma of the lung with pilomatricoma-like features. Histopathology 2002; 40:201–202.

298. Flieder DB, Koss MN, Nicholson A, et al. Solitary pulmonary papillomas in adults: A clinicopathologic and in situ hybridization study of 14 cases combined with 27 cases in the literature. Am J Surg Pathol 1998; 22:1328–1342.

299. Dulmet-Brender E, Jaubert F, Huchon G. Exophytic endobronchial epidermoid carcinoma. Cancer 1986; 57:1358–1364.

300. Katzenstein A-L, Prioleau PG, Askin FB. The histologic spectrum and significance of clear-cell change in lung carcinoma. Cancer 1980; 45: 943–947.

301. Churg A, Johnston WH, Stulbarg M. Small cell squamous and mixed small cell squamous-small cell anaplastic carcinomas of the lung. Am J Surg Pathol 1980; 4:255–263.

302. Brambilla E, Moro D, Veale D, et al. Basal cell (basaloid) carcinoma of the lung – a new morphologic and phenotypic entity with separate prognostic significance. Hum Pathol 1992; 23:993–1003.

303. Moro D, Brichon PY, Brambilla E, et al. Basaloid bronchial carcinoma – a histologic group with a poor prognosis. Cancer 1994; 73:2734–2739.

304. Kim DJ, Kim KD, Shin DH, Ro JY, Chung KY. Basaloid carcinoma of the lung: a really dismal histologic variant? Ann Thorac Surg 2003; 76:1833–1837.

305. Said JW, Nash G, Banks-Schlegel S, et al. Keratin in human lung tumors. Patterns of localization of different-molecular-weight keratin proteins. Am J Pathol 1983; 113:27–31.

306. Wilson TS, McDowell EM, McIntire R, Trump BF. Elaboration of human chorionic gonadotropin by lung tumors. Arch Pathol Lab Med 1981; 105:169–173.

307. Miyake M, Ito M, Mitsuoka A, et al. Alpha-fetoprotein and human chorionic gonadotropin-producing lung cancer. Cancer 1987; 59: 227–232.

308. Dirnhofer S, Freund M, Rogatsch H, Krabichler S, Berger P. Selective expression of trophoblastic hormones by lung carcinoma: Neuroendocrine tumors exclusively produce human chorionic gonadotropin alpha-subunit (HCG alpha). Hum Pathol 2000; 31:966–972.

309. Dingemans KP, Mooi WJ. Ultrastructure of squamous cell carcinoma of the lung. Pathol Annu 1984; 19:249–273.

310. Romagosa V, Bella MR, Truchero C, Moya J. Necrotizing sialometaplasia (adenometaplasia) of the trachea. Histopathology 1992; 21:280–282.

311. Littman CD. Necrotizing sialometaplasia (adenometaplasia) of the trachea. Histopathology 1993; 22:298–299.

312. Sturm N, Lantuejoul S, Laverriere MH, et al. Thyroid transcription factor 1 and cytokeratins 1, 5, 10, 14 (34 beta E12) expression in basaloid and large-cell neuroendocrine carcinomas of the lung. Hum Pathol 2001; 32:918–925.

Adenocarcinoma

313. Zang EA, Wynder EL. Cumulative tar exposure – a new index for estimating lung cancer risk among cigarette smokers. Cancer 1992; 70:69–76.

314. Bourke W, Milstein D, Giura R, et al. Lung cancer in young adults. Chest 1992; 102:1723–1729.

315. Kodama T, Shimosato Y, Kameya T. Histology and ultrastructure of bronchogenic and bronchial gland adenocarcinomas (including adenoid cystic and mucoepidermoid carcinomas) in relation to histogenesis. In: Shimosato Y, Melamed MR, Nettesheim P, eds. Morphogenesis of Lung Cancer. Boca Raton, FL: CRC Press; 1982:147–166.

316. Edwards CW. Pulmonary adenocarcinoma: review of 106 cases and proposed new classification. J Clin Pathol 1987; 40:125–135.

317. Harwood TR, Gracey DR, Yokoo H. Pseudomesotheliomatous carcinoma of the lung – a variant of peripheral lung cancer. Am J Clin Pathol 1976; 65:159–167.

318. Alvarez-Fernandez E. Alveolar trapping in pulmonary carcinomas. Diag Histopathol 1982; 5:59–64.

319. Silver SA, Askin FB. True papillary carcinoma of the lung: a distinct clinicopathologic entity. Am J Surg Pathol 1997; 21:43–51.

320. Amin MB, Tamboli P, Merchant SH, et al. Micropapillary component in lung adenocarcinoma – A distinctive histologic feature with possible prognostic significance. Am J Surg Pathol 2002; 26:358–364.

321. Miyoshi T, Satoh Y, Okumura S, et al. Early-stage lung adenocarcinomas with a micropapillary pattern, a distinct pathologic marker for a significantly poor prognosis. Am J Surg Pathol 2003; 27:101–109.

322. Roh MS, Lee JI, Choi PJ, Hong YS. Relationship between micropapillary component and micrometastasis in the regional lymph nodes of patients with stage I lung adenocarcinoma. Histopathology 2004; 45:580–586.

322a. Makimoto Y, Nabeshima K, Iwasaki H, et al. Micropapillary pattern: a distinct pathological marker to subclassify tumours with a significantly poor prognosis within small peripheral lung adenocarcinoma (≤20 mm) with mixed bronchioalveolar and invasive subtypes (Noguchi's type C tumours). Histopathology 2005; 46:677–684.

323. Herrera GA, Alexander B, DeMoraes HP. Ultrastructural subtypes of pulmonary adenocarcinoma. A correlation with patient survival. Chest 1983; 84:581–586.

324. Herrera GA, Turbat-Herrera EA, Alexander CB. Ultrastructural heterogeneity of pulmonary scar adenocarcinomas: correlation with patients' survival. Ultrastruct Pathol 1988; 12:265–277.

325. Nakajima T, Kodama T, Tsumuraya M, Shimosato Y, Kameya T. S-100 protein-positive Langerhans' cells in various human lung cancers especially in peripheral adenocarcinomas. Virchows Arch A Pathol Anat Histopathol 1985; 407:177–189.

326. Dammrich J, Buchwald J, Papadopoulos T, Muller-Hermelink HK. Special subtypes of pulmonary adenocarcinomas indicated by different tumor cell HLA-expression and stromal infiltrates – a light, electron microscopic and immunohistologic study. Virchows Arch B Cell Pathol 1991; 61:9–18.

327. Raab SS, Berg LC, Swanson PE, Wick MR. Adenocarcinoma in the lung in patients with breast cancer – a prospective analysis of the discriminatory value of immunohistology. Am J Clin Pathol 1993; 100:27–35.

328. Clover J, Oates J, Edwards C. Anti-cytokeratin 5/6: A positive marker for epithelioid mesothelioma. Histopathology 1997; 31:140–143.

329. Singh G, Katyal SL, Torikata C. Carcinoma of type II pneumocytes. Immunodiagnosis of a subtype of 'bronchioloalveolar carcinomas'. Am J Pathol 1981; 102:195–208.

330. Mizutani Y, Nakajima T, Morinaga S, et al. Immunohistochemical localization of pulmonary surfactant apoproteins in various lung tumours. Special reference to nonmucus-producing lung adenocarcinomas. Cancer 1988; 61:532–540.

331. Linnoila RI, Jensen SM, Steinberg SM, et al. Peripheral airway cell marker expression in non-small-cell lung carcinoma – association with distinct clinicopathologic features. Am J Clin Pathol 1992; 97:233–243.

332. Dairaku M, Sueishi K, Tanaka K, Horie A. Immunohistological analysis of surfactant-apoprotein in the bronchiolo-alveolar carcinoma. Virchows Arch B Cell Pathol 1983; 400:223–234.

333. Nicholson AG, McCormick CJ, Shimosato Y, Butcher DN, Sheppard MN. The value of PE-10, a monoclonal antibody against pulmonary surfactant, in distinguishing primary and metastatic lung tumours. Histopathology 1995; 27:57–60.

334. DiLoreto C, DiLauro V, Puglisi F, et al. Immunocytochemical expression of tissue specific transcription factor-1 in lung carcinoma. J Clin Pathol 1997; 50:30–32.

335. Tan DF, Li Q, Deeb G, et al. Thyroid transcription factor-1 expression prevalence and its clinical implications in non-small cell lung cancer: A high-throughput tissue microarray and immunohistochemistry study. Hum Pathol 2003; 34:597–604.

336. Skov BG, Sorensen JB, Hirsch FR, Larsson LI, Hansen HH. Prognostic impact of histologic demonstration of chromogranin A and neuron specific enolase in pulmonary adenocarcinoma. Ann Oncol 1991; 2:355–360.

337. Kimula Y. A histochemical and ultrastructural study of adenocarcinoma of the lung. Am J Surg Pathol 1978; 2:253–264.

338. Marcus PB, Martin JH, Green RH, Krouse MA. Glycocalyceal bodies and microvillous core rootlets, their value in tumour typing. Arch Pathol Lab Med 1979; 103:89–92.

339. Tsao MS, Fraser RS. Primary pulmonary adenocarcinoma with enteric differentiation. Cancer 1991; 68:1754–1757.

340. Weidner N. Intriguing case – pulmonary adenocarcinoma with intestinal-type differentiation. Ultrastruct Pathol 1992; 16:7–10.

341. Tsutahara S, Shijubo N, Hirasawa M, et al. Lung adenocarcinoma with type-II pneumocyte characteristics. Eur Respir J 1993; 6:135–137.

342. Ogata T, Endo K. Clara cell granules of peripheral lung cancers. Cancer 1984; 54:1635–1644.

343. Dekmezian R, Ordonez NG, Mackay B. Bronchioloalveolar adenocarcinoma with myoepithelial cells. Cancer 1991; 67:2356–2360.

344. Hiroshima K, Toyozaki T, Iyoda A, et al. Ultrastructural study of intranuclear inclusion bodies of pulmonary adenocarcinoma. Ultrastruct Pathol 1999; 23:383–389.

345. Tsumuraya M, Kodama T, Kameya T, et al. Light and electron microscopic analysis of intranuclear inclusions in papillary adenocarcinoma of the lung. Acta Cytol 1981; 25:523–532.

346. Edwards CW. Alveolar carcinoma: a review. Thorax 1984; 39:166–174.

347. Clayton F. The spectrum and significance of bronchioloalveolar carcinomas. Pathol Annu 1988; 23(Part 2):361–394.

347a. Travis WD, Garg K, Franklin WA, et al. Evolving concepts in the pathology and computed tomography imaging of lung adenocarcinoma and bronchioalveolar carcinoma. J Clin Oncol 2005; 23:3279–3287.

348. Manning JT, Spjut HJ, Tschen JA. Bronchioloalveolar carcinoma: the significance of two histopathologic types. Cancer 1984; 54:525–534.

349. Clayton F. Bronchioloalveolar carcinomas. Cell types, patterns of growth, and prognostic correlates. Cancer 1986; 57:1555–1564.

350. Albertine KH, Steiner RM, Radack DM, et al. Analysis of cell type and radiographic presentation as predictors of the clinical course of patients with bronchioloalveolar cell carcinoma. Chest 1998; 113:997–1006.

351. Goldstein NS, Thomas M. Mucinous and nonmucinous bronchioloalveolar adenocarcinomas have distinct staining patterns with thyroid transcription factor and cytokeratin 20 antibodies. Am J Clin Pathol 2001; 116:319–325.

352. Lau SK, Desrochers MJ, Luthringer DJ. Expression of thyroid transcription factor-1, cytokeratin 7, and cytokeratin 20 in bronchioloalveolar carcinomas: an immunohistochemical evaluation of 67 cases. Mod Pathol 2002; 15:538–542.

353. Simsir A, Wei XJ, Yee H, Moreira A, Cangiarella J. Differential expression of cytokeratins 7 and 20 and thyroid transcription factor-1 in bronchioloalveolar carcinoma – An immunohistochemical study in fine-needle aspiration biopsy specimens. Am J Clin Pathol 2004; 121:350–357.

354. Saad RS, Liu YL, Han H, Landreneau RJ, Silverman JF. Prognostic significance of thyroid transcription factor-1 expression in both early-stage conventional adenocarcinoma and bronchioloalveolar carcinoma of the lung. Hum Pathol 2004; 35:3–7.

355. Copin MC, Buisine MP, Leteurtre E, et al. Mucinous bronchioloalveolar carcinomas display a specific pattern of mucin gene expression among primary lung adenocarcinomas. Hum Pathol 2001; 32:274–281.

356. Nakano K, Iyama K, Mori T, et al. Loss of alveolar basement membrane type IV collagen alpha 3, alpha 4, and alpha 5 chains in bronchioloalveolar carcinoma of the lung. J Pathol 2001; 194:420–427.

357. Kumaki F, Matsui K, Kawai T, et al. Expression of matrix metalloproteinases in invasive pulmonary adenocarcinoma with bronchioloalveolar component and atypical adenomatous hyperplasia. Am J Pathol 2001; 159:2125–2135.

358. Ohori NP, Yousem SA, Griffin J, et al. Comparison of extracellular matrix antigens in subtypes of bronchioloalveolar carcinoma and conventional pulmonary adenocarcinoma – an immunohistochemical study. Am J Surg Pathol 1992; 16:675–686.

359. Noguchi M, Morikawa A, Kawasaki M, et al. Small adenocarcinoma of the lung: histologic characteristics and prognosis. Cancer 1995; 75:2844–2852.

360. Suzuki K, Yokose T, Yoshida J, et al. Prognostic significance of the size of central fibrosis in peripheral adenocarcinoma of the lung. Ann Thorac Surg 2000; 69:893–897.

361. Terasaki H, Niki T, Matsuno Y, et al. Lung adenocarcinoma with mixed bronchioloalveolar and invasive components – Clinicopathological features, subclassification by extent of invasive foci, and immunohistochemical characterization. Am J Surg Pathol 2003; 27:937–951.

362. Kodama T, Kameya T, Shimosato Y, et al. Cell incohesiveness and pattern of extension in a rare case of bronchioloalveolar carcinoma. Ultrastruct Pathol 1980; 1:177–188.

363. Barsky SH, Grossman DA, Ho J, Holmes EC. The multifocality of bronchioloalveolar lung carcinoma: evidence and implications of a multiclonal origin. Mod Pathol 1994; 7:633–640.

364. Holst VA, Finkelstein S, Yousem SA. Bronchioloalveolar adenocarcinoma of lung: Monoclonal origin for multifocal disease. Am J Surg Pathol 1998; 22:1343–1350.

365. Kodama T, Biyajima S, Watanabe S, Shimosato Y. Morphometric study of adenocarcinomas and hyperplastic epithelial lesions in the peripheral lung. Am J Clin Pathol 1986; 85:146–151.

366. Nakamura S, Koshikawa T, Sato T, Hayashi K, Suchi T. Extremely well-differentiated papillary adenocarcinoma of the lung with prominent cilia formation. Acta Pathol Jpn 1992; 42:745–750.

367. Hewer TF. The metastatic origin of alveolar cell tumour of the lung. J Pathol Bacteriol 1961; 81:323–330.

368. Rosenblatt MB, Lisa JR, Collier F. Primary and metastatic bronchiolo-alveolar carcinoma. Dis Chest 1967; 52:147–152.

369. Barbareschi M, Murer B, Colby TV, et al. CDX-2 homeobox gene expression is a reliable marker of colorectal adenocarcinoma metastases to the lungs. Am J Surg Pathol 2003; 27:141–149.

370. Rossi G, Murer B, Cavazza A, et al. Primary mucinous (so-called colloid) carcinomas of the lung – A clinicopathologic and immunohistochemical study with special reference to CDX-2 homeobox gene and MUC2 expression. Am J Surg Pathol 2004; 28:442–452.

371. Platt JA, Kraipowich N, Villafane F, DeMartini JC. Alveolar type II cells expressing jaagsiekte sheep retrovirus capsid protein and surfactant proteins are the predominant neoplastic cell type in ovine pulmonary adenocarcinoma. Vet Pathol 2002; 39:341–352.

372. Delas-Heras M, Barsky SH, Hasleton P, et al. Evidence for a protein related immunologically to the jaagsiekte sheep retrovirus in some human lung tumours. Eur Resp J 2000; 16:330–332.

373. Yousem SA, Finkelstein SD, Swalsky PA, Bakker A, Ohori NP. Absence of jaagsiekte sheep retrovirus DNA and RNA in bronchioloalveolar and conventional human pulmonary adenocarcinoma by PCR and RT-PCR analysis. Hum Pathol 2001; 32:1039–1042.

374. Moran CA, Hochholzer L, Fishback N, Travis WD. Koss MN. Mucinous (so-called colloid) carcinomas of lung. Mod Pathol 1992; 5:634–638.

375. Hayashi H, Kitamura H, Nakatani Y, Inayama Y, Ito T. Primary signet-ring cell carcinoma of the lung: Histochemical and immunohistochemical characterization. Hum Pathol 1999; 30:378–383.

376. Castro CY, Moran CA, Flieder DG, Suster S. Primary signet ring cell adenocarcinoma of the lung: a clinicopathological study of 15 cases. Histopathology 2001; 39:397–401.

377. Kragel PJ, Devaney KO, Meth BM, et al. Mucinous cystadenoma of the lung. A report of two cases with immunohistochemical and ultrastructural analysis. Arch Pathol Lab Med 1990; 114:1053–1056.

378. Roux FJ, Lantuejoul S, Brambilla E, Brambilla C. Mucinous cystadenoma of the lung. Cancer 1995; 76:1540–1544.

379. Graeme-Cook F, Mark EJ. Pulmonary mucinous cystic tumors of borderline malignancy. Hum Pathol 1991; 22:185–190.

380. Davison AM, Lowe JW, DaCosta P. Adenocarcinoma arising in a mucinous cystadenoma of the lung. Thorax 1992; 47:129–130.

381. Dixon AY, Moran JF, Wesselius LJ, McGregor DH. Pulmonary mucinous cystic tumor – case report with review of the literature. Am J Surg Pathol 1993; 17:722–728.

382. Gowar FJS. An unusual mucous cyst of the lung. Thorax 1978; 33:796–799.

383. Kradin RL, Young RH, Dickerson GR, Kirkham SE, Mark EJ. Pulmonary blastoma with argyrophil cells and lacking sarcomatous features (pulmonary endodermal tumour resembling fetal lung). Am J Surg Pathol 1982; 6:165–172.

384. Kodama T, Shimosato Y, Watanabe S, et al. Six cases of well-differentiated adenocarcinoma simulating fetal lung tubules in pseudoglandular stage: comparison with pulmonary blastoma. Am J Surg Pathol 1984; 8:735–744.

385. Nakatani Y, Dickersin GR, Mark EJ. Pulmonary endodermal tumor resembling fetal lung – a clinicopathologic study of five cases with immunohistochemical and ultrastructural characterization. Hum Pathol 1990; 21:1097–1107.

386. Mardini G, Pai U, Chavez AM, Tomashefski JF. Endobronchial adenocarcinoma with endometrioid features and prominent neuroendocrine differentiation – a variant of fetal adenocarcinoma. Cancer 1994; 73:1383–1389.

387. Nakatani Y, Kitamura H, Inayama Y, Ogawa N. Pulmonary endodermal tumor resembling fetal lung – the optically clear nucleus is rich in biotin. Am J Surg Pathol 1994; 18:637–642.

388. Koss MN, Hochholzer L, O'Leary T. Pulmonary blastomas. Cancer 1991; 67:2368–2381.

389. Nakatani Y, Kitamura H, Inayama Y, et al. Pulmonary adenocarcinomas of the fetal lung type: A clinicopathologic study indicating differences in histology, epidemiology, and natural history of low-grade and high-grade forms. Am J Surg Pathol 1998; 22:399–411.

390. Babycos PB, Daroca PJ. Polypoid pulmonary endodermal tumor resembling fetal lung: report of a case. Mod Pathol 1995; 8:303–306.

391. Yang P, Morizumi H, Sano T, et al. Pulmonary blastoma: an ultrastructural and immunohistochemical study with special reference to nuclear filament aggregation. Ultrastruct Pathol 1995; 19:501–509.

392. Sekine S, Shibata T, Matsuno Y, et al. β-catenin mutations in pulmonary blastomas: association with morule formation. J Pathol 2003; 200: 214–221.

393. Bakris GL, Mulopulos GP, Korchik R, et al. Pulmonary scar carcinoma. A clinicopathologic analysis. Cancer 1983; 52:493–497.

394. Suzuki A. Growth characteristics of peripheral type adenocarcinoma of the lung in terms of roentgenological findings. In: Shimosato Y, Melamed MR, Nettesheim P, eds. Morphogenesis of Lung Cancer. Boca Raton, FL: CRC Press; 1982:91–110.

395. Shimosato Y, Hashimoto T, Kodama T, et al. Prognostic implication of fibrotic focus (scar) in small peripheral lung cancers. Am J Surg Pathol 1980; 4:365–373.

396. Barsky SH, Huang SJ, Bhuta S. The extracellular matrix of pulmonary scar carcinomas is suggestive of a desmoplastic origin. Am J Pathol 1986; 124:412–419.

397. Madri JA, Carter D. Scar cancers of the lung: origin and significance. Hum Pathol 1984; 15:625–631.

398. Kung ITM, Lui IOI, Loke SL, et al. Pulmonary scar cancer. A pathologic reappraisal. Am J Surg Pathol 1985; 9:391–400.

399. Kolin A, Koutoulakis A. Role of arterial occlusion in pulmonary scar cancers. Hum Pathol 1988; 19:1161–1167.

400. Goldstein NS, Mani A, Chmielewski G, Welsh R, Pursel S. Prognostic factors in T1 N0 M0 adenocarcinomas and bronchioloalveolar carcinomas of the lung. Am J Clin Pathol 1999; 112:391–402.

Small cell carcinoma

401. Souhami RL, Law K. Longevity in small cell lung cancer – A report to the Lung Cancer Subcommittee of the United Kingdom Coordinating Committee for Cancer Research. Br J Cancer 1990; 61:584–589.

402. Shore DF, Paneth M. Survival after resection of small cell carcinoma of the bronchus. Thorax 1980; 35:819–822.

403. Prasad US, Naylor AR, Walker WS, et al. Long term survival after pulmonary resection for small cell carcinoma of the lung. Thorax 1989; 44:784–787.

404. Smit EF, Groen HJM, Timens W, Deboer WJ, Postmus PE. Surgical resection for small cell carcinoma of the lung – a retrospective study. Thorax 1994; 49:20–22.

405. World Health Organization. Histological Typing of Lung Tumours. Geneva, Switzerland: World Health Organization; 1981.

406. Hirsch FR, Osterlind K, Hansen HH. The prognostic significance of histopathologic subtyping of small cell carcinoma of the lung according to the classification of the World Health Organization. A study of 375 consecutive patients. Cancer 1983; 52:2144–2150.

407. Choi H, Byhardt RW, Clowry LJ, et al. The prognostic significance of histologic subtyping in small cell carcinoma of the lung. Am J Clin Oncol 1984; 7:389–397.

408. Bepler G, Neumann K, Holle R, Havemann K, Kalbfleisch H. Clinical relevance of histologic subtyping in small cell lung cancer. Cancer 1989; 64:74–79.

409. Ewing SL, Sumner HW, Ophoven JJ, Mayer JE, Humphrey EW. Small cell anaplastic carcinoma with differentiation: a report of 14 cases. Lab Invest 1980; 42:115.

410. Nicholson SA, Beasley MB, Brambilla E, et al. Small cell lung carcinoma (SCLC) – A clinicopathologic study of 100 cases with surgical specimens. Am J Surg Pathol 2002; 26:1184–1197.

411. Hirsch FR, Matthews MJ, Aisner S, et al. Histopathologic classification of small cell lung cancer. Changing concepts and terminology. Cancer 1988; 62:973–977.

412. Azzopardi JG. Oat-cell carcinoma of the bronchus. J Pathol Bacteriol 1959; 78:513–519.

413. Carter D. Small-cell carcinoma of the lung. Am J Surg Pathol 1983; 7:787–795.

414. Sturgis CD, Nassar DL. DAntonio JA, Raab SS. Cytologic features useful for distinguishing small cell from non-small cell carcinoma in bronchial brush and wash specimens. Am J Clin Pathol 2000; 114:197–202.

415. Vollmer RT. The effect of cell size on the pathologic diagnosis of small and large cell carcinoma of the lung. Cancer 1982; 50:1380–1383.

416. Marchevsky AM, Gal AA, Shah S, Koss MN. Morphometry confirms the presence of considerable nuclear size overlap between 'small cells' and 'large cells' in high-grade pulmonary neuroendocrine neoplasms. Am J Clin Pathol 2001; 116:466–472.

417. Brambilla E, Moro D, Gazzeri S, et al. Cytotoxic chemotherapy induces cell differentiation in small-cell lung carcinoma. J Clin Oncol 1991; 9:50–61.

418. Yesner R. Small cell tumors of the lung. Am J Surg Pathol 1983; 8:775–785.

419. Vollmer RT, Ogden L, Crissman JD. Separation of small-cell from non-small-cell lung cancer. Arch Pathol Lab Med 1984; 108:792–794.

420. Maloney DJL, Morritt GN, Walbaum PR, Lamb D. Histological features of small-cell carcinomas and survival after surgical resection. Thorax 1983; 38:715.

421. Mooi WJ, Dingemans KP, Zandwijk N van. Prevalence of neuroendocrine granules in small cell lung carcinomas: usefulness of electron microscopy in lung cancer classification. J Pathol 1986; 149:41–47.

422. Thunnissen FBJM, Diegenbach PC, Vanhattum AH, et al. Further evaluation of quantitative nuclear image features for classification of lung carcinomas. Pathol Res Pr 1992; 188:531–535.

423. Bensch KG, Corrin B, Pariente R, Spencer H. Oat cell carcinoma of the lung: its origin and relationship to bronchial carcinoid. Cancer 1968; 22:1163–1172.

424. Hattori S, Matsuda M, Tateishi R, Tatsumi N, Terazawa T. Oat-cell carcinoma of the lung containing serotonin granules. Gann 1968; 59:123–129.

425. McDowell EM, Trump BF. Pulmonary small cell carcinoma showing tripartite differentiation in individual cells. Hum Pathol 1981; 12:286–294.

426. Leong AS-Y, Canny AR. Small cell anaplastic carcinoma of the lung with glandular and squamous differentiation. Am J Surg Pathol 1981; 5:307–309.

427. Saba SR, Azar HA, Richman AV, et al. Dual differentiation in small cell carcinoma (oat cell carcinoma) of the lung. Ultrastruct Pathol 1981; 2:131–138.

428. Bolen JW, Thorning D. Histogenetic classification of lung carcinomas. Small cell carcinomas studied by light and electron microscopy. J Submicrosc Cytol Pathol 1982; 149:499–514.

429. Jiminez C, Dardick I, McCaughey WTE, et al. Practical value of electron microscopy diagnoses in biopsies of lung carcinoma patients. Lab Invest 1982; 46:41A–42A.

430. Neal MH, Kosinski R, Cohen P, Ohrenstein JM. Atypical endocrine tumours of the lung. A clinicopathologic study of 19 cases. Hum Pathol 1986; 17:1264–1277.

431. Broers JLV, Ramaekers FCS, Klein Rot M, et al. Cytokeratin in different types of human lung cancer as monitored by chain-specific monoclonal antibodies. Cancer Res 1988; 48:3221–3229.

432. Moss F, Bobrow LG, Sheppard MN, et al. Expression of epithelial and neural antigens in small cell and non small cell lung carcinoma. J Pathol 1986; 149:103–111.

433. Gosney JR, Gosney MA, Lye M, Butt SA. Reliability of commercially available immunocytochemical markers for identification of neuroendocrine differentiation in bronchoscopic biopsies of bronchial carcinoma. Thorax 1995; 50:116–120.

434. Lyda MH, Weiss LM. Immunoreactivity for epithelial and neuroendocrine antibodies are useful in the differential diagnosis of lung carcinomas. Hum Pathol 2000; 31:980–987.

435. Wong KF, Chan JK, Ng CS, et al. CD56 (NKH1)-positive hematolymphoid malignancies: an aggressive neoplasm featuring frequent cutaneous/mucosal involvement, cytoplasmic azurophilic granules, and angiocentricity. Hum Pathol 1992; 23:798–804.

436. Lantuejoul S, Laverriere MH, Sturm N, et al. NCAM (neural cell adhesion molecules) expression in malignant mesotheliomas. Hum Pathol 2001; 31:415–421.

437. Hamid Q, Corrin B, Sheppard MN, Huttner WB, Polak JM. Expression of chromogranin A mRNA in small cell carcinoma of the lung. J Pathol 1991; 163:293–297.

438. Patriarca C, Pruneri G, Alfano RM, et al. Polysialylated N-CAM, chromogranin A and B, and secretogranin II in neuroendocrine tumours of the lung. Virchows Arch 1997; 430:455–460.

439. Lantuejoul S, Moro D, Michalides RJAM, Brambilla C, Brambilla E. Neural cell adhesion molecules (NCAM) and NCAM-PSA expression in neuroendocrine lung tumors. Am J Surg Pathol 1998; 22:1267–1276.

440. Lauweryns JM, Ranst L Van. Leu-7 immunoreactivity in human, monkey, and pig bronchopulmonary neuroepithelial bodies and neuroendocrine cells. J Histochem Cytochem 1987; 35:687–691.

441. Ariza A, Mate JL, Isamat M, et al. Standard and variant CD44 isoforms are commonly expressed in lung cancer of the non-small cell type but not of the small cell type. J Pathol 1995; 177:363–368.

Large cell carcinoma

442. Downey RS, Sewell CW, Mansour KA. Large cell carcinoma of the lung: a highly aggressive tumor with dismal prognosis. Ann Thorac Surg 1989; 47:806–808.

443. Rossi G, Marchioni A, Milani M, et al. TTF-1, cytokeratin 7, 34betaE12, and CD56/NCAM immunostaining in the subclassification of large cell carcinomas of the lung. Am J Clin Pathol 2004; 122:884–893.

444. Churg A. The fine structure of large cell undifferentiated carcinoma of the lung. Evidence for its relation to squamous cell carcinomas and adenocarcinomas. Hum Pathol 1978; 9:143–156.

445. Carter N, Nelson F, Gosney JR. Ultrastructural heterogeneity in undifferentiated bronchial carcinoma. J Pathol 1993; 171:53–57.

446. Edwards C, Carlile A. Clear cell carcinoma of the lung. J Clin Pathol 1985; 38:880–885.

447. Morgan A, MacKenzie D. Clear cell carcinoma of the lung. J Pathol Bacteriol 1964; 87:25–29.

448. McNamee CJ, Simpson RHW, Pagliero KM, Meyns B, Hamilton-Wood C. Primary clear-cell carcinoma of the lung. Respir Med 1993; 87:471–473.

449. Hamid QA, Corrin B, Dewar A, Hoefler H, Sheppard MN. Expression of gastrin-releasing peptide (human bombesin) gene in large cell undifferentiated carcinoma of the lung. J Pathol 1990; 161:145–151.

450. Travis WD, Linnoila RI, Tsokos MG, et al. Neuroendocrine tumors of the lung with proposed criteria for large-cell neuroendocrine carcinoma – an ultrastructural, immunohistochemical, and flow cytometric study of 35 cases. Am J Surg Pathol 1991; 15:529–553.

451. Brambilla E, Veale D, Moro D, et al. Neuroendocrine phenotype in lung cancers – comparison of immunohistochemistry with biochemical determination of enolase isoenzymes. Am J Clin Pathol 1992; 98:88–97.

452. Jiang SX, Kameya T, Shoji M, et al. Large cell neuroendocrine carcinoma of the lung: A histologic and immunohistochemical study of 22 cases. Am J Surg Pathol 1998; 22:526–537.

453. Mooi WJ, Dewar A, Springall DR, Polak JM, Addis BJ. Non-small cell lung carcinomas with neuroendocrine features. A light microscopic, immunohistochemical and ultrastructural study of 11 cases. Histopathology 1988; 13:329–337.

454. Hammond ME, Sause WT. Large cell neuroendocrine tumors of the lung. Cancer 1985; 56:1624–1629.

455. Linnoila RI, Mulshine JL, Steinberg SM, et al. Neuroendocrine differentiation in endocrine and nonendocrine lung carcinoma. Am J Clin Pathol 1988; 90:641–652.

456. Wick MR, Berg LC, Hertz MI. Large cell carcinoma of the lung with neuroendocrine differentiation – a comparison with large cell undifferentiated pulmonary tumors. Am J Clin Pathol 1992; 97:796–805.

457. Travis WD, Gal AA, Colby TV, et al. Reproducibility of neuroendocrine lung tumor classification. Hum Pathol 1998; 29:272–279.

458. Graziano SL, Mazid R, Newman N, et al. The use of neuroendocrine immunoperoxidase markers to predict chemotherapy response in patients with non-small-cell lung cancer. J Clin Oncol 1989; 7:1398–1406.

459. Moertel CG, Kvols LK, O'Connell MJ, Rubin J. Treatment of neuroendocrine carcinomas with combined etoposide and cisplatin – evidence of major therapeutic activity in the anaplastic variants of these neoplasms. Cancer 1991; 68:227–232.

460. Souquet PJ, Chauvin F, Boissel JP, et al. Polychemotherapy in advanced non-small-cell lung cancer – a meta-analysis. Lancet 1993; 342:19–21.

461. Ruckdeschel J, Linnoila RI, Mulshine JL, et al. The impact of neuroendocrine and epithelial differentiation on recurrence and survival in patients with lung cancer. Lung Cancer 1991; 7(Suppl):56.

462. Schleusener JT, Tazelaar HD, Jung SH, et al. Neuroendocrine differentiation is an independent prognostic factor in chemotherapy-treated nonsmall cell lung carcinoma. Cancer 1996; 77:1284–1291.

463. Warren WH, Faber LP, Gould VE. Neuroendocrine neoplasms of the lung. A clinicopathologic update. J Thorac Cardiovasc Surg 1989; 98:321–332.

464. Berendsen HH, Leij L De, Poppema S, et al. Clinical characterization of non-small-cell lung cancer tumors showing neuroendocrine differentiation features. J Clin Oncol 1989; 7:1614–1620.

465. Kibbelaar RE, Moolenaar KEC, Michalides RJAM, et al. Neural cell adhesion molecule expression, neuroendocrine differentiation and prognosis in lung carcinoma. Eur J Cancer 1991; 27:431–435.

466. Pujol JL, Simony J, Demoly P, et al. Neural cell adhesion molecule and prognosis of surgically resected lung cancer. Am Rev Respir Dis 1993; 148:1071–1075.

467. Sunday ME, Choi N, Spindel ER, Chin WW, Mark EJ. Gastrin-releasing peptide gene expression in small cell and large cell undifferentiated lung carcinomas. Hum Pathol 1991; 22:1030–1039.

468. Sundaresan V, Reeve JG, Stenning S, Stewart S, Bleehen NM. Neuroendocrine differentiation and clinical behaviour in non-small cell lung tumours. Br J Cancer 1991; 64:333–338.

469. Graziano SL, Tatum AT, Newman NB, et al. The prognostic significance of neuroendocrine markers and carcinoembryonic antigen in patients with resected stage I and II non-small cell lung cancer. Cancer Res 1994; 54:2908–2913.

470. Abbona G, Papotti M, Viberti L, et al. Chromogranin A gene expression in non-small cell lung carcinomas. J Pathol 1998; 186:151–156.

470a. Howe MC, Chapman A, Kerr K, et al. Neuroendocrine differentiation in non-small cell lung cancer and its relation to prognosis and therapy. Histopathology 2005; 46:195–201.

471. Carles J, Rosell R, Ariza A, et al. Neuroendocrine differentiation as a prognostic factor in non-small cell lung cancer. Lung Cancer 1993; 10:209–219.

472. Brambilla E. Basaloid carcinoma of the lung. In: Corrin B, ed. Pathology of Lung Tumors. Edinburgh, UK: Churchill Livingstone; 1997:71–82.

473. Kim DJ, Kim KD, Shin DH, et al. Basaloid carcinoma of the lung: a really dismal histologic variant? Ann Thorac Surg 2003; 76:1833–1837.

474. Foroulis CN, Iliadis KH, Mauroudis PM, Kosmidis PA. Basaloid carcinoma, a rare primary lung neoplasm: report of a case and review of the literature. Lung Cancer 2002; 35:335–338.

475. Lin O, Harkin TJ, Jagirdar J. Basaloid-squamous cell carcinoma of the bronchus: report of a case with review of the literature. Arch Pathol Lab Med 1995; 119:1167–1170.

476. Begin LR, Eskandari J, Joncas J, Panasci L. Epstein–Barr virus related lymphoepithelioma-like carcinoma of lung. J Surg Oncol 1987; 36: 280–283.

477. Wong MP, Chung LP, Yuen ST, et al. In situ detection of Epstein-Barr virus in non-small cell lung carcinomas. J Pathol 1995; 177:233–240.

478. Chen FF, Yan JJ, Lai WW, Jin YT, Su IJ. Epstein-Barr virus-associated nonsmall cell lung carcinoma: Undifferentiated 'lymphoepithelioma-like' carcinoma as a distinct entity with better prognosis. Cancer 1998; 82:2334–2342.

479. Han AJ, Xiong M, Gu YY, Lin SX, Xiong M. Lymphoepithelioma-like carcinoma of the lung with a better prognosis. A clinicopathologic study of 32 cases. Am J Clin Pathol 2001; 115:841–850.

480. Chang YL, Wu CT, Shih JY, Lee YC. New aspects in clinicopathologic and oncogene studies of 23 pulmonary lymphoepithelioma-like carcinomas. Am J Surg Pathol 2002; 26:715–723.

481. Wockel W, Hofler G, Popper HH, Morresi A. Lymphoepithelioma-like carcinoma of the lung. Pathol Res Pr 1995; 191:1170–1174.

482. Morbini P, Riboni R, Tomaselli S, Rossi A, Magrini U. EBER- and LMP-1-expressing pulmonary lymphoepithelioma-like carcinoma in a Caucasian patient. Hum Pathol 2003; 34:623–625.

483. Chan ATC, Teo PML, Lam KC, et al. Multimodality treatment of primary lymphoepithelioma-like carcinoma of the lung. Cancer 1998; 83:925–929.

484. Cavazza A, Colby TV, Tsokos M, Rush W, Travis WD. Lung tumors with a rhabdoid phenotype. Am J Clin Pathol 1996; 105:182–188.

485. Rubenchik I, Dardick I, Auger M. Cytopathology and ultrastructure of primary rhabdoid tumor of lung. Ultrastruct Pathol 1996; 20:355–360.

486. Itakura E, Tamiya S, Morita K, et al. Subcellular distribution of cytokeratin and vimentin in malignant rhabdoid tumor: Three-dimensional imaging with confocal laser scanning microscopy and double immunofluorescence. Mod Pathol 2001; 14:854–861.

487. Chetty R. Combined large cell neuroendocrine, small cell and squamous carcinomas of the lung with rhabdoid cells. Pathology 2000; 32:209–212.

488. Miyagi J, Tsuhako K, Kinjo T, et al. Rhabdoid tumour of the lung is a dedifferentiated phenotype of pulmonary adenocarcinoma. Histopathology 2000; 37:37–44.

489. Tamboli P, Toprani TH, Amin MB, et al. Carcinoma of lung with rhabdoid features. Hum Pathol 2004; 35:8–13.

490. Shimazaki H, Aida S, Sato M, et al. Lung carcinoma with rhabdoid cells: a clinicopathological study and survival analysis of 14 cases. Histopathology 2001; 38:425–434.

Adenosquamous carcinoma

491. Fitzgibbons PL, Kern WH. Adenosquamous carcinoma of the lung: a clinical and pathological study of seven cases. Hum Pathol 1985; 16:463–466.

492. Naunheim KS, Taylor JR, Skosey C, et al. Adenosquamous lung carcinoma: clinical characteristics, treatment, and prognosis. Ann Thorac Surg 1987; 44:462–466.

493. Takamori S, Noguchi M, Morinaga S, et al. Clinicopathologic characteristics of adenosquamous carcinoma of the lung. Cancer 1991; 67:649–654.

494. Shimizu J, Oda M, Hayashi Y, Nonomura A, Watanabe Y. A clinicopathological study of resected cases of adenosquamous carcinoma of the lung. Chest 1996; 109:989–994.

495. Sridhar KS, Bounassi MJ, Raub W, Richman SP. Clinical features of adenosquamous lung carcinoma in 127 patients. Am Rev Respir Dis 1990; 142:19–23.

Sarcomatoid carcinoma

496. Battifora H. Spindle cell carcinoma. Ultrastructural evidence of squamous origin and collagen production by tumor cells. Cancer 1976; 37:2275–2282.

497. Addis BJ, Corrin B. Pulmonary blastoma, carcinosarcoma and spindle cell carcinoma: an immunohistochemical study of keratin intermediate filaments. J Pathol 1985; 147:291–301.

498. Humphrey PA, Scroggs MW, Roggli VL, Shelburne JD. Pulmonary carcinomas with a sarcomatoid element: an immunocytochemical and ultrastructural analysis. Hum Pathol 1988; 19:155–165.

499. Lucas DR, Pass HI, Madan SK, et al. Sarcomatoid mesothelioma and its histological mimics: a comparative immunohistochemical study. Histopathology 2003; 42:270–279.

500. Holst VA, Finkelstein S, Colby TV, Myers JL, Yousem SA. p53 and K-ras mutational genotyping in pulmonary carcinosarcoma, spindle cell carcinoma, and pulmonary blastoma: Implications for histogenesis. Am J Surg Pathol 1997; 21:801–811.

501. Dacic S, Finkelstein SD, Sasatomi E, Swalsky PA, Yousem SA. Molecular pathogenesis of pulmonary carcinosarcoma as determined by microdissection-based allelotyping. Am J Surg Pathol 2002; 26:510–516.

502. Fishback NF, Travis WD, Moran CA, Guinee DG, McCarthy WF. Koss MN. Pleomorphic (spindle/giant cell) carcinoma of the lung – a clinicopathologic correlation of 78 cases. Cancer 1994; 73:2936–2945.

503. Rossi G, Cavazza A, Sturm N, et al. Pulmonary carcinomas with pleomorphic, sarcomatoid, or sarcomatous elements – A clinicopathologic and immunohistochemical study of 75 cases. Am J Surg Pathol 2003; 27:311–324.

504. Nappi O, Glasner SD, Swanson PE, Wick MR. Biphasic and monophasic sarcomatoid carcinomas of the lung – a reappraisal of 'carcinosarcomas' and 'spindle-cell carcinomas'. Am J Clin Pathol 1994; 102:331–340.

505. Wick MR, Ritter JH, Humphrey PA. Sarcomatoid carcinomas of the lung: A clinicopathologic review. Am J Clin Pathol 1997; 108:40–53.

506. Pelosi G, Fraggetta F, Nappi O, et al. Pleomorphic carcinomas of the lung show a selective distribution of gene products involved in cell differentiation, cell cycle control, tumor growth, and tumor cell motility – A clinicopothologic and immunohistochemical study of 31 cases. Am J Surg Pathol 2003; 27:1203–1215.

507. Ro JY, Chen JL, Lee JS, et al. Sarcomatoid carcinoma of the lung – immunohistochemical and ultrastructural studies of 14 cases. Cancer 1992; 69:376–386.

508. Nash AD, Stout AP. Giant cell carcinoma of the lung. Report of 5 cases. Cancer 1958; 11:369–376.

509. Wang N-S, Seemayer TA, Ahmed MN, Knaack J. Giant cell carcinoma of the lung. A light and electron microscopic study. Hum Pathol 1976; 7:3–16.

510. Addis BJ, Dewar A, Thurlow NP. Giant cell carcinoma of the lung – immunohistochemical and ultrastructural evidence of dedifferentiation. J Pathol 1988; 155:231–240.

511. Kika 1908 cited by Herxheimer G. Reinke G. Carcinoma sarcomatodes (Pathologie des Krebses). Ergeb Allg Path Pathol Anatom 1912; 16:280–282.

512. Thompson L, Chang B, Barsky SH. Monoclonal origins of malignant mixed tumors (carcinosarcomas): evidence for a divergent histogenesis. Am J Surg Pathol 1996; 20:277–285.

513. Stewart HL, Grady HG, Andervont HB. Development of sarcoma at site of serial transplantation of pulmonary tumours in inbred mice. J Natl Cancer Inst 1947; 7:207–225.

514. Davis MP, Eagen RT, Weiland LH, Pairolero PC. Carcinosarcoma of the lung: Mayo Clinic experience and response to chemotherapy. Mayo Clin Proc 1984; 59:598–603.

515. Cabarcos A, Dorrojnsoro MG, Beristain JLL. Pulmonary carcinosarcoma: a case study and review of the literature. Br J Dis Chest 1985; 79:83–94.

516. Koss MN, Hochholzer L, Frommelt RA. Carcinosarcomas of the lung – A clinicopathologic study of 66 patients. Am J Surg Pathol 1999; 23:1514–1526.

517. Cohen-Salmon D, Michel RP, Wang N-S, Eddy D, Hanson R. Pulmonary carcinosarcoma and carcinoma: report of a case studied by electron microscopy, with critical review of the literature. Ann Pathol 1985; 5:115–124.

518. Rainosek DE, Ro JY, Ordonez NG, Kulaga AD, Ayala AG. Sarcomatoid carcinoma of the lung: a case with atypical carcinoid and rhabdomyosarcomatous components. Am J Clin Pathol 1994; 102: 360–364.

519. Mayall FG, Gibbs AR. Pleural and pulmonary carcinosarcomas. J Pathol 1992; 167:305–311.

520. Huszar M, Herczog E, Lieberman Y, Geiger B. Distinctive immunofluorescent labeling of epithelial and mesenchymal elements of carcinosarcoma with antibodies specific for different intermediate filaments. Hum Pathol 1984; 15:532–538.

521. Gatter KC, Dunnill MS, Muijan GNP van, Mason DY. Human lung tumours may coexpress different classes of intermediate filaments. J Clin Pathol 1986; 39:950–954.

522. Cupples J, Wright J. An immunohistological comparison of primary lung carcinosarcoma and sarcoma. Pathol Res Pr 1990; 186:326–329.

523. Stackhouse EM, Harrison EG, Ellis FH. Primary mixed malignancies of lung: carcinosarcoma and blastoma. J Thorac Cardiovasc Surg 1969; 57:385–399.

524. Spencer H. Pulmonary blastomas. J Pathol Bacteriol 1961; 82:161–165.

525. Barrett NK, Barnard WG. Some unusual thoracic tumours. Br J Surg 1945; 32:447–457.

526. Barnard WG. Embryoma of lung. Thorax 1952; 7:299–301.

527. Roth JA, Elguezabal A. Pulmonary blastoma evolving into carcinosarcoma. Am J Surg Pathol 1978; 2:407–413.

528. Edwards CW, Saunders AM, Collins F. Mixed malignant tumour of the lung. Thorax 1979; 34:629–639.

529. Olenick SJ, Fan CC, Ryoo JW. Mixed pulmonary blastoma and carcinosarcoma. Histopathology 1994; 25:171–174.

530. Francis D, Jacobsen M. Pulmonary blastoma. In: Muller K-M, ed. Pulmonary Diseases – Clinicopathological Correlations Current Topics in Pathology No 73. Berlin: Springer; 1983:265–294.

531. Yousem SA, Wick MR, Randhawa P, Manivel JC. Pulmonary blastoma. An immunohistochemical analysis with comparison with fetal lung in its pseudoglandular stage. Am J Clin Pathol 1990; 93:167–175.

532. Inoue H, Kasai K, Shinada J, Yoshimura H, Kameya T. Pulmonary blastoma – comparison between its epithelial components and fetal bronchial epithelium. Acta Pathol Jpn 1992; 42:884–892.

533. Heckman CJ, Truang LD, Cagle PT, Font RL. Pulmonary blastoma with rhabdomyosarcomatous differentiation: an electron microscopic and immunohistochemical study. Am J Surg Pathol 1988; 12:35–40.

534. Cohen RE, Weaver MG, Montenegro HD, Abdul-Karim FW. Pulmonary blastoma with malignant melanoma component. Arch Pathol Lab Med 1990; 114:1076–1078.

535. Scully RE, Mark EJ, McNeely BU. Case records of the Massachusetts General Hospital: case 3 – 1984, pulmonary blastoma with major component of small cell carcinoma. N Engl J Med 1984; 310:178–187.

536. Siegel RJ, Bueso-Ramos C, Cohen C, et al. Pulmonary blastoma with germ cell (yolk sac) differentiation: report of two cases. Mod Pathol 1992; 4:566–570.

537. Jackson MD, Albrecht R, Roggli VL, Shelbourne JD. Pulmonary blastoma: an ultrastructural and histochemical study. Ultrastruct Pathol 1984; 7:259–268.

538. Tamai S, Kameya T, Shimosato Y, Tsumuraya M, Wada T. Pulmonary blastoma: an ultrastructural study of a case and its transplanted tumour in athymic nude mice. Cancer 1980; 46:1389–1396.

539. Berean K, Truong LD, Dudley AW, Cagle PT. Immunohistochemical characteristics of pulmonary blastoma. Am J Clin Pathol 1988; 89:773–777.

540. Garcia-Escudero A, Gonzalez-Campora R, Villar-Rodriguez JL, Lag-Asturiano E. Thyroid transcription factor-1 expression in pulmonary blastoma. Histopathology 2004; 44:507–508.

Prognostic factors

541. Buccheri G, Ferrigno D. Prognostic factors in lung cancer – tables and comments. Eur Respir J 1994; 7:1350–1364.

542. Greenberg SD, Fraire AE, Kinner BM, Johnson EH. Tumor cell type versus staging in the prognosis of carcinoma of the lung. Pathol Annu 1987; 2:387–405.

543. Wetzels RH, Velden LA van der, Schaafsma HE, et al. Immunohistochemical localization of basement membrane type VII collagen and laminin in neoplasms of the head and neck. Histopathology 1992; 21:459–464.

544. Kerr KM, Lamb D, Wathen CG, Walker WS, Douglas NJ. Pathological assessment of mediastinal lymph nodes in lung cancer – implications for non-invasive mediastinal staging. Thorax 1992; 47:337–341.

545. Prenzel KL, Monig SP, Sinning JM, et al. Lymph node size and metastatic infiltration in non-small cell lung cancer. Chest 2003; 123:463–467.

546. Passlick B, Izbicki JR, Kubuschak B, et al. Immunohistochemical assessment of individual tumour cells in lymph nodes of patients with non-small-cell lung cancer. J Clin Oncol 1994; 12:1827–1832.

547. Passlick B, Izbicki JR, Kubuschok B, Thetter O, Pantel K. Detection of disseminated lung cancer cells in lymph nodes: impact on staging and prognosis. Ann Thorac Surg 1996; 61:177–183.

548. Salerno CT, Frizelle S, Niehans GA, et al. Detection of occult micrometastases in non-small cell lung carcinoma by reverse transcriptase-polymerase chain reaction. Chest 1998; 113:1526–1532.

549. Nicholson AG, Graham ANJ, Pezzella F, et al. Does the use of immunohistochemistry to identify micrometastases provide useful information in the staging of node-negative non-small cell lung carcinomas? Lung Cancer 1997; 18:231–240.

550. Goldstein NS, Mani A, Chmielewski G, Welsh R, Pursel S. Immunohistochemically detected micrometastases in peribronchial and mediastinal lymph nodes from patients with T1, N0, M0 pulmonary adenocarcinomas. Am J Surg Pathol 2000; 24:274–279.

551. Kitaichi M, Asamoto H, Izumi T, Furuta M. Histological classification of regional lymph nodes in relation to postoperative survival in primary lung cancer. Hum Pathol 1981; 12:1000–1005.

552. Fernando HC, Goldstraw P. The accuracy of clinical evaluative intrathoracic staging in lung cancer as assessed by postsurgical pathologic staging. Cancer 1990; 65:2503–2506.

553. Nash G, Hutter RVP, Henson DE. Practice protocol for the examination of specimens from patients with lung cancer. Arch Pathol Lab Med 1995; 119:695–700.

554. Mountain CF. Revisions in the International System for Staging Lung Cancer. Chest 1997; 111:1710–1717.

555. Mountain CF. A new international staging system for lung cancer. Chest 1986; 89(Suppl):225S–233S.

556. Bunker ML, Raab SS, Landreneau RJ, Silverman JF. The diagnosis and significance of visceral pleural invasion in lung carcinoma – Histologic predictors and the role of elastic stains. Am J Clin Pathol 1999; 112:777–783.

557. Mountain CF, Dresler CM. Regional lymph node classification for lung cancer staging. Chest 1997; 111:1718–1723.

558. Velzen E van, Snijder RJ, Brutel dlR, Elbers HJ, van den Bosch JM. Type of lymph node involvement influences survival rates in T1N1M0 non-small cell lung carcinoma. Lymph node involvement by direct extension compared with lobar and hilar node metastases. Chest 1996; 110:1469–1473.

559. Riquet M. Manac'h D, Pimpec-Barthes F, Dujon A, Chehab A. Prognostic significance of surgical-pathologic N1 disease in non-small cell carcinoma of the lung. Ann Thorac Surg 1999; 67:1572–1576.

560. Lipford EH, Eggleston JC, Lillemore KD, et al. Prognostic factors in surgically resected limited-state, nonsmall cell carcinoma of the lung. Am J Surg Pathol 1984; 8:357–365.

561. Fraire AE, Johnson EH, Yesner R, et al. Prognostic significance of histopathologic subtype and stage in small cell lung cancer. Hum Pathol 1992; 23:520–528.

562. Carriaga MT, Henson DE. The histologic grading of cancer. Cancer 1995; 75:406–421.

563. Ladekarl M, Boekhansen T, Henriknielsen R, et al. Objective malignancy grading of squamous cell carcinoma of the lung: stereologic estimates of mean nuclear size are of prognostic value, independent of clinical stage of disease. Cancer 1995; 76:797–802.

564. Pastorino U. Benefits of neoadjuvant chemotherapy in NSCLC. Chest 1996; 109:S96–S101.

565. Smit EF, Groen HJM, Splinter TAW, Ebels T, Postmus PE. New prognostic factors in resectable non-small cell lung cancer. Thorax 1996; 51:638–646.

566. Kimura T, Sato T, Onodera K. Clinical significance of DNA measurements in small cell lung cancer. Cancer 1993; 72:3216–3222.

567. Tanaka I, Masuda R, Furuhata Y, et al. Flow cytometric analysis of the DNA content of adenocarcinoma of the lung, especially for patients with stage 1 disease with long term follow-up. Cancer 1995; 75:2461–2465.

568. Asamura H, Ando M, Matsuno Y, Shimosato Y. Histopathologic prognostic factors in resected adenocarcinomas – Is nuclear DNA content prognostic? Chest 1999; 115:1018–1024.

569. Zimmerman PV, Hawson GAT, Bint MH, Parsons PG. Ploidy as a prognostic determinant in surgically treated lung cancer. Lancet 1987; 2:530–533.

570. Yasushira K. Flow cytometric analysis of DNA ploidy level in paraffin-embedded tissue of non-small-cell lung cancer. Eur J Cancer Clin Oncol 1988; 24:455–460.

571. Ogawa J, Tsurumi T, Inoue H, Shohtsu A. Relationship between tumor DNA ploidy and regional lymph node changes in lung cancer. Cancer 1992; 69:1688–1695.

572. Battlehner CN, Saldiva PHN, Carvalho CRR, et al. Nuclear/cytoplasmic ratio correlates strongly with survival in non-disseminated neuroendocrine carcinoma of the lung. Histopathology 1993; 22: 31–34.

573. Tungekar MF, Gatter KC, Dunnill MS, Mason DY. Ki-67 immunostaining and survival in operable lung cancer. Histopathology 1991; 19:545–550.

574. Theunissen PHMH, Leers MPG, Bollen ECM. Proliferating cell nuclear antigen (PCNA) expression in formalin-fixed tissue of non-small-cell lung carcinoma. Histopathology 1992; 20:251–255.

575. Shiba M, Kohno H, Kakizawa K, et al. Ki-67 immunostaining and other prognostic factors including tobacco smoking in patients with resected nonsmall cell lung carcinoma. Cancer 2000; 89:1457–1465.

576. Poleri C, Morero JL, Nieva B, et al. Risk of recurrence in patients with surgically resected stage I non-small cell lung carcinoma – Histopathologic and immunohistochemical analysis. Chest 2003; 123:1858–1867.

577. Boldy DAR, Ayres JG, Crocker J, Waterhouse JAH, Gilthorpe M. Interphase nucleolar organiser regions and survival in squamous cell carcinoma of the bronchus – a ten year follow up study of 138 cases. Thorax 1991; 46:871–877.

578. Ogura S, Abe S, Sukoh N, et al. Correlation between nucleolar organizer regions visualized by silver staining and the growth rate in lung adenocarcinoma. Cancer 1992; 70:63–68.

579. Antonangelo L, Bernardi FD, Capelozzi VL, et al. Morphometric evaluation of argyrophilic nucleolar organizer region is useful in predicting long-term survival in squamous cell carcinoma of the lung. Chest 1997; 111:110–114.

580. Fujiwara M, Okayasu I, Takemura T, et al. Telomerase activity significantly correlates with chromosome alterations, cell differentiation, and proliferation in lung adenocarcinomas. Mod Pathol 2000; 13: 723–729.

581. Ghosh M, Crocker J, Morris A. Apoptosis in squamous cell carcinoma of the lung: correlation with survival and clinicopathological features. J Clin Pathol 2001; 54:111–115.

582. Usuda K, Saito Y, Sagawa M, et al. Tumor doubling time and prognostic assessment of patients with primary lung cancer. Cancer 1994; 74:2239–2244.

583. Battifora H, Sorensen HR, Mehta P, et al. Tumor-associated antigen 43-9f is of prognostic value in squamous cell carcinoma of the lung – a retrospective immunohistochemical study. Cancer 1992; 70:1867–1872.

584. Clarke MR, Landreneau RJ, Resnick NM, et al. Prognostic significance of CD44 expression in adenocarcinoma of the lung. J Clin Pathol Clin Mol Pathol 1995; 48:M200–M204.

585. Vargas SO, Leslie KO, Vacek PM, Socinski MA, Weaver DL. Estrogen-receptor-related protein p29 in primary nonsmall cell lung carcinoma: Pathologic and prognostic correlations. Cancer 1998; 82:1495–1500.

586. Furukawa T, Watanabe S, Kodama T, et al. T-zone histiocytes in adenocarcinoma of the lung in relation to postoperative prognosis. Cancer 1985; 56:2651–2656.

587. Takise A, Kodama T, Shimosato Y, Watanabe S, Suemasu K. Histopathologic prognostic factors in adenocarcinomas of the peripheral lung less than 2 cm in diameter. Cancer 1992; 61:2083–2088.

588. Zeid NA, Muller HK. S100 positive dendritic cells in human lung tumours associated with cell differentiation and enhanced survival. Pathology 1993; 25:338–343.

589. Yuan A, Yang PC, Yu CJ, et al. Tumor angiogenesis correlates with histologic type and metastasis in non-small-cell lung cancer. Am J Respir Crit Care Med 1995; 152:2157–2162.

590. Giatromanolaki A, Koukourakis M, Obyrne K, et al. Prognostic value of angiogenesis in operable non-small cell lung cancer. J Pathol 1996; 179:80–88.

591. Fontanini G, Lucchi M, Vignati S, et al. Angiogenesis as a prognostic indicator of survival in non-small-cell lung carcinoma: A prospective study. J Nat Cancer Inst 1997; 89:881–886.

592. Kayser G, Baumhakel JD, Szoke T, et al. Vascular diffusion density and survival of patients with primary lung carcinomas. Virchows Arch 2003; 442:462–467.

593. Fujisawa T, Yamaguchi Y, Saitoh Y, Hiroshima K, Ohwada H. Blood and lymphatic vessel invasion as prognostic factors for patients with primary resected nonsmall cell carcinoma of the lung with intrapulmonary metastases. Cancer 1995; 76:2464–2470.

594. Brechot JM, Chevret S, Charpentier MC, et al. Blood vessel and lymphatic vessel invasion in resected nonsmall cell lung carcinoma: correlation with TNM stage and disease free and overall survival. Cancer 1996; 78:2111–2118.

595. Sulzer MA, Leers MPG, Vannoord JA, Bollen ECM, Theunissen PHMH. Reduced E-cadherin expression is associated with increased lymph node metastasis and unfavorable prognosis in non-small cell lung cancer. Am J Respir Crit Care Med 1998; 157:1319–1323.

596. Salon C, Moro D, Lantuejoul S, et al. E-cadherin-[beta]-catenin adhesion complex in neuroendocrine tumors of the lung: a suggested role upon local invasion and metastasis. Hum Pathol 2004; 35:1148–1155.

597. Smith DR, Kunkel SL, Burdick MD, et al. Production of interleukin-10 by human bronchogenic carcinoma. Am J Pathol 1994; 145:18–25.

598. Watanabe N, Nakajima I, Abe S, et al. Staining pattern of type IV collagen and prognosis in early stage adenocarcinoma of the lung. J Clin Pathol 1994; 47:613–615.

599. Matsui K, Kitagawa M, Sugiyama S, Yamamoto K. Distribution pattern of the basement membrane components is one of the significant prognostic correlates in peripheral lung adenocarcinomas. Hum Pathol 1995; 26:186–194.

600. Kodate M, Kasai T, Hashimoto H, et al. Expression of matrix metalloproteinase (gelatinase) in T1 adenocarcinoma of the lung. Pathol Int 1997; 47:461–469.

601. KarAmis A, Panagou P, Tsilalis T, Bouros D. Association of expression of metalloproteinases and their inhibitors with the metastatic potential of squamous-cell lung carcinomas – A molecular and immunohistochemical study. Am J Respir Crit Care Med 1997; 156:1930–1936.

602. Thomas P, Khokha R, Shepherd FA, Feld R, Tsao MS. Differential expression of matrix metalloproteinases and their inhibitors in non-small cell lung cancer. J Pathol 2000; 190:150–156.

603. Carey FA, Fabbroni G, Lamb D. Expression of proliferating cell nuclear antigen in lung cancer – a systematic study and correlation with DNA ploidy. Histopathology 1992; 20:499–503.

604. Brown DC, Gatter KC. Comparison of proliferation rates assessed using multiblock and conventional tissue blocks of lung carcinoma. J Clin Pathol 1992; 45:579–582.

605. Maniwa Y, Yoshimura M, Obayashi C, et al. Association of p53 gene mutation and telomerase activity in resectable non-small cell lung cancer. Chest 2001; 120:589–594.

606. Han H, Landreneau RJ, Santucci TS, et al. Prognostic value of immunohistochemical expressions of p53, HER-2/neu, and bcl-2 in stage I non-small-cell lung cancer. Hum Pathol 2002; 33:105–110.

607. Gessner C, Liebers U, Kuhn H, et al. BAX and p16INK4A are independent positive prognostic markers for advance tumour stage of nonsmall cell lung cancer. Eur Resp J 2002; 19:134–140.

608. Brechot JM, Molina T, Theobald S, et al. [2000 Standards, options and recommendations for prognostic value of oncogenes and tumor suppressor genes in non small cell lung cancer.] Bull Cancer 2002; 89:857–867.

609. Greatens TM, Niehans GA, Rubins JB, et al. Do molecular markers predict survival in non-small-cell lung cancer? Am J Respir Crit Care Med 1998; 157:1093–1097.

610. Silvestrini R, Costa A, Lequaglie C, et al. Bcl-2 protein and prognosis in patients with potentially curable nonsmall-cell lung cancer. Virchows Arch 1998; 432:441–444.

611. Meert AP, Martin B, Delmotte P, et al. The role of EGF-R expression on patient survival in lung cancer: a systematic review with meta-analysis. Eur Resp J 2002; 20:975–981.

612. Harada M, Dosakaakita H, Miyamoto H, Kuzumaki N, Kawakami Y. Prognostic significance of the expression of ras oncogene product in non-small-cell lung cancer. Cancer 1992; 69:72–77.

613. Silini EM, Bosi F, Pellegata NS, et al. K-ras gene mutations: an unfavorable prognostic marker in stage I lung adenocarcinoma. Virchows Arch 1994; 424:367–373.

614. Fujino M, Dosakaakita H, Harada M, et al. Prognostic significance of p53 and ras p21 expression in nonsmall cell lung cancer. Cancer 1995; 76:2457–2463.

615. Fukuyama Y, Mitsudomi T, Sugio K, et al. K-ras and p53 mutations are an independent unfavourable prognostic indicator in patients with non-small-cell lung cancer. Br J Cancer 1997; 75:1125–1130.

616. Korkolopoulou P, Oates J, Crocker J, Edwards C. p53 expression in oat and non-oat small cell lung carcinomas – correlations with proliferating cell nuclear antigen. J Clin Pathol 1993; 46:1093–1096.

617. Marchett I, Buttitta F, Merlo G, et al. p53 alterations in non-small cell lung cancers correlate with metastatic involvement of hilar and mediastinal lymph nodes. Cancer Res 1993; 53:2846–2851.

618. Jiang SX, Sato YC, Kuwao S, Kameya T. Expression of bcl-2 oncogene protein is prevalent in small cell lung carcinomas. J Pathol 1995; 177:135–138.

619. Dalquen P, Sauter G, Torhorst J, et al. Nuclear p53 overexpression is an independent prognostic parameter in node-negative non-small cell lung carcinoma. J Pathol 1996; 178:53–58.

620. Laudanski J, Niklinska W, Burzykowski T, Chyczewski L, Niklinski J. Prognostic significance of p53 and bcl-2 abnormalities in operable nonsmall cell lung cancer. Eur Resp J 2001; 17:660–666.

621. Groeger AM, Esposito V, DeLuca A, et al. Prognostic value of immunohistochemical expression of p53, bax, Bcl-2 and Bcl-x(L) in resected non-small-cell lung cancers. Histopathology 2004; 44:54–63.

622. Johnson BE, Inde DC, Makuch RW, et al. Myc family oncogene amplification in tumor cell lines established from small cell lung cancer patients and its relationship to clinical status and course. J Clin Invest 1987; 79:1629–1634.

623. Biedler JL. Genetic aspects of multidrug resistance. Cancer 1992; 70:1799–1809.

624. Wright SR, Boag AH, Valdimarsson G, et al. Immunohistochemical detection of multidrug resistance protein in human lung cancer and normal lung. Clin Cancer Res 1998; 4:2279–2289.

625. Scheffer GL, Pijnenborg ACLM, Smit EF, et al. Multidrug resistance related molecules in human and murine lung. J Clin Pathol 2002; 55:332–339.

626. Takanami I, Imamura T, Hashizume T, et al. Transforming growth factor beta[1] as a prognostic factor in pulmonary adenocarcinoma. J Clin Pathol 1994; 47:1098–1100.

627. Woll PJ. New perspectives in lung cancer. 2. Growth factors and lung cancer. Thorax 1991; 46:924–929.

628. Weber S, Zuckerman JE, Bostwick DG, et al. Gastrin-releasing peptide is a selective mitogen for small cell carcinoma in vitro. J Clin Invest 1985; 75:306–309.

629. Cuttita F, Carney DN, Mulshine J, et al. Bombesin-like peptides can function as autocrine growth factors in human small cell lung cancer. Nature 1985; 316:823–826.

Future developments in treatment

630. Cullen M. Lung cancer – 4: Chemotherapy for non-small cell lung cancer: the end of the beginning. Thorax 2003; 58:352–356.

631. Taller A, Chilevers ER, Dransfield I, et al. Inhibition of neuropeptide stimulated tyrosine phosphorylation and tyrosine kinase activity stimulates apoptosis in small cell lung cancer cells. Cancer Res 1996; 56:4255–4263.

632. Krystal GW, Hines SJ, Organ CP. Autocrine growth of small cell lung cancer mediated by coexpression of c-kit and stem cell factor. Cancer Res 1996; 56:370–376.

633. Krystal GW, Honsawek S, Litz J, Buchdunger E. The selective tyrosine kinase inhibitor STI571 inhibits small cell lung cancer growth. Clin Cancer Res 2000; 6:3319–3326.

634. Wang WL, Healy ME, Sattler M, et al. Growth inhibition and modulation of kinase pathways of small cell lung cancer cell lines by the novel tyrosine kinase inhibitor STI 571. Oncogene 2000; 19:3521–3528.

635. Shapiro GI, Supko JG, Patterson A, et al. A phase II trial of the cyclin-dependent kinase inhibitor flavopiridol in patients with previously untreated stage IV non-small cell lung cancer. Clin Cancer Res 2001; 7:1590–1599.

636. Hainsworth JD, Lennington WJ, Greco FA. Overexpression of Her-2 in patients with poorly-differentiated carcinoma or poorly-differentiated adenocarcinoma of unknown primary site. J Clin Oncol 2000; 18: 632–635.

637. Lynch TJ, Bell DW, Sordella R, et al. Activating mutations in the epidermal growth factor receptor underlying responsiveness of non-small-cell lung cancer to gefitinib. N Engl J Med 2004; 350:2129–2139.

638. Paez JG, et al. EGFR mutations in lung cancer: correlation with clinical response to gefitinib therapy. Science 2004; 304:1497–1500.

639. Woll PJ, Rozengurt E. Bombesin and bombesin antagonists: studies in Swiss 3T3 cells and human small cell lung cancer. Br J Cancer 1992; 57:579–586.

640. Trepel JB, Moyer JD, Cuttita F, et al. A novel bombesin receptor antagonist inhibits autocrine signals in a small cell carcinoma cell line. Biochem Biophys Res Commun 1992; 156:1383–1389.

641. Karp JE, Kaufmann SH, Adjei AA, et al. Current status of clinical trials of farnesyltransferase inhibitors. Curr Opin Oncol 2001; 13:470–476.

642. Darnell RB, Deangelis LM. Regression of small-cell lung carcinoma in patients with paraneoplastic neuronal antibodies. Lancet 1993; 341: 21–22.

643. Baselga J, Pfister D, Cooper MR, et al. Phase I studies of anti-epidermal growth factor receptor chimeric antibody C225 alone and in combination with cisplatin. J Clin Oncol 2000; 18:904–914.

644. Agus DB, Bunn PA, Jr., Franklin W, Garcia M, Ozols RF. HER-2/neu as a therapeutic target in non-small cell lung cancer, prostate cancer, and ovarian cancer. Semin Oncol 2000; 27:53–63.

645. Stahel RA, Gilks WR, Schenker T. Antigens of lung cancer: results of the third international workshop on lung tumor and differentiation antigens. J Natl Cancer Inst 1994; 86:669–702.

646. Streiter RM, Polverizi PJ, Arenberg DA, et al. Role of c-x-c chemokines as regulators of angiogenesis in lung cancer. J Leukocyte Biol 1995; 57:752–762.

647. Brock CS, Lee SM. Anti-angiogenic strategies and vascular targeting in the treatment of lung cancer. Eur Resp J 2002; 19:557–570.

648. Gazdar AF, Miyajima K, Reddy J, et al. Molecular targets for cancer therapy and prevention. Chest 2004; 125:97S–97a.

649. Bunn PA, Soriano A, Johnson G, Heasley L. New therapeutic strategies for lung cancer – Biology and molecular biology come of age. Chest 2000; 117:163S–168S.

650. Weill D, Mack M, Roth J, et al. Adenoviral-mediated p53 gene transfer to non-small cell lung cancer through endobronchial injection. Chest 2000; 118:966–970.

651. Fong KM, Sekido Y, Gazdar AF, Minna JD. Lung cancer – 9: Molecular biology of lung cancer: clinical implications. Thorax 2003; 58:892–900.

652. Roth JA, Grammer SF, Swisher SG, et al. Gene therapy approaches for the management of non-small cell lung cancer. Semin Oncol 2001; 28:50–56.

653. Elenitoba-Johnson KS. Complex regulation of telomerase activity – Implications for cancer therapy. Am J Pathol 2001; 159:405–410.

654. White LK, Wright WE, Shay JW. Telomerase inhibitors. Trends Biotechnol 2001; 19:114–120.

12

Tumours

12.2

Other epithelial tumours

CARCINOID TUMOURS, TUMOURLETS AND NEUROENDOCRINE CELL HYPERPLASIA

Carcinoid tumours

The term carcinoid was introduced in 1907 to distinguish certain previously described low-grade intestinal neoplasms from adenocarcinomas.[1,2] Bronchial carcinoids were subsequently described, together with 'cylindromas' (adenoid cystic carcinomas of tracheobronchial gland origin, see p. 591), as well differentiated bronchial tumours.[3] These two tumours came to be known as the carcinoid and cylindromatous types of bronchial adenoma, but this nomenclature was abandoned when it was realised that their histogenesis differed and that both were of at least low-grade malignancy.

It is now appreciated that carcinoid tumours are neuroendocrine neoplasms of low-grade malignancy, related to a variety of more malignant bronchopulmonary tumours that also show evidence of such differentiation.[4-6] These include small cell carcinoma, atypical carcinoid and large cell neuroendocrine carcinoma. Evidence of neuroendocrine differentiation can also be found in occasional squamous cell and adenocarcinomas. These tumours can all generally be distinguished with ease but together they form a spectrum and occasional examples are difficult to classify precisely. Carcinoids, the microscopic tumour-like hyperplasias of the bronchopulmonary neuroendocrine cells known as tumourlets, and neuroendocrine cell hyperplasia are considered in this chapter while carcinomas showing neuroendocrine differentiation are dealt with in Chapter 12.1.

About 12% of all carcinoids arise in the lung but less than 1% of lung tumours are carcinoids.[7] The sex incidence is equal and they occur over a wide age range.[8,9] The mean age is about 55 years, significantly lower than that for carcinoma of the lung. About 8% develop in the second decade, making them the most common primary pulmonary tumour of childhood.[10,11] Carcinoid tumours are not related to smoking or environmental pollution: it is not known what promotes their formation but they are sometimes associated with multiple foci of neuroendocrine cell hyperplasia and tumourlets.[12,13] They do not appear to dedifferentiate into small cell or large cell neuroendocrine carcinomas although focal carcinoid differentiation is sometimes observed within otherwise classic small cell carcinoma.

Clinical features

Most patients with bronchopulmonary carcinoid tumours present with cough, haemoptysis or symptoms referable to the consequences of collapse or pneumonia distal to airway obstruction.[8,9] Sometimes there is wheezing, or even stridor, and these features have occasionally been mistaken for asthma. Small central tumours and those in the periphery of the lung may be asymptomatic and only discovered by chance. Occasionally a polypoid carcinoid may be coughed up spontaneously and no trace of its origin found on bronchoscopy.

Very occasionally, bronchial carcinoids present with metastatic deposits or with a variety of paraneoplastic endocrine syndromes, including Cushing's syndrome, acromegaly or the carcinoid syndrome.[14–18] In contrast to their gastrointestinal counterparts, bronchopulmonary carcinoids may cause the carcinoid syndrome in the absence of metastases, although these are usually present. This is because they release their secretions directly into the systemic circulation rather than into portal vessels. For the same reason, the endocarditis that forms part of the carcinoid syndrome affects valves on the left side of the heart rather than the right. Bronchopulmonary carcinoids may also be associated with pituitary, parathyroid and pancreatic islet cell tumours as part of a multiple endocrine neoplasia syndrome known as MEN1.

Gross appearances

Most bronchopulmonary carcinoids arise in the walls of central airways where they are seen on bronchoscopy as smooth cherry-red nodules that protrude into the airway. The bulk of the tumour often extends between the bronchial cartilages to invade the adjacent lung but sometimes the tumour grows entirely into the lumen of the airway, forming an endobronchial polyp. A combination of endobronchial and intrapulmonary growth may also be found, giving the tumour a dumb-bell or cottage-loaf appearance (Fig. 12.2.1). Those that extend into the lung usually have a well-defined, rounded border. Bronchopulmonary carcinoids are notorious for bleeding profusely if biopsied, although this is not the experience of all groups.[8] The cut surface of the tumour has a soft pinkish-tan or yellow appearance, and may be focally haemorrhagic. A minority of bronchopulmonary carcinoids arise in the periphery of the lung.[19] Occasionally there are multiple tumours.[20,21] These are particularly likely to be associated with multiple tumourlets and hyperplasia of bronchiolar neuroendocrine cells.[12,13]

Microscopy

Microscopy shows that carcinoid tumours have a thin fibrous capsule that is often incomplete; they may also exhibit infiltra-

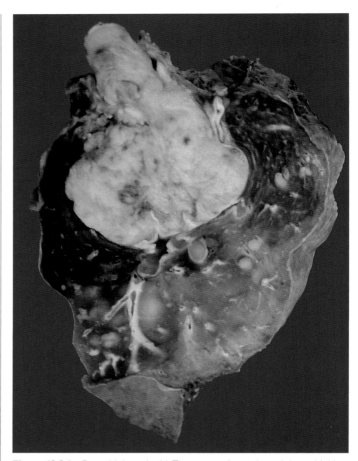

Figure 12.2.1 Bronchial carcinoid. The tumour is partly endobronchial but the bulk of it has grown into the surrounding lung. Note its well-circumscribed edge.

Box 12.2.1 Histological patterns of bronchopulmonary carcinoid tumours

Classic patterns:
  Mosaic (insular)
  Trabecular
Variants:
  Paraganglioid
  Adenopapillary
  Clear cell
  Oncocytic
  Melaninogenic
  Spindle cell

The pattern may vary within a tumour but to a limited degree histological pattern correlates with site, central tumours tending to be trabecular and peripheral growths mosaic or spindle cell.[19]

---

tive activity (Fig. 12.2.2). Several histological patterns, which may be present in combination, are recognised (Box 12.2.1).[22] The most common patterns are the trabecular and the mosaic.[23,24] In the former the tumour cells are arranged in interlocking cords or ribbons while in the latter they form nests or

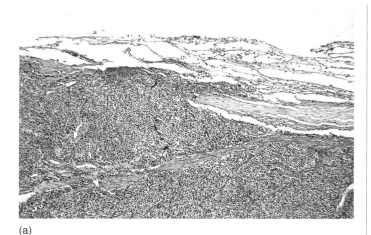

(a)

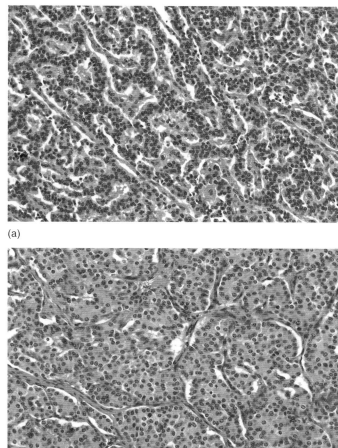

(a)

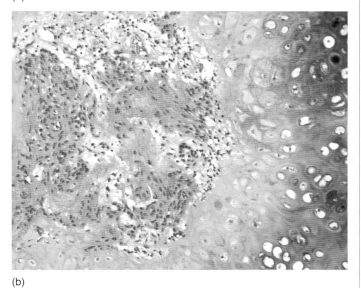

(b)

(b)

Figure 12.2.3 Bronchial carcinoid tumours. (a) Trabecular pattern, in which the tumour cells form anastomosing cords. (b) Mosaic pattern, in which the tumour cells are arranged in nests. In both patterns the groups of tumour cells are separated by a delicate vascular stroma, nuclei are regular and there are no atypical features.

Figure 12.2.2 Bronchial carcinoid tumours showing infiltrative activity. (a) Typical carcinoid tumours have a thin fibrous capsule that is often incomplete. (b) Infiltration of cartilage may be seen in typical carcinoids.

islands separated by a delicate fibrovascular stroma (Fig. 12.2.3). The tumour cells are uniform and generally polygonal, with a moderate amount of eosinophilic cytoplasm and round nuclei having finely granular chromatin and inconspicuous nucleoli. Necrosis is not seen and mitoses are not readily evident, numbering less than $2/2\,mm.^2$ If either necrosis or a higher mitotic rate is identified, the tumour is classified as an atypical carcinoid (see below) or, if 11 or more mitoses per $2\,mm^2$ are evident, a large cell neuroendocrine carcinoma (see p. 556).

About 40% of bronchial carcinoids are biphasic, being made up of groups of neuroendocrine cells surrounded by S-100 positive sustentacular cells, a feature that is also found in chemodectomas and which has caused these carcinoids to be termed 'paraganglioid'.[25,26] An alternative view is that these tumours are not carcinoids at all but paragangliomas. Support for this

view comes from the identification of scanty ganglion cells in a few examples, leading to the introduction of the term pulmonary gangliocytic paraganglioma (see also p. 627).[27,28] Sustentacular cells are less common in the more malignant neuroendocrine tumours.[26]

Some carcinoid tumours have an adenopapillary pattern, with small amounts of mucin contained within either tumour cells or gland lumina (Fig. 12.2.4).[22,24,29] Peripheral tumours tend to show a spindle cell pattern in which groups of fusiform cells are separated by a rich network of blood vessels (Fig. 12.2.5).[19,23,30] Other carcinoid tumours have abundant clear[31,32] (Fig. 12.2.6) or eosinophilic cytoplasm (Fig. 12.2.7),[33–35] the latter representing oncocytic change, something that may also be seen in occasional tracheobronchial gland tumours and in glomangiomas. Clear cell carcinoids may be confused with benign clear cell tumours (see p. 613),[31] but the immunohistochemical and

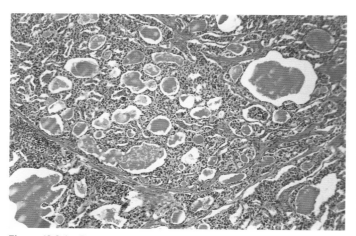

Figure 12.2.4 Bronchial carcinoid tumour of adenopapillary pattern.

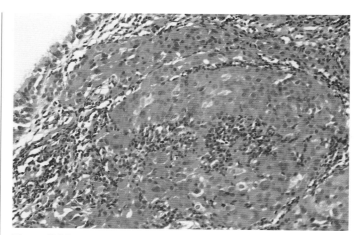

Figure 12.2.7 An oncocytic bronchial carcinoid tumour. The tumour cells have abundant deeply eosinophilic cytoplasm.

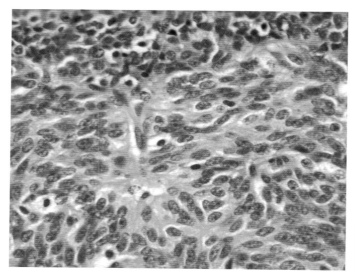

Figure 12.2.5 A peripheral pulmonary carcinoid tumour of spindle cell pattern.

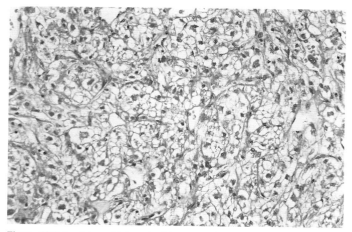

Figure 12.2.6 A bronchial carcinoid tumour of clear cell pattern.

ultrastructural features, which are outlined below, are very different. Melanin is occasionally evident within the tumour cells[36–41] and rare examples contain rod-shaped crystalloid cytoplasmic inclusions.[42] Argentaffin stains are seldom positive but argyrophilia can often be demonstrated.

Cartilage and bone may form in the stroma of bronchial carcinoid tumours (Fig. 12.2.8). This has been variously ascribed to the tumour infiltrating the perichondrium of the bronchial cartilage or to release of various growth factors by the tumour. Apudamyloid is also occasionally found in the stroma of carcinoid tumours.[43,44] Stromal vascularity may be very marked, with dilated sinusoidal vessels separating groups of tumour cells to give an appearance resembling that of a chemodectoma, the distinction from which is based on the immunocytochemical demonstration of cytokeratin (see below). Alternatively, the hypervascularity may suggest a glomus tumour, which is distinguished by immunocytochemistry and electron microscopy.[45]

Electron microscopy shows that the cytoplasm contains abundant dense-core neurosecretory granules, which range from 100–250 nm in diameter and vary in shape and electron density (Fig. 12.2.9).[4–6,46–49] Epithelial features include desmosomes and occasional bundles of tonofilaments. Oncocytic tumours are characterised by closely packed mitochondria in addition to neurosecretory granules, but it may not be possible to demonstrate both in the same cells.[33–35]

Immunohistochemistry may be used to identify markers of neuroendocrine differentiation.[46,48,50,51] Unfortunately, none of the antibodies currently available is totally specific,[52] the best probably being synaptophysin, chromogranin and CD56.[53–58] Other specific components of the neurosecretory granules include biologically active amines and peptides such as serotonin, calcitonin, gastrin-releasing peptide (human bombesin), ACTH, vasoactive intestinal polypeptide and leu-enkephalin. Differences between central and peripheral carcinoids are described, the latter more frequently expressing immunoreac-

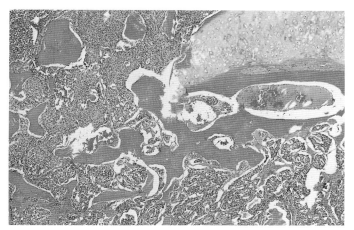

Figure 12.2.8 A bronchial carcinoid tumour in which there is stromal bone formation.

tivity for gastrin-releasing peptide, calcitonin and ACTH.[51,59] One bronchial carcinoid contained eight different hormones.[60] The ability to produce more than one hormone may account for variations in granule size seen in a single cell.[49] However, neuroendocrine tumours may even store multiple peptides within a single granule.[61] Occasional tumours show evidence of dual exocrine and endocrine (so-called amphicrine[62]) differentiation; for example, neuroendocrine granules have been identified in the same tumour cells as type II pneumocyte lamellar bodies, Clara cell granules and mucus vacuoles.[63,64] The intermediate filaments in the neuroendocrine cells consist of cytokeratin.[65] Although the lung marker TTF-1 is expressed by small cell carcinoma and large cell neuroendocrine carcinoma, reports of its expression by carcinoid tumours, tumourlets and neuroendocrine cell hyperplasia vary.[66,67]

Behaviour

Typical carcinoids are of low-grade malignancy and infiltration of adjacent lung or bronchus is often seen. However, it is important to distinguish typical and atypical carcinoids as the latter carry a worse prognosis (see below). Nuclear pleomorphism is sometimes apparent in typical carcinoids but, as with other endocrine tumours, this is a poor indicator of metastatic potential. It is likely that most early series failed to exclude tumours that would now be regarded as atypical carcinoids, and therefore over-estimated the tendency for them to metastasise. In a series of 101 bronchial carcinoids, 10 of the 12 that metastasised were histologically atypical.[9] Typical carcinoid tumours metastasise to hilar nodes in only 6–10% of cases,[51,68,69] and distant metastases, which may involve liver, lung, brain, adrenal or bone, are even less common. Deposits in bone may be osteosclerotic. Treatment usually requires lobectomy or, if the tumour involves the main bronchus, pneumonectomy. However, more limited procedures are sometimes feasible and a correct biopsy diagnosis is therefore important.

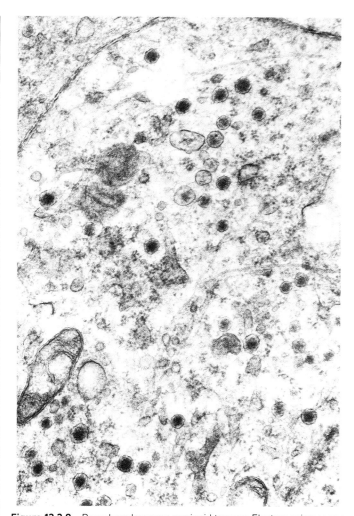

Figure 12.2.9 Bronchopulmonary carcinoid tumour. Electron microscopy shows a wealth of dense-core neuroendocrine granules.

Atypical carcinoid tumours

Atypical carcinoids make up about 11% of bronchopulmonary carcinoid tumours.[19] Most are peripheral in location,[70] and up to 70% eventually metastasise.[19,51,68,69,71,72] There is little effective treatment for metastatic disease as carcinoid tumours lack the chemosensitivity of small cell carcinomas[73] and the somatostatin analogues that are successfully employed in controlling the advance of metastatic islet cell tumours are only occasionally effective.[74] The five year survival rate is about 60%, which is closer to that of typical carcinoids (95%) than that of large cell neuroendocrine carcinomas and small cell carcinomas (2%). The peak age incidence (56 years, range 19–75 years) is also intermediate between that of typical carcinoid tumours (50 years, range 19–75 years) and small cell carcinoma (62 years, range 30–79 years) and they are more often seen in smokers than are their more benign counterparts. Ectopic endocrine activity is commoner with atypical than typical carcinoids.

Atypical carcinoid tumours are recognised by increased mitotic activity and necrosis being seen in a tumour with the

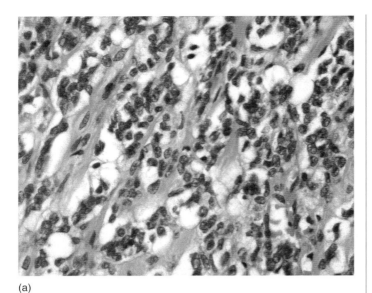

(a)

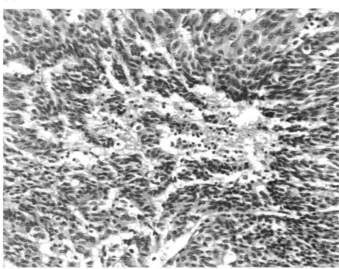

(b)

Figure 12.2.10 Atypical carcinoid. (a) Increased malignant potential is suggested by (a) mitoses numbering more than 2/2mm² and (b) foci of punctate necrosis (right of centre).

characteristic cellular make-up and trabecular or mosaic architecture of a carcinoid (Fig. 12.2.10). The necrosis is usually punctate and confined to the centres of cell groups, but it may be more extensive and it may lead to focal dystrophic calcification. The atypical features may not be apparent in small biopsies as they are often focal. Atypical tumours were originally defined as carcinoids that showed any one or a combination of features that included pleomorphism, prominent nucleoli, hyperchromasia, hypercellularity and disorganisation, as well as the aforementioned necrosis and increased mitotic activity,[68] but some of these additional features are of little prognostic importance. Nuclear pleomorphism for example may be found in otherwise unexceptional carcinoids that behave in an indolent manner.

Necrosis and increased mitotic activity are the most reliable pointers to atypical behaviour. Mitoses number 3–10 per 2mm² (about 10 high power fields); more than 10 indicates large cell neuroendocrine or small cell carcinoma (see Table 12.1.13, p. 556).[75] Within a group of atypical carcinoids, those with 6–10 mitoses per 2mm² were more aggressive than those with 2–5, and patients with tumours measuring over 3.5cm also fared badly.[76]

Electron microscopy shows that atypical carcinoids contain fewer dense-core granules than typical carcinoids, but more than small cell carcinomas. The immunohistochemical features are generally similar to those of typical carcinoids, but with increasing malignancy there is a progressive loss of chromogranin positivity, loss of heterozygosity and increased incidence of gene abnormalities.[77,78] Also, the C-terminal peptide of human pre-bombesin is detectable in the majority of atypical tumours whereas it can only be shown in a small number of typical carcinoids.[79] Increasing atypicality is also associated with loss of the S100-positive sustentacular cells that characterise many typical carcinoid tumours.[25,80] Aneuploidy occurs in both typical and atypical carcinoids but is commoner in the latter.[81–84] Proliferative activity assessed by expression of the Ki-67 antigen is higher in atypical than in typical carcinoids.[85] All these features correlate with the observed behaviour of atypical carcinoids, which is intermediate between that of typical carcinoids and small cell carcinoma. Thus, in the spectrum of neuroendocrine tumours of the lung, atypical carcinoids come between typical carcinoid and the neuroendocrine carcinomas in terms of their pathological features, natural history and prognosis (Table 12.2.1).

Molecular biology and genetics of carcinoids

Comparative genomic hybridisation has shown frequent chromosomal abnormalities at 11q (the site of the MEN1 gene) in both typical and atypical carcinoids. Loss of heterozygosity at 3p, 13q, 9p21 and 17p has also been described. Other chromosomal abnormalities are rare in typical carcinoids but atypical carcinoids have also shown DNA under-representation at 10q and 13q.[86] In general, atypical carcinoids show more extensive genetic alterations than typical carcinoids. However, these genetic abnormalities differ from those seen in large cell neuroendocrine carcinoma and small cell carcinoma, possibly because typical carcinoids are not associated with smoking. Examples of this include different mutations of the p53 gene and differences in the ratio of bcl2 : bax proteins.[87] However, other than their relative frequencies in relation to atypical versus typical carcinoids, these data as yet carry no prognostic significance. Nevertheless, they support the opinion that typical and atypical carcinoids are more closely related to each other than to large cell neuroendocrine carcinoma and small cell carcinoma.[78,86,88–92]

Tumourlets and neuroendocrine cell hyperplasia

While neuroendocrine cells are abundant in fetal lung, few are found in adult lungs where they are normally scattered singly

Table 12.2.1 A comparison of typical carcinoid, atypical carcinoid, large cell neuroendocrine carcinoma and small cell carcinoma

	Typical carcinoid	Atypical carcinoid	Large cell neuroendocrine carcinoma	Small cell carcinoma
Behaviour				
Local invasion	Present	Present	Present	Present
Lymphatic metastases	Occasional	Not infrequent	Frequent	Usual
Distant metastases	Rare	45–70%	>50%	95–100%
5-year survival	95%	60%	27–35%	2%
Histology				
Architecture	Well organised	Focal loss	Moderate loss	Poor
Necrosis	None	Focal	Abundant	Abundant
DNA deposition on vessels	None	None	None	Frequent
Cytology				
Mitoses	Not seen (≤2/10HPF)	Common (>2–10/10HPF)	Numerous (>10/10HPF)	Numerous (>10/10HPF)
Pleomorphism	Usually absent	Moderate	Marked	Small cell
Argyrophilia	Common	Variable	–	Rare
Neuroendocrine markers	Common, diffuse	Common, diffuse	Common, Often patchy	Common, Often patchy
Aetiology				
Role of smoking	None	Weak	Strong	Strong
Male/female ratio	0.8:1	2:1	2.5:1	Declining[a]
Mean age (years)	50	56	63	62
Ultrastructure				
Granule numbers	Many	Moderate numbers	–	Scanty
Granule size (nm)	150–250	80–140	–	80–140

[a]The male/female ratio of small cell carcinoma was formerly high but has been constantly dropping as more women smoke.

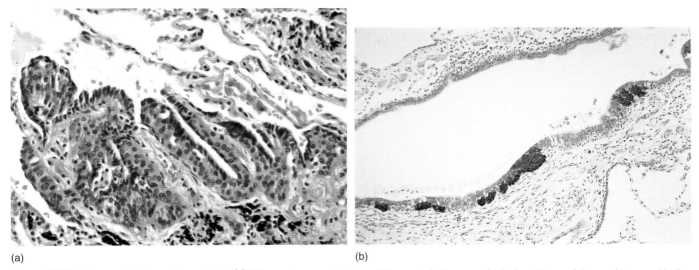

(a)　　　　　　　　　　　　　　　　　　　　(b)

Figure 12.2.11 Neuroendocrine cell hyperplasia. (a) A focus of neuroendocrine cell hyperplasia is present in the basal layer of the respiratory epithelium, limited by the basement membrane. (b) The hyperplastic cells are more easily seen by immunohistochemistry and are demonstrated here with an immunoperoxidase stain for chromogranin.

and sparsely along the bronchial basement membrane. Occasionally however, aggregates of neuroendocrine cells are encountered in adult lungs, occurring either as clusters of cells or as linear arrays along the basement membrane. If such aggregates are confined by the basement membrane the process is termed neuroendocrine cell hyperplasia, whereas if they penetrate the basement membrane the term tumourlet is used (for lesions up to a size of 5 mm; beyond 5 mm they are regarded as carcinoid tumours) (Figs 12.2.11, 12.2.12).[93]

The term tumourlet was coined by Whitwell,[94] but Liebow had earlier noted their histological resemblance to carcinoid tumours and referred to them, perhaps more accurately, as atypical carcinoid proliferations.[95] However, Whitwell's term tumourlet is in more general use. Opinion is divided as to

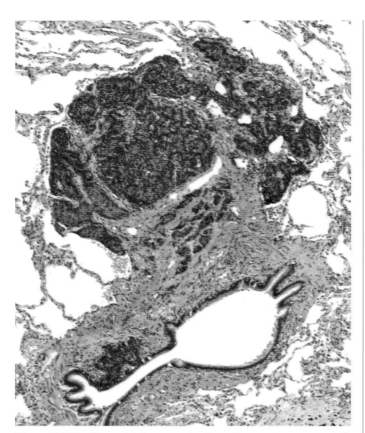

Figure 12.2.12 Tumourlet. A neuroendocrine cell aggregate composed of small, oval cells has infiltrated the peribronchiolar lung parenchyma.

whether they represent hyperplasia or neoplasia, with the former view generally being favoured. They seldom, if ever, metastasise and if similar deposits are found in the hilar lymph nodes[96,97] or the pulmonary lesions are larger than 5mm, they should be classified as carcinoid tumours.

Clinical features

Tumourlets are most frequently associated with bronchiectasis and are often multiple.[98] Other conditions associated with neuroendocrine cell hyperplasia and tumourlets include pulmonary hypertension,[99] bronchopulmonary dysplasia[100] and various causes of focal pulmonary scarring.[101,102] However, they are not particularly associated with diffuse interstitial fibrosis.

It has generally been assumed that diffuse neuroendocrine cell hyperplasia and tumourlets are pathological curiosities devoid of any clinical import but this view has had to be revised following reports of their association with clinically significant obstructive airway disease.[12,103–105] Histological examination in such cases has shown fibrous obliteration of bronchioles associated with diffuse idiopathic neuroendocrine cell hyperplasia and multiple tumourlets. This syndrome has been termed

diffuse idiopathic pulmonary neuroendocrine cell hyperplasia. It is suggested that in these cases the tumourlets are the cause rather than an effect of the fibrosis, and that the fibrosis is mediated by the secretion of fibrogenic cytokines such as gastrin-releasing peptide (human bombesin).[103] Similar postulates were advanced in a report of interstitial pulmonary fibrosis associated with diffuse neuroendocrine hyperplasia that extended out from the bronchioles to fill many alveoli.[106] It is now considered that diffuse idiopathic pulmonary neuroendocrine cell hyperplasia represents a pre-invasive precursor of peripheral typical carcinoid tumours, although not of other neuroendocrine tumours. However, no genetic markers have been identified that might distinguish diffuse idiopathic pulmonary neuroendocrine cell hyperplasia from neuroendocrine cell hyperplasia secondary to lung damage.

Microscopy

Tumourlets are minute, tumour-like proliferations that are generally only detectable by microscopy and discovered incidentally. They arise in close proximity to bronchioles as multiple nests of cells separated by narrow connective tissue septa (Fig. 12.2.12). Their cells are uniform and have regular, round, oval or spindle-shaped nuclei with finely dispersed chromatin. Electron microscopy shows that the cytoplasm contains granules of typical dense-core type averaging 100nm in diameter.[107] The immunohistochemical features are identical to those of normal bronchopulmonary neuroendocrine cells and of carcinoid tumours (see above).[50,51,108]

The relationship between tumourlets and bronchioles can often be clearly seen and it is likely that tumourlets arise from bronchiolar neuroendocrine cells.[109,110] Bronchiolar epithelium may directly overlie the cell clusters, or the bronchiole may be distended by the tumourlet. In lungs in which tumourlets have been identified, markers such as synaptophysin or chromogranin usually reveal many more but smaller clusters of cells within the basal layer of the bronchiolar epithelium. Examination of lungs resected for carcinoid tumours or carcinoma may also show a significant increase in the number of neuroendocrine cells, including clusters large enough to disturb and narrow small airways (Fig. 12.2.13).[13,103] Occasionally, otherwise typical carcinoid tumours may be accompanied by multiple fully formed tumourlets.[12]

Differential diagnosis

Tumourlets differ from carcinoid tumours only in their size. An arbitrary upper size limit of 5mm has been adopted.[93] Tumourlets may be confused with meningothelioid nodules (see p. 688). Unlike tumourlets, the latter are not related to airspaces but are situated within the interstitium, generally near septal veins: they lack neuroendocrine features. Localised regenerative proliferations of bronchiolar epithelium have sometimes been termed tumourlets, but they usually consist of

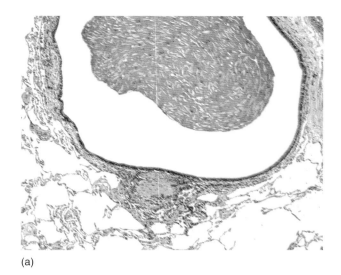

(a)

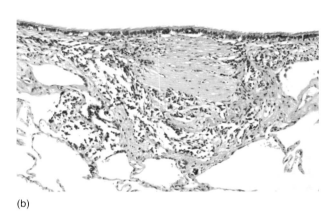

(b)

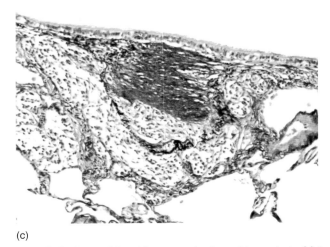

(c)

Figure 12.2.13 Diffuse idiopathic neuroendocrine cell hyperplasia. (a) A dilated bronchiole shows chronic obstructive changes. (b) At the lower border of Fig. (a) there is a small focus of neuroendocrine cell hyperplasia and fibrosis. (c) An elastin stain shows that this represents fibrous obliteration of a branching bronchiole. This was just one of many such foci identified throughout a surgical lung biopsy undertaken because of unexplained obstructive lung disease.

stratified squamous epithelium and lack the pattern of a true tumourlet; they also are devoid of any neuroendocrine features.

Prognosis

Diffuse idiopathic neuroendocrine cell hyperplasia generally pursues a benign course but the condition is slowly progressive and the subsequent obliterative bronchiolitis has occasionally necessitated transplantation.[104]

SALIVARY GLAND-TYPE TUMOURS

The mixed seromucous glands of the trachea and bronchi are similar to the minor salivary glands and give rise to the same range of tumours.[111] Many are of low-grade malignancy and the term bronchial adenoma, previously used to cover both tracheobronchial gland tumours and bronchial carcinoid tumours,[3] has therefore been abandoned despite them very rarely occurring in combination.[112] Salivary gland-type tumours are less common than bronchial carcinoids, in a ratio of 1 : 10, and most are either adenoid cystic carcinomas or mucoepidermoid tumours. Pleomorphic adenoma, the most common tumour of the major salivary glands, is rare in the lower respiratory tract. It is probable that some central adenocarcinomas arise in tracheobronchial glands although the site of origin of these aggressive tumours can rarely be identified with confidence and claims that they have a distinctive morphological pattern[113,114] are not entirely convincing.

Salivary gland-type tumours are usually central lesions that tend to protrude into the airway lumen, causing such symptoms as cough and haemoptysis, possibly of long duration. Alternatively, there may be a history of repeated episodes of pneumonia. Occasionally a salivary gland-type tumour is coughed up spontaneously.[115] Clinical evaluation to exclude metastasis from a salivary gland primary is always prudent, particularly if the lung tumour is peripheral or one of many.

Adenoid cystic carcinoma

Adenoid cystic carcinoma, formerly known as cylindroma, has an equal sex incidence and is a tumour of middle age (mean about 50 years), being extremely rare under the age of 30.[111,116,117] Clinical features are as outlined above.

Pathological features

Adenoid cystic carcinomas most often involve the lower trachea or large bronchi but some are peripheral, presumably derived from glands in small bronchi.[118,119] They are slowly growing infiltrative tumours that thicken and narrow the airway wall. They form poorly defined, sessile, nodular growths that may ulcerate centrally but more usually infiltrate extensively beneath an intact mucosa, ultimately involving adjacent lung tissue and hilar lymph nodes by direct invasion.[119] Perineural infiltration is a characteristic feature.

Pulmonary adenoid cystic carcinomas are identical in their microscopical appearances to those encountered in other sites, which include salivary gland, breast, skin, oesophagus, cervix uteri and prostate. The tumour cells form well-demarcated groups within which small cysts give a cribriform or tubular appearance (Fig. 12.2.14). The cysts may contain alcianophilic connective tissue mucin, secreted by their lining myoepithelial cells. Serial sections show that these spaces are continuous with the stroma of the tumour. While most of this secretion is mucoid and haematoxyphil, in places it becomes eosinophilic and hyaline, forming connective tissue cylinders that gave the tumour its former name cylindroma. Closely packed, small, dark myoepithelial cells form the dominant cell population, but there are also true ducts lined by slightly larger cells that secrete periodic acid-Schiff positive epithelial mucin.[120] As in the salivary glands, these tumours may occasionally be more solid and of higher grade. The immunocytochemical profile of adenoid cystic carcinoma reflects its myoepithelial nature, the tumour cells staining for cytokeratin, vimentin and actin; S-100 staining may also be positive (Table 12.2.2). The cysts contain components of basement membrane which may stain for laminin, fibronectin and type IV collagen.[117,121,122]

Differential diagnosis

The histological features are usually sufficiently distinctive to allow a confident diagnosis but in small biopsies it may be difficult to distinguish adenoid cystic carcinoma from adenocarcinoma, basaloid carcinoma, small cell carcinoma and lymphoma. Identification of a myoepithelial phenotype is then helpful.

Treatment and prognosis

The central location of adenoid cystic carcinomas and their predilection for submucosal and perineural spread make it difficult to treat these tumours effectively. Despite this, resection is the treatment of choice, with stenting, local ablation and radiotherapy forming alternative options for tumours that cannot be completely resected. Because of their growth pattern it is particularly important that the resection margins are checked by frozen section before closure. Nevertheless, local recurrence is frequent, often after a period of years, and may eventually lead to fatal pulmonary infection due to obstruction. Metastases are uncommon but may develop in lymph nodes, bone, kidney, liver, brain and lung.[118]

Mucoepidermoid carcinoma

Clinical features

Mucoepidermoid carcinomas comprise 0.1–0.2% of primary lung tumours.[123] All ages are affected, although approximately 50% of cases present before 30 years of age and 20% before

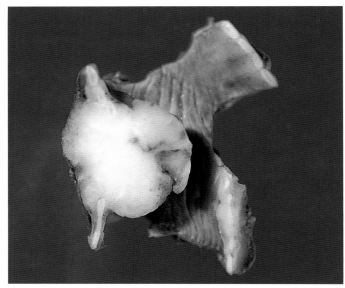

(a)

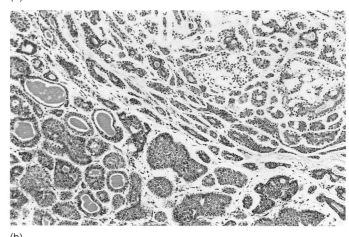

(b)

Figure 12.2.14 Adenoid cystic carcinoma of bronchial gland origin. (a) The tumour is almost wholly endobronchial. (b) Histologically, these tumours are identical to those that arise in the salivary glands. Microcysts give the tumour a cribriform pattern.

Table 12.2.2 Immunohistochemistry of salivary gland-type tumours				
	Adenoid cystic carcinoma	*Mucoepidermoid carcinoma*	*Pleomorphic adenoma*	*Acinic cell carcinoma*
Cytokeratin	+++	+++	+++	+++
S-100 protein	+	–	++	–
Actin	+++	–	++	–
Vimentin	++	–	++	–
Glial fibrillary protein	–	–	++	–
Chromogranin	–	–	–	–

20 years. There is a female sex predominance.[124] Muco-epidermoid carcinoma shows a spectrum of malignancy.[111,116,123–131] Low- and high-grade variants are recognised, the former comprising about 80% of these neoplasms. The younger patients generally have low-grade tumours, most of which are cured by surgical resection. The high-grade tumours are generally found in patients over the age of 30 years and prove fatal in 23% of cases.[124] Although typically presenting with symptoms of obstruction, occasional patients may be misdiagnosed as having asthma.[132] Imaging classically reflects airway obstruction and an endobronchial mass, sometimes with punctate calcification.[133]

Gross features

Mucoepidermoid carcinoma may be found at any location in the respiratory tract, but is most common in the main, lobar or segmental bronchi. Very rarely, the tumour is peripheral[130] or has a papillary stucture.[131] The gross appearances vary according to the degree of malignancy. Low-grade tumours form smooth, partly cystic, polypoid masses that project into the lumen of the bronchus (Fig. 12.2.15). They grow by expansion and compress surrounding tissue. The overlying bronchial mucosa, which may show squamous metaplasia, is generally intact. More aggressive tumours tend to be less clearly defined, irregular and solid: they infiltrate surrounding lung and more closely resemble the commoner carcinomas of the lung.

Microscopy

The essential microscopic feature of mucoepidermoid carcinomas is that they contain both glands and squamous elements (Fig. 12.2.15). The glands are lined by a mixture of mucous and non-secretory columnar cells, and contain epithelial mucus that may calcify or even ossify.[124] The mucous cells are also found mixed with the squamous cells in a sheet-like arrangement. The squamous cells are linked by intercellular bridges but keratinization is not seen.[125] Sheets of regular, polygonal cells with abundant eosinophilic cytoplasm and known as transitional or intermediate cells merge with the mucous and squamous cells and may be the dominant component. In some tumours the cells have abundant clear cytoplasm or, rarely, show oncocytic change.[134] Low-grade tumours lack cellular atypia and mitoses, features that are seen particularly in the squamous component of the more malignant tumours. Genetic analysis has shown t(11;19) mutation in two cases.[133,135]

Differential diagnosis

The histological features are usually sufficiently distinctive to permit a confident diagnosis but separation from mucus gland adenoma and carcinoid may be difficult in small biopsies or on frozen section. Immunohistochemistry may help exclude carcinoid tumours but, in practice, as long as the surgeons are aware that they are dealing with a low-grade malignancy or benign tumour and that bronchoplastic resection is an option, defini-

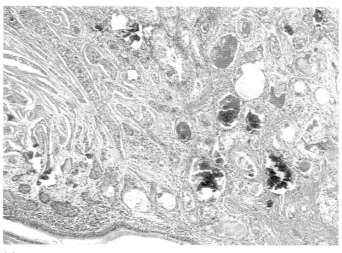

(a)

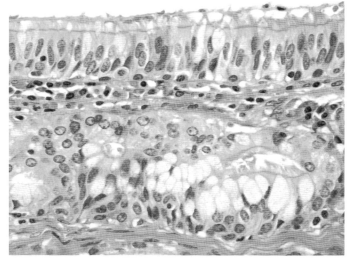

(b)

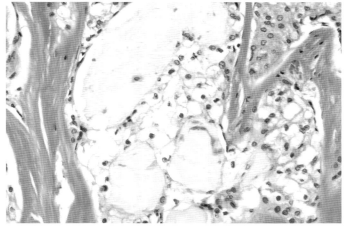

(c)

Figure 12.2.15 Low-grade mucoepidermoid carcinoma. (a) At low power, this endobronchial tumour shows a mixed solid and glandular pattern. Many of the tumour acini are distended by mucus, in which there is focal dystrophic calcification. (b) An island of tumour beneath the surface epithelium consists of intermediate and goblet cells. (c) Focal clear cell change may also be present.

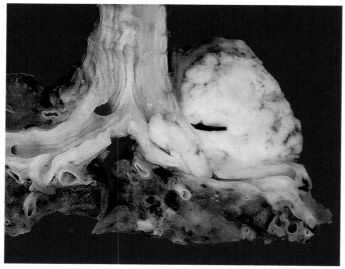

(a)

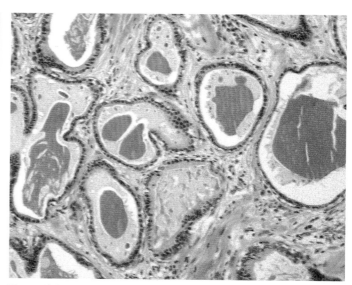

Figure 12.2.17 Mucus gland adenoma. An endobronchial tumour consists solely of glands lined by cytologically bland mucus-secreting columnar cells.

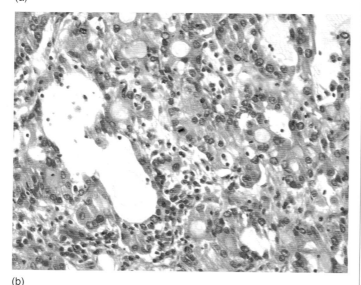

(b)

Figure 12.2.16 High-grade mucoepidermoid carcinoma. (a) An endobronchial tumour occludes a segmental bronchus and an adjacent lymph node is greatly enlarged by a metastatic tumour. (b) The intermediate cells are pleomorphic and mitotically active, and there is some resemblance to an adenocarcinoma.

pattern and a lack of *in situ* carcinoma in the overlying epithelium all favour mucoepidermoid carcinoma. The differential diagnosis also includes necrotizing sialometaplasia, a reactive, non-invasive process that generally follows prolonged tracheal intubation.[136]

Treatment and prognosis

Surgical resection is the treatment of choice for both low-grade and high-grade tumours, with bronchoplastic surgery an option in low-grade cases. The prognosis of low-grade tumours is generally excellent although nodal involvement and metastases have been reported.[124,128,137] The prognosis in children appears to be slightly better than in adults, probably reflecting a higher incidence of low-grade tumours in younger patients.[10,126] The prognosis for high-grade tumours is variably reported[123,124,138] but about 25% of patients with these tumours develop metastases, typically in lymph nodes, bone or skin.

Mucous gland adenoma

Mucous gland adenoma, or cystadenoma, is one of the rarest tumours of tracheobronchial glands and one that has no direct counterpart in the salivary glands.[111,115,139–141] Reported examples cover a wide age range, including childhood. They arise in main, lobar or segmental bronchi as smooth, rounded, polypoid tumours. The overlying bronchial mucosa is usually intact and the cut surface may show irregular microcystic spaces filled with mucus. Invasion of bronchial wall or lung parenchyma is not seen and these tumours tend to remain superficial to the bronchial cartilage. Surgical resection, ideally by bronchoplastic resection, is curative.

Microscopically, glands, which sometimes form small cysts, are lined by columnar or cuboidal mucous cells and contain mucin (Fig. 12.2.17). The intermediate and squamous cells of a

tive classification may wait until examination of the resection specimen.

High-grade tumours show a more infiltrative growth pattern (Fig. 12.2.16) and it is difficult to draw absolute distinctions between high-grade mucoepidermoid carcinoma and adenosquamous carcinoma, both of which have a dual cell population. However, adenosquamous carcinomas tend to arise in the periphery of the lung whereas mucoepidermoid carcinomas arise in major airways. Frank keratinisation with the formation of keratin pearls suggests adenosquamous carcinoma rather than mucoepidermoid carcinoma whereas the presence of abundant cells that are transitional in appearance between squamous and mucous cells, foci of the more characteristic low-grade

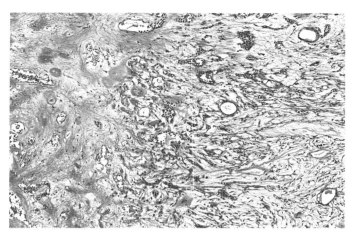

Figure 12.2.18 Pleomorphic adenoma of the bronchus, a glandular tumour with an abundant myxoid stroma showing chondroid differentiation.

mucoepidermoid carcinoma are not seen but the identification by electron microscopy of occasional squamous, myoepithelial and oncocytic elements indicates a possible overlap with low-grade mucoepidermoid carcinoma.[140,141]

Oncocytoma

Oncocytes, or oxyphil cells, have abundant, finely granular, eosinophilic cytoplasm due to the presence of numerous closely packed mitochondria. These organelles are very striking when examined by electron microscopy but may also be demonstrated by their affinity for phosphotungstic acid haematoxylin, with which they stain dark blue. Oncocytes are also distinguished by their strong expression of cytokeratin 14.[142] Oncocytes occur in the thyroid, parathyroid and salivary glands and give rise to oncocytic tumours in all these sites. In normal bronchial glands, oncocytic change affects small groups of cells in ducts and acini and is seen more frequently with increasing age (see Fig. 1.18).[143] Bronchial carcinoids, glomus tumours, mucoepidermoid carcinomas and acinic cell carcinomas are all occasionally oncocytic, and recognition of their true nature may depend upon the use of mucus stains, immunocytochemistry or electron microscopy.[144]

Pure oncocytomas are exceedingly rare in the airways.[111,144–146] Some reported cases have been very small incidental lesions in which the oncocytes formed acinar or tubulopapillary patterns.[111,145] Grossly, oncocytomas usually form well-demarcated, solid nodules ranging in size from 1 to 3.5 cm. They are generally solitary but multiple pulmonary oncocytomas have been described.[147] Histologically, the oncocytic tumour cells are arranged in sheets or nests. They show little mitotic activity and no necrosis. Focal infiltrative growth may be noted at the periphery of lesions but this is not regarded as indicating malignancy.[146] The tumour cells stain focally for cytokeratin and vimentin, but not for actin, S-100 or neuroendocrine markers.[146] The absence of neuroendocrine markers helps exclude oncocytic carcinoid. Granular cell tumours

resemble oncocytomas but are S-100 positive and cytokeratin negative.

Oncocytoma carries an excellent prognosis. Lymph node metastasis is recorded in one case but 2 years after lobectomy the patient was free of disease.[148]

Pleomorphic adenoma

Pleomorphic adenoma, which is the most common tumour of major salivary glands, is rare in the lower respiratory tract.[149–153] The histological features are similar to those seen in the salivary gland tumour except that ducts are relatively sparse: microscopy shows epithelial and myoepithelial cells in a myxoid or chondroid stroma (Fig. 12.2.18). The tumour cells react strongly with antibodies to cytokeratin and variably for vimentin, actin, S-100 protein and glial fibrillary acidic protein (Table 12.2.2).[150] Occasional tumours show cytological atypia or local infiltrative activity and these tumours are prone to metastasize.[111,150,154] Frankly carcinomatous elements may also be seen arising from a pleomorphic adenoma (carcinoma ex pleomorphic adenoma). Some rare malignant endobronchial myxoid tumours probably represent a variant of pleomorphic adenoma.[155]

Epithelial-myoepithelial carcinoma

Terms such as adenomyoepithelioma and myoepithelioma have been previously applied to this tracheobronchial gland tumour but it is of low malignant potential and the name epithelial-myoepithelial carcinoma is therefore recommended.[93] It is particularly rare in the lower respiratory tract, no more than 20 cases being recorded.[156–162] Age at presentation ranges from 33 to 71 years, with no sex predominance.

Pathological features

Grossly, the tumour either protrudes into the bronchus or forms a large intrapulmonary mass. The cut surface may be solid or gelatinous. Microscopically, both epithelial and myoepithelial elements are usually present, although purely myoepithelial tumours also occur. The typical tubule is lined by two cell types, an inner layer of cytokeratin-positive epithelial cells surrounded by an outer mantle of myoepithelial cells, the latter expressing smooth muscle actin and S-100 antigen. The outer cells may in turn be surrounded by a rim of PAS-positive basement membrane material (Fig. 12.2.19). In purely myoepithelial areas, the tumour cells vary from polygonal to spindle-shaped and generally form solid nodules separated by a hyaline stroma (Fig. 12.2.19).[163–167]

Differential diagnosis

The differential diagnosis includes several other types of tracheobronchial gland neoplasm. Pleomorphic adenomas often contain myoepithelial cells and ducts, but chondroid or myxochondroid elements usually predominate.[150] Adenoid

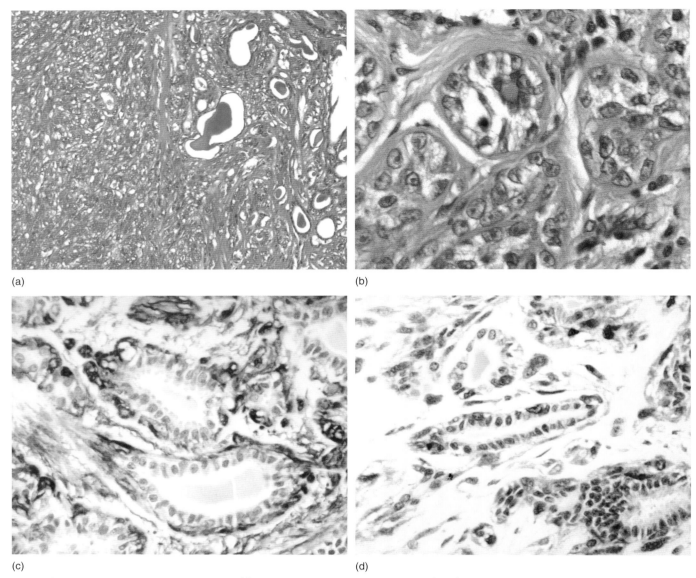

Figure 12.2.19 Epithelial–myoepithelial carcinoma. (a) The tumour shows a mixture of tubules (right) and a more solid spindle cell proliferation (left). (b) The tubules are lined by an inner layer of epithelial cells surrounded by an outer layer of myoepithelial cells which have a clear cytoplasm. The myoepithelial cells stain for both S-100 (c) and smooth muscle actin (d).

cystic carcinomas may resemble epithelial-myoepithelial carcinomas with a predominantly ductal pattern, but are more infiltrative and cribriform areas are usually also present. Epithelial-myoepithelial carcinoma may also enter the differential diagnosis of pulmonary clear cell tumours (see Table 12.3.1, p. 615).[166]

Treatment and prognosis

Surgical resection is the treatment of choice. Epithelial-myoepithelial carcinomas are generally indolent growths but recurrence or metastasis has been recorded in purely myoepitheliomatous cases that showed brisk mitotic activity, necrosis and atypia.[165,166]

Acinic cell carcinoma

The histological appearances of this rare tumour are identical to those of its salivary gland counterpart. It is an indolent growth and the prognosis is good. Of the 15 cases reported by 1999 only one had metastasised and this only to the local lymph nodes.[168] The pattern is generally solid but reticulin surrounds groups of tumour cells and outlines an acinar pattern. Lumen formation may be apparent. The tumour cells are regular and have a poorly staining slightly basophilic, vacuolated or granular cytoplasm.[169,170] Periodic acid-Schiff reactions after diastase digestion are variable but generally weak. Electron microscopy shows dense cytoplasmic granules of about 500 nm diameter, as seen in the serous acini of the tracheobronchial glands.[169,170] The differential diagnosis includes carcinoid tumour, chemodectoma and benign clear cell tumour.

PAPILLOMAS

Several types of tumour show a tendency to endobronchial growth, by which is meant that they grow predominantly into the lumen of the airways. They include squamous cell carcinomas,[171] basaloid carcinomas, carcinoids,[29] some tracheobronchial gland neoplasms,[131] carcinosarcomas, occasional metastases, and the papillomas that are dealt with here. These neoplasms need to be distinguished from inflammatory polyps, which are dealt with in Ch. 12.7, p. 686.

Solitary papilloma

Solitary papillomas are generally squamous cell in type but glandular papillomas and mixed squamous and glandular papillomas are also recognised.[172] Sometimes a bronchial papilloma of mixed squamous and mucous cell type is continuous with a mucous cell adenoma of an underlying bronchial gland.[173]

Aetiological factors concerned in the development of solitary squamous cell papillomas include human papilloma virus, which is found in over 50% of cases,[172,174–177] and cigarette smoking, perhaps acting in combination. The patients are generally middle-aged or elderly men. Types 16 and 18 papilloma virus are involved in these solitary tumours rather than the types 6 and 11 found in papillomatosis.[175,176] About one-third show cytologic atypia and there is a spectrum of microscopic appearances, ranging from a simple benign, cytologically bland papilloma with or without an inflamed hyaline stroma to the invasive papillary squamous cell carcinoma discussed in Chapter 12.1.[173] In solitary squamous papillomas, the epithelial covering may show the whole range of changes described in the development of squamous cell carcinoma in flat bronchial epithelium: squamous metaplasia, dysplasia, carcinoma-*in-situ* and invasive tumour. In general, older patients are more likely to have lesions that are malignant. Most are cured by excision, but about 20% recur.[172]

Papillomas clothed entirely by mucous, simple columnar or ciliated cells are termed glandular (or columnar cell) papillomas (Fig. 12.2.20).[93,178] They develop in the larger conductive airways and generally affect middle-aged patients, with a slight female preponderance. The age range is wide – 26 to 74 years.[179] Most are cured by excision, but occasional cases recur.[172]

Mixed squamous and columnar cell papillomas are rare. They are commoner in male smokers, as with squamous papillomas, and may show cytologic atypia. No such cases have recurred.[172]

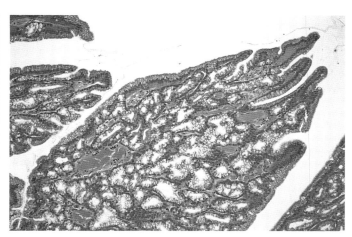

Figure 12.2.20 A bronchial papilloma of glandular type in which the epithelium consists of columnar mucous cells.

Some bronchial tumours resemble papillary urothelial tumours and have been called transitional cell papillomas.[173,180] Tumours of this name are well known in the nose, where they are also known as Schneiderian, Ringertz or inverted papilloma. Earlier editions of the World Health Organization's histological classification of lung tumours referred to transitional cell papillomas[181] whereas the current edition uses the term inverted papilloma.[93] However, specialists in nasal pathology do not accept that the bronchial tumours are the same as those seen in the nose, where they are regarded as polyps showing squamous metaplasia:[182] those in the bronchi are a subtype of squamous cell papilloma and comparing them to tumours of the nose or urinary tract is probably best avoided.

Recurrent respiratory papillomatosis

Recurrent respiratory papillomatosis most commonly affects the larynx. Only 5% of patients have involvement of the trachea or large bronchi, and fewer than 1% have more distal lung involvement.[183,184] The onset is generally before the age of 11 years and most examples regress before puberty. However, repeated laser therapy may first be required because the lesions are prone to recur. If left untreated, the lesions may enlarge, spread, and endanger the airway. Multiple laryngeal, tracheal and bronchial papillomas cause hoarseness, stridor and respiratory obstruction, while the rare pulmonary lesions appear on chest radiographs as solid or cystic rounded nodules.[185] The human papilloma virus is an aetiological factor and types 6 and 11 have been identified in the lesions.[185–189] However, since orofacial papilloma virus infection is common and recurrent respiratory papillomatosis is rare, other host and/or viral factors probably contribute to pathogenesis. For example, an association with HLA DRB1*0301 has recently been reported.[185,187–190]

The papillomas have a narrow connective tissue stalk covered by non-keratinising stratified squamous epithelium. There is no atypia but certain cytological changes typical of a

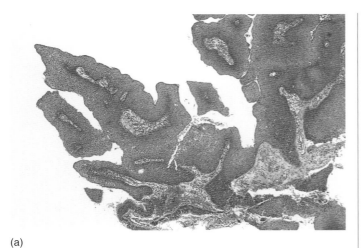

(a)

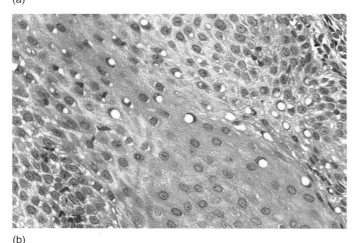

(b)

Figure 12.2.21 Bronchial papillomatosis. (a) The papillae are covered by well-differentiated non-keratinising squamous epithelium. (b) High magnification shows nuclear shrinkage with perinuclear vacuolation indicative of papilloma virus infection.

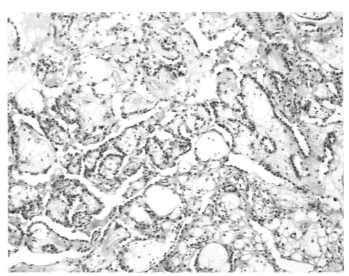

Figure 12.2.22 Papillary adenoma. The tumour consist of papillae lined by cytologically bland pneumocyte-like cells. It differs from sclerosing pneumocytoma by its lack of stromal cells.

genital condyloma caused by the human papilloma virus may be found, namely koilocytosis, which is characterised by irregular nuclear shrinkage, binucleation and perinuclear clearing (Fig. 12.2.21).[191] The papillomatous proliferation may extend into the soft tissues surrounding the airways, even though there are no cytological features of malignancy. Such extension has been termed invasive papillomatosis.[192] In the lung such lesions form clusters of squamous cells that fill several adjacent alveoli without destroying their walls. Continued growth leads to expansion of the alveoli and compression of the surrounding lung. In larger invasive lesions, central cavitation occurs, with the danger of secondary infection.

Frank malignant change to squamous cell carcinoma, characterised by atypia, keratinisation and infiltrative growth, supervenes in about 2% of cases. Smoking and irradiation, the latter used in the past to treat the papillomatosis, appear to promote this complication, which has been recorded in patients whose ages have ranged from 6 to 35 years.[191,193–198] Malignant change

has been associated with type 11 papilloma virus infection followed by increased expression of p53 and Rb proteins.[199]

ADENOMAS

Papillary adenoma

Papillary adenomas are rare well-circumscribed parenchymal lesions. Affected patients are usually asymptomatic, the lesions being found incidentally on imaging. The tumours may be encapsulated and are typically soft solid masses that range from 1–4 cm in size. Multiple type II cell papillary adenomas are recorded in a child with neurofibromatosis.[200]

The lining cells are cuboidal or columnar (Fig. 12.2.22). They stain for cytokeratins, TTF-1, surfactant apoproteins, CEA and EMA and have the ultrastructural features of either Clara cells or type II alveolar epithelial cells or both these cell types.[173,201–206]

Papillary adenomas are distinguished from sclerosing pneumocytoma by lacking the varied architecture of the latter and by the TTF-1 and EMA staining being limited to the surface epithelium. They are distinguished from alveolar adenoma by their papillary growth pattern and focal ciliated or Clara cell morphology. Metastases also need to be excluded, especially those from the thyroid. Occasionally, papillary adenomas show infiltrative growth, in which case their distinction from papillary adenocarcinoma is uncertain and they are probably best classified as low-grade adenocarcinomas.

Alveolar adenoma

This tumour often resembles a lymphangioma microscopically and some examples have probably been reported as such.[207,208] Its epithelial nature was established in 1986 by a combination

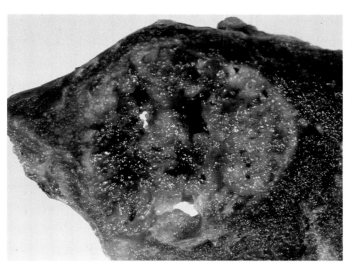

Figure 12.2.23 Alveolar adenoma forming a well-circumscribed 13 mm peripheral nodule. (Illustration provided by Dr M Jagusch, formerly of Auckland, New Zealand.)

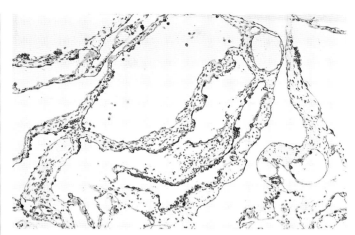

Figure 12.2.25 Alveolar adenoma. The cells lining the spaces stain for cytokeratin, showing that the tumour is an adenoma rather than a lymphangioma (Immunoperoxidase stain).

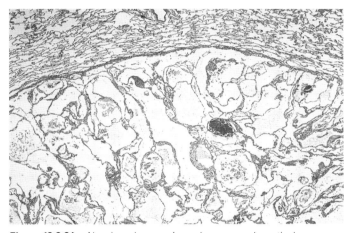

Figure 12.2.24 Alveolar adenoma. Irregular spaces, deceptively resembling lymphatics, are separated by fibrous septa of varying thickness with flattened lining cells. (Case of Dr M Jagusch, formerly of Auckland, New Zealand.)

of electron microscopy and immunocytochemistry.[209] Only a few have been reported since.[210–214] One group compared the lesion to the sclerosing pneumocytoma described below and suggested that it was a variant of the latter.[215]

The mean age of the patients reported to date is about 60 years. They have all had solitary peripheral lung lesions, measuring up to 2 cm in diameter, most of which were discovered incidentally as a radiographic 'coin lesion'.[209,210] None has recurred after local excision or lobectomy.[214]

Alveolar adenomas are well-circumscribed tumours with a solid grey or haemorrhagic appearance on the cut surface (Fig. 12.2.23). Microscopy typically shows irregular spaces, empty or filled with periodic acid-Schiff positive, eosinophilic material (Fig. 12.2.24). Occasional lesions may be solid and mimic a scle-

rosing pneumocytoma.[215–217] The spaces are lined by flattened or cuboidal cytokeratin-positive cells that have the ultrastructural features of type I and II alveolar epithelial cells (Fig. 12.2.25). They also stain for surfactant apoprotein and TTF-1. However they are negative for the Clara cell marker, CC10[214] and they do not express endothelial markers. This latter finding helps exclude lymphangioma, which the tumour may mimic morphologically. The spaces are separated by fibrous septa that are generally thin but may show exuberant connective tissue proliferation so that a mesenchymal neoplasm with cystic change enters the differential diagnosis. There may also be focal lymphoid infiltration or central stellate scarring.

SCLEROSING PNEUMOCYTOMA (SCLEROSING 'HAEMANGIOMA')

This unusual lung tumour was first described in 1956[218] under the name sclerosing haemangioma, a term that reflects two common histological features, sclerosis and vascular proliferation, that are both now thought to represent secondary changes in an essentially epithelial neoplasm. This view is based on immunohistochemical and ultrastructural evidence that the tumour cells are akin to type II pneumocytes: they stain for epithelial rather than endothelial markers and have ultrastructural features characteristic of type II cells.

The term sclerosing pneumocytoma is therefore more appropriate than sclerosing haemangioma[219] although the latter is still preferred by the World Health Organization for historic reasons.[93] It is suggested that these tumours are related to the peripheral papillary adenoma and the alveolar adenoma described above.[210] Several authors have proposed that they are hamartomatous[216,220,221] but rare reports of them metastasising to hilar lymph nodes[215–217,222] and evidence of clonality supports them being neoplastic.[223]

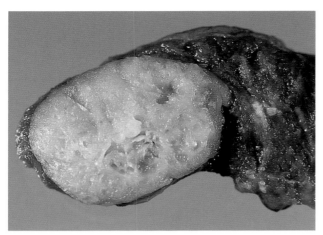

Figure 12.2.26 Sclerosing pneumocytoma forming a well-circumscribed peripheral tumour. It shows microcystic change and is yellow because of its high lipid content. (Illustration provided by Dr M Jagusch, formerly of Auckland, New Zealand.)

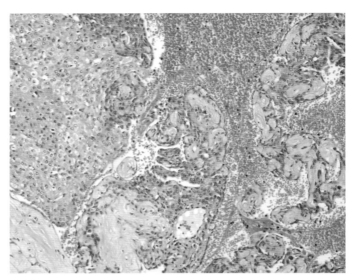

Figure 12.2.27 Sclerosing pneumocytoma showing a typically mixed solid, papillary, haemorrhagic and sclerotic architecture.

Clinical features

Patients with sclerosing pneumocytoma range from 13–83 years of age, with a peak incidence in the fifth decade and the ratio of females to males being about 5 to 1.[216,219,224–226] The preponderance of females is reflected in the demonstration of oestrogen and progesterone receptors on the tumour.[227,228] Most of the patients with these receptors have been Asian.[229] Most patients are asymptomatic, but some complain of cough or haemoptysis. Imaging shows a solitary circumscribed mass that may rarely be calcified or cystic while the haemorrhagic variants are sometimes identifiable by nuclear magnetic resonance. The tumours are generally benign but, as noted above, hilar lymph node metastasis is recorded.[215–217] One example was observed over a period of 47 years, at which stage it occupied the whole of the left thoracic cavity but had not metastasised.[230]

Pathological features

Sclerosing pneumocytomas are well circumscribed but not encapsulated tumours: they show expansile growth and compress rather than infiltrate the adjacent lung. The cut surface is variegated, with red well-vascularised areas and yellow foci amid firmer grey tissue (Fig. 12.2.26). Most tumours are peripheral and solitary, but multiple lesions have been reported.[224,231,232] Rare cystic examples are also recorded.[233]

Histologically, the tumours may be papillary, solid, sclerotic or angiomatoid. One of these patterns may predominate but they are more commonly seen in combination (Fig. 12.2.27).[234] In the papillary areas the covering cells have moderate amounts of lightly eosinophilic cytoplasm and oval, slightly irregular nuclei with a single nucleolus (Fig. 12.2.28). Mitoses are rare and atypia is unusual. These cells may be continuous with normal bronchiolar epithelium. They stain for cytokeratin, epithelial membrane antigen and thyroid transcription factor-1 (Fig. 12.2.29).[235] A second cell type forms the stroma of the papillae

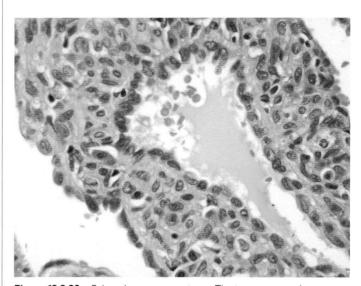

Figure 12.2.28 Sclerosing pneumocytoma. The tumour comprises cuboidal lining cells, which have eosinophilic cytoplasm, and more rounded stromal cells that have either eosinophilic or clear cytoplasm.

and often fills the interpapillary spaces. These cells are rounded and uniform with distinct cell borders. They contain centrally located cytologically bland nuclei with fine chromatin. Their cytoplasm is either eosinophilic or clear (Fig. 12.2.28). These cells, like those covering the surface of the papillae, express epithelial membrane antigen and thyroid transcription factor-1 but not cytokeratin (Fig. 12.2.29).[215,234–237] The two cell types show an identical pattern of monoclonality.[223]

Secondary changes include haemorrhage, haemosiderosis, foamy macrophage accumulation, sclerosis, focal dystrophic calcification, cystic degeneration and even a granulomatous

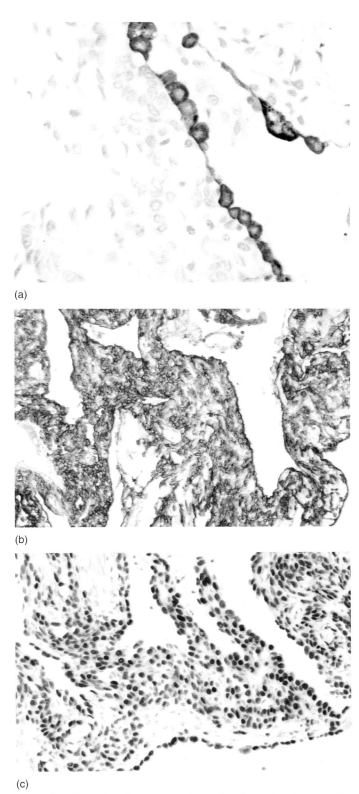

(a)

(b)

(c)

Figure 12.2.29 Sclerosing pneumocytoma. Only the surface tumour cells stain for cytokeratins (a) but both surface and stromal cells stain for epithelial membrane antigen (b) and thyroid transcription factor-1 (c).

reaction (Fig. 12.2.30).[238] The formation of 'giant lamellar bodies' is a further secondary change. These structures represent extracellular accumulations of surfactant material arranged in lamellar fashion and forming roughly spherical bodies that measure up to 25 μm in diameter.[239] They are not specific to sclerosing pneumocytomas but are encountered most frequently in these tumours.

Differential diagnosis

The relationship between sclerosing pneumocytoma and the inflammatory myofibroblastic tumour described on p. 609 was formerly confused by the application of terms such as histiocytoma and xanthoma to both. However, the two entities are quite distinct.[240] Although both may show fibrosis and xanthomatous change, they are usually distinguishable by the marked plasma cell and lymphocytic infiltrate of the inflammatory myofibroblastic tumour and the basic papillary structure of a sclerosing pneumocytoma.

Epithelioid haemangioendothelioma is another tumour characterised by sclerosis and a papillary structure, but it is generally multifocal and differs in its radiographic appearances and natural history as well as microscopically: furthermore, its stromal cells express endothelial rather than epithelial markers (see p. 625) and staining of TTF-1 is also negative.

Sclerosing pneumocytomas characterised by sheets of clear cells may be mistaken for the benign clear cell tumour of the lung described on p. 613 and also for metastatic renal cell carcinoma but they are distinguished from both these tumours by their TTF-1 and EMA positivity. Clear cell carcinoma of the lung is distinguished by showing malignant features and lacking the two cell types seen in sclerosing pneumocytoma. Papillary adenoma and alveolar adenoma similarly lack these two cell types. Separation of sclerosing pneumocytoma from papillary adenocarcinoma and adenoma may be difficult but the former generally shows atypia and both lack the distinctive stromal cells of a sclerosing pneumocytoma.[241]

PULMONARY THYMOMA

It is rare to encounter primary thymomas outside the mediastinum but examples have been described in the neck, trachea, thyroid, lung and pleura, sometimes associated with thymic rests in these tissues.[242–250] The diagnosis of thymoma in such sites requires careful review of the clinical and radiological findings to exclude metastasis or direct spread from a primary mediastinal lesion (see Fig. 12.6.15, p. 678).

Patients with pulmonary or pleural thymomas may be asymptomatic or complain of chest pain, weight loss or breathlessness. One patient with an intrapulmonary thymoma had myasthenia gravis.[242] Radiology shows a circumscribed central or peripheral pulmonary nodule, a pleural nodule, pleural thickening or pleural effusion. Occasionally there are multiple intrapulmonary tumours, or a thymoma may involve the pleura diffusely in the manner of a mesothelioma.[249]

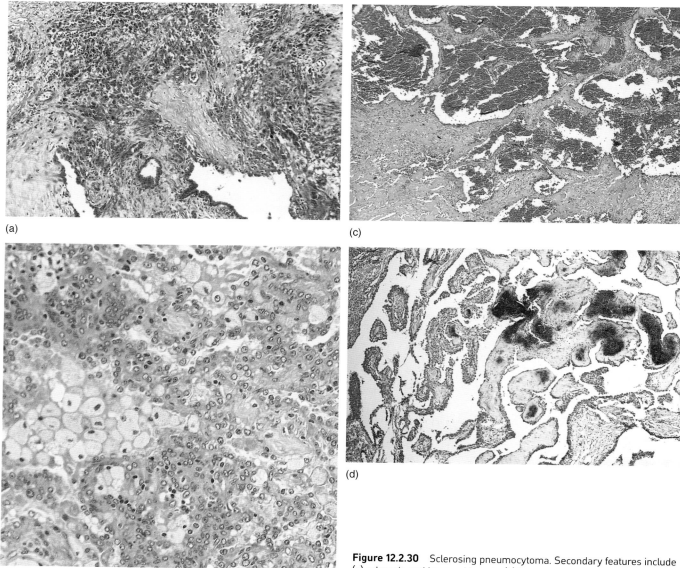

(a)

(c)

(b)

(d)

Figure 12.2.30 Sclerosing pneumocytoma. Secondary features include (a) sclerosis and haemosiderosis, (b) foamy macrophage accumulation, (c) angiomatoid change and (d) dystrophic calcification.

Pulmonary thymomas are identical to those that arise in the thymus but are not so clearly encapsulated. Infiltrative growth is therefore more difficult to assess. Some invasive tumours prove to be inoperable and others have metastasised.[248] However, most pulmonary thymomas are slowly growing tumours that can be cured by surgical resection.

Predominantly epithelial thymomas arising in the lung are likely to be mistaken for carcinoma, those of mixed cellularity for lymphoepithelial carcinoma, those predominantly lymphocytic for lymphoma or small cell carcinoma, and those of spindle cell pattern for localised fibrous tumour. Thymoma carries a better prognosis than many of these and a correct histological diagnosis is therefore important. Except in the case of lymphoepithelial carcinoma, the mixed cellularity of a thymoma is helpful in suggesting the correct diagnosis but sometimes electron microscopy is necessary.[245] The lymphocytes

within a thymoma express CD1a whereas those within a lymphoepithelial carcinoma or those reacting to a carcinoma do not. TTF-1 staining would indicate carcinoma of the lung, being found in about 30% of pulmonary large cell undifferentiated carcinomas but not in thymomas, while CD5 is more commonly expressed in thymomas.[251,252] Positive immunostaining for cytokeratin generally distinguishes spindle cell thymomas from both localised fibrous tumour and lymphoma.

REFERENCES

Carcinoid tumours, tumourlets and neuroendocrine cell hyperplasia

1. Lubarsch O. Ueber den primaren Krebs des Ileum nebst Bemerkungen uber das gleichzeitige Vorkommen Von Krebs und Tuberculose. Virchows Arch A Pathol Anat Histopathol 1888; 111:280–317.

2. Oberndorfer S. Karzinoide Tumoren des Dunndarmes. Frankf Z Pathol 1907; 1:426–432.

3. Hamperl H. Uber gutartige Bronchialtumoren (Cylindrome und Carcinoide). Virchows Arch A Pathol Anat Histopathol 1937; 300:46–88.

4. Bensch KG, Gordon GB, Miller LR. Electron microscopic and biochemical studies on the bronchial carcinoid tumor. Cancer 1965; 18:592–602.

5. Gmelich JT, Bensch KG, Liebow AA. Cells of Kultchitzsky type in bronchioles and their relation to the origin of peripheral carcinoid tumor. Lab Invest 1967; 17:88–98.

6. Bensch KG, Corrin B, Pariente R, Spencer H. Oat cell carcinoma of the lung: its origin and relationship to bronchial carcinoid. Cancer 1968; 22:1163–1172.

7. Godwin JD. Carcinoid tumors. Cancer 1975; 36:560–569.

8. Hurt R, Bates M. Carcinoid tumours of the bronchus: a 33 year experience. Thorax 1984; 39:617–623.

9. McCaughan BC, Martini N, Bains MS. Bronchial carcinoids. Review of 124 cases. J Thorac Cardiovasc Surg 1985; 89:8–17.

10. Hartman GE, Shochat SJ. Primary pulmonary neoplasms of childhood: a review. Ann Thorac Surg 1983; 36:108–119.

11. Wang LT, Wilkins EW, Bode HH. Bronchial carcinoid tumors in pediatric patients. Chest 1993; 103:1426–1428.

12. Miller MA, Mark GJ, Kanarek D. Multiple peripheral pulmonary carcinoids and tumorlets of carcinoid type, with restrictive and obstructive lung disease. Am J Med 1978; 65:373–378.

13. Gould VE, Linnoila I, Memoli VA, Warren WH. Neuroendocrine components of the bronchopulmonary tract in hyperplasias, dysplasias and neoplasms. Lab Invest 1983; 15:519–537.

14. Melmon KL, Sjoerdsma A, Mason DT. Distinctive clinical and therapeutic aspects of the syndrome associated with bronchial carcinoid tumors. Am J Med 1965; 39:568–581.

15. Ricci C, Patrassi N, Massa R, Mineo C, Benedetti-Valentini F. Carcinoid syndrome in bronchial adenoma. Am J Surg 1973; 126:671–677.

16. Sonksen PH, Ayres AB, Braimbridge M, et al. Acromegaly caused by pulmonary carcinoid tumours. Clin Endocrinol 1976; 5:503–513.

17. Okike N, Bernatz PE, Woolner LB. Carcinoid tumors of the lung. Ann Thorac Surg 1976; 22:270–277.

18. Huber RM, Schopohl J, Losa M, et al. Growth-hormone releasing hormone in a bronchial carcinoid. Cancer 1991; 67:2538–2542.

19. Bonikos DS, Bensch KG, Jamplis RW. Peripheral pulmonary carcinoid tumours. Cancer 1976; 37:1977–1998.

20. Felton WL, Liebow AA, Lindskog GF. Peripheral and multiple bronchial adenomas. Cancer 1953; 6:555–566.

21. Skinner C, Ewen SWB. Carcinoid lung: diffuse pulmonary infiltration by a multifocal bronchial carcinoid. Thorax 1976; 31:212–219.

22. Wise WS, Bonder D, Aikawa M, Hsieh CL. Carcinoid tumour of lung with varied histology. Am J Surg Pathol 1982; 6:261–267.

23. Salyer DC, Salyer WR, Eggleston JC. Bronchial carcinoid tumours. Cancer 1975; 36:1522–1537.

24. Jones RA, Dawson IMP. Morphology and staining patterns of endocrine tumours in the gut, pancreas and bronchus and their possible significance. Histopathology 1977; 1:137–150.

25. Barbareschi M, Frigo B, Mosca L, et al. Bronchial carcinoids with S-100 positive sustentacular cells. A comparative study with gastrointestinal carcinoids, pheochromocytomas and paragangliomas. Pathol Res Pr 1990; 186:212–222.

26. Gosney JR, Denley H, Resi M. Sustentacular cells in pulmonary neuroendocrine tumours. Histopathology 1999; 34:211–215.

27. Hironaka M, Fukayama M, Takayashiki N, et al. Pulmonary gangliocytic paraganglioma - Case report and comparative immunohistochemical study of related neuroendocrine neoplasms. Am J Surg Pathol 2001; 25:688–693.

28. Min KW. Spindle cell carcinoids of the lung with paraganglioid features: a reappraisal of their histogenetic origin from paraganglia using immunohistochemical and electronmicroscopic techniques. Ultrastruct Pathol 2001; 25:207–217.

29. Mark EJ, Quay SC, Dickerson GR. Papillary carcinoid tumor of lung. Cancer 1981; 48:316–324.

30. Ranchod M, Levine GD. Spindle-cell carcinoid tumours of the lung. Am J Surg Pathol 1980; 4:315–331.

31. Becker NH, Soifer I. Benign clear cell tumour ('sugar tumor') of the lung. Cancer 1971; 27:712–719.

32. Gaffey MJ, Mills SE, Frierson HF, Askin FB, Maygarden SJ. Pulmonary clear cell carcinoid tumor: Another entity in the differential diagnosis of pulmonary clear cell neoplasia. Am J Surg Pathol 1998; 22:1020–1025.

33. Sklar JL, Churg A, Bensch KG. Oncocytic carcinoid tumor of the lung. Am J Surg Pathol 1980; 4:287–292.

34. Scharifker D, Marchevsky A. Oncocytic carcinoid of lung: an ultrastructural analysis. Cancer 1981; 47:530–532.

35. Alvarez-Fernandez E, Folque-Gomez E. Atypical bronchial carcinoid with oncocytoid features. Arch Pathol Lab Med 1981; 105:428–431.

36. Cebelin MS. Melanocytic bronchial carcinoid tumor. Cancer 1980; 46:1843–1848.

37. Gould VE, Memoli VE, Dardi LE, et al. Neuroendocrine carcinomas with multiple immunoreactive peptides and melanin production. Ultrastruct Pathol 1981; 2:199–217.

38. Grazer R, Cohen SM, Jacobs JB, Lucas P. Melanin-containing peripheral carcinoid of the lung. Am J Surg Pathol 1982; 6:73–78.

39. Carlson JA, Dickersin GR. Melanotic paragangliod carcinoid tumor – a case report and review of the literature. Ultrastruct Pathol 1993; 17:353–372.

40. Fukuda T, Kobayashi H, Kamishima T, et al. Peripheral carcinoid tumor of the lung with focal melanin production. Pathol Int 1994; 44:309–316.

41. Iihara K, Yamaguchi K, Fujioka Y, Uno S. Pigmented neuroendocrine tumor of the lung, showing neuromelanin. Pathol Int 2002; 52:734–739.

42. Grogg KL, Padmalatha C, Leslie KO. Bronchial carcinoid tumor with crystalloid cytoplasmic inclusions. Arch Pathol Lab Med 2002; 126:93–96.

43. Gordon HW, Miller R, Mittman C. Medullary carcinoma of the lung with amyloid stroma: a counterpart of medullary carcinoma of the thyroid. Hum Pathol 1973; 4:431–436.

44. Abe Y, Utsunomiya H, Tsutsumi Y. Atypical carcinoid tumor of the lung with amyloid stroma. Acta Pathol Jpn 1992; 42:286–292.

45. Heard BE, Dewar A, Firmin RK, Lennox SC. One very rare and one new tracheal tumour found by electron microscopy: glomus tumour and acinic cell tumour resembling carcinoid tumours by light microscopy. Thorax 1982; 37:97–103.

46. Hage E. Histochemistry and fine structure of bronchial carcinoid tumours. Virchows Arch A Pathol Anat Histopathol 1973; 361:121–128.

47. Capella C, Gabrielli M, Polak JM, et al. Ultrastructural and histological study of 11 bronchial carcinoids. Virchows Arch A Pathol Anat Histopathol 1979; 381:313–329.

48. Fisher ER, Palekar A, Paulson JD. Comparative histopathologic histochemical, electron microscopic and tissue culture studies of bronchial carcinoids and oat cell carcinomas of lung. Am J Clin Pathol 1978; 69:165–172.

49. Warren WH, Memoli VA, Gould VE. Immunohistochemical and ultrastructural analysis of bronchopulmonary neuroendocrine neoplasms. I Carcinoids Ultrastruct Pathol 1984; 6:15–27.

50. Cutz E, Chan W, Kay JM, Chamberlain DW. Immunoperoxidase staining for serotonin, bombesin, calcitonin and leu-enkephalin in pulmonary tumourlets, bronchial carcinoids and oat cell carcinomas. Lab Invest 1982; 46:16A.

51. Bonato M, Cerati M, Pagani A, et al. Differential diagnostic patterns of lung neuroendocrine tumours – a clinico-pathological and immunohistochemical study of 122 cases. Virchows Arch A Pathol Anat Histopathol 1992; 420:201–211.

52. Loy TS, Darkow GVD, Quesenberry JT. Immunostaining in the diagnosis of pulmonary neuroendocrine carcinomas: an immunohistochemical study with ultrastructural correlations. Am J Surg Pathol 1995; 19:173–182.

53. Totsch M, Muller LC, Hittmair A, et al. Immunohistochemical demonstration of chromogranin-A and chromogranin-B in neuroendocrine tumors of the lung. Hum Pathol 1992; 23:312–316.

54. Gould VE, Wiedenmann B, Lee I, et al. Synaptophysin expression in neuroendocrine neoplasms as determined by immunocytochemistry. Am J Pathol 1987; 126:243–257.

55. Gosney JR, Gosney MA, Lye M, Butt SA. Reliability of commercially available immunocytochemical markers for identification of neuroendocrine differentiation in bronchoscopic biopsies of bronchial carcinoma. Thorax 1995; 50:116–120.

56. Boers JE, Denbrok JLM, Koudstaal J, Arends JW, Thunnissen FBJM. Number and proliferation of neuroendocrine cells in normal human airway epithelium. Am J Respir Crit Care Med 1996; 154:758–763.

57. Lantuejoul S, Moro D, Michalides RJAM, Brambilla C, Brambilla E. Neural cell adhesion molecules (NCAM) and NCAM-PSA expression in neuroendocrine lung tumors. Am J Surg Pathol 1998; 22:1267–1276.

58. Lyda MH, Weiss LM. Immunoreactivity for epithelial and neuroendocrine antibodies are useful in the differential diagnosis of lung carcinomas. Hum Pathol 2000; 31:980–987.

59. Roth KA, Ritter J, Mazoujian G. Central and peripheral bronchial carcinoids possess distinct peptide immunostaining patterns. In: Fenoglio-Preiser CM, Wolff M, Rilke F, eds. Progress in Surgical Pathology. Philadelphia: Field and Wood; 1992:241–250.

60. Rees LH, Bloomfield GA, Rees GM, et al. Multiple hormones in a bronchial tumor. J Clin Endocrinol Metab 1974; 38:1090–1097.

61. Erlandson RA, Nesland JM. Tumors of the endocrine/neuroendocrine system – an overview. Ultrastruct Pathol 1994; 18:149–170.

62. Chejfec G, Capella C, Solcia E, Jao W, Gould VE. Amphicrine cells, dysplasias and neoplasias. Cancer 1985; 56:2683–2690.

63. Geller SA, Gordon RE. Peripheral spindle-cell carcinoid tumour of the lung with type II pneumocyte features. Am J Surg Pathol 1984; 8:145–150.

64. Sheppard MN, Thurlow NP, Dewar A. Amphicrine differentiation in bronchioloalveolar cell carcinoma. Ultrastruct Pathol 1994; 18:437–441.

65. Blobel GA, Gould VE, Moll R, et al. Coexpression of neuroendocrine markers and epithelial cytoskeletal proteins in bronchopulmonary neuroendocrine neoplasms. Lab Invest 1985; 52:39–51.

66. Sturm N, Rossi G, Lantuejoul S, et al. Expression of thyroid transcription factor-1 in the spectrum of neuroendocrine cell lung proliferations with special interest in carcinoids. Hum Pathol 2002; 33:175–182.

67. Du E, Goldstraw P, Zacharias Z, et al. TTF-1 expression in tumorlets, typical and atypical carcinoids, and large cell neuroendocrine carcinomas. Hum Pathol 2004; 35:825–831.

68. Arrigoni MG, Woolner LB, Bernatz PE. Atypical carcinoid tumours of the lung. J Thorac Cardiovasc Surg 1972; 64:413–421.

69. Fink G, Krelbaum T, Yellin A, et al. Pulmonary carcinoid – Presentation, diagnosis, and outcome in 142 cases in Israel and review of 640 cases from the literature. Chest 2001; 119:1647–1651.

70. Mark EJ, Ramirez JF. Peripheral small-cell carcinoma of the lung resembling carcinoid tumour. Arch Pathol Lab Med 1985; 109:263–269.

71. Mills SE, Cooper PH, Walker AN, Kron IL. Atypical carcinoid tumor of the lung. Am J Surg Pathol 1982; 6:643–654.

72. Lequaglie C, Patriarca C, Cataldo I, et al. Prognosis of resected well-differentiated neuroendocrine carcinoma of the lung. Chest 1991; 100:1053–1056.

73. Struyf NJA, Vanmeerbeeck JPA, Ramael MRL, et al. Atypical bronchial carcinoid tumours. Respir Med 1995; 89:133–138.

74. Christinmaitre S, Chabbertbuffet N, Mure A, Boukhris R, Bouchard P. Use of somatostatin analog for localization and treatment of ACTH secreting bronchial carcinoid tumor. Chest 1996; 109:845–846.

75. Travis WD, Rush W, Flieder DB, et al. Survival analysis of 200 pulmonary neuroendocrine tumors with clarification of criteria for atypical carcinoid and its separation from typical carcinoid. Am J Surg Pathol 1998; 22:934–944.

76. Beasley MB, Thunnissen FBJ, Brambilla E, et al. Pulmonary atypical carcinoid: Predictors of survival in 106 cases. Hum Pathol 2000; 31:1255–1265.

77. Przygodzki RM, Finkelstein SD, Langer JC, et al. Analysis of p53, K-ras-2, and C-raf-1 in pulmonary neuroendocrine tumors: correlation with histological subtype and clinical outcome. Am J Pathol 1996; 148:1531–1541.

78. Onuki N, Wistuba II, Travis WD, et al. Genetic changes in the spectrum of neuroendocrine lung tumors. Cancer 1999; 85:600–607.

79. Addis BJ, Hamid Q, Ibrahim NBN, et al. Immunohistochemical markers of small cell carcinoma and related neuroendocrine tumours of the lung. J Pathol 1987; 153:137–150.

80. Barbareschi M, Detassis C, Palma PD, Arrigoni GL. Atypical bronchial carcinoids lack S-100 positive sustentacular cells. Pathol Res Pr 1991; 187:856.

81. Jackson-York GL, Davis BH, Warren WH, Gould VE, Memoli VA. Flow cytometric DNA content analysis in neuroendocrine carcinoma of the lung – correlation with survival and histologic subtype. Cancer 1991; 68:374–379.

82. Travis WD, Linnoila RI, Tsokos MG, et al. Neuroendocrine tumors of the lung with proposed criteria for large-cell neuroendocrine carcinoma – an ultrastructural, immunohistochemical, and flow cytometric study of 35 cases. Am J Surg Pathol 1991; 15:529–553.

83. Caulet S, Capron F, Ghorra C, et al. Flow cytometric DNA analysis of 20 bronchopulmonary neuroendocrine tumours. Eur Respir J 1993; 6:83–89.

84. Padberg BC, Woenchkhaus J, Hilger G, et al. DNA cytophotometry and prognosis in typical and atypical bronchopulmonary carcinoids: a clinicomorphologic study of 100 neuroendocrine lung tumors. Am J Surg Pathol 1996; 20:815–822.

85. Costes V, Martyane C, Picot MC, et al. Typical and atypical bronchopulmonary carcinoid tumors: a clinicopathologic and KI-67-labeling study. Hum Pathol 1995; 26:740–745.

86. Walch AK, Zitzelsberger HF, Aubele MM, et al. Typical and atypical carcinoid tumors of the lung are characterized by 11q deletions as detected by comparative genomic hybridization. Am J Pathol 1998; 153:1089–1098.

87. Brambilla E, Negoescu A, Gazzeri S, et al. Apoptosis-related factors p53, Bcl,2 and Bax in neuroendocrine lung tumors. Am J Pathol 1996; 149:1941–1952.

88. Ullmann R, Schwendel A, Klemen H, et al. Unbalanced chromosomal aberrations in neuroendocrine lung tumors as detected by comparative genomic hybridization. Hum Pathol 1998; 29:1145–1149.

89. Finkelstein SD, Hasegawa T, Colby T, Yousem SA. 11q13 allelic imbalance discriminates pulmonary carcinoids from tumorlets – A microdissection-based genotyping approach useful in clinical practice. Am J Pathol 1999; 155:633–640.

90. Ullmann R, Petzmann S, Klemen H, et al. The position of pulmonary carcinoids within the spectrum of neuroendocrine tumors of the lung and other tissues. Genes Chromosomes Cancer 2002; 34:78–85.

91. Petzmann S, Ullmann R, Klemen H, Renner H, Popper HH. Loss of heterozygosity on chromosome arm 11q in lung carcinoids. Hum Pathol 2001; 32:333–338.

92. Gugger M, Burckhardt E, Kappeler A, et al. Quantitative expansion of structural genomic alterations in the spectrum of neuroendocrine lung carcinomas. J Pathol 2002; 196:408–415.

93. World Health Organization. Tumours of the lung, pleura, thymus and heart. Lyons: IARC Press; 2004:

94. Whitwell F. Tumourlets of the lung. J Pathol Bacteriol 1955; 70:529–541.

95. Liebow AA. Tumours of the lower respiratory tract. Atlas of Tumor Pathology. Washington: Armed Forces Institute of Pathology; 1952:16.

96. Hausman DH, Weimann RB. Pulmonary tumorlet with hilar lymph node metastasis. Cancer 1967; 20:1515–1519.

97. D'Agati VD, Perzin KH. Carcinoid tumorlets of the lung with metastasis to a peribronchial lymph node. Cancer 1985; 55:2472–2476.

98. Canessa PA, Santini D, Zanelli M, Capecchi V. Pulmonary tumourlets and microcarcinoids in bronchiectasis. Monaldi Arch Chest Dis 1997; 52:138–139.

99. Heath D, Yacoub M, Gosney JR, et al. Pulmonary endocrine cells in hypertensive pulmonary vascular disease. Histopathology 1990; 16:21–28.

100. Johnson DE, Lock JE, Elde RP, Thompson TR. Pulmonary neuroendocrine cells in hyaline membrane disease and bronchopulmonary dysplasia. Pediatr Res 1982; 16:446–454.

101. Churg A, Warnock ML. Pulmonary tumorlet: a form of peripheral carcinoid. Cancer 1976; 37:1469–1477.

102. Pelosi G, Zancanaro C, Sbabo L, et al. Development of innumerable neuroendocrine tumorlets in pulmonary lobe scarred by intralobar

sequestration – immunohistochemical and ultrastructural study of an unusual case. Arch Pathol Lab Med 1992; 116:1167–1174.

103. Aguayo SM, Miller YE, Waldron JA, et al. Brief report – idiopathic diffuse hyperplasia of pulmonary neuroendocrine cells and airways disease. N Engl J Med 1992; 327:1285–1288.

104. Sheerin N, Harrison NK, Sheppard MN, et al. Obliterative bronchiolitis caused by multiple tumourlets and microcarcinoids successfully treated by single lung transplantation. Thorax 1995; 50:207–209.

105. Miller RR, Muller NL. Neuroendocrine cell hyperplasia and obliterative bronchiolitis in patients with peripheral carcinoid tumors. Am J Surg Pathol 1995; 19:653–658.

106. Armas OA, White DA, Erlandson RA, Rosai J. Diffuse idiopathic pulmonary neuroendocrine cell proliferation presenting as interstitial lung disease. Am J Surg Pathol 1995; 19:963–970.

107. Torikata C. Tumorlets of the lung – an ultrastructural study. Ultrastruct Pathol 1991; 15:189–195.

108. Gosney J, Green ART, Taylor W. Appropriate and inappropriate neuroendocrine products in pulmonary tumourlets. Thorax 1990; 45:679–683.

109. Ranchod M. The histogenesis and development of pulmonary tumorlets. Cancer 1977; 39:1135–1145.

110. Bonikos DS, Archibald R, Bensch KE. On the origin of the so-called tumourlets of the lung. Hum Pathol 1976; 7:461–469.

Salivary gland-type tumours

111. Spencer H. Bronchial mucous gland tumours. Virchows Arch A Pathol Anat Histopathol 1979; 383:101–115.

112. Rodriguez J, Diment J, Lombardi L, et al. Combined typical carcinoid and acinic cell tumor of the lung: A heretofore unreported occurrence. Hum Pathol 2003; 34:1061–1065.

113. Kimula Y. A histochemical and ultrastructural study of adenocarcinoma of the lung. Am J Surg Pathol 1978; 2:253–264.

114. Edwards CW. Pulmonary adenocarcinoma: review of 106 cases and proposed new classification. J Clin Pathol 1987; 40:125–135.

115. Terashima M, Nishimura Y, Nakata H, Iwai Y, Yokoyama M. Spontaneous coughing up of a polyp. Respiration 2000; 67:101–103.

116. Conlan AA, Payne WS, Woolner LB, Sanderson DR. Adenoid cystic carcinoma (cylindroma) and mucoepidermoid carcinoma of the bronchus. J Thorac Cardiovasc Surg 1978; 76:370–377.

117. Moran CA, Suster S, Koss MN. Primary adenoid cystic carcinoma of the lung - a clinicopathologic and immunohistochemical study of 16 cases. Cancer 1994; 73:1390–1397.

118. Gallagher CG, Stark R, Teskey J, Kryger M. Atypical manifestations of pulmonary adenoid cystic carcinoma. Br J Dis Chest 1986; 80:396–399.

119. Inoue H, Iwashita A, Kanegae H, et al. Peripheral pulmonary adenoid cystic carcinoma with substantial submucosal extension to the proximal bronchus. Thorax 1991; 46:147–148.

120. Azumi N, Battifora H. The cellular composition of adenoid cystic carcinoma. Cancer 1987; 60:1589–1598.

121. Nomori H, Kaseda S, Kobayashi K, et al. Adenoid cystic carcinoma of the trachea and main-stem bronchus. A clinical, histopathologic, and immunohistochemical study. J Thorac Cardiovasc Surg 1988; 96:271–277.

122. Tsubochi H, Suzuki T, Suzuki S, et al. Immunohistochemical study of basaloid squamous cell carcinoma, adenoid cystic and mucoepidermoid carcinoma in the upper aerodigestive tract. Anticancer Res 2000; 20:1205–1211.

123. Heitmiller RF, Mathisen DJ, Ferry JA, Mark EJ, Grillo HC. Mucoepidermoid lung tumours. Ann Thorac Surg 1989; 47:394–399.

124. Yousem SA, Hochholzer L. Mucoepidermoid tumours of the lung. Cancer 1987; 60:1346–1352.

125. Klacsmann PG, Olson JL, Eggleston JC. Mucoepidermoid carcinoma of the bronchus: an electron microscopic study of the low-grade and high-grade variants. Cancer 1979; 43:1720–1733.

126. Mullins JD, Barnes RP. Childhood bronchial mucoepidermoid tumours: a case report and review of the literature. Cancer 1979; 44:315–322.

127. Lack EE, Harris GBC, Eraklis AJ, Vawter GF. Primary bronchial tumours in childhood. Cancer 1983; 51:492–497.

128. Metcalf JS, Maize JC, Shaw EB. Bronchial mucoepidermoid carcinoma metastatic to skin. Report of a case and review of the literature. Cancer 1986; 58:2556–2559.

129. Wolf KM, Mehta D, Claypool WD. Mucoepidermoid carcinoma of the lung with intracranial metastases. Chest 1988; 94:435–438.

130. Green LK, Gallion TL, Gyorkey F. Peripheral mucoepidermoid tumour of the lung. Thorax 1991; 46:65–66.

131. Guillou L, Deluze P, Zysset F, Costa J. Papillary variant of low-grade mucoepidermoid carcinoma - an unusual bronchial neoplasm – a light microscopic, ultrastructural and immunohistochemical study. Am J Clin Pathol 1994; 101:269–274.

132. Cicutto LC, Chapman KR, Chamberlain D, Downey GP. Difficult asthma: consider all of the possibilities. Can Respir J 2000; 7:415–418.

133. Johansson M, Mandahl N, Johansson L, et al. Translocation 11; 19 in a mucoepidermoid tumor of the lung. Cancer Genet Cytogenet 1995; 80:85–86.

134. LopezTerrada D. Bloom MGK, Cagle PT, Ostrowski ML. Oncocytic mucoepidermoid carcinoma of the trachea. Arch Pathol Lab Med 1999; 123:635–637.

135. Stenman G, Petursdottir V, Mellgren G, Mark J. A child with a t(11;19)(Q14-21;p12) in a pulmonary mucoepidermoid carcinoma. Virchows Arch 1998; 433:579–581.

136. Romagosa V, Bella MR, Truchero C, Moya J. Necrotizing sialometaplasia (adenometaplasia) of the trachea. Histopathology 1992; 21:280–282.

137. Barsky SH, Martin SE, Matthews M, Gazdar A. Costa JC. 'Low-grade' mucoepidermoid carcinoma of the bronchus with 'high-grade' biological behavior. Cancer 1983; 51:1505–1509.

138. Vadasz P, Egervary M. Mucoepidermoid bronchial tumors: a review of 34 operated cases. Eur J Cardiothorac Surg 2000; 17:566–569.

139. Edwards CW, Matthews HR. Mucous gland adenoma of the bronchus. Thorax 1981; 36:147–148.

140. Heard BE, Corrin B, Dewar A. Pathology of seven mucous cell adenomas of the bronchial glands with particular reference to ultrastructure. Histopathology 1985; 9:687–701.

141. England DM, Hochholzer L. Truly benign 'bronchial adenoma' – report of 10 cases of mucous gland adenoma with immunohistochemical and ultrastructural findings. Am J Surg Pathol 1995; 19:887–899.

142. Chu PG, Weiss LM. Cytokeratin 14 immunoreactivity distinguishes oncocytic tumour from its renal mimics: an immunohistochemical study of 63 cases. Histopathology 2001; 39:455–462.

143. Matsuba K, Takizawa T, Thurlbeck W. Oncocytes in human bronchial mucous glands. Thorax 1972; 27:181–184.

144. Fechner RE, Bentinck BR. Ultrastructure of bronchial oncocytoma. Cancer 1973; 31:1451–1457.

145. Warter A, Walter P, Saboutchi M, Jory A. Oncocytic bronchial adenoma. Virchows Arch A Pathol Anat Histopathol 1981; 392:231–239.

146. Tashiro Y, Iwata Y, Nabae T, Manabe H. Pulmonary oncocytoma: report of a case in conjunction with an immunohistochemical and ultrastructural study. Pathol Int 1995; 45:448–451.

147. Laforga JB, Aranda FI. Multicentric oncocytoma of the lung diagnosed by fine-needle aspiration. Diagn Cytopathol 1999; 21:51–54.

148. Nielsen AL. Malignant bronchial oncocytoma: case report and review of the literature. Hum Pathol 1985; 16:852–854.

149. Sakamoto H, Uda H, Tanaka T, et al. Pleomorphic adenoma in the periphery of the lung – report of a case and review of the literature. Arch Pathol Lab Med 1991; 115:393–396.

150. Moran CA, Suster S, Askin FB, Koss MN. Benign and malignant salivary gland-type mixed tumors of the lung – clinicopathologic and immunohistochemical study of eight cases. Cancer 1994; 73:2481–2490.

151. Sweeney EC, McDermott M. Pleomorphic adenoma of the bronchus. J Clin Pathol 1996; 49:87–89.

152. Pomp J, Pannekoek BJM, Overdiep SH. Pleomorphic adenoma and severe tracheal obstruction. Resp Med 1998; 92:889–891.

153. Ang KL, Dhannapuneni VR, Morgan WE, Soomro IN. Primary pulmonary pleomorphic adenoma – An immunohistochemical study and review of the literature. Arch Pathol Lab Med 2003; 127:621–622.

154. Payne WS, Schier J, Woolner JB. Mixed tumors of the bronchus (salivary gland type). J Thorac Cardiovasc Surg 1965; 49:663–668.

155. Nicholson AG, Baandrup U, Florio R, Sheppard MN, Fisher C. Malignant myxoid endobronchial tumour: a report of two cases with a unique histological pattern. Histopathology 1999; 35:313–318.

156. Nistal M, Garciaviera M, Martinezgarcia C, Paniagua R. Epithelial myoepithelial tumor of the bronchus. Am J Surg Pathol 1994; 18:421–425.

157. Tsuji N, Tateishi R, Ishiguro S, Terao T, Higashiyama M. Adenomyoepithelioma of the lung. Am J Surg Pathol 1995; 19:956–962.

158. Wilson RW, Moran CA. Epithelial-myoepithelial carcinoma of the lung: Immunohistochemical and ultrastructural observations and review of the literature. Hum Pathol 1997; 28:631–635.

159. Shanks JH, Hasleton PS, Curry A, Rahman A. Bronchial epithelial-myoepithelial carcinoma. Histopathology 1998; 33:90–91.

160. Ryska A, Kerekes Z, Hovorkova E, Barton P. Epithelial-myoepithelial carcinoma of the bronchus. Pathol Res Pr 1998; 194:431–435.

161. Pelosi G, Fraggetta F, Maffini F, et al. Pulmonary epithelial-myoepithelial tumor of unproven malignant potential: Report of a case and review of the literature. Mod Pathol 2001; 14:521–526.

162. Fulford LG, Kamata Y, Okudera K, et al. Epithelial-myoepithelial carcinomas of the bronchus. Am J Surg Pathol 2001; 25:1508–1514.

163. Strickler JG, Hegstrom J, Thomas MJ, Yousem SA. Myoepithelioma of the lung. Hum Pathol 1987; 111:1082–1085.

164. Strickler JG, Hegstrom J, Thomas MJ, et al. Myoepithelioma of the lung. Arch Pathol Lab Med 1991; 111:1082–1085.

165. Higashiyama M, Kodama K, Yokouchi H, et al. Myoepithelioma of the lung: report of two cases and review of the literature. Lung Cancer 1998; 20:47–56.

166. Miura K, Harada H, Aiba S, Tsutsui Y. Myoepithelial carcinoma of the lung arising from bronchial submucosa. Am J Surg Pathol 2000; 24:1300–1304.

167. Veeramachaneni R, Gulick J, Halldorsson AO, Van TT, Zhang PL, Herrera GA. Benign myoepithelioma of the lung – A case report and review of the literature. Arch Pathol Lab Med 2001; 125:1494–1496.

168. Ukoha OO, Quartararo P, Carter D, Kashgarian M, Ponn RB. Acinic cell carcinoma of the lung with metastasis to lymph nodes. Chest 1999; 115:591–595.

169. Fechner RE, Bentinck BR, Askew JB. Acinic cell tumor of the lung. Cancer 1972; 29:501–508.

170. Moran CA, Suster S, Koss MN. Acinic cell carcinoma of the lung (Fechner tumor) – a clinicopathologic, immunohistochemical, and ultrastructural study of five cases. Am J Surg Pathol 1992; 16:1039–1050.

Papillomas

171. Dulmet-Brender E, Jaubert F, Huchon G. Exophytic endobronchial epidermoid carcinoma. Cancer 1986; 57:1358–1364.

172. Flieder DB, Koss MN, Nicholson A, et al. Solitary pulmonary papillomas in adults: A clinicopathologic and in situ hybridization study of 14 cases combined with 27 cases in the literature. Am J Surg Pathol 1998; 22:1328–1342.

173. Spencer H, Dail DH, Areaud AJ. Non-invasive bronchial epithelial papillary tumors. Cancer 1980; 45:1486–1497.

174. Trillo A, Guha A. Solitary condylomatous papilloma of the bronchus. Arch Pathol Lab Med 1988; 112:731–733.

175. Popper HH, Wirnsberger G, Juttner-Smolle FM, Pongratz MG, Sommersgutter M. The predictive value of human papilloma virus (HPV) typing in the prognosis of bronchial squamous cell papillomas. Histopathology 1992; 21:323–330.

176. Popper HH, Elshabrawi Y, Wockel W, et al. Prognostic importance of human papilloma virus typing in squamous cell papilloma of the bronchus: comparison of in situ hybridization and the polymerase chain reaction. Hum Pathol 1994; 25:1191–1197.

177. Syrjanen KJ. HPV infections and lung cancer. J Clin Pathol 2002; 55:885–891.

178. Henry M, Landers R, Kealy WF, Bredin CP. Solitary columnar bronchial papilloma: a rare endoscopic finding. Resp Med 1998; 92:878–879.

179. Basheda S, Gephardt GN, Stoller JK. Columnar papilloma of the bronchus – case report and literature review. Am Rev Respir Dis 1991; 144:1400–1402.

180. Assor D. A papillary transitional cell tumor of the bronchus. Am J Clin Pathol 1971; 55:761–764.

181. World Health Organization. Histological typing of lung tumours. Geneva, Switzerland: World Health Organization; 1981.

182. Michaels L, Young M. Histogenesis of papillomas of the nose and paranasal sinuses. Arch Pathol Lab Med 1995; 119:821–826.

183. Singer DB, Greenberg SD, Harrison GM. Papillomatosis of the lung. Am Rev Respir Dis 1966; 94:777–783.

184. Kramer SS, Wehunt WD, Kashima H. Pulmonary manifestations of juvenile laryngotracheal papillomatosis. AJR Am J Roentgenol 1985; 144:687–694.

185. Harada H, Miura K, Tsutsui Y, et al. Solitary squamous cell papilloma of the lung in a 40-year-old woman with recurrent laryngeal papillomatosis. Pathol Int 2000; 50:431–439.

186. Mounts P, Kashima H. Association of human papilloma virus subtype and clinical course in respiratory papillomatosis. Laryngoscope 1984; 94:28–33.

187. Terry RM, Lewis FA, Griffiths S, Wells M, Bird CC. Demonstration of human papillomavirus types 6 and 11 in juvenile laryngeal papillomatosis by in-situ hybridization. J Pathol 1987; 153:245–248.

188. Carey FA, Salter DM, Kerr KM, Lamb D. An investigation into the role of human papillomavirus in endobronchial papillary squamous tumours. Respir Med 1990; 84:445–447.

189. Yousem SA, Ohori NP, Sonmezalpan E. Occurrence of human papillomavirus DNA in primary lung neoplasms. Cancer 1992; 69:693–697.

190. Gelder CM, Williams OM, Hart KW, et al. HLA class II polymorphisms and susceptibility to recurrent respiratory papillomatosis. J Virol 2003; 77:1927–1939.

191. Helmuth RA, Strate RW. Squamous carcinoma of the lung in a nonirradiated, nonsmoking patient with juvenile laryngotracheal papillomatosis. Am J Surg Pathol 1987; 11:643–650.

192. Fechner RE, Goepfert H, Alford BR. Invasive laryngeal papillomatosis. Arch Otolaryngol 1974; 99:147–151.

193. Runckel D, Kessler S. Bronchogenic squamous carcinoma in nonirradiated juvenile laryngotracheal papillomatosis. Am J Surg Pathol 1980; 4:293–296.

194. Dallimore NS. Squamous bronchial carcinoma arising in a case of multiple juvenile papillomatosis. Thorax 1985; 40:797–798.

195. Guillou L, Sahli R, Chaubert P, et al. Squamous cell carcinoma of the lung in a non-smoking, nonirradiated patient with juvenile laryngotracheal papillomatosis – evidence of human papillomavirus-11 DNA in both carcinoma and papillomas. Am J Surg Pathol 1991; 15:891–898.

196. Wilde E, Duggan MA, Field SK. Bronchogenic squamous cell carcinoma complicating localized recurrent respiratory papillomatosis. Chest 1994; 105:1887–1888.

197. Orphanidou D, Dimakou K, Latsi P, et al. Recurrent respiratory papillomatosis with malignant transformation in a young adult. Respir Med 1996; 90:53–55.

198. Cook JR, Hill DA, Humphrey PA, Pfeifer JD, ElMofty SK. Squamous cell carcinoma arising in recurrent respiratory papillomatosis with pulmonary involvement: Emerging common pattern of clinical features and human papillomavirus serotype association. Mod Pathol 2000; 13:914–918.

199. Lele SM, Pou AM, Ventura K, Gatalica Z, Payne D. Molecular events in the progression of recurrent respiratory papillomatosis to carcinoma. Arch Pathol Lab Med 2002; 126:1184–1188.

Adenomas

200. Kurotaki H, Kamata Y, Kimura M, Nagai K. Multiple papillary adenomas of type-II pneumocytes found in a 13-year-old boy with von Recklinghausen's disease. Virchows Arch A Pathol Anat Histopathol 1993; 423:319–322.

201. Fantone JC, Geisinger KR, Appelman HD. Papillary adenoma of the lung with lamellar and electron dense granules. Cancer 1982; 50:2839–2844.

202. Noguchi M, Kodama T, Shimosato Y, et al. Papillary adenoma of type 2 pneumocytes. Am J Surg Pathol 1986; 10:134–139.

203. Fine G, Chang CH. Adenoma of type-2 pneumocytes with oncocytic features. Arch Pathol Lab Med 1991; 115:797–801.

204. Fukuda T, Ohnishi Y, Kanai I, et al. Papillary adenoma of the lung - histological and ultrastructural findings in 2 cases. Acta Pathol Jpn 1992; 42:56–61.

205. Hegg CA, Flint A, Singh G. Papillary adenoma of the lung. Am J Clin Pathol 1992; 97:393–397.

206. Dessy E, Braidotti P, DelCurto B, et al. Peripheral papillary tumor of type-II pneumocytes: a rare neoplasm of undetermined malignant potential. Virchows Arch 2000; 436:289–295.

207. Wada A, Tateishi R, Terazawa T, Matsuda M, Hattori S. Lymphangioma of the lung. Arch Pathol Lab Med 1974; 98:211–213.

208. Al-Hilli F. Lymphangioma (or alveolar adenoma?) of the lung. Histopathology 1987; 11:979–980.

209. Yousem SA, Hochholzer L. Alveolar adenoma. Hum Pathol 1986; 17:1066–1071.

210. Semeraro D, Gibbs AR. Pulmonary adenoma: a variant of sclerosing haemangioma of lung? J Clin Pathol 1989; 42:1222–1223.

211. Siebenmann RE, Odermatt B, Hegglin J. Binswanger RO. Das Alveolarzelladenom. Ein neu erkannter gutartiger Lungentumor. Pathologie 1990; 11:48–54.

212. Oliveira P, Nunes JFM, Clode AL, Dacosta JD, Almeida MO. Alveolar adenoma of the lung: further characterization of this uncommon tumour. Virchows Arch 1996; 429:101–108.

213. Bohm J, Fellbaum C, Bautz W, Prauer HW, Hofler H. Pulmonary nodule caused by an alveolar adenoma of the lung. Virchows Arch 1997; 430:181–184.

214. Burke LM, Rush WI, Khoor A, et al. Alveolar adenoma: A histochemical, immunohistochemical, and ultrastructural analysis of 17 cases. Hum Pathol 1999; 30:158–167.

215. Nicholson AG, Magkou C, Snead D, et al. Unusual sclerosing haemangiomas and sclerosing haemangioma-like lesions, and the value of TTF-1 in making the diagnosis. Histopathology 2002; 41:404–413.

216. Spencer H, Nambu S. Sclerosing haemangiomas of the lung. Histopathology 1986; 10:477–487.

217. Tanaka I, Inoue M, Matsui Y, et al. A case of pneumocytoma (so-called sclerosing hemangioma) with lymph node metastasis. Jpn J Clin Oncol 1986; 16:77–86.

Sclerosing pneumocytoma (sclerosing 'haemangioma')

218. Liebow AA, Hubbell DS. Sclerosing haemangioma (histiocytoma, xanthoma) of the lung. Cancer 1956; 9:53–75.

219. Chan K-W, Gibbs AR, Lo WS, Newman GR. Benign sclerosing pneumocytoma of lung (sclerosing haemangioma). Thorax 1982; 37:404–412.

220. Hill GS, Eggleston JC. Electron microscopic study of so-called pulmonary sclerosing haemangioma. Report of a case suggesting epithelial origin. Cancer 1972; 30:1092–1106.

221. Kennedy A. Sclerosing haemangioma of the lung: an alternative view of its development. J Clin Pathol 1973; 26:792–799.

222. Miyagawa-Hayashino A. Tazelaar HD, Langel DI, Colby TV. Pulmonary sclerosing Hemangioma with lymph node metastases – Report of 4 cases. Arch Pathol Lab Med 2003; 127:321–325.

223. Niho S, Suzuki K, Yokose T, et al. Monoclonality of both pale cells and cuboidal cells of sclerosing hemangioma of the lung. Am J Pathol 1998; 152:1065–1069.

224. Katzenstein A-LA, Gmelich JT, Carrington CB. Sclerosing hemangioma of the lung. A clinicopathologic study of 51 cases. Am J Surg Pathol 1980; 4:343–356.

225. Nagata N, Dairaku M, Ishida T, Sueishi K, Tanaka K. Sclerosing haemangioma of the lung. Cancer 1985; 55:116–123.

226. Yousem SA, Wick MR, Singh G, et al. So-called sclerosing hemangiomas of the lung. Am J Surg Pathol 1988; 12:582–590.

227. Ohori NP, Yousem SA, Sonmezalpan E, Colby TV. Estrogen and progesterone receptors in lymphangioleiomyomatosis, epithelioid hemangioendothelioma, and sclerosing hemangioma of the lung. Am J Clin Pathol 1991; 96:529–535.

228. Aihara T, Nakajima T. Sclerosing hemangioma of the lung - pathological study and enzyme immunoassay for estrogen and progesterone receptors. Acta Pathol Jpn 1993; 43:507–515.

229. Leong ASY, Chan KW, Seneviratne HSK. A morphological and immunohistochemical study of 25 cases of so-called sclerosing haemangioma of the lung. Histopathology 1995; 27:121–128.

230. Shibata R, Mukai M, Okada Y, et al. A case of sclerosing hemangioma of the lung presenting as a gigantic tumor occupying the left thoracic cavity. Virchows Arch 2003; 442:409–411.

231. Noguchi M, Kodama T, Morinaga S, et al. Multiple sclerosing haemangiomas of the lung. Am J Surg Pathol 1986; 10:429–435.

232. Lee ST, Lee YC, Hsu CY, Lin CC. Bilateral multiple sclerosing hemangiomas of the lung. Chest 1992; 101:572–573.

233. Khoury JD, Shephard MN, Moran CA. Cystic sclerosing haemangioma of the lung. Histopathology 2003; 43:239–243.

234. Devouassoux-Shisheboran M, Hayashi T, Linnoila RI, Koss MN, Travis WD. A clinicopathologic study of 100 cases of pulmonary sclerosing hemangioma with immunohistochemical studies – TTF-1 is expressed in both round and surface cells, suggesting an origin from primitive respiratory epithelium. Am J Surg Pathol 2000; 24:906–916.

235. RodriguezSoto J. Colby TV, Rouse RV. A critical examination of the immunophenotype of pulmonary sclerosing hemangioma. Am J Surg Pathol 2000; 24:442–450.

236. Chan ACL, Chan JKC. Pulmonary sclerosing hemangioma consistently expresses thyroid transcription factor-1 (TTF-1) – A new clue to its histogenesis. Am J Surg Pathol 2000; 24:1531–1536.

237. Illei PB, Rosai J, Klimstra DS. Expression of thyroid transcription factor-1 and other markers in sclerosing hemangioma of the lung. Arch Pathol Lab Med 2001; 125:1335–1339.

238. Moran CA, Zeren H, Koss MN. Sclerosing hemangioma of the lung – granulomatous variant. Arch Pathol Lab Med 1994; 118:1028–1030.

239. Perry LJ, Florio R, Dewar A, Nicholson AG. Giant lamellar bodies as a feature of pulmonary low-grade MALT lymphomas. Histopathology 2000; 36:240–244.

240. Arean WM, Wheat MW. Sclerosing hemangiomas of the lung. Am Rev Respir Dis 1962; 85:261–271.

241. Chan AC, Chan JK. Can pulmonary sclerosing haemangioma be accurately diagnosed by intra-operative frozen section? Histopathology 2002; 41:392–403.

Pulmonary thymoma

242. McBurney R, Clagget O, McDonald JR. Primary intrapulmonary neoplasms (thymoma?) associated with myasthenia gravis. Mayo Clin Proc 1951; 26:354–356.

243. Yeoh CB, Ford JM, Lattes R, Wylie RH. Intrapulmonary thymoma. J Thorac Cardiovasc Surg 1966; 51:131–136.

244. Kung ITM, Loke SL, So SY, et al. Intrapulmonary thymoma: report of two cases. Thorax 1985; 40:471–474.

245. Green WR, Pressoir R, Gumbs RV, et al. Intrapulmonary thymoma. Arch Pathol Lab Med 1987; 111:1074–1076.

246. James CL, Iyer PV, Leong AS-Y. Intrapulmonary thymoma. Histopathology 1992; 21:175–177.

247. Marchevsky AM. Lung tumors derived from ectopic tissues. Semin Diagn Pathol 1995; 12:172–184.

248. Moran CA, Suster S, Fishback NF, Koss MN. Primary intrapulmonary thymoma: a clinicopathologic and immunohistochemical study of eight cases. Am J Surg Pathol 1995; 19:304–312.

249. Payne CB, Morningstar WA, Chester EH. Thymoma of the pleura masquerading as diffuse mesothelioma. Am Rev Respir Dis 1960; 94:441–446.

250. Shih DF, Wang JS, Tseng HH, Tiao WM. Primary pleural thymoma. Arch Pathol Lab Med 1997; 121:79–82.

251. Pomplun S, Wotherspoon AC, Shah G, et al. Immunohistochemical markers in the differentiation of thymic and pulmonary neoplasms. Histopathology 2002; 40:152–158.

252. Fukayama M, Maeda Y, Funata N, et al. Pulmonary and pleural thymoma. Diagnostic application of lymphocyte markers to the thymoma of unusual site. Am J Clin Pathol 1988; 89:617–621.

12

Tumours

12.3

Soft tissue tumours

INFLAMMATORY MYOFIBROBLASTIC TUMOUR

A wide variety of names has been applied to this tumour, reflecting its varied cellular composition on the one hand and the confusion that exists over its nature on the other. It has been variously named plasma cell granuloma,[1,2] inflammatory pseudotumour,[3] xanthoma, xanthomatous pseudotumour, fibrous histiocytoma or histiocytoma,[2,4,5] mast cell tumour or mast cell granuloma,[6,7] and the currently favoured term, inflammatory myofibroblastic tumour.[8,8a] Most examples are pulmonary but these tumours have also been reported in many other sites, including the mesentery, mediastinum, soft tissue, larynx, stomach, oesophagus, intestine, liver, genitourinary tract, central nervous system, nerve, heart, skin and breast.

Clinical features

The age range stretches from the first year of life to the eighth decade but most patients are less than 40 years old and many are children.[1,2,9] This lesion is one of the most common primary lung tumours seen in young people.[10] The sexes are affected equally and there are no significant racial or geographical differences.

About half the patients are asymptomatic, the lesion being discovered as a chance radiological finding. Other patients complain of cough, haemoptysis, chest pain or dyspnoea, sometimes accompanied by systemic features that are possibly related to interleukin production by the lesion, namely low grade pyrexia, weight loss, microcytic hypochromic anaemia, polyclonal hyperglobulinaemia and a raised erythrocyte sedimentation rate.[11] Hypercalcaemia has also been recorded, apparently caused by the tumour secreting calcitriol.[12] HRCT typically shows a solitary mass with sharp regular borders, or if the tumour is endobronchial, obstructive pneumonia or atelectasis.[13]

Aetiology[14]

Inflammatory myofibroblastic tumours form a neoplastic subgroup of the rather nebulous and broad category 'inflammatory pseudotumours', which also includes several non-neoplastic fibroinflammatory mass lesions. Previous reports that they can be induced experimentally by irritants[15,16] and in man represent organising pneumonia[17] or antecedent infection[2,2,3,18,19] probably relate to the non-neoplastic varieties of inflammatory pseudotumour rather than inflammatory myofibroblastic tumour. However, some infective agents,[19–21] particularly human herpes-8 virus, may play a role in the development of these neoplasms.[22,23]

In a review of 118 cases, no instances of malignant change were identified[24] but there are examples of vascular invasion[25] and sarcomatous change with distant metastasis.[2,26,27] Chromosomal translocations, aneuploidy and monoclonality are being increasingly described.[28–33] The identification of 2p23 chromosomal aberrations associated with expression of anaplastic lymphoma kinase (ALK) in 33% of pulmonary examples favours a neoplastic basis.[32] Moreover, identical clonality in separate lesions supports a metastatic process.[34] Considerable weight is attached to these recent molecular findings and the predominant view today is that these tumours are either myofibroblastic or fibroblastic reticulum cell neoplasms of low malignant potential.[8,8a]

Pathology

The lesions occur with equal frequency on the two sides and are slightly more common in the lower lobes. There are instances of bilateral tumours, multiple lesions in the same lung, satellite nodules about the main mass and the simultaneous occurrence of pulmonary and extrapulmonary lesions.[1,9,25,35–37] There may be endobronchial extension with disruption of bronchial cartilage and polypoid protrusion into the lumen.[1,4,5,38] The lesions form rounded masses that can measure less than 1 cm or occupy the whole hemithorax.[1,2,39] They are sharply circumscribed and generally of firm consistency with a yellow, tan or grey cut surface (Fig. 12.3.1). Other examples may be softer and more fleshy, or even mucoid. Focal calcification may be apparent in the larger examples.

Microscopically, there are two major patterns, fibrous and inflammatory, but these are the ends of a spectrum and both are often seen in the same tumour. Generally, the tumours are composed of cellular or collagenised fibrous tissue heavily infiltrated by plasma cells, histiocytes, lymphocytes and foam cells in varying proportion (Fig. 12.3.2).[1,2,16,38,40] Mast cells occasionally predominate.[6,7] Eosinophils and neutrophils are infrequent. There is often hyalinisation, occasionally calcification and rarely ossification.[1,41] Central necrosis with the formation of a small cavity is occasionally seen. In more cellular areas, there may be a woven or 'storiform' pattern and mitoses may be seen. Plasma cells and lymphocytes tend to be most conspicuous at the periphery of the lesion where they often extend into adjacent lung as an interstitial infiltrate and sometimes form lymphoid follicles.

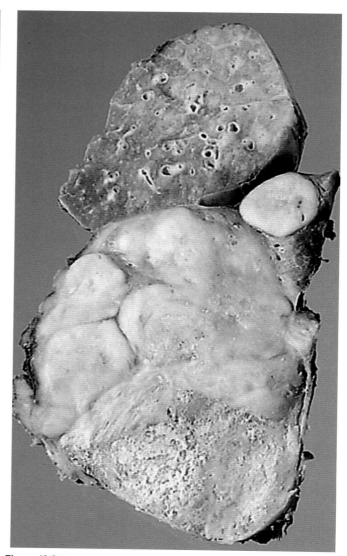

Figure 12.3.1 Inflammatory myofibroblastic tumour occupying the major part of the lower lobe with a satellite nodule at the hilum.

Russell bodies are often found in areas rich in plasma cells. There is no capsule and incorporation of lung tissue into the expanding mass may result in the presence of epithelial inclusions. The pulmonary architecture is generally effaced but vascular, perineural and bronchiolar invasion may be evident (Fig. 12.3.3). Histiocytes and foam cells, together with Touton giant cells, may either be interspersed with spindle cells or form discrete clusters. Some inflammatory myofibroblastic tumours consist largely of plump histiocytes set in a loose myxoid stroma in which there are few inflammatory cells. Some such examples have been incorrectly termed histiocytomas or xanthomas[3,16,38,40,42–44] but it is important that such examples are diagnosed correctly so that clinicians are aware of their more malignant growth potential.

Immunocytochemistry demonstrates the presence of vimentin and actin in most cases, and cytokeratin in one-third, consistent with the spindle cells being myofibroblasts.[8]

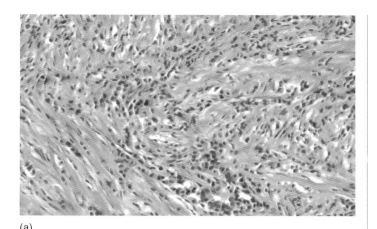

(a)

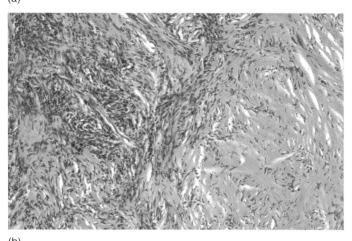

(b)

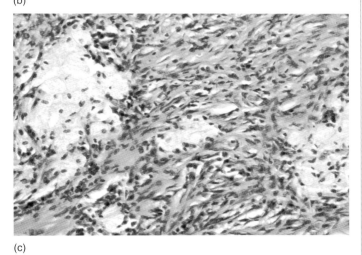

(c)

Figure 12.3.2 Inflammatory myofibroblastic tumour – variations in morphology. (a) Many plasma cells and lymphocytes are mixed with the myofibroblastic cells. (b) Inflammatory areas merge with areas of dense hyaline fibrosis. (c) Focal collections of foam cells are seen.

Immunocytochemistry also demonstrates the polytypic nature of the plasma cells[45–47] and in about half the cases cytoplasmic anaplastic lymphoma kinase (ALK), which correlates well with the presence of ALK gene rearrangements detected by *in situ* hybridisation.[32,48,49]

Ultrastructural studies[15,16,38–40,44,45,50,51] confirm that the spindle cells have the features of myofibroblasts, uncommitted mesenchymal cells or fibroblasts, and that the histiocytes may contain numerous myelin figures resulting from phagosomal activity.

Differential diagnosis

The differential diagnosis includes mycobacterial spindle cell tumour, sclerosing pneumocytoma, lymphoma, plasmacytoma, localised organising pneumonia, amyloid tumour, hyalinising granuloma, intrapulmonary localised fibrous tumour, malignant fibrous histiocytoma, follicular dendritic cell tumour, lymphoepithelial carcinoma, spindle cell carcinoma, localised fibromuscular scars and invasive fibrous tumour of the trachea.

Mycobacterial spindle cell tumours, as seen in AIDS patients (see p. 209), resemble the lesion now being considered but the spindle cells contain numerous mycobacteria and have the phenotype of macrophages rather than myofibroblasts. In a sclerosing pneumocytoma (see p. 599), large numbers of foam cells and fibrosis may produce an appearance similar to the xanthomatous variety of inflammatory myofibroblastic tumour but there are also papillary formations and angiomatoid areas that are not seen in the latter and the stromal cells stain for EMA and TTF-1. Lymphomas (see p. 648) are not so well circumscribed as inflammatory myofibroblastic tumours and like plasmacytomas (see p. 655), comprise a dense and often monotonous infiltrate of atypical monoclonal cells. In the most common primary lymphoma of the lung, marginal zone lymphoma of MALT origin, lymphoepithelial lesions are often prominent and the dense infiltrate mainly comprises CD20-positive B-lymphocytes. Organising pneumonia may produce a chronic inflammatory mass but this is generally irregular in outline, and a connective tissue stain will reveal the underlying lung architecture to be intact. Although hyaline areas resemble amyloid, stains for this substance are negative.[1] Hyalinising granuloma (see p. 687) is less cellular than inflammatory myofibroblastic tumour and affected patients are older while histologically, the inflammation is less intense and is more pronounced peripherally. The possibility that hyalinising granuloma represents an aged inflammatory myofibroblastic tumour cannot be excluded but the different geographical distribution of the two diseases is against this. However, progression to calcifying fibrous pseudotumour (see p. 717) is suggested by a unique case that showed such a combination of patterns.[52]

When fibrohistiocytic elements predominate, inflammatory myofibroblastic tumour needs to be distinguished from malignant fibrous histiocytomas and on addressing this problem one group found necrosis, bizarre giant cells, numerous mitoses, high cellularity and poor circumscription to be more significant histological features of malignancy than nuclear pleomorphism and atypical mitoses.[53] Others rely on inflammatory myofibroblastic tumours lacking cytological atypia, pleomorphism and abnormal mitoses,[46] or recommend p53 oncogene identification as an indicator of malignancy.[54] Occasional cases may however undergo sarcomatous transforma-

epithelial carcinoma and inflammatory sarcomatoid carcinoma (see pp. 558, 561) are both distinguished by their epithelial markers and cytological atypia.

Course of the disease

In most cases, growth is slow and occasional instances of arrested growth[56] or spontaneous resolution are recorded.[9] Indeed, some cases of calcified fibrous pseudotumour of the lung may represent involuted inflammatory myofibroblastic tumours.[52] The majority of lesions are resected before the diagnosis has been established and this is usually curative. Attempts at enucleation may be followed by recurrence,[24] possibly with mediastinal extension mimicking sclerosing mediastinitis.[1] If the pleural surface is involved and the tumour is adherent to chest wall or mediastinum, excision may be difficult and the usual good prognosis adversely affected. Infiltration of vessels at a distance from the main tumour mass has been reported and occasionally death is due to extension into pulmonary veins or oesophagus.[18,25,45,51] Exceptional instances of sarcomatous change have been referred to above.[2,27,57]

The histological features provide a poor prediction of behaviour. Aneuploidy appears to correlate better with a more aggressive course[58] while in one series of extrapulmonary inflammatory myofibroblastic tumours a combination of aneuploidy, atypia, ganglion-like cells and p53 expression was identified as providing the best predictor of aggressive behaviour.[59]

PLEUROPULMONARY BLASTOMA

Unlike other tumours that have been termed pulmonary blastoma (see pp. 551, 563) pleuropulmonary blastoma lacks an epithelial component and consists entirely of primitive blastema showing varying lines of sarcomatous differentiation. These tumours may be pulmonary, pleural or mediastinal and are largely confined to childhood.[60–64] They appear to be the true embryonic tumour or blastoma of the lung. This is supported by cytogenetic analysis, which has revealed partial trisomy of chromosome 2q, an abnormality that has also been reported in hepatoblastoma and embryonal rhabdomyosarcoma.[65,66] It is also noteworthy that pleuropulmonary blastoma has been reported in association with familial cystic nephroma.[67] In the past, pleuropulmonary blastoma has been reported under a variety of terms, including cystic blastoma and sarcomas or malignant mesenchymoma arising in congenital cysts.[68–75]

Clinical features

Patients are usually less than 12 years old and of either sex but rare cases have been reported in adults.[76] The patient may be asymptomatic but there is usually chest pain, breathlessness and fever. Imaging shows a cystic or solid peripheral mass, possibly accompanied by pneumothorax.[60–62,64,77,78] The cystic tumours are generally found in the youngest patients.[64]

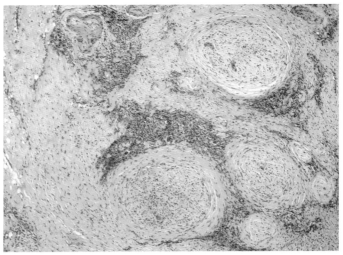

(a)

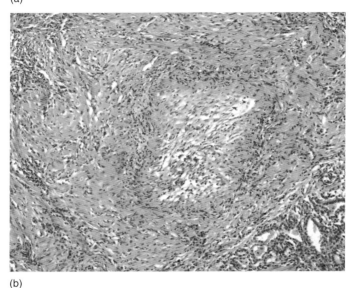

(b)

Figure 12.3.3 Inflammatory myofibroblastic tumour. (a) Invasion of the chest wall with widespread perineural infiltration. (b) Vascular invasion may also be seen, in this instance within the lung parenchyma.

tion. Follicular dendritic cell tumours, which may extend into the lungs from the mediastinum, closely resemble the fibrohistiocytic variant of inflammatory myofibroblastic tumour and may only be distinguished by the use of dendritic cell markers such as CD21 and CD35; confusion between these two entities may have led to some reports of malignant change in extrapulmonary inflammatory myofibroblastic tumours.

Intrapulmonary localised fibrous tumours are identical to those that occur in the pleura (see p. 714) and are usually subpleural. They also lack the inflammatory component of myofibroblastic tumours and their CD34 positivity is a further distinguishing feature. Invasive fibrous tumour of the trachea[55] is not a well-defined entity and some examples may have represented inflammatory myofibroblastic tumours. Lympho-

Pathological features

Pleuropulmonary blastomas form large multilobed masses that may be difficult to resect. Cystic (type 1), partly cystic (type 2) and solid (type 3) varieties are described.[64] The cysts may be unilocular or multilocular. In the type 2 lesions, the solid component may be limited to a nodule of tumour protruding into the cyst. The solid areas sometimes show necrosis and haemorrhage.

Microscopically, small round or spindle-shaped blastomatous cells comprise the malignant component and in the cystic varieties these cells are typically concentrated immediately beneath a lining epithelium in a so-called cambium layer (Fig. 12.3.4). The cysts are lined by a non-neoplastic epithelium. Solid areas consist of sheets of a similar blastema, but often with a greater degree of pleomorphism, mitotic activity and divergent sarcomatous differentiation resulting in foci of rhabdomyosarcoma or chondrosarcoma (Fig. 12.3.5). Very cellular areas alternating with others composed of looser myxoid tissue may result in an appearance resembling that of a Wilms tumour.

Differential diagnosis

Low-grade cystic examples resemble both mesenchymal cystic hamartoma and type 4 congenital cystic adenomatoid malformation (see pp. 71, 62). Indeed, type 4 congenital cystic adenomatoid malformation may be a precursor of pleuropulmonary blastoma in the way that type 1 congenital cystic adenomatoid malformations give rise to adenocarcinoma and nephrogenic rests antedate Wilms' tumour. In the few published cases of type 4 congenital cystic adenomatoid malformation small areas of cellular blastomatous proliferation may be seen[79] and it is arguable that such cases are better classified as type 1 pleuropulmonary blastomas.[64] Staining with desmin may be helpful as focal areas are sometimes positive in pleuropulmonary blastoma.[64,79,80] Well-differentiated fetal adenocarcinoma and pulmonary blastoma are excluded by the absence of malignant epithelial elements. Pleuropulmonary blastoma is distinguished from malignant small cell tumour of the thoracopulmonary region (Askin tumour, see p. 720) by its location in the periphery of the lung rather than the chest wall, cystic nature and focal sarcomatous differentiation, while in doubtful cases CD99 staining and chromosomal analysis may be helpful.

Treatment and prognosis

The long-term survival is 25–50%,[60] with the solid variety and those involving the pleura or mediastinum having a particularly poor prognosis.[64] The 5-year survival rate for type 1 pleuropulmonary blastoma is 83% compared with 42% for types 2 and 3.[64] Younger patients are more likely to have surgically resectable lower grade tumours. Complete surgical resection is important as these tumours tend to recur in a more malignant form.[81,82]

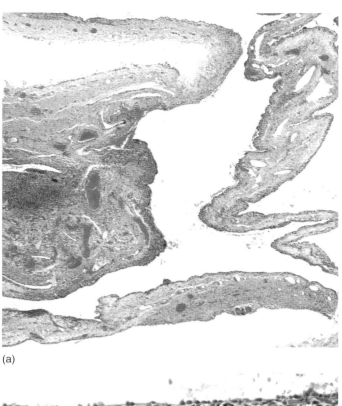

(a)

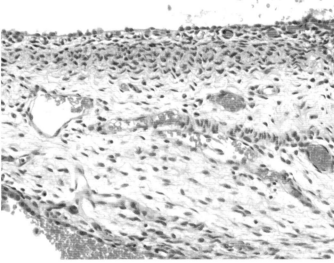

(b)

Figure 12.3.4 Pleuropulmonary blastoma. Cystic (type 1) variant. (a) The tumour forms a multiloculated cyst. Even at low power, foci of stromal cellularity are identifiable. (b) Stromal hypercellularity sometimes forms a subepithelial 'cambium' layer.

BENIGN CLEAR CELL TUMOUR ('SUGAR TUMOUR')

This is a particularly rare tumour of uncertain nature that was first described in abstract form in 1963 and in full in 1971.[83,84] About 50 cases have been described to date.[83–98] They span a wide age range (8–73 years, mean 49 years) and have an equal

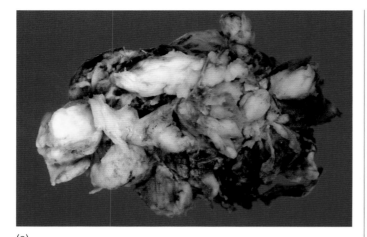

(a)

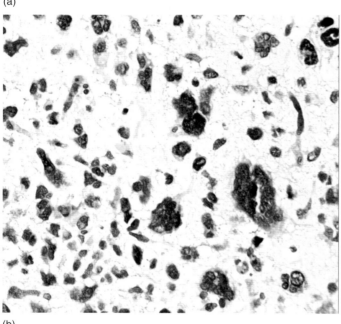

(b)

Figure 12.3.5 Pleuropulmonary blastoma. Solid (type 3) variant (a) Recurrence of a cystic type 1 pleuropulmonary blastoma in solid form. (b) Microscopy shows undifferentiated sarcoma with marked pleomorphism.

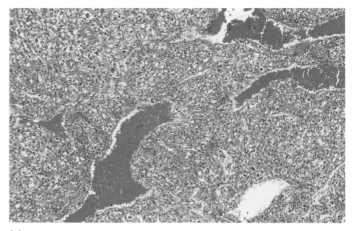

(a)

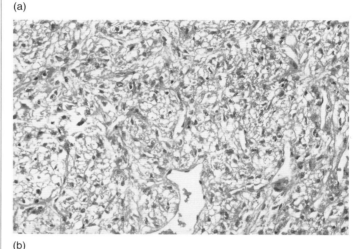

(b)

Figure 12.3.6 Benign clear cell tumour. Trabeculae of cells with clear cytoplasm are separated by thin-walled sinusoidal vessels. (a) low power; (b) high power.

sex incidence. Most patients are asymptomatic and the tumour is often an incidental finding in chest radiographs, where it is seen as a solitary 'coin lesion' in the periphery of the lung. Upper and lower lobes are equally affected. Although initially believed to be unique to the lung, examples of clear cell tumour have now been reported in the trachea, pancreas, ligamentum teres hepatis, rectum, uterus, vulva, breast and heart, a few of which have exhibited aggressive behaviour, sometimes metastasising to the lungs.[99-106] Certain abdominopelvic sarcomas of perivascular epithelioid cells appear to represent further malignant examples of extrapulmonary clear cell tumours.[107] In the lungs, lobectomy, wedge resection or even simple enucleation is generally curative, but in one case widespread metastases resulted in death 17 years after resection.[91,108]

Pathology

On gross inspection, the tumour has a sharp outline and lacks any obvious connection with major airways, blood vessels or pleura. The cut surface is often haemorrhagic: otherwise it is a translucent pinkish-grey and not yellow, as are many renal carcinomas. Necrosis is rare; it was only present in the case that metastasised and may therefore augur malignancy.[91,108-110]

The microscopic appearances are rather uniform, consisting of sheets and cords of large polygonal or spindle cells with distinct outlines and abundant clear cytoplasm that is generally rich in glycogen (Fig. 12.3.6), a feature that has given rise to the colloquial term 'sugar tumour'. A few reticulin fibres representing type IV collagen surround individual tumour cells.[98] Nuclei are hyperchromatic and often have irregular outlines. Binucleate, or even multinucleate, cells may be present. Mitoses are generally absent. Although the cytoplasm is characteristically clear it may contain fine eosinophil granules which sometimes appear to radiate from the nucleus. Lipochrome is found

Table 12.3.1 Features of benign clear cell tumour and other pulmonary clear cell tumours

Tumour markers	Glycogen	Fat	Mucin	Vessels	NE	HMB45	S-100	CK	EMA	TTF-1
Benign clear cell tumour	+	−	−	Sinusoidal	−	+	+	−	−	−
Metastatic renal carcinoma	+	+	−	Arterial	−	−	−	+	+	−
Clear cell carcinoma of the lung	−	−	+ or −	Arterial	−	−	−	+	+	+/−
Clear cell carcinoid	−	−	−	Sinusoidal	+	−	−/+*	+	+	−/+
Sclerosing pneumocytoma	−	+	−	Arterial	−	−	−	+	+	+

+, present; −, absent. CK, cytokeratins; NE, neuroendocrines.
*Positive in sustentacular cells.

in some tumour cells. A rich blood supply is evident in many parts of the tumour, taking the form of large thin-walled sinusoidal vessels that lack a muscle coat (Fig. 12.3.6). Hyaline connective tissue may form around or within vessel walls and occasionally this progresses to more extensive fibrosis with calcification. Inclusions lined by bronchiolar or alveolar epithelium probably represent entrapment of adjacent lung tissue.

Histogenesis

Firm agreement has yet to be reached regarding the nature of the benign clear cell tumour but there is increasing evidence that it represents a 'PEComa' (a tumour of 'perivascular epithelioid cells' – see below). Previously suggested lines of derivation or differentiation include neuroendocrine cell,[85,87,93,109] Clara cell,[89] melanocyte,[94] smooth muscle and pericyte.[86,90,97] Immunocytochemical stains for epithelial markers are negative[89,93,95] while neuron specific enolase, synaptophysin, CD56 actin, S-100, vimentin and CD34 are variably expressed.[93,94,98] Electron microscopy generally confirms the presence of glycogen but reports are otherwise inconsistent.[86,89,92,98] However, ultrastructural evidence of melanogenesis[94] is in line with reports that HMB45 (human melanin black-45) is consistently and diffusely expressed, a feature that benign clear cell tumours share with lymphangioleiomyomatosis (see p. 295) and angiomyolipoma (see p. 619).[98,111–113] This has led to suggestions that these lesions all derive from a putative 'perivascular epithelioid cell'[113,114] and raise the possibility that benign clear cell tumour should be added to the spectrum of pulmonary manifestations of tuberous sclerosis (see p. 488).[96,115] A unique hybrid lesion in which the features of a benign clear cell tumour were intermingled with those of lymphangioleiomyomatosis is described in a woman lacking any other features of tuberous sclerosis,[116] while two patients have been reported with benign clear cell tumours of the uterus associated with lymphangioleiomyomatosis of the pelvic lymph nodes, and in one of them tuberous sclerosis.[104]

Differential diagnosis

The importance of this lesion lies in its distinction from clear cell carcinoma of the lung, either primary (see p. 556) or metastatic from the kidney or elsewhere.[117] The major differences are outlined in Table 12.3.1. The characteristic vascular pattern is helpful, the wide thin-walled sinusoids of the benign tumour contrasting with the thick-walled narrow arterioles of a carcinoma. Renal carcinomas owe their seemingly empty cytoplasm to the presence of both glycogen and fat and it is useful to be able to demonstrate the latter if reserve tissue is available. A diastase-controlled periodic acid-Schiff stain is also useful in distinguishing mucus-secreting adenocarcinomas of solid pattern from the glycogen-rich benign tumour. Chemodectoma, carcinoid and haemangiopericytoma all contain sinusoidal vessels on occasion but lack significant quantities of glycogen and only haemangiopericytoma has reticulin surrounding individual cells.

'HAMARTOMA' (CHONDROID HAMARTOMA, ADENOCHONDROMA, MIXED MESENCHYMOMA)

Despite their popular name – chondroid hamartoma – it is likely that these lesions are benign connective tissue neoplasms rather than tumour-like malformations.[118–121] They are widely regarded as being hamartomatous because of their disorganised mix of the various connective and epithelial tissues normally found in the lung but their rarity in childhood and continued growth in adult life favour them being neoplasms, albeit benign. The identification of chromosomal rearrangements (6p21 and 12q14-15) similar to those found in lipomas and leiomyomas[122,123] also favours neoplasia rather than malformation. Terms such as adenochondroma, adenofibroma[124] and fibroadenoma[125] imply a benign mixed neoplasm but it is now appreciated that epithelial structures are commonly entrapped in many lung tumours, both primary and metastatic,[126,127] and this is how the epithelial clefts of the so-called adenochondroma or chondroid hamartoma should be regarded. A name that reflects a purely mesenchymal nature appears appropriate and, since these tumours display a variety of connective tissues, the term mesenchymoma has been recommended.[120] However, the term 'hamartoma' is well-entrenched and continues to be used.

Clinical features

These tumours are fairly common, constituting about 8% of all 'coin' lesions in chest radiographs (see Table 12.1.6, p. 537). In an unselected post mortem series, an incidence of 1 in 400 was

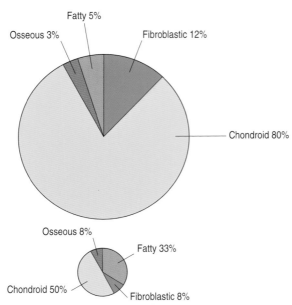

Fatty 5%

Osseous 3%

Fibroblastic 12%

Chondroid 80%

Osseous 8%

Fatty 33%

Chondroid 50%

Fibroblastic 8%

Figure 12.3.7 The predominant tissue in a series of 154 'hamartomas' comprising 142 parenchymal (top) and 12 endobronchial (bottom) tumours.[120]

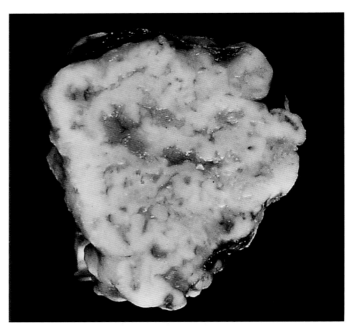

Figure 12.3.8 A 'hamartoma' of the lung forming a 4.5 cm tumour that 'shelled out' at operation.

found.[128] The age range is wide but they are rare in children; the peak age incidence is the sixth decade and they are more common in men.[120] Sequential radiographs show that most first develop in adult life and slowly increase in size thereafter. Most are parenchymal and asymptomatic but about 8% are endobronchial[120] and cause coughing, dyspnoea, haemoptysis, obstructive pneumonia or collapse.[129,130] Multiple lesions are uncommon, as is involvement of the trachea;[120,131–134] multiplicity raises the possibility of Carney's triad (see below).[135] An accompanying carcinoma of the lung is encountered more frequently than expected[120,136] but this may be fortuitous, the carcinoma causing the chest to be investigated so that an asymptomatic 'hamartoma' is revealed. Sarcomatous change is recorded but is exceptionally rare.[137] One study identified a high incidence of associated congenital anomalies and benign tumours, prompting the authors to envisage a 'pulmonary hamartoma syndrome'.[138]

Pathological features[119–121]

There are no significant pathological differences between parenchymal and endobronchial growths, although the proportions in which the various connective tissues are represented differ (Fig. 12.3.7) and epithelial clefts are less prominent in endobronchial than parenchymal tumours.[119,139,140] Most measure 1–3 cm in diameter but they range up to 9 cm. They lack a capsule but are sharply circumscribed and shell out easily at operation (Fig. 12.3.8), after which there is little risk of recurrence. Most are lobulated and the predominant tissue is cartilage (Fig. 12.3.9), which may calcify or undergo osseous change.

Other connective tissues commonly found include fat, fibrous tissue and loose mesenchyme with a myxoid appearance (Fig. 12.3.10). These various components are usually present in combination, together with cells of transitional form.[121] The lesions may come close to the bronchial cartilage but there is no continuity with this tissue, as there is in tracheobronchopathia osteochondroplastica; fibromyxoid spindle cells probably represent the progenitor mesenchymal element.[121] The connective tissue components are quite regular cytologically and show no evidence of malignancy. Intersecting the connective tissue lobules are clefts lined by ciliated pseudostratified columnar epithelium, which is quite normal cytologically. The retention of cilia is notable, as these are usually lost when respiratory epithelium becomes neoplastic.

Differential diagnosis

There is a close genetic relationship between 'hamartoma' and other benign mesenchymal tumours such as lipoma, chondroma and fibroma (which are discussed below) but these entities can be excluded histologically because they consist of just one mesenchymal tissue. More difficulty may be encountered if metastatic teratoma is removed from the lung following successful chemotherapy and submitted for pathological examination with inadequate clinical information (see p. 677).

Treatment and prognosis

The parenchymal tumours are often enucleated or removed by wedge resection but lobectomy may be undertaken if there is

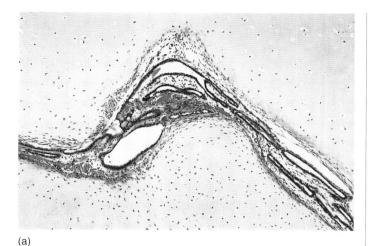

(a)

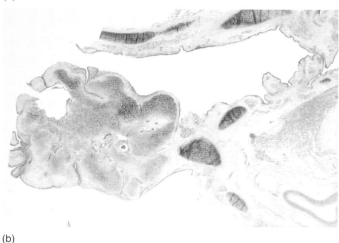

(b)

Figure 12.3.9 (a) A 'hamartoma' composed of mature cartilage intersected by clefts lined by respiratory epithelium. (b) A polypoid endobronchial 'hamartoma', which is also predominantly composed of cartilage.

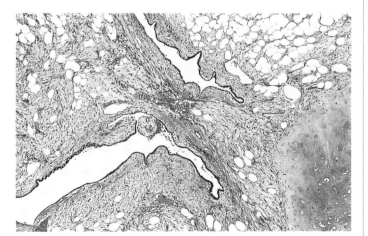

Figure 12.3.10 A 'hamartoma' formed of myxoid fibrous tissue and fat as well as cartilage.

chronic parenchymal damage. Endobronchial lesions are generally treated by bronchoplastic resection. Recurrence is rare[120] and sarcomatous transformation even rarer.[137]

LIPOMA, CHONDROMA AND FIBROMA

If the proposed nature of the 'hamartomas' (mixed mesenchymomas) outlined above is accepted, they are obviously closely related to benign connective tissue neoplasms composed of a single tissue – lipomas,[141–144] chondromas[145,146] and fibromas[147] for example – none of which is common in the lungs.[119] Like the mixed mesenchymomas, all these neoplasms may either lie entirely within the lung substance or protrude into major bronchi (Fig. 12.3.11), but the proportion of lipomas and chondromas that are endobronchial is higher than the 8% found with the so-called hamartomas. Epithelial clefts are not found in single tissue benign mesenchymal tumours, which resemble in every way their counterparts that occur more commonly in other parts of the body. Like chondroid hamartomas, they appear to have no malignant potential: the rare primary pulmonary fibrosarcomas, liposarcomas, chondrosarcomas and osteosarcomas (dealt with below) are believed to be sarcomatous from their outset.

Carney's triad

This is a rare combination of three unusual neoplasms that affects young women.[145,146,148–150] The patients are generally in the second or third decade, the youngest recorded being a girl aged 9 years. The three tumours are pulmonary chondromas, extraadrenal paragangliomas (chemodectomas) and gastric stromal tumours (epithelioid leiomyosarcoma). In a review of 79 patients, 85% were female, 22% presented with three tumours and 78% with two. The most common combination was one that included gastric and pulmonary tumours. Intervals up to 26 years between detection of the first and second components were noted but the mean is 8 years. A total of 13% of patients died of the disorder and some cases are familial.[151] Early recognition of the syndrome is important in view of the malignant potential of the gastric lesions and paragangliomas. Pulmonary metastases from one or other of these may be difficult to distinguish from chondromas clinically but calcification in pulmonary opacities is a useful radiographic pointer to the opacities being chondromas. The chondromas have no malignant potential. They differ from chondroid 'hamartomas' in lacking both epithelial clefts and other connective tissue components (Fig. 12.3.12) and in being encapsulated. They are generally peripheral growths.[146] Concurrent duodenal stromal tumour, pulmonary chondromatous 'hamartoma' and pancreatic islet cell tumour in a 63-year-old man has been reported as a possible variant of Carney's triad.[152] Adrenocortical adenomas may also be associated with Carney's triad[151] but the significance of this observation is uncertain as these tumours are very common in the general population.

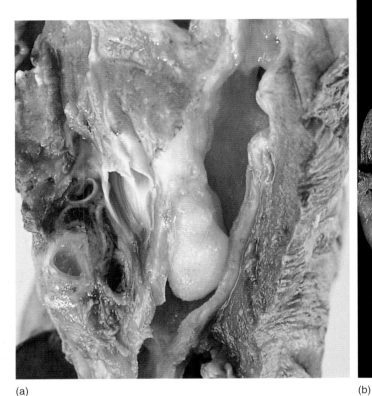

(a)

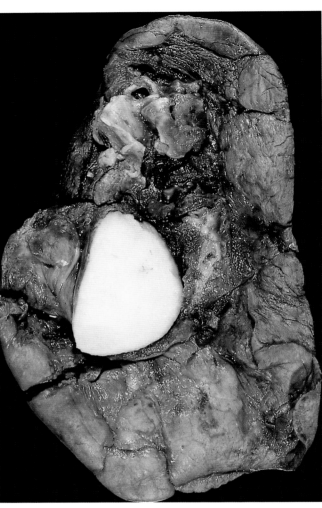

(b)

Figure 12.3.11 Examples of endobronchial (a) and parenchymal (b) lipomas. (Illustration of the parenchymal lesion provided by Dr JT Gmelich, Pasadena, USA.)

HISTIOCYTOMA

Pulmonary lesions that have all the features of benign fibrous histiocytomas, as described in other sites, have been widely regarded as forming part of a plasma cell granuloma/histiocytoma complex but most would now be regarded as inflammatory myofibroblastic tumours (see p. 609) and every effort should be made to confirm this diagnosis. Nevertheless, true fibrous histiocytomas very rarely occur in the lungs whereas most 'cystic fibrohistiocytic tumours' of the lungs are metastases from low-grade cellular fibrous histiocytomas (see Ch. 12.5).[153]

LEIOMYOMA AND FIBROLEIOMYOMA

A diagnosis of primary pulmonary leiomyoma or fibroleiomyoma should be advanced only with caution. Pulmonary tumours corresponding to these terms often prove to be multiple and confined to middle-aged women with uterine fibroids, representing examples of so-called benign metastasising leiomyomas of the uterus (see p. 676). In the rare instances in which the patient is male, a history of previous surgery for a 'soft tissue tumour' can often be elicited. True primary leiomyomas that develop in the lungs are distinctly rare.[154–159]

Patients with a pulmonary leiomyoma may be of any age, from infancy onwards. The sex incidence is equal. The tumours may involve the airways or be peripheral, the former usually giving rise to symptoms resulting from obstruction while the latter are often discovered by chance in an asymptomatic person. Pulmonary leiomyosarcomas developing in AIDS are referred to below under miscellaneous sarcomas.

Pulmonary leiomyomas resemble those encountered in other sites in every way (Fig. 12.3.13). They show a well-developed fascicular pattern and lack features suggesting malignancy, such as atypia, haemorrhage and necrosis. Immunostaining for smooth muscle actin supports the diagnosis.

Leiomyomas of the lung are well-circumscribed tumours, in contrast to the more frequently seen fibromuscular scars that are stellate in outline and lack a definite edge. These may be rich in smooth muscle and are often considered to be smooth muscle hamartomas but if there is any appreciable degree of fibrosis a more likely explanation is that they represent old scars in which there is prominent reactive smooth muscle hyperplasia. Diffuse changes of this nature are often seen in end-stage diffuse pulmonary fibrosis and the term 'muscular cirrhosis of the lung' has been used for this (see p. 272). A case reported as 'diffuse fibro-leiomyomatous hamartomatosis'[160] is possibly just a further example of 'muscular cirrhosis'. Pulmonary lymphangioleiomyomatosis is another diffuse infiltrative process rather than a circumscribed tumour (see p. 295). Other conditions to be distinguished from leiomyoma include the CD34 positive intrapulmonary localised fibrous tumour (see p. 714), nerve sheath tumours, which are S100 positive, inflammatory myofibroblastic tumour, which generally shows a lymphoplasmacytic infiltrate, and epithelial-myoepithelial carcinoma (see p. 595), which expresses epithelial as well as muscle markers.

ANGIOMYOLIPOMA

Angiomyolipomas are rare benign tumours composed of a mixture of small to medium-sized blood vessels, smooth muscle and fat, all of which appear quite mature. They are most commonly found in the kidney, but have been reported in a variety of other sites, including the lung.[161–163] One pulmonary angiomyolipoma has been reported in a patient suffering from tuberous sclerosis but not lymphangioleiomyomatosis, two conditions that are sometimes associated with extrapulmonary angiomyolipomas (see p. 298).[164] Angiomyolipomas express the melanocyte marker HMB45, which is also found in the 'perivascular epithelioid cells' of lymphangioleiomyomatosis (see p. 295) and the benign clear cell tumour of the lung that is dealt with above.[165] Angiomyolipomas have been regarded as hamartomas rather than neoplasms but the demonstration of clonality casts doubt upon this.[166]

MISCELLANEOUS SARCOMAS

Bronchopulmonary sarcomas are rare, outnumbered by carcinomas 700 to 1.[167] They generally appear to arise without antecedent lesions but occasional examples have developed in bronchial cysts[70,168] and arteriovenous fistulas,[169] or after radiation therapy.[170] However, some of those 'arising' in bronchial cysts would now be recognised to be pleuropulmonary blastomas (see above). More recently, leiomyosarcomas have been encountered in many organs, including the lung, in association with Epstein–Barr virus in AIDS[171,172] and following transplantation.[173]

Except for a few notable exceptions that have arisen in children,[70,171,174] sarcomas of the lung generally affect the middle-aged and elderly. Many varieties are described, all of which

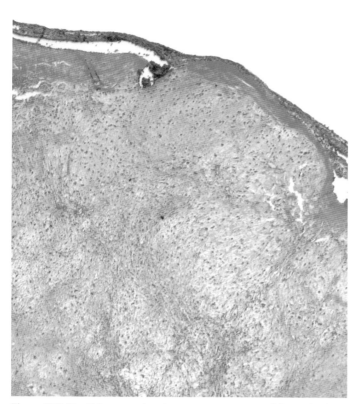

Figure 12.3.12 Pulmonary chondroma as a component of Carney's triad. The tumour is composed solely of benign chondroid elements. (Section provided by Dr TV Colby, Scottsdale, USA.)

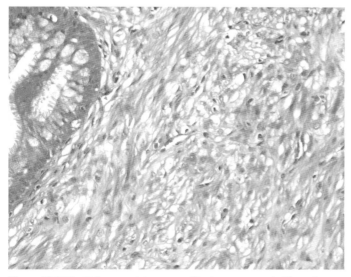

Figure 12.3.13 Pulmonary leiomyoma. The tumour, resected from the lung of a male patient, comprises cytologically bland spindle cells with abundant eosinophilic cytoplasm, as seen in leiomyomas arising at other sites.

resemble their counterparts elsewhere in the body. They should be categorised according to current criteria for soft tissue tumours independent of their origin in the lungs.

Most pulmonary sarcomas derive from smooth muscle or fibrous tissue[175–178] or are anaplastic. In recent years malignant fibrous histiocytoma has been separated from fibrosarcoma, and examples have been reported in the lung.[170,179–187] The most common histological subtype is storiform-pleomorphic but the inflammatory and giant cell subtypes may also be encountered in the lung.[179,188] They contain foam cells, giant cells and myofibroblasts as well as fibroblasts. They have to be distinguished from inflammatory myofibroblastic tumour (see above) by the usual cytological criteria of malignancy and from spindle cell carcinoma by their lack of epithelial markers such as cytokeratin.

It is likely that certain low-grade fibrous tumours, some of which have been reported as haemangiopericytomas, are intrapulmonary examples of the localised fibrous tumours more usually encountered in the pleura (see p. 714) despite lacking a pleural connection.[189,190] Support for this comes from their growth pattern in tissue culture[191] and CD34 positivity.[192]

Malignant nerve sheath tumours arising in the lung as opposed to other intrathoracic sites are particularly rare[193,194] and, in the absence of von Recklinghausen's disease, may be mistaken for fibrosarcoma. They are dealt with more fully on p. 629. Other rare varieties include liposarcoma,[195] rhabdomyosarcoma,[196] chondrosarcoma,[197–200] osteosarcoma,[201] giant cell tumour,[202] alveolar soft part sarcoma[203] and angiosarcoma.[204,205] Myxoid change may be prominent in several of these sarcomas.[206,207] Synovial sarcomas of both monophasic spindle cell and biphasic pattern have been described as arising in the lung:[187,208–211] they express cytokeratins, EMA and the bcl-2 oncogene and show the t(X;18)(p11.2;q11.2) translocation seen in synovial sarcomas of soft tissues (Fig. 12.3.14). Sarcomas arising in the major pulmonary blood vessels are described on p. 627. Occasionally a pulmonary sarcoma may elaborate multiple mesenchymal elements such as bone, cartilage and striated muscle and is best described as a malignant mesenchymoma.[212]

A distinction is generally made between endobronchial and intrapulmonary sarcomas, at least as far as the most common varieties, leiomyosarcoma and fibrosarcoma, are concerned: the endobronchial tumours present earlier and have the better prognosis.[175,199] Small intrapulmonary sarcomas may metastasise early but large intrapulmonary growths are equally lethal due to direct invasion of the chest wall and mediastinum. Tumour grade and mitotic activity give a good indication of the degree of malignancy.[176,177]

VASCULAR TUMOURS AND PROLIFERATIONS

Haemangioma and lymphangioma

Haemangiomas and lymphangiomas of the lung are very rare.[213–223] Some of the cases reported before immunocytochem-

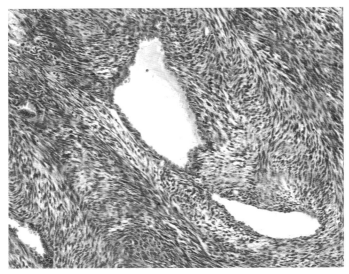

(a)

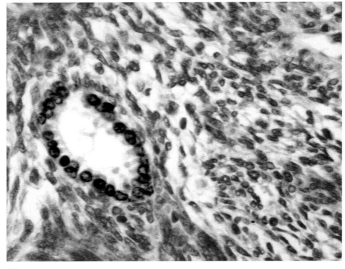

(b)

Figure 12.3.14 Synovial sarcoma of the lung. (a) A monophasic synovial sarcoma surrounds residual entrapped air spaces. (b) Staining for TTF-1 confirms that gland-like structures are indeed entrapped lung elements and not part of a biphasic synovial sarcoma.

istry was available were possibly examples of alveolar adenoma (see p. 598) or sclerosing pneumocytoma (see p. 599), the distinction from which can generally be made by immunohistochemical staining for endothelial markers (factor VIII and CD31), cytokeratins, EMA and TTF-1. Pulmonary haemangiomas and lymphangiomas resemble the commoner such tumours found elsewhere: they form circumscribed lesions consisting of dilated, closely apposed, endothelium-lined vascular spaces which share adventitial connective tissue but lack a media (Fig. 12.3.15). Histologically, they differ only in their content – blood or lymph, but it is notoriously difficult to tell whether the presence of blood is genuine or artefactual, justify-

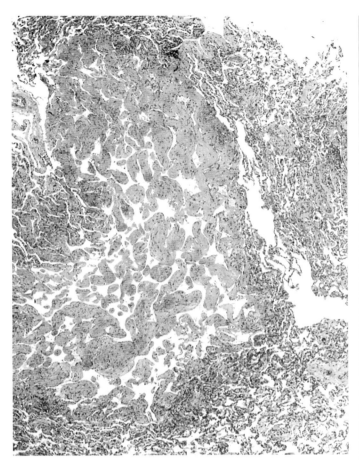

Figure 12.3.15 Lymphangioma of the lung. A localised mass composed interweaving vascular channels devoid of blood.

ing the use of the non-committal term angioma. Sometimes a haemangioma forms a pedunculated endobronchial tumour.[224] More often it is an asymptomatic parenchymal mass but there is always the danger of life-threatening haemorrhage.

Haemangiomatosis and lymphangiomatosis

Pulmonary haemangiomatosis is a rare condition in which the lungs may be affected diffusely (Fig. 12.3.16) or by multifocal nodules. The diffuse form is most frequently encountered in very young children as part of a generalised vascular malformation affecting many viscera and soft tissues.[225,226] The multifocal form is more often confined to the lungs and may present in later life. Pulmonary lesions manifest themselves by causing haemoptysis, shortness of breath, haemorrhagic pleural effusions and pneumonia. Vascular fragility and thrombocytopenia due to platelet trapping both contribute to the haemorrhage. The lungs are infiltrated diffusely or in a multifocal manner by a network of vascular spaces of varying size. The infiltration is particularly prominent where there is abundant connective tissue – beneath the pleura, in interlobular septa and around airways. Arteriovenous communication is not a feature and the

disease is not hereditary. It thus differs from arteriovenous fistula and hereditary haemorrhagic telangiectasia (see below). It should also be distinguished from pulmonary peliosis (see below), and from capillary haemangiomatosis (see p. 429). Tracheobronchial haemangiomatosis is recorded in blue rubber bleb disease accompanying the more usual cavernous haemangiomas of the skin and gastrointestinal tract.[227]

A similar condition involving lymphatic channels is known as lymphangiomatosis (Figs 12.3.17, 12.3.18),[219,228–230] while if the nature of the vascular channels is uncertain the term angiomatosis may be used.[231] Although generally a disorder of children, lymphangiomatosis may first present in adult life.[232] It causes shortness of breath, tiredness and chylous effusions. Chest radiographs show bilateral reticular infiltrates, often more marked in the lower lobes. The lung markings represent a proliferation of anastomosing endothelium-lined channels along pulmonary lymphatic routes, especially the pleura and interlobular septa, accompanied by spindle cells, which stain for smooth muscle actin. The histological appearances resemble those of congenital lymphangiectasia (see p. 75) but differ in the greater number of lymphatics while the prominent vascular lumina distinguish the condition from lymphangioleiomyomatosis (see p. 295). There may be associated abnormalities of the thoracic and retroperitoneal lymphatics.[232,233] In one example the lungs were compressed by a mass of dense connective tissue containing numerous dilated lymphatic pathways which invaded the chest wall and diaphragm.[234] Pulmonary lymphangiomatosis may also form part of the Klippel–Trenaunay syndrome, the more common manifestations of which are soft tissue hypertrophy, angiomas and varicosities (see p. 483).

Pulmonary telangiectasia

Telangiectasias are localised dilatations of small precapillary blood vessels, which in the lungs may be so small that they are not evident on chest radiographs. Multiple pulmonary telangiectasias occur in two unrelated conditions, hereditary haemorrhagic telangiectasia (Rendu–Osler–Weber disease, see p. 483) and cirrhosis of the liver. Patients with liver failure due to cirrhosis occasionally present with hypoxia due to pulmonary shunts through vascular lesions analogous to cutaneous spider naevii, casts of which show them to consist of both dilated existing vessels and newly formed channels.[235–238]

Pulmonary peliosis

Peliosis is well known in the liver as a rare vascular anomaly of uncertain aetiology. Extrahepatic peliosis is exceptional but very rarely, pulmonary involvement has been reported in association with similar lesions in the liver and spleen.[239,240] One such patient was receiving anabolic steroids, which is often the case with peliosis hepatis. The pulmonary lesion was an unexpected postmortem finding in one case but another patient died of haemoptysis from rupture of a peliotic lesion in the lungs. Pulmonary peliosis consists of multiple, irregularly distributed, thin-walled blood spaces of variable size.

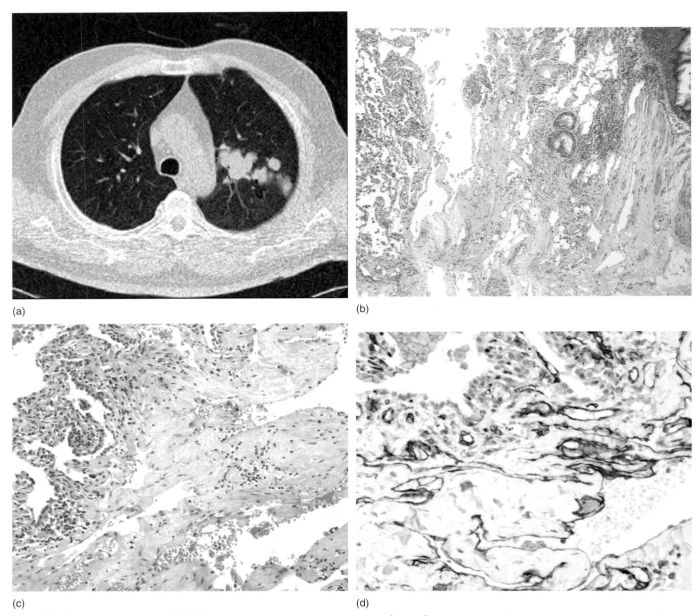

(a)

(b)

(c)

(d)

Figure 12.3.16 Haemangiomatosis. (a) HRCT shows a serpiginous mass in the lung. (b and c) The bronchial wall and alveolar parenchyma are infiltrated by anastomosing vascular channels. (d) CD31 stain demonstrates that the channels have an endothelial lining.

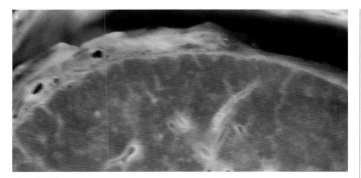

Figure 12.3.17 Lymphangiomatosis. The pleura is markedly thickened and the interlobular septa are unduly prominent.

Haemangiopericytoma

The histological boundaries between haemangiopericytoma and localised fibrous tumour have become increasingly blurred and it is likely that most of the tumours reported as pulmonary haemangiopericytomas[176,241–247] were intrapulmonary localised fibrous tumours. The latter are described on p. 714 and no further attention will be paid to haemangiopericytoma.

Glomus tumour

Rare instances of glomus tumour (glomangioma) have been reported in the trachea[248–254] and lung,[255–260] suggesting that the

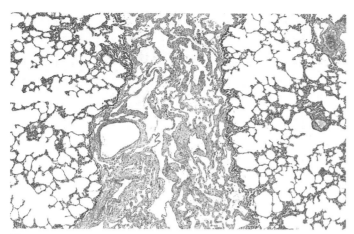

Figure 12.3.18 Lymphangiomatosis. An interlobular septum is thickened by the presence of numerous lymphatics.

specialised arteriovenous anastomoses familiar in the nailbeds also exist in the lower respiratory tract. The histological appearances are identical to those of glomus tumours elsewhere and for the most part they are similarly benign in their behaviour. The affected patients were adults who were asymptomatic or presented with cough or non-specific symptoms and were found to have well demarcated nodules in their major airways or lungs.

Pathology

Glomus tumours consist of a network of vessels of capillary size surrounded by small, uniform, rounded cells with moderate amounts of eosinophilic or clear cytoplasm, set in a hyaline or myxoid stroma. Occasionally they undergo oncocytic transformation.[251] The nuclei are round with finely dispersed chromatin and indistinct nucleoli (Fig. 12.3.19). A reticulin or periodic acid-Schiff stain reveals a fine basement membrane network surrounding individual tumour cells. Immunohistochemical stains are positive for vimentin and actin, weakly so for desmin and negative for cytokeratins, melanocytic markers (HMB-45, S-100 protein) and CD31. Markers of endothelium (factor VIII-related antigen, CD34) stain the vasculature but not the tumour cells. On electron microscopy there is abundant basement membrane and the cells contain prominent cytoplasmic filaments with dense bodies and rows of pinocytotic vesicles,[248,249,255] features very similar to those of smooth muscle although there is little resemblance on light microscopy.

Differential diagnosis

Many of the immunohistochemical and ultrastructural features of glomus cells are also seen in pericytes but these cells are more elongated, have long processes and far fewer myofilaments and dense bodies. Glomus cells, pericytes and smooth muscle cells are closely related[261] but the differential diagnosis is unlikely to include haemangiopericytoma and leiomyoma. However, the distinction from carcinoid tumour (see p. 583)

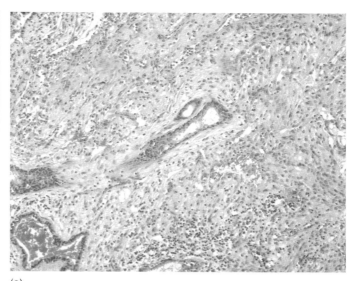

(a)

(b)

Figure 12.3.19 An endobronchial glomus tumour. (a) The tumour surrounds entrapped gland ducts. (b) The tumour cells have clear cytoplasm, are cytologically bland and are in close apposition to capillaries.

may be difficult by light microscopy, particularly in a small biopsy.[260] Helpful histological features are the distinctive reticulin pattern of a glomus tumour and the absence of immunohistochemical staining for cytokeratins and neuroendocrine differentiation.

Prognosis

Most pulmonary glomus tumors are benign. Only a few glomangiosarcomas are recorded in the lung, some disseminating widely to extrapulmonary sites.[258,262] Their malignant nature is evidenced by brisk mitotic activity, cytological atypia and necrosis.

Kaposi's sarcoma

Epidemiology and aetiology

Kaposi's sarcoma was initially known as a rare sporadic disease of elderly European men, usually of Italian or Jewish ancestry, and as a more frequent disease affecting younger men, and occasionally women and children in central and east Africa. More recently the disease has become more widespread and immunodeficiency has been recognised as a risk factor. Groups at particular risk now include transplant recipients, patients being treated for leukaemia or lymphoma, and those suffering from AIDS.[263–267,287,288] These patients suffer from a particularly aggressive disseminated form of the disease. Up to 70% of AIDS patients in the USA formerly developed Kaposi's sarcoma,[268–270] but the proportion is now less. A notable feature is that these cases are almost all men who acquired their HIV by homosexual contact whereas the tumour is rare in AIDS patients infected with HIV by intravenous injection.[263,271–274] This suggests sexual transmission of a causative agent, presumably a virus distinct from but often transmitted with HIV.[275] This is supported by a reduction in the incidence of the tumour as homosexual promiscuity lessens and by the identification of human herpes virus 8 in lesional tissue from patients with all forms of Kaposi's sarcoma.[276–283] DNA sequences unique to this virus appear to be preferentially associated with Kaposi's sarcoma, serosal lymphoma, some inflammatory myofibroblastic tumours and multicentric Castleman's disease.[284] Their identification in bronchoalveolar lavage fluid appears to be highly sensitive and specific for pulmonary involvement by Kaposi's sarcoma.[285]

Following the identification of human herpes virus 8-associated Kaposi sarcoma in the Uygurs of Xinjiang, Northwest China, a serological survey of the region identified the virus in a high proportion of the population, leading to speculation that it had been carried thither (or thence) by travellers on the ancient silk road connecting Europe and China.[286]

Clinical features

The sporadic European form of the disease is characterised by purple macules on the skin of the legs and feet. It generally runs an indolent course. Visceral lesions are present in 10 to 20% of patients, with lymph nodes, gastrointestinal tract, liver, lungs, heart, bone and spleen involved in descending order of frequency.[289] Very rarely, predominantly pulmonary involvement is seen without skin lesions.[265,290–292] In Africa, Kaposi's sarcoma accounts for up to 15% of all tumours and is more aggressive: lymphadenopathy and pulmonary involvement are common.[293,294]

Pulmonary involvement by Kaposi's sarcoma is often overlooked, partly because co-existing opportunistic infections blur the clinical and radiographic appearances and partly because open lung biopsy is often thought necessary to make the diagnosis. In most cases, visceral lesions are preceded by cutaneous disease but this is not always the case.[287,288,290,292,293] About 16% of one group of HIV-positive patients had bronchial lesions but no mucocutaneous disease.[295]

The most common symptom of pulmonary Kaposi's sarcoma is breathlessness, which may be accompanied by cough, wheezing or haemoptysis. Pleural effusion is frequently present. Chest radiographs show either diffuse pulmonary infiltrates, fine nodularity or a combination of the two. The changes are often bilateral.[296] Mucosal lesions may be seen at bronchoscopy as bright red raised areas. The prognosis in AIDS is adversely affected by the development of pulmonary Kaposi's sarcoma as this introduces the added risks of pulmonary haemorrhage, pulmonary oedema due to lymphatic obstruction and airway narrowing.

Pathology[291,293,297,298]

At autopsy, multiple small haemorrhagic nodules are found scattered throughout the lungs and visible in the tracheobronchial mucosa or on the visceral pleura. The nodules may aggregate to form larger masses.

Histologically, there is often interstitial infiltration in addition to the nodules visible macroscopically. Low power microscopy reveals a characteristic distribution of the infiltrative disease along lymphatic pathways: the interlobular septa and visceral pleura are thickened and a cuff of neoplastic tissue forms around arteries and their accompanying airways (Fig. 12.3.20). The infiltrate consists of spindle cells and variable numbers of inflammatory cells, particularly plasma cells. The spindle cells closely resemble fibroblasts or endothelial cells and may form a network of irregular vascular channels. Red blood cells are often scattered between the spindle cells or be present in the vascular spaces. Obvious features of malignancy are often lacking but scanty mitoses are usually evident. The histogenesis of Kaposi's sarcoma is still debated but it is likely that the malignant cells are endothelial, originating either in lymphatics or in blood vessels.[299–301] The tumour cells express the vascular markers CD31, CD34 and factor VIII. The infiltrate extends into the walls of airways but the bronchial epithelium usually remains intact. Arteries and veins appear to offer more resistance although some separation of muscle fibres may occur. The intervening lung shows non-specific features such as alveolar oedema, haemosiderosis and the development of lymphoid aggregates. A variant of Kaposi's sarcoma, described as 'inflammatory'[270] or 'polymorphous',[297] is characterised by a predominant infiltrate of lymphocytes and plasma cells with inconspicuous spindle cells: in contrast to other forms of the disease it forms a diffuse infiltrate and seldom produces a mass lesion. The inflammatory form is particularly common in AIDS patients.

Diagnosis by bronchial or transbronchial biopsies requires a high index of suspicion.[297,298] The inflammatory form of Kaposi's sarcoma is particularly likely to be mistaken for inflammatory granulation tissue, but with a knowledge of the different variants of the disease and of its distribution, the diagnosis should be evident. Mycobacterial spindle cell pseudotumour also enters the differential diagnosis and as both conditions are predisposed to by severe immunodeficiency they may coexist. The mycobacterial lesion consists of shorter spindle-shaped or even

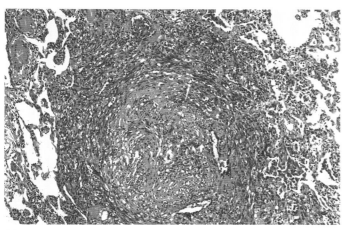

(a)

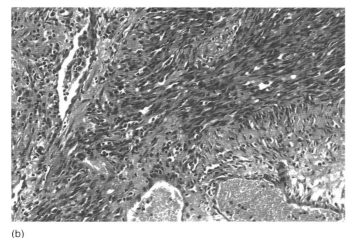

(b)

Figure 12.3.20 (a) Kaposi's sarcoma surrounds and infiltrates a pulmonary artery and its accompanying bronchiole in an AIDS patient. (b) Higher magnification shows the tumour to consist of spindle cells separated by slit-like vascular spaces.

polygonal cells with voluminous eosinophilic cytoplasm. It lacks the blood-filled slit-like spaces seen in Kaposi's sarcoma and mitoses are not observed. The component cells are histiocytic, staining for CD68 and strongly with the Ziehl–Nielsen method, but not for the vascular markers such as CD31 and CD34, which are evinced by Kaposi's sarcoma.

Epithelioid haemangioendothelioma ('intravascular bronchiolo-alveolar tumour')

Dail and Liebow provided the first comprehensive description of this tumour but mistakenly believed it to be epithelial in type and introduced the term 'intravascular bronchioloalveolar tumour'.[302,303] Earlier reports had suggested a possible decidual origin[304] and other examples had been mistaken for chondrosarcoma. The endothelial nature of the neoplastic cells was established by the identification of Weibel–Palade bodies in the cytoplasm by electron microscopy[305,306] and the later demonstration of immunoreactivity for factor VIII-related

antigen.[303,307,308] This led to the introduction of terms such as sclerosing angiogenic tumour,[306] sclerosing interstitial vascular sarcoma[309] sclerosing epithelial angiosarcoma[310] and low-grade sclerosing angiosarcoma.[308] The neoplasm was also included among the so-called 'histiocytoid haemangiomas'.[311] Soft tissue[312,313] and hepatic[308,314,315] counterparts were then recognised, and nomenclature was standardised by the adoption of the term epithelioid haemangioendothelioma.

Clinical features

Although pulmonary epithelioid haemangioendothelioma occurs over a wide age range (12–71 years) and in both sexes, about 50% of patients are less than 40 years of age and 80% are female.[303,316] Oestrogen receptors have been detected in a minority of tumours.[317] Symptoms are slight at first but shortness of breath slowly increases. Occasionally the tumour presents as a solitary pulmonary nodule[318] but initial chest radiographs usually show numerous small nodular opacities, mostly less than 1 cm in diameter, scattered throughout both lungs. They enlarge only slowly and patients may survive for as long as 15 years after diagnosis before dying of restrictive pulmonary failure. One patient presented with hypertrophic pulmonary osteoarthropathy and following treatment with azathioprine remained well with no apparent progression for 16 years.[319] Unusual intrathoracic forms of the disease include an anterior mediastinal mass, diffuse pleural thickening resembling malignant mesothelioma,[320,321] and a solitary peripheral calcified nodule.[322] Widespread involvement of the lungs may also result in pulmonary hypertension.[323] Alveolar haemorrhage and pleural effusion are further unusual manifestations of the disease.[324]

Pathology

At autopsy, the lungs are studded by multiple hard nodules and the pleura may be diffusely thickened (Fig. 12.3.21). Microscopically, the nodules have a central core of myxoid or hyaline connective tissue, which may show central calcification, chondrification or ossification (Fig. 12.3.22). Elastin stains reveal compressed alveolar walls and obliterated vessels. Congo red staining may be positive but the characteristic birefringence and dichroism of amyloid are absent. The nodules are more cellular at the periphery where the stroma contains single, or small clusters of tumour cells. Tumour cell nuclei are oval with dispersed granular chromatin and a small nucleolus; they lack atypia and mitoses are infrequent. The cytoplasm is abundant, eosinophilic and often contains vacuoles, which may coalesce to form an intracellular lumen (Fig. 12.3.23). These miniature lumina sometimes contain a few red blood cells but if not they are apt to be confused with the mucin vacuoles of an adenocarcinoma.

At the periphery, the nodules extend into adjacent bronchioles and alveoli as papillary processes that are often clothed by cuboidal cells (Fig. 12.3.23). In paraffin sections these are not clearly distinguishable from stromal cells but marked differ-

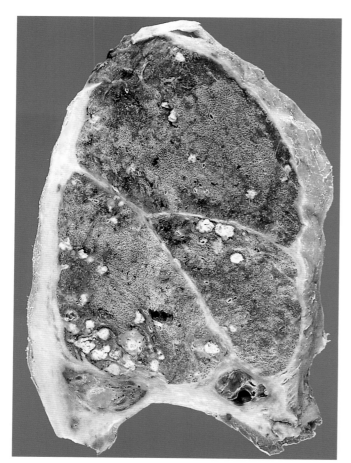

Figure 12.3.21 Epithelioid haemangioendothelioma forming multiple pulmonary nodules and thickening the pleura diffusely in the manner of a mesothelioma. (Illustration provided by Dr CGB Simpson, Aberystwyth, UK.[320])

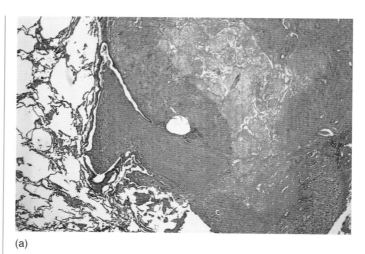

(a)

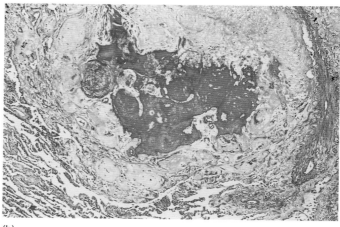

(b)

Figure 12.3.22 Epithelioid haemangioendothelioma. The tumour nodules are more cellular at the periphery, where they (a) protrude into neighbouring airspaces giving them a micropolypoid structure. (b) The centres of the nodules show hyaline sclerosis, and sometimes calcification.

ences are evident on electron microscopy.[305,306] The surface cells are type II alveolar epithelial cells and are presumably reactive. The tumour cells have ultrastructural features more suggestive of vasoformative cells, and immunoreactive factor VIII-related antigen is demonstrable both in the cytoplasm and within vacuoles (Fig. 12.3.24).[303,307,308]

Extension within the lung may occur by lymphatic spread, producing appearances similar to those seen in cases of lymphatic permeation by carcinoma (so-called carcinomatous 'lymphangitis' – see p. 672),[322] and the pleura may be involved diffusely, resulting in a gross appearance that resembles that of a mesothelioma (Fig. 12.3.21).[320–322] Extrathoracic spread is rare but extrapulmonary deposits are recorded in sites such as the liver, bone and skin.[303,308,314,317,318,325] The characteristic micropolypoid structure is not seen outside the lung and is evidently a product of the alveolar architecture.

With such a slow-growing multifocal tumour, the identification of a solitary deposit in the liver raises the question whether the pulmonary lesions are metastases from an occult hepatic primary.[326,327] Based on a study of basement membrane compo-

sition it has been claimed that the pulmonary tumours represent multicentric primary growths rather than metastases,[328] but this issue is unsettled.[317] There are cases in which the multiple pulmonary lesions have developed long after epithelioid haemangioendothelioma has been diagnosed in an extrapulmonary site.[320,329]

Differential diagnosis

The differential diagnosis includes lesions containing cartilage or myxoid connective tissue, such as chondroid 'hamartoma', chondrosarcoma and sclerosing pneumocytoma. The latter is typically a solitary lesion and contains sclerotic areas and papillary processes that may resemble those of epithelioid haemangioendothelioma, but the presence of prominent vascular spaces in the sclerosing pneumocytoma usually enables the distinction to be made.

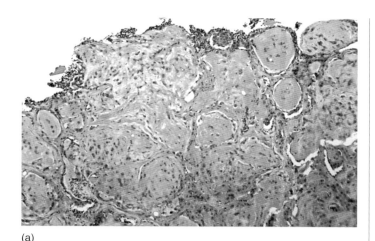

(a)

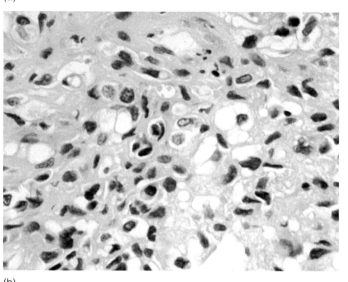

(b)

Figure 12.3.23 Epithelioid haemangioendothelioma. (a) The tumour nodules have a micropolypoid structure at their periphery. (b) Vacuolation of tumour cells is sometimes evident, probably representing primitive angiogenesis.

Chemodectoma (non-chromaffin paraganglioma)

The existence of chemoreceptors on intrapulmonary blood vessels is based on functional observations[330] backed up by a single morphological description of glomera (paraganglia, chemoreceptors) in the outer coats of pulmonary arteries at their branching points closely related to adjacent nerves.[331] Primary pulmonary chemodectomas could develop from such structures. However, most intrathoracic chemodectomas arise outside the lung[332–335] or if intrapulmonary eventually prove to be metastases from an occult growth in the neck. Apart from the so-called multiple minute chemodectomas of the lung described separately (see meningiothelioid nodules, p. 688), few cases of primary pulmonary chemodectoma have been reported, and it is debatable whether these represent chemodectomas or carcinoids.[336–342] Reticulin stains often show that the cell cords of a carcinoid intercommunicate, in contrast to the non-

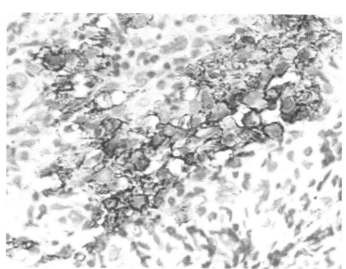

Figure 12.3.24 Epithelioid haemangioendothelioma. The tumour cells stain for the endothelial marker CD31.

communicating *Zellballen* of a chemodectoma, but occasionally both these patterns are found within a single tumour indicating that this is not a reliable point of distinction. Carcinoids and chemodectomas both contain dense-core granules, which are indistinguishable in size and structure. The nature of the dense-core granules is obscure but one reputed pulmonary chemodectoma was shown to contain noradrenaline,[343] while a few others have secreted catecholamines.[344,345] Cytokeratin immunocytochemistry was formerly thought to provide a clear means of distinguishing carcinoids from chemodectomas but it is now recognised that positive reactions may be obtained with both.[346–349] Chemodectomas are characterised by S100-positive sustentacular cells surrounding cells with neuroendocrine characteristics but this feature is also described in a substantial number of bronchopulmonary carcinoids. However, some workers prefer to regard tumours of this description as chemodectomas and have substantiated this claim by demonstrating scanty ganglion cells in occasional examples, which they term gangliocytic paragangliomas rather than paragangliod carcinoids.[350,351] These few examples have included both a central peribronchial tumour of *Zellballen* pattern and peripheral spindle cell growths. All have been benign.

Sarcomas of the major pulmonary blood vessels

A rare form of sarcoma arises within the pulmonary trunk, the main pulmonary arteries or the right side of the heart and gives rise to multiple pulmonary tumours.[352–360] Less commonly, similar tumours arise in the pulmonary veins, the chambers on the left side of the heart or the aorta and metastasise via the systemic circulation.[156,203,359,361–364]

Clinical features

Patients with sarcoma of the pulmonary arteries cover a wide age range, from 21 to 80 years, but most tumours occur between

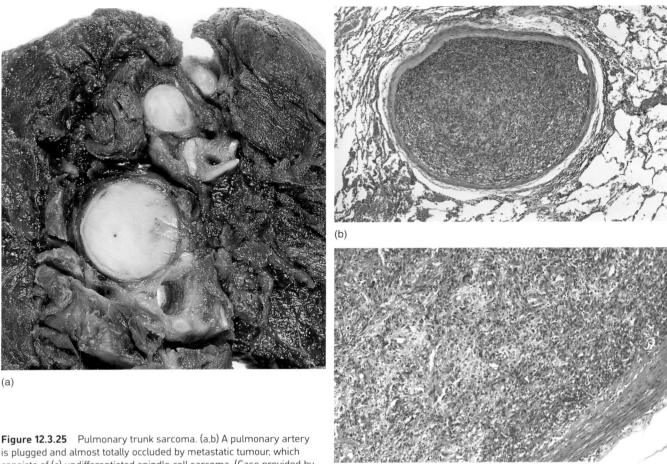

Figure 12.3.25 Pulmonary trunk sarcoma. (a,b) A pulmonary artery is plugged and almost totally occluded by metastatic tumour, which consists of (c) undifferentiated spindle cell sarcoma. (Case provided by Dr W Kenyon, Liverpool, UK.)

the ages or 45 and 65 and there appears to be a predominance of females. An association with radiation is recorded.[181] Dyspnoea, chest pain and cough may be accompanied by episodes of haemoptysis, syncope, a systolic murmur or right ventricular dilatation and failure.[365] Plain chest radiography shows increased hilar shadowing and hypoperfusion of the lung fields, often leading to a mistaken diagnosis of pulmonary thromboembolism.[182,366,367] Weight loss, fever and anaemia are additional features more suggestive of malignancy.[368] Diagnosis during life has been unusual but modern imaging techniques, such as angiography and computerised tomography, make this possible.[369,370] Fragmentation and tumour embolisation result in multiple pulmonary metastases, which appear as peripheral rounded nodules or masses. Metastatic sites beyond the lungs include lymph nodes, brain, diaphragm, thyroid and pancreas.

Pathology

At surgery or autopsy, the pulmonary trunk is distended by soft, grey, polypoid tumour, often mixed with thrombus. This frequently extends distally into one or both main pulmonary arteries and, less often, proximally to involve the pulmonary valve and right ventricular outflow tract. Sometimes the tumour appears to arise in the right ventricle or atrium. The intima and media of the pulmonary trunk are infiltrated but often quite superficially. In about half the cases tumour extends directly into smaller intrapulmonary branches (Fig. 12.3.25a,b). It may spread from the arteries to present as a diffuse pulmonary infiltrate.[205]

In biopsy material, pathologists often misinterpret the pulmonary deposits as infarcts, haemorrhagic pneumonia or haemorrhage as many are well vascularised and liable to bleed. Other deposits, however, are more solid. Some tumours consist of a fairly uniform population of polygonal or spindle cells whereas others show marked pleomorphism and giant tumour cells (Fig. 12.3.25c). They are most frequently termed undifferentiated, pleomorphic or intimal sarcomas but other terms reflect their ability to differentiate in a number of directions and include, in descending order of frequency, leiomyosarcoma, rhabdomyosarcoma, chondrosarcoma, fibromyxosarcoma, mesenchymoma (containing mixed elements), osteosarcoma, myxosarcoma, angiosarcoma and malignant fibrous histiocytoma.[183]

Thus, some tumours show the formation of bone or cartilage. The few examples subjected to electron microscopy have shown striated[352] or smooth muscle[356,371] or have been undifferentiated.[372] Occasional cases are examples of epithelioid angiosarcoma,[358] and are likely to be confused with poorly differentiated carcinoma, particularly pseudovascular variants:[373] both carcinoma and epithelioid angiosarcoma express cytokeratin[374] but only the latter expresses endothelial markers. Rare tumours of the pulmonary trunk appear to be benign and have been reported under terms such as myxoma.[375]

NEURAL TUMOURS

Nerve sheath tumours

Posterior mediastinal or paravertebral nerve sheath tumours are fairly common but in the lower respiratory tract tumours of nerve sheath origin are distinctly rare.[176,194,376–380] They develop in both sexes and may be endobronchial or parenchymal.[176] They comprise both neurofibromas and neurilemmomas (Schwannomas), some of which are malignant. Neurofibromas are more frequent in men, whereas schwannomas are more common in women. The gross, microscopical, immunocytochemical and ultrastructural appearances are identical to those of nerve sheath tumours elsewhere (Fig. 12.3.26). Melanin production is described in one malignant Schwannoma of the bronchus[381] and rhabdomyoblastic differentiation is recorded in rare malignant nerve sheath tumours (so-called 'triton' tumours) of the lung.[382]

It is uncertain what proportion of patients with intrapulmonary nerve sheath tumours have neurofibromatosis but most have no other features of the disease. Such patients are often asymptomatic, their tumours having reached a considerable size by the time they are discovered on a routine chest radiograph. Others have chest symptoms attributable to the obstructive effect of the tumour. Some lesions are visible bronchoscopically as a polypoid mass bulging into the lumen of an airway, and this may cause bronchiectasis.[383] The airways may also be affected diffusely and require stenting.[380] A unique case of multiple neurofibromas has been described with severe hypoxaemia due to right to left shunts within the tumours.[384]

Granular cell tumour

Granular cell tumours were first described by Abrikossoff in 1926 and in the respiratory tract shortly afterwards.[385–387] They were initially considered to be of striated muscle origin but a neural derivation is now thought more likely[388–391] and the original term granular cell myoblastoma has therefore been modified. The tongue is the most common site but they also occur in many other locations, including the lip, skin, breast, muscle, neurohypophysis and other viscera. A small proportion, about 8%, arise in the tracheobronchial tree or the periphery of the lung.[392–398]

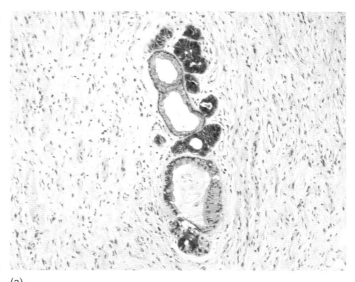

(a)

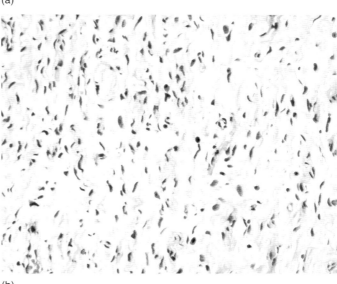

(b)

Figure 12.3.26 Neurofibroma, (a) As in the skin, the tumour surrounds rather than destroys glands. (b) The tumour consists of cytologically bland wavy spindle cells, and mast cells are evident in the stroma. (Case provided by Dr A Herbert, London, UK.)

Clinical features

Patients with bronchopulmonary granular cell tumour range in age from 20 to 47 years (median 45 years) and show no sex predilection.[395,398] The tumours are either incidental findings or cause obstructive symptoms or haemoptysis. A small number of patients have multiple pulmonary lesions[394] and some have associated soft tissue granular cell tumours.[394,396] Imaging usually shows obstructive changes. At bronchoscopy, granular cell tumours usually appear as endobronchial nodules at points of bifurcation but others are plaque-like. They range in size up to 6.5 cm in diameter.

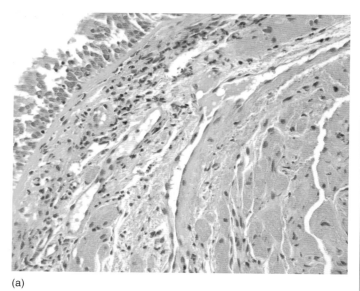

(a)

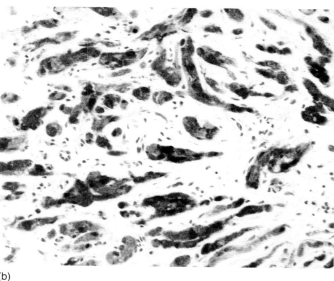

(b)

Figure 12.3.27 A granular cell tumour that formed a bronchial polyp. (a) The tumour is composed of polygonal cells with abundant eosinophilic cytoplasm. (b) The tumour cells are strongly positive for S-100 protein.

Pathology

Bronchoscopic biopsy is usually diagnostic, showing the characteristic cells lying directly beneath the epithelium, which may undergo squamous metaplasia. The tumour cells are closely packed in cords, sheets or nests. They are polygonal or spindle-shaped and have small, densely staining nuclei and abundant, coarsely granular, eosinophilic and PAS-positive cytoplasm (Fig. 12.3.27a). Nerve fibres may be seen among the tumour cells. Infiltration of the adjacent lung is often seen and lymph nodes may be directly involved but metastasis is not a feature.

Ultrastructurally, the cytoplasmic granules are consistent with them being of lysosomal autophagic or cell membrane

origin[388,389,399] and the presence of axons and an incomplete basement membrane around the cells is thought to point to a Schwann cell origin.[400] This is supported by the immuno-histochemical demonstration S-100 neural protein (Fig. 12.3.27b).[388,398,401] Negative reactions are obtained for cytokeratin and neuroendocrine markers.

Differential diagnosis

Granular cell tumours may, be confused with oncocytic carcinoid tumours (see p. 585) or oncocytic tumours of bronchial gland origin (see p. 595). Carcinoid tumours are typically much more vascular than granular cell tumours. Electron microscopy of oncocytic tumours shows closely packed mitochondria rather than the autophagic granules of granular cell tumours. Some carcinoid tumours may stain weakly for S-100 protein but both carcinoid tumours and bronchial gland tumours also stain for cytokeratin whereas granular cell tumours do not.

Prognosis

Granular cell tumours generally grow slowly and no malignant examples are described in the lung. Nevertheless, effective therapy usually requires formal resection.

Meningioma

Occasional meningiomas, identical to those found within the cranium but apparently primary to the lungs, have been described.[402-413] It has been suggested that they arise from ectopic arachnoid cells,[408] but it is likely that arachnoid-like cells are an inherent part of the normal lung (see p. 23) and that this is the source of the pulmonary tumours. This relates them to the meningothelioid nodules (so-called multiple minute chemodectomas, see p. 688) but pulmonary meningiomas are generally solitary and are not minute.

Clinical features

The reported cases have ranged from 51 to 70 years of age. The patients have generally been asymptomatic, their tumour being discovered on routine chest examination. The tumours have generally been solitary but in one case there were multiple pulmonary meningiomas and the patient also had neurofibromatosis.[404]

Pathology

The tumours are well circumscribed but are not encapsulated. They have no obvious connection with airways, blood vessels or pleura. Histologically, they consist of sheets of regular ovoid or spindle cells forming the 'meningothelial whorls' and psammoma bodies characteristic of the intracranial growths (Fig. 12.3.28). Immunohistochemistry shows that the tumour cells stain positively for vimentin and epithelial membrane antigen but negatively for cytokeratin and S-100 protein. Electron

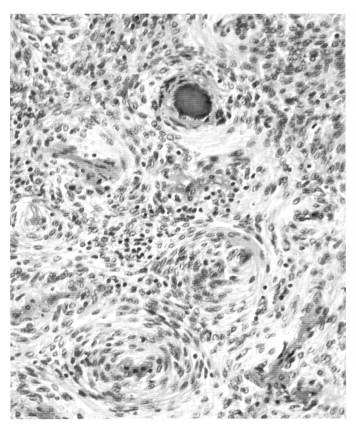

Figure 12.3.28 Meningioma of the lung. There was no evidence of an intracranial lesion. (Section provided by Dr TV Colby, Scottsdale, USA.)

microscopy shows complex cellular interdigitations and many desmosomes.

Differential diagnosis

An occult primary in the cranium obviously needs to be excluded before the diagnosis of primary pulmonary meningioma can be countenanced. The degree of atypia is of no significance as some metastases appear quite benign histologically, giving rise to the term 'benign metastasising meningioma'.[414]

Treatment and prognosis

Treatment is by surgical resection, following which recurrence is very rare.[412]

Ependymoma

Rare examples of ependymomas occurring outside the central nervous system have been described in the pelvis and posterior mediastinum and in one patient only, the lung.[415] This was an elderly woman who also had a small cell carcinoma treated by chemotherapy and it is uncertain whether the ependymoma

represented metaplastic change in the carcinoma, perhaps due to the chemotherapy, or whether it arose in ectopic ependyma. The tumour had the usual morphology of a malignant ependymoma and showed strong immunoreactivity for glial fibrillary protein with less intense staining for vimentin, epithelial membrane antigen and S-100 protein.

REFERENCES

Inflammatory myofibroblastic tumour

1. Bahadori M, Liebow AA. Plasma cell granulomas of the lung. Cancer 1973; 31:191–208.
2. Spencer H. The pulmonary plasma cell/histiocytoma complex. Histopathology 1984; 8:903–916.
3. Umiker WO, Iverson L. Postinflammatory 'tumors' of the lung. Report of four cases simulating xanthoma, fibroma or plasma cell tumor. J Thorac Surg 1954; 28:55–63.
4. Bates T, Hull OH. Histiocytoma of the bronchus. A report of a case in a six-year-old child. Am J Dis Child 1958; 95:53–56.
5. Bates HR, Buis LJ, Johns TNP. Endobronchial histiocytoma. Chest 1976; 69:705–706.
6. Sherwin RP, Kern WH, Jones JC. Solitary mast cell granuloma (histiocytoma) of the lung. Cancer 1965; 18:634–641.
7. Charette EE, Mariano AV, LaForet EG. Solitary mast cell 'tumour' of the lung. Arch Intern Med 1966; 118:358–362.
8. Coffin CM, Watterson J, Priest JR, Dehner LP. Extrapulmonary inflammatory myofibroblastic tumor (inflammatory pseudotumor) – a clinicopathologic and immunohistochemical study of 84 cases. Am J Surg Pathol 1995; 19:859–872.
8a. Nonaka D, Birbe R, Rosai J. So-called inflammatory myofibroblastic tumour: a proliferative lesion of fibroblastic reticulum cells? Histopathology 2005; 46:604–613.
9. Mandalbaum I, Brashear RE, Hull MT. Surgical treatment and course of pulmonary pseudotumour (plasma cell granuloma). J Thorac Cardiovasc Surg 1981; 82:77–82.
10. Hartman GE, Shochat SJ. Primary pulmonary neoplasms of childhood: a review. Ann Thorac Surg 1983; 36:108–119.
11. Rohrlich P, Peuchmaur M, Cocci SD, et al. Interleukin-6 and interleukin-1 beta production in a pediatric plasma cell granuloma of the lung. Am J Surg Pathol 1995; 19:590–595.
12. Helikson MA, Havey AD, Zerwekh JE, Breslau NA, Gardner DW. Plasma cell granuloma producing calcitriol and hypercalcemia. Ann Intern Med 1986; 105:379–381.
13. Agrons GA, Rosado-de-Christenson ML, Kirejczyk WM, Conran RM, Stocker JT. Pulmonary inflammatory pseudotumor: radiologic features. Radiology 1998; 206:511–518.
14. Dehner LP. The enigmatic inflammatory pseudotumours: the current state of our understanding, or misunderstanding. J Pathol 2000; 192:277–279.
15. Alvarez-Fernandez E, Escalona-Zapata J. Pulmonary plasma cell granuloma - an electron microscopic and tissue culture study. Histopathology 1983; 7:279–286.
16. Chen HP, Lee SS, Berardi RS. Inflammatory pseudotumor of the lung. Ultrastructural and light microscopic study of a myxomatous variant. Cancer 1984; 54:861–865.
17. Matsubara O, Tan-Liu NS, Kenney RM, Mark EJ. Inflammatory pseudotumors of the lung: progression from organizing pneumonia to fibrous histiocytoma or to plasma cell granuloma in 32 cases. Hum Pathol 1988; 19:807–814.
18. Kubicz ST, Paradowska W, Czarnowska-Nastula B, Boroworiczowa D. Pseudo-tumor of the lung in children. Ann Radiol (Paris) 1975; 18:447–452.
19. Janigan DJ, Marrie TJ. An inflammatory pseudotumor of the lung in Q fever pneumonia. N Engl J Med 1983; 308:86–87.
20. Lipton JH, Fong TC, Gill MJ, Burgess K, Elliott PD. Q fever inflammatory pseudotumor of the lung. Chest 1987; 92:756–757.

21. Arber DA, Kamel OW, Vanderijn M, et al. Frequent presence of the Epstein–Barr virus in inflammatory pseudotumor. Hum Pathol 1995; 26:1093–1098.

22. Gomez-Roman JJ, Ocejo-Vinyals G, Sanchez-Velasco P, Nieto EH, Leyva-Cobian F, Val-Bernal JF. Presence of human herpesvirus-8 DNA sequences and overexpression of human IL-6 and cyclin D1 in inflammatory myofibroblastic tumor (inflammatory pseudotumor). Lab Invest 2000; 80:1121–1126.

23. Gomez-Roman JJ, Sanchez-Velasco P, Ocejo-Vinyals G, Hernandez-Nieto E, Leyva-Cobian F, Val-Bernal JF. Human herpesvirus-8 genes are expressed in pulmonary inflammatory myofibroblastic tumor (inflammatory pseudotumor). Am J Surg Pathol 2001; 25:624–629.

24. Berardi RS, Lee SS, Chen HP, Stines GJ. Inflammatory pseudotumors of the lung. Surg Gynecol Obstet 1988; 156:89–96.

25. Warter A, Satge D, Roeslin N. Angioinvasive plasma cell granulomas of the lung. Cancer 1987; 59:435–443.

26. Saitoh K, Shindo N, Toh Y, Yoshizawa A, Kudo K. Electron microscopic study of chronic eosinophilic pneumonia. Pathol Int 1996; 46:855–861.

27. Donner LR, Trompler RA, White RR. Progression of inflammatory myofibroblastic tumor (inflammatory pseudotumor) or soft tissue into sarcoma after several recurrences. Hum Pathol 1996; 27:1095–1098.

28. Treissman SP, Gillis DA, Lee CLY, Giacomoantonio M, Resch L. Omental-mesenteric inflammatory pseudotumor. Cytogenetic demonstration of genetic changes and monoclonality in one tumor. Cancer 1994; 73:1433–1437.

29. Snyder CS, Dellaquila M, Haghighi P, Baergen RN, Suh YK, Yi ES. Clonal changes in inflammatory pseudotumor of the lung: a case report. Cancer 1995; 76:1545–1549.

30. Biselli R, Ferlini C, Fattorossi A, Boldrini R, Bosman C. Inflammatory myofibroblastic tumor (inflammatory pseudotumor): DNA flow cytometric analysis of nine pediatric cases. Cancer 1996; 77:778–784.

31. Su LD, Atayde-Perez A, Sheldon S, Fletcher JA, Weiss SW. Inflammatory myofibroblastic tumor: cytogenetic evidence supporting clonal origin. Mod Pathol 1998; 11:364–368.

32. Yousem SA, Shaw H, Cieply K. Involvement of 2p23 in pulmonary inflammatory pseudotumors. Hum Pathol 2001; 32:428–433.

33. Bridge JA, Kanamori M, Ma ZG, et al. Fusion of the ALK gene to the clathrin heavy chain gene, CLTC, in inflammatory myofibroblastic tumor. Am J Pathol 2001; 159:411–415.

34. Debelenko LV, Arthur DC, Pack SD, Helman LJ, Schrump DS, Tsokos M. Identification of CARS-ALK fusion in primary and metastatic lesions of an inflammatory myofibroblastic tumor. Lab Invest 2003; 83: 1255–1265.

35. Titus JL, Harrison EG, Clagett OT, Anderson MW, Knatt LJ. Xanthomatous and inflammatory pseudotumors of the lung. Cancer 1962; 15:522–538.

36. Strutynsky N, Balthazar EJ, Klein RM. Inflammatory pseudotumours of the lung. Br J Radiol 1974; 47:94–96.

37. Lemarchadour F, Lavielle JP, Guilcher C, et al. Coexistence of plasma cell granulomas of lung and central nervous system – a case report. Pathol Res Pract 1995; 191:1038–1045.

38. Buell R, Wang N-S, Seemayer TA, Ahmed MN. Endobronchial plasma cell granuloma (xanthomatous pseudotumor). A light and electron microscopic study. Hum Pathol 1976; 7:411–426.

39. Shirakusa T, Miyazaki N, Kitagawa T, Sugiyama K. Ultrastructural study of pulmonary plasma cell granuloma – report of a case. Br J Dis Chest 1979; 73:289–296.

40. Katzenstein A-LA, Maurer JJ. Benign histiocytic tumor of the lung. A light and electron-microscopic study. Am J Surg Pathol 1979; 3:61–68.

41. Tomita T, Dixon A, Watanabe I, Mantz F, Richany S. Sclerosing vascular variant of plasma cell granuloma. Hum Pathol 1980; 11:197–202.

42. Fisher ER, Beyer FD. Post-inflammatory tumour (xanthoma) of lung. Dis Chest 1959; 36:43–48.

43. Narodick BG. Fibrous histiocytoma or xanthoma of the lung with bronchial involvement. J Thorac Cardiovasc Surg 1973; 65:653–657.

44. Dentworth P, Lynch MJ, Fallis JC. Xanthomatous pseudotumor of lung: a case report with electron microscope and lipid studies. Cancer 1968; 22:345–355.

45. Muraoka S, Sato T, Takahashi T, Ando M, Shimoda A. Plasma cell granuloma of the lung with extrapulmonal extension. Immunohistochemical and electron microscopic studies. Acta Pathol Jpn 1985; 35:933–944.

46. Ramachandra S, Hollowood K, Bisceglia M, Fletcher CDM. Inflammatory pseudotumour of soft tissues: a clinicopathological and immunohistochemical analysis of 18 cases. Histopathology 1995; 27:313–323.

47. Rose AG, McCormick S, Cooper K, Titus JL. Inflammatory pseudotumor (plasma cell granuloma) of the heart: report of two cases and literature review. Arch Pathol Lab Med 1996; 120:549–554.

48. Cook JR, Dehner LP, Collins MH, et al. Anaplastic lymphoma kinase (ALK) expression in the inflammatory myofibroblastic tumor. A comparative immunohistochemical study. Am J Surg Pathol 2001; 25:1364–1371.

49. Cessna MH, Zhou H, Sanger WG, et al. Expression of ALK1 and p80 in inflammatory myofibroblastic tumor and its mesenchymal mimics: A study of 135 cases. Modern Pathol 2002; 15:931–938.

50. Kuzela DC. Ultrastructural study of postinflammatory 'tumor' of the lung. Cancer 1975; 36:149–156.

51. Pettinato G, Manivel JC, De Rosa N, Dehner LP. Inflammatory myofibroblastic tumor (plasma cell granuloma) – clinicopathologic study of 20 cases with immunohistochemical and ultrastructural observations. Am J Clin Pathol 1990; 94:538–546.

52. Pomplun S, Goldstraw P, Davies SE, Burke MM, Nicholson AG. Calcifying fibrous pseudotumour arising within an inflammatory pseudotumour: evidence of progression from one lesion to the other? Histopathology 2000; 37:380–382.

53. Gal AA, Koss MN, McCarthy WF, Hochholzer L. Prognostic factors in pulmonary fibrohistiocytic lesions. Cancer 1994; 73:1817–1824.

54. Ledet SC, Brown RW, Cagle PT. p53 immunostaining in the differentiation of inflammatory pseudotumor from sarcoma involving the lung. Mod Pathol 1995; 8:282–286.

55. Tan-Liu NS, Matsubara O, Grillo HC, Mark EJ. Invasive fibrous tumor of the tracheobronchial tree: clinical and pathologic study of seven cases. Hum Pathol 1989; 20:180–184.

56. Bush A, Sheppard MN, Wahn U, Warner JO. Spontaneous arrest of growth of a plasma cell granuloma. Respir Med 1992; 86:161–164.

57. Maier HC, Sommers SC. Recurrent and metastatic pulmonary fibrous histiocytoma/plasma cell granuloma in a child. Cancer 1987; 60: 1073–1076.

58. Biselli R, Boldrini R, Ferlini C, Boglino C, Inserra A, Bosman C. Myofibroblastic tumours: neoplasias with divergent behaviour. Ultrastructural and flow cytometric analysis. Pathol Res Pract 1999; 195:619–632.

59. Hussong JW, Brown M, Perkins SL, Dehner LP, Coffin CM. Comparison of DNA ploidy, histologic, and immunohistochemical findings with clinical outcome in inflammatory myofibroblastic tumors. Mod Pathol 1999; 12:279–286.

Pleuropulmonary blastoma

60. Manivel JC, Priest JR, Watterson J, et al. Pleuropulmonary blastoma. The so-called pulmonary blastoma of childhood. Cancer 1988; 62:1516–1526.

61. Cohen M, Emms M, Kaschula R. Childhood pulmonary blastoma: a pleuropulmonary variant of the adult-type pulmonary blastoma. Pediatr Pathol 1991; 11:737–749.

62. Hachitanda Y, Aoyama C, Sato JK, Shimada H. Pleuropulmonary blastoma in childhood – a tumor of divergent differentiation. Am J Surg Pathol 1993; 17:382–391.

63. Pacinda SJ, Ledet SC, Gondo MM, et al. p53 and MDM2 immunostaining in pulmonary blastomas and bronchogenic carcinomas. Hum Pathol 1996; 27:542–546.

64. Priest JR, McDermott MB, Bhatia S, Watterson J, Manivel JC, Dehner LP. Pleuropulmonary blastoma: A clinicopathologic study of 50 cases. Cancer 1997; 80:147–161.

65. Sciot R, Cin PD, Brock P, et al. Pleuropulmonary blastoma (pulmonary blastoma of childhood): genetic link with other embryonal malignancies? Histopathology 1994; 24:559–563.

66. Yang P, Hasegawa T, Hirose T, et al. Pleuropulmonary blastoma: Fluorescence in situ hybridisation analysis indicating trisomy 2. Am J Surg Pathol 1997; 21:854–859.

67. Delahunt B, Thomson KJ, Ferguson AF, Neale TJ, Meffan PJ, Nacey JN. Familial cystic nephroma and pleuropulmonary blastoma. Cancer 1993; 71:1338–1342.

68. Weinblatt ME, Siegel SE, Isaacs H. Pulmonary blastoma associated with cystic lung disease. Cancer 1982; 49:669–671.

69. Ueda K, Gruppo R, Unger F, Martin M, Bove K. Rhabdomyosarcoma of lung arising in congenital cystic adenomatoid malformation. Cancer 1977; 40:383–388.

70. Hedlund GL, Bisset GSI, Bove KE. Malignant neoplasms arising in cystic hamartomas of the lung in childhood. Radiology 1989; 173:77–79.

71. d'Agostino S, Bonoldi E, Dante S, Meli S, Cappellari F, Musi L. Embryonal rhabdomyosarcoma of the lung arising in cystic adenomatoid malformation: case report and review of the literature. J Pediatr Surg 1997; 32:1381–1383.

72. Ozcan C, Celik A, Ural Z, Veral A, Kandiloglu G, Balik E. Primary pulmonary rhabdomyosarcoma arising within cystic adenomatoid malformation: a case report and review of the literature. J Pediatr Surg 2001; 36:1062–1065.

73. Domizio P, Liesner RJ, Dicks-Mireaux C, Risdon RA. Malignant mesenchymoma associated with a congenital lung cyst in a child: case report and review of the literature. Pediatr Pathol 1990; 10:785–797.

74. Krous HF, Sexauer CL. Embryonal rhabdomyosarcoma arising within a congenital bronchogenic cyst in a child. J Pediatr Surg 1981; 16:506–508.

75. Weinberg AG, Currarino G, Moore GC, Votteler TP. Mesenchymal neoplasia and congenital pulmonary cysts. Pediatr Radiol 1980; 9:179–182.

76. Hill DA, Sadeghi S, Schultz MZ, Burr JS, Dehner LP. Pleuropulmonary blastoma in an adult: an initial case report. Cancer 1999; 85:2368–2374.

77. Indolfi P, Casale F, Carli M, et al. Pleuropulmonary blastoma: management and prognosis of 11 cases. Cancer 2000; 89:1396–1401.

78. Dehner LP. Pleuropulmonary blastoma is THE pulmonary blastoma of childhood. Semin Diagn Pathol 1994; 11:144–151.

79. MacSweeney F, Papagiannopoulos K, Goldstraw P, Sheppard MN, Corrin B, Nicholson AG. An assessment of the expanded classification of congenital cystic adenomatoid malformations and their relationship to malignant transformation. Am J Surg Pathol 2003; 27:1139–1146.

80. Hill DA, Dehner LP. A cautionary note about congenital cystic adenomatoid malformation (CCAM) type 4. Am J Surg Pathol 2004; 28:554–555.

81. Wright JR, Jr. Pleuropulmonary blastoma: A case report documenting transition from type I (cystic) to type III (solid). Cancer 2000; 88:2853–2858.

82. Papagiannopoulos KA, Sheppard M, Bush A, Goldstraw P. Pleuropulmonary blastoma: is prophylactic resection of congenital lung cysts effective? Ann Thorac Surg 2001; 72:604–605.

Benign clear cell tumour ('sugar tumour')

83. Liebow AA, Castleman B. Benign 'clear cell tumors' of the lung. Am J Pathol 1963; 43:13a-14a.

84. Liebow AA, Castleman B. Benign clear cell ('sugar') tumors of the lung. Yale J Biol Med 1971; 43:213–222.

85. Becker NH, Soifer I. Benign clear cell tumour ('sugar tumor') of the lung. Cancer 1971; 27:712–719.

86. Hoch WS, Patchefsky AS, Takeda M, Gordon G. Benign clear cell tumor of the lung. Cancer 1974; 33:1328–1336.

87. Harbin WP, Mark GJ, Greene RE. Benign clear cell tumor ('sugar tumor') of the lung: case report and review of the literature. Radiology 1978; 129:595–596.

88. Zolliker A, Jacques J, Goldstein AS. Benign clear cell tumor of the lung. Arch Pathol Lab Med 1979; 103:526–530.

89. Andrion A, Mazzucco G, Gugliotta P, Monga G. Benign clear cell ('sugar') tumor of the lung. A light microscopic, histochemical and ultrastructural study with a review of the literature. Cancer 1985; 56:2657–2663.

90. Fukuda T, Machinami R, Jashita T, Nagashima K. Benign clear cell tumor of the lung in an 8-year-old girl. Arch Pathol Lab Med 1986; 110:664–666.

91. Sale GE, Kulander BG. 'Benign' clear-cell tumor (sugar tumor) of the lung with hepatic metastases ten years after resection of pulmonary primary tumor. Arch Pathol Lab Med 1988; 112:1177–1178.

92. Nguyen G-K. Aspiration biopsy cytology of benign clear cell ('sugar') tumor of the lung. Acta Cytol 1989; 33:511–515.

93. Gaffey MJ, Mills SE, Askin FB, et al. Clear cell tumor of the lung. A clinicopathologic, immunohistochemical and ultrastructural study of eight cases. Am J Surg Pathol 1990; 14:248–259.

94. Gaffey MJ, Mills SE, Zarbo RJ, Weiss LM, Gown AM. Clear cell tumor of the lung – immunohistochemical and ultrastructural evidence of melanogenesis. Am J Surg Pathol 1991; 15:644–653.

95. Gal AA, Koss MN, Hochholzer L, Chejfec G. An immunohistochemical study of benign clear cell (sugar) tumor of the lung. Arch Pathol Lab Med 1991; 115:1034–1038.

96. Flieder DB, Travis WD. Clear cell "Sugar" tumor of the lung: Association with lymphangioleiomyomatosis and multifocal micronodular pneumocyte hyperplasia in a patient with tuberous sclerosis. Am J Surg Pathol 1997; 21:1242–1247.

97. Lantuejoul S, Isaac S, Pinel N, Negoescu A, Guibert B, Brambilla E. Clear cell tumor of the lung: An immunohistochemical and ultrastructural study supporting a pericytic differentiation. Modern Pathol 1997; 10:1001–1008.

98. Hashimoto T, Oka K, Hakozaki H, et al. Benign clear cell tumor of the lung. Ultrastruct Pathol 2001; 25:479–483.

99. Kung M, Landa JF, Lubin J. Benign clear cell tumor (sugar tumor) of the trachea. Cancer 1984; 54:517–519.

100. Zamboni G, Pea M, Martignoni G, et al. Clear cell 'sugar' tumor of the pancreas: a novel member of the family of lesions characterized by the presence of perivascular epithelioid cells. Am J Surg Pathol 1996; 20:722–730.

101. Folpe AL, Goodman ZD, Ishak KG, et al. Clear cell myomelanocytic tumor of the falciform ligament/ligamentum teres: a novel member of the perivascular epithelioid clear cell family of tumors with a predilection for children and young adults. Am J Surg Pathol 2000; 24:1239–1246.

102. Tanaka Y, Ijiri R, Kato K, et al. HMB-45/melan-A and smooth muscle actin-positive clear-cell epithelioid tumor arising in the ligamentum teres hepatis: additional example of clear cell 'sugar' tumors. Am J Surg Pathol 2000; 24:1295–1299.

103. Tazelaar HD, Batts KP, Srigley JR. Primary extrapulmonary sugar tumor (PEST): A report of four cases. Modern Pathol 2001; 14:615–622.

104. Vang R, Kempson RL. Perivascular epithelioid cell tumor ('PEComa') of the uterus – A subset of HMB-45-positive epithelioid mesenchymal neoplasms with an uncertain relationship to pure smooth muscle tumors. Amer J Surg Pathol 2002; 26:1–13.

105. Govender D, Sabaratnam RM, Essa AS. Clear cell 'sugar' tumor of the breast – Another extrapulmonary site and review of the literature. Amer J Surg Pathol 2002; 26:670–675.

106. Dimmler A, Seitz G, Hohenberger W, Kirchner T, Faller G. Late pulmonary metastasis in uterine PEComa. J Clin Pathol 2003; 56:627–628.

107. Bonetti F, Martignoni G, Colato C, et al. Abdominopelvic sarcoma of perivascular epithelioid cells. Report of four cases in young women, one with tuberous sclerosis. Modern Pathol 2001; 14:563–568.

108. Sale GE, Kulander BG. Benign clear cell tumor of lung with necrosis. Cancer 1976; 37:2355–2358.

109. Ozdemir A, Zaman NU, Rullis I, Webb WR. Benign clear cell tumor of the lung. J Thorac Cardiovasc Surg 1974; 68:131–133.

110. Dahms BB. Benign clear cell tumor of lung with necrosis. Cancer 1976; 37:2355–2358.

111. Pea M, Bonetti F, Zamboni G, Martignoni G, Fiore-Donati L, Doglioni C. Clear cell tumour and angiomyolipoma. Am J Surg Pathol 1991; 15:199–202.

112. Kaiserling E, Krober S, Xiao JC, Schaumburg-Lever G. Angiomyolipoma of the kidney. immunoreactivity with HMB- 45 light- and electron-microscopic findings. Histopathology 1994; 25:41–48.

113. Bonetti F, Pea M, Martignoni G, et al. Clear cell ('sugar') tumor of the lung is a lesion strictly related to angiomyolipoma - the concept of a family of lesions characterized by the presence of the perivascular epithelioid cells (PEC). Pathology 1995; 26:230–236.

114. Pea M, Martignoni G, Zamboni G, Bonetti F. Perivascular epithelioid cell. Am J Surg Pathol 1996; 20:1149–1153.

115. Chuah KL, Tan PH. Multifocal micronodular pneumocyte hyperplasia, lymphangiomyomatosis and clear cell micronodules of the lung in a Chinese female patient with tuberous sclerosis. Pathology 1998; 30:242–246.

116. Hironaka M, Fukayama M. Regional proliferation of HMB-45-positive clear cells of the lung with lymphangioleiomyomatosis-like distribution, replacing the lobes with multiple cysts and a nodule. Am J Surg Pathol 1999; 23:1288–1293.

117. Leong AS-Y, Meredith DJ. Clear cell tumors of the lung. In Corrin B, ed. Pathology of Lung Tumors. London: Churchill Livingstone, 1997; 159–174.

'Hamartoma' (chondroid hamartoma, adenochondroma, mixed mesenchymoma)

118. Bateson EM. So-called hamartoma of the lung – a true neoplasm of fibrous connective tissue of the bronchi. Cancer 1973; 31:1458–1467.

119. Tomashefski JF. Benign endobronchial mesenchymal tumors. Their relationship to parenchymal pulmonary hamartomas. Am J Surg Pathol 1982; 6:531–540.

120. van den Bosch JMM, Wagenaar SjSc, Corrin B, Elbers JRJ, Knaepen PJ, Westermann CJJ. Mesenchymoma of the lung (so called hamartoma): a review of 154 parenchymal and endobronchial cases. Thorax 1987; 42:790–793.

121. Takemura T, Kusafuka K, Fujiwara M, et al. An immunohistochemical study of the mesenchymal and epithelial components of pulmonary chondromatous hamartomas. Pathol Int 1999; 49:938–946.

122. Xiao S, Lux ML, Reeves R, Hudson TJ, Fletcher JA. HMGI(Y) activation by chromosome 6p21 rearrangements in multilineage mesenchymal cells from pulmonary hamartoma. Am J Pathol 1997; 150:901–910.

123. Tallini G, Vanni R, Manfioletti G, et al. HMGI-C and HMGI(Y) immunoreactivity correlates with cytogenetic abnormalities in lipomas, pulmonary chondroid hamartomas, endometrial polyps, and uterine leiomyomas and is compatible with rearrangement of the HMGI-C and HMGI(Y) genes. Lab Invest 2000; 80:359–369.

124. Suster S, Moran CA. Pulmonary adenofibroma – report of two cases of an unusual type of hamartomatous lesion of the lung. Histopathology 1993; 23:547–551.

125. Scarff RW, Gowar FJS. Fibroadenoma of the lung. J Pathol Bacteriol 1944; 56:257–259.

126. Wolff M, Kaye G, Silva F. Pulmonary metastases (with admixed epithelial elements) from smooth muscle neoplasms. Report of nine cases, including three males. Am J Surg Pathol 1979; 3:325–342.

127. Alvarez-Fernandez E. Alveolar trapping in pulmonary carcinomas. Diag Histopathol 1982; 5:59–64.

128. McDonald JR, Harrington SW, Clagett OT. Hamartoma (often called chondroma) of the lung. J Thorac Surg 1945; 14:128–143.

129. Sharkey RA, Mulloy EMT, O'Neil S. Endobronchial hamartoma presenting as massive haemoptysis. Eur Respir J 1996; 9:2179–2180.

130. Cosio BG, Villena V, EchaveSustaeta J, et al. Endobronchial hamartoma. Chest 2002; 122:202–205.

131. King TE, Christopher KL, Schwarz MI. Multiple pulmonary chondromatous hamartomas. Hum Pathol 1982; 13:496–497.

132. Laroche CM, Stewart S, Wells F, Shneerson J. Multiple recurrent intrapulmonary and endobronchial mesenchymomas (hamartomas). Thorax 1993; 48:572–573.

133. Suzuki N, Ohno S, Ishii Y, Kitamura S. Peripheral intrapulmonary hamartoma accompanied by a similar endotracheal lesion. Chest 1994; 106:1291–1293.

134. Dominguez H, Hariri J, Pless S. Multiple pulmonary chondrohamartomas in trachea, bronchi and lung parenchyma. Review of the literature. Respir Med 1996; 90:111–114.

135. Kiryu T, Kawaguchi S, Matsui E, Hoshi H, Kokubo M, Shimokawa K. Multiple chondromatous hamartomas of the lung – A case report and review of the literature with special reference to Carney syndrome. Cancer 1999; 85:2557–2561.

136. Karasik A, Modan M, Jacob CO, Lieberman Y. Increased risk of lung cancer in patients with chondromatous hamartoma. J Thorac Cardiovasc Surg 1980; 80:217–220.

137. Basile A, Gregoris A, Antoci B, Romanelli M. Malignant change in a benign pulmonary hamartoma. Thorax 1989; 44:232–233.

138. Gabrail NY, Zara BY. Pulmonary hamartoma syndrome. Chest 1990; 97:962–965.

139. Bateson EM. Cartilage-containing tumours of the lung. Relationship between the purely cartilaginous type (chondroma) and the mixed type (so-called hamartoma): an unusual case of multiple tumours. Thorax 1967; 22:256–259.

140. Bateson EM. Histogenesis of intrapulmonary and endobronchial hamartomas and chondromas (cartilage-containing tumours): a hypothesis. J Pathol 1970; 101:77–83.

Lipoma, chondroma and fibroma

141. Moran CA, Suster S, Koss MN. Endobronchial lipomas – a clinicopathologic study of four cases. Mod Pathol 1994; 7:212–214.

142. Huisman C, vanKralingen KW, Postmus PE, Sutedja TG. Endobronchial lipoma: A series of three cases and the role of electrocautery. Respiration 2000; 67:689–692.

143. Muraoka M, Oka T, Akamine S, et al. Endobronchial lipoma – Review of 64 cases reported Japan. Chest 2003; 123:293–296.

144. Kim NR, Kim HJ, Kim JK, Han J. Intrapulmonary lipomas: report of four cases. Histopathology 2003; 42:305–306.

145. Carney JA, Sheps SG, Go VLW, Gordon H. The triad of gastric leiomyosarcoma, functioning extra-adrenal paraganglioma and pulmonary chondroma. N Engl J Med 1977; 296:1517–1518.

146. Carney JA. The triad of gastric epithelioid leiomyosarcoma, functioning extra-adrenal paraganglioma, and pulmonary chondroma. Cancer 1979; 43:374–382.

147. Engelman RM. Pulmonary fibroma: a rare benign tumor. Am Rev Respir Dis 1967; 96:1242–1245.

148. Margulies KB, Sheps SG. Carney's triad: guidelines for management. Mayo Clin Proc 1988; 63:496–502.

149. Raafat F, Salman WD, Roberts K, Ingram L, Rees R, Mann JR. Carney's triad: gastric leiomyosarcoma, pulmonary chondroma and extra-adrenal paraganglioma in young females. Histopathology 1986; 10:1325–1333.

150. Carney JA. The triad of gastric epithelioid leiomyosarcoma, pulmonary chondroma, and functioning extra-adrenal paraganglioma: a five-year review. Medicine (Baltimore) 1983; 62:159–169.

151. Carney JA. Gastric stromal sarcoma, pulmonary chondroma, and extra-adrenal paraganglioma (Carney Triad): natural history, adrenocortical component, and possible familial occurrence. Mayo Clin Proc 1999; 74:543–552.

152. Ngadiman S, Horenstein MG, Campbell WG. The concurrence of duodenal epithelioid stromal sarcoma, pulmonary chondromatous hamartoma, and nonfunctioning pancreatic islet cell tumor – a possible analogue of Carney's triad? Arch Pathol Lab Med 1994; 118:840–843.

Histiocytoma

153. Osborn M, Mandys V, Beddow E, et al. Cystic fibrohistiocytic tumours presenting in the lung: primary or metastatic disease? Histopathology 2003; 43:556–562.

Leiomyoma and fibroleiomyoma

154. Williams RB, Daniel RA. Leiomyoma of the lung. J Thorac Surg 1950; 19:806–810.

155. Vera-Roman JM, Sobonya RE, Gomez-Garcia JL, Sanz-Bondia JR, Paris-Romeu F. Leiomyoma of the lung. Cancer 1983; 52:936–941.

156. Peters P, Trotter SE, Sheppard MN, Goldstraw P. Primary leiomyoma of the pulmonary vein. Thorax 1992; 47:393–394.

157. Naresh KN, Pai SA, Vyas JJ, Soman CS. Leiomyoma of the bronchus – a case report. Histopathology 1993; 22:288–289.

158. Ozcelik U, Kotiloglu E, Gocmen A, Senocak ME, Kiper N. Endobronchial leiomyoma: a case report. Thorax 1995; 50:101–102.

159. Olgun N, Ozaksoy D, Ucan ES, et al. Paediatric endobronchial leiomyoma mimicking asthma. Respir Med 1995; 89:581–582.

160. Cruickshank DB, Harrison GK. Diffuse fibro-leiomyomatous hamartomatosis of the lung. Thorax 1953; 8:316–318.

Angiomyolipoma

161. Guinee DG, Thornberry DS, Azumi N, Przygodzki RM, Koss MN, Travis WD. Unique pulmonary presentation of an angiomyolipoma: analysis of clinical, radiographic, and histopathologic features. Am J Surg Pathol 1995; 19:476–480.

162. Ito M, Sugamura Y, Ikari H, Sekine I. Angiomyolipoma of the lung. Arch Pathol Lab Med 1998; 122:1023–1025.

163. Garcia TR, deJuan MJM. Angiomyolipoma of the liver and lung: A case explained by the presence of perivascular epithelioid cells. Pathol Res Pract 2002; 198:363–367.

164. Wu K, Tazelaar HD. Pulmonary angiomyolipoma and multifocal micronodular pneumocyte hyperplasia associated with tuberous sclerosis. Hum Pathol 1999; 30:1266–1268.

165. Stone CH, Lee MW, Amin MB, et al. Renal angiomyolipoma – Further immunophenotypic characterisation of an expanding morphologic spectrum. Arch Pathol Lab Med 2001; 125:751–758.

166. Paradis V, Laurendeau I, Vieillefond A, et al. Clonal analysis of renal sporadic angiomyolipomas. Hum Pathol 1998; 29:1063–1067.

Miscellaneous sarcomas

167. Cameron EWJ. Primary sarcoma of the lung. Thorax 1975; 30:516–520.

168. Bernheim J, Griffel B, Versano S, Bruderman I, Saba K. Mediastinal leiomyosarcoma in the wall of a bronchial cyst. Arch Pathol Lab Med 1980; 104:221.

169. Wang N-S, Seemayer TA, Ahmed MN, Morin J. Pulmonary leiomyosarcoma associated with an arteriovenous fistula. Arch Pathol 1974; 98:100–105.

170. Chowdhury LN, Swerdlow MA, Jao W, Kathpalia S, Desser RK. Postirradiation malignant fibrous histiocytoma of the lung. Am J Clin Pathol 1980; 74:820–826.

171. McClain KL, Leach CT, Jenson HB, et al. Association of Epstein-Barr virus with leiomyosarcomas in young people with AIDS. N Engl J Med 1995; 332:12–18.

172. Bluhm JM, Yi ES, Diaz G, Colby TV, Colt HG. Multicentric endobronchial smooth muscle tumors associated with the Epstein-Barr virus in an adult patient with the acquired immunodeficiency syndrome: A case report. Cancer 1997; 80:1910–1913.

173. Somers CR, Tesoriero AA, Hartland E, Robertson CF, Robinson PJ, Chow CW. Multiple leiomyosarcomas of both donor and recipient origin arising in a heart-lung transplant patient. Am J Surg Pathol 1998; 22:1423–1428.

174. Pettinato G, Manivel JC, Saldana MJ, Peyser J, Dehner LP. Primary bronchopulmonary fibrosarcoma of childhood and adolescence: reassessment of a low-grade malignancy. Clinicopathologic study of five cases and review of the literature. Hum Pathol 1989; 20:463–471.

175. Guccion JG, Rosen SH. Bronchopulmonary leiomyosarcoma and fibrosarcoma. A study of 32 cases and review of the literature. Cancer 1972; 30:836–847.

176. Attanoos RL, Appleton MAC, Gibbs AR. Primary sarcomas of the lung: a clinicopathological and immunohistochemical study of 14 cases. Histopathology 1996; 29:29–36.

177. Moran CA, Suster S, Abbondanzo SL, Koss MN. Primary leiomyosarcomas of the lung: a clinicopathologic and immunohistochemical study of 18 cases. Mod Pathol 1997; 10:121–128.

178. Shimizu J, Sasaki M, Nakamura Y, et al. Simultaneous lung and liver resection for primary pulmonary leiomyosarcoma. Respiration 1997; 64:179–181.

179. Yousem SA, Hochholzer L. Malignant fibrous histiocytoma of the lung. Cancer 1987; 60:2532–2541.

180. McDonnell T, Kyriakos M, Roper C, Mazoujian G. Malignant fibrous histiocytoma of the lung. Cancer 1988; 61:137–145.

181. Shah IA, Kurtz SM, Simonsen RL. Radiation-induced malignant fibrous histiocytoma of the pulmonary artery. Arch Pathol Lab Med 1991; 115:921–925.

182. Sleyster TJW, Heystraten FMJ. Malignant fibrous histiocytoma mimicking pulmonary embolism. Thorax 1988; 43:580–581.

183. Lamuraglia GM, McLoud TC, Mark EJ, Kazemi H. A 54-year-old woman with intermittent hemoptysis, increasing exertional dyspnea, and a left mediastinal mass – malignant fibrous histiocytoma of pulmonary artery, with embolism and pulmonary infarcts. N Engl J Med 1994; 330: 997–1002.

184. Shijubo N, Sugaya F, Imada A, et al. Malignant fibrous histiocytoma presenting as an endobronchial polyp of the carina. Eur Respir J 1995; 8:1430–1431.

185. Halyard MY, Camoriano JK, Culligan JA, et al. Malignant fibrous histiocytoma of the lung - report of four cases and review of the literature. Cancer 1996; 78:2492–2497.

186. Nistal M, Jimenez Heffernan JA, Hardisson D, Viguer JM, Bueno J, Garcia Miguel P. Malignant fibrous histiocytoma of the lung in a child. An unusual neoplasm that can mimick inflammatory pseudotumour. Eur J Pediatr 1997; 156:107–109.

187. Keel SB, Bacha E, Mark EJ, Nielsen GP, Rosenberg AE. Primary pulmonary sarcoma: A clinicopathologic study of 26 cases. Modern Pathol 1999; 12:1124–1131.

188. Kimizuka G, Okuzawa K, Yarita T. Primary giant cell malignant fibrous histiocytoma of the lung: A case report. Pathol Int 1999; 49:342–346.

189. Abrahamson JR, Friedman NB. Intrapulmonary stromal mesothelioma. J Thorac Cardiovasc Surg 1966; 51:300–306.

190. Goodlad JR, Fletcher CDM. Solitary fibrous tumour arising at unusual sites – analysis of a series. Histopathology 1991; 19:515–522.

191. Alvarez-Fernandez E, Escalona-Zapata J. Intrapulmonary mesotheliomas: their identification by tissue culture. Virchows Arch A Pathol Anat Histopathol 1982; 395:331–343.

192. van de Rijn M, Lombard CM, Rouse RV. Expression of CD34 by solitary fibrous tumors of the pleura, mediastinum, and lung. Am J Surg Pathol 1994; 18:814–820.

193. Bartley TD, Arean VM. Intrapulmonary neurogenic tumours. J Thorac Cardiovasc Surg 1965; 50:114–123.

194. Oosterwijk WM, Swierenga J. Neurogenic tumours with an intrathoracic localisation. Thorax 1968; 23:374–384.

195. Ruiz-Palomo F, Calleja JL, Fogue L. Primary liposarcoma of the lung in a young woman. Thorax 1990; 45:298–299.

196. Comin CE, Santucci M, Novelli L, Dini S. Primary pulmonary rhabdomyosarcoma: Report of a case in an adult and review of the literature. Ultrastruct Pathol 2001; 25:269–273.

197. Sun C-CJ, Kroll M, Miller JE. Primary chondrosarcoma of the lung. Cancer 1982; 50:1864–1866.

198. Kurotaki H, Tateoka H, Takeuchi M, Yagihashi S, Kamata Y, Nagai K. Primary mesenchymal chondrosarcoma of the lung - a case report with immunohistochemical and ultrastructural studies. Acta Pathol Jpn 1992; 42:364–371.

199. Hayashi T, Tsuda N, Iseki M, Kishikawa M, Shinozaki T, Hasumoto M. Primary chondrosarcoma of the lung - a clinicopathologic study. Cancer 1993; 72:69–74.

200. Azimullah PC, Teengs JP, Boerma EJ. Chondrosarcoma of the lobar bronchus with prolonged postoperative survival. Eur Respir J 1994; 7:1537–1538.

201. Reingold IM, Amromin GD. Extraosseous osteosarcoma of the lung. Cancer 1971; 28:491–498.

202. Kuroda M, Oka T, Horiuchi H, Ishida T, Machinami R, Hebisawa A. Giant cell tumor of the lung – an autopsy case report with immunohistochemical observations. Pathol Int 1994; 44:158–163.

203. Tsutsumi Y, Deng YL. Alveolar soft part sarcoma of the pulmonary vein. Acta Pathol Jpn 1991; 41:771–777.

204. Tralka GA, Katz S. Hemangioendothelioma of the lung. Am Rev Respir Dis 1963; 87:107–115.

205. Yousem SA. Angiosarcoma presenting in the lung. Arch Pathol Lab Med 1986; 110:112–115.

206. Koizumi N, Fukuda T, Ohnishi Y, et al. Pulmonary myxoid leiomyosarcoma. Pathol Int 1995; 45:879–884.

207. Inayama Y, Hayashi H, Ogawa N, Mitsui H, Nakatani Y. Low-grade pulmonary myxoid sarcoma of uncertain histogenesis. Pathol Int 2001; 51:204–210.

208. Zeren H, Moran CA, Suster S, Fishback NF, Koss MN. Primary pulmonary sarcomas with features of monophasic synovial sarcoma: a clinicopathological, immunohistochemical, and ultrastructural study of 25 cases. Hum Pathol 1995; 26:474–480.

209. Kaplan MA, Goodman MD, Satish J, Bhagavan BS, Travis WD. Primary pulmonary sarcoma with morphologic features of monophasic synovial sarcoma and chromosome translocation t(x; 18). Am J Clin Pathol 1996; 105:195–199.

210. Hisaoka M, Hashimoto H, Iwamasa T, Ishikawa K, Aoki T. Primary synovial sarcoma of the lung: report of two cases confirmed by molecular detection of SYT-SSX fusion gene transcripts. Histopathology 1999; 34:205–210.

211. Mikami Y, Nakajima M, Hashimoto H, Kuwabara K, Sasao Y, Manabe T. Primary poorly differentiated monophasic synovial sarcoma of the lung. A case report with immunohistochemical and genetic studies. Pathol Res Pract 2003; 199:827–833.

212. Kalus M, Rahman F, Jenkins DE, Beall AC. Malignant mesenchymoma of the lung. Arch Pathol 1973; 95:199–202.

Vascular tumours and proliferations

213. Paul KP, Borner C, Muller KM, Vogt-Moykopf I. Capillary hemangioma of the right main bronchus treated by sleeve resection in infancy. Am Rev Respir Dis 1991; 143:876–879.

214. Bowyer JJ, Sheppard M. Capillary haemangioma presenting as a lung pseudocyst. Arch Dis Child 1990; 65:1162–1164.

215. Hamada K, Ishii Y, Nakaya M, Sawabata N, Fukuda K, Suzuki H. Solitary lymphangioma of the lung. Histopathology 1995; 27:482–483.

216. Wada A, Tateishi R, Terazawa T, Matsuda M, Hattori S. Lymphangioma of the lung. Arch Pathol Lab Med 1974; 98:211–213.

217. Al-Hilli F. Lymphangioma (or alveolar adenoma?) of the lung. Histopathology 1987; 11:979–980.

218. Holden WE, Morris JF, Antonovic R, Gill TH, Kessler S. Adult intrapulmonary and mediastinal lymphangioma causing haemoptysis. Thorax 1987; 42:635–636.

219. Faul JL, Berry GJ, Colby TV, et al. Thoracic lymphangiomas, lymphangiectasis, lymphangiomatosis, and lymphatic dysplasia syndrome. Am J Respir Crit Care Med 2000; 161:1037–1046.

220. Wilson C, Askin FB, Heitmiller RF. Solitary pulmonary lymphangioma. Ann Thorac Surg 2001; 71:1337–1338.

221. Nagayasu T, Hayashi T, Ashizawa K, et al. A case of solitary pulmonary lymphangioma. J Clin Pathol 2003; 56:396–398.

222. Irani S, Brack T, Pfaltz M, Russi EW. Tracheal lobular capillary hemangioma – A rare cause of recurrent hemoptysis. Chest 2003; 123:2148–2149.

223. Kobayashi A, Ohno S, Bando M, Oshikawa K, Sugiyama Y. Cavernous hemangiomas of lungs and liver in an asymptomatic girl. Respiration 2003; 70:647–650.

224. Harding JR, Williams J, Seal RME. Pedunculated capillary haemangioma of the bronchus. Br J Dis Chest 1978; 72:336–342.

225. Holden KR, Alexander F. Diffuse neonatal hemangiomatosis. Pediatrics 1970; 46:411–421.

226. Rowen M, Thompson JR, Williamson RA, Wood BJ. Diffuse pulmonary hemangiomatosis. Radiology 1978; 127:445–451.

227. Gilbey LK, Girod CE. Blue rubber bleb nevus syndrome – Endobronchial involvement presenting as chronic cough. Chest 2003; 124:760–763.

228. Swank DW, Hepper NGG, Folkert KE, Colby TV. Intrathoracic lymphangiomatosis mimicking lymphangioleiomyomatosis in a young woman. Mayo Clin Proc 1989; 64:1264–1268.

229. Ramani P, Shah A. Lymphangiomatosis – histologic and immunohistochemical analysis of four cases. Am J Surg Pathol 1993; 17:329–335.

230. Tazelaar HD, Kerr D, Yousem SA, Saldana MJ, Langston C, Colby TV. Diffuse pulmonary lymphangiomatosis. Hum Pathol 1993; 24:1313–1322.

231. Canny GJ, Cutz E, Maclusky IB, Levison H. Diffuse pulmonary angiomatosis. Thorax 1991; 46:851–853.

232. Takahashi K, Takahashi H, Maeda K, et al. An adult case of lymphangiomatosis of the mediastinum, pulmonary interstitium and retroperitoneum complicated by chronic disseminated intravascular coagulation. Eur Respir J 1995; 8:1799–1802.

233. Joshi M, Cole S, Knibbs D, Diana D. Pulmonary abnormalities in Klippel-Trenaunay syndrome – a histologic, ultrastructural, and immunocytochemical study. Chest 1992; 102:1274–1277.

234. Carlson KC, Parnassus WN, Klatt CC. Thoracic lymphangiomatosis. Arch Pathol Lab Med 1987; 111:475–477.

235. Rydell R, Hoffbauer FW. Multiple pulmonary arteriovenous fistulas in juvenile cirrhosis. Am J Med 1956; 21:450–460.

236. Berthelot P, Walker JG, Sherlock S, Reid L. Arterial changes in the lungs in cirrhosis of the liver – lung spider nevi. N Engl J Med 1966; 274:291–298.

237. Stanley NN, Williams AJ, Dewar CA, Blendis LM, Reid L. Hypoxia and hydrothoraces in a case of liver cirrhosis: correlation of physiological, radiographic, scintigraphic, and pathological findings. Thorax 1977; 32:457–471.

238. Macnee W, Buist TAS, Finlayson NDC, et al. Multiple microscopic pulmonary arteriovenous connections in the lungs presenting as cyanosis. Thorax 1985; 40:316–318.

239. Ichijima K, Kobashi Y, Yamabe H, Fujii Y, Inoue Y. Peliosis hepatis: an unusual case involving multiple organs. Acta Pathol Jpn 1980; 30:109–120.

240. Lie JT. Pulmonary peliosis. Arch Pathol Lab Med 1985; 109:878–879.

241. Davis Z, Berliner WP, Weiland LH, Clagett OT. Primary pulmonary hemangiopericytoma. J Thorac Cardiovasc Surg 1972; 64:882–825.

242. Meade JB, Whitwell F, Bickford BJ, Waddington JKB. Primary haemangiopericytoma of lung. Thorax 1974; 29:1–15.

243. Razzuk MA, Nassur A, Gardner MA, Martin J, Gohara SF, Urschel HC. Primary pulmonary hemangiopericytoma. J Thorac Cardiovasc Surg 1977; 74:227–229.

244. Shin MS, Ho K-J. Primary hemangiopericytoma of the lung: radiography and pathology. Am J Roentgenol 1979; 133:1077–1083.

245. Yousem SA, Hochholzer L. Primary pulmonary hemangiopericytoma. Cancer 1987; 59:549–555.

246. Rusch VW, Shuman WP, Schmidt R, Laramore GE. Massive pulmonary hemangiopericytoma. An innovative approach to evaluation and treatment. Cancer 1989; 64:1928–1936.

247. Rothe TB, Karrer W, Gebbers JO. Recurrent haemoptysis in a young woman – a case of a malignant haemangiopericytoma of the lung. Thorax 1994; 49:188–189.

248. Fabich DR, Hafez G-R. Glomangioma of the trachea. Cancer 1980; 45:2337–2341.

249. Heard BE, Dewar A, Firmin RK, Lennox SC. One very rare and one new tracheal tumour found by electron microscopy: glomus tumour and acinic cell tumour resembling carcinoid tumours by light microscopy. Thorax 1982; 37:97–103.

250. Sheffield EA, Dewar A, Corrin B, Addis BJ, Conroy B. Glomus tumour of the trachea. Histopathology 1988; 13:234–236.

251. Shin DH, Park SS, Lee JH, Park MH, Lee JD. Oncocytic glomus tumor of the trachea. Chest 1990; 98:1021–1023.

252. Garcia-Prats MD, Sotelo-Rodriguez MT, Ballestin C, et al. Glomus tumour of the trachea – report of a case with microscopic, ultrastructural and immunohistochemical examination and review of the literature. Histopathology 1991; 19:459–464.

253. Arapantoni-Dadioti P, Panayiotides J, Fatsis M, Antypas G. Tracheal glomus tumour. Respiration 1995; 62:160–162.

254. Menaissy YM, Gal AA, Mansour KA. Glomus tumor of the trachea. Ann Thorac Surg 2000; 70:295–297.

255. Tang C, Toker CK, Foris NP,, et al. Glomangioma of the lung. Am J Surg Pathol 1978; 2:103–109.

256. Brooks JJ, Miettinen M, Virtanen I. Desmin immunoreactivity in glomus tumors. Am J Clin Pathol 1987; 87:292–294.

257. Koss MN, Hochholzer L, Moran CA. Primary pulmonary glomus tumor: A clinicopathologic and immunohistochemical study of two cases. Modern Pathol 1998; 11:253–258.

258. Gaertner EM, Steinberg DM, Huber M, et al. Pulmonary and mediastinal glomus tumors – Report of five cases including a pulmonary glomangiosarcoma: A clinicopathologic study with literature review. Am J Surg Pathol 2000; 24:1105–1114.

259. Oizumi S, Kon Y, Ishida T, et al. A rare case of bronchial glomus tumor. Respiration 2001; 68:95–98.

260. Yilmaz A, Bayramgurler B, Aksoy F, Tuncer LY, Selvi A, Uzman O. Pulmonary glomus tumour: a case initially diagnosed as carcinoid tumour. Respirology 2002; 7:369–371.

261. Granter SR, Badizadegan K, Fletcher CDM. Myofibromatosis in adults, glomangiopericytoma, and myopericytoma : A spectrum of tumors showing perivascular myoid differentiation. Am J Surg Pathol 1998; 22:513–525.

262. Hishida T, Hasegawa T, Asamura H, et al. Malignant glomus tumor of the lung. Pathol Int 2003; 53:632–636.

263. Gottlieb GJ, Ackerman AB. Kaposi's sarcoma: an extensively disseminated form in young homosexual men. Hum Pathol 1982; 13:882–842.

264. Gunawardena KA, Al-Hasani MK, Haleem A, Al-Suleiman M, Al-Khader AA. Pulmonary Kaposi's sarcoma in two recipients of renal transplants. Thorax 1988; 43:653–656.

265. Khan GA, Klapper P. Pulmonary haemorrhage following renal transplantation. Thorax 1995; 50:98–99.

266. Yousem SA. Lung tumors in the immunocompromised host. In: Corrin B, ed. Pathology of Lung Tumors. London: Churchill Livingstone; 1997:189–212.

267. Aboulafia DM. The epidemiologic, pathologic, and clinical features of AIDS-associated pulmonary Kaposi's sarcoma. Chest 2000; 117:1128–1145.

268. Reichert CM, O'Leary TJ, Levens DL, Simrell CR, Macher AM. Autopsy pathology in the acquired immune deficiency syndrome. Am J Pathol 1983; 112:357–382.

269. Guarda LA, Luna MA, Smith JL, Mansett PWA, Gyorkey F, Roca AN. Acquired immune deficiency syndrome and postmortem findings. Am J Clin Pathol 1984; 81:549–557.

270. Moskowitz LB, Hensley GT, Gould EW, Weiss SD. Frequency and anatomic distribution of lymphadenopathic Kaposi's sarcoma in the acquired immunodeficiency syndrome. Hum Pathol 1985; 16:447–456.

271. Farber HW, Mark EJ, Moore EH, Michael NL, Weinstein DF. A 29-year-old man with a positive test for HIV and a reticulonodular pulmonary infiltrate – pulmonary Kaposi's sarcoma – acquired immunodeficiency syndrome (AIDS). N Engl J Med 1990; 322:43–51.

272. Beral V, Peterman TA, Berkelman R, Jaffe HW. Kaposi's sarcoma among persons with AIDS: a sexually transmitted infection? Lancet 1990; 335:123–128.

273. Nash G, Said JW, Nash SV, Degirolami U. The pathology of AIDS – Kaposi's sarcoma. Mod Pathol 1995; 8:208–209.

274. Cadranel J, Mayaud C. Intrathoracic Kaposi's sarcoma in patients with AIDS. Thorax 1995; 50:407–414.

275. Siegal B, Levinton-Kriss S, Schiffer A, et al. Kaposi's sarcoma in immunosuppression. Possibly the result of a dual viral infection. Cancer 1990; 65:492–498.

276. Chang Y, Cesarman E, Pessin MS, et al. Identification of herpesvirus-like DNA sequences in AIDS-associated Kaposi's sarcoma. Science 1994; 266:1865–1869.

277. Moore PS, Chang YA. Detection of herpesvirus-like DNA sequences in Kaposi's sarcoma in patients with those and without HIV infection. N Engl J Med 1995; 332:1181–1185.

278. Cesarman E, Chang YA, Moore PS, Said JW, Knowles DM. Kaposi's sarcoma-associated herpesvirus-like DNA sequences in AIDS-related body-cavity-based lymphomas. N Engl J Med 1995; 332:1186–1191.

279. Roizman B. New viral footprints in Kaposi's sarcoma. N Engl J Med 1995; 332:1227–1228.

280. Jin YT, Tsai ST, Yan JJ, Hsiao JH, Lee YY, Su IJ. Detection of Kaposi's sarcoma-associated herpesvirus-like DNA sequence in vascular lesions: a reliable diagnostic marker for Kaposi's sarcoma. Am J Clin Pathol 1996; 105:360–363.

281. Li JJ, Huang YQ, Cockerell CJ, Friedmankien AE. Localisation of human herpes-like virus type 8 in vascular endothelial cells and perivascular spindle-shaped cells of Kaposi's sarcoma lesions by in situ hybridisation. Am J Pathol 1996; 148:1741–1748.

282. Dictor M, Rambech E, Way D, Witte M, Bendsoe N. Human herpesvirus 8 (Kaposi's sarcoma-associated herpesvirus) DNA in Kaposi's sarcoma lesions, AIDS Kaposi's sarcoma cell lines, endothelial Kaposi's sarcoma simulators, and the skin of immunosuppressed patients. Am J Pathol 1996; 148:2009–2016.

283. Kennedy MM, Cooper K, Howells DD, et al. Identification of HHV8 in early Kaposi's sarcoma: implications for Kaposi's sarcoma pathogenesis. J Clin Pathol Mol Pathol 1998; 51:14–20.

284. Chadburn A, Cesarman E, Nador RG, Liu YF, Knowles DM. Kaposi's sarcoma-associated herpesvirus sequences in benign lymphoid proliferations not associated with human immunodeficiency virus. Cancer 1997; 80:788–797.

285. Tamm M, Reichenberger F, McGandy CE, et al. Diagnosis of pulmonary Kaposi's sarcoma by detection of human herpes virus 8 in bronchoalveolar lavage. Am J Respir Crit Care Med 1998; 157:458–463.

286. Dilnur P, Katano H, Wang ZH, et al. Classic type of Kaposi's sarcoma and human herpesvirus 8 infection in Xinjiang, China. Pathol Int 2001; 51:845–852.

287. Miller RF, Tomlinson MC, Cottrill CP, Donald JJ, Spittle MF, Semple SJG. Bronchopulmonary Kaposi's sarcoma in patients with AIDS. Thorax 1992; 47:721–725.

288. Mitchell DM, McCarty M, Fleming J, Moss FM. Bronchopulmonary Kaposi's sarcoma in patients with AIDS. Thorax 1992; 47:726–729.

289. Dantzig PI, Richardson D, Rayhanzadeh S, Mauro J, Shoss R. Thoracic involvement of non-African Kaposi's sarcoma. Chest 1974; 66:522–525.

290. Loring WE, Wolman SR. Idiopathic multiple hemorrhagic sarcoma of lung (Kaposi's sarcoma). N Y State J Med 1965; 65:668–675.

291. Misra DP, Sunderrajan EV, Hurst DJ, Maltby JD. Kaposi's sarcoma of the lung: radiography and pathology. Thorax 1982; 37:155–156.

292. Chin R, Jones DF, Pegram PS, Haponik EF. Complete endobronchial occlusion by Kaposi's sarcoma in the absence of cutaneous involvement. Chest 1994; 105:1581–1582.

293. Templeton AC. Studies in Kaposi's sarcoma: post mortem findings and disease patterns in women. Cancer 1972; 30:854–867.

294. Pozniak AL, Latif AS, Neill P, Houston S, Chen K, Robertson V. Pulmonary Kaposi's sarcoma in Africa. Thorax 1992; 47:730–733.

295. Schnapp LM, Gruden JF, Hopewell PC, Stansell JD. Presentation of AIDS-related pulmonary Kaposi's sarcoma diagnosed by bronchoscopy. Am J Respir Crit Care Med 1996; 153:1385–1390.

296. Maduri GU, Stover DE, Lee M, Myskowski PL, Caravelli JF, Zaman MB. Pulmonary Kaposi's sarcoma in the acquired immune deficiency syndrome. Am J Med 1986; 81:11–18.

297. Purdy LJ, Colby TV, Yousem SA, Battifora H. Pulmonary Kaposi's sarcoma: premortem histologic diagnosis. Am J Surg Pathol 1986; 10:301–311.

298. Hamm PG, Judson MA, Aranda CP. Diagnosis of pulmonary Kaposi's sarcoma with fiberoptic bronchoscopy and endobronchial biopsy: a report of five cases. Cancer 1987; 59:807–810.

299. Russell Jones R, Paull JS, Spry C, Wilson Jones E. Histogenesis of Kaposi's sarcoma in patients with and without acquired immune deficiency syndrome (AIDS). J Clin Pathol 1986; 39:742–749.

300. Marguart KH. Weibel-Palade bodies in Kaposi's sarcoma. J Clin Pathol 1987; 40:933.

301. Kostianovsky M, Lamy Y, Greco MA. Immunohistochemical and electron microscopic profiles of cutaneous Kaposi's sarcoma and bacillary angiomatosis. Ultrastruct Pathol 1992; 16:629–640.

302. Dail DH, Liebow AA. Intravascular bronchioloalveolar tumour. Am J Pathol 1975; 78:6a-7a.

303. Dail DH, Liebow AA, Gmelich JT, et al. Intravascular, bronchiolar and alveolar tumour of the lung (IVBAT). Cancer 1983; 51:452–464.

304. Farinacci CJ, Blauw MD, Jennings EM. Multifocal pulmonary lesions of possible decidual origin (so-called pulmonary deciduosis): report of a case. Am J Clin Pathol 1973; 59:508–514.

305. Corrin B, Manners B, Millard M, Weaver L. Histogenesis of the so-called 'intravascular bronchioloalveolar tumour'. J Pathol 1979; 128:163–167.

306. Weldon-Linne CM, Victor TA, Christ ML, Fry WA. Angiogenic nature of the 'intravascular tumor' of the lung: an electron microscopic study. Arch Pathol Lab Med 1981; 105:174–179.

307. Weldon-Linne CM, Victor TA, Christ ML. Immunohistochemical identification of factor VIII-related antigen in the intravascular bronchioloalveolar tumor of the lung. Arch Pathol Lab Med 1981; 105:628–629.

308. Corrin B, Harrison WJ, Wright DH. The so-called intravascular bronchioloalveolar tumour of the lung (low-grade sclerosing angiosarcoma): presentation with extrapulmonary deposits. Diag Histopathol 1983; 6:229–237.

309. Azumi N, Churg A. Intravascular and sclerosing bronchioloalveolar tumour: a pulmonary sarcoma of probable vascular origin. Am J Surg Pathol 1981; 5:587–596.

310. Bhagavan BS, Dorfman HD, Murthy MSN. Intravascular bronchioloalveolar tumor (IVBAT). Am J Surg Pathol 1982; 6:41–52.

311. Rosai J, Gold J, Landy R. The histiocytoid hemangiomas. A unifying concept embracing several previously described entities of skin, soft tissues, large vessels, bone and heart. Hum Pathol 1979; 10:707–730.

312. Weidner N. Intriguing case – atypical tumor of the mediastinum – epithelioid hemangioendothelioma containing metaplastic bone and osteoclast-like giant cells. Ultrastruct Pathol 1991; 15:481–488.

313. Weiss SW, Enzinger FM. Epithelioid hemangioendothelioma. A vascular tumor often mistaken for carcinoma. Cancer 1982; 50:970–981.

314. Gledhill A, Kay JM. Hepatic metastases in a case of intravascular bronchioloalveolar tumour. J Clin Pathol 1984; 37:279–282.

315. Ishak KG, Sesterhenn IA, Goodman ZD, Rabin L, Stromayer FW. Epithelioid hemangioendothelioma of the liver. Hum Pathol 1984; 15:839–852.

316. Kitaichi M, Nagai S, Nishimura K, et al. Pulmonary epithelioid haemangioendothelioma in 21 patients, including three with partial spontaneous regression. Eur Resp J 1998; 12:89–96.

317. Bollinger BK, Laskin WB, Knight CB. Epithelioid hemangioendothelioma with multiple site involvement – literature review and observations. Cancer 1994; 73:610–615.

318. Nagata N, Takatsu H, Sato Y, Yoshimatsu T, Urabe M, Kido M. Metastatic pulmonary epithelioid hemangioendothelioma with peculiar radiographic features. Respiration 1999; 66:78–80.

319. Ledson MJ, Convery R, Carty A, Evans CC. Epithelioid haemangioendothelioma. Thorax 1999; 54:560–561.

320. Corrin B, Dewar A, Simpson CGB. Epithelioid haemangioendothelioma of the lung. Ultrastruct Pathol 1996; 20:345–347.

321. Lin BTY, Colby T, Gown AM, et al. Malignant vascular tumors of the serous membranes mimicking mesothelioma: a report of 14 cases. Am J Surg Pathol 1996; 20:1431–1439.

322. Yousem SA, Hochholzer L. Unusual thoracic manifestations of epithelioid hemangioendothelioma. Arch Pathol Lab Med 1981; 111:459–463.

323. Yi ES, Auger WR, Friedman PJ, Morris TA, Shin SS. Intravascular bronchioloalveolar tumor of the lung presenting as pulmonary thromboembolic disease and pulmonary hypertension. Arch Pathol Lab Med 1995; 119:255–260.

324. Kradin RL, Aquino S, Christiani DC, Mark EJ, Spitzer TR, Amatruda JF. Hemoptysis in a 20-year-old man with multiple pulmonary nodules. Epithelioid hemangioendothelioma of the lung (Intravascular, sclerosing bronchioloalveolar tumor) with lymph-node metastasis. N Engl J Med 2000; 342:572–578.

325. Yanagawa H, Hashimoto Y, Bando H, Takishita Y, Nagano T. Intravascular bronchioloalveolar tumor with skin metastases. Chest 1994; 105:1882–1884.

326. Echevarria RA. Angiogenic nature of 'intravascular bronchioloalveolar tumor'. Arch Pathol Lab Med 1981; 105:627–628.

327. Verbeken E, Bayls J, Moerman P, Knockaert D, Goddeeris P, Lauweryns JM. Lung metastasis of malignant epithelioid hemangioendothelioma mimicking a primary intravascular bronchioalveolar tumor. A histologic, ultrastructural, and immunohistochemical study. Cancer 1985; 55:1741–1746.

328. Nerlich A, Berndt R, Schleicher E. Differential basement membrane composition in multiple epithelioid haemangioendotheliomas of liver and lung. Histopathology 1991; 18:303–307.

329. Theurillat JPP, Vavricka SR, Went P, et al. Morphologic changes and altered gene expression in an epithelioid hemangioendothelioma during a ten-year course of disease. Pathol Res Pract 2003; 199:165–170.

330. Dawes GS, Comroe JH. Chemoreflexes from the heart and lungs. Physiol Rev 1954; 34:167–201.

331. Blessing MH, Hora BI. Glomera in der lunge des menschen. Zeitschrift fur Zellforschung 1968; 87:562–570.

332. Ashley DJB, Evans CJ. Intrathoracic carotid-body tumour (chemodectoma). Thorax 1966; 21:184–185.

333. Assaf HM, Almomen AA, Martin JG. Aorticopulmonary paraganglioma - a case report with immunohistochemical studies and literature review. Arch Pathol Lab Med 1992; 116:1085–1087.

334. Gallimore AP, Goldstraw P. Tracheal paraganglioma. Thorax 1993; 48:866–867.

335. Sing TMYS, Wong KP, Young N, Despas P. Chemodectoma of the trachea. Thorax 1996; 51:341–342.

336. Heppleston AG. A carotid-body-like tumour in the lung. J Path Bact 1958; 75:461–464.

337. Mostecky H, Lichtenberg J, Kalus M. A non-chromaffin paraganglioma of the lung. Thorax 1966; 21:205–208.

338. Fawcett FJ, Husband EM. Chemodectoma of lung. J Clin Pathol 1967; 20:260–262.

339. Goodman ML, LaForet EG. Solitary primary chemodectomas of the lung. Chest 1972; 61:48–50.

340. Hagemeyer O, Gabius HJ, Kayser K. Paraganglioma of the lung – developed after exposure to nuclear radiation by the Tschernobyl atomic reactor accident? Respiration 1994; 61:236–239.

341. Singh G, Lee RE, Brooks DH. Primary pulmonary paraganglioma. Cancer 1977; 40:2286–2289.

342. Medalie NS, Mendelsohn MG, Esposito M. Multicentric metachronous pulmonary and intravagal paraganglioma: A case report with immunohistochemical findings. Arch Pathol Lab Med 1996; 120:1137–1140.

343. Blessing MH, Borchard F, Lenz W. Glomustumor (sog. chemodektom) der lunge. Virchows Arch A Pathol Anat Histopathol 1973; 359:315–329.

344. Hamid Q, Varndell IM, Ibrahim NB, Mingazzini P, Polak JM. Extraadrenal paragangliomas. An immunocytochemical and ultrastructural report. Cancer 1987; 60:1776–1781.

345. Shibahara J, Goto A, Niki T, Tanaka M, Nakajima A, Fukayama M. Primary pulmonary paraganglioma – Report of a functioning case with immunohistochemical and ultrastructural study. Am J Surg Pathol 2004; 28:825–829.

346. Blobel GA, Gould VE, Moll R, et al. Coexpression of neuroendocrine markers and epithelial cytoskeletal proteins in bronchopulmonary neuroendocrine neoplasms. Lab Invest 1985; 52:39–51.

347. Johnson TL, Zarbo RJ, Lloyd RV, Crissman JD. Paragangliomas of the head and neck: immunohistochemical neuroendocrine and intermediate filament typing. Mod Pathol 1988; 1:216–223.

348. Moran CA, Rush W, Mena H. Primary spinal paragangliomas: a clinicopathological and immunohistochemical study of 30 cases. Histopathology 1997; 31:167–173.

349. Chetty R, Pillay P, Jaichand V. Cytokeratin expression in adrenal phaeochromocytomas and extra-adrenal paragangliomas. J Clin Pathol 1998; 51:477–478.

350. Hironaka M, Fukayama M, Takayashiki N, Saito K, Sohara Y, Funata N. Pulmonary gangliocytic paraganglioma – Case report and comparative immunohistochemical study of related neuroendocrine neoplasms. Am J Surg Pathol 2001; 25:688–693.

351. Min KW. Spindle cell carcinoids of the lung with paraganglioid features: a reappraisal of their histogenetic origin from paraganglia using immunohistochemical and electron microscopic techniques. Ultrastruct Pathol 2001; 25:207–217.

352. Bleisch VR, Kraus FT. Polypoid sarcoma of the pulmonary trunk. Cancer 1980; 46:314–324.

353. Nonomura A, Kurumaya H, Kono H, et al. Primary pulmonary artery sarcoma. Report of two autopsy cases studied by immunohistochemistry and electron microscopy, and review of 110 cases reported in the literature. Acta Pathol Jpn 1988; 38:883–896.

354. van Damme H, Vancerdeweg W, Schoofs E. Malignant fibrous histiocytoma of the pulmonary artery. Ann Surg 1987; 205:203–207.

355. Sanderson M, Britton M. Pulmonary artery leiomyosarcoma. Respir Med 1991; 85:337–338.

356. Johansson L, Carlen B. Sarcoma of the pulmonary artery: report of four cases with electron microscopic and immunohistochemical examinations, and review of the literature. Virchows Arch 1994; 424:217–224.

357. Emmertbuck MR, Stay EJ, Tsokos M, Travis WD. Pleomorphic rhabdomyosarcoma arising in association with the right pulmonary artery. Arch Pathol Lab Med 1994; 118:1220–1222.

358. Goldblum JR, Rice TW. Epithelioid angiosarcoma of the pulmonary artery. Hum Pathol 1995; 26:1275–1277.

359. Herrmann MA, Shankerman RA, Edwards WD, Shub C, Schaff HV. Primary cardiac angiosarcoma: a clinicopathologic study of six cases. J Thorac Cardiovasc Surg 1992; 103:655–664.

360. Mandel J, Mark EJ, McLoud TC, Hales CA. A 69-year-old woman with pleuritic pain and pulmonary arterial obstruction – Sarcoma of the intima of the pulmonary artery. N Engl J Med 2000; 343:493–500.

361. Fitzmaurice RJ, McClure J. Aortic intimal sarcoma: an unusual case with pulmonary vasculature involvement. Histopathology 1990; 17:457–462.

362. Katoh M, Shigematsu H. Leiomyosarcoma of the heart and its pulmonary metastasis, both with prominent osteoclast-like multinucleated giant cells expressing tartrate-resistant acid phosphatase activity. Pathol Int 1999; 49:74–78.

363. Oliai BR, Tazelaar HD, Lloyd RV, Doria MI, Trastek VF. Leiomyosarcoma of the pulmonary veins. Am J Surg Pathol 1999; 23:1082–1088.

364. Okuno T, Matsuda K, Ueyama K, et al. Leiomyosarcoma of the pulmonary vein. Pathol Int 2000; 50:839–846.

365. Shmookler BM, Marsh HB, Roberts WC. Primary sarcoma of the pulmonary trunk and/or right or left main pulmonary artery: a rare cause of obstruction of right ventricular outflow. Am J Med 1977; 63:263–272.

366. Madu EC, Taylor DC, Durzinsky DS, Fraker TDJr. Primary intimal sarcoma of the pulmonary trunk simulating pulmonary embolism. Am Heart J 1993; 125:1790–1792.

367. Kaplinsky EJ, Favaloro RR, Pombo G, et al. Primary pulmonary artery sarcoma resembling chronic thromboembolic pulmonary disease. Eur Resp J 2000; 16:1202–1204.

368. Parish JM, Rosenow EC, Swensen SJ, Crotty TB. Pulmonary artery sarcoma – clinical features. Chest 1996; 110:1480–1488.

369. Gosalbez F, Gudin C, Miralles M, Naya J, Valle JM. Intimal sarcoma of the left pulmonary artery: diagnosis, treatment and survival. Cardiovascular Surgery 1993; 1:447–448.

370. Mattoo A, Fedullo PF, Kapelanski D, Ilowite JS. Pulmonary artery sarcoma – A case report of surgical cure and 5-year follow-up. Chest 2002; 122:745–747.

371. Hayata T, Sato E. Primary leiomyosarcoma of the pulmonary artery. Acta Pathol Jpn 1977; 27:137–143.

372. Hiroshima K, Uruma T, Ishibashi M, Ohwada H, Hayashi Y. A case of primary sarcoma of the pulmonary artery. Acta Pathol Jpn 1992; 42:755–759.

373. Nappi O, Swanson PE, Wick MR. Pseudovascular adenoid squamous cell carcinoma of the lung: clinicopathologic study of three cases and comparison with true pleuropulmonary angiosarcoma. Hum Pathol 1994; 25:373–378.

374. Gray MH, Rosenberg AE, Dickersin GR, Bhan AK. Cytokeratin expression in epithelioid vascular neoplasms. Hum Pathol 1990; 21:212–217.

375. Huang CY, Huang CH, Yang AH, Wu MH, Ding YA, Yu WC. Solitary pulmonary artery myxoma manifesting as pulmonary embolism and subacute cor pulmonale. Am J Med 2003; 115:680–681.

Neural tumours

376. Crofts NF, Forbes GB. Malignant neurilemmoma of the lung metastasizing to the heart. Thorax 1964; 19:334–337.

377. Kitamura H. Primary epithelioid malignant schwannoma of the lung. Pathol Int 1994; 44:317–324.

378. McCluggage WG, Bharucha H. Primary pulmonary tumours of nerve sheath origin. Histopathology 1995; 26:247–254.

379. Nesbitt JC, Vega DM, Burke T, Mackay B. Cellular Schwannoma of the bronchus. Ultrastruct Pathol 1996; 20:349–354.

380. Cranshaw JH, Morgan C, Knowles G, Nicholson AG, Goldstraw P. Intramural neurofibroma of the trachea treated by multiple stents. Thorax 2001; 56:583–584.

381. Rowlands D, Edwards C, Collins F. Malignant melanotic schwannoma of the bronchus. J Clin Pathol 1987; 40:1449–1455.

382. Moran CA, Suster S, Koss MN. Primary malignant 'triton' tumour of the lung. Histopathology 1997; 30:140–144.

383. Miura H, Kato H, Hayata Y, Ebihara Y, Gonullu U. Solitary bronchial mucosal neuroma. Chest 1989; 95:245–247.

384. O'Donohue WJ, Edland J, Mohiuddin SM, Schultz RD. Multiple pulmonary neurofibromas with hypoxaemia. Arch Intern Med 1986; 146:1618–1619.

385. Abrikossof A. Uber Myome ausgehend von der guergestreiften willkuerlichen Muskulatur. Virchows Arch A Pathol Anat Histopathol 1926; 260:215–233.

386. Frenckner P. The occurrence of so-called myoblastomas in the mouth and upper air passages. Report of five cases. Acta Otolaryngol (Stockh) 1938; 26:689–701.

387. Kramer R. Myoblastoma of the bronchus. Ann Otol Rhinol Laryngol 1939; 48:1083–1086.

388. Buley ID, Gatter KC, Kelly PMA, Heryet A, Millard PR. Granular cell tumours revisited. An immunohistological and ultrastructural study. Histopathology 1988; 12:263–274.

389. Mittal KR, True LD. Origin of granules in granular cell tumor. Intracellular myelin formation with autodigestion. Arch Pathol Lab Med 1988; 112:302–303.

390. Filie AC, Lage JM, Azumi N. Immunoreactivity of S100 protein, alpha-1-antitrypsin, and CD68 in adult and congenital granular cell tumors. Mod Pathol 1996; 9:888–892.

391. Ordonez NG, Mackay B. Granular cell tumor: A review of the pathology and histogenesis. Ultrastruct Pathol 1999; 23:207–222.

392. Lack EE, Harris GBC, Eraklis AJ, Vawter GF. Primary bronchial tumours in childhood. Cancer 1983; 51:492–497.

393. Schulster PL, Khan FA, Azueta V. Asymptomatic pulmonary granular cell tumour presenting as a coin lesion. Chest 1975; 68:256–258.

394. Young CD, Gay RM. Multiple endobronchial granular cell myoblastomas discovered at bronchoscopy. Hum Pathol 1984; 15:193–194.

395. Hernandez OG, Haponik EF, Summer WR. Granular cell tumour of the bronchus: bronchoscopic and clinical features. Thorax 1986; 41:927–931.

396. Chen KTK. Cytology of bronchial benign granular-cell tumor. Acta Cytol 1991; 35:381–384.

397. Demontpreville VT, Dulmet EM. Granular cell tumours of the lower respiratory tract. Histopathology 1995; 27:257–262.

398. Deavers M, Guinee D, Koss MN, Travis WD. Granular cell tumors of the lung: clinicopathologic study of 20 cases. Am J Surg Pathol 1995; 19:627–635.

399. Sobel HJ, Schwartz R, Marquet E. Light and electron microscopic study of the origin of granular cell myoblastoma. J Pathol 1973; 109:101–111.

400. Gorancis JC, Komarovsky RA, Kuzina LF. Granular cell myoblastoma. Cancer 1970; 25:542–550.

401. Stefansson K, Wollman R, Jerkovic M. S-100 protein in granular cell tumors (granular cell myoblastomas). Cancer 1982; 49:1834–1838.

402. Kemnitz P, Spormann H, Heinrich P. Meningioma of lung: first report with light and electron microscopic findings. Ultrastruct Pathol 1982; 3:359–365.

403. Chumas JC, Lorelle CA. Pulmonary meningioma: a light- and electron-microscopic study. Am J Surg Pathol 1982; 6:795–801.

404. Unger PD, Geller SA, Anderson PJ. Pulmonary lesions in a patient with neurofibromatosis. Arch Pathol Lab Med 1984; 108:654–657.

405. Kodama K, Doi O, Higashiyama M, Horai T, Tateishi R, Nakagawa H. Primary and metastatic pulmonary meningioma. Cancer 1991; 67:1412–1417.

406. Flynn SD, Yousem SA. Pulmonary meningiomas: a report of two cases. Hum Pathol 1991; 22:469–474.

407. Drlicek M, Grisold W, Lorber J, Hackl H, Wuketich S, Jellinger K. Pulmonary meningioma - immunohistochemical and ultrastructural features. Am J Surg Pathol 1991; 15:455–459.

408. Robinson PG. Pulmonary meningioma - report of a case with electron microscopic and immunohistochemical findings. Am J Clin Pathol 1992; 97:814–817.

409. Moran CA, Hochholzer L, Rush W, Koss MN. Primary intrapulmonary meningiomas: a clinicopathologic and immunohistochemical study of ten cases. Cancer 1996; 78:2328–2333.

410. Lockett L, Chiang V, Scully N. Primary pulmonary meningioma: Report of a case and review of the literature. Am J Surg Pathol 1997; 21:453–460.

411. Kaleem Z, Fitzpatrick MM, Ritter JH. Primary pulmonary meningioma: Report of a case and review of the literature. Arch Pathol Lab Med 1997; 121:631–636.

412. Prayson RA, Farver CF. Primary pulmonary malignant meningioma. Am J Surg Pathol 1999; 23:722–726.

413. Falleni M, Roz E, Dessy E, et al. Primary intrathoracic meningioma: histopathological, immunohistochemical and ultrastructural study of two cases. Virchows Archiv 2001; 439:196–200.

414. Cerda-Nicolas M, Lopez-Gines C, Perez-Bacete M, Roldan P, Talamantes F, Barbera J. Histologically benign metastatic meningioma: morphological and cytogenetic study. Case report. J Neurosurg 2003; 98:194–198.

415. Crotty TB, Hooker RP, Swensen SJ, Scheithauer BW, Myers JL. Primary malignant ependymoma of the lung. Mayo Clin Proc 1992; 67:373–378.

12

Tumours

12.4

Lymphoproliferative disease

Lymphoproliferative disease is a useful term as it covers lymphoid infiltrates of the lung of questionable status as well as those that are evidently reactive or neoplastic. Until recently, those of questionable status included lymphoid interstitial pneumonia and so-called pseudolymphoma but the application of modern laboratory techniques has clarified the nature of both these conditions. However, the emergence of apparently monoclonal post-transplantation lymphoproliferative lesions (see Ch. 11) that regress when immunosuppression is reduced has again blurred the distinction between lymphoid hyperplasia and neoplasia. However, consistent application of the latest WHO classifications of extranodal lymphomas will ensure uniformity in terminology.[1,2]

INTRAPULMONARY LYMPH NODES

The lymphoid elements of the lung consist of intrapulmonary lymph nodes and airway-associated lymphoid tissue, details of which are provided on p. 25. The two are best considered separately. Intrapulmonary lymph nodes have a normal follicular and sinusoidal architecture, and may undergo all those changes encountered in lymph nodes elsewhere. In the lungs, they are often heavily pigmented with carbon. Most are situated at the hilum but they may be found anywhere in the lung, occasionally as far out as the pleura (Fig. 12.4.1). In one necropsy study intrapulmonary lymph nodes were identified in 18% of patients.[3] They are generally asymptomatic and discovered incidentally on chest radiographs, following which they may be excised to exclude cancer, increasingly so since the advent of high resolution computed tomography (HRCT).[3a,3b] Otherwise they are of no clinical significance.

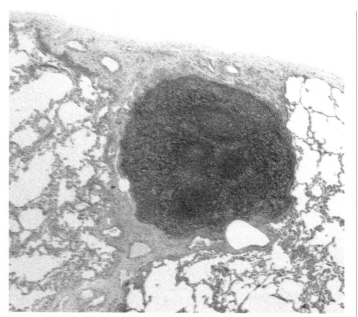

Figure 12.4.1 An intrapulmonary lymph node lies just beneath the pleura.

LYMPHOID HYPERPLASIA

Hyperplasia of the airway-associated lymphoid tissue may be seen in a variety of diseases and is often no more than an epiphenomenon. Thus, lung tumours and many focal pulmonary infections are often attended by a chronic inflammatory infiltrate comprising a mixture of lymphocytes, plasma cells and histiocytes, sometimes with lymphoid follicles. Such an infiltrate is also a general feature of viral, rickettsial and mycoplasma pneumonia. Similarly, extrinsic allergic alveolitis is characterised by an interstitial lymphoid infiltrate that histologically may closely resemble lymphoid interstitial pneumonia. Chronic interstitial inflammation is particularly marked in obstructive pneumonitis. It is also a component of all patterns of chronic idiopathic interstitial pneumonia, although the intensity of the infiltrate variously considerably, being light in desquamative interstitial pneumonia, moderate in cellular non-specific interstitial pneumonia and heavy in lymphoid interstitial pneumonia. Expansion of the bronchial mucosa-associated lymphoid tissue is particularly conspicuous in follicular bronchiectasis. However, all these conditions have their own specific features that facilitate their recognition.

Hyperplasia of the pulmonary lymphoid tissue also occurs in the absence of any accompanying morphological pointers to its aetiology, although the conditions with which it is associated often provide a clue to its causation. Three forms are recognised, follicular bronchiolitis, lymphoid interstitial pneumonia and nodular lymphoid hyperplasia.[4,5] The first of these is centriacinar, the second diffuse and the last forms a localised tumour-like nodule. Castleman's disease may also present as primary pulmonary disease, but more commonly involves the lung as part of a multi-organ disorder and is discussed below under secondary involvement.

The term 'diffuse pulmonary lymphoid hyperplasia' has been used for a pattern of disease intermediate between follicular bronchiolitis and lymphoid interstitial pneumonia, as well as a synonym for lymphoid interstitial pneumonia.[6] However, we view it as a global term encompassing both follicular bronchiolitis and lymphoid interstitial pneumonia.

Follicular bronchiolitis

Follicular bronchitis/bronchiolitis is a predominantly peribronchial lymphocytic infiltrate with abundant germinal centres, often associated with various systemic disorders. It represents an expansion of the normally sparse peribronchiolar lymphoid tissue.[4,6,7] There may be extension of the process into the bronchiolar epithelium and into the walls of neighbouring alveoli but the air spaces are spared. In extreme cases the lymphoid follicles are evenly distributed throughout the lung, perhaps even involving the pleura, when the term diffuse lymphoid hyperplasia has sometimes been applied,[8] but this process does not otherwise differ materially from follicular bronchiolitis.[4,9]

Clinical features

Patients with follicular bronchiolitis commonly present in middle age. They complain of breathlessness and cough and suffer from recurrent episodes of fever or pneumonia.[6] There are several clinical associations, which are listed in Box 12.4.1. The sexes are affected equally apart from the patients in whom follicular bronchiolitis is associated with connective tissue disorders, in which females predominate.[6,10–13] Chest X-ray findings are similar to those seen in lymphocytic interstitial pneumonia, but HRCT typically shows bilateral centrilobular and peribronchial nodules rather than ground glass opacification (Fig. 12.4.2).[10,11,13,14]

Box 12.4.1 Conditions associated with follicular bronchiolitis and lymphoid interstitial pneumonia

Immunological disorders[15]
  Sjögren's syndrome[16,18]
  Hashimoto's thyroiditis[21]
  Pernicious anaemia[19]
  Autoimmune haemolytic anaemia[16,17]
  Chronic active hepatitis[20]
  Primary biliary cirrhosis[25]
  Myasthenia gravis[16]
Immunodeficiency
  AIDS, particularly AIDS affecting children[22,23,26,27]
Allergy, including asthma[a]
Allogeneic bone marrow transplantation[b]

[a]Only reported for follicular bronchiolitis.[6]
[b]Only reported for lymphoid interstitial pneumonia.[24]

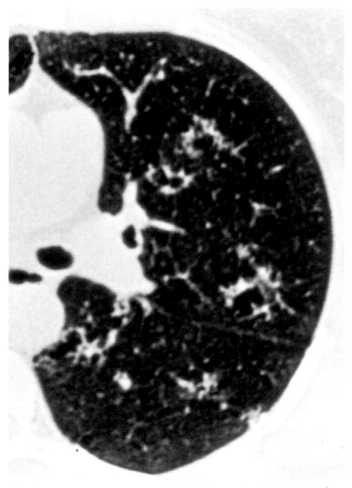

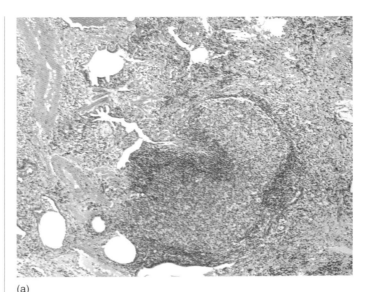

(a)

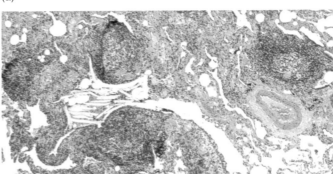

(b)

Figure 12.4.2 Follicular bronchiolitis. HRCT shows focal bronchocentric nodules.

Figure 12.4.3 Follicular bronchiolitis. (a) A lymphoid follicle is closely related to a bronchiole, compressing the lumen. (b) The bronchiolar lumen contains retained proteinaceous debris and cholesterol because of narrowing by hyperplastic lymphoid follicles.

Aetiology

Follicular bronchiolitis is associated with a range of conditions similar to that found with lymphoid interstitial pneumonia and their aetiology is therefore probably similar (see below).

Pathological features

Follicular bronchiolitis is characterised by prominent peribronchial and peribronchiolar lymphoid follicles with only a minor interstitial component (Fig. 12.4.3). Hyperplastic follicles may also been seen in the interlobular septa and the visceral pleura. Compression of the airways may lead to an obstructive endogenous lipoid pneumonia or secondary infection so that pus may be seen in the bronchioles and focal organising pneumonia more distally.

Differential diagnosis

The differential diagnosis of follicular bronchiolitis is from the other forms of bronchiolitis described in Chapter 3. It also has

to be distinguished from follicular bronchiectasis, a term used when prominent follicular hyperplasia accompanies airway dilatation. Lymphoid follicles may also be prominent in the middle lobe syndrome (see p. 89), but this is a localised disease. Extrinsic allergic alveolitis may also show prominent peribronchial lymphoid follicles, but there are usually granulomas and a significant interstitial inflammatory component.

Treatment and prognosis

Most patients respond well to steroid therapy, although non-resolving alveolar collapse, fibrosis and even bulla formation may occur. Occasional cases show obliterative bronchiolitis but this probably represents an independent manifestation of an associated connective tissue disorder rather than progression of the follicular bronchiolitis.

Lymphoid interstitial pneumonia

Lymphoid (or lymphocytic or lymphoplasmacytic) interstitial pneumonia is characterised by a prominent, diffuse, alveolar infiltrate of lymphocytes and plasma cells.[15] Occasional cases are idiopathic but it is generally associated with a variety of clinical conditions that generally reflect impaired immunity (Box 12.4.1).[16–27]

Clinical features

The age and sex distribution tend to reflect the associated diseases listed in Box 12.4.1, with most cases occurring in middle age and there being a slight female preponderance. In some cases there is a familial pattern of inheritance.[28] Most patients complain of cough and dyspnoea accompanied by systemic features such as weight loss and low-grade pyrexia. They often have gammaglobulinemia.[16,25,29–31] Pulmonary function tests show a restrictive defect. Chest X-rays show reticular, coarse reticulonodular or fine reticulonodular opacities[4,16,25,30] while HRCTs may show cystically dilated air-spaces.[32–34]

Aetiology

The aetiology of lymphoid interstitial pneumonia is probably multifactorial as there is evidence that both viruses and immune processes contribute. The viruses include Epstein–Barr virus and, in children particularly, HIV.[35–41] The identification of monoclonal gammopathy in some patients[29] and of clones of lymphoid cells with high sequence homology to auto-reactive lymphocytes[42] suggests autoimmunity while an association with congenital immunodeficiency suggests further pathways of lymphocyte dysregulation.[31,43] In the acquired immunodeficiency of HIV infection, high levels of chemokines such as IL-18 may be in part responsible for recruitment of inflammatory cells into the interstitium.[44]

Pathological features

The involved lung tissue may appear consolidated on gross inspection but microscopy shows that it is the alveolar walls that are affected rather than the air spaces, being expanded by an interstitial infiltrate. The infiltrate is predominantly composed of small lymphocytes but these are mixed with plasma cells, a few larger mononuclear cells and histiocytes (Fig. 12.4.4). There is little peribronchial involvement. The distribution may be similar to that encountered in the more diffuse forms of pulmonary lymphoma, being particularly prominent in relation to lymphatics and thus most marked around bronchovascular bundles, bordering interlobular septa and beneath the pleura. It also forms rounded nodular aggregates about small intralobular vessels but the alveolar walls are nevertheless considerably thickened. The term diffuse lymphoid hyperplasia has been applied to this pattern. Lymphoid follicles are frequent and there may be poorly formed granulomas.[8,16] The follicles largely consist of B cells but the interstitial lymphocytes pre-dominantly comprise T cells. Occasionally there is local deposition of amyloid (Fig. 12.4.5).[7,12] Molecular studies show no immunoglobulin heavy chain restriction or gene re-arrangement.[4,7,8,21,25,45] Lymphoid interstitial pneumonia may occasionally overlap with follicular bronchiolitis (see above), these two conditions representing different patterns of lymphoid hyperplasia, particularly in patients with connective tissue disorders (Fig. 12.4.6).[4,7,9]

Differential diagnosis

The infiltrate of lymphoid interstitial pneumonia is much denser than that seen in the other interstitial pneumonias and is generally not accompanied by any significant degree of fibrosis.[15] It most closely resembles cellular non-specific interstitial pneumonia from which it is only distinguished by a subjective assessment of the intensity of the infiltrate, this being less marked in non-specific interstitial pneumonia. Extrinsic allergic alveolitis is also characterised by a predominantly T-cell infiltrate with occasional granulomas, but a peribronchiolar concentration of the infiltrate and the presence of organising pneumonia distinguish it from lymphoid interstitial pneumonia.[46] Extrinsic allergic alveolitis, sarcoidosis and lymphoid interstitial pneumonia are compared in Table 6.1.3 (p. 283). Distinguishing these conditions is greatly facilitated by correlation with clinical data, especially the HRCT findings (Tables 12.4.1, 12.4.2).[47,48] The distinction of lymphoid interstitial pneumonia from marginal zone lymphomas of MALT origin is considered on p. 651.

Treatment and prognosis

Older reports probably included cases that were lymphomatous from the outset, which would explain why the condition has been regarded as having a propensity to evolve into frank lymphoma. More recent studies, taking advantage of molecular techniques, suggest that apart from the cases complicating AIDS[35,36,49] lymphomatous change is unusual. The prognosis is therefore better than was formerly believed, although it remains unpredictable.[30] Some patients recover completely, others remain stable[31] or slowly progress to end-stage fibrosis[34] and some die within months.[4,25,30] Treatment is usually with corticosteroids, with or without cytotoxic therapy. Recently, patients with symptomatic HIV-related lymphoid interstitial pneumonia have improved following highly active antiretroviral therapy.[50]

Nodular lymphoid hyperplasia[8,51]

Over the last two decades, it has become apparent that most localised lymphoid lesions arising in the lung are marginal zone non-Hodgkin's lymphomas.[52–54] However, a few prove to be polyclonal and reactive in nature and the term nodular lymphoid hyperplasia is now applied to these, having superseded pseudolymphoma, as being more histogenetically accurate.

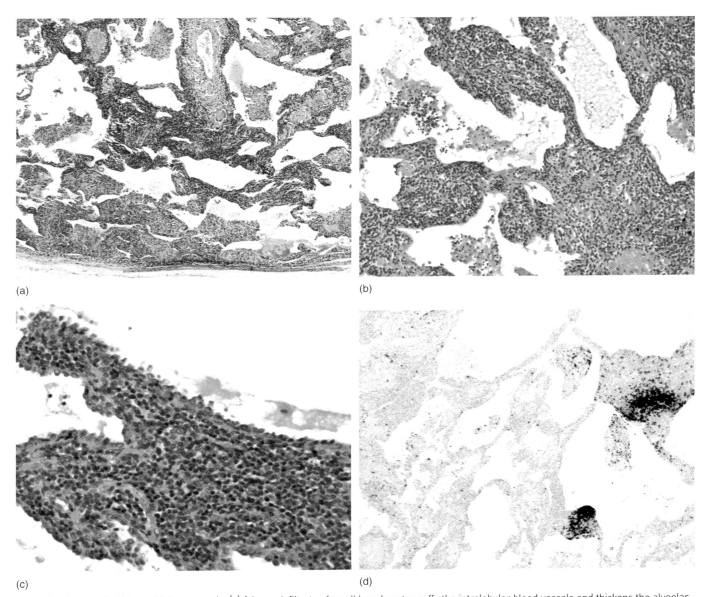

Figure 12.4.4 Lymphoid interstitial pneumonia. (a) A heavy infiltrate of small lymphocytes cuffs the intralobular blood vessels and thickens the alveolar walls. (b) Although the alveolar walls are markedly expanded, there is little involvement of the air spaces. (c) The interstitial infiltrate comprises small round lymphocytes, plasma cells and histiocytes. (d) Most of the lymphocytes are T-cells and CD20 staining shows only tight aggregates of B-cells, mainly within follicles (compare with the lymphomatous infiltration in Fig. 12.4.12d).

Clinical features

Patients range in age from 19–80 years (mean 65) and show a slight female preponderance.[51] The lesions are generally a chance radiographic finding but patients may complain of cough, shortness of breath and pleuritic pain. Most lesions are solitary and if multiple, unilateral. Surgical resection is curative.

Pathological features

Nodular lymphoid hyperplasia forms well-circumscribed nodules measuring up to 6 cm, which are of fleshy or rubbery consistence and usually subpleural. Histologically, lymphoid

follicles are well developed and plasma cells are prominent between the follicles (Fig. 12.4.7). There may be extensive central scarring. Any infiltrative activity at the periphery is quite limited. Atypical cells are not seen. Immunochemistry shows a mixture of B and T cells, with the former expressing both κ and λ light chains. Staining for bcl-2 is negative and no immunoglobulin heavy chain gene rearrangement is detectable when sought by the polymerase chain reaction.

Differential diagnosis

Nodular lymphoid hyperplasia differs from lymphoid interstitial pneumonia in being focal rather than diffuse and the

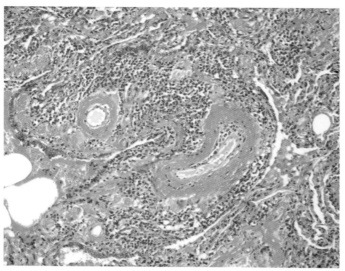

Figure 12.4.5 Lymphoid interstitial pneumonia. Rare cases show deposition of amyloid or, as in this case, light chains.

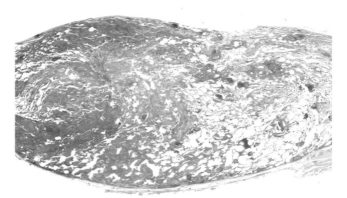

Figure 12.4.6 Histological overlap in lymphoid hyperplasia. On the left, the process consists of a diffuse interstitial infiltrate, whereas on the right there is follicular bronchiolitis.

Table 12.4.1 Clinical and pathological characteristics of LIP, cellular NSIP and extrinsic allergic alveolitis

	LIP	Cellular NSIP	Extrinsic allergic alveolitis
Age	Wide age range	26–50 years	Wide age range
Sex	In adults, female preponderance	Male preponderance	Dependent on causative agent
Associated diseases			
Autoimmunity	Common	Fairly common	No
Immunodeficiency	Common (especially in HIV +ve children)	May be seen in HIV infected patients.[48]	No
Idiopathic disease	Rare	Fairly common	No
Amyloidosis	Rare	No	No
Environmental allergen	No	No	Yes
Hypogammaglobulinaemia	Common	No	No
Lavage lymphocytosis	Common	Common	Common
Imaging			
Chest radiograph	Ground-glass or reticulonodular shadowing. Occasionally normal	Non-specific, variable shadowing. May be normal	Variable shadowing (dependent on stage of disease). May wax and wane on serial radiographs
HRCT	Spectrum of randomly distributed nodules (1–4 mm) through to ground-glass opacification with the latter sometimes accompanied by thin-walled cystic air-spaces	Ground-glass opacification without architectural disturbance or honeycombing.	Subacute disease is characterised by ground-glass opacification and poorly-defined centrilobular nodularity; expiratory scans show air-trapping reflecting bronchiolitis. Chronic disease shows fibrosis of non-specific pattern and distribution
Histopathology			
Distribution	Diffuse	Diffuse	Often centriacinar
Inflammation	Severe interstitial infiltrate	Mild interstitial infiltrate	Mild to severe interstitial infiltrate
Architecture	Little architectural destruction	No architectural destruction	May be lost in chronic disease
Interstitial fibrosis	Rare	None	May be present in chronic disease
Interstitial cell types	Small round lymphocytes, plasma cells, histiocytes.	Small round lymphocytes, plasma cells, histiocytes, some fibroblasts	Small round lymphocytes, plasma cells, Histiocytes, some fibroblasts
Granulomas	Rare	No	Common
Organising pneumonia	Rare	Rare (less than 10% of cases)	Common (70% of cases)

From Nicholson 2001.[47] LIP, lymphoid interstitial pneumonia; NSIP, non-specific interstitial pneumonia.

Table 12.4.2   Clinical and pathological characteristics of LIP, MALT lymphoma and nodular lymphoid hyperplasia

	LIP	MALT lymphoma	Nodular lymphoid hyperplasia	Lymphomatoid granulomatosis
Age	Wide age range	Usually 50–70 years	19–80 years	4–80 years
Sex	In adults, female preponderance	Slight male preponderance	Slight male preponderance	Male preponderance
Associated diseases				
Autoimmunity	Common	Rare	None	None
Immunodeficiency	Common (especially HIV +ve children)	Rare	None	Occasional
Amyloidosis	Rare	Rare	None	None
Imaging				
Chest radiograph	Ground-glass or reticulonodular shadowing. Occasionally normal	Consolidation (single or multifocal). Air bronchograms	Variably sized nodules (occasionally multiple)	Multiple bilateral nodules (may be cavitating)
HRCT	Spectrum of randomly distributed nodules (1–4 mm) through to ground-glass opacification with the latter sometimes accompanied by thin-walled cystic airspaces	Consolidation (single or multifocal) with ground-glass at periphery of lesions. Air bronchograms	Not known	Cavitating nodules, sometimes with peripheral ground-glass attenuation
Histopathology				
Architecture	Diffuse severe interstitial infiltrate. Little architectural destruction	Consolidated mass (alveolar + interstitial). May be multifocal, or rarely diffuse	Single or multiple nodules	Multiple nodules, usually with focal necrosis. Infiltrate usually angiocentric
Cell type	Mainly T-lymphocytes, with lesser numbers of plasma cells and histiocytes	Mainly B-lymphocytes (lymphocyte-like, plasmacytoid, and/or monocytoid)	Mainly T-lymphocytes with some plasma cells and histiocytes.	Mainly T-lymphocytes with some plasma cells and histiocytes, and a variable population of atypical B cells
Germinal centres	Yes	Yes	Yes	Occasional (secondary reactive phenomenon)
Dutcher bodies	No	Yes	No	No
Monoclonality	No	Yes	No	Yes

From Nicholson 2001.[47] LIP, lymphoid interstitial pneumonia; MALT, mucosa-associated lymphoid tissue.

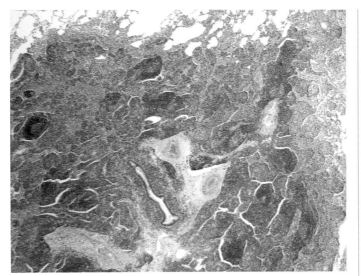

Figure 12.4.7   Nodular lymphoid hyperplasia. A pulmonary nodule is composed of hyperplastic germinal centres interspersed by a mixed infiltrate of plasma cells and small lymphocytes. The features are similar to those of marginal zone lymphomas of MALT origin, but no evidence of clonality was found on immunohistochemistry or molecular analysis.

principal alternatives are inflammatory myofibroblastic tumour (see p. 609) and marginal zone non-Hodgkin's lymphoma of MALT-type (see below). It differs from inflammatory myofibroblastic tumour in lacking the spindle cell background seen in the latter. The distinction from marginal zone non-Hodgkin's lymphoma of MALT-type is particularly difficult and often uncertain without molecular studies but any significant degree of infiltrative activity along adjacent lymphatics would favour lymphoma.

LYMPHOPROLIFERATIVE DISEASE COMPLICATING SEVERE IMMUNE IMPAIRMENT

The spread of AIDS and the development of organ transplantation have both seen the appearance of a remarkable spectrum of lymphoproliferative disease from which the lungs have not been spared. The chief pulmonary manifestations have been lymphoid hyperplasia, including lymphoid interstitial pneumonia (see above), and a variety of lesions that have many of the features of lymphoma.[55–58] In the case of post-transplantation lymphoproliferative disease, some of these lesions regress when immunosuppressive therapy is withdrawn or even reduced, while in the case of AIDS-related lymphomas tumour grade appears to vary with the patient's immune status, the more severely immunodepleted developing more aggressive neoplasms.[59]

Lymphoproliferative disease complicating profound immunosuppression generally involves B cells; T cells are poorly represented. The B-cell proliferation is probably attributable to T-lymphocyte deficiency for in normal individuals T cells control the division of B cells. T-cell deficiency also permits the proliferation of latent Epstein–Barr virus infection. This virus is a further stimulus to B-cell proliferation and its constituents have been identified in most of the resultant tumours.[60–63] It would appear that after a period of unchecked polyclonal B-lymphocyte proliferation, a clone of malignant cells may emerge. The resultant B-cell tumours are often high-grade and notable for affecting extranodal tissues, including the lungs on occasion.[60,64,65] There is a particularly high risk of pulmonary involvement, around 60%, after heart–lung transplantation. Transplantation of lungs alone carries less of a risk. AIDS-related lymphoma of the pleura is considered separately (see p. 718).

PRIMARY PULMONARY LYMPHOMA

The lungs are often involved in disseminated nodal lymphomas of all types, but primary pulmonary lymphoma of the lung is relatively rare, accounting for less than 0.5% of all primary lung neoplasms. Nevertheless, several large series have been reported.[52–54,66–71] They were originally categorised in the same way as nodal lymphomas and later as low and high grade MALT lymphomas but the WHO classification is now followed. This recommends the terms marginal zone non-Hodgkin lymphoma of MALT origin and diffuse large B-cell non-Hodgkin lymphoma respectively for the pulmonary lymphomas previously classified as low- and high-grade. The low-grade tumours have the characteristic histology of marginal zone non-Hodgkin lymphomas arising at other sites and, although the rarer high-grade tumours usually lack these distinctive morphological features, some contain low-grade areas, making it likely that they also arise from MALT.[53,54]

These two lesions form approximately 95% of primary pulmonary lymphomas, the other 5% comprising lymphomatoid granulomatosis, plasmacytoma, Hodgkin lymphoma, anaplastic large cell lymphoma, CD56-positive (natural killer cell) lymphoma,[72] the CD21- and CD35-positive follicular dendritic cell tumour,[73] solitary mast cell tumour[74,75] and exceptional cases that appear to be of follicle centre cell origin and are therefore directly comparable to nodal lymphomas.[53]

Marginal zone B-cell lymphoma of MALT type

Clinical features

More than 80% of patients with these tumours are over 40 years of age, with a mean age of about 55 years; children are rarely affected.[53] There is a slight male preponderance. Over half the patients are asymptomatic at presentation, the disease being first detected on routine radiographs. Other patients suffer from cough, dyspnoea, chest pain and haemoptysis, sometimes accompanied by malaise, weight loss or pyrexia.[68] Paraproteinaemia is present in up to 20% of cases and this is usually of IgM type (macroglobulinaemia).[76] Evidence of Sjögren's syndrome or, less often, another connective tissue disorder such as lupus erythematosus, may be present,[18] and there may be a history of lymphoma in other extranodal sites, such as the gastrointestinal tract, salivary glands, orbit or skin. Some patients have systemic ('B') symptoms. Imaging shows variable patterns, with unilateral or bilateral disease, isolated or multiple opacities, diffuse infiltration, reticulonodular shadowing and pleural effusions all being described. HRCT typically shows multiple or solitary areas of consolidation, with associated air bronchograms and haloes of ground glass shadowing at lesion margins (Fig. 12.4.8).[77] Diagnosis is possible with cytological specimens (Fig. 12.4.9) or small biopsies,[54,78,79] although immunohistochemistry, flow cytometry and molecular analysis may be required,[80–82] together with HRCT correlation. More often a surgical lung biopsy is needed.

Aetiology

Whereas gastric marginal zone lymphomas of MALT origin show a strong relation to *Helicobacter pylori* infection, less is known of the aetiology of the comparable tumours arising in

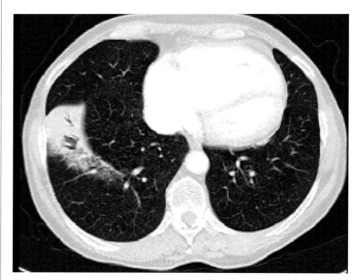

Figure 12.4.8 Marginal zone lymphoma of MALT origin. HRCT shows an area of consolidation with ground-glass changes at its periphery. Air bronchograms are present within the consolidation.

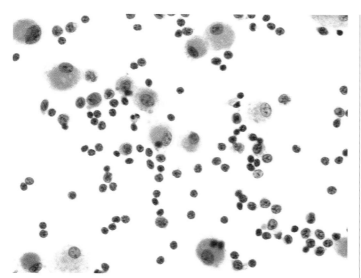

Figure 12.4.9 Marginal zone lymphoma of MALT origin. Bronchial washings show many small lymphocytes, which proved to be of B-cell phenotype.

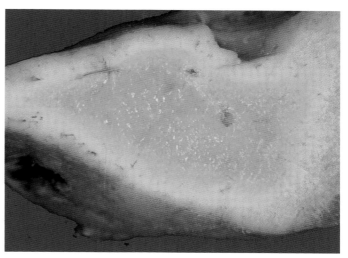

Figure 12.4.10 Marginal zone lymphoma of MALT origin. The lung shows diffuse fleshy consolidation.

the lungs. However, there is evidence that smoking[83] auto-immune disorders,[61,84] immunosuppressive therapy,[85,86] AIDS, co-existent tuberculosis[87] and hepatitis C[88] may all play a role. Neoplastic change in the bronchus-associated lymphoid tissue is therefore likely to be multifactorial. Molecular studies have shown various translocations,[89,90] trisomy of chromosome 3[91] and mutation of the bcl-10 gene.[92] How these chromosomal abnormalities relate to lymphomagenesis remains obscure, but the high incidence of trisomy 3 in both extranodal and nodal marginal zone lymphomas supports the view that they are distinct from other types of non-Hodgkin lymphomas.

Pathological features

The macroscopic appearances vary from a localised tan or grey tumour to areas of apparent pulmonary consolidation (Fig. 12.4.10). Preserved bronchovascular bundles can sometimes be seen on the cut surface.

Microscopically, the tumours consist of small lymphocytes, which may be centrocyte-like, lymphocyte-like or monocytoid although all are thought to be variations of the same neoplastic cell (Fig. 12.4.11). Some of the lymphocytes contain nuclear inclusion immunoglobulin known as Dutcher bodies. The lymphocytes first proliferate around the bronchovascular bundles and then spread out in the connective tissue planes alongside blood vessels and their accompanying lymphatics. At this stage, there is prominent involvement of the interlobular septa (Fig. 12.4.12a). As the disease progresses there is invasion of the alveolar walls, which are first expanded and then destroyed leading to filling of the air spaces and obliteration of the alveolar architecture. This ultimately results in a tumour mass in which only the larger airways and blood vessels are spared. The

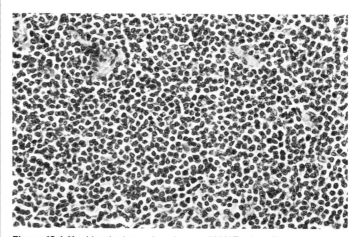

Figure 12.4.11 Marginal zone lymphoma of MALT origin. The tumour is composed of a monotonous sheet of small mature lymphocytes.

latter may be infiltrated[93] but not on the scale seen with lymphomatoid granulomatosis. Ultimately, the tumour cells also infiltrate the pleura and bronchial cartilage. Hyaline sclerosis is common and lymphoid follicles are often evident, particularly when stains for the CD21 marker of follicular dendritic cells are employed (Fig. 12.4.13). Epithelioid and giant cell granulomas may be observed on occasion (Fig. 12.4.14) and lymphoepithelial lesions are often present: recognition of the latter is facilitated by cytokeratin staining (Fig. 12.4.15). Giant lamellar bodies derived from type II pneumocytes may be seen within the tumour, possibly related to airway obstruction.[94] Necrosis is rare. Amyloid is present in up to 10% of cases.[70,71,95,96]

B-lymphocytes can be identified with stains for CD20 or CD79a and the background reactive T-cells with CD3 (Fig. 12.4.12d,e). Immunostains for κ and λ light chains may provide

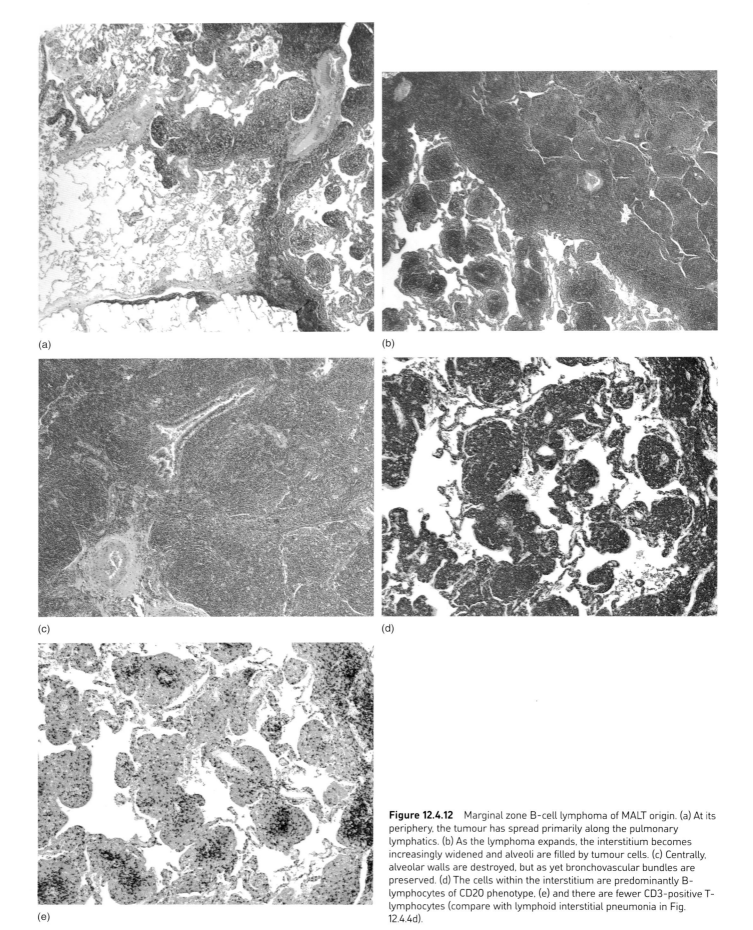

Figure 12.4.12 Marginal zone B-cell lymphoma of MALT origin. (a) At its periphery, the tumour has spread primarily along the pulmonary lymphatics. (b) As the lymphoma expands, the interstitium becomes increasingly widened and alveoli are filled by tumour cells. (c) Centrally, alveolar walls are destroyed, but as yet bronchovascular bundles are preserved. (d) The cells within the interstitium are predominantly B-lymphocytes of CD20 phenotype, (e) and there are fewer CD3-positive T-lymphocytes (compare with lymphoid interstitial pneumonia in Fig. 12.4.4d).

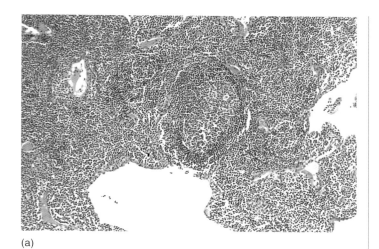

(a)

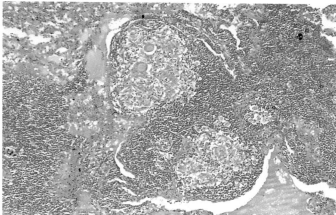

Figure 12.4.14 Tuberculoid granulomas in a marginal zone lymphoma of MALT origin.

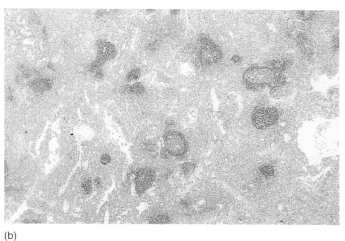

(b)

Figure 12.4.13 (a) Marginal zone lymphoma of MALT origin in which there are prominent reactive lymphoid follicles. (b) The follicles are particularly well demonstrated with the CD21 marker of follicular dendritic cells.

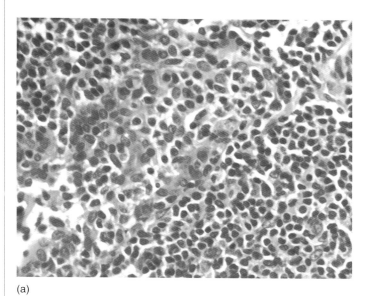

(a)

evidence of clonality but are not always successful. However, amplification of the immunoglobulin heavy chain gene by the polymerase chain reaction may provide firmer evidence of monoclonality.[54] The bcl-2 oncogene is not expressed in the follicle centre cells but is positive in the colonising neoplastic lymphocytes. The neoplastic cells are also CD5 and CD10 negative. If there is nodal involvement the features there are those of nodal marginal zone B-cell non-Hodgkin lymphomas.[97,98]

Differential diagnosis

The principal histological difficulty lies in distinguishing marginal zone lymphoma from lymphoid interstitial pneumonia. These conditions share many histological features but involvement of alveolar spaces, destruction of alveolar walls, the presence of giant lamellar bodies and infiltration of the pleura and

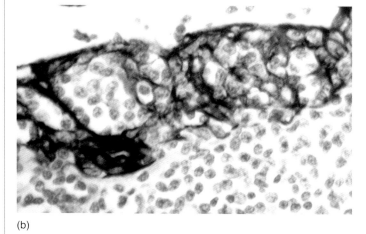

(b)

Figure 12.4.15 Lymphoepithelial lesions in a marginal zone lymphoma of MALT origin. These lesions may be difficult to recognise in haematoxylin and eosin stains (a) but are readily apparent in sections immunostained for cytokeratin (b).

bronchial cartilage all favour lymphoma. Immunohistochemical characterisation of the infiltrate is of considerable help for whereas the small lymphocytes in lymphoid interstitial pneumonia are predominantly T cells, the interstitial infiltrate in marginal zone lymphoma has a predominantly B-cell phenotype (compare Fig. 12.4.4 and Fig. 12.4.12).[4,7,54,71,71] Finally, molecular studies may provide firm supportive evidence, amplification of the immunoglobulin heavy chain gene favouring lymphoma.

Distinguishing lymphoma from nodular lymphoid hyperplasia is described above. Distinguishing primary from secondary lymphoma depends upon clinical data. Lymphocyte-rich variants of thymoma (WHO type B1) involving the lung may resemble lymphoma but are easily recognised by cytokeratin, CD3 and CD1a positivity.[99]

Clinically, the differential diagnosis often includes bronchioloalveolar cell carcinoma and organising pneumonia, in which case a cytological specimen or endoscopic biopsy showing a dense lymphocytic infiltrate with the appropriate immunophenotype may be sufficient to identify marginal zone lymphoma.

Treatment and prognosis

These tumours are either Stage Ie (confined to the lungs) or IIe (Ie plus hilar/mediastinal involvement) and resection has often resulted in prolonged remission.[100]

In some elderly patients with asymptomatic disease, a 'wait and watch' policy is often appropriate for these indolent tumours. The five-year survival is greater than 90%.[53,54,69] Metastases involve other mucosal sites rather than lymph nodes.[54,68] Recurrence is associated with a tendency towards transition to diffuse large B-cell lymphoma.[53] Extensive pulmonary involvement that is not amenable to resection carries a worse prognosis.

Diffuse large B-cell non-Hodgkin lymphoma

Clinical features

Diffuse large B-cell non-Hodgkin lymphoma forms about 20% of pulmonary lymphomas. The age range is similar to that of marginal zone non-Hodgkin lymphoma of MALT origin, but the patients are usually symptomatic at presentation, complaining of cough, hemoptysis, dyspnoea and systemic ('B') symptoms. Imaging shows solid masses, which are often multiple.

Aetiology

It is likely that these tumours represent blastic transformation of marginal zone non-Hodgkin lymphomas of MALT origin,[54,61,84,101] probably through further mutation. There is a rare association with fibrosing alveolitis and connective tissue diseases.[54,61,84,101] Diffuse large B-cell lymphomas are also found in immunodeficient individuals, notably those undergoing

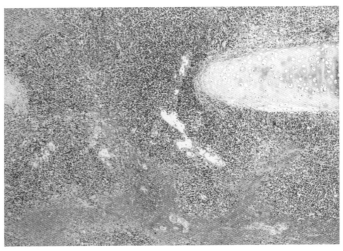

(a)

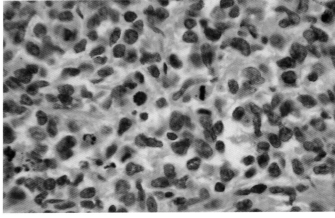

(b)

Figure 12.4.16 A diffuse large B-cell lymphoma shows necrosis (bottom of a) and considerable cellular pleomorphism (b).

immunosuppression following organ transplantation or suffering from AIDS.

Pathological features

Macroscopically, areas of pulmonary involvement typically form solid or necrotising cream-coloured masses. Microscopically, the lung architecture is destroyed by sheets of tumour cells that have large irregular vesicular nuclei and moderate amounts of cytoplasm. The cells are pleomorphic and there are many mitoses (Fig. 12.4.16). Lymphoid follicles, lymphoepithelial lesions and granulomas are seldom evident but hyperplastic bronchial MALT may be found in the distant non-involved lung. Foci of marginal zone non-Hodgkin lymphomas of MALT origin may be seen.[54] The neoplastic cells are of B-cell phenotype, mixed with reactive T cells. Evidence of monoclonality is occasionally obtained by demonstrating heavy chain gene amplification with the polymerase chain reaction.[54]

Differential diagnosis

There are few difficulties in identifying the confluent sheets of blast cells of a large cell lymphoma, other than distinguishing the condition from other undifferentiated neoplasms, which may be accomplished by applying stains for lymphocyte markers (CD45), cytokeratins, α-fetoprotein, and epithelial membrane antigen. A surgical lung biopsy may be required to identify the angiocentric lesions of lymphomatoid granulomatosis but, although both are B-cell proliferations, B cells are comparatively scarce in lymphomatoid granulomatosis and the few present are usually positive for Epstein–Barr virus, while those in immunocompetent patients with diffuse large B-cell non-Hodgkin's lymphoma are negative.[102]

Treatment and prognosis

Extensive involvement of the lung usually precludes resection and most patients require combination chemotherapy. The 5-year survival figures range from 0–60%.[53,54,69]

Lymphomatoid granulomatosis

Aetiology and nomenclature

Lymphomatoid granulomatosis is a rare disease characterised by a necrotising, angiocentric, polymorphous and usually atypical lymphoid infiltrate that typically forms tumour-like masses in the lungs, brain, skin and other tissues. It was first described by Liebow in 1972, the rather ambiguous term chosen reflecting initial uncertainty concerning the nature of the condition.[103–105]

Early attempts to characterise the lymphoid cells established that the majority were T cells and the condition was therefore included, together with polymorphic reticulosis (lethal midline granuloma of the nose), in a spectrum of so-called post-thymic T-cell proliferations.[106,107] However, although further studies substantiated the predominant T-cell phenotype, rearrangement of the T-cell receptor genes could be identified in only a minority of cases.[107–111] and it was subsequently shown that the scanty atypical cells were of B-cell phenotype, often with rearrangement of the immunoglobulin heavy chain gene.[112–115] Epstein–Barr virus (EBV) was localised to the atypical B cells[65,111,116,117] and lymphomatoid granulomatosis is currently regarded as representing a T-cell rich, EBV-driven, angiocentric B-cell proliferation, distinct from polymorphic reticulosis.[112]

Note has to be taken however, of occasional cases that are histologically identical to lymphomatoid granulomatosis yet consist entirely of T cells. These are generally not associated with the Epstein–Barr virus and may represent peripheral T-cell lymphomas.[113] Other lymphomas may also show an angiocentric pattern resembling that seen in lymphomatoid granulomatosis.[72] Thus, what appears to be a distinct morphological entity, may be mimicked by various lymphoproliferative diseases showing angiocentricity and secondarily involving the lung, the identification of which will probably become important as treatment evolves.[7]

Conversely, what were initially described as separate conditions are now regarded as merely different grades of lymphomatoid granulomatosis. Thus, based on the degree of atypia and necrosis, benign lymphocytic angiitis and granulomatosis[118–120] is now considered to be the lowest grade of lymphomatoid granulomatosis, while the highest grade conforms to what has been termed angiocentric lymphoma.[93,107,121]

Clinical features

Patients with lymphomatoid granulomatosis cover a wide age range but most are middle-aged with the median age at diagnosis being in the sixth decade: men are affected twice as frequently as women.[122–125] Most patients present with pyrexia, weight loss and general malaise in addition to chest symptoms such as cough, chest pain and dyspnoea. About a quarter have neurological symptoms at presentation and half develop an erythematous, macular rash or subcutaneous nodules some time during their illness.[126] CD4 lymphocyte counts may be low.[123] Chest radiographs and HRCT typically reveal bilateral, multiple, rounded masses, predominantly located in the middle and lower zones.[127] These vary in size and may coalesce or cavitate; they are frequently mistaken for metastases. Unilateral lesions or a diffuse infiltrative process are less often seen. Hilar node enlargement is not a feature in the early stages of the disease although lymph node involvement is present in 22% of cases at autopsy[105] and can be more readily recognised as malignant than the lesions in the lungs.

Lymphomatoid granulomatosis may also present in other organs. Neurological symptoms may result either from similar involvement of small vessels in the central nervous system or peripheral nerves or from the formation of tumour-like masses in the brain. In the kidney, there may be a diffuse interstitial infiltrate or distinct tumours[128] but, in contrast to Wegener's granulomatosis, there is no glomerulonephritis. Other affected sites include skin, liver, spleen, adrenals, heart, pancreas, gastrointestinal tract and pancreas.[105] Extrapulmonary lesions generally resemble those in the lungs but in the skin it is unusual to find cells bearing the EBV genome. This has led to suggestions that the skin lesions may be caused by cytokines released by lesions elsewhere rather than direct involvement.[129] Extrapulmonary involvement is unusual in benign lymphocytic angiitis and granulomatosis.

Aetiology

Apart from its close association with EBV, the aetiology of lymphomatoid granulomatosis is obscure, although the patients sometimes have obvious underlying defects in their cell-mediated immunity. These may be congenital, as in the Wiskott-Aldrich syndrome,[130] or acquired, as in AIDS,[131] agnogenic myeloid metaplasia[132] and the treatment of other forms of lymphoma.[133,134] There is also some similarity between lymphomatoid granulomatosis and post-transplantation lymphoproliferative disorders (see Ch. 11, p. 519): both are essentially angiocentric B-cell proliferations, both bear the EBV genome and both vary in their clonality, but they differ in the proportion of reactive T cells.[135,136] These are plentiful in lymphomatoid granulomatosis but typically sparse in the post-transplantation lymphoproliferative disorders. It appears likely that impaired immunity underlies the development of both these diseases.

Pathological features

Macroscopically, the lungs contain nodules of pinkish-grey tissue, the largest of which show central necrosis and cavitation (Fig. 12.4.17). Alternatively, areas of confluent consolidation may be seen. The pleura is frequently thickened but effusions are unusual.

Microscopically, most cases show broad tracts of necrosis separated by a mixed angiocentric infiltrate that includes usually scanty pleomorphic atypical lymphoid cells. The vessel walls are expanded but not destroyed by the infiltrate (Fig. 12.4.18). While most of the lymphocytes stain for T-cell markers, the atypical lymphoid cells stain as B cells, analogous to the findings in T-cell-rich B-cell lymphomas. The B cells may also be positive for CD30 but are negative for CD15. The background T cells are predominantly CD8-positive.[137] The degree of cellular atypia varies considerably, and includes lymphocytes with irregular, folded nuclei and larger blast-like cells with promi-

nent nucleoli and condensed marginal chromatin. The lesions are graded 1–3 on the degree of lymphocytic atypia, the presence of necrosis and the polymorphic/monomorphic nature of the infiltrate, grade 3 lesions being synonymous with angiocentric lymphomas.[107] The B-cell proliferation index correlates well with histological grade.[138] Eosinophils and giant cells are not usually present in significant numbers and sarcoid-like granulomas are not a feature.

Differential diagnosis

In contrast to true vasculitis, in which the vessel wall is destroyed by a necrotising inflammatory process, vascular involvement is characterised by separation of the components of the wall by the infiltrating cells. This is usually best seen in the intima, which becomes greatly thickened as the infiltrate lifts the endothelium and obliterates the lumen (Fig. 12.4.18). Similar cells infiltrate the alveolar and bronchiolar walls, giving

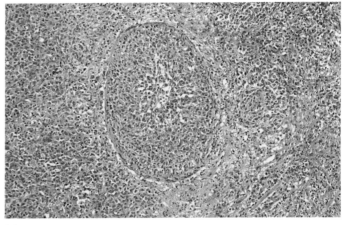

(a)

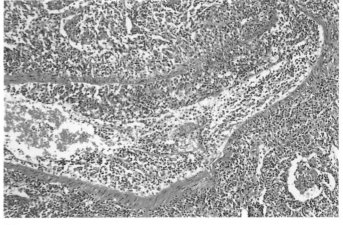

(b)

Figure 12.4.18 Lymphomatoid granulomatosis. (a and b) The walls of small pulmonary blood vessels are heavily infiltrated by atypical lymphoid cells. Immunostaining shows that although many T cells are present the atypical cells are B cells.

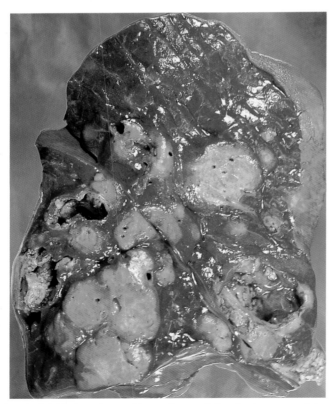

Figure 12.4.17 Lymphomatoid granulomatosis forming large necrotising fleshy masses within the lung. (Case of Dr P King, Johannesburg, South Africa.)

rise to additional non-specific reactive changes, such as organising alveolar fibrinous exudates, proliferation of alveolar epithelial cells and bronchiolitis obliterans. However, the cardinal feature that distinguishes lymphomatoid granulomatosis from other granulomatous vasculitides is the presence of the atypical B-lymphocytes. Gene rearrangement studies may be of value if there is any doubt.[114] Distinction from diffuse large B-cell non-Hodgkin lymphomas is discussed above.

Treatment and prognosis

Survival is generally short, but varies from a few months to many years according to grade.[105,113,114] High-dose steroids and cyclophosphamide and combination chemotherapy have been used, and good responses to interferon-α 2b[139] and bone marrow transplantation have been described.[140]

Hodgkin disease

Primary pulmonary Hodgkin disease is very uncommon and much rarer than secondary involvement.[141] The diagnosis is only justified if hilar lymph nodes are uninvolved and disease elsewhere has been excluded.

Clinical features, treatment and prognosis

Reported cases cover a wide age range (18–82 years, mean 43 years) and there is a slight female predominance.[142–147] Most patients complain of breathlessness and cough and about half also have systemic symptoms such as weight loss and fever. Chest radiographs may show multiple nodules or solitary tumours and there may be cavitation in the larger lesions. Following treatment, relapse occurs in the majority of cases, either in the lungs or elsewhere. Solitary tumours are less frequently associated with systemic symptoms and have a better prognosis than bilateral growths.[145]

Pathological features

The microscopic appearances are typical of Hodgkin disease, usually of either nodular sclerosing or mixed cellularity type. Bronchi are frequently involved, with resultant obstructive changes distally, but presentation as an endobronchial lesion is rare.[148] Larger lesions usually undergo extensive central necrosis. Away from the nodules, a lymphatic or vascular distribution of spread is discernible, the pleura may be infiltrated and atypical cells may be found in air spaces.[143] As in other organs, the lesions of Hodgkin disease may be accompanied by sarcoid-like epithelioid and giant cell granulomas.[149]

Differential diagnosis

The differential diagnosis of pulmonary Hodgkin disease includes necrotising granulomatous inflammation, particularly Wegener's granulomatosis, sarcoidosis and infection, Langerhans cell histiocytosis, undifferentiated carcinoma and other forms of malignant lymphoma. Wegener's granulomatosis can be excluded if clearly atypical lymphoid cells are present. Large numbers of eosinophils may cause Langerhans cell histiocytosis to be considered, but the extensive necrosis is not a feature of this disorder and the Langerhans cells lack the malignant characteristics of mononuclear Hodgkin cells and Reed-Sternberg cells. Undifferentiated carcinomas occasionally appear extremely pleomorphic: in the giant cell variant nuclei may have the multilobed appearance and large nucleoli of Reed–Sternberg cells. Neutrophils are frequently present in undifferentiated carcinomas but eosinophils are seldom a feature. In debatable cases, immunostaining for cytokeratins, CD30 and CD15 can be decisive.

Exclusion of other forms of malignant lymphoma may be impossible when only standard histological preparations are available: immunocytochemistry, which has often been lacking in reported cases, may be required. Some forms of T-cell lymphoma may simulate Hodgkin disease by showing extreme degrees of cellular pleomorphism and a background of reactive inflammatory cells.

Plasmacytoma

Extramedullary plasmacytomas are rare tumours. The majority occur in the upper respiratory tract and few are recorded in the lung or bronchus, these forming about 6% of all extramedullary plasmacytomas.[150–155] Some earlier cases may have represented inflammatory myofibroblastic tumours,[156,157] while others were probably marginal zone lymphomas of MALT origin showing predominantly plasmacytoid differentiation.

Only about 7% of patients with multiple myeloma have intrathoracic disease[158] and this is rarely confined to the lung. However, pulmonary plasmacytoma occasionally precedes or accompanies other manifestations of disseminated disease.[159,160] The presence of a paraprotein is not necessarily indicative of multifocal disease: resection of a solitary intrapulmonary plasmacytoma may be followed by disappearance of a circulating paraprotein,[161] or of urinary Bence Jones protein.[162] However, as in myelomatosis, the gammopathy may lead to renal failure.[155]

Pathological features

Microscopically, plasmacytomas consist of sheets of plasma cells: many may appear normal but others have multiple nuclei and some show nuclear pleomorphism. The spindle-shaped and inflammatory cells seen in inflammatory myofibroblastic tumours are lacking. Immunohistochemical investigation confirms the diagnosis by demonstrating a monoclonal population. Occasionally, amyloid is found in the stroma,[150] or there is material that resembles amyloid but lacks the typical staining reactions of amyloid and consists of monotypic immunoglobulin.[153,163] Sometimes the plasma cells are overshadowed by numerous macrophages distended by large amounts of ingested immunoglobulin (crystal-storing histiocytosis), which renders the cytoplasm eosinophilic and can be shown to be monoclonal.[164,165] Monoclonality needs to be verified as similar appearances can be produced by reactive conditions that result in excessive immunoglobulin production.[166]

Prognosis

The overall 2- and 5-year survival rates of pulmonary plasmacytomas are 66% and 40%, respectively.[167]

Large cell anaplastic lymphoma

Large cell anaplastic lymphoma characteristically involves the lymph nodes or skin, but rare cases are limited to the lungs.[168,169] Patient ages range from 27 to 66 years and the sexes are affected equally. In one patient the lymphoma complicated HIV infection. The morphology and immunophenotype are the same as at other sites, the tumour cells being CD30 positive, CD15 negative and sometimes EMA positive. Epstein-Barr virus is not detected. Most patients have died of their disease.

SECONDARY PULMONARY LYMPHOMA

Secondary involvement of the lung in patients with malignant lymphoma is common and may be due to direct invasion from involved mediastinal lymph nodes or metastasis via the bloodstream or lymphatics.[141] At presentation, only about 12% of patients with Hodgkin disease and 4% of patients with non-Hodgkin lymphoma have radiographic evidence of lung involvement[170] but the figure exceeds 50% in patients dying with disseminated disease. Whereas non-Hodgkin lymphomas tend to involve the lungs in a diffuse fashion, suggesting that they follow lymphatic pathways, the pulmonary lesions of Hodgkin disease are often nodular, and polypoid endobronchial masses are occasionally seen.[148]

Patients with peripheral T-cell lymphomas frequently have evidence of extranodal spread. Involvement of lung or pleura is present in 20% of cases at presentation and develops in a further 20% during the course of the disease.[171] Some current classifications of peripheral T-cell lymphomas include *angioimmunoblastic lymphadenopathy* and pulmonary infiltrates may be apparent in this condition at presentation.[172,173] The microscopic features are similar to those in the lymph nodes: a mixed infiltrate, which includes plasma cells and immunoblasts is present in the interstitium, and capillaries with hyperplastic endothelium are prominent.[172,174] *Multiple myelomatosis* may involve the lungs and be associated there with the deposition of material similar to that better known in the renal tubules.[175] Lymphocytic infiltrates of the lung, pleura and hilar lymph nodes are also described in *Waldenström's macroglobulinaemia*.[176,177] *Systemic mast cell disease* has also presented as diffuse parenchymal lung disease.[178]

Cutaneous T-cell lymphoma (mycosis fungoides or Sézary syndrome) involves the lungs in about two-thirds of cases at autopsy. The interstitial infiltrate of convoluted or cerebriform

cells follows the bronchovascular bundles in a lymphatic distribution and may form nodular aggregates[179] or simulate pneumonia.[180] A similar lymphatic distribution is described in cases of *malignant histiocytosis*[181–183] and *leukaemia*[184,185] with pulmonary involvement.

Intravascular lymphoma (angiotropic lymphoma)

Intravascular (or angiotropic) lymphoma is to be distinguished from the angiocentric lymphoma described above. It was originally considered to represent a form of malignant 'angioendotheliomatosis'[186] but is now recognised to be a lymphoma of unusual distribution, the malignant cells being almost exclusively confined to the lumen of capillaries and small arteries and veins throughout the body.[187,188] The neoplastic cells generally exhibit a B-cell phenotype but occasional cases composed of T cells have been reported. The neoplastic cells have been shown to lack CD29 (beta1-integrin), a molecule integral to lymphocyte trafficking.[189] Gene mutations on chromosome 1 and trisomy 18 have also been reported.[190] Most cases are diagnosed post mortem but the disease is relatively sensitive to combination chemotherapy if treated early.[191]

Clinical features

Intravascular lymphoma usually presents with fever and features referable to the skin or central nervous system.[187] The lung is generally involved at a late stage of the disease but rare cases are reported in which the process is apparently confined to the lungs.[186,191–193] Involvement of the pulmonary vasculature is sometimes so extensive that pulmonary hypertension is the presenting feature.[194] Alternatively, the process may present as interstitial lung disease[192,195] or even obstructive airway disease with air trapping.[196] Affected patients are usually in the fifth to seventh decades of life. Chest radiographs may be normal or show non-specific infiltrates. Laboratory findings are also often unhelpful. Despite the presence of numerous malignant cells within small blood vessels, only rarely are they identified in blood films.

Pathological features

Microscopic examination shows a proliferation of neoplastic round or spindle-shaped cells that is confined to capillaries and small arteries and veins throughout the body. Affected vessels may show intimal fibrosis. The neoplastic cells have large, vesicular, indented nuclei, eosinophilic nucleoli and moderate amounts of cytoplasm. They are usually B cells and stain for the appropriate lymphoid markers (Fig. 12.4.19). Occasional cases have been reported to have a T-cell phenotype. Monoclonality may be demonstrated with immunohistochemical stains for κ and λ chains and by gene rearrangement studies.[193,197]

Differential diagnosis

The differential diagnosis of angiotropic lymphoma includes metastatic carcinoma and melanoma, leukaemia and lymphoid

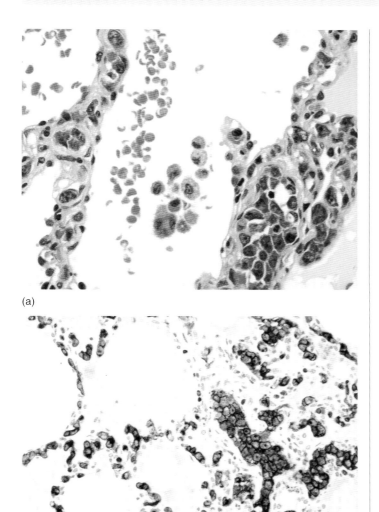

(a)

(b)

Figure 12.4.19 Intravascular lymphoma. (a) Atypical lymphoid cells are evident within small pulmonary blood vessels. (b) With CD 20 staining the tumour is categorised as an intravascular large B-cell lymphoma. (Case provided by Dr AC Wotherspoon, London, UK.)

interstitial pneumonia. The first of these are distinguished by immunohistochemical identification of lymphoid (CD45), epithelial (cytokeratin) and melanocyte (S100 and HMB45) markers. Leukaemia may be distinguished by reference to blood counts and bone marrow examination and lymphoid interstitial pneumonia by the intravascular rather than interstitial location of the cells.

ANGIOFOLLICULAR LYMPH NODE HYPERPLASIA (GIANT LYMPH NODE HYPERPLASIA, CASTLEMAN'S DISEASE)

Clinical features, treatment and prognosis

Angiofollicular lymph node hyperplasia typically affects mediastinal lymph nodes but has also been reported in the lung,[198,199] the pleura[200] and the chest wall,[201] in addition to many extrathoracic sites. Some patients have multicentric disease. Two histological patterns are described – hyaline-vascular and plasma cell. The hyaline-vascular pattern is much more common; it is seen more often in the localised form of the disease and is generally either asymptomatic or presents because of pressure effects. The plasma cell pattern is more often seen in multicentric disease. This is a systemic disease that is characterised by fever, sweating, fatigue, anaemia, lymphadenopathy, hepatosplenomegaly, skin rashes, an elevated erythrocyte sedimentation rate, polyclonal hypergammaglobulinaemia and bone marrow plasmacytosis. In contrast to the solitary form of the disease, which is quite benign and usually cured by surgery, the multicentric variety has an aggressive course with a mean survival of 5 years: some patients with multicentric disease develop lymphoma.[202–204a] Others are AIDS patients who are also suffering from Kaposi's sarcoma and in these patients DNA sequences of the Kaposi sarcoma virus (human herpes virus 8) have been identified within the Castleman's disease, raising the possibility of this virus playing a causative role in both diseases.[205] The same virus is incriminated in body cavity-based lymphoma (see p. 718), which is also recorded in association with multicentric Castleman's disease.[206]

Pathological features

In the hyaline-vascular variant, which is the type most likely to be seen in the lungs, there are prominent lymphoid follicles of abnormal pattern. The germinal centres are reduced in size and contain increased numbers of follicular dendritic cells and reduced numbers of follicular centre cells. The reduced germinal centres are surrounded by an expanded layer of mantle cells arranged in concentric layers, resulting in an onion-skin appearance. Blood vessels enter the germinal centres while between the follicles there are increased numbers of high-endothelial venules and clusters of plasmacytoid monocytes (Fig. 12.4.20). The plasma cell variant overlaps histologically with both lymphoid interstitial pneumonia and marginal zone lymphoma of MALT origin (Fig. 12.4.21). Ancillary investigations are required to exclude the latter, along the line of those undertaken for nodular lymphoid hyperplasia, as the lesions may form solid masses that are rich in plasma cells and therefore mimic plasmacytoid variants of lymphoma. Such nodularity argues against lymphoid interstitial pneumonia, which does not usually have aggregations of plasma cells, although some imaging studies have classified the plasma cell variant of Castleman's as a form of lymphoid interstitial pneumonia. Ultimately

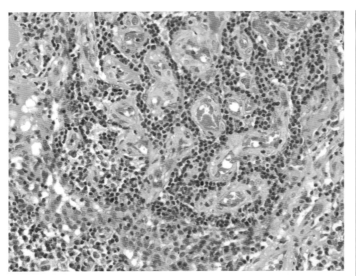

Figure 12.4.20 Hyaline vascular variant of Castleman's disease. Germinal centres within the bronchial MALT contain prominent hyalinised capillaries.

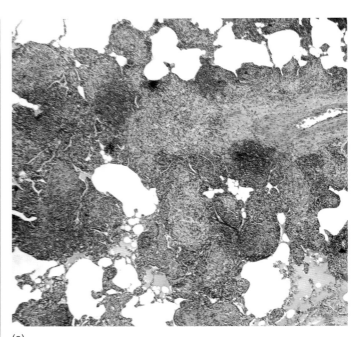

(a)

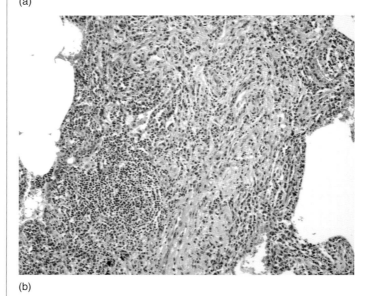

(b)

Figure 12.4.21 Plasma cell variant of Castleman's disease. (a) Lymphoid cells infiltrate the parenchymal interstitium and an interlobular septum. (b) The infiltrate includes many plasma cells, which proved to be polyclonal.

the diagnosis may be easier to make on any lymph nodes that may be involved.

PULMONARY PROBLEMS IN LEUKAEMIA

Respiratory distress often develops in advanced leukaemia and in these circumstances it can be difficult clinically to distinguish leukaemic infiltration of the lungs from opportunistic infection and from the cytotoxic effects of antileukaemic chemotherapy.[207] Furthermore, the chemotherapy may well have been augmented with bone marrow transplantation.[207–209a] Post-transplantation lymphoproliferative disease is rare with bone marrow transplantation and, although usually extranodal, seldom affects the lungs.[210] However, bone marrow transplantation is preceded by whole body irradiation and introduces the possibility of both radiation injury and graft-versus-host disease. Haemostasis may also be impaired and these patients are liable to suffer diffuse alveolar haemorrhage. There are therefore six possible conditions to consider when such patients complain of breathlessness (Box 12.4.2).

The chest radiograph is generally non-specific and seldom of help in distinguishing these conditions and even after full haematological and microbiological investigations the diagnosis may remain uncertain. However, bronchoalveolar lavage is generally of value in diagnosing leukaemic infiltration, opportunistic infections and haemorrhage, the last of these being characterised by haemosiderin-laden macrophages as well as fresh blood. If bronchoalveolar lavage is not diagnostic, the histopathological appearances of leukaemic infiltration, infection and cytotoxic damage are sufficiently distinctive to make biopsy a worthwhile procedure,[211–215] particularly as these

---

Box 12.4.2 Causes of breathlessness in leukaemia

Leukaemic infiltration
Infection
Cytotoxic drug damage
Irradiation injury
Graft-versus-host disease
Alveolar haemorrhage

three categories of disease fit well with the therapeutic regimens available to the clinician, namely, further antileukaemic drugs, antimicrobials and steroids respectively. It matters little that the pathological changes induced by radiotherapy and antileukaemic drugs are virtually identical, or that they are difficult to distinguish from some of the features of graft-versus-host disease.

Leukaemic involvement of the lungs consists of an interstitial infiltrate that predominantly involves the bronchopulmonary bundles, interlobular septa and the pleura, wherein run the lymphatics, but also spilling out into the air spaces. Micronodular aggregates of leukaemic cells may form, as in secondary involvement of the lung by lymphoma.[185] In many cases of myeloid leukaemia coming to autopsy, diffuse accumulations of leukaemic cells are found filling minor blood vessels, especially those of the lungs, a process known as leukostasis.[216] Chronic lymphocytic leukaemia occasionally extends into the lung parenchyma in a bronchiolocentric fashion, mimicking bronchiolitis.[217] High-grade transformation (Richter syndrome) is also described.[218]

The spectrum of opportunistic infection is wide but as well as the common bacterial pneumonias, invasive aspergillosis, cytomegalovirus infection and pneumocystis pneumonia are particularly common.[214,219,220] Herpes, parainfluenza and respiratory syncytial virus pneumonias are also recorded.[221–224] Infection is a likely cause of some cases of organising pneumonia that have been reported in bone marrow recipients.[225–227]

The pathology in the cytotoxic group consists of interstitial pneumonitis, diffuse alveolar damage and vascular disease.[24,211–214] It carries a high mortality.[228] Biopsy shows lymphocytic infiltration and fibrosis of the alveolar walls, oedema, fibrinous exudates, haemorrhage and hyaline membranes. Regenerating alveolar epithelium may show atypia, regardless of whether cytomegalovirus is present.[229] Small blood vessels show organising thrombus and intimal thickening, sometimes resulting in pulmonary veno-occlusive disease.[230,231] It is probable that such changes reflect the toxicity of antileukaemic drugs or whole-body irradiation rather than graft-versus-host disease for they occur in the absence of the better known extrapulmonary manifestations of this condition and occur with syngeneic as well as allogeneic grafts.[232,233] However, some patients develop obstructive airway disease a year or more after the marrow transplant, and this may be a manifestation of graft-versus-host disease[208,234–239] mediated by tumour necrosis factor.[240] Biopsy shows lymphocytic bronchiolitis and constrictive obliterative bronchiolitis (see p. 119).[227,234,236,238,241] Lymphoid interstitial pneumonia is also recorded and it is suggested that this is also a manifestation of graft-versus-host disease.[24,242]

Late manifestations of bone marrow transplantation include the development of solid tumours but the risk of lung cancer does not appear to be increased.[243] However, impaired lung function of uncertain nature can be detected in many long-term survivors who are free of respiratory symptoms.[244]

REFERENCES

Intrapulmonary lymph nodes

1. World Health Organization. Tumours of haematopoietic and lymphoid tissues. Lyons: IARC Press, 2001.
2. World Health Organization. Tumours of the lung, pleura, thymus and heart. Lyons: IARC Press, 2004.
3. Trapnell DH. Recognition and incidence of intrapulmonary lymph nodes. Thorax 1964; 19:44–50.
3a. Kradin RI, Spirn PW, Mark EJ. Intrapulmonary lymph nodes. Clinical, radiologic and pathologic features. Chest 1985; 87:662–667.
3b. Yokomise H, Mizuno H, Ike O, Wada H, Hitomi S, Itoh H. Importance of intrapulmonary lymph nodes in the differential diagnosis of small pulmonary nodular shadows. Chest 1998; 113:703–706.
4. Nicholson AG, Wotherspoon AC, Diss TC, et al. Reactive pulmonary lymphoid disorders. Histopathology 1995; 26:405–412.
5. Travis WD, Galvin JR. Non-neoplastic pulmonary lymphoid lesions. Thorax 2001; 56:964–971.
6. Yousem SA, Colby TV, Carrington CB. Follicular bronchitis/bronchiolitis. Hum Pathol 1985; 16:700–706.
7. Nicholson AG. Lymphoproliferative lung disease. In: Corrin B, ed. Pathology of Lung Tumors. London: Churchill Livingstone; 1997: 213–224.
8. Kradin RL, Mark EJ. Benign lymphoid disorders of the lung with a theory regarding their development. Hum Pathol 1983; 14:857–867.
9. Scully RE, McNeely WF, McNeely BU, et al. A 30-year-old man with a dry cough, dyspnea, and nodular pulmonary lesions – diffuse lymphoid hyperplasia of lungs, peribronchiolar (follicular bronchiolitis) and interstitial (lymphocytic interstitial pneumonitis). N Engl J Med 1993; 328:1696–1705.
10. Chatte G, Streichenberger N, Boillot O, Gille D, Loire R, Cordier JF. Lymphocytic bronchitis/bronchiolitis in a patient with primary biliary cirrhosis. Eur Respir J 1995; 8:176–179.
11. Fortoul TI, Cano Valle F, Oliva E, Barrios R. Follicular bronchiolitis in association with connective tissue diseases. Lung 1985; 163:305–314.
12. Kradin RL, Young RH, Kradin LA, Mark EJ. Immunoblastic lymphoma arising in chronic lymphoid hyperplasia of the pulmonary interstitium. Cancer 1982; 50:1339–1343.
13. Howling SJ, Hansell DM, Wells AU, Nicholson AG, Flint JD, Muller NL. Follicular bronchiolitis: thin-section CT and histologic findings. Radiology 1999; 212:637–642.
14. Romero S, Barroso E, Gil J, Aranda I, Alonso S, Garciapachon E. Follicular bronchiolitis: Clinical and pathologic findings in six patients. Lung 2003; 181:309–319.
15. Liebow AA, Carrington CB. The interstitial pneumonias. In: Simon M, ed. Frontiers of Pulmonary Radiology. New York: Grune & Stratton; 1969:102–141.
16. Liebow AA, Carrington CB. Diffuse pulmonary lymphoreticular infiltrations associated with dysproteinaemia. Med Clin North Am 1973; 57:809–843.
17. DeCouteau WE, Tourville D, Ambrus JL, Montes M, Adler R, Tomasi TB. Lymphoid interstitial pneumonia and autoerythrocyte sensitisation syndrome. Arch Intern Med 1974; 134:519–522.
18. Strimlan CV, Rosenov EC, Divertie MB, Harrison EG. Pulmonary manifestations of Sjogren's syndrome. Chest 1976; 70:354–361.
19. Levison AI, Hopewell PC, Stites DP, Spitler LE, Fudenburg HH. Coexistent lymphoid interstitial pneumonia, pernicious anaemia and agammaglobulinaemia; comment on autoimmune pathogenesis. Arch Intern Med 1976; 136:213–216.
20. Helman CA, Keeton GR, Benatar SR. Lymphoid interstitial pneumonia with associated chronic active hepatitis and renal tubular acidosis. Am Rev Respir Dis 1977; 115:161–164.
21. Julsrud PR, Brown LR, Li C-Y, Rosenow EC, Crowe JK. Pulmonary processes of mature-appearing lymphocytes: pseudolymphoma, well-differentiated lymphocytic lymphoma and lymphocytic interstitial pneumonitis. Diag Radiology 1978; 127:289–296.

22. Solal-Celigny P, Couderc LJ, Herman P, et al. Lymphoid interstitial pneumonitis in acquired immunodeficiency syndrome-related complex. Am Rev Respir Dis 1985; 131:956–960.

23. Grieco MH, Chinoy-Achara P. Lymphocytic interstitial pneumonia associated with the acquired immune deficiency syndrome. Am Rev Respir Dis 1985; 131:952–955.

24. Perreault C, Cousineau S, D'Angelo G, et al. Lymphoid interstitial pneumonia after allogeneic bone marrow transplantation: a possible manifestation of chronic graft-versus-host disease. Cancer 1985; 55:1–9.

25. Koss MN, Hochholzer L, Langloss JM, Wehart WD, Lazarus AA. Lymphoid interstitial pneumonia: clinicopathological and immunopathological findings in 18 cases. Pathology 1987; 19:178–185.

26. Morris JC, Rosen MJ, Marchevsky A, Teirstein AS. Lymphocytic interstitial pneumonia in patients at risk from the acquired immune deficiency syndrome. Chest 1987; 91:63–67.

27. Joshi VV. Pathology of AIDS in children. Pathol Annu 1989; 24(Part1):355–381.

28. O'Brodovich HM, Moser MM, Lu L. Familial lymphoid interstitial pneumonia: a long-term follow up. Pediatrics 1980; 65:523–528.

29. Montes T, Tomasi TB, Noebreu TH, Culver GJ. Lymphoid interstitial pneumonia with monoclonal gammopathy. Am Rev Respir Dis 1968; 98:277–280.

30. Strimlan CV, Rosenow EC, Weiland LH, Brown LR. Lymphocytic interstitial pneumonitis. Ann Intern Med 1978; 88:616–621.

31. Church JA, Isaacs H, Saxon A, Keens TG, Richards W. Lymphoid interstitial pneumonitis and hypogammaglobulinemia. Am Rev Respir Dis 1981; 124:491–498.

32. Desai SR, Nicholson AG, Stewart S, Twentyman OM, Flower CD, Hansell DM. Benign pulmonary lymphocytic infiltration and amyloidosis: computed tomographic and pathologic features in three cases. J Thorac Imaging 1997; 12:215–220.

33. Johkoh T, Muller NL, Pickford HA, et al. Lymphocytic interstitial pneumonia: thin-section CT findings in 22 patients. Radiology 1999; 212:567–572.

34. Johkoh T, Ichikado K, Akira M, et al. Lymphocytic interstitial pneumonia: follow-up CT findings in 14 patients. J Thorac Imaging 2000; 15:162–167.

35. Kramer MR, Saldana MJ, Ramos M, Pitchenik AE. High titers of Epstein–Barr virus antibodies in adult patients with lymphocytic interstitial pneumonitis associated with AIDS. Respir Med 1992; 86: 49–52.

36. Barbera JA, Hayashi S, Hegele RG, Hogg JC. Detection of Epstein–Barr virus in lymphocytic interstitial pneumonia by in situ hybridization. Am Rev Respir Dis 1992; 145:940–946.

37. Kaan PM, Hegele RG, Hayashi S, Hogg JC. Expression of bcl-2 and Epstein–Barr virus LMP1 in lymphocytic interstitial pneumonia. Thorax 1997; 52:12–16.

38. Itescu S, Brancato LJ, Winchester R. A sicca syndrome in HIV infection: association with HLA-DR5 and CD8 lymphocytosis. Lancet 1989; ii:466–468.

39. Travis WD, Fox CH, Devaney KO, et al. Lymphoid pneumonitis in 50 adult patients infected with the human immunodeficiency virus – lymphocytic interstitial pneumonitis versus nonspecific interstitial pneumonitis. Hum Pathol 1992; 23:529–541.

40. Koga M, Umemoto Y, Nishikawa M, Nakashima K, Ishihara T, Furukawa S. A case of lymphoid interstitial pneumonia in a 3-month-old boy not associated with HIV infection: Immunohistochemistry of lung biopsy specimens and serum transforming growth factor-beta 1 assay. Pathol Int 1997; 47:698–702.

41. Kurosu K, Yumoto N, Rom WN, et al. Aberrant expression of immunoglobulin heavy chain genes in Epstein–Barr virus-negative, human immunodeficiency virus-related lymphoid interstitial pneumonia. Lab Invest 2000; 80:1891–1903.

42. Kurosu K, Yumoto N, Furukawa M, Kuriyama T, Mikata A. Third complementarity-determining-region sequence analysis of lymphocytic interstitial pneumonia: most cases demonstrate a minor monoclonal population hidden among normal lymphocyte clones. Am J Respir Crit Care Med 1997; 155:1453–1460.

43. Nicholson AG, Kim H, Corrin B, et al. The value of classifying interstitial pneumonitis in childhood according to defined histological patterns. Histopathology 1998; 33:203–211.

44. TeruyaFeldstein J, Kingma DW, Weiss A, et al. Chemokine gene expression and clonal analysis of B cells in tissues involved by lymphoid interstitial pneumonitis from HIV-infected pediatric patients. Modern Pathol 2001; 14:929–936.

45. Kawabuchi B, Tsuchiya S, Nakagawa K, et al. Immunophenotypic and molecular analysis of a case of lymphocytic interstitial pneumonia. Acta Pathol Jpn 1993; 43:260–264.

46. Colby TV, Coleman A. The histologic diagnosis of extrinsic allergic alveolitis and its differential diagnosis. Prog Surg Pathol 1989; 10: 11–25.

47. Nicholson AG. Lymphocytic interstitial pneumonia and other lymphoproliferative disorders in the lung. Seminars in Respiratory and Critical Care Medicine 2001; 22:409–422.

48. Koyama M, Johkoh T, Honda O, et al. Chronic cystic lung disease: diagnostic accuracy of high-resolution CT in 92 patients. Am J Roentgenol 2003; 180:827–835.

49. Teruya-Feldstein J, Temeck BK, Sloas MM, et al. Pulmonary malignant lymphoma of mucosa-associated lymphoid tissue (MALT) arising in a pediatric HIV-positive patient. Am J Surg Pathol 1995; 19:357–363.

50. Dufour V, Wislez M, Bergot E, Mayaud C, Cadranel J. Improvement of symptomatic human immunodeficiency virus-related lymphoid interstitial pneumonia in patients receiving highly active antiretroviral therapy. Clin Infect Dis 2003; 36:e127-e130.

51. Abbondanzo SL, Rush W, Bijwaard KE, Koss MN. Nodular lymphoid hyperplasia of the lung – A clinicopathologic study of 14 cases. Amer J Surg Pathol 2000; 24:587–597.

52. Addis BJ, Hyjek E, Isaacson PG. Primary pulmonary lymphoma: a re-appraisal of its histogenesis and its relationship to pseudolymphoma and lymphoid interstitial pneumonia. Histopathology 1988; 13:1–17.

53. Li G, Hansmann M-L, Zwingers T, Lennert K. Primary lymphomas of the lung: morphological, immunohistochemical and clinical features. Histopathology 1990; 16:519–531.

54. Nicholson AG, Wotherspoon AC, Diss TC, et al. Pulmonary B-cell non-Hodgkin's lymphomas. The value of immunohistochemistry and gene analysis in diagnosis. Histopathology 1995; 26:395–403.

Lymphoproliferative disease complicating severe immune impairment

55. Di Carlo EF, Amberson JB, Metroka CE, Ballard P, Moore A, Mouradian JA. Malignant lymphomas and the acquired immunodeficiency syndrome. Evaluation of 30 cases using a working formulation. Arch Pathol Lab Med 1986; 110:1012–1016.

56. Nalesnik MA, Jaffe R, Starzl TE, et al. The pathology of posttransplant lymphoproliferative disorders occurring in the setting of cyclosporine A-prednisone immunosuppression. Am J Pathol 1988; 133:173–192.

57. Yousem SA, Randhawa P, Locker J, et al. Posttransplant lymphoproliferative disorders in heart-lung transplant recipients: primary presentation in the allograft. Hum Pathol 1989; 20:361–369.

58. Ray P, Antoine M, MaryKrause M, et al. AIDS-related primary pulmonary lymphoma. Am J Respir Crit Care Med 1998; 158:1221–1229.

59. Gaidano G, Carbone A, DallaFavera R. Pathogenesis of AIDS-related lymphomas: Molecular and histogenetic heterogeneity. Am J Pathol 1998; 152:623–630.

60. Hamilton-Dutoit SJ, Pallesen G, Franzmann MB, et al. AIDS-related lymphoma – histopathology, immunophenotype, and association with Epstein–Barr virus as demonstrated by in situ nucleic acid hybridization. Am J Pathol 1991; 138:149–163.

61. Kamel OW, van de Rijn M, Lebrun DP, Weiss LM, Warnke RA, Dorfman RF. Lymphoid neoplasms in patients with rheumatoid arthritis and dermatomyositis: frequency of Epstein–Barr virus and other features associated with immunosuppression. Hum Pathol 1994; 25:638–643.

62. Thomas JA, Crawford DH, Burke M. Clinicopathologic implications of Epstein–Barr virus related B cell lymphoma in immunocompromised patients. J Clin Pathol 1995; 48:287–290.

63. Baumforth KRN, Young LS, Flavell KJ, Constandinou C, Murray PG. Demystified. The Epstein-Barr virus and its association with human cancers. J Clin Pathol Mol Pathol 1999; 52:307–322.

64. Ioachim HL, Dorsett B, Cronin W, Maya M, Wahl S. Acquired immunodeficiency syndrome-associated lymphomas – clinical, pathologic, immunologic, and viral characteristics of 111 cases. Hum Pathol 1991; 22:659–673.

65. Haque AK, Myers JL, Hudnall SD, et al. Pulmonary lymphomatoid granulomatosis in acquired immunodeficiency syndrome: lesions with Epstein-Barr virus infection. Modern Pathol 1998; 11:347–356.

Primary pulmonary lymphoma

66. Herbert A, Wright DH, Isaacson P, Smith JL. Primary malignant lymphoma of the lung. Hum Pathol 1984; 15:415–422.

67. Kennedy JL, Nathwani BN, Burke JS, Hill LR, Rappaport H. Pulmonary lymphomas and other pulmonary lymphoid lesions. Cancer 1985; 56:539–552.

68. Cordier JF, Chailleux E, Lauque D, et al. Primary pulmonary lymphomas – a clinical study of 70 cases in nonimmunocompromised patients. Chest 1993; 103:201–208.

69. Fiche M, Capron F, Berger F, et al. Primary pulmonary non-Hodgkin's lymphomas. Histopathology 1995; 26:529–537.

70. Kurtin PJ, Myers JL, Adlakha H, et al. Pathologic and clinical features of primary pulmonary extranodal marginal zone B-cell lymphoma of MALT type. Am J Surg Pathol 2001; 25:997–1008.

71. Begueret H, Vergier B, Parrens M, et al. Primary lung small B-cell lymphoma versus lymphoid hyperplasia – Evaluation of diagnostic criteria in 26 cases. Am J Surg Pathol 2002; 26:76–81.

72. Wong KF, Chan JK, Ng CS, Lee KC, Tsang WY, Cheung MM. CD56 (NKH1)-positive hematolymphoid malignancies: an aggressive neoplasm featuring frequent cutaneous/mucosal involvement, cytoplasmic azurophilic granules, and angiocentricity. Hum Pathol 1992; 23:798–804.

73. Shah RN, Ozden O, Yeldandi A, Peterson L, Rao S, Laskin WB. Follicular dendritic cell tumor presenting in the lung: A case report. Hum Pathol 2001; 32:745–749.

74. Kudo H, Morinaga S, Shimosato Y, et al. Solitary mast cell tumor of the lung. Cancer 1988; 61:2089–2094.

75. Li XH. Case for the panel. Microvillous structure in a mast cell tumor of lung. Ultrastruct Pathol 1990; 14:95–100.

76. Valdez R, Finn WG, Ross CW, Singleton TP, Tworek JA, Schnitzer B. Waldenstrom macroglobulinemia caused by extranodal marginal zone B-cell lymphoma – A report of six cases. Am J Clin Pathol 2001; 116:683–690.

77. King LJ, Padley SP, Wotherspoon AC, Nicholson AG. Pulmonary MALT lymphoma: imaging findings in 24 cases. Eur Radiol 2000; 10:1932–1938.

78. Davis WB, Gadek JE. Detection of pulmonary lymphoma by bronchoalveolar lavage. Chest 1987; 91:787–790.

79. Sprague RI, deBlois GG. Small lymphocytic pulmonary lymphoma. Diagnosis by transthoracic fine needle aspiration. Chest 1989; 96:929–930.

80. Betsuyaku T, Munakata M, Yamaguchi E, et al. Establishing diagnosis of pulmonary malignant lymphoma by gene rearrangement analysis of lymphocytes in bronchoalveolar lavage fluid. Am J Respir Crit Care Med 1994; 149:526–529.

81. Meda BA, Buss DH, Woodruff RD, et al. Diagnosis and subclassification of primary and recurrent lymphoma. The usefulness and limitations of combined fine-needle aspiration cytomorphology and flow cytometry. Am J Clin Pathol 2000; 113:688–699.

82. Murphy BA, Meda BA, Buss DH, Geisinger KR. Marginal zone and mantle cell lymphomas: assessment of cytomorphology in subtyping small B-cell lymphomas. Diagn Cytopathol 2003; 28:126–130.

83. Richmond I, Pritchard GE, Ashcroft T, Avery A, Corris PA, Walters EH. Bronchus associated lymphoid tissue (BALT) in human lung – its distribution in smokers and non-smokers. Thorax 1993; 48:1130–1134.

84. Nicholson AG, Wotherspoon AC, Jones AL, Sheppard MN, Isaacson PG, Corrin B. Pulmonary B-cell non-Hodgkin's lymphoma associated with autoimmune disorders: a clinicopathological review of six cases. Eur Respir J 1996; 9:2022–2025.

85. Symmons DP. Neoplasms of the immune system in rheumatoid arthritis. Am J Med 1985; 78:22–28.

86. Frizzera G. Immunosuppression, autoimmunity, and lymphoproliferative disorders. Hum Pathol 1994; 25:627–629.

87. Inadome Y, Ikezawa T, Oyasu R, Noguchi M. Malignant lymphoma of bronchus-associated lymphoid tissue (BALT) coexistent with pulmonary tuberculosis. Pathol Int 2001; 51:807–811.

88. Luppi M, Longo G, Ferrari MG, et al. Additional neoplasms and HCV infection in low-grade lymphoma of MALT type. Br J Haematol 1996; 94:373–375.

89. Kubonishi I, Sugito S, Kobayashi M, et al. A unique chromosome translocation, t(11; 12; 18)(q21; q13; q21) [correction of t(11; 12; 18)(q13; q13; q12)], in primary lung lymphoma. Cancer Genet Cytogenet 1995; 82:54–56.

90. Ye H, Liu H, Attygalle A, et al. Variable frequencies of t(11; 18)(q21; q21) in MALT lymphomas of different sites: significant association with CagA strains of H pylori in gastric MALT lymphoma. Blood 2003; 102:1012–1018.

91. Wotherspoon AC, Finn TM, Isaacson PG. Trisomy 3 in low-grade B-cell lymphomas of mucosa-associated lymphoid tissue. Blood 1995; 85:2000–2004.

92. Ohshima K, Muta H, Kawasaki C, et al. Bcl10 expression, rearrangement and mutation in MALT lymphoma: correlation with expression of nuclear factor-kappaB. Int J Oncol 2001; 19:283–289.

93. Colby TV, Carrington CB. Pulmonary lymphomas simulating lymphomatoid granulomatosis. Am J Surg Pathol 1982; 6:19–32.

94. Perry LJ, Florio R, Dewar A, Nicholson AG. Giant lamellar bodies as a feature of pulmonary low-grade MALT lymphomas. Histopathology 2000; 36:240–244.

95. Dacic S, Colby TV, Yousem SA. Nodular amyloidoma and primary pulmonary lymphoma with amyloid production: A differential diagnostic problem. Modern Pathol 2000; 13:934–940.

96. Lim JK, Lacy MQ, Kurtin PJ, Kyle RA, Gertz MA. Pulmonary marginal zone lymphoma of MALT type as a cause of localised pulmonary amyloidosis. J Clin Pathol 2001; 54:642–646.

97. Ortiz-Hidalgo C, Wright DH. The morphological spectrum of monocytoid B-cell lymphoma and its relationship to lymphomas of mucosa-associated lymphoid tissue. Histopathology 1992; 21:555–561.

98. Ngan BY, Warnke RA, Wilson M, Takagi K, Cleary ML, Dorfman RF. Monocytoid B-cell lymphoma: a study of 36 cases. Hum Pathol 1991; 22:409–421.

99. Moran CA, Suster S, Fishback NF, Koss MN. Primary intrapulmonary thymoma: a clinicopathologic and immunohistochemical study of eight cases. Am J Surg Pathol 1995; 19:304–312.

100. Uppal R, Goldstraw P. Primary pulmonary lymphoma. Lung Cancer 1992; 8:95–100.

101. Orchard TR, Eraut CD, Davison AG. Non-Hodgkin's lymphoma arising in cryptogenic fibrosing alveolitis. Thorax 1998; 53:228–229.

102. Sabourin JC, Kanavaros P, Briere J, et al. Epstein-Barr virus (EBV) genomes and EBV-encoded latent membrane protein (LMP) in pulmonary lymphomas occurring in nonimmunocompromised patients. Am J Surg Pathol 1993; 17:995–1002.

103. Liebow AA, Carrington CRB, Friedman PJ. Lymphomatoid granulomatosis. Hum Pathol 1972; 3:457–558.

104. Liebow AA. Pulmonary angiitis and granulomatosis. Am Rev Respir Dis 1973; 108:1–18.

105. Katzenstein ALA, Carrington CB, Liebow AA. Lymphomatoid granulomatosis. A clinicopathologic study of 152 cases. Cancer 1979; 43:360–373.

106. Jaffe ES. Post-thymic lymphoid neoplasia. Surgical Pathology of the Lymph Nodes and Related Organs Major Problems in Pathology No 16. Philadelphia: Saunders; 1985.

107. Lipford EH, Margolick JB, Longo DL, Fauci AS, Jaffe ES. Angiocentric immunoproliferative lesions: a clinicopathologic spectrum of post-thymic T-cell proliferations. Blood 1988; 72:1674–1681.

108. Harris TJ, Bhan AK, Murphy GF, Sanchez NP, Mihm MC. Lymphomatoid papulosis and lymphomatoid granulomatosis: T cell subset populations. Am J Invest Dermatol 1981; 76:326.

109. Gaulard P, Henni T, Marolleau J-P, et al. Lethal midline granuloma (polymorphic reticulosis) and lymphomatoid granulomatosis – evidence for a monoclonal T-cell lymphoproliferative disorder. Cancer 1988; 62:705–710.

110. Nichols PW, Koss M, Levine AM, Lukes RJ. Lymphomatoid granulomatosis: A T-cell disorder. Am J Med 1982; 72:467–471.

111. Tanaka Y, Sasaki Y, Kurozumi H, et al. Angiocentric immunoproliferative lesion associated with chronic active Epstein-Barr virus infection in an 11-year-old boy. Clonotopic proliferation of Epstein–Barr virus-bearing CD4+ T lymphocytes. Am J Surg Pathol 1994; 18:623–631.

112. Guinee D, Jaffe E, Kingma D, et al. Pulmonary lymphomatoid granulomatosis – evidence for a proliferation of Epstein-Barr virus infected B-lymphocytes with a prominent T-cell component and vasculitis. Am J Surg Pathol 1994; 18:753–764.

113. Myers JL, Kurtin PJ, Katzenstein ALA, et al. Lymphomatoid granulomatosis: evidence of immunophenotypic diversity and relationship to Epstein–Barr virus infection. Am J Surg Pathol 1995; 19:1300–1312.

114. Nicholson AG, Wotherspoon AC, Diss TC, et al. Lymphomatoid granulomatosis: evidence that some cases represent Epstein–Barr virus-associated B-cell lymphoma. Histopathology 1996; 29:317–324.

115. Taniere P, Thivolet-Bejui F, Vitrey D, et al. Lymphomatoid granulomatosis – a report on four cases: evidence for B phenotype of the tumoral cells. Eur Resp J 1998; 12:102–106.

116. Katzenstein AA, Peiper SC. Detection of Epstein-Barr virus genomes in lymphomatoid granulomatosis: analysis of 29 cases by the polymerase chain reaction. Mod Pathol 1990; 3:435–441.

117. Peiper SC. Angiocentric lymphoproliferative disorders of the respiratory system: incrimination of Epstein-Barr virus in pathogenesis. Blood 1993; 82:687–690.

118. Saldana MJ, Patchefsky AS, Israel HI, Atkinson GW. Pulmonary angiitis and granulomatosis: the relationship between histological features, organ involvement and response to treatment. Hum Pathol 1977; 8:391–409.

119. Israel HL, Patchefsky AJ, Saldana MJ. Wegener's granulomatosis, lymphomatoid granulomatosis and benign lymphocytic angiitis and granulomatosis. Ann Intern Med 1977; 87:691–699.

120. Gracey DR, DeRemee RA, Colby TV, Unni KK, Weiland LH. Benign lymphocytic angiitis and granulomatosis: experience with three cases. Mayo Clin Proc 1988; 63:323–331.

121. Norton AJ. Angiocentric lymphoma. Current Diagn Pathol 1994; 1:158–166.

122. Bone RC, Vernon M, Sobonya RE, Rendon H. Lymphomatoid granulomatosis: report of a case and review of the literature. Am J Med 1978; 65:709–716.

123. Sordillo PP, Epremian B, Koziner B, Lacher M, Lieberman P. Lymphomatoid granulomatosis. An analysis of clinical and immunologic characteristics. Cancer 1982; 49:2070–2076.

124. Fauci AS, Haynes BF, Costa J, Katz P, Wolff SM. Lymphomatoid granulomatosis. Prospective clinical and therapeutic experience over 10 years. N Engl J Med 1982; 306:68–74.

125. Koss MN, Hochholzer L, Langloss JM, Wehunt WD, Lazarus AA. Lymphomatoid granulomatosis: a clinicopathologic and immunopathologic study of 42 patients. Pathology 1986; 18:283–288.

126. Key S, Fu Y-S, Minars N, Brady JW. Lymphomatoid granulomatosis of the skin: light microscopic and ultrastructural studies. Cancer 1974; 34:1675–1682.

127. Frazier AA, Rosado-de-Christenson ML, Galvin JR, Fleming MV. Pulmonary angiitis and granulomatosis: radiologic-pathologic correlation. Radiographics 1998; 18:687–710.

128. Klein FA. Lymphomatoid granulomatosis masquerading as hypernephroma with lung masses. J Urol 1984; 131:942–944.

129. Teruya-Feldstein J, Jaffe ES, Burd PR, et al. The role of Mig, the monokine induced by interferon-gamma, and IP-10, the interferon-gamma-inducible protein-10, in tissue necrosis and vascular damage associated with Epstein-Barr virus-positive lymphoproliferative disease. Blood 1997; 90:4099–4105.

130. Ilowite NT, Fligner CL, Ochs HD, et al. Pulmonary angiitis with atypical lymphoreticular infiltrates in Wiskott-Aldrich syndrome: possible relationship to lymphomatoid granulomatosis and EBV infection. Clin Immunol Immunopathol 1986; 41:479–484.

131. Colby TV. Central nervous system lymphomatoid granulomatosis in AIDS? Hum Pathol 1989; 20:301–302.

132. Naschitz JE, Yeshurun D, Grishkan A, Boss JH. Lymphomatoid granulomatosis of the lung in a patient with agnogenic myeloid metaplasia. Respiration 1984; 45:316–320.

133. Bekassy AN, Cameron R, Garwicz S, Laurin S, Wiebe T. Lymphomatoid granulomatosis during treatment of acute lymphoblastic lymphoma in a 6 year old girl. Am J Paed Hematol-Oncol 1985; 7:377–380.

134. Imai Y, Yamamoto K, Suzuki K, et al. Lymphomatoid granulomatosis (LYG) occurring in a patient with follicular lymphoma during remission. Jpn J Clin Hematol 1992; 33:507–513.

135. Swerdlow SH. Post-transplant lymphoproliferative disorders: a morphologic, phenotypic and genotypic spectrum of disease. Histopathology 1992; 20:373–385.

136. Burke MM. Complications of heart and lung transplantation and of cardiac surgery. In Anthony PP, MacSween RNM eds. Recent Advances in Histopathology, vol. 16. New York: Churchill Livingstone; 1994:95–122.

137. Morice WG, Kurtin PJ, Myers JL. Expression of cytolytic lymphocyte-associated antigens in pulmonary lymphomatoid granulomatosis. Am J Clin Pathol 2002; 118:391–398.

138. Guinee DG, Jr., Perkins SL, Travis WD, Holden JA, Tripp SR, Koss MN. Proliferation and cellular phenotype in lymphomatoid granulomatosis: implications of a higher proliferation index in B cells. Am J Surg Pathol 1998; 22:1093–1100.

139. Wilson WH, Kingma DW, Raffeld M, Wittes RE, Jaffe ES. Association of lymphomatoid granulomatosis with Epstein–Barr viral infection of B lymphocytes and response to interferon-alpha 2b. Blood 1996; 87:4531–4537.

140. Bernstein ML, Reece ER, de Chadarevian JP, Koch PA. Bone marrow transplantation in lymphomatoid granulomatosis. Report of a case. Cancer 1986; 58:969–972.

141. Berkman N, Breuer R. Pulmonary involvement in lymphoma. Respir Med 1993; 87:85–92.

142. Kern WGH, Crepeau AG, Jones JC. Primary Hodgkin's disease of the lung. Cancer 1961; 14:1151–1165.

143. Yousem SA, Weiss LM, Colby TV. Primary pulmonary Hodgkin's disease. Cancer 1986; 57:1217–1224.

144. Radin AI. Primary pulmonary Hodgkin's disease. Cancer 1990; 65: 550–563.

145. Schee ACvd, Dinkla BA, Knapen Av. Primary pulmonary manifestation of Hodgkin's disease. Respiration 1990; 57:127–128.

146. Pinson P, Joos G, Praet M, Pauwels R. Primary pulmonary Hodgkin's disease. Respiration 1992; 59:314–316.

147. Boshnakova T, Michailova V, Koss M, Georgiev C, Todorov T, Sarbinova M. Primary pulmonary Hodgkin's disease – Report of two cases. Resp Med 2000; 94:830–831.

148. Harper PG, Fisher C, McLennan K, Souhami RL. Presentation of Hodgkin's disease as an endobronchial lesion. Cancer 1984; 53:147–150.

149. Daly PA, O'Brian DS, Robinson I. Hodgkin's disease with a granulomatous pulmonary presentation mimicking sarcoidosis. Thorax 1988; 43:407–409.

150. Okada S, Ohtsuki H, Midorikawa O, Hashimoto K. Bronchial plasmacytoma identified by immunoperoxidase technique on paraffin embedded section. Acta Pathol Jpn 1982; 32:149–155.

151. Dux S, Pitlik S, Rosenfeld JB, Pick J, Ben-Bassat M. Localised visceral immunocytoma associated with serological findings suggesting systemic lupus erythematosus. BMJ 1984; 288:898–899.

152. Roikjaer O, Thomsen JK. Plasmacytoma of the lung. A case report describing two tumors of different immunologic type in a single patient. Cancer 1986; 58:2671–2674.

153. Morinaga S, Watanabe H, Gemma A, et al. Plasmacytoma of the lung associated with nodular deposits of immunoglobulin. Am J Surg Pathol 1987; 11:989–995.

154. Brackett LE, Myers JR, Sherman CB. Laser treatment of endobronchial extramedullary plasmacytoma. Chest 1994; 106:1276–1277.

155. Wise JN, Schaefer RF, Read RC. Primary pulmonary plasmacytoma – A case report. Chest 2001; 120:1405.

156. Childness WG, Adie GC. Plasma cell tumors of the mediastinum and lung. J Thorac Surg 1950; 19:794–799.

157. Cotton BM, Pinedo JR. Plasma cell tumours of the lung: report of a case. Dis Chest 1952; 21:218–221.

158. Herskovic T, Anderson HA, Bayrd ED. Intrathoracic plasmacytomas. Dis Chest 1952; 47:1–6.

159. Kernan JA, Meyer BW. Malignant plasmacytoma of the lung with metastases. J Thorac Cardiovasc Surg 1966; 51:739–744.

160. Amin R. Extramedullary plasmacytoma of the lung. Cancer 1985; 56:152–156.

161. Baroni CD, Mineo TC, Ricci C, Guarino S, Mandelli F. Solitary secretory plasmacytoma of the lung in a 14 year old boy. Cancer 1977; 40:2329–2332.

162. Wile A, Olinger G, Peter JB, Dornfield L. Solitary intraparenchymal pulmonary plasmacytoma associated with production of an M-protein. Cancer 1976; 37:2338–2342.

163. Piard F, et al. Solitary plasmacytoma of the lung with light chain extracellular deposits: a case report and review of the literature. Histopathology 1998; 32:356–361.

164. Kazzaz B, Dewar A, Corrin B. An unusual pulmonary plasmacytoma. Histopathology 1992; 21:285–287.

165. Prasad ML, Charney DA, Sarlin J, Keller SM. Pulmonary immunocytoma with massive crystal storing histiocytosis: A case report with review of literature. Am J Surg Pathol 1998; 22:1148–1153.

166. Jones D, Renshaw AA. Recurrent crystal-storing histiocytosis of the lung in a patient without a clonal lymphoproliferative disorder. Arch Pathol Lab Med 1996; 120:978–980.

167. Koss MN, Hochholzer L, Moran CA, Frizzera G. Pulmonary plasmacytomas: a clinicopathologic and immunohistochemical study of five cases. Ann Diagn Pathol 1998; 2:1–11.

168. Rush WL, Andriko JAW, Taubenberger JK, et al. Primary anaplastic large cell lymphoma of the lung: A clinicopathologic study of five patients. Modern Pathol 2000; 13:1285–1292.

169. Beltran S, Tomas Labat ME, Ferreras FP. Primary Ki-1 positive anaplastic large cell non-Hodgkin's lymphoma of the lung. A case study and review of the literature. An Med Interna 2001; 18:587–590.

Secondary pulmonary lymphoma

170. Filly R, Blauk N, Castellino RA. Radiographic distribution of intrathoracic disease in previously untreated patients with Hodgkin's disease and non-Hodgkin's lymphoma. Radiology 1976; 120:277–281.

171. Weis JW, Winter MW, Phyliky RL, Banks DM. Peripheral T-cell lymphomas: histologic, immunohistologic and clinical characterisation. Mayo Clin Proc 1986; 61:411–426.

172. Zylak CJ, Banerjee R, Galbraith PA, McCarthy DS. Lung involvement in angioimmunoblastic lymphadenopathy (AIL). Radiology 1976; 121:513–519.

173. Myers TJ, Cole SR, Pastuszak WT. Angioimmunoblastic lymphadenopathy: pleural-pulmonary disease. Cancer 1978; 40:266–271.

174. Iseman MD, Schwarz MI, Stanford RE. Interstitial pneumonia in angio-immunoblastic lymphadenopathy with dysproteinaemia: a case report with special histologic studies. Ann Intern Med 1976; 85:752–755.

175. Chejfec G, Natarelli J, Gould VE. 'Myeloma lung' – A previously unreported complication of multiple myeloma. Hum Pathol 1983; 14:558–561.

176. Rausch PG, Herion JC. Pulmonary manifestations of Waldenstroms's macroglobulinaemia. Am J Hematol 1980; 9:201–209.

177. Lin P, Bueso-Ramos C, Wilson CS, Mansoor A, Medeiros LJ. Waldenstrom macroglobulinemia involving extramedullary sites: morphologic and immunophenotypic findings in 44 patients. Am J Surg Pathol 2003; 27:1104–1113.

178. Schmidt M, Dercken C, Loke O, et al. Pulmonary manifestation of systemic mast cell disease. Eur Resp J 2000; 15:623–625.

179. Rappaport H, Thomas LB. Mycosis fungoides: the pathology of extracutaneous involvement. Cancer 1974; 34:1198–1229.

180. Rubin DL, Blank N. Rapid pulmonary dissemination in mycosis fungoides simulating pneumonia. A case report and review of the literature. Cancer 1985; 56:649–651.

181. Colby TV, Carrington CB, Mark GJ. Pulmonary involvement in malignant histiocytosis. A clinicopathologic spectrum. Am J Surg Pathol 1981; 5:61–73.

182. Wongchaowart B, Kennealy JA, Crissman J, Hawkins H. Respiratory failure in malignant histiocytosis. Am Rev Respir Dis 1981; 124:640–642.

183. Stempel DA, Volberg FM, Parker BR, Lewiston NJ. Malignant histiocytosis presenting as interstitial pulmonary disease. Am Rev Respir Dis 1982; 126:726–728.

184. Colby TV, Carrington CB. Lymphoreticular tumours and infiltrates of the lung. Pathol Annu 1983; 18:27–70.

185. Rollins SD, Colby TV. Lung biopsy in chronic lymphocytic leukemia. Arch Pathol Lab Med 1988; 112:607–611.

186. Remberger K, Nawrath-Koll I, Gokel JM, Haider M. Systemic angioendotheliomatosis of the lung. Pathol Res Pract 1987; 182:265–270.

187. Wick MR, Mills SE, Scheithauer BW, Cooper PH, Davitz MA, Parkinson K. Reassessment of malignant angioendotheliomatosis. Am J Surg Pathol 1986; 10:112–113.

188. Theaker JM, Gatter KC, Esiri MM, Easterbrook P. Neoplastic angioendotheliomatosis – further evidence supporting a lymphoid origin. Histopathology 1986; 10:1261–1270.

189. Owa M, Koyama J, Asakawa K, Hikita H, Kubo K, Ikeda SI. Intravascular lymphomatosis presenting as reversible severe pulmonary hypertension. Int J Cardiol 2000; 75:283–284.

190. Tsukadaira A, Okubo Y, Ogasawara H, et al. Chromosomal aberrations in intravascular lymphomatosis. Am J Clin Oncol 2002; 25:178–181.

191. Takamura K, Nasuhara Y, Mishina T, et al. Intravascular lymphomatosis diagnosed by transbronchial lung biopsy. Eur Respir J 1997; 10:955–957.

192. Tan TB, Spaander PJ, Blaisse M, Gerritzen FM. Angiotropic large cell lymphoma presenting as interstitial lung disease. Thorax 1988; 43:578–579.

193. Yousem SA, Colby TV. Intravascular lymphomatosis presenting in the lung. Cancer 1990; 65:349–353.

194. Snyder LS, Harmon KR, Estensen RD. Intravascular lymphomatosis (malignant angioendotheliomatosis) presenting as pulmonary hypertension. Chest 1989; 96:1199–1200.

195. Ko YH, Han JH, Go JH, et al. Intravascular lymphomatosis: a clinicopathological study of two cases presenting as an interstitial lung disease. Histopathology 1997; 31:555–562.

196. Walls JG, Hong G, Cox JE, et al. Pulmonary intravascular lymphomatosis. Presentation with dyspnea and air trapping. Chest 1999; 115:1207–1210.

197. Demirer T, Dail DH, Aboulafia DM. Four varied cases of intravascular lymphomatosis and a literature review. Cancer 1994; 73:1738–1745.

Angiofollicular lymph node hyperplasia (giant lymph node hyperplasia, Castleman's disease)

198. Awotedu AA, Otulana BA, Ukoli CO. Giant lymph node hyperplasia of the lung (Castleman's disease) associated with recurrent pleural effusion. Thorax 1990; 45:775–776.

199. Barrie JR, English JC, Muller N. Castleman's disease of the lung: radiographic, high-resolution CT, and pathologic findings. AJR Am J Roentgenol 1996; 166:1055–1056.

200. Mohamedani AA, Bennett MK. Angiofollicular lymphoid hyperplasia in a pulmonary fissure. Thorax 1985; 40:686–687.

201. Matsuda H, Mori M, Yasumoto K, Sugimachi K. Angiofollicular lymph node hyperplasia arising from the intercostal space. Thorax 1988; 43:337–338.

202. Weisenburger DD, Nathwani BN, Winberg CD, Rappaport H. Multicentric angiofollicular lymph node hyperplasia: A clinicopathologic study of 16 cases. Hum Pathol 1985; 16:162–172.

203. Baruch Y, Ben-Arie Y, Kerner H, Lorber M, Best LA, Gershoni-Baruch R. Giant lymph node hyperplasia (Castleman's disease): a clinical study of eight patients. Postgrad Med J 1991; 67:366–370.

204. Abdelreheim FA, Koss W, Rappaport ES, Arber DA. Coexistence of Hodgkin's disease and giant lymph node hyperplasia of the plasma-cell type (Castleman's disease). Arch Pathol Lab Med 1996; 120:91–96.

204a. Guihot A, Couderc LJ, Agbalika F, et al. Pulmonary manifestations of multicentric Castleman's disease in HIV infection: a clinical, biological and radiological study. Eur Respir J 2005; 26:118–125.

205. Dupin N, Gorin I, Deleuze J, Agut H, Huraux J-M, Escande J-P. Herpes-like DNA sequences, AIDS-related tumors, and Castleman's disease. New Engl J Med 1995; 333:798–799.

206. Teruya-Feldstein J, Zauber P, Setsuda JE, et al. Expression of human herpesvirus-8 oncogene and cytokine homologues in an HIV-seronegative patient with multicentric Castleman's disease and primary effusion lymphoma. Lab Invest 1998; 78:1637–1642.

Pulmonary problems in leukaemia

207. Breuer R, Lossos IS, Berkman N, Or R. Pulmonary complications of bone marrow transplantation. Respir Med 1993; 87:571–579.

208. Sloane JP, Norton J. Invited review – the pathology of bone marrow transplantation. Histopathology 1993; 22:201–209.

209. Soubani AO, Miller KB, Hassoun PM. Pulmonary complications of bone marrow transplantation. Chest 1996; 109:1066–1077.

209a. Roychowdhury M, Pambuccian SE, Aslan DL, et al. Pulmonary complications after bone marrow transplantation: an autopsy study from a large transplantation center. Arch Pathol Lab Med 2005; 129:366–371.

210. Orazi A, Hromas RA, Neiman RS, et al. Posttransplantation lymphoproliferative disorders in bone marrow transplant recipients are aggressive diseases with a high incidence of adverse histologic and immunobiologic features. Am J Clin Pathol 1997; 107:419–429.

211. Moir DH, Turner JJ, Ma DDF, Biggs JC, St Vincent's Hospital bone marrow transplantation team. Autopsy findings in bone marrow transplantation. Pathology 1982; 14:197–204.

212. Sloane JP, Depledge MH, Powles RL, Morgenstern GR, Trickey BS, Dady PJ. Histopathology of the lung after bone marrow transplantation. J Clin Pathol 1983; 36:546–554.

213. Bombi JA, Cardesa A, Llebaria C, et al. Main autopsy findings in bone marrow transplant patients. Arch Pathol Lab Med 1987; 111:125–129.

214. Doran HM, Sheppard MN, Collins PW, Jones L, Newland AC, Vanderwalt JD. Pathology of the lung in leukaemia and lymphoma – a study of 87 autopsies. Histopathology 1991; 18:211–219.

215. White DA, Wong PW, Downey R. The utility of open lung biopsy in patients with hematologic malignancies. Am J Respir Crit Care Med 2000; 161:723–729.

216. van Buchem MA, Wondergem JH, Kool LJ, et al. Pulmonary leukostasis: radiologic-pathologic study. Radiology 1987; 165:739–741.

217. Trisolini R, Lazzari AL, Poletti V. Bronchiolocentric pulmonary involvement due to chronic lymphocytic leukemia. Haematologica 2000; 85:1097.

218. Snyder LS, Cherwitz DL, Dykoski RK, Rice KL. Endobronchial Richter's syndrome. A rare manifestation of chronic lymphocytic leukemia. Am Rev Respir Dis 1988; 138:980–983.

219. Beschorner WE, Hutchins GM, Burns WH, Saral R, Tutschka PJ, Santos GW. Cytomegalovirus pneumonia in bone marrow transplant recipients: miliary and diffuse patterns. Am Rev Respir Dis 1980; 122:107–114.

220. Stals FS, Steinhoff G, Wagenaar SS, et al. Cytomegalovirus induces interstitial lung disease in allogeneic bone marrow transplant recipient rats independent of acute graft-versus-host response. Lab Invest 1996; 74:343–352.

221. Harrington SW, Hooton TM, Hackman RC, et al. An outbreak of respiratory syncytial virus in a bone marrow transplant center. J Infect Dis 1989; 158:987–993.

222. Carrigan DR, Drobyski WR, Russler SK, Tapper MA, Knox KK, Ash RC. Interstitial pneumonitis associated with human herpesvirus-6 infection after marrow transplantation. Lancet 1991; 338:147–149.

223. Wendt CH, Weisdorf DJ, Jordan MC, Balfour HH, Hertz MI. Parainfluenza virus respiratory infection after bone marrow transplantation. N Engl J Med 1992; 326:921–926.

224. Cone RW, Hackman RC, Huang MLW, et al. Human herpesvirus-6 in lung tissue from patients with pneumonitis after bone marrow transplantation. N Engl J Med 1993; 329:156–161.

225. Thirman MJ, Devine SM, O'Toole K, et al. Bronchiolitis obliterans organizing pneumonia as a complication of allogeneic bone marrow transplantation. Bone Marrow Transplantation 1992; 10:307–311.

226. Thirman MJ, Devine SM, O'Toole K, et al. Bronchiolitis obliterans organizing pneumonia as a complication of allogeneic bone marrow transplantation. Bone Marrow Transplantation 1992; 10:307–311.

227. Yousem SA. The histological spectrum of pulmonary graft versus host disease in bone marrow transplant recipients. Hum Pathol 1995; 26:668–675.

228. Crawford SW, Hackman RC. Clinical course of idiopathic pneumonia after bone marrow transplantation. Am Rev Respir Dis 1993; 147:1393–1400.

229. Elias AD, Mark EJ, Trotman-Dickenson B. A 60-year-old man with pulmonary infiltrates after a bone marrow transplantation – Busulfan pneumonitis. N Engl J Med 1997; 337:480–489.

230. Williams LM, Fussell S, Veith RW, Nelson S, Mason CM. Pulmonary veno-occlusive disease in an adult following bone marrow transplantation: case report and review of the literature. Chest 1996; 109:1388–1391.

231. Hackman RC, Madtes DK, Petersen FB, Clark JG. Pulmonary veno-occlusive disease following bone marrow transplantation. Transplantation 1989; 47:989–992.

232. Appelbaum FR, Meyers JD, Fefer A, et al. Nonbacterial nonfungal pneumonia following marrow transplantation in 100 identical twins. Transplantation 1982; 33:265–268.

233. Clark JG, Hansen JA, Hertz MI, Parkman R, Jensen L, Peavy HH. Idiopathic pneumonia syndrome after bone marrow transplantation. Am Rev Respir Dis 1993; 147:1601–1606.

234. Roca J, Granena A, Rodriguez-Roisin R, Alvarez P, Agusti-Vidal A, Rozman C. Fatal airway disease in an adult with chronic graft-versus-host disease. Thorax 1982; 37:77–78.

235. Ralph DD, Springmeyer SC, Sullivan KM, Hackman RC, Storb R, Thomas ED. Rapidly progressive air-flow obstruction in marrow transplant recipients. Possible association between obliterative bronchiolitis and chronic graft-versus-host disease. Am Rev Respir Dis 1984; 129:641–644.

236. Urbanski SJ, Kossakowska AE, Curtis J, et al. Idiopathic small airways pathology in patients with graft-versus-host disease following allogeneic bone marrow transplantation. Am J Surg Pathol 1987; 11:965–971.

237. Epler GR. Bronchiolitis obliterans and airway obstruction associated with graft-versus-host disease. Clin Chest Med 1988; 9:551–556.

238. Ralph DD, Springmeyer SC, Sullivan KM, Hackman RC, Storb R, Thomas ED. Rapidly progressive air-flow obstruction in marrow transplant recipients. Possible association between obliterative bronchiolitis and chronic graft-versus-host disease. Am Rev Respir Dis 1994; 129:641–644.

239. Paz HL, Crilley P, Topolsky DL, Coll WX, Patchefsky A, Brodsky I. Bronchiolitis obliterans after bone marrow transplantation – the effect of preconditioning. Respiration 1993; 60:109–114.

240. Piguet PF, Grau GE, Collart MA, Vassalli P, Kapanci Y. Pneumopathies of the graft-versus-host reaction. Alveolitis associated with an increased level of tumor necrosis factor mRNA and chronic interstitial pneumonitis. Lab Invest 1989; 61:37.

241. Yokoi T, Hirabayashi N, Ito M, et al. Broncho-bronchiolitis obliterans as a complication of bone marrow transplantation: a clinicopathological study of eight autopsy cases. Virchows Archiv 1997; 431:275–282.

242. Perreault C, Coosineau S, D'Angelo G, et al. Lymphoid interstitial pneumonia after allogeneic bone marrow transplantation. Cancer 1985; 55:1–9.

243. Curtis RE, Rowlings PA, Deeg HJ, et al. Solid cancers after bone marrow transplantation. N Engl J Med 1997; 336:897–904.

244. Cerveri I, Zoia MC, Fulgoni P, et al. Late pulmonary sequelae after childhood bone marrow transplantation. Thorax 1999; 54:131–135.

12

Tumours

12.5

Miscellaneous tumours

Table 12.5.1 compares the successive WHO/IASLC classifications of miscellaneous lung tumours with the plan adopted here. In this book, hamartoma and clear cell tumour are discussed under mesenchymal tumours and sclerosing haemangioma and thymoma under epithelial tumours, as we believe this reflects their histogenesis more accurately. This leaves only melanoma and germ cell tumours to be dealt with in this chapter.

MELANOMA

Melanocytes are not a normal feature of the lower respiratory tract and descriptions of a blue naevus[1] and primary melanomas[2–6] of the bronchi are therefore surprising. Whether these tumours can be presumed to arise from ectopic melanocytes is not entirely clear since melanin production is documented in bronchopulmonary carcinoid tumours,[7–11] which are thought to be of endodermal rather than neural crest origin. Melanin pigmentation has also been recorded in a bronchial Schwannoma,[12] a benign clear cell tumour of the lung[13] and a pulmonary blastoma.[14]

Clinical features, treatment and prognosis

Primary melanomas of the lower respiratory tract are very rare. Age at presentation ranges from 29–80 years and there is no sex predilection.[3,15] The tumours nearly always involve large bronchi or the trachea and the patients complain of persistent cough and haemoptysis or symptoms attributable to obstructive pneumonia. Treatment is surgical but the prognosis is poor.[6]

Pathological features

Tracheobronchial melanomas are generally polypoid but occasional 'flat' examples are reported. Microscopically, they are identical to those that occur elsewhere, being predominantly pigmented, probably because amelanotic melanomas in the lung are likely to be interpreted as anaplastic carcinomas

Table 12.5.1 Progressive classifications of miscellaneous tumours of the lung

1981 WHO classification	1999 and 2004 WHO/IASLC classifications	2005 Pathology of the Lung
Carcinosarcoma (carcinoma)	Hamartoma (mesenchymal)	
Pulmonary blastoma (carcinoma)	Sclerosing haemangioma (other epithelial)	
Malignant melanoma	Clear cell tumour (mesenchymal)	
Malignant lymphomas (lymphoproliferative disease)	Thymoma (other epithelial)	
Others	Melanoma	Melanoma
	Teratoma	Germ cell tumours

Text in parentheses shows the classification adopted in this book.
WHO, World Health Organization; IASLC, International Association for the Study of Lung Cancer.

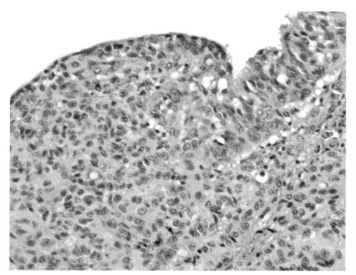

Figure 12.5.1 Melanoma. A primary endobronchial lesion shows malignant polygonal cells, within which melanin pigment can be seen. (Section provided by Dr TV Colby, Scottsdale, USA.)

(Fig. 12.5.1). If there is no pigmentation, or if pigmented carcinoid tumour is suspected, the presence of S-100 protein and HMB-45 antigen, the absence of cytokeratin expression and neuroendocrine markers, and the identification of melanosomes by electron microscopy are helpful diagnostic features.

Differential diagnosis

Strict criteria must be applied before a diagnosis of primary malignant melanoma of the lower respiratory tract can be accepted.[4] Very few reported cases withstand close scrutiny. There should be no evidence of a current or previous primary melanoma elsewhere and any previously resected lesions of the skin, adjacent mucosal surfaces or the eye should be reviewed. The phenomenon of spontaneous regression of an extrapulmonary melanoma after metastasis has occurred bedevils the exclusion of a bronchial melanoma having such an origin. Junctional change in bronchial epithelium is regarded as the best histological evidence of a primary bronchial origin, particularly if it is well away from the tumour because neoplastic melanocytes may directly infiltrate the overlying epithelium and mimic

junctional activity. True junctional change has been well described in only a few melanomas of the lower respiratory tract.[2,5,16,17] In a review of 18 previously published cases, only two were considered to be proven, eight were thought to be near proven, four probable and four improbable.[2]

GERM CELL TUMOURS

Primary germ cell tumours of the lung (teratoma and choriocarcinoma) are extremely rare[18–28] and the possibility of metastasis should always be excluded. Germ cell tumours of the anterior mediastinum arise in the thymus and the presence of thymic tissue in several reported cases of intrapulmonary teratoma suggests that these may have originated in heterotopic thymic tissue.[20,21]

Clinical features, treatment and prognosis

Pulmonary germ cell tumours show a wide age range (3 months–68 years) and a slight female preponderance.[21] They are also more prevalent in the upper lobes and on the left side.[28,29] The presenting symptoms are usually not specific, apart from the expectoration of hair, a dramatic but rare manifestation.[22] Surgical treatment is the treatment of choice. Prognosis depends on tumour type.

Pathological features and differential diagnosis

Pulmonary teratomas tend to be large and cystic, and may be partly or entirely endobronchial, resulting in bronchiectasis.[29] The cysts are often in continuity with the bronchi. About two thirds are benign and consist solely of mature tissues such as skin (with its usual appendages, including hair), bronchus, pancreas (which is also a frequent feature of mediastinal teratomas), cartilage and neural tissue. Malignant primary teratomas of the lung show the usual variety of differentiated and anaplastic tissues.

Some of the reported malignant germ cell tumours have been choriocarcinomas associated with elevated levels of serum human chorionic gonadotrophin,[24–27] and a few of these have arisen in infants[18] or men.[26,30,31] They have displayed the usual mixture of cytotrophoblastic and syncytiotrophoblastic elements.

Other pulmonary germ cell tumours have contained yolk sac elements and secreted α-fetoprotein.[32,33] Mixed yolk sac and blastomatous differentiation is also described.[34,35] The immunohistochemical demonstration of β-human chorionic gonadotrophin and α-fetoprotein is of little value as these trophoblastic markers may be seen in carcinoma of the lung.[36] It is notable that some of the few primary choriocarcinomas of the lung reported in men have been combined with carcinoma of more conventional pattern.[31]

The differential diagnosis includes metastatic teratoma, either by direct (see Fig. 12.6.14) or distant spread. In the latter context, it is important to remember that chemotherapy may ablate all the malignant elements of the tumour so that the pulmonary metastases may only contain totally mature elements and appear quite benign (see p. 677).[37,38] Pleuropulmonary blastoma, pulmonary blastoma and carcinosarcoma do not form the organoid structures seen in a teratoma.

REFERENCES

Melanoma

1. Ferrara G, Boscaino A, Derosa G. Bronchial blue naevus. A previously unreported entity. Histopathology 1995; 26:581–583.
2. Herbert A. Primary malignant melanoma of the lung. In: Williams CJ, Krikorian JG, Green MR, Raghavan D, eds. Textbook of Uncommon Cancer. Chichester: John Wiley; 1988:383–397.
3. Jennings TA, Axiotis CA, Kress Y, Carter D. Primary malignant melanoma of the lower respiratory tract – report of a case and literature review. Am J Clin Pathol 1990; 94:649–655.
4. Littman CD. Metastatic melanoma mimicking primary bronchial melanoma. Histopathology 1991; 18:561–563.
5. Farrell DJ, Kashyap AP, Ashcroft T, Morritt GN. Primary malignant melanoma of the bronchus. Thorax 1996; 51:223–224.
6. Wilson RW, Moran CA. Primary melanoma of the lung: A clinicopathologic and immunohistochemical study of eight cases. Am J Surg Pathol 1997; 21:1196–1202.
7. Cebelin MS. Melanocytic bronchial carcinoid tumor. Cancer 1980; 46:1843–1848.
8. Gould VE, Memoli VE, Dardi LE, Sobel HJ, Somers SC, Johannessen JV. Neuroendocrine carcinomas with multiple immunoreactive peptides and melanin production. Ultrastruct Pathol 1981; 2:199–217.
9. Grazer R, Cohen SM, Jacobs JB, Lucas P. Melanin-containing peripheral carcinoid of the lung. Am J Surg Pathol 1982; 6:73–78.
10. Carlson JA, Dickersin GR. Melanotic paraganglioid carcinoid tumor – a case report and review of the literature. Ultrastruct Pathol 1993; 17:353–372.
11. Fukuda T, Kobayashi H, Kamishima T, et al. Peripheral carcinoid tumor of the lung with focal melanin production. Pathol Int 1994; 44:309–316.
12. Rowlands D, Edwards C, Collins F. Malignant melanotic schwannoma of the bronchus. J Clin Pathol 1987; 40:1449–1455.
13. Gaffey MJ, Mills SE, Zarbo RJ, Weiss LM, Gown AM. Clear cell tumor of the lung – immunohistochemical and ultrastructural evidence of melanogenesis. Am J Surg Pathol 1991; 15:644–653.
14. Cohen RE, Weaver MG, Montenegro HD, Abdul-Karim FW. Pulmonary blastoma with malignant melanoma component. Arch Pathol Lab Med 1990; 114:1076–1078.
15. Ost D, Joseph C, Sogoloff H, Menezes G. Primary pulmonary melanoma: case report and literature review. Mayo Clin Proc 1999; 74:62–66.
16. Reid JD, Mehta VT. Melanoma of the lower respiratory tract. Cancer 1966; 19:627–631.
17. Mori K, Cho H, Som M. Primary 'flat' melanoma of the trachea. J Pathol Bacteriol 1977; 121:101–105.

Germ cell tumours

18. Kay S, Reed WG. Chorioepithelioma of the lung in a female infant seven months old. Am J Pathol 1955; 29:555–560.
19. Pound AW, Willis RA. A malignant teratoma of the lung in an infant. J Pathol 1969; 98:111–114.
20. Day DW, Taylor SA. An intrapulmonary teratoma associated with thymic tissue. Thorax 1975; 30:582–586.
21. Holt S, Deverall PB, Boddy JE. A teratoma of the lung containing thymic tissue. J Pathol 1978; 126:85–89.
22. Filho JCC, Coehlo JCMR. Teratomas pulmonares benignos. Relato de dois casos. Benign lung teratomas. Report of two cases. J Pneumologia 1985; 11:82–88.
23. Jamieson MPG, McGowan AR. Endobronchial teratoma. Thorax 1982; 37:157–159.
24. Tanimura A, Natsuyama H, Kawano M, et al. Primary choriocarcinoma of the lung. Hum Pathol 1985; 16:1281–1284.
25. Pushchak MJ, Farhi DC. Primary choriocarcinoma of the lung. Arch Pathol Lab Med 1987; 111:477–479.
26. Sullivan LG. Primary choriocarcinoma of the lung in a man. Arch Pathol Lab Med 1989; 113:82–83.
27. Aparicio J, Oltra A, Martinez-Moragon E, Llorca C, Gomez-Aldaravi L, Pastor M. Extragonadal nongestational choriocarcinoma involving the lung: a report of three cases. Respiration 1996; 63:251–253.
28. Asano S, Hoshikawa Y, Yamane Y, Ikeda M, Wakasa H. An intrapulmonary teratoma associated with bronchiectasis containing various kinds of primordium: a case report and review of the literature. Virchows Archiv 2000; 436:384–388.
29. Morgan DE, Sanders C, McElvein RB, Nath H, Alexander CB. Intrapulmonary teratoma: a case report and review of the literature. J Thorac Imaging 1992; 7:70–77.
30. Hayakawa K, Takahashi M, Sasaki K, et al. Primary choriocarcinoma of the lung. Acta Pathol Jpn 1977; 27:123–135.
31. Chen FS, Tatsumi A, Numoto S. Combined choriocarcinoma and adenocarcinoma of the lung occurring in a man – Case report and review of the literature. Cancer 2001; 91:123–129. .
32. Hunter S, Hewan-Lowe K, Costa MJ. Primary pulmonary alpha-fetoprotein-producing malignant germ cell tumor. Hum Pathol 1990; 21:1074–1076.
33. Kakkar N, Vasishta RK, Banerjee AK, Garewal G, Deodhar SD, Bambery P. Primary pulmonary malignant teratoma with yolk sac element associated with hematologic neoplasia. Respiration 1996; 63:52–54.
34. Siegel RJ, Bueso-Ramos C, Cohen C, et al. Pulmonary blastoma with germ cell (yolk sac) differentiation: report of two cases. Mod Pathol 1992; 4:566–570.
35. Miller RR, Champagne K, Murray RCN. Primary pulmonary germ cell tumor with blastomatous differentiation. Chest 1994; 106:1595–1596.
36. Boucher LD, Yoneda K. The expression of trophoblastic cell markers by lung carcinomas. Hum Pathol 1995; 26:1201–1206.
37. Madden M, Goldstraw P, Corrin B. Effect of chemotherapy on the histological appearances of testicular teratoma metastatic to the lung: correlation with patient survival. J Clin Pathol 1984; 37:1212–1214.
38. Cagini L, Nicholson AG, Horwich A, Goldstraw P, Pastorino U. Thoracic metastasectomy for germ cell tumours: long term survival and prognostic factors. Ann Oncol 1998; 9:1185–1191.

12

Tumours

12.6

Secondary tumours of the lungs

ROUTES OF TUMOUR SPREAD TO THE LUNGS

Extrapulmonary neoplasms may involve the lungs by direct extension or by metastasis. Direct extension may be through the pleura or along lymphatic or blood vessels. Metastasis is by way of the pulmonary or bronchial arteries and possibly within the lungs via the airways (aerial metastasis).

Direct extension

Direct invasion of the lungs through the pleura complicates primary or metastatic growths in the pleura, mediastinal lymph nodes, thymus, oesophagus, chest wall, breast, thyroid or abdomen. No particular route is followed, other than penetration of the fused pleurae. Alternatively, there may be retrograde spread through pulmonary lymphatics once the lymphatic pathway is obstructed by tumour emboli in the mediastinal lymph nodes. Further dissemination within pulmonary lymphatics may be widespread and this is one route (but not the most common) by which secondary tumours produce the characteristic appearances of so-called 'lymphangitis carcinomatosa' (see below).

Direct invasion of the lungs along veins is rare, as this entails invasion of pulmonary veins between the lungs and the left atrium and retrograde venous extension into the lungs. Direct extension along the pulmonary arteries is also rare but is occasionally seen with sarcomas originating in the pulmonary trunk or the right side of the heart (see p. 627).

Metastasis

With their vast capillary network and unique position in the circulation it is not surprising that the lungs are frequently the site of metastatic tumours. The incidence of lung involvement in

Box 12.6.1 Primary tumour sites

Primary tumour sites ranked in descending order of frequency according to the propensity of their tumours to metastasise to the lungs (left) and the likelihood of a pulmonary metastasis having originated in a particular site (right). The difference between the two columns is largely accounted for by differences in the frequency of cancer developing in these sites: thus tumours of the kidney frequently metastasise to the lungs but are not as common as tumours of the breast, colon, pancreas, stomach or skin. Other factors include selective attachment of tumour cells to endothelium based on particular cell surface components.

1	Kidney	1	Breast
2	Skin	2	Colon
3	Breast	3	Pancreas
4	Thyroid	4	Stomach
5	Pancreas	5	Skin
6	Prostate	6	Kidney
7	Stomach	7	Ovary
8	Uterus	8	Prostate
9	Colon	9	Uterus

Box 12.6.2 Patterns of secondary tumour growth in the lungs

Blood-borne metastases
   Solitary nodule
   Multiple nodules
   Massive tumour embolism
   Microangiopathy
Diffuse lymphatic permeation (lymphangitis carcinomatosa)
Endobronchial metastases
Intra-alveolar spread
   Diffuse airspace
   Lepidic growth (bronchioloalveolar cell carcinoma pattern)
Interstitial growth

metastatic disease is second only to that of the liver, pulmonary metastases being found at necropsy in 30–50% of patients dying of cancer.[1] The commoner extrathoracic tumours may be ranked in the following descending order in regard to the frequency with which they metastasise to the lungs: kidney, skin, breast, thyroid, pancreas, prostate, stomach, uterus and colon (Box 12.6.1). Tumours of the lung itself and certain rare tumours, notably choriocarcinoma and osteosarcoma, also commonly metastasise to the lungs. Some tumours with a high tendency to metastasise to the lungs are not themselves common. Therefore they are not the first to be considered when trying to identify the origin of pulmonary metastases. Thus, an order of frequency different from the above applies when considering possible sites of origin following the identification of pulmonary metastases (Box 12.6.1). If these organs are grouped regionally, it is found that the genitourinary tract accounts for 28% of pulmonary metastases, the gastrointestinal tract for 28%, the breasts for 17% and sarcomas for 11%.[2]

Metastases in the lung almost all arise from tumour emboli arrested in small pulmonary arteries.[3] Bronchial arterial dissemination is far less common but may account for some endobronchial metastases. Groups of tumour cells enter the circulation by invasion of small peripheral veins or through the thoracic duct, and generally come to rest in pulmonary arteries of between 400 and 800 μm in diameter.[4] Occasionally, there is widespread occlusion of medium-sized pulmonary arteries by tumour or tumour-associated thrombus (see below, p. 671).

Pulmonary arteries are less resistant to invasion by malignant tumour than their counterparts in the systemic circulation.[5] Nevertheless, although microscopic emboli are very common in the lungs, most fail to establish themselves. In many cases of abdominal carcinoma, malignant cells in the lungs are only to be found in thrombus within the pulmonary arteries, and many of these intraluminal malignant cells are degenerate.[1] Although viable cells within tumour emboli are in the minority, it is of

course these which invade the walls of the pulmonary arteries to form secondary lung tumours, and then promote further tumour dissemination via the pulmonary veins and systemic arteries. It is very unusual to encounter widespread systemic metastases in the total absence of tumour deposits in the lungs. Systemic dissemination is dependent as much on pulmonary metastases invading pulmonary venules than single cancer cells traversing the lung capillaries.

Although the high incidence of lung involvement in metastatic disease owes much to the special position of the lungs in the circulation, other factors are also involved. Many cancers display characteristic organ colonisation patterns that do not conform to simple mechanical trapping. Organ preferences of metastatic spread appear to be influenced by selective attachment of tumour cells to endothelium, based on particular cell surface components.[6] On the other hand hyperoxic injury to the pulmonary endothelium increases the number of pulmonary metastases.[7] An intriguing correlation between cigarette smoking and a high risk of breast cancer metastasising to the lungs has been noted.[8]

PATTERNS OF TUMOUR SPREAD WITHIN THE LUNGS

Secondary growth in the lung may take the form of discrete nodules, diffuse lymphatic permeation, diffuse consolidation, endobronchial growth, or massive tumour embolism (Box 12.6.2).[9–11] Metastases in the pleura are usually multinodular but occasionally form a continuous sheet and mimic the appearances of a mesothelioma. They are dealt with in Chapter 13 (see p. 719).

Blood-borne metastases

Discrete tumour nodules

Metastases in the lung commonly take the form of discrete nodules or well-circumscribed masses, which are generally multiple and bilateral (Fig. 12.6.1). They affect the lower lobes more often than the upper, and are most common in the outer parts of the lungs, all this in accordance with the distribution of blood within the lungs and with the sites of embolic lodge-

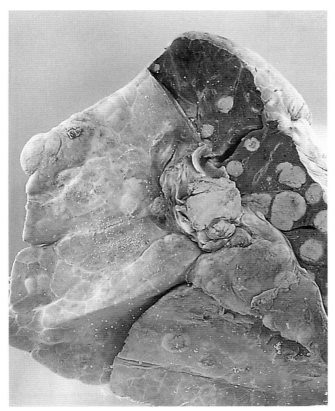

Figure 12.6.1 Pulmonary metastases forming well-circumscribed masses.

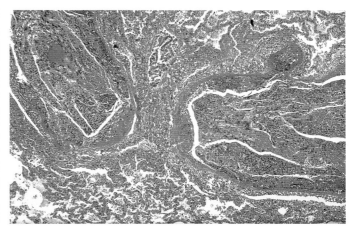

Figure 12.6.2 Embolic choriocarcinoma occludes the pulmonary arteries.

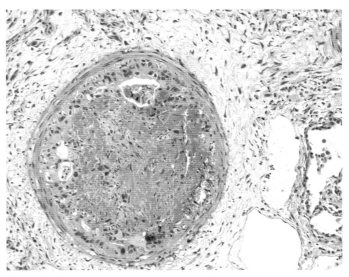

Figure 12.6.3 Carcinomatous microangiopathy in a man with occult gastric carcinoma who died of rapidly progressive pulmonary hypertension. Metastatic tumour and thrombus fills the lumen of a small pulmonary artery.

ment.[1,4,12,13] Metastatic deposits may be of any size, and whereas they are sometimes all the same size, in other cases, growths of many different sizes are seen. Although metastatic tumours are generally multiple, solitary deposits forming 'coin lesions' may be encountered (see Box 12.1.6, p. 537). Pulmonary metastases generally have well-circumscribed margins, in contrast to the ill-defined infiltrating edge usually seen with primary malignant lung tumours. On its cut surface, a metastasis is generally white and opaque but may show necrosis and haemorrhage. Cavitation and calcification are occasionally seen.[14] Appearances indicative of the site of origin are considered below.

Massive tumour embolism

Tumour emboli occluding the main pulmonary arteries are rare[10] but tumours such as renal cell carcinomas and hepatocellular carcinomas have a propensity to invade the systemic veins and may present with massive tumour embolism. This may also occur with tumours arising in the right side of the heart and pulmonary trunk.

Microscopic tumour angiopathy

Microscopic tumour emboli are found in up to 26% of cancer patients coming to autopsy,[10,15–17] typically occluding small muscular pulmonary arteries and arterioles (Fig. 12.6.2). Symptoms are generally similar to those seen with lymphangitic spread (see below)[9] but rarely the emboli may be sufficiently extensive to cause pulmonary hypertension and right ventricular failure.[18–21] This is alternatively termed *carcinomatous arteriopathy* or *carcinomatous pulmonary endarteritis* (Fig. 12.6.3).[17] Carcinomas of the stomach and breast are the most common tumours to have this effect but it may also be seen with tumours of the liver and placenta. The emboli may consist purely of tumour cells, a mixture of cells and fibrin, or show severe fibrointimal hyperplasia with scanty tumour cells, the last of these being particularly characteristic of metastatic gastric adenocarcinoma.[11] Such arteriopathy is generally first diagnosed *post mortem* but is sometimes detected by lung biopsy or from examining material obtained at pulmonary artery catheterisation.[22] Survival in such patients has seldom exceeded 12 weeks.[17–21]

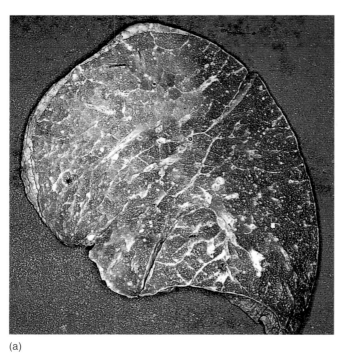

(a)

(b)

(c)

Figure 12.6.4 'Lymphangitis carcinomatosa' (a) Tumour fills lymphatics throughout the lung, thickening the interlobular septa and periarterial sheaths. (b) Pleural lymphatics permeated by tumour. (c) Microscopy shows tumour filling the periarterial lymphatics. (Fig. (b) provided by Dr GA Russell, Tunbridge Wells, UK.)

Lymphatic spread within the lung

The major route of spread within the lung of both metastatic and primary tumours is along lymphatics. When very marked this results in so-called '*lymphangitis carcinomatosa*' a condition in which the entire lymphatic system of the lungs is brought into sharp relief by pale threads of tumour tissue filling these vessels (Fig. 12.6.4).[23] A network of occluded lymph channels is clearly visible on the visceral pleural surface, while on the cut surface the broncho-arterial bundles in the centres of the acini and the veins in the interlobular septa are cuffed by tumour spreading along their accompanying lymphatics. Although this picture may be produced by direct extension from tumour deposits in hilar lymph nodes, a more common source of involvement is multiple minute tumour emboli reaching the lungs via the pulmonary arteries and subsequently invading the lymphatics.[1,4,24] The main evidence for this is the high incidence of tumour emboli within small pulmonary arteries and the frequent absence of marked hilar lymph node enlargement in lymphangitis carcinomatosa. There is also a high incidence of minute blood-borne tumour emboli in organs other than the lung in this condition, notably in the bone marrow. In one case,

previous thoracoplasty, which reduces pulmonary perfusion as well as ventilation, appeared to have caused the lung on that side to be spared the widespread lymphatic permeation present in the other.[25] Tumours most likely to give rise to lymphangitis carcinomatosa are those arising in the stomach, pancreas, breast and colon and in the lung itself.

Endobronchial metastases

In following lymphatics to the hilum of the lung, neoplastic cells may occlude mucosal lymph channels and thereby develop into secondary tumours in the main air passages, so simulating primary growths of the bronchus. Sometimes these metastases protrude into the lumen of the bronchus (Fig. 12.6.5).[26,27] Such endobronchial metastases are encountered with a wide variety of tumours but most commonly originate from growths in the intestine, cervix uteri and breast.[26] Primary tumours of the bronchus with a propensity to grow in this way include carcinosarcomas, carcinoids and bronchial gland tumours. Fibreoptic bronchial biopsy may detect lymphatic permeation even when bronchoscopy is normal.[28]

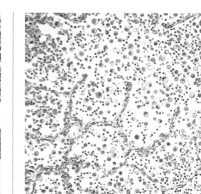

Figure 12.6.5 Metastatic osteosarcoma showing endobronchial growth.

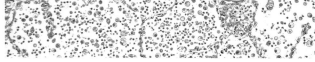

Figure 12.6.7 Poorly cohesive cells of metastatic carcinoma fill the alveolar spaces, mimicking desquamative interstitial pneumonia.

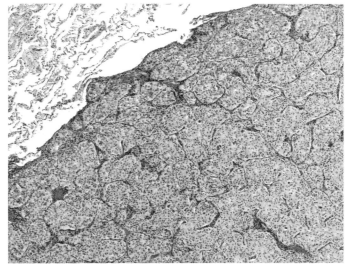

Figure 12.6.6 Metastatic carcinoma growing from one alveolus to the next without disturbing the alveolar architecture.

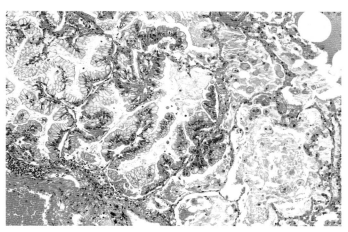

Figure 12.6.8 Metastatic adenocarcinoma of the pancreas growing along the alveolar walls in the manner of a primary bronchioloalveolar cell carcinoma.

Intra-alveolar spread

Microscopical examination of the growing edge may show tumour extending into the lumen of neighbouring alveoli by which means it spreads from one air space to the next (Fig. 12.6.6). When this occurs, the alveolar septa are generally compressed and in older parts eventually obliterated. Elastin stains often demonstrate the skeletal remains of alveolar septa in what appears to be solid tumour tissue.

Alternatively, non-cohesive tumour cells may fill many alveoli without affecting the alveolar walls, resulting in appearances that simulate desquamative interstitial pneumonia (Fig. 12.6.7). This is distinguished by careful attention to the cytological features of the free cells, aided by the immunocytochemical demonstration of cytokeratin, which is present in carcinoma cells but not in the macrophages of desquamative interstitial pneumonia.[29] This pattern has been shown to be non-angiogenic, the tumour cells depending on the pre-existent

alveolar capillaries rather than inducing neo-angiogenesis.[30] Some metastatic breast carcinomas showing such non-angiogenic alveolar spread have apparently been confined to the lungs, with obvious implications regarding prognosis and treatment.[31] Such non-angiogenic spread is also seen with some primary pulmonary tumours, where it again carries a favourable prognosis.[30,32–34]

Lepidic spread

A further route of tumour spread within the alveolar tissues of the lung is one in which the tumour cells grow along the surface of alveolar walls. The tumour replaces the alveolar epithelium, usually in a layer no more than one cell thick. Neither the alveolar walls nor the air spaces are obliterated, the tumour using the alveolar walls as a supporting scaffold (Fig. 12.6.8). This is termed a lepidic growth pattern. It is the pattern of growth found with primary bronchioloalveolar cell carcinomas (see

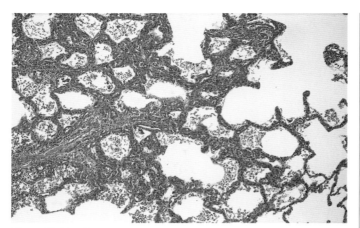

Figure 12.6.9 Metastatic mesothelioma growing within the alveolar walls.

p. 548), but is one that may be adopted by any adenocarcinoma, either primary or metastatic.[35,36] Pancreatic, gastric and colorectal growths are the most common metastatic tumours to grow in this way in the lungs. Because it does not destroy the lung tissue, this growth is likely to mimic an area of pneumonic consolidation both radiographically and on macroscopical examination of the cut surface of the lung. There may be a single area of diffuse involvement or multiple foci may develop in both lungs. A mucoid appearance may be evident, depending on the secretory status of the tumour. Considerable controversy attends the possibility of aerial metastases accounting for the frequent multifocal distribution of primary lung tumours, which evince this pattern of growth (see p. 549) but in cases of metastatic tumour vascular dissemination provides an adequate explanation.

Interstitial spread

Another extralymphatic route of tumour spread in the alveolar tissues of the lung is within the alveolar interstitium, which is correspondingly thickened (Fig. 12.6.9). The air spaces are eventually obliterated by this encroachment. Total destruction of the alveolar architecture may take place in the older parts of the tumour as with intra-alveolar growth.

PRIMARY OR METASTATIC TUMOUR?

The development of metastatic disease long after the primary growth has been eradicated is well recognised[37] but mention of previous operations is often neglected when a new specimen is submitted to the laboratory.

A multiplicity of growths in the lungs always suggests metastatic disease but solitary metastases are not uncommon and the question whether a given tumour is primary or metastatic arises particularly in patients with a solitary lung nodule. Up to 9% of solitary lung nodules prove to be metastases (see Box 12.1.6, p. 537).

Whether the lung is the site of single or multiple growths, recognition of the site of origin assumes particular clinical importance where there is site-specific therapy. Testicular teratoma and carcinoma of the breast, ovary, prostate and thyroid fall into this category. Familiarity with the histological appearances of tumours is of limited help in the hunt for the primary site for there can be no certainty in distinguishing, for example, one adenocarcinoma from another by this means.

The gross appearances are seldom informative with regard to the tissue of origin but obvious mucin secretion, melanin production or bone or cartilage formation may be helpful on occasions. Similarly, the metastases of choriocarcinomas and angiosarcomas are often grossly haemorrhagic and smooth muscle tumours may display a recognisable fascicular pattern.

Sometimes the microscopic pattern gives a clear indication of an extrapulmonary derivation, but often the tumour is anaplastic or the pattern of differentiation is one seen in both pulmonary and extrapulmonary primary growths. All the common carcinomas of the lung may be mimicked microscopically by metastases. Adenocarcinomas are broadly similar whether they arise in lung, alimentary tract or the female genital tract. Adenosquamous carcinomas of lung and uterus are similar histologically while squamous cell carcinomas are identical regardless of origin. Similarly, recognising the source of anaplastic large cell carcinomas is a common histopathological problem wherever they are encountered, and even small cell carcinomas may arise outside the lungs. However, there are some purely morphological characteristics that may point to particular types of tumour arising in the lungs themselves rather than in some other parts of the body and these will now be described.

Squamous cell carcinoma of the bronchus arises in foci of dysplasia and develops through an *in situ* phase (see p. 531). Such lesions are multifocal and recognition of these premalignant changes in the surface epithelium of neighbouring airways may help in deciding that a squamous cell carcinoma is primary rather than metastatic. Continuity between invasive and apparently *in situ* carcinoma is less helpful because metastases can erode a bronchus and replace the surface epithelium to mimic pre-existent *in situ* carcinoma. Immunocytochemistry is helpful in determining the origin of a squamous cell carcinoma in the lung as cytokeratin 5/6 is a sensitive and specific marker for primary growths of this phenotype.[38]

Adenocarcinoma presents particular difficulties in distinguishing primary from secondary growths.[39,40] Scarring may suggest the possibility of a primary scar cancer but it is notoriously difficult to prove that such fibrosis antedates the tumour (see p. 551). Central fibrosis may be a consequence of tissue destruction in either primary or metastatic pulmonary tumours, rather than the cause of the tumour, while metastases sometimes develop in lung scars. However, premalignant epithelial atypia suggests that a tumour is a primary scar cancer rather than a metastasis.

Electron microscopy is unhelpful if the tumour is composed only of mucous or undifferentiated cells but the identification of Clara cell granules or lamellar (surfactant) bodies is indica-

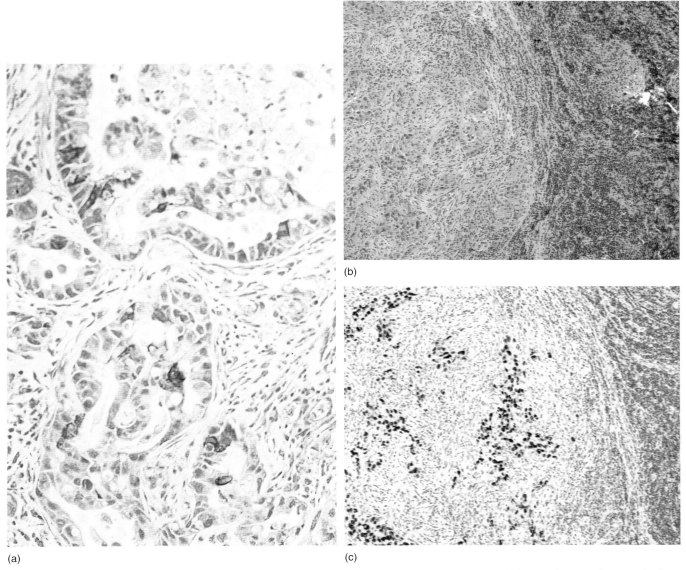

(a)

(b)

(c)

Figure 12.6.10 (a) A positive immunoperoxidase reaction for surfactant apoprotein enables this pleural deposit of adenocarcinoma to be recognised as having originated in the lung. (b) Non-small cell carcinoma in a hilar node in a patient with a pulmonary mass and a history of previous breast carcinoma. (c) The tumour cells seen in (b) stain for TTF-1, indicating metastasis from the lung.

tive of a primary origin in the lung: conversely, terminal webs are diagnostic of intestinal carcinomas.[41] Glycocalyceal bodies and microvillous core rootlets are characteristic of adenocarcinomas of the gastrointestinal tract but on occasion are also found in primary lung carcinomas.[42–44]

Cytochemical characterisation of mucin has been utilised to distinguish primary and secondary mucus-secreting adenocarcinomas[45,46] but the specificity is low. Immunocytochemistry is more helpful. Primary adenocarcinoma may be recognised by the immunocytochemical demonstration of surfactant apoprotein, thyroid transcription factor-1 (TTF-1) (Fig. 12.6.10) or Clara cell antigens.[47–56] Conversely, these markers enable the lungs to be recognised as the origin of tumours in other organs.[57] TTF-1 is a more sensitive lung marker than surfactant apoprotein and its

antibody is the method of choice for establishing origin in the lung.[49,54] Attention should be confined to the nuclei as cytoplasmic TTF-1 immunoreactivity is occasionally encountered as a non-specific feature in various neoplasms.[58] TTF-1 is highly specific for lung and thyroid[52,53,55] and in primary carcinomas of the lung it is reported to be positive in the nuclei of up to 76% of adenocarcinomas (but seldom in mucinous varieties) and 40% of large cell carcinomas.[55] Some report that it is positive in 38% of squamous cell carcinomas but our experience of this is to the contrary. TTF-1 positivity is variously reported in bronchopulmonary carcinoids: 69% in one series[59] and none in two others.[60,61]

Immunocytochemical markers specific for other organs occasionally help in identifying an extrapulmonary origin, e.g. thyroglobulin, prostate-specific antigen and hepatocyte paraffin-1, while a mammary origin is likely if a lung tumour expresses oestrogen receptors and cystic disease fluid protein-15.[62–65] Similarly, the immunocytochemical demonstration of CDX-2 strongly favours an adenocarcinoma as having originated in the large bowel[66,67] (except in the case of primary colloid carcinoma of the lung, which also expresses CDX-2),[68] while calcitonin is a strong pointer to metastatic medullary carcinoma of the thyroid rather than a primary carcinoid tumour. Studies on renal markers are ongoing.[69]

However, some proposed discriminants are of less value. For example, villin is expressed in a substantial proportion of pulmonary as well as gastrointestinal adenocarcinomas,[70,71] while the Wilms tumour suppressor gene WT-1 is expressed in pulmonary adenocarcinomas as well as renal, ovarian and mesothelial neoplasms.[72] A useful website for assessing the specificities and sensitivities of antibodies in relation to primary sites is available at www.ipox.org.

Individual cytokeratins can be helpful: there is a high chance that a squamous cell carcinoma positive for cytokeratin 7 has originated in the uterine cervix, most other squamous cell carcinomas failing to express this epitope.[73] A combination of cytokeratins 7 and 20 also affords a limited degree of confidence in distinguishing groups of adenocarcinomas.[74] Thus, adenocarcinomas arising in the lung, endometrium, thyroid and breast are generally cytokeratin 7 positive and cytokeratin 20 negative whereas the converse is seen with colonic carcinomas. These patterns also help to distinguish bronchopulmonary and gastrointestinal carcinoids.[59] However, mucinous bronchioloalveolar cell carcinoma differs from other adenocarcinomas of the lung in that it is generally cytokeratin 20 positive (and TTF-1 negative).[75] The combination of cytokeratins 7 and 20 does not distinguish pulmonary adenocarcinoma from pleural mesothelioma of epithelioid pattern, techniques for which are considered on p. 709.

In future, immunocytochemistry will be augmented by molecular techniques: organ specific gene profiles that enable adenocarcinomas of the lung, colon and ovary to be distinguished have already been identified[76] and the recognition of cytogenetic aberrations may enable synovial sarcomas metastasising to the lung to be correctly categorised.[77]

Specific tumour patterns

Clear cell carcinoma in the lung raises the possibility of metastatic renal carcinoma. A diastase-controlled periodic acid-Schiff stain is helpful in this context as the renal tumours contain glycogen and fat but no mucin whereas some pulmonary clear cell carcinomas are mucin-rich. If features of malignancy such as excessive mitotic activity and necrosis are not evident, the possibility of benign clear cell tumour of the lung (see p. 613) arises: like a renal metastasis this stains for glycogen rather than mucin. In this case any available reserve tissue should be utilised for a fat stain, a positive reaction favouring a renal origin. There are also vascular differences between these tumours, the metastases of a renal carcinoma

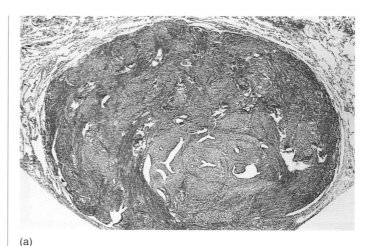

(a)

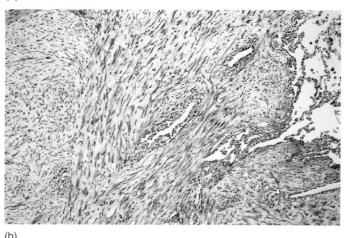

(b)

Figure 12.6.11 (a,b) 'Benign metastasising leiomyoma' of the uterus. This was one of many pulmonary nodules in a woman with uterine fibroids. No cytological evidence of malignancy was apparent in any of the uterine or pulmonary tumours.

lacking the thin-walled wide sinusoids that characterise the benign clear cell tumour of lung (see Table 12.3.1, p. 615).

'Benign metastasising leiomyoma' of the uterus[78–82] provides an example of well-differentiated metastases being confused with benign primary lung tumours. Obviously, a tumour that metastasises to the lung cannot be truly benign but in this entity neither the primary growth nor its metastases shows any microscopic evidence of malignancy whatsoever (Fig. 12.6.11). Despite suggestions that the condition represents multifocal origin,[83] molecular studies confirm that the pulmonary lesions are indeed metastatic.[84] Primary leiomyoma of the lung is rare and before such a diagnosis is contemplated, metastatic tumour must be excluded, particularly in a middle-aged woman with multiple lung tumours. Some may evolve from benign tumour emboli released at myomectomy, some from intravenous leiomyomatosis of the myometrium[85] and some may represent metastases of a very well-differentiated leiomyosarcoma. Very rarely, the patient is male, the primary tumour then arising in sites such as the skin.[86] The metastases may be discovered by

chance radiographically, appearing as multiple rounded opacities in an individual with no respiratory complaints. They grow quite slowly in the lungs, leading to gradually increasing breathlessness and eventually fatal respiratory failure. The median survival is quoted as 94 months after excision of the pulmonary metastases, compared with 22 months with metastatic leiomyosarcoma.[82] During pregnancy or after oophorectomy or the menopause, growth is even slower or may stop completely.[87,88] Anti-oestrogen drugs may be beneficial; in this, and the almost exclusively female predilection, the condition resembles pulmonary lymphangioleiomyomatosis (see p. 295) but the latter is characterised radiographically by an interstitial infiltrate rather than multiple discrete opacities, and is a primary lung disease. Other tumours that have metastasised despite entirely benign histological appearances include *thymoma*,[89] *giant cell tumours of bone*,[90] *cellular fibrous histiocytoma*[91] (see below) and *meningioma*.[92]

In a patient with *sarcoma* or *melanoma* elsewhere, even a solitary pulmonary lesion is most often a metastasis. Conversely, if the patient has a nodal *lymphoma*, a solitary parenchymal lesion in the lung is more likely to be an independent primary carcinoma.[39]

Paraganglioma is distinctly rare in the lung (see p. 627). Usually when a patient appears to have a primary paraganglioma of the lung, cytokeratin positivity indicates that it is a carcinoid or subsequent events suggest that it is a metastasis from sites such as the glomus jugulare. When considering the possibility of carcinoid tumour or any neuroendocrine tumour of cribriform pattern, metastatic *adenocarcinoma of the prostate* needs to be kept in mind.[93]

Metastases in the lung often engulf pre-existent structures and the survival of entrapped airspaces in a metastatic sarcoma must not be mistaken for the epithelial component of a *primary sarcomatoid carcinoma*.[86,94] Obstruction of engulfed airspaces may lead to marked cystic change,[95–100] occasionally resulting in haemopneumothorax or pneumomediastinum.[101] This change appears to be particularly common in the condition known as '*benign metastasising leiomyoma*', which is described above, and may have led to some low-grade metastatic soft tissue tumours being described as primary pulmonary tumours under terms such as *cystic fibrohistiocytic tumour*.[97,98] Most cases classified as such have been shown to represent metastatic cellular fibrous histiocytomas. They show a male predominance and long-term survival despite extensive disease (Fig. 12.6.12).[102]

A further trap for the pathologist arises from the surgeon withholding information that the patient has had a testicular *teratoma* treated by chemotherapy. Subsequent metastases are thought to be worth excising and the pathologist can give useful prognostic information, or, if ignorant of the clinical circumstances, make a totally wrong diagnosis. Anaplastic areas of these tumours are often completely necrotic, having been destroyed by chemotherapy. Alternatively, fibrous scars may be the only remnants of successfully treated metastases. In other cases, metastases consist only of well-differentiated tissues with limited growth potential. All these findings indicate that chemotherapy has been successful, whereas viable malignant

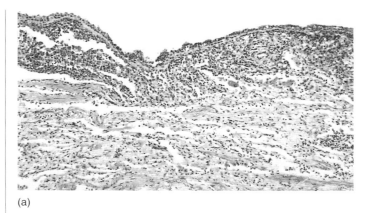

(a)

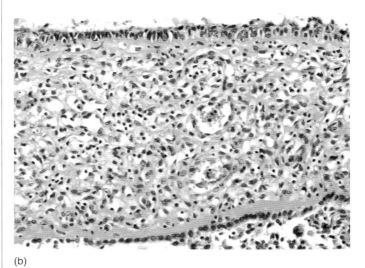

(b)

Figure 12.6.12 Metastatic cellular fibrous histiocytoma (cystic fibrohistiocytic tumour of lung). (a) Multiple thin-walled cystic masses within the lung were originally diagnosed as cystic mesenchymal hamartoma but it was later found that the patient had had a cellular fibrous histiocytoma resected over a decade earlier. (b) The walls of the cysts comprise a cytologically bland fibrohistiocytic proliferation and the diagnosis was revised to metastatic cellular fibrous histiocytoma.

tumour indicates that it has failed.[103,104] Chemotherapy may also result in an arteriovenous fistula developing in an ablated pulmonary metastasis.[105] On occasion, chemotherapy results in metastatic teratoma being reduced to such well differentiated cartilage and respiratory epithelium that the residual tumour closely mimics a chondroid 'hamartoma' (Fig. 12.6.13).[103,106] Teratomas spreading directly from the mediastinum need also to be considered (Fig. 12.6.14), as does direct spread from a thymoma into the lung (Fig. 12.6.15).

Other metastatic tumours that may mimic primary lung growths include low-grade *endometrial stromal sarcoma*[95,100,107,108] and *clear cell odontogenic carcinoma*.[109]

Finally, there is the possibility that the multifocal lesions of pulmonary *epithelioid haemangioendothelioma* (see p. 625) may

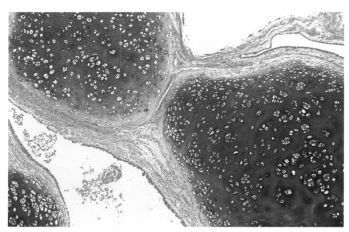

Figure 12.6.13 Pulmonary metastasis of testicular teratoma excised after chemotherapy. Histologically, the tumour appears entirely benign, this indicating that the chemotherapy has been successful and that the prognosis is favourable. In this example, the predominant component of the tumour is cartilage and it is easy to see how the lesion could be erroneously diagnosed as a chondroid hamartoma if the necessary clinical information was lacking.

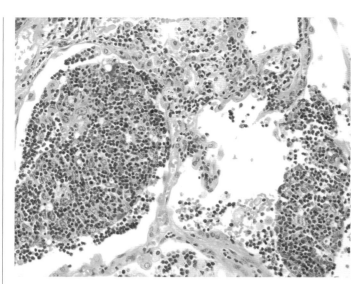

Figure 12.6.15 Secondary thymoma that infiltrated the lung directly from the thymus. Islands of epithelial cells mixed with lymphocytes are seen in alveoli.

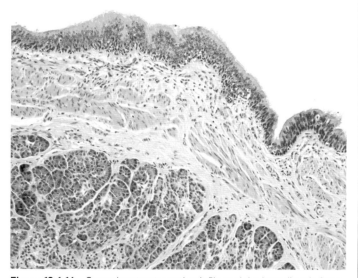

Figure 12.6.14 Secondary teratoma that infiltrated the lung directly from the mediastinum. The tumour is well differentiated and in this area has formed both respiratory (top) and pancreatic (bottom) tissue.

represent metastases from a clinically silent primary growth in an organ such as the liver.[110,111]

EFFECTS OF SECONDARY LUNG TUMOURS

The capillary bed of the lungs is an effective filter of tumour emboli, and secondary tumours in the lungs are therefore the usual immediate source of metastases in other organs, except of course those that reach the liver via the portal circulation. Pulmonary metastases, like primary tumours in the lung, may also result in non-neoplastic systemic disturbances, such as hypertrophic pulmonary osteoarthropathy and blood eosinophilia.[112]

Local effects on the lung are inevitable if there is extensive replacement of lung tissue, but it is remarkable how few symptoms pulmonary metastases generally cause. The most common effects are compression of the lung and mediastinal shift by an effusion caused by pleural rather than pulmonary metastases and terminal bronchopneumonia. The latter is largely attributable to general debility but pneumonia and abscess formation may also follow airway obstruction by secondary lung tumours. Haemoptysis is seldom severe except with metastatic choriocarcinoma or angiosarcoma. Massive pulmonary metastases result in a significant reduction in lung volume, while lymphangitis carcinomatosa renders the lung stiff and impairs gas transfer, but is only occasionally severe enough to cause respiratory failure.[113] Widespread pulmonary artery occlusion may cause pulmonary hypertension (see patterns of spread above)[4,114–119] while repeated episodes of tumour embolism may result in recurrent infarction.[120] Even fatal massive tumour embolism has been recorded[121,122] or necessitated emergency embolectomy.[123]

PROLONGED SURVIVAL DESPITE METASTATIC DISEASE

The prognosis in patients with secondary lung tumours is of course very poor but instances of prolonged survival[124] and even spontaneous regression are well known. Spontaneous regression of metastatic tumours is most common with renal carcinomas:[125,126] it sometimes follows resection of the primary tumour,[127] whilst in other cases hormonal influences are possibly responsible.[88,125]

Although chemotherapy and radiotherapy are the mainstays of treatment of metastatic disease, there is increasing interest in the resection of solitary and even multiple pulmonary metastases.[104,128–131] An International Registry for Lung Metastases has shown an actuarial survival after complete metastasectomy of 36% at 5 years, 26% at 10 years, and 22% at 15 years.[132] Favourable prognostic indicators are solitary metastases, prolonged interval between primary tumour and metastasis, completeness of resection and certain tumour types such as metastatic teratoma, breast carcinoma and melanoma.[104,132–134] Incomplete resection does not usually offer any survival advantage but the 'debulking' of certain tumours, for example metastatic thyroid tumours resistant to chemotherapy, helps control symptoms and may also prolong survival.[135]

REFERENCES

Routes of tumour spread to the lungs

1. Willis RA. The spread of tumours in the human body. London: Butterworth; 1973:170.
2. Shepherd MP. Thoracic metastases. Thorax 1982; 37:366–370.
3. Wong CW, Song C, Grimes MM, et al. Intravascular location of breast cancer cells after spontaneous metastasis to the lung. Am J Pathol 2002; 161:749–753.
4. Morgan AD. The pathology of subacute cor pulmonale in diffuse carcinomatosis of the lungs. J Pathol Bacteriol 1949; 61:75–84.
5. Kolin A, Koutoulakis T. Invasion of pulmonary arteries by bronchial carcinomas. Hum Pathol 1987; 18:1165–1171.
6. Pauli BU, Lee C-C. Organ preference of metastasis. The role of organ-specifically modulated endothelial cells. Lab Invest 1988; 58:379–387.
7. Adamson IYR, Young L, Orr FW. Tumor metastasis after hyperoxic injury and repair of the pulmonary endothelium. Lab Invest 1987; 57:71–77.
8. Murin S, Inciardi J. Cigarette smoking and the risk of pulmonary metastasis from breast cancer. Chest 2001; 119:1635–1640.

Patterns of tumour spread within the lungs

9. Soares FA, Pinto AP, Landell GA, de Oliveira JA. Pulmonary tumor embolism to arterial vessels and carcinomatous lymphangitis. A comparative clinicopathological study. Arch Pathol Lab Med 1993; 117:827–831.
10. Winterbauer RH, Elfenbein IB, Ball WC, Jr. Incidence and clinical significance of tumor embolisation to the lungs. Am J Med 1968; 45:271–290.
11. Shields DJ, Edwards WD. Pulmonary hypertension attributable to neoplastic emboli: an autopsy study of 20 cases and a review of the literature. Cardiovasc Pathol 1992; 1:279–287.
12. Pryce DM, Heard BE. The distribution of experimental pulmonary emboli in the rabbit. J Pathol Bacteriol 1956; 71:15–25.
13. Crow J, Slavin G, Kreel L. Pulmonary metastasis: A pathologic and radiologic study. Cancer 1981; 47:2595–2602.
14. Semple J, West LR. Calcified pulmonary metastases from testicular and ovarian tumours. Thorax 1955; 10:287–292.
15. Filderman AE, Coppage L, Shaw C, Matthay RA. Pulmonary and pleural manifestations of extrathoracic malignancies. Clin Chest Med 1989; 10:747–807.
16. Le Cam Y, Tuel N, Zimbacca F, Bousser J, Guivarch G. Neoplastic pulmonary embolism. An uncommon cause of acute respiratory distress with normal pulmonary radiography. Rev Pneumol Clin 1997; 53:355–359.

17. Kupari M, Laitinen L, Hekali P, Luomanmaki K. Cor pulmonale due to tumor cell embolisation. Report of a case and a brief review of the literature. Acta Med Scand 1981; 210:507–510.
18. von Herbay A, Illes A, Waldherr R, Otto HF. Pulmonary tumor thrombotic microangiopathy with pulmonary hypertension. Cancer 1990; 66:587–592.
19. Sato Y, Marutsuka K, Asada Y, Yamada M, Setoguchi T, Sumiyoshi A. Pulmonary tumor thrombotic microangiopathy. Pathol Int 1995; 45:436–440.
20. Yao DX, Flieder DB, Hoda SA. Pulmonary tumor thrombotic microangiopathy: an often missed antemortem diagnosis. Arch Pathol Lab Med 2001; 125:304–305.
21. Yutani C, Imakita M, Ishibashiueda H, Katsuragi M, Yoshioka T, Kunieda T. Pulmonary hypertension due to tumor emboli – a report of 3 autopsy cases with morphological correlations to radiological findings. Acta Pathol Jpn 1993; 43:135–141.
22. Abati A, Landucci D, Solomon D. Diagnosis of pulmonary microvascular metastases by cytologic evaluation of pulmonary artery catheter-derived blood specimens. Hum Pathol 1994; 25:257–262.
23. Wu TT. Generalised lymphatic carcinosis ('lymphangitis carcinoma') of the lungs. J Pathol Bacteriol 1936; 43:61–76.
24. Harold JT. Lymphangitis carcinomatosis of the lungs. Q J Med 1952; 21:353–360.
25. Hauser TE, Steer A. Lymphangitic carcinomatosis of the lungs: six case reports and a review of the literature. Ann Intern Med 1951; 34:881–898.
26. Shepherd MP. Endobronchial metastatic disease. Thorax 1982; 37:362–365.
27. Ormerod LP, Horsfield N, Alani FSS. How frequently do endobronchial secondaries occur in an unselected series? Respir Med 1998; 92:599–600.
28. Chuang MT, Marchevsky A, Teirstein A, Kirschner PA, Kleinerman J. Diagnosis of lung cancer by fibreoptic bronchoscopy: problems in the histological classification of non-small carcinomas. Thorax 1984; 39:175–178.
29. Mutton AE, Hasleton PS, Curry A, et al. Differentiation of desquamative interstitial pneumonia (DIP) from pulmonary adenocarcinoma by immunocytochemistry. Histopathology 1998; 33:129–135.
30. Pezzella F, Di Bacco A, Andreola S, et al. Angiogenesis in primary lung cancer and lung secondaries. Eur J Cancer 1996; 32A:2494–2500.
31. Pezzella F, Manzotti M, DiBacco A, et al. Evidence for novel non-angiogenic pathway in breast-cancer metastasis. Lancet 2000; 355:1787–1788.
32. Passalidou E, Trivella M, Singh N, et al. Vascular phenotype in angiogenic and non-angiogenic lung non-small cell carcinomas. Br J Cancer 2002; 86:244–249.
33. Pezzella F, Pastorino U, Tagliabue E, et al. Non-small-cell lung carcinoma tumor growth without morphological evidence of neo-angiogenesis. Am J Pathol 1997; 151:1417–1423.
34. Offersen BV, Pfeiffer P, Hamilton-Dutoit S, Overgaard J. Patterns of angiogenesis in non-small-cell lung carcinoma. Cancer 2001; 91:1500–1509.
35. Hewer TF. The metastatic origin of alveolar cell tumour of the lung. J Pathol Bacteriol 1961; 81:323–330.
36. Rosenblatt MB, Lisa JR, Collier F. Primary and metastatic bronchiolo-alveolar carcinoma. Dis Chest 1967; 52:147–152.

Primary or metastatic tumour?

37. Inayama Y, Shoji A, Odagiri S, et al. Detection of pulmonary metastasis of low-grade endometrial stromal sarcoma 25 years after hysterectomy. Pathol Res Pract 2000; 196:129–134.
38. Jerome Marson V, Mazieres J, Groussard O, et al. Expression of TTF-1 and cytokeratins in primary and secondary epithelial lung tumours: correlation with histological type and grade. Histopathology 2004; 45:125–134.
39. Cahan WG, Castro EB, Hajdu SI. The significance of a solitary lung shadow in patients with colon carcinoma. Cancer 1974; 33:414–421.
40. Flint A, Lloyd RV. Pulmonary metastases of colonic carcinoma – distinction from pulmonary adenocarcinoma. Arch Pathol Lab Med 1992; 116:39–42.
41. Dvorak AM, Monahan RA. Metastatic adenocarcinoma of unknown primary site. Diagnostic electron microscopy to determine the site of tumor origin. Arch Pathol Lab Med 1982; 106:21–24.

42. Marcus PB, Martin JH, Green RH, Krouse MA. Glycocalyceal bodies and microvillous core rootlets, their value in tumour typing. Arch Pathol Lab Med 1979; 103:89–92.

43. Marcus PB. Glycocalyceal bodies and their role in tumor typing. J Submicrosc Cytol Pathol 1981; 13:483–500.

44. Weidner N. Intriguing case – pulmonary adenocarcinoma with intestinal-type differentiation. Ultrastruct Pathol 1992; 16:7–10.

45. Foster CS. Mucus-secreting 'alveolar-cell' tumour of the lung: a histochemical comparison of tumours arising within and outside the lung. Histopathology 1980; 4:567–577.

46. Alvarez-Fernandez E. Histochemical classification of mucin-producing pulmonary carcinomas based on the qualitative characteristics of the mucin and its relationship to histogenesis. Histochemistry 1981; 71:117–123.

47. Nicholson AG, McCormick CJ, Shimosato Y, Butcher DN, Sheppard MN. The value of PE-10, a monoclonal antibody against pulmonary surfactant, in distinguishing primary and metastatic lung tumours. Histopathology 1995; 27:57–60.

48. Khoor A, Whitsett JA, Stahlman MT, Halter SA. Expression of surfactant protein B precursor and surfactant protein B mRNA in adenocarcinoma of the lung. Mod Pathol 1997; 10:62–67.

49. Bejarano PA, Baughman RP, Biddinger PW, et al. Surfactant proteins and thyroid transcription factor-1 in pulmonary and breast carcinomas. Mod Pathol 1996; 9:445–452.

50. Kaufmann O, Dietel M. Thyroid transcription factor-1 is the superior immunohistochemical marker for pulmonary adenocarcinomas and large cell carcinomas compared to surfactant proteins A and B. Histopathology 2000; 36:8–16.

51. Khoor A, Whitsett JA, Stahlman MT, Olson SJ, Cagle PT. Utility of surfactant protein B precursor and thyroid transcription factor 1 in differentiating adenocarcinoma of the lung from malignant mesothelioma. Hum Pathol 1999; 30:695–700.

52. Ordonez NG. Value of thyroid transcription factor-1 immunostaining in distinguishing small cell lung carcinomas from other small cell carcinomas. Am J Surg Pathol 2000; 24:1217–1223.

53. Agoff SN, Lamps LW, Philip AT, et al. Thyroid transcription factor-1 is expressed in extrapulmonary small cell carcinomas but not in other extrapulmonary neuroendocrine tumors. Modern Pathol 2000; 13: 238–242.

54. Kaufmann O, Dietel M. Expression of thyroid transcription factor-1 in pulmonary and extrapulmonary small cell carcinomas and other neuroendocrine carcinomas of various primary sites. Histopathology 2000; 36:415–420.

55. Pelosi G, Fraggetta F, Pasini F, et al. Immunoreactivity for thyroid transcription factor-1 in stage I non-small cell carcinomas of the lung. Am J Surg Pathol 2001; 25:363–372.

56. Oliveira AM, Tazelaar HD, Myers JL, Erickson LA, Lloyd RV. Thyroid transcription factor-1 distinguishes metastatic pulmonary from well-differentiated neuroendocrine tumors of other sites. Am J Surg Pathol 2001; 25:815–819.

57. Srodon M, Westra WH. Immunohistochemical staining for thyroid transcription factor-1: A helpful aid in discerning primary site of tumor origin in patients with brain metastases. Hum Pathol 2002; 33:642–645.

58. Bejarano PA, Mousavi F. Incidence and significance of cytoplasmic thyroid transcription factor-1 immunoreactivity. Arch Pathol Lab Med 2003; 127:193–195.

59. Cai YC, Banner B, Glickman J, Odze RD. Cytokeratin 7 and 20 and thyroid transcription factor 1 can help distinguish pulmonary from gastrointestinal carcinoid and pancreatic endocrine tumors. Hum Pathol 2001; 32:1087–1093.

60. Sturm N, Rossi G, Lantuejoul S, et al. Expression of thyroid transcription factor-1 in the spectrum of neuroendocrine cell lung proliferations with special interest in carcinoids. Hum Pathol 2002; 33:175–182.

61. Du E, Goldstraw P, Zacharias Z, et al. TTF-1 expression in tumorlets, typical and atypical carcinoids, and large cell neuroendocrine carcinomas. Human Pathology 2004; 35:825–831.

62. Chaubert P, Hurlimann J. Mammary origin of metastases – immunohistochemical determination. Arch Pathol Lab Med 1992; 116:1181–1188.

63. Raab SS, Berg LC, Swanson PE, Wick MR. Adenocarcinoma in the lung in patients with breast cancer – a prospective analysis of the discriminatory value of immunohistology. Am J Clin Pathol 1993; 100:27–35.

64. Canver CC, Memoli VA, Vanderveer PL, Dingivan CA, Mentzer RM. Sex hormone receptors in non-small cell lung cancer in human beings. J Thorac Cardiovasc Surg 1994; 108:153–157.

65. Ollayos CW, Riordan P, Rushin JM. Estrogen receptor detection in paraffin sections of adenocarcinoma of the colon, pancreas and lung. Arch Pathol Lab Med 1994; 118:630–632.

66. Barbareschi M, Murer B, Colby TV, et al. CDX-2 homeobox gene expression is a reliable marker of colorectal adenocarcinoma metastases to the lungs. Am J Surg Pathol 2003; 27:141–149.

67. Saad RS, Cho P, Silverman JF, Liu Y. Usefulness of Cdx2 in separating mucinous bronchioloalveolar adenocarcinoma of the lung from metastatic mucinous colorectal adenocarcinoma. Am J Clin Pathol 2004; 122:421–427.

68. Rossi G, Murer B, Cavazza A, et al. Primary mucinous (so-called colloid) carcinomas of the lung – A clinicopathologic and immunohistochemical study with special reference to CDX-2 homeobox gene and MUC2 expression. Am J Surg Pathol 2004; 28:442–452.

69. Ordonez NG. The diagnostic utility of immunohistochemistry in distinguishing between mesothelioma and renal cell carcinoma: a comparative study. Hum Pathol 2004; 35:697–710.

70. Tan JY, Sidhu G, Greco MA, Ballard H, Wieczorek R. Villin, cytokeratin 7, and cytokeratin 20 expression in pulmonary adenocarcinoma with ultrastructural evidence of microvilli with rootlets. Hum Pathol 1998; 29:390–396.

71. Sharma S, Tan JY, Sidhu G, Wieczorek R, Miller DC, Cassai ND. Lung adenocarcinomas metastatic to the brain with and without ultrastructural evidence of rootlets: An electron microscopic and immunohistochemical study using cytokeratins 7 and 20 and villin. Ultrastruct Pathol 1998; 22:385–391.

72. Oates J, Edwards C. HBME-1, MOC-31, WT1 and calretinin: an assessment of recently described markers for mesothelioma and adenocarcinoma. Histopathology 2000; 36:341–347.

73. Chu P, Wu E, Weiss LM. Cytokeratin 7 and cytokeratin 20 expression in epithelial neoplasms: A survey of 435 cases. Modern Pathol 2000; 13:962–972.

74. Chu PG, Weiss LM. Keratin expression in human tissues and neoplasms. Histopathology 2002; 40:403–439.

75. Goldstein NS, Thomas M. Mucinous and nonmucinous bronchioloalveolar adenocarcinomas have distinct staining patterns with thyroid transcription factor and cytokeratin 20 antibodies. Am J Clin Pathol 2001; 116:319–325.

76. Giordano TJ, Shedden KA, Schwartz DR, et al. Organ-specific molecular classification of primary lung, colon, and ovarian adenocarcinomas using gene expression profiles. Am J Pathol 2001; 159:1231–1238.

77. van de Rijn M, Barr FG, Collins MH et al. Absence of SYT-SSX fusion products in soft tissue tumors other than synovial sarcoma. Am J Clin Pathol 1999; 112:43–49.

78. Steiner PE. Metastasizing fibroleiomyoma of the uterus – report of a case and review of the literature. Am J Pathol 1939; 15:89–109.

79. Spiro RH, McPeak CJ. On the so-called metastasizing leiomyoma. Cancer 1966; 19:544–548.

80. Parenti DJ, Morley TF, Giudice JC. Benign metastasizing leiomyoma – a case report and review of the literature. Respiration 1992; 59:347–350.

81. Canzonieri V, Damore ESG, Bartoloni G, Piazza M, Blandamura S, Carbone A. Leiomyomatosis with vascular invasion. a unified pathogenesis regarding leiomyoma with vascular microinvasion, benign metastasizing leiomyoma and intravenous leiomyomatosis. Virchows Arch 1994; 425:541–545.

82. Kayser K, Zink S, Schneider T, et al. Benign metastasizing leiomyoma of the uterus: documentation of clinical, immunohistochemical and lectin-histochemical data of ten cases. Virchows Archiv 2000; 437: 284–292.

83. Cho KR, Woodruff JD, Epstein JI. Leiomyoma of the uterus with multiple extrauterine smooth muscle tumors: a case report suggesting multifocal origin. Hum Pathol 1989; 20:80–83.

84. Tietze L, Gunther K, Horbe A, et al. Benign metastasizing leiomyoma: A cytogenetically balanced but clonal disease. Hum Pathol 2000; 31:126–128.

85. Clement PB. Intravenous leiomyomatosis of the uterus. Pathol Annu 1988; 23(Pt 2):153–183.

86. Wolff M, Kaye G, Silva F. Pulmonary metastases (with admixed epithelial elements) from smooth muscle neoplasms. Report of nine cases, including three males. Am J Surg Pathol 1979; 3:325–342.

87. Horstmann JP, Pietra GG, Harman JA, Cole NG, Grinspan S. Spontaneous regression of pulmonary leiomyomas during pregnancy. Cancer 1977; 39:314–321.

88. Banner A, Carrington CB, Emory WB, et al. Efficacy of oophorectomy in lymphangioleiomyomatosis and benign metastasizing leiomyoma. N Engl J Med 1981; 305:204–209.

89. Levine GD, Rosai J. Thymic hyperplasia and neoplasia: a review of current concepts. Hum Pathol 1978; 9:495–515.

90. Dyke SC. Metastases of the 'benign' giant cell tumor of bone (osteoclastoma). J Pathol Bacteriol 1981; 34:259–263.

91. Colby TV. Metastasizing dermatofibroma. Am J Surg Pathol 1997; 21:976.

92. Miller DC, Ojemann RG, Proppe KH, et al. Benign metastasizing meningioma. J Neurosurg 1985; 62:763–766.

93. Anton RC, Schwartz MR, Kessler ML, Cagle PT. Metastatic carcinoma of the prostate mimicking primary carcinoid tumor of the lung and mediastinum. Pathol Res Pract 1998; 194:753–758.

94. Alvarez-Fernandez E. Alveolar trapping in pulmonary carcinomas. Diag Histopathol 1982; 5:59–64.

95. Itoh T, Mochizuki M, Kumazaki S, Ishihara T, Fukayama M. Cystic pulmonary metastases of endometrial stromal sarcoma of the uterus, mimicking lymphangiomyomatosis: A case report with immunohistochemistry of HMB45. Pathol Int 1997; 47:725–729.

96. Hasegawa S, Inui K, Kamakari K, Kotoura Y, Suzuki K, Fukumoto M. Pulmonary cysts as the sole metastatic manifestation of soft tissue sarcoma – Case report and consideration of the pathogenesis. Chest 1999; 116:263–265.

97. Holden WE, Mulkey DD, Kessler S. Multiple peripheral lung cysts and hemoptysis in an otherwise asymptomatic adult. Am Rev Respir Dis 1982; 126:930–932.

98. Joseph MG, Colby TV, Swensen SJ, Mikus JP, Gaensler EA. Multiple cystic fibrohistiocytic tumors of the lung: report of two cases. Mayo Clin Proc 1990; 65:192–197.

99. Matsumoto K, Yamamoto T, Hisayoshi T, Asano G. Intravenous leiomyomatosis of the uterus with multiple pulmonary metastases associated with large bullae-like cyst formation. Pathol Int 2001; 51:396–401.

100. Aubry MC, Myers JL, Colby TV, Leslie KO, Tazelaar HD. Endometrial stromal sarcoma metastatic to the lung – A detailed analysis of 16 patients. Am J Surg Pathol 2002; 26:440–449.

101. Park SI, Choi E, Lee HB, Rhee YK, Chung MJ, Lee YC. Spontaneous pneumomediastinum and hemopneumothoraces secondary to cystic lung metastasis. Respiration 2003; 70:211–213.

102. Osborn M, Mandys V, Beddow E, et al. Cystic fibrohistiocytic tumours presenting in the lung: primary or metastatic disease? Histopathology 2003; 43:556–562

103. Madden M, Goldstraw P, Corrin B. Effect of chemotherapy on the histological appearances of testicular teratoma metastatic to the lung: correlation with patient survival. J Clin Pathol 1984; 37:1212–1214.

104. Cagini L, Nicholson AG, Horwich A, Goldstraw P, Pastorino U. Thoracic metastasectomy for germ cell tumours: long term survival and prognostic factors. Ann Oncol 1998; 9:1185–1191.

105. Casson AG, McCormack D, Craig I, Inculet R, Levin L. A persistent pulmonary lesion following chemotherapy for metastatic choriocarcinoma. Chest 1993; 103:269–270.

106. Moran CA, Travis WD, Carter D, Koss MN. Metastatic mature teratoma in lung following testicular embryonal carcinoma and teratocarcinoma. Arch Pathol Lab Med 1993; 117:641–644.

107. Abrams J, Talcott J, Corson JM. Pulmonary metastases in patients with low-grade endometrial stromal sarcoma. Clinicopathologic findings with immunohistochemical characterisation. Am J Surg Pathol 1989; 13:133–140.

108. Chang KL, Crabtree GS, Lim-Tan SK, Kempson RL, Hendrickson MR. Primary uterine endometrial stromal neoplasms. A clinicopathologic study of 117 cases. Am J Surg Pathol 1990; 14:415–438.

109. Brinck U, Gunawan B, Schulten HJ, Pinzon W, Fischer U, Fuzesi L. Clear-cell odontogenic carcinoma with pulmonary metastases resembling pulmonary meningothelial-like nodules. Virchows Archiv 2001; 438:412–417.

110. Echevarria RA. Angiogenic nature of 'intravascular bronchioloalveolar tumor'. Arch Pathol Lab Med 1981; 105:627–628.

111. Verbeken E, Bayls J, Moerman P, Knockaert D, Goddeeris P, Lauweryns JM. Lung metastasis of malignant epithelioid hemangioendothelioma mimicking a primary intravascular bronchioalveolar tumor. A histologic, ultrastructural, and immunohistochemical study. Cancer 1985; 55:1741–1746.

Effects of secondary lung tumours

112. Lowe D, Fletcher CDM. Eosinophilia in squamous cell carcinoma of the oral cavity, external genitalia and anus – clinical correlations. Histopathology 1984; 8:627–632.

113. Fujita J, Yamagishi Y, Kubo A, Takigawa K, Yamaji Y, Takahara J. Respiratory failure due to pulmonary lymphangitis carcinomatosis. Chest 1993; 103:967–968.

114. Bagshawe KD, Brooks WDW. Subacute pulmonary hypertension due to chorionepithelioma. Lancet 1959; 1:653–658.

115. He XW, Tang YH, Luo ZQ, Cheng TO. Subacute cor pulmonale due to tumor embolisation to the lungs. Angiology 1989; 40:11–17.

116. Seckl MJ, Rustin GJS, Newlands ES, Gwyther SJ, Bomanji J. Pulmonary embolism, pulmonary hypertension, and choriocarcinoma. Lancet 1991; 338:1313–1315.

117. Veinot JP, Ford SE, Price RG. Subacute cor pulmonale due to tumor embolisation. Arch Pathol Lab Med 1992; 116:131–134.

118. Soares FA, Landell GAM, Deoliveira JAM. Pulmonary tumor embolism to alveolar septal capillaries – an unusual cause of sudden cor pulmonale. Arch Pathol Lab Med 1992; 116:187–188.

119. Hibbert M, Braude S. Tumour microembolism presenting as 'primary pulmonary hypertension'. Thorax 1997; 52:1016–1017.

120. Edmondstone WM. Flitting radiographic shadows: an unusual presentation of cancer in the lungs. Thorax 1998; 53:906–908.

121. Storey PD, Goldstein W. Pulmonary embolisation from primary hepatic carcinoma. Arch Intern Med 1962; 110:262–269.

122. Wakasa K, Sakurai M, Uchida A, Yoshikawa H, Maeda A. Massive pulmonary tumor emboli in osteosarcoma: occult and fatal complication. Cancer 1990; 66:583–586.

123. Watanabe S, Shimokawa S, Sakasegawa K, Masuda H, Sakata R, Higashi M. Choriocarcinoma in the pulmonary artery treated with emergency pulmonary embolectomy. Chest 2002; 121:654–656.

Prolonged survival despite metastatic disease

124. Casciato DA, Nagurka C, Tabbarah HJ. Prolonged survival with unresected pulmonary metastases. Ann Thorac Surg 1983; 36:202–208.

125. Bloom HJG, Wallace DM. Hormones and the kidney: possible therapeutic role of testosterone in a patient with regression of metastases from renal adenocarcinoma. BMJ 1964; 2:476–480.

126. Palmer MA, Viswanath S, Desmond AD. Spontaneous regression of metastatic renal cell carcinoma. J R Soc Med 1993; 86:113–114.

127. Everson TC. Spontaneous regression of cancer. Ann N Y Acad Sci 1964; 14:721–735.

128. Casson AG, Putnam JB, Natarajan G, et al. Five-year survival after pulmonary metastasectomy for adult soft tissue sarcoma. Cancer 1992; 69: 662–668.

129. Matthay RA, Arroliga AC. Resection of pulmonary metastases. Am Rev Respir Dis 1993; 148:1691–1696.

130. Sakamoto T, Tsubota N, Iwanaga K, Yuki T, Matsuoka H, Yoshimura M. Pulmonary resection for metastases from colorectal cancer. Chest 2001; 119:1069–1072.

131. Davidson RS, Nwogu CE, Brentjens MJ, Anderson TM. The surgical management of pulmonary metastasis: current concepts. Surg Oncol 2001; 10:35–42.

132. Long-term results of lung metastasectomy: prognostic analyses based on 5206 cases. The International Registry of Lung Metastases. J Thorac Cardiovasc Surg 1997; 113:37–49.

133. Leo F, Cagini L, Rocmans P, et al. Lung metastases from melanoma: when is surgical treatment warranted? Br J Cancer 2000; 83:569–572.

134. Friedel G, Pastorino U, Ginsberg RJ, et al. Results of lung metastasectomy from breast cancer: prognostic criteria on the basis of 467 cases of the International Registry of Lung Metastases. Eur J Cardiothorac Surg 2002; 22:335–344.

135. Protopapas AD, Nicholson AG, Vini L, Harmer CL, Goldstraw P. Thoracic metastasectomy in thyroid malignancies. Ann Thorac Surg 2001; 72:1906–1908.

12

Tumours

12.7

Tumour-like conditions

This chapter deals with certain tumour-like lesions of the lower respiratory tract, these being non-neoplastic processes that present as masses or nodules within the lung and thereby simulate true neoplasms. Table 12.7.1 shows how these lesions have been categorised over the past 25 years. Many entities listed as tumour-like in the 1981 WHO classification of lung tumours were re-classified as neoplasms in 1999, but the tumour-like category nevertheless grew because several new tumour-like entities had been identified in the interim. The 2004 WHO classification of lung tumours did not include tumour-like lesions as it was limited to neoplasms but it is notable that some lesions classified as tumour-like in 1999 were included. For example, inflammatory pseudotumour, regarded as a tumour-like lesion in 1999 was included as inflammatory myofibroblastic tumour in the mesenchymal tumour section of the 2004 classification. Similarly, several lesions that appeared in the tumour-like section of the previous edition of this book are now dealt with in other sections, for example pleuropulmonary endometriosis now comes under systemic disorders, while localised areas of organising pneumonia, Langerhans cell histiocytosis and lymphangioleiomyomatosis are considered in the diffuse parenchymal diseases section. Tumourlets are not considered to be neoplastic but are nevertheless considered with the related carcinoid tumours. Other terms, e.g. pseudolymphoma, have simply become obsolete.

REGENERATION PROCESSES MIMICKING NEOPLASIA

Throughout the lower respiratory tract, regenerative processes may be so atypical that carcinomatous transformation has to be considered in the differential diagnosis. This impression is often augmented by excessive mitotic activity and metaplasia. Thus, at the alveolar level, necrotising lesions such as infarcts and the granulomatoses may be bordered by foci of atypical squamous hyperplasia that are easily mistaken for squamous cell carcinoma. Similarly, damage to the bronchial epithelium is often followed by atypical regeneration that is easily mistaken for

Table 12.7.1 Successive classifications of tumour-like lesions involving the lung

1981 WHO classification	1999 WHO/IASLC classification[a]	2005 Pathology of the Lungs 2nd edn.	
	Amyloid tumour	Chapter 12.7	Amyloid tumour
	Bronchial inflammatory polyp		Bronchial inflammatory polyp
	Hyalinising granuloma		Hyalinising granuloma
	Minute meningothelioid nodules		Minute meningothelioid nodules
	Multifocal micronodular pneumocyte hyperplasia		Multifocal micronodular pneumocyte hyperplasia
		Other Chapters	Congenital peribronchial myofibroblastic tumour (Ch. 2)
			Bacillary angiomatosis (Ch. 5.3)
			Actinomycosis (Ch. 5.3)
Eosinophilic granuloma	Langerhans cell histiocytosis		Langerhans cell histiocytosis (Ch. 6.1)
	Lymphangioleiomyomatosis		Lymphangioleiomyomatosis (Ch. 6.1)
	Organising pneumonia		Organising pneumonia (Ch. 6.2)
	Endometriosis		Endometriosis (Ch. 10)
Tumourlet	Tumourlet		Tumourlet (Ch. 12.2)
Sclerosing haemangioma			Sclerosing pneumocytoma (Ch. 12.2)
Hamartoma			Hamartoma (Ch. 12.3)
Inflammatory pseudotumour	Inflammatory pseudotumour		Inflammatory myofibroblastic tumour (Ch. 12.3)
Lymphoproliferative lesions			Lymphoproliferative disease (Ch. 12.4)
			Rheumatoid nodules (Ch. 10)
			Splenosis (Ch. 13)
			Folded lung (Ch. 13)

[a]The 2004 WHO/IASLC classification is restricted to neoplasms and does not include tumour-like lesions. IASLC, International Association for the Study of Lung Cancer.

Table 12.7.2 Bronchopulmonary amyloidosis

Amyloid type	Distribution of amyloid (Radiology ± bronchoscopy)	Clinical significance
AL	Intrathoracic lymphadenopathy	Usually a manifestation of systemic AL amyloidosis
AL	Laryngeal	Nodular or diffuse infiltrative form. Usually localised but sometimes extends into trachea. Associated with focal clonal immunocyte dyscrasia
AL	Tracheobronchial	Nodular or diffuse infiltrative form. Usually confined to the respiratory tract. Associated with focal clonal immunocyte dyscrasia
AL	Parenchymal: Nodular	Solitary or multiple nodules, usually confined to respiratory tract in association with focal clonal immunocyte dyscrasia
AL	Parenchymal: Diffuse alveolar septal	Diffuse alveolar septal distribution usually a manifestation of systemic amyloidosis associated with low-grade monoclonal gammopathy, myeloma etc.
ATTR, AA, others	Parenchymal: Diffuse alveolar septal	Usually an incidental histological finding. Clinically evident disease and radiological abnormalities rare

AA, serum amyloid A protein; AL, light chain; ATTR, transthyretin. (Adapted from Gillmore JD, Hawkins PN. Amyloidosis and the respiratory tract. Thorax 1999; 54:444–451.[5] With permission from British Medical Association.)

carcinoma, particularly when exfoliated cells are being examined. Bronchoscopy inevitably involves bronchial injury and cytopathologists have to be aware of the atypicalities that follow this procedure. Necrotising lesions of the larynx are sometimes accompanied by atypical regeneration that involves both the surface epithelium and the submucosal glands: the term *necrotising sialometaplasia* has been applied to this and to a similar process involving the trachea in patients with herpetic tracheitis undergoing repeated intubation (see p. 93).

AMYLOID TUMOUR

Amyloidosis of the lower respiratory tract may develop as part of generalised amyloidosis or in isolation (Table 12.7.2).[1–5] Pul-

monary involvement in generalised amyloidosis is dealt with on p. 489 and this section deals only with amyloidosis confined to the lower respiratory tract. This takes the form of either multifocal nodules or solitary tumour masses. The disease is usually confined to either the lung parenchyma or the major airways but occasionally affects both.[6] In the airways, the tumours may be solitary or multifocal, whereas parenchymal tumours are usually solitary. Rarely however, there may be extensive pulmonary involvement with extension to the hilar lymph nodes and involvement of adjacent structures,[7,8] including the pleura.[9–11] Other forms of amyloid confined to the lower respiratory tract include rare examples of amyloid in the stroma of tumours – apudamyloid in the case of neuroendocrine tumours[12–14] and immunoamyloid in the case of lymphomas.[15–20] Amyloid has also been described in the lymphoid interstitial pneumonia associated with Sjögren's syndrome,[21,22] in similar pulmonary infiltrates associated with macroglobulinaemia[23] and in association with localised light-chain deposition.[24] The corpora amylacea described on p. 321 also consist of amyloid.

Clinical features

The age range of patients with amyloid tumours is wide but most are middle-aged. There is no sex predilection and the lesions are not related to smoking. Tracheobronchial and parenchymal forms of amyloid are distinguished because they differ markedly in their symptomatology, but pathologically, amyloid tumours of the main airways are identical to those situated in the periphery of the lung. The former obstruct major airways and cause coughing, breathlessness, wheezing and even stridor, whereas the latter often form an asymptomatic mass that is discovered by chance radiographically, and is then suspected of being malignant.

Pathology

Amyloid tumours consist of crumbling eosinophilic amorphous material that exhibits the characteristic dichroism and birefringence of amyloid when stained with Congo red. The amyloid is often partly calcified or even ossified and is surrounded by foreign body giant cells, lymphocytes and plasma cells (Figs 12.7.1–12.7.3).[2,8] The plasma cells are polyclonal, and the amyloid is of the immune or AL type, as it typically is when the lungs are involved in generalised amyloidosis (Table 12.7.2).[25] This may be confirmed by the congophilia being resistant to prior potassium permanganate treatment,[2,26] immuno-histochemistry[27,28] or full chemical analysis.[29] As there is no evidence of generalised disease, it is likely that the immunoamyloid is formed locally by the surrounding plasma cells rather than resulting from circulating immunoglobulin light chains. Support for this is provided by a case in which amyloid nodules were associated with polyclonal light chain deposits, both of which were confined to the lungs.[30] The polyclonality of the associated plasma cells favours the likelihood that isolated pulmonary amyloid represents a local hyperimmune response to an unknown antigen.

Differential diagnosis

The calcification and ossification that is often evident in amyloid tumours (Fig. 12.7.3) probably underlies erroneous suggestions that tracheobronchopathia osteochondroplastica develops from multifocal tracheobronchial amyloidosis.[31–33] Although their bronchoscopic appearances may be similar, the two conditions are in fact quite different. Apart from the characteristic features of tracheobronchopathia, described on p. 90, Congo red staining is generally reliable in distinguishing the two. Caseous tuberculosis may also be suspected, but the correct diagnosis can be made without Congo red and Ziehl–Neelsen stains from the nature of the surrounding reac-

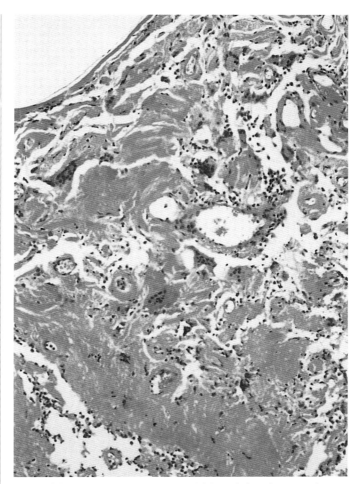

Figure 12.7.1 Localised pulmonary amyloid consisting of a mass of eosinophilic amorphous material.

tion. The foreign body giant cells engulfing the amyloid are a very characteristic feature, whereas the epithelioid and giant cell granulomas of tuberculosis are lacking. A more difficult distinction is that from amyloid-producing lymphomas, particularly plasmacytomas.[15–20] Features suggesting lymphoma include lymphatic tracking by the cellular infiltrate, sheet-like clusters of plasma cells and light chain restriction.[19] Amyloid-like nodules associated with light-chain deposition consist of electron-dense granular material, rather than the fibrils seen in amyloidosis and fail to stain with Congo red.[24] Pulmonary hyalinising granuloma may also mimic an amyloid tumour but is composed of dense lamellar collagen rather than amorphous material and does not stain with Congo red.

Treatment and prognosis

Tracheobronchial amyloid tumours are generally removed piecemeal and incompletely, so that they require repeated surgery whereas recurrence of a resected parenchymal tumour, although recorded,[34] is unusual. Laser therapy has also been used for extensive airway involvement. Localised amyloidosis

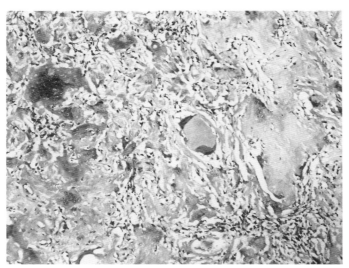

Figure 12.7.2 Pulmonary amyloid tumour showing a vigorous foreign body giant cell reaction to the amyloid and a lymphoplasmacytic infiltrate.

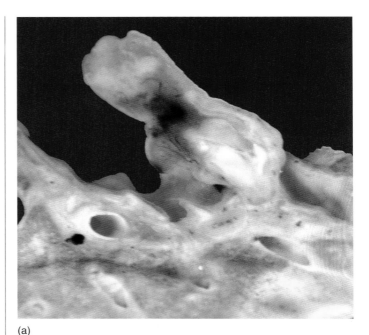

(a)

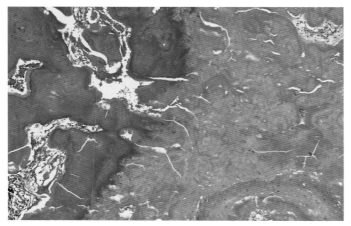

Figure 12.7.3 A pulmonary amyloid tumour showing prominent dystrophic calcification. Together with ossification, this has led to erroneous claims that tracheobronchopathia osteochondroplastica represents a form of tracheobronchial amyloidosis.

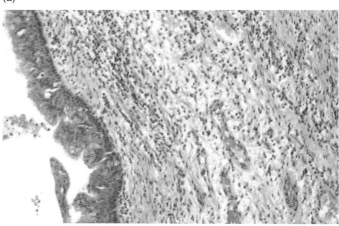

(b)

Figure 12.7.4 Inflammatory polyp. (a) A myxoid polyp protrudes into a segmental bronchus. (b) The polyp is lined by respiratory epithelium and there is moderate chronic inflammation of the stroma.

has a much better prognosis than systemic amyloidosis and it is therefore important to exclude involvement of other organs. It is also important to ensure that the amyloid is of AL type as other types require different treatment and might also require relatives to be screened for inherited forms of the disease.[11]

BRONCHIAL INFLAMMATORY POLYP

Inflammatory polyps of the bronchus have a core of oedematous connective tissue covered by respiratory epithelium (Fig. 12.7.4). They are reactive and often show a heavy acute or chronic inflammatory infiltrate. In infancy they may be caused

by trauma from suction at the time of delivery.[35] The surface epithelium may be replaced by granulation tissue or show squamous metaplasia or goblet cell hyperplasia but these changes are focal, unlike the squamous, glandular and mixed papillomas described on p. 597.

Inflammatory polyps may cause collapse or hyperexpansion, the latter more common in infancy. They are usually solitary but inflammatory polyposis complicating bronchiectasis is recorded in a patient with cystic fibrosis.[36] Inflammatory polyps have no malignant potential and may resolve with antibiotic treatment.[37] Alternatively, they may be excised at bronchoscopy while chronic lung damage has occasionally necessitated lobectomy.[35]

HYALINISING GRANULOMA

Hyalinising granuloma is a rare condition of unknown aetiology. Most cases have been reported from the New World.[38–43] There are few reports from Europe[44] or Asia.[45]

Clinical features

Most patients are middle-aged, with a mean between 40 and 45 years. They are either asymptomatic or have mild breathlessness, low-grade pyrexia and general malaise. The radiographic appearances, those of single or multiple pulmonary nodules, are usually interpreted as representing primary or secondary neoplasms. The nodules tend to enlarge slowly and the disease has a benign course.

Aetiology

The microscopical appearances of hyalinising granuloma have been likened to those of sclerosing mediastinitis and a common aetiology is suggested by the simultaneous occurrence of pulmonary hyalinising granuloma and sclerosing mediastinitis or retroperitoneal fibrosis, or sometimes all three conditions.[38,41,44,45] Associated immunological abnormalities include the presence of antinuclear antibodies, rheumatoid factor, anti-microsomal and anti-smooth-muscle antibodies, circulating immune complexes and Coombs-positive haemolytic anaemia.[38–40] Other clinical associations include systemic idiopathic fibrosis,[45] synchronous lymphoma,[46,47] Castleman's disease[48] and multiple sclerosis.[49]

An abnormal response to chronic infection, such as tuberculosis or histoplasmosis, has been suggested as the cause of hyalinising granuloma but, although skin tests may be positive, culture and stains for microbes are invariably negative.[38,41] The apparent predilection of this condition for North America is compatible with there being an unusual infective agent but it may denote unwillingness to make the diagnosis of an unfamiliar and debatable entity in other countries.

Pathology

The nodules may be single (about one-third of cases), or multiple and bilateral, and vary from a few millimetres to 15 cm in diameter.[38] They are well-circumscribed and may be subpleural or lie deep within the lung parenchyma. Cavitation and calcification are unusual features.[38,41,42]

Microscopically, the centre generally consists of hyaline collagen arranged in a distinctive pattern of concentric lamellae, sometimes with focal calcification or ossification (Fig. 12.7.5).[41] The periphery is more cellular, showing an infiltrate of lymphocytes, plasma cells, histiocytes, fibroblasts and occasional giant cells. Blood vessels may be infiltrated by the inflammatory cells or incorporated into the sclerotic area where they are encircled by the hyaline lamellae. The original report included lesions that stained for amyloid[38] but subsequent workers have excluded such cases[41] and electron microscopy has not confirmed the presence of amyloid.[40]

Differential diagnosis

Hyalinising granuloma is to be distinguished from amyloidosis (see above), necrobiotic (rheumatoid) nodules (see p. 473) and Wegener's granulomatosis (see p. 438). The necrosis seen in active examples of the last two of these entities is lacking but

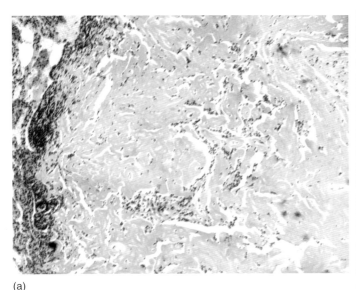
(a)

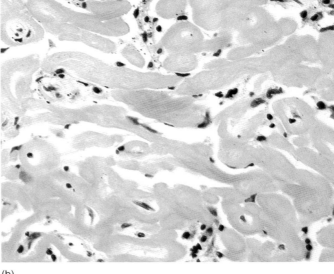
(b)

Figure 12.7.5 Pulmonary hyalinising granuloma. (a) The lesion forms a mass of densely fibrotic tissue with a peripheral rim of chronic inflammation. (b) The fibrotic tissue consists of thick interweaving collagen bundles.

their healed lesions can closely resemble hyalinising granuloma. Sclerosing lymphomas may be excluded by immunohistochemistry. Infections such as tuberculosis and histoplasmosis need to be excluded as far as is possible by culture and appropriate stains. Inflammatory myofibroblastic tumour may have densely sclerotic foci, rendering its distinction difficult in small biopsies, but in resection specimens the myofibroblastic areas characteristic of this tumour are generally evident, while in hyalinising granuloma inflammation is confined to the periphery of the lesion.

Treatment and prognosis

There is no specific treatment but symptomatic lesions may be resected. The prognosis is good and morbidity may be more frequently encountered in relation to fibrosis at other sites.

MULTIPLE MINUTE MENINGOTHELIOID NODULES (MULTIPLE MINUTE PULMONARY 'CHEMODECTOMAS')

Histogenesis and epidemiology

Multiple microscopic lung tumours that resembled chemodectomas (paragangliomas) were first described in 1960[50] and were long known as minute pulmonary chemodectomas or chemodectomatosis.[51] However, electron microscopy fails to show the dense-core granules of chemoreceptor cells but demonstrates complex interdigitating cell processes, prominent desmosomes and cytoplasmic tangles of fibrils. There is a marked ultrastructural and immunohistochemical resemblance to meningeal arachnoid granulations and meningiomas,[52–56] in which context it is of interest that a few primary pulmonary meningiomas have been reported (see p. 630). The term meningothelioid (or

arachnoid) nodules is therefore preferred to minute pulmonary chemodectomas. Some authors suggest that that they have a similar function to the meningeal arachnoid granulations that absorb cerebrospinal fluid and return it to the dural veins: it is suggested that in the lung they may return interstitial fluid to the pulmonary veins and so minimise the danger of pulmonary oedema.[57] Clonality and loss of heterozygosity have been reported but not so frequently as in meningiomas.[56] Reported increases in their number and size probably represent hyperplasia induced by local changes in perfusion, rather than neoplasia.

These lesions are generally found fortuitously at autopsy or in surgical samples. An incidence of 1 in every 200–300 autopsies is reported, but this can be increased to around 1 in 25 if a specific search is made.[50,52,58,59] They are more common in patients with thromboembolic disease, other forms of chronic pulmonary disease in which scarring occurs, and cardiac failure.[58,59] They also appear to be commoner in people who reside at high altitude.[57] A tendency to pulmonary oedema may be the linking factor. The age range is wide but most patients are in their fifth or sixth decades. There is a female preponderance of about five to one, in connection with which it is notable that the lesions bear a progesterone receptor.[60]

Pathology

Meningothelioid nodules measure up to 3 mm in diameter. They are occasionally visible beneath the pleura or on the cut surface of the lung but most are discovered only when randomly selected tissue is examined microscopically. They are situated in the pulmonary interstitium close to the walls of veins, causing distension of adjacent alveoli. They consist of aggregated small nests of closely packed cells separated by collagen and elastic tissue (Fig. 12.7.6). The cells have moderate amounts of lightly

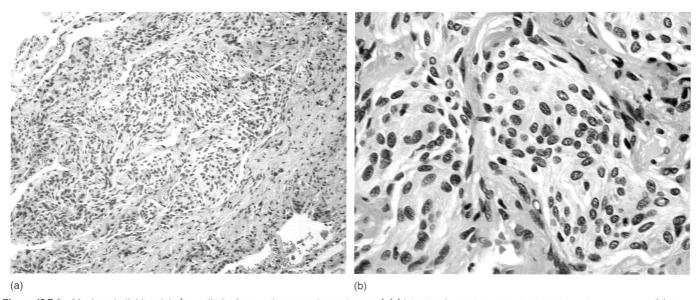

(a)   (b)

Figure 12.7.6 Meningothelioid nodule (so-called minute pulmonary chemodectoma). (a) Islands of round to oval cells lie within a fibrous stroma. (b) The cells have oval nuclei and eosinophilic cytoplasm without clear cell boundaries.

eosinophilic cytoplasm and often appear elongated. Nuclei are oval or reniform, and vesicular, with a small nucleolus. They are confined to the lung and have no malignant potential.

Unlike true chemodectomas, sustentacular cells are not present and, unlike tumourlets, argyrophilia and immunohistochemical stains for neuroendocrine markers are negative. Meningothelioid nodules stain for epithelial membrane antigen, progesterone receptor[60] and vimentin but not for cytokeratin, neuron specific enolase, S-100 or actin. The location of tumourlets adjacent to small airways rather than veins is another helpful point of distinction.

MULTIFOCAL MICRONODULAR TYPE II PNEUMOCYTE HYPERPLASIA

Micronodular type II pneumocyte hyperplasia is largely though not exclusively confined to patients with tuberous sclerosis, of which it is a particularly rare manifestation.[61-69] It may be seen in otherwise normal lungs or in association with pulmonary lymphangioleiomyomatosis. Unlike lymphangioleiomyomato-

sis, it affects tuberous sclerosis patients of either sex and the hyperplastic type II cells fail to stain for HMB-45.[68] The condition is multifocal and microscopic and usually of no clinical significance. However, in rare cases the lesions are of an appreciable size and so numerous that pulmonary function is severely compromised.[70] The hyperplastic cells stain for cytokeratin surfactant apoprotein and epithelial membrane antigen unlike meningothelioid nodules. They show no atypia and appear to be devoid of any malignant potential (Fig. 12.7.7).

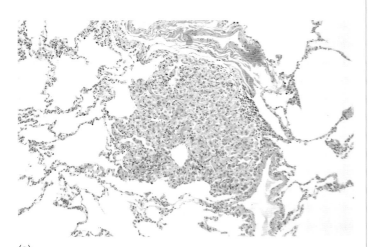

(a)

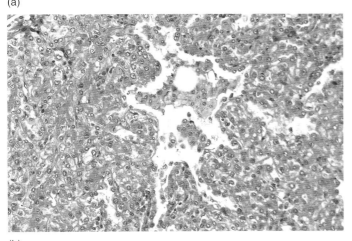

(b)

Figure 12.7.7   (a) Low- and (b) high-power views of micronodular type II cell hyperplasia in tuberous sclerosis.

REFERENCES

Amyloid tumour

1. Thompson PJ, Citron KM. Amyloid and the lower respiratory tract. Thorax 1983; 38:84–87.
2. Hui AN, Koss MN, Hochholzer L, Wehunt WD. Amyloidosis presenting in the lower respiratory tract. Arch Pathol Lab Med 1986; 110:212–218.
3. Cordier JF, Loire R, Brune J. Amyloidosis of the lower respiratory tract. Chest 1986; 90:827–831.
4. Utz JP, Swensen SJ, Gertz MA. Pulmonary amyloidosis. The Mayo Clinic experience from 1980 to 1993. Ann Intern Med 1996; 124:407–413.
5. Gillmore JD, Hawkins PN. Amyloidosis and the respiratory tract. Thorax 1999; 54:444–451.
6. Schulz C, Hauck RW, Nathrath WBJ, Prauer HW, Linke RP, Emslander HP. Combined amyloidosis of the upper and lower respiratory tract. Respiration 1995; 62:163–166.
7. Thompson PJ, Jewkes J, Corrin B, Citron KM. Primary bronchopulmonary amyloid tumour with massive hilar lymphadenopathy. Thorax 1983; 38:153–154.
8. Laden SA, Cohen ML, Harley RA. Nodular pulmonary amyloidosis with extrapulmonary involvement. Hum Pathol 1984; 15:594–597.
9. Knapp MJ, Roggli VL, Kim J, Moore JO, Shelbourne JD. Pleural amyloidosis. Arch Pathol Lab Med 1988; 112:57–60.
10. Adams AL, Castro CY, Singh SP, Moran CA. Pleural amyloidosis mimicking mesothelioma: a clinicopathologic study of two cases. Ann Diagn Pathol 2001; 5:229–232.
11. Shah PL, Gillmore JD, Copley SJ, et al. The importance of complete screening for amyloid fibril type and systemic disease in patients with amyloidosis in the respiratory tract. Sarcoidosis Vasc Diffuse Lung Dis 2002; 19:134–142.
12. Gordon HW, Miller R, Mittman C. Medullary carcinoma of the lung with amyloid stroma: a counterpart of medullary carcinoma of the thyroid. Hum Pathol 1973; 4:431–436.
13. Al-Kaisi N, Abdul-Karim FW, Mendelsohn G, Jacobs G. Bronchial carcinoid tumour with amyloid stroma. Arch Pathol Lab Med 1988; 112:211–214.
14. Abe Y, Utsunomiya H, Tsutsumi Y. Atypical carcinoid tumor of the lung with amyloid stroma. Acta Pathol Jpn 1992; 42:286–292.
15. Davis CJ, Butchart EG, Gibbs AR. Nodular pulmonary amyloidosis occurring in association with pulmonary lymphoma. Thorax 1991; 46:217–218.
16. Michaels L, Hyams VJ. Amyloid in localised deposits and plasmacytomas of the respiratory tract. J Pathol 1979; 128:29–38.
17. Jenkins MCF, Potter M. Calcified pseudotumoural mediastinal amyloidosis. Thorax 1991; 46:686–687.
18. Ihling C, Weirich G, Gaa A, Schaefer HE. Amyloid tumours of the lung – an immunocytoma? Pathol Res Pract 1996; 192:446–452.
19. Dacic S, Colby TV, Yousem SA. Nodular amyloidoma and primary pulmonary lymphoma with amyloid production: A differential diagnostic problem. Modern Pathol 2000; 13: 934–940.
20. Lim JK, Lacy MQ, Kurtin PJ, Kyle RA, Gertz MA. Pulmonary marginal zone lymphoma of MALT type as a cause of localised pulmonary amyloidosis. J Clin Pathol 2001; 54:642–646.
21. Bonner H, Ennis RS, Geelhoed GW, Tarpley TM. Lymphoid infiltration and amyloidosis of lung in Sjögren's syndrome. Arch Pathol Lab Med 1973; 95:42–44.

22. Kobayashi H, Matsuoka R, Kitamura S, Tsunoda N, Saito K. Sjögren's syndrome with multiple bullae and pulmonary nodular amyloidosis. Chest 1988; 94:438–440.

23. Zatloukal P, Bezdicek P, Schimonova M, Havlicek F, Tesarova P, Slovakova A. Waldenstrom's macroglobulinemia with pulmonary amyloidosis. Respiration 1998; 65:414–416.

24. Khoor A, Myers JL, Tazelaar HD, Kurtin PJ. Amyloid-like pulmonary nodules, including localized light-chain deposition. Am J Clin Pathol 2004; 121, 200–204.

25. Smith RRL, Hutchins GM, Moore GW, Humphrey RL. Type and distribution of pulmonary parenchymal and vascular amyloid: correlation with cardiac amyloidosis. Am J Med 1979; 66:96–104.

26. DaCosta P, Corrin B. Amyloidosis localized to the lower respiratory tract: probable immunoamyloid nature of the tracheobronchial and nodular pulmonary forms. Histopathology 1985; 9:703–710.

27. Miura K, Shirasawa H. Lambda III subgroup immunoglobulin light chains are precursor proteins of nodular pulmonary amyloidosis. Am J Clin Pathol 1993; 100:561–566.

28. Toyoda M, Ebihara Y, Kato H, Kita S. Tracheobronchial AL amyloidosis - histologic, immunohistochemical, ultrastructural, and immunoelectron microscopic observations. Hum Pathol 1993; 24:970–976.

29. Page DL, Isersky C, Harada M, Glenner GG. Immunoglobulin origin of localized nodular pulmonary amyloidosis. Res Exp Med 1972; 159:75–86.

30. Stokes MB, Jagirdar J, Burchstin O, Kornacki S, Kumar A, Gallo G. Nodular pulmonary immunoglobulin light chain deposits with coexistent amyloid and nonamyloid features in an HIV- infected patient. Modern Pathol 1997; 10:1059–1065.

31. Sakula A. Tracheobronchopathia osteoplastica. Its relationship to primary tracheobronchial amyloidosis. Thorax 1968; 23:105–110.

32. Alroy GG, Lichtig C, Kaftori JK. Tracheobronchopathia osteoplastica: end stage of primary lung amyloidosis? Chest 1972; 61:465–468.

33. Jones AW, Chatterji AN. Primary tracheobronchial amyloidosis with tracheobronchopathia osteoplastica. Br J Dis Chest 1977; 71:268–272.

34. Dyke PC, Demaray MJ, Delavan JW, Rasmussen RA. Pulmonary amyloidoma. Am J Clin Pathol 1974; 61:301–305.

Bronchial inflammatory polyp

35. McShane D, Nicholson AG, Goldstraw P, et al. Inflammatory endobronchial polyps in childhood: clinical spectrum and possible link to mechanical ventilation. Pediatr Pulmonol 2002; 34:79–84.

36. Roberts C, Devenny AM, Brooker R, Cockburn JS, Kerr KM. Inflammatory endobronchial polyposis with bronchiectasis in cystic fibrosis. Eur Resp J 2001; 18:612–615.

37. Yamagishi M, Harada H, Kurihara M, et al. Inflammatory endotracheal polyp resolved after antibiotic treatment. Respiration 1993; 60:193–196.

Hyalinising granuloma

38. Engleman P, Liebow AA, Gmelich J, Friedman PJ. Pulmonary hyalinizing granuloma. Am Rev Respir Dis 1977; 115:997–1008.

39. Schlosnagle DC, Check IJ, Sewell CW, Plummer A, York RM, Hunter RL. Immunologic abnormalities in two patients with pulmonary hyalinizing granuloma. Am J Clin Pathol 1982; 78:231–235.

40. Guccion JG, Rohatgi PK, Saini N. Pulmonary hyalinizing granuloma. Electron microscopic and immunologic studies. Chest 1984; 85:571–573.

41. Yousem SA, Hochholzer L. Pulmonary hyalinizing granuloma. Am J Clin Pathol 1987; 87:1–6.

42. Patel Y, Ishikawa S, Macdonnell KF. Pulmonary hyalinizing granuloma presenting as multiple cavitary calcified nodules. Chest 1991; 100: 1720–1721.

43. Russell AFR, Suggit RIC, Kazzi JC. Pulmonary hyalinising granuloma: a case report and literature review. Pathology 2000; 32:290–293.

44. Dent RG, Godden DJ, Stovin PGI, Stark JE. Pulmonary hyalinising granuloma in association with retroperitoneal fibrosis. Thorax 1983; 38:955–956.

45. Kuramochi S, Kawai T, Yakumaru K, et al. Multiple pulmonary hyalinizing granulomas associated with systemic idiopathic fibrosis. Acta Pathol Jpn 1991; 41:375–382.

46. Drasin H, Blume MR, Rosenbaum EH, Klein HZ. Pulmonary hyalinizing granulomas in a patient with malignant lymphoma, with development nine years later of multiple myeloma and systemic amyloidosis. Cancer 1979; 44:215–220.

47. Ren YF, Raitz EN, Lee KR, Pingleton SK, Tawfik O. Pulmonary small lymphocytic lymphoma (mucosa-associated lymphoid tissue type) associated with pulmonary hyalinizing granuloma. Chest 2001; 120:1027–1030.

48. Atagi S, Sakatani M, Akira M, Yamamoto S, Ueda E. Pulmonary hyalinizing granuloma with Castleman's disease. Intern Med 1994; 33:689–691.

49. John PG, Rahman J, Payne CB. Pulmonary hyalinizing granuloma: an unusual association with multiple sclerosis. South Med J 1995; 88:1076–1077.

Multiple minute meningothelioid nodules

50. Korn D, Bensch K, Liebow AA, Castleman B. Multiple minute pulmonary tumours resembling chemodectomas. Am J Pathol 1960; 37:641–672.

51. Zak FG, Chabes A. Pulmonary chemodectomatosis. JAMA 1963; 183:887–889.

52. Churg AM, Warnock ML. So-called 'minute pulmonary chemodectoma'. A tumour not related to paragangliomas. Cancer 1976; 37:1759–1769.

53. Kuhn C, Askin FB. The fine structure of so-called minute pulmonary chemodectomas. Hum Pathol 1975; 6:681–691.

54. Gaffey MJ, Mills SE, Askin FB. Minute pulmonary meningothelial-like nodules. A clinicopathologic study of so-called minute pulmonary chemodectoma. Am J Surg Pathol 1988; 12:167–175.

55. Torikata C, Mukai M. So-called minute chemodectoma of the lung. An electron microscopic and immunohistochemical study. Virchows Arch A Pathol Anat Histopathol 1990; 417:113–118.

56. Niho S, Yokose T, Nishiwaki Y, Mukai K. Immunohistochemical and clonal analysis of minute pulmonary meningothelial-like nodules. Hum Pathol 1999; 30:425–429.

57. Heath D, Williams D. Arachnoid nodules in the lungs of high altitude Indians. Thorax 1993; 48:743–745.

58. Spain DM. Intrapulmonary chemodectomas in subjects with organising pulmonary thromboemboli. Am Rev Respir Dis 1967; 96:1158–1164.

59. Ichinose H, Hewitt RL, Drapanas T. Minute pulmonary chemodectoma. Cancer 1971; 28:692–700.

60. Pelosi G, Maffini F, Decarli N, Viale G. Progesterone receptor immunoreactivity in minute meningothelioid nodules of the lung. Virchows Archiv 2002; 440:543–546.

Multifocal micronodular Type II pneumocyte hyperplasia

61. Corrin B, Liebow AA, Friedman PJ. Pulmonary lymphangiomyomatosis. Am J Pathol 1975; 79:347–382.

62. Lie JT, Miller RD, Williams DE. Cystic disease of the lungs in tuberous sclerosis. Clinicopathologic correlation, including body plethysmographic lung function tests. Mayo Clin Proc 1980; 55:547–553.

63. Popper HH, Juettner-Smolle FM, Pongratz MG. Micronodular hyperplasia of type-II pneumocytes – a new lung lesion associated with tuberous sclerosis. Histopathology 1991; 18:347–354.

64. Popper HH. Micronodular hyperplasia of type-II pneumocytes. Histopathology 1992; 20:281.

65. Guinee D, Singh R, Azumi N, et al. Multifocal micronodular pneumocyte hyperplasia: a distinctive pulmonary manifestation of tuberous sclerosis. Mod Pathol 1995; 8:902–906.

66. Bonetti F, Chiodera P. The lung in tuberous sclerosis. In: Corrin B, ed. Pathology of Lung Tumors. London: Churchill Livingstone; 1997:225–240.

67. Lantuejoul S, Ferretti G, Negoescu A, Parent B, Brambilla E. Multifocal alveolar hyperplasia associated with lymphangioleiomyomatosis in tuberous sclerosis. Histopathology 1997; 30:570–575.

68. Muir TE, Leslie KO, Popper H, et al. Micronodular pneumocyte hyperplasia. Am J Surg Pathol 1998; 22:465–472.

69. Yamanaka A, Kitaichi M, Fujimoto T, Hirai T, Hori H, Konishi F. Multifocal micronodular pneumocyte hyperplasia in a postmenopausal woman with tuberous sclerosis. Virchows Archiv 2000; 436:389–392.

70. Cancellieri A, Poletti V, Corrin B. Respiratory failure due to micronodular type II pneumocyte hyperplasia. Histopathology 2002; 41:263–265.

13

Pleura and chest wall

NORMAL STRUCTURE AND FUNCTION OF THE PLEURA

The lung is surrounded by a smooth glistening membrane, the visceral pleura, which is reflected at the hilum over the mediastinum and the inside of the chest wall as the parietal pleura. The potential space thus created extends from the root of the neck, 3 cm above the mid-point of the clavicle, down behind the abdominal cavity and the kidney as the costodiaphragmatic recess, as far as the 12th rib. The two layers of the pleura are in close contact and slide easily over each other because of a thin mucinous film between them. Although this facilitates respiratory movements, there is little respiratory embarrassment if the pleural space is obliterated. Indeed, elephants and other large animals that generate large negative intrathoracic pressures lose their pleural cavities early in development without suffering any evident respiratory disability. The pleural cavities have therefore been called 'an anatomical luxury and a pathological hazard'.[1]

Each pleural surface consists of connective tissue covered by a single layer of flattened mesothelial cells, which secrete fluid rich in hyaluronic acid. However, most of the pleural fluid (which normally amounts to no more than a few millilitres) is a transudate of blood plasma with a protein concentration of less than 2 g/dl, mainly albumin. Although the parietal and visceral layers of the pleura both receive blood from systemic arteries – distal branches of the intercostal and bronchial arteries respectively – the latter are sparse and most of the pleural fluid enters through the parietal pleura. Initial views that it was absorbed by the visceral pleura were based on the false assumption that the two pleurae were morphologically similar and that Starling principles would apply. In fact the parietal and visceral pleurae differ considerably in structure.[2,3] Whereas the connective tissue of the parietal pleura is thin and capillaries and lymphatics within this tissue are no more than a few microns from the pleural space, the connective tissue of the visceral pleura is relatively thick; it constitutes the lung capsule and the underlying pulmonary blood vessels are separated from the pleural space by as much as 60–70 μm (Fig. 13.1). Furthermore, the parietal pleura is equipped with specialised stomata, described below, which provide a direct exit from the pleural space.[4] Most of the fluid therefore both enters and is absorbed from the pleural space through the parietal pleura (Fig. 13.2).

The uptake of macromolecules and particles less than 4 nm in diameter probably takes place by passive diffusion through the gap junctions that connect many mesothelial cells[5] and by active vesicular transport across the mesothelial cytoplasm.[6,7] Larger particles are mainly cleared in the caudal portions of the parietal pleura. The systemic lymphatic network is particularly rich here, and mesothelial and lymphatic endothelial cells are in direct apposition, without an intervening basement membrane. Here too, stomata in the parietal pleura provide a direct connection between the pleural cavity and the underlying lymphatics.[8] Over the lower mediastinum the stomata are associated with collections of macrophages and lymphoid cells, visible macroscopically as pale spots known as Kampmeier's foci. Particles up to about 10 μm are absorbed by the stomata-membrana-cribriformis complex, a process that is monitored by the lymphoreticular cells of Kampmeier's foci. Many particles are rapidly cleared by this route[9] but some are retained in Kampmeier's foci to form what are termed black spots.[10–12]

The mesothelial cells are joined by either tight or gap junctions and desmosomes, or in places merely overlap, like lymphatic endothelial cells. Pinocytotic vesicles are plentiful in the cytoplasm, which also contains rough endoplasmic reticulum and bundles of fine filaments. Mesothelial cells express epithelial markers such as cytokeratin. The mesothelial cell surface is not smooth but bears long, slender microvilli measuring up to 3 μm in length and 0.3 μm in width, suggesting an absorptive function. The numbers of microvilli vary from cell to cell. They are sparse over the ribs but increase towards the base of the lung and are more numerous on the visceral than the parietal pleura.[13] With their surface mucopolysaccharide coat, microvilli may also counter frictional forces.[14] Except at the specialised points in the parietal pleura described above, both layers of mesothelium rest upon a continuous basement membrane, beneath which there is a connective tissue network. In the visceral pleura this contains a thin inner and a thick outer elastic lamina (Fig. 13.1).

Mesothelial cells are readily damaged and desquamate in large numbers in many pathological conditions. Unlike epithelium, mesothelial repair does not solely involve centripetal migration of adjacent cells, as evidenced by the fact that large and small pleural lesions heal in exactly the same time. Mesothelial repair depends upon the differentiation of submesothelial connective tissue cells[15–19] and exfoliated mesothelial cells resettling on the denuded areas[20,21] as well as the centripetal migration of adjacent mesothelial cells.[21,22] Macrophages also settle out from the pleural fluid[23,24] but do not appear to differentiate into mesothelial cells.[15,25] Differentiation of proliferating submesothelial cells involves the acquisition of cytokeratin antigens, markers of mesothelial cells not normally found in connective tissue; this complicates the interpretation of immunocytochemical stains used to distinguish granulation tissue from mesothelioma of sarcomatous pattern (see p. 713).[17,18]

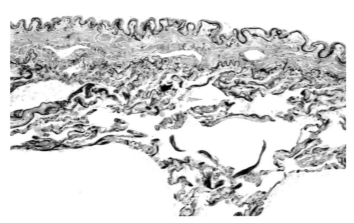

Figure 13.1 The normal visceral pleura. This comprises thin inner and thicker outer layers of elastin separated by collagen. (Elastin van Gieson stain.)

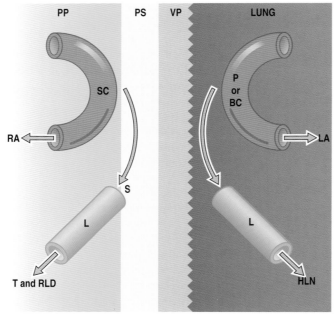

Figure 13.2 The normal formation and drainage of pleural fluid. Pleural fluid is normally derived from the high pressure systemic blood vessels in the parietal pleura and most of it leaves the pleural space through stomata in the parietal pleura. This changes when the pulmonary venous pressure rises (as in left heart failure) and when the pulmonary vasculature is unduly leaky (as in pneumonia), in which circumstances fluid enters the pleural space through the visceral pleura. PP, parietal pleura; PS, pleural space; VP, visceral pleura; SC, systemic capillary; P or BC, pulmonary or bronchial capillary; RA, right atrium; LA, left atrium; S, pleuro-lymphatic stroma; L, lymphatic; T and RLD, thoracic and right lymphatic ducts; HLN, hilar lymphatic nodes.

Test	Sensitivity for exudate (%)	Specificity for exudates (%)
Light's criteria (one or more of the following)	98	83
1 Ratio of pleural fluid protein level to serum protein level >0.5	86	84
2 Ratio of pleural fluid LDH level to serum LDH level >0.6	90	82
3 Pleural fluid LDH level >two-thirds the upper limit of normal for serum LDH level	82	89
Pleural fluid cholesterol level >60 mg/dl	54	92
Pleural fluid cholesterol level >43 mg/dl	75	80
Ratio of pleural fluid cholesterol level to serum cholesterol level >0.3	89	81
Serum albumin level – pleural fluid albumin level ≤ 1.2 g/dl	87	92

LDH denotes lactic dehydrogenase.

PLEURAL EFFUSIONS

Pleural effusions may be serous (hydrothorax), bloody (haemothorax) or chylous (chylothorax), or consist of frank pus (pyothorax or empyema thoracis). Most are caused by malignancy or infection.[26] Their rapid therapeutic removal occasionally alters pulmonary haemodynamics to such an extent that pulmonary oedema or even pulmonary haemorrhage results.[27,28]

Hydrothorax

Serous effusions may be clear or cloudy, the former usually denoting a transudate low in protein content and the latter a protein-rich exudate: 3 g protein/dl is the traditional demarcation point between transudates and exudates but pleural fluid/serum ratios of protein, lactic dehydrogenase and cholesterol are now widely used (Box 13.1).[29–31]

Transudates develop in cardiac failure, overhydration, constrictive pericarditis and fibrosing mediastinitis, the fluid accumulation resulting from an imbalance between hydrostatic and osmotic forces in each case. In cardiac failure the effusion is commonly unilateral. It is often stated that the right side is more frequently involved than the left but several studies have failed to confirm this. However, pleural effusion is more likely to develop when the cardiac failure is accompanied by pulmonary venous hypertension than when there is systemic venous hypertension; thus pleural effusion is common with left ventricular failure but rare with cor pulmonale.

Exudates are of varying aetiology, being the result of pleural or pulmonary irritation from any cause. The irritation is often due to acute infection, which is usually pneumonic but may be a pulmonary or subdiaphragmatic abscess. Other causes include acute pancreatitis,[32] rheumatoid disease, lupus erythematosus, tuberculosis, pulmonary infarction, a drug reaction (notably to practolol, methysergide and bromocriptine), nonmalignant asbestos pleurisy, cancer and lymphatic obstruction or deficiency, and even pleural amyloidosis.[33] Acute irritation typically leads to an accumulation of neutrophils in the fluid and chronic disease to increased numbers of lymphocytes. A predominance of eosinophils is occasionally found, even in the absence of blood eosinophilia: there is no very strong causal relationship but air in the pleural cavity may excite an eosinophilic reaction. Exudates caused by cancer and pulmonary infarction are commonly blood-stained.[26] The presence of tumour markers in the exudate may contribute to the diagnosis.[34] Pleural exudates due to defective lymphatic drainage are rich in lymphocytes and, if the obstruction involves the thoracic duct, are likely to be chylous. They may be part of a generalised disorder, as in the heritable *yellow nail syndrome* (lymphoedema of varied distribution due to lymphatic hypoplasia, accompanied by yellow discolouration and distortion of the nails, usually manifest in later life and often associated with an immunological disorder such as lymphopenia, hypogammaglobulinaemia or macroglobulinaemia, Fig. 13.3).[35–39]

Ascites may also result in pleural effusion due to ascitic fluid crossing the diaphragm, in which case the nature of the pleural effusion is similar to that of the ascitic fluid from which it derives. The passage is through mesothelium-lined channels, which are generally microscopic but may measure up to 5 mm.[40] The sudden development of a pleural effusion in association with ascites secondary to a pelvic tumour is known as Meig's syndrome (see p. 494). Hydrothorax is also recorded in patients with ascites secondary to cirrhosis[40] and in those undergoing peritoneal dialysis.[41] Ovarian stimulation undertaken for *in vitro* fertilisation is a more recently recognised cause of pleural effusion accompanying ascites.[42]

Chylothorax

Serous exudates due to lymphatic obstruction should be distinguished from the collection of chyle in the pleural space. The latter is due to obstruction or rupture of the thoracic duct. Chyle is rich in dietary fat and a chylous effusion appears milky (Fig. 13.3). Rupture of the thoracic duct is usually traumatic, while obstruction may be developmental, neoplastic or surgical, or due to rare conditions such as lymphangioleiomyomatosis (see p. 295), angiofollicular lymphoid hyperplasia (Castleman's disease, see p. 657) or the yellow-nail syndrome (see p. 75).[43] Pseudochylothorax may develop in a long standing serous exudate: this also looks milky and has a high content of cholesterol but it lacks the triglycerides and chylomicrons found in chyle.[44]

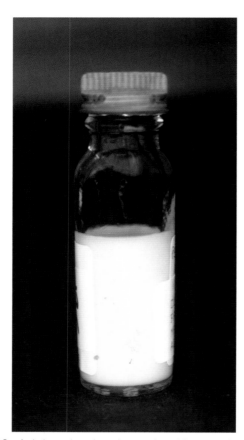

Figure 13.3   A chylous pleural exudate, aspirated from a patient with the yellow-nail syndrome.

Haemothorax

Haemorrhage into a pleural sac may follow trauma to the chest, pulmonary embolism or spontaneous rupture of an aneurysm of the thoracic aorta.[45] Occasionally, rupture of an emphysematous bulla is followed by haemopneumothorax, blood and air escaping simultaneously from the damaged lung into the sac.[46] Thoracic endometriosis may also cause haemopneumothorax (see p. 494).

Biliothorax (thoracobilia)

The removal of gallstones from the pleural cavity is one of the more unusual thoracic operations.[47] Such calculi enter the thorax by producing a cholecystopleural fistula. The accompanying bile is liable to cause a chemical pleuritis resulting in severe respiratory insufficiency.

PNEUMOTHORAX

Air may enter the pleural sac either through the chest wall or the visceral pleura. In the former case the condition is almost always due to trauma, a fractured clavicle or rib lacerating the parietal pleura and allowing the ingress of air through an associated wound of the skin. Sometimes, the local blood vessels may also be damaged and the condition becomes one of haemopneumothorax. In surgical operations on the thorax the pleural sac is often opened and allowed to fill with air. Formerly, air was deliberately introduced into the pleural sac in the treatment of chronic respiratory tuberculosis, to collapse and thus rest the lung (artificial pneumothorax). Further consideration will be limited to air entering the pleural sac through the visceral pleura.

Clinical features

Pneumothorax is usually sudden in onset, and often occurs during physical exertion. It is generally unilateral. Bilateral pneumothorax, which is not uncommon, is more serious since there is interference with the inflation of both lungs. The onset is painful, and quickly followed by shortness of breath, especially in patients with emphysema or other extensive chronic pulmonary disease that already impairs their respiratory capacity. In the cases in which the tissues create a valve at the site of perforation, the pneumothorax may build up slowly without any sudden symptoms; in these instances the displacement of the mediastinum is apt to be greater.

Epidemiology

Epidemiological studies show that men are affected more than women (in a ratio of 2.4 : 1), that there is a biphasic age distribution and that most deaths occur in older patients.[48] The reasons for this become apparent when one considers the pathogenesis of the condition.

Pathogenesis and pathological features

Escape of air into the pleural space from the lungs may be due to trauma or some pathological change in the lungs, usually emphysema. It causes the lung to collapse and if bilateral may prove fatal (see Fig. 7.2.5, p. 378). Rare conditions in which pneumothorax occurs particularly frequently include Langerhans cell histiocytosis of the lung (see p. 290), pulmonary lymphangioleiomyomatosis, (see p. 295) cystic fibrosis (see p. 65) and thoracic endometriosis (see p. 494). More recently, cystic necrosis of the lung resulting from advanced pneumocystis pneumonia (see p. 223) has been recognised as a cause of pneumothorax.[49]

Pneumothorax also occurs in healthy young individuals who appear to have normal lungs. This is known as spontaneous pneumothorax. When treatment in such cases has necessitated thoracotomy it has usually been found that at the apex of the lung there is an area of fibrosis, 2–3 cm in its greatest dimension, surmounted by one or more bullae up to 1 cm or so in diameter, the so-called apical cap.[50,51] A hole may be found in the pleural surface adjoining the bullae, or one of the latter may have a tear in its wall. Microscopy shows subpleural alveolar collapse and fibrosis, and an accumulation of chronic inflam-

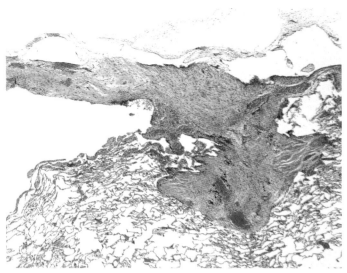

Figure 13.4 A bulla, rupture of which had caused pneumothorax, associated with a focus of subpleural alveolar collapse and fibrosis, the so-called apical cap. The overlying visceral pleura show reactive mesothelial hyperplasia and oedema.

matory cells (Fig. 13.4), but no evidence of tuberculosis or other specific disease. It has been suggested that, since most of these patients are tall, thin men, the changes in the apical region of the lungs – demonstrably affected bilaterally in some cases – may be developmental in origin and possibly related to rapid somatic growth. Their tall build will result in the apices of these individuals' lungs being particularly poorly perfused when they stand erect. This ischaemia may damage the apices directly or contribute to the fibrosis by impairing the resolution of any inflammatory process.[52] A developmental anomaly is suggested by the observation that spontaneous pneumothorax is often associated with minor anatomical anomalies of the bronchi[53] and rare familial cases are recorded.[54] Because the apical changes are frequently bilateral, there is often recurrence on the opposite side.

Irrespective of its initial pathogenesis, a pneumothorax may be *open* or *closed*: in the former, the aperture remains patent, so that air can pass freely into and out of the sac; in the latter, the opening soon becomes sealed, and thus traps the air that has entered. Once the air leak has been sealed, the air in the pleural sac is gradually absorbed over the ensuing weeks – oxygen first and nitrogen later. Occasionally – particularly in older people – the tissues near the orifice act as a valve, allowing air to enter but not to escape. In these cases pressure builds up in the sac, displacing the structures of the mediastinum to the opposite side, with consequent grave embarrassment of respiration. This is known as pressure or tension pneumothorax.

Pneumothorax causes a reactive mesothelial hyperplasia associated with an inflammatory infiltrate that is frequently rich in eosinophils and is sometimes called *'reactive eosinophilic pleuritis'*.[55,56] The infiltrate is superficial, penetrating only a short distance into the substance of the lung beneath the pleura: this distinguishes the process from eosinophilic granuloma of the lung (see p. 290) and eosinophilic pneumonia (see p. 461). Small

blood vessels may be involved but limitation of the process to the subpleural region of the lung distinguishes it from a true vasculitis.

If air is maintained in the pleural cavity for many months, as was once customary in the treatment of pulmonary tuberculosis, the mesothelium may undergo extensive squamous change. It is uncertain whether this represents metaplasia of the mesothelium, extension of metaplastic bronchial epithelium through a bronchopleural fistula or implantation of skin, but progression to malignancy has been noted.[57] In cystic fibrosis, focal replacement of the visceral pleural mesothelium by ciliated columnar or squamous epithelium has been described, possibly due to rupture of bronchiectatic abscesses[58] and perhaps contributing to the pathogenesis of pneumothorax in this condition.[59] Unexplained columnar or mucous cell metaplasia of the pleura has also been reported.[60]

Pleurodesis

If a patient suffers from repeated pneumothoraces, it may be necessary to obliterate the pleural cavity, a procedure termed *pleurodesis*. This may be effected surgically, by stripping the pleura, or by the instillation of sclerosing substances such as talc or tetracycline. Intractable pleural effusions may also require such treatment, especially in the palliation of malignant effusions. However, before performing pleurodesis consideration should be given to the possibility of the underlying condition requiring lung transplantation at some future date as pleurodesis would make this extremely difficult technically. The histological observation of a numerous birefringent crystals in a fibrotic pleura indicates that pleurodesis has been undertaken in the past. Neoplasia involving the chest wall 2 years after talc pleurodesis is recorded but the tumour was an adenocarcinoma of the peripheral lung rather than a pleural mesothelioma[61] and is therefore likely to have been coincidental, particularly as no mesotheliomas developed in any of 80 patients who had undergone talc pleurodesis 22–35 years previously.[62] Although commercial talc is often contaminated by tremolite asbestos and talc miners have developed mesothelioma, cosmetic talc and that used in medicine are rigorously screened to ensure their purity; they appear to be entirely non-carcinogenic.[63]

INFLAMMATION OF THE PLEURA (PLEURITIS, PLEURISY)

Inflammation of the pleural sac can develop in many conditions (Box 13.2). Usually, it is secondary to inflammation of one of the adjoining thoracic or subdiaphragmatic structures, particularly the lungs. Sometimes, it is a manifestation of systemic lupus erythematosus or another connective tissue disorder (see below). Asbestos causes pleural inflammation (see below) and certain drugs may also cause pleural inflammation and fibrosis (see p. 392). Eosinophilic pleuritis as a reaction to air in the pleural cavity has been mentioned above.

Box 13.2 Causes of pleural inflammation and fibrosis

Infection, particularly of the lungs
Other pulmonary lesions, e.g. infarction
Connective tissue disease
Drug reaction
Asbestos
Pneumothorax
Sarcoidosis
Pancreatitis
Post-cardiac injury (Dressler's syndrome)
Radiation
Renal failure
Trauma
Malignancy

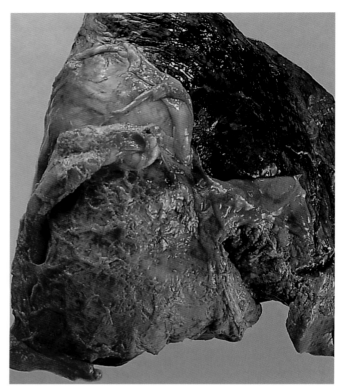

Figure 13.5 Empyema thoracis. There is shaggy fibrinopurulent thickening of both pleural surfaces over the lower lobe.

Acute inflammation of the pleura commences with hyperaemia, which is followed by exudation of fluid and leukocytes into the sac. Initially, before the exudate has fully formed, the pleurisy is dry (fibrinous pleurisy). This is accompanied by considerable pain on breathing and a rub that is audible on auscultation. With the development of an exudate (serofibrinous pleurisy) the visceral and parietal pleural surfaces separate and the pain and rub diminish. Should the cause be bacterial, the serofibrinous exudate may be replaced by a suppurative one, the cavity becoming filled by pus – the condition known as empyema thoracis or pyothorax (see below).

In many cases of serofibrinous pleurisy the inflammation regresses as time or treatment brings about recovery from the underlying disease. In such cases, the exudate is absorbed, and unless the pleura has been extensively denuded of its mesothelium the sac recovers its smooth lining. Where mesothelium has been lost, adhesions may form between the lung and the chest wall: at first the adhesions are fibrinous, but later, through organisation, they become fibrous. In this way, part or all of the cavity may be obliterated. This occasions no great disadvantage. However, an appreciable degree of diffuse fibrous thickening of the pleura of any cause impairs movement of the chest. Accordingly, bilateral diffuse pleural fibrosis has important clinical consequences. The causes are as numerous as those of pleuritis (Box 13.2) but asbestos is particularly important and the condition is therefore dealt with below under the heading of non-malignant asbestos-induced pleural disease.

The organisation of surface fibrin often involves the development of abundant granulation tissue and this may mimic sarcomatoid mesothelioma. The expression of keratin by spindle cell is generally taken as evidence that they are mesothelial rather than fibroblastic, and therefore indicative of mesothelioma, but the demonstration that reactive submesothelial spindle cells stain similarly[17] throws doubt on this. However, the supposition may remain valid if attention is confined to the deeper parts of the process for as granulation tissue matures away from the surface the intensity of the cytokeratin staining lessens.

Empyema thoracis (pyothorax)

Empyema thoracis represents a collection of pus in the pleural space (Fig. 13.5). It is usually a complication of pneumonia and with the widespread use of antibiotics is now rare. When it does occur there is usually some underlying debilitating condition such as diabetes or alcoholism, chronic lung disease such as bronchiectasis or carcinoma, or the patient is on long-term immunosuppressive therapy. In about one-third of cases the condition is associated with a necrotising pneumonia or 'primary' lung abscess, due to aspirated anaerobes (see p. 88). Often there is a mixture of bacteria, the predominant ones being the anaerobic or microaerophilic *Streptococcus milleri*, *Peptostreptococci*, *Peptococci*, *Fusobacterium nucleatum*, *Bacteroides melaninogenicus*, *Bacteroides fragilis*, clostridia, *Escherichia coli* and *Pseudomonas aeruginosa*.[64–67] *Klebsiella pneumoniae* is common in patients with diabetes mellitus,[68] whereas in children *Staphylococcus aureus* is common, the empyema generally complicating underlying staphylococcal pneumonia or pneumatocele (see p. 179). If it complicates a staphylococcal pneumatocele the empyema may be associated with pneumothorax. This combination is known as pyopneumothorax and may also develop when a cavitating rheumatoid nodule establishes a bronchopleural fistula.[69,70] Empyema may also follow thoracotomy, or less commonly thoracocentesis, penetrating injuries or rupture of the oesophagus during instrumentation or by a sharp foreign body. Blood-borne and transdiaphragmatic infection are rare causes of empyema.

In empyema thoracis, the whole of the sac or merely a part, usually the lower part, may be filled with thick viscous pus (Fig. 13.5). Sometimes the pus is confined to an interlobar fissure. Organisation of parts of the exudate leads to the formation of firm adhesions that restrict spread of the infection and localise the pus. Alternatively, the pus may extend into the lung and rupture into a bronchus leading to the sudden dissemination of infected material throughout the bronchial tree. If the patient survives this, there remains a chronic bronchopleural fistula. Occasionally, the pleural infection erodes the chest wall leading to discharge of pus through the skin (*empyema necessitans*).

Empyema thoracis is a serious condition which, if inadequately treated, has a high mortality. Sometimes infection is overcome without intervention, and the pus is eventually replaced by granulation tissue and fibrous tissue. Even in favourable cases the damage to the serosa is severe: when the suppuration subsides, fibrous adhesions develop and eventually obliterate the cavity. The lining of the cavity may undergo calcification during the succeeding years.

Tuberculosis of the pleura

Pleural involvement is common in tuberculosis, usually taking the form of an effusion in an apparently healthy young person soon after the primary infection. Pleural involvement may also complicate obvious active pulmonary tuberculosis or even apparently healed disease. The effusion is usually clear but occasionally blood-tinged. It contains numerous lymphocytes. Tubercle bacilli may be demonstrable, for the condition is truly infective rather than an allergic reaction as was once thought. Occasionally there is a dry painful pleurisy.

The pleura may be infected directly or by blood-borne spread from either the Ghon focus or caseous hilar lymph nodes. Bilateral effusion suggests blood spread but one pleural cavity may be infected directly from the other, as may the pericardium.

In the early stages of a tuberculous pleurisy, the appearance of the visceral and parietal serosal surfaces does not differ greatly from that seen in the usual serofibrinous form of pleurisy. Discrete miliary granulomas may stud the pleura but more often there is diffuse surface involvement. However, typical tubercles can be seen histologically. Pleural biopsy with both histological and bacteriological examination has a sensitivity of greater than 90%,[71] which is one reason why the condition is believed to be infective rather than allergic. Ultimately, there is caseation and in time, this may undergo calcification.

Even before effective antituberculosis drugs were available, such an effusion usually disappeared within 3–4 months, leaving at most a minor degree of obliteration of the costophrenic angle in the radiographs. However, some patients developed extensive thick rigid adhesions with consequent restriction of pulmonary ventilation.

A more severe form of tuberculous infection of the pleura may develop in the course of post-primary tuberculosis if a tuberculous cavity erodes into the pleural sac. The result is the

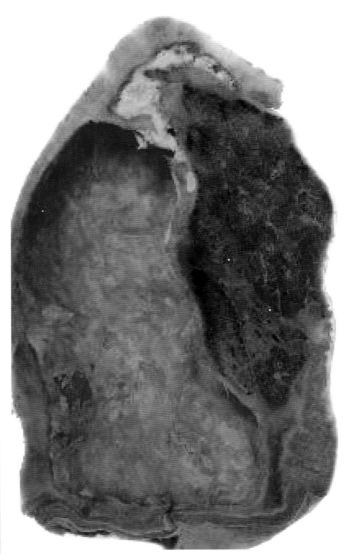

Figure 13.6 Tuberculous empyema. There is an extensive area of caseation between the thickened visceral and parietal layers of the pleura over the apex of the lung; elsewhere, the two layers are separated by fluid exudate that filled the large space between them. Compressed lung is seen on the right. (Reproduced by permission of the curator of the Gordon Museum, Guy's Hospital, London, UK.)

condition conventionally described as a *tuberculous empyema* (Fig. 13.6), although the semifluid matter that collects is caseous and not true pus, except when there is a simultaneous or subsequent infection by pyogenic bacteria. The exudate in the pleural sac becomes encased in a thick, fibrosing layer of tuberculous granulation tissue. The same condition may result from rupture of a juxtavertebral abscess in cases of tuberculosis of the thoracic spine. Similarly, tuberculosis of a rib may be complicated by pleural effusion or 'empyema'. Bronchopleural fistula may be present in association with tuberculous 'empyema'. This increases the liability to secondary infection, which in some cases is caused by fungi.[72]

The formerly common establishment of an artificial pneumothorax to rest a tuberculous lung has been mentioned above.

Other manipulations favoured in the past for the same purpose included the resection of several ribs (*thoracoplasty*) or the introduction of some inert material into the pleural sac, a procedure known as *plombage*: decades later, the patient may find worm-like threads of wax in his sputum,[73] or pathologists unfamiliar with this outdated procedure may be surprised to find one side of a deceased elderly patient's chest largely filled with what look remarkably like white billiard balls. More often, complications such as infection led to the removal of the plomb within a few years of its insertion.[74] Various forms of plombage material were favoured: plastic in the form of sponge or lucite spheres, packets of shredded plastic, and injections of paraffin wax or vegetable oil (*oleothorax*).[75] The development of carcinoma of the lung underlying lucite spheres is mentioned on p. 719.

Connective tissue disorders

Pleural involvement is common in rheumatoid disease and systemic lupus erythematosus, but rare in systemic sclerosis, polymyositis and dermatomyositis.[76]

Rheumatoid disease

Pleurisy and pleural effusions are the most common of the several respiratory manifestations of rheumatoid disease (see Box 10.1, p. 472). The pleural inflammation may be non-specific or represented by classic rheumatoid nodules.[77] Sometimes a subpleural rheumatoid nodule discharges into the pleural space and the characteristic palisade of cells forms a linear pattern over the surface of the pleura (Fig. 13.7).[78] An effusion, unilateral or bilateral, generally forms. This is an exudate, rich in immunoglobulins and other proteins, and sometimes cloudy or opalescent due to a high cholesterol content. Glucose levels in the fluid are low, apparently due to impaired glucose transport.[79] Lymphocytes are the predominant leukocytes, but sometimes there is a unique microscopical pattern – a combination of large elongated multinucleate cells, cholesterol crystals, clumps of eosinophilic granular material and a dearth of mesothelial cells.[80-82] The elongated cells are believed to come from the palisade layer of the granuloma. Their bizarre shape makes them liable to be mistaken for carcinoma cells. Rheumatoid pleural effusions are liable to become infected, sometimes resulting in empyema. At other times a cavitating intra-pulmonary rheumatoid nodule leads to the development of a bronchopleural fistula and pyopneumothorax.[69,70]

Systemic lupus erythematosus

Pleurisy, with or without effusion, is among the most common visceral manifestations of systemic lupus erythematosus, far exceeding pulmonary involvement in frequency. The pleural effusions are usually bilateral and the fluid is an exudate rich in proteins. Glucose concentrations are normal. The cells are usually unremarkable but occasionally lupus erythematosus

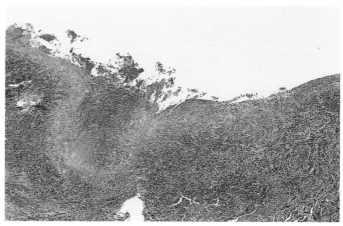

(a)

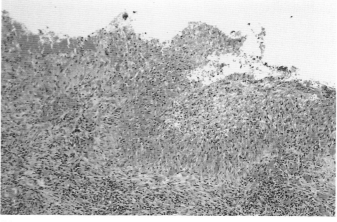

(b)

Figure 13.7 A rheumatoid nodule is seen discharging into the pleural space (a), following which the palisade of histiocytes fronts the pleural space rather than the centre of a granuloma (b).

(LE) cells may form. These are phagocytes that have taken up effete nuclear material so that their own nuclei are stretched around a large haemotoxyphil inclusion. Biopsy shows non-specific chronic inflammation or fibrosis.

NON-MALIGNANT ASBESTOS-INDUCED PLEURAL DISEASE

Besides asbestosis, carcinoma of the lung and pleural mesothelioma, respiratory disease attributable to the inhalation of asbestos includes pleurisy, which is generally accompanied by an effusion, and pleural fibrosis.[83] The latter takes several forms: distinctive plaques and less distinct pleural fibrosis that may be focal or diffuse.

In contrast to asbestosis and asbestos-induced lung cancer, both of which generally require relatively high exposure levels, all pleural diseases attributable to asbestos are associated with relatively low asbestos burdens in the lung.[84] Furthermore, it is very difficult to identify asbestos in the pleural lesions themselves although they are attributable to asbestos inhalation.

Benign asbestos pleurisy and pleural effusion

An exudative pleurisy may develop within 10 years of first contact with asbestos and therefore be found in persons currently at work in the industry. The effusion may be asymptomatic[83] or the patient may complain of pleuritic pain, sometimes accompanied by fever, leukocytosis and an elevated blood sedimentation rate.[85] The effusion is usually small and bloodstained, giving rise to suspicion of malignancy. It often resolves spontaneously, only to recur, perhaps on the other side. It may progress to diffuse pleural fibrosis that requires decortication.[85] Asbestos-induced pleurisy is thought to play no part in the development of pleural mesothelioma.

Asbestos-induced pleural fibrosis

Bilateral obliteration of the costophrenic angles is a common radiographic finding in healthy asbestos workers. It presumably reflects the organisation of previous asymptomatic effusions. Pleural fibrosis of non-specific character is common in such workers, and in those suffering from asbestosis a diffuse but thin fibrous thickening of the visceral pleura is almost invariably present. Indeed, apart from the presence of asbestos in the lungs, this is one of the few pathological features that distinguish asbestosis from idiopathic pulmonary fibrosis.

This thin fibrous thickening of the visceral pleura is of no clinical consequence but occasionally asbestos-exposed individuals develop extensive, thick fibrosis of the pleura in the absence of asbestosis (Fig. 13.8) and this may severely compromise expansion of the chest.[24,86–90] It may be bilateral or limited to one side.[91] If bilateral, the resultant restrictive defect in lung function is responsible for incapacitating breathlessness and this form of pleural fibrosis is one of the industrial diseases recognised by the British government for compensation purposes. Somewhat surprisingly in view of the comparatively small amounts of asbestos required to produce diffuse pleural fibrosis, carcinoma of the lung is also recognised as a prescribed industrial disease when it complicates such pleural fibrosis, but this is peculiar to the UK. Mesothelioma may develop in patients with such restrictive pleural fibrosis but the tumour is thought to arise independently. Diffuse pleural fibrosis is diagnosed when it is bilateral, over 5 mm thick and affects more than 25% of the pleura.[92] Although generally limited to the pleura, it occasionally extends into the chest wall[93] and mediastinum.[94] The lung parenchyma immediately beneath the thickened pleura may show diffuse interstitial fibrosis but this should not be interpreted as asbestosis unless there is also evidence of substantial asbestos exposure.

Asbestos-induced pleural fibrosis has to be distinguished from pleural plaque, which is described below, and from a cryptogenic form of bilateral fibrosing pleuritis that has been

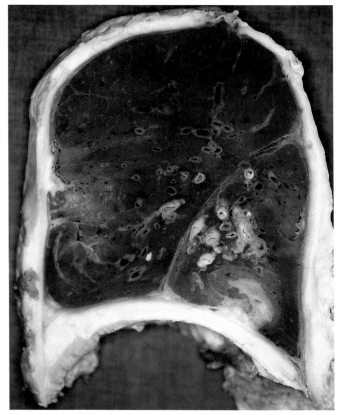

Figure 13.8 Diffuse thick fibrous thickening of the pleura in an asbestos worker. At the base of the lower lobe there is also a localised area of pleural thickening (Blesovsky's disease).

reported in a few patients in whom asbestos, systemic connective tissue disorders, tuberculosis and all other recognised causes of pleural fibrosis have been excluded.[95] Such cryptogenic diffuse pleural fibrosis has been reported in three sisters.[96] In other patients it has been associated with a thin rim of subpleural fibrosis.[97]

Blesovsky's disease (folded lung, rounded atelectasis)

Localised patches of pleural fibrosis may be important clinically, not for their functional effects, but because they may mimic a peripheral lung tumour radiographically. The contracture of the pleural scar draws the adjacent lung tissue to it, causing a localised area of collapse. The bases of the lungs are particularly affected (Table 13.1 and see Fig. 13.8).[98] The collapsed lung often appears to be folded upon itself and the resultant radiographic opacity has a comet's tail appearance. The condition is variously known as Blesovsky's disease, folded lung or rounded atelectasis.[24,98–102] In 25% of cases the lesion is bilateral.[91] There is often a history of asbestos exposure, but like the other forms of asbestos-induced pleural fibrosis, the condition is thought to play no part in the pathogenesis of mesothelioma.

Table 13.1 Lobar distribution of Blesovsky's disease in 100 reported cases[98]

	Right	Left
Upper lobe	2	3
Middle lobe/lingual	11	10
Lower lobe	47	27

Pleural plaques

Pleural plaques are a further form of asbestos-induced pleural fibrosis, described separately because of their distinctive pathological appearance.[24] Although they are occasionally found in persons with no history of asbestos exposure, the association with asbestos is a firm one, based on both epidemiological evidence[103,104] and the identification of asbestos in the underlying lung.[105] Pleural plaques therefore provide strong evidence of asbestos exposure, which may be occupational or environmental. They occur after exposure to all types of asbestos but anthophyllite is particularly potent. Plaques are common in areas where the soil is contaminated with asbestiform minerals, for example parts of Finland and Greece.[106,107] The longer and heavier the exposure, the more extensive the plaques, but even slight exposure can be sufficient. Very few develop within 15 years of first exposure and most appear after thirty years. Post mortem studies show that plaques are more common than can be appreciated from radiological examination in life.[103] Pleural plaques are harmless and have no relationship to mesothelioma, or lung cancer, other than their association with asbestos.[108]

Pathology

Plaques are localised raised areas that are generally multifocal and bilateral. They may occur on the visceral pleura or even the peritoneum[109] but usually affect the parietal pleura, particularly in relation to the ribs and the central tendon of the diaphragm. They have an irregular outline, a smooth shiny pearly-grey surface and a low profile, typically about 5 mm in height: their other dimensions are very variable (Fig. 13.9a). Microscopically, plaques are hyaline, avascular and almost acellular (Fig. 13.9b). In a pleural biopsy, even a small number of spindle cells in a hyaline lesion should suggest the possibility of paucicellular hyaline mesothelioma rather than plaque. The hyaline collagen bundles have a characteristic pattern that is often likened to basket weave. Calcification is common. Inflammation is not found, except at the periphery and there it is mild.

Pathogenesis

Although the connection between asbestos and plaques is firmly established, the pathogenetic mechanism is obscure. Organisation of exudates probably underlies the other less distinctive forms of pleural fibrosis found in asbestos workers but it is difficult to envisage a special type of exudate that may give rise to plaques. Furthermore, the plaques are covered by an

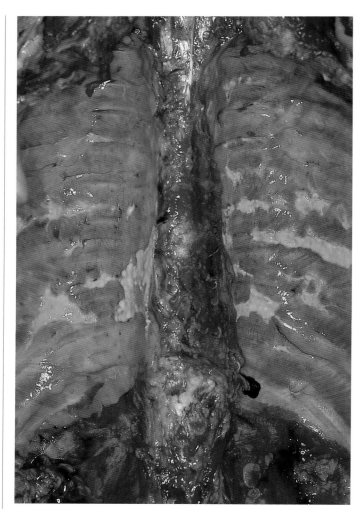

(a)

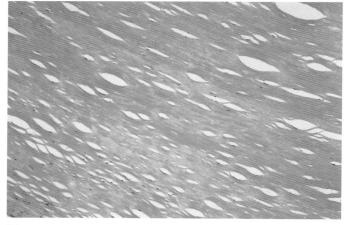

(b)

Figure 13.9 Pleural plaques. (a) The eviscerated thoracic cavity showing pearly white and irregular plaques on the inner side of the chest wall. (b) Microscopically, the plaques are practically acellular, consisting of hyaline collagen that has a 'basket-weave' pattern. They provide strong evidence of asbestos exposure.

intact mesothelium and are not usually attended by adhesions. It has been suggested that the parietal pleura is particularly affected because it is abraded by asbestos fibres projecting through the visceral pleura, but no such projections have been identified. A further possibility derives from consideration of the lymphatic drainage of the pleural cavity, which is largely through the parietal pleura. Short asbestos fibres have been identified in the visceral pleura[110] and indeed, in small numbers as ferruginous bodies in plaques.[111] It is likely that some short asbestos fibres reach the pleural cavity, whence their disposal would be by the stomata and lymphatics of the parietal pleura (see p. 691). Any fibres arrested by the ribs or the tendinous portion of the diaphragm would elicit submesothelial fibrosis at these sites.[24]

PLEURAL TUMOURS

Pleuropulmonary blastoma is dealt with on p. 612 and this section will consider only those tumours that are initially confined to the pleura, of which mesothelioma is by far the most important.

Mesothelioma

Mesotheliomas arise most commonly in the pleura but also develop in the peritoneum and occasionally in the pericardium or tunica vaginalis of the testis.[112,113] They are malignant neoplasms: the terms benign fibrous mesothelioma and multicystic mesothelioma are misnomers in that the former is not of mesothelial origin and the latter is not neoplastic (see localised fibrous tumour on p. 714 and multicystic mesothelioma on p. 714). A benign mesothelial neoplasm is encountered in the peritoneum and rarely in the pleura but is termed adenomatoid tumour rather than benign mesothelioma (see p. 714). Well-differentiated papillary mesothelioma is a low-grade mesothelioma that warrants separate consideration (see p. 713).

Incidence

Mesothelioma was very rare in the nineteenth and early twentieth centuries. Indeed, as late as the 1950s, some eminent authorities denied its existence. However, it is now recognised to be one of the most important occupational diseases. Its incidence has been steadily rising and in industrialised countries mesothelioma now accounts for about 1% of all cancer deaths. Measures to curtail exposure to its principal cause, asbestos, were introduced and progressively strengthened in many countries in the latter half of the twentieth century but such is the long latent interval between exposure and disease that these do not have an effect for several decades. The durability of asbestos is another factor hampering efforts to reduce the incidence of mesothelioma. It is calculated that the numbers in Britain will triple between 1991 and 2020 and only then decline.[114] In contrast, there is already a decline in the incidence of mesothelioma in the USA where the use of amphibole asbestos was restricted as early as the 1960s.[115]

Aetiology

In the mid-twentieth century, it was increasingly suspected that mesothelioma was related to asbestos exposure and substance was given to this in 1960, when Wagner and colleagues showed a high incidence of the tumour in the area near Kimberley, northern Cape province, South Africa where blue asbestos is mined.[116] The relationship between asbestos exposure and mesothelioma was subsequently confirmed in other countries where asbestos is mined and in those that import and process the ore.[117–121] Asbestos and similar fibrous substances are virtually the only recognised causes of mesothelioma. Smoking does not increase the risk of mesothelioma. Cases that can be attributed to causes such as radiation, chronic inflammation and scarring are exceptionally rare.[116,122-127] However, there is evidence suggesting that simian virus 40 (SV40) promotes the development of mesothelioma, acting either independently or synergistically with asbestos. This virus contaminated monkey kidney cells used in the manufacture of early batches of poliomyelitis vaccine and may have reached man in this way. SV40 sequences are selectively expressed in many mesotheliomas, the development of which has been attributed to the ability of the sequences to inactivate the p53 and Rb tumour suppressor genes and promote the secretion of various growth factors.[128–130] However, subsequent investigations have resulted in both supportive and contrary findings[131–136] and the relationship of SV40 infection to development of mesotheliomas remains uncertain.

The risk of mesothelioma is substantial in the mining, transportation and processing of asbestos but is dose-related and can be minimised by precautionary measures based on good industrial hygiene. The principal manufacturing industries using asbestos are those producing items such as specialised cement products, insulating materials and brake linings. All industries applying and re-fitting asbestos insulation carry a potential risk and many cases have been seen in construction and demolition work, ship-fitting and other dockyard work, and railway carriage maintenance. Many joiners, heating engineers, boilermen, railwaymen and former naval servicemen have been exposed unknowingly,[137] while some exposure is para-occupational, incurred by men such as shipyard welders who work alongside those applying or stripping asbestos. The families of asbestos workers are also at increased risk through being exposed to asbestos dust carried home on work clothes. Such exposure may occur very early in life.[138] Others appear to have developed mesothelioma because they live in the vicinity of asbestos mines or factories, but it is always difficult to exclude occupational, para-occupational or domestic exposure in such cases.[139,140] However, environmental exposure undoubtedly occurs in parts of the world such as Turkey and the Metsovo region of Greece where the soil contains asbestos,[106,107,141,142] and town dwellers are subjected to continuous low levels of asbestos exposure from such sources as brake linings. Thus, exposure to asbestos may be:

- direct, from the handling of asbestos ore or its products
- paraoccupational, from working alongside asbestos workers, as in shipyards
- household, for example from the clothes of an asbestos worker
- neighbourhood, from living near an asbestos mine or factory
- ambient.

The carcinogenicity of asbestos depends on its physical properties and it is notable that not all forms of asbestos carry the same risk of mesothelioma.[143] The various types of asbestos have been described on p. 345 where a broad division was drawn between the serpentine chrysotile (white asbestos) and the straight-fibred amphiboles, crocidolite (blue asbestos), amosite (brown asbestos), anthophyllite, tremolite and actinolite. Chrysotile accounts for more than 90% of all asbestos used and of the others only crocidolite and amosite are now produced commercially. The principal cause of mesothelioma in Britain is crocidolite, while in North America, it is amosite. Chrysotile is thought not to cause mesothelioma[144,145] and the few mesotheliomas associated with this form of asbestos are probably due to contamination of the chrysotile by tremolite.[146-148] Contamination with tremolite is also the probable explanation of the occasional mesotheliomas observed in talc and vermiculate miners[146] and of mesotheliomas reported in Southeast Turkey amongst inhabitants of houses whitewashed with a non-asbestiform ore.[149]

The particular physical properties of asbestos that determine its carcinogenicity are fibre diameter, length and biodegradability. Its dimensions determine whether a fibre reaches the lung and all three factors determine whether it is retained there or cleared. Fibres thinner than $0.25\,\mu m$ and longer than $5\,\mu m$ carry the greatest risk of mesothelioma.[150] The curly chrysotile fibres tend to settle in large airways and to be eliminated by ciliary action, while those that reach the lung break up more readily than the amphiboles and are cleared more rapidly. Because of this, a former chrysotile miner may ultimately have more tremolite than chrysotile in his lungs although the tremolite is only a contaminant of the mined ore.

The physical properties of asbestos not only govern whether it reaches, and is cleared from the lung but are also responsible for its carcinogenicity. Thus, whereas the injection of fibrous tremolite into the pleural cavity of rats produced mesotheliomas, an equal dose of non-asbestiform tremolite did not.[151]

Fibrous minerals other than asbestos may have fibres of the same shape and size as the dangerous amphibole forms of asbestos. In central Turkey a high incidence of mesothelioma is associated with environmental exposure to erionite, which is a fine fibrous form of the volcanic silicate, zeolite.[110] In inhalation experiments, erionite exceeds asbestos in its ability to induce mesotheliomas.[152] Much attention therefore centres on the many other naturally occurring fibrous minerals, some of which are in commercial use as oil absorbents or cat litter, and on man-made fibres.[153] Fortunately, many of these fibres are not in the respirable range but the potential dangers are shown by the high incidence of mesothelioma in rats injected with fibreglass particles of respirable size.[154,155] A variety of bronchopulmonary abnormalities is reported in workers exposed to fine fibreglass[156] but so far at least there have been no convincing reports of man-made fibres causing cancer in man.[157-159]

Susceptibility to mesothelioma is probably influenced by genetic factors. Thus, the prevalence of mesotheliomas induced experimentally with asbestos was found to vary according to the strain of mice studied.[160] Genetic factors are also suggested by the development of mesothelioma in families[161,162] but it must be remembered that one family member may inadvertently expose others to asbestos, for example by bringing home soiled work clothes.

The age incidence of mesothelioma is largely determined by the time at which an individual is first exposed to asbestos and the latent interval between exposure and presentation, which is generally over 20 years with a mean of about 40 years, but may be as short as 15 years.[163-165] Where environmental exposure occurs from birth, mesotheliomas start to develop from about the age of 14.[166] The cause of mesotheliomas occurring in younger children is unknown.[167-170] Cases without evidence of asbestos exposure are touched upon again below.

The sex incidence of mesothelioma is also largely determined by asbestos exposure, men greatly outnumbering women, a difference that is not so marked in the rare cases where asbestos does not appear to be involved. In all other respects mesothelioma in women is identical to mesothelioma in men.[171]

The cumulative dose of asbestos is of greater importance than the duration of exposure: short periods of high exposure can be very hazardous. Some women who developed mesotheliomas after making military gas masks in Nottingham during the Second World War had only short periods of exposure, in some cases as little as three months, but their exposure was heavy. Nevertheless, the level of exposure necessary to cause pleural mesothelioma is far less than that required to cause asbestosis (see Table 7.1.3, p. 349). Peritoneal tumours are generally associated with heavy exposure and the proportion of mesotheliomas arising in the peritoneum diminishes as occupational hygiene improves: in one asbestos manufacturing company the ratio of peritoneal to pleural tumours fell from 5 : 1 before 1921 to 1 : 3 after 1950.[172] The proportion of peritoneal cases has always been low in mining. Ingested asbestos fibres do not penetrate the walls of the gastrointestinal tract, and peritoneal mesothelioma is presumed to be caused by inhaled asbestos crossing both the pleura and the diaphragm.[173]

The assessment of asbestos load is described on p. 347 but a simple first step is to examine thick ($20-30\,\mu m$) unstained sections of the lungs for asbestos bodies. In cases of mesothelioma, the presence of as few as one asbestos body in a standard $5\,\mu m$ thick section of lung is regarded as evidence of substantial exposure,[174-176] obviating the need for more sophisticated procedures. However, an inability to identify asbestos bodies in histological sections does not exclude asbestos causation.

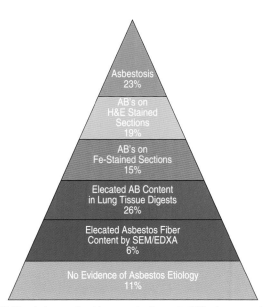

Figure 13.10 Asbestos load in mesothelioma. In 23% of cases asbestosis is evident, in another 19% there is no pulmonary fibrosis but asbestos bodies can be identified in standard sections, in a further 15% asbestos bodies are detected when iron stains are employed, in a further 26% asbestos body counts in lung digests are elevated, in a further 6% excess asbestos fibre is found when lung digests are examined by scanning electron microscopy, leaving 11% in which a link with asbestos cannot be established.[181,183] (Figure provided by Professor V Roggli, Durham, USA.)

Even after an exhaustive occupational history and the most detailed analysis, some mesotheliomas provide no evidence of asbestos exposure or other cause whatsoever. The proportion of such cases varies considerably, probably depending upon the degree of industrialisation so that in a non-industrialised country the low background incidence becomes important. In Britain and the USA, 10–20% of mesotheliomas appear to be unrelated to asbestos exposure.[177–182] One group reported that asbestos bodies were identified in histological sections in 57% of mesothelioma cases, that the figure reached 83% when asbestos bodies were sought in lung digests by light microscopy and 89% when electron microscopy was used to identify coated and uncoated fibres in lung digests (Fig. 13.10).[181,183] Another group, which confined their attention to a careful occupational history or the presence of asbestos bodies in lung sections, identified asbestos exposure in 87% of cases.[182]

Evidence that there is a low background of mesothelioma unrelated to asbestos derives from several sources:

- mortality trends in industrialised countries record an equal sex incidence in the early twentieth century
- the subsequent increase is largely confined to men
- mesothelioma in childhood is rare, but well established[169,170]
- non-asbestos fibrous minerals of the type known to cause mesothelioma in Turkey are widespread and could conceivably cause sporadic disease elsewhere
- although rare, associations with possible causes such as radiotherapy and chronic infection are recorded.[121–126]

Clinical features

Mesothelioma is more common in men, reflecting their greater exposure to asbestos. It generally presents after the age of 50 years but may arise at any age.

Patients with pleural mesothelioma complain of continuous chest pain due to infiltration of the chest wall and dyspnoea due to pleural effusion or encasement of the lung by tumour restricting chest movement. The effusion is often blood-stained. Mediastinal infiltration may result in superior vena caval compression, Horner's syndrome or recurrent laryngeal nerve palsy.[184] Invasion of the spinal canal may cause paraplegia.[185] Chest radiographs typically show diffuse pleural thickening on the affected side but at first the tumour may be localised or multifocal. Symptoms due to metastases generally develop only terminally, if at all, but rarely they are the initial manifestation of the disease.[186–188]

Pleural aspiration

As well as relieving breathlessness, aspiration of pleural fluid can be helpful diagnostically, particularly in the recognition of metastatic tumour:[189,190] its sensitivity in the diagnosis of mesothelioma depends upon the expertise of the cytologist and a biopsy is often preferred.[191]

Exfoliated cells may be examined in films in the conventional way or concentrated into cell blocks, which may be sectioned for light or electron microscopy. Immunocytochemical procedures (see below) may be applied to either smears or sections of these cells.[192–194] Pleural fluid is particularly suitable for flow cytometry, cytogenetic and molecular studies and scanning electron microscopy.[195,196]

The cytological diagnosis of adenocarcinoma or other types of metastatic tumour in serous effusions is often relatively straightforward for in addition to reactive mesothelial cells, recognisable by their microvillous border and denser perinuclear staining, a separate population of malignant cells can be recognised.[197–199] However, the distinction between benign and malignant mesothelial cells is notoriously difficult.[191] Reactive mesothelial cells can be alarmingly large and binucleate or multinucleate. The nuclear-cytoplasmic ratio is often not significantly increased in mesothelioma but nuclear irregularity and prominent multiple nucleoli may suggest malignancy. A feature particularly suggestive of epithelioid mesothelioma is the presence of papillary aggregates or morulae containing up to a hundred or so cells and having a scalloped edge (Fig. 13.11).

Although attention is usually concentrated on the cellular component, the supernatant fluid can also be informative. Many mesotheliomas, but not carcinomas, secrete hyaluronic acid which can then reach high levels in the pleural fluid.[200] Conversely, the demonstration of carcinoembryonic antigen in a pleural effusion favours metastatic carcinoma.[201–203]

Macroscopic features

Pleural mesothelioma is commoner on the right than the left, in a ratio of 3:2.[182] The reason for this is poorly understood but may

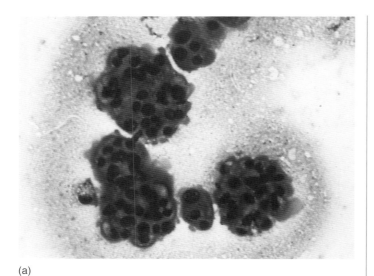

(a)

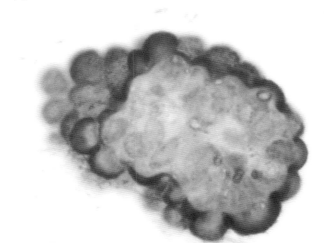

(b)

Figure 13.11 Mesothelioma in a pleural aspirate. (a) The exfoliated malignant cells are clumped together in so-called morulae. (b) The cells stain strongly for epithelial membrane antigen, a feature supportive but not diagnostic of malignancy.

depend upon differences in fibre burden, pleural area and chest wall movement on the two sides.

Asbestos fibres reaching the pleural cavity are concentrated in Kampmeier's foci (see p. 692)[10] and thoracoscopy has shown that mesothelioma typically first involves the parietal pleura where these foci are found, appearing there as multiple small grape-like nodules: involvement of the visceral pleura follows.[204] Progression of the tumour results in coalescence of the nodules to form plaques and, ultimately, a continuous sheet of tumour fusing the visceral and parietal pleura and obliterating the pleural space (Fig. 13.12), except for occasional residual loculi containing glairy fluid or blood. Areas of necrosis or haemorrhage and softer areas of mucoid consistency may be seen and occasionally the whole tumour appears gelatinous. In

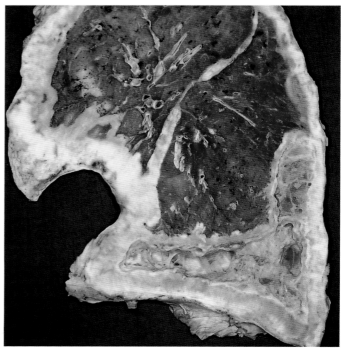

Figure 13.12 Pleural mesothelioma. Dense white tumour encases the lung and spreads along a fissure.

the late stage, tumour encases the lung as a layer of dense white tissue up to several centimetres thick, which extends into fissures and infiltrates the peripheral lung parenchyma so that at autopsy the lung has to be forcibly dissected from the chest wall. It is very rare for a mesothelioma to remain localised and form a solitary mass.[205–209] A feature of mesothelioma that is often stressed is a supposed predilection to infiltrate along biopsy tracks or surgical incisions, but this is a feature of all malignant tumours.[210] Metastasis is late but at death may be widespread (see below).

Microscopic features

Needle biopsy of the pleura is often disappointing and a firm diagnosis of mesothelioma is sometimes not possible until thoracoscopic or open biopsy, or rarely autopsy is undertaken. Reactive mesothelial cells may form loose aggregates and it is important that in small biopsies these are not mistaken for true papillae, which are suggestive but not pathognomonic of mesothelioma.[198,211]

Despite their epithelioid appearance, mesothelial cells are of mesodermal origin and their malignant counterparts display a wide diversity of differentiation, which has led to the alternative name of mesodermoma being suggested.[212–214] This diversity is reflected in the traditional histological classification of mesotheliomas as epithelioid, sarcomatoid (or fibrous) and biphasic (or mixed).[215] The epithelioid type is the commonest in

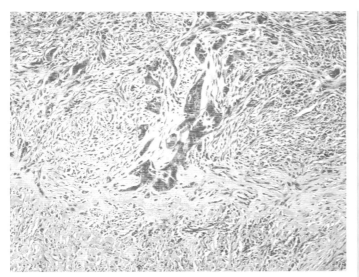

Figure 13.13 Biphasic mesothelioma comprising both epithelioid and sarcomatoid elements.

most series[216,217] but widespread sampling of the tumour, which is possible post mortem, increases the proportion of biphasic tumours.[218]

A mixed (biphasic) pattern combining the epithelioid and sarcomatoid features described below is the classic pattern of mesothelioma (Fig. 13.13). The two components often merge where they meet and the combination makes a distinctive picture that presents few diagnostic problems (which are considered below).

In well-differentiated tumours of purely epithelioid type a tubulopapillary pattern is most commonly seen (Fig. 13.14), but the pattern may be purely tubular, composed of well-formed glandular spaces, or papillary, in which small, irregular, cystic spaces are lined by tumour cells and filled by papillary projections with delicate cores of connective tissue and a covering of tumour cells. As in other papillary neoplasms, psammoma bodies (calcospherites) may be formed. Mesothelioma may also be strikingly glandular in morphology (Fig. 13.15) Individual tumour cells are generally cuboidal or polygonal with moderate amounts of eosinophilic cytoplasm and round nuclei containing a single nucleolus. Sometimes they are peg-shaped, with only a narrow base (Fig. 13.16). In many cases mitoses are infrequent and there may be little cellular pleomorphism. Occasionally there is atypia but no evidence of invasive activity: this appears to be a premalignant state.[219] The term mesothelioma-*in-situ* has been introduced to describe such changes but it is recommended by its originator that the term should only be used when the surface changes are accompanied by invasive tumour (Fig. 13.17).[220] Vacuoles may develop within the cytoplasm of tumour cells, compressing the nuclei and simulating signet-ring cell carcinoma.[221] In some tumours the glands are lined by flattened cells, giving the tumour a lace-like microcystic appearance (Fig. 13.18). The stroma around the tumour cells is typically myxoid and may be abundant, with wide

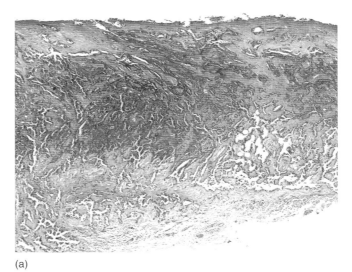

(a)

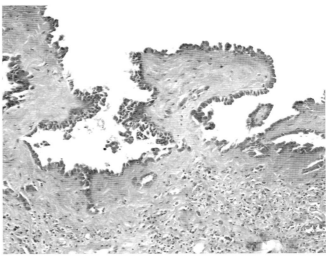

(b)

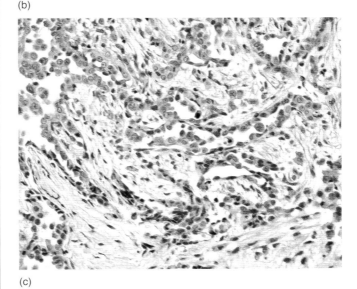

(c)

Figure 13.14 Variants of epithelioid mesothelioma. (a) Tubulopapillary, the most commonly seen pattern. (b) Papillary foci are seen on the surface. (c) with a tubular pattern invading the stroma.

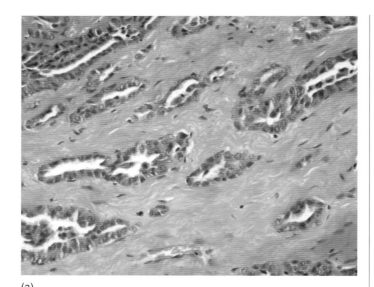

(a)

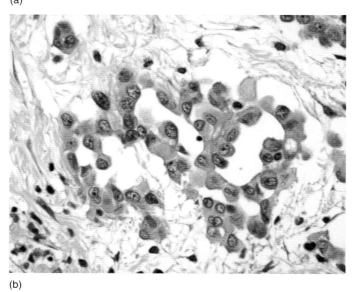

(b)

Figure 13.15 Variants of epithelioid mesothelioma. The mesotheliomatous glands closely resemble those of an adenocarcinoma. In (a) the stroma is fibrous while in (b) it is myxoid.

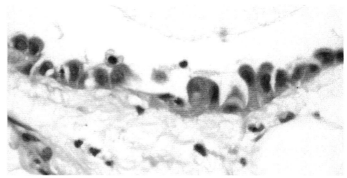

Figure 13.16 Mesothelioma of epithelioid pattern. Note that some of the tumour cells are peg-shaped.

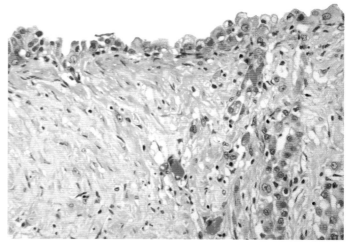

Figure 13.17 Mesothelioma-*in-situ*. This term should only be used when there is unequivocal invasion adjacent to the surface proliferation (as there is on the right).

separation of the gland spaces, although it may also show sclerosis (see Fig. 13.15). Undifferentiated epithelioid mesotheliomas often consist of sheets of cells with abundant eosinophilic cytoplasm but few other characteristic features and little intervening stroma (Fig. 13.17). Alternatively, there may be little cytoplasm and a focal resemblance to small cell carcinoma.[222,223] The diversity of these tumours is shown by reports of focal trophoblastic differentiation and chorionic gonadotrophin secretion,[224,225] or the tumour having a deciduoid,[226–229a] small cell,[222] rhabdoid[230] or clear cell[231,232] phenotype (Fig. 13.18). Their diversity is further emphasised by reports of chromogranin being demonstrated immunocytochemically in mesotheliomas of glandular pattern.[233]

In the sarcomatoid (fibrous) type of mesothelioma the cells are spindle-shaped and set in a varying amount of collagenised stroma so that the cellularity varies greatly. Markedly pleomorphic, cellular foci showing mitotic activity are indistinguishable from other forms of undifferentiated sarcoma or the tumour may consist of bland spindle cells widely scattered in a densely collagenised stroma constituting the so-called desmoplastic variant, which may be very difficult to distinguish from scar tissue (Fig. 13.19). Cartilaginous, osseous, muscular or fatty differentiation is occasionally seen and, if no epithelioid elements are present, the tumour may resemble a primary sarcoma of one of these tissues (Fig. 13.20).[212,213,234–237] However, it is uncommon for these heterologous patterns to dominate the histological picture and the adoption of nomenclature such as osteosarcoma of the pleura for an otherwise typical mesothelioma in an asbestos worker is inappropriate and may prejudice a justifiable claim for industrial compensation. Rare cases showing a

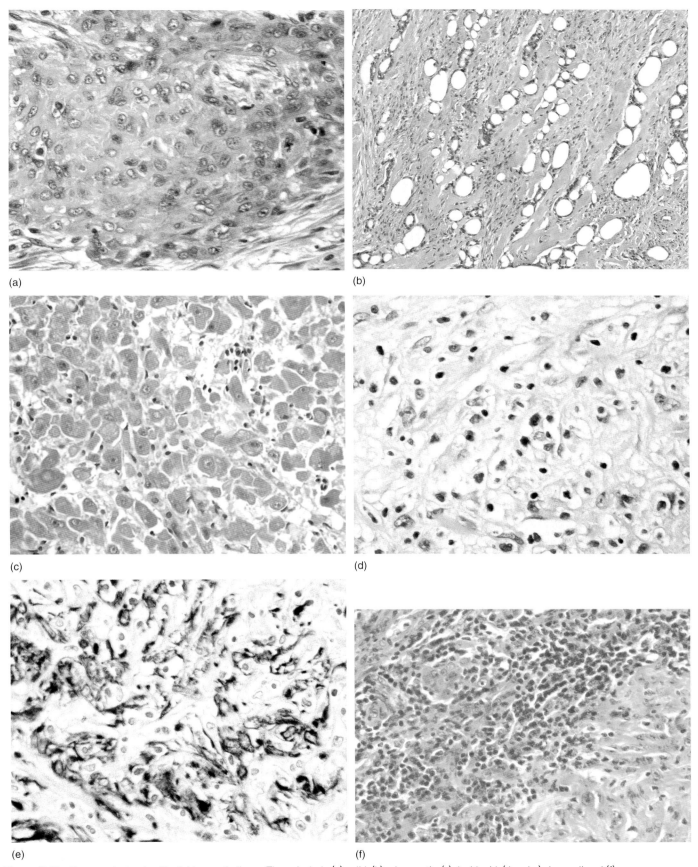

Figure 13.18 Rarer variants of epithelioid mesothelioma. These include (a) solid, (b) microcystic, (c) deciduoid, (d and e) clear cell and (f) lymphohistiocytoid. (Fig. (e), cytokeratin stain).

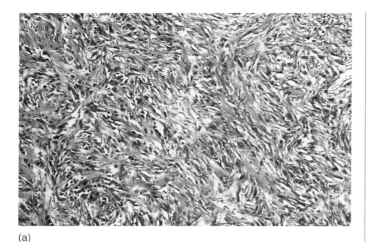

(a)

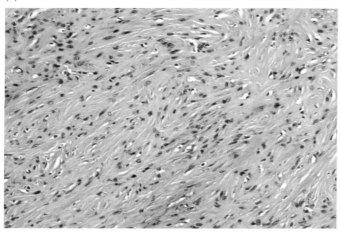

(b)

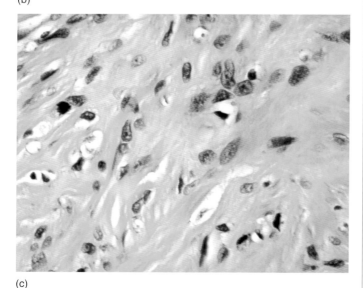

(c)

Figure 13.19 Sarcomatoid (fibrous) mesothelioma. (a) A cellular spindle cell tumour showing pleomorphism and other cytological features of malignancy. (b) The desmoplastic variant showing densely hyaline fibrosis and little cellularity. The distinction from scar tissue depends on finding atypical cytokeratin-positive spindle cells. A lack of zonation, a storiform pattern, numerous mitoses (c) and foci of necrosis are further features suggestive of malignancy.

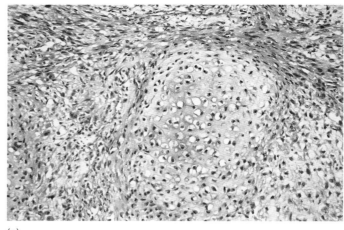

(a)

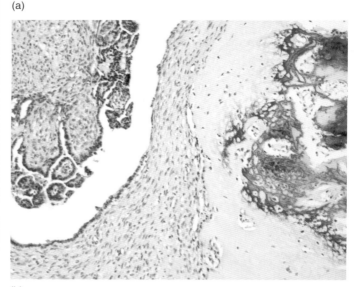

(b)

Figure 13.20 (a) Cartilaginous and (b) osseous differentiation in a sarcomatoid mesothelioma.

marked lymphohistiocytoid reactive infiltrate have been mistakenly diagnosed as lymphomas.[238,239]

Mesotheliomas frequently evince distinctive features when stained for mucus or examined by immunocytochemistry or electron microscopy. These procedures are often invaluable in the differential diagnosis of a tumour involving the serous cavities of the body and will now be considered.

Differential diagnosis of mesothelioma

The classic gross appearance of a pleural mesothelioma, that of a firm pale tumour encasing the lung, may be mimicked by extensive pleural fibrosis or by a peripheral carcinoma of the lung growing along the pleura – so-called pseudomesotheliomatous carcinoma of the lung,[240–242] as well as other tumours growing in a similar manner (see Fig. 12.3.21, p. 626).[243,244] Each

is glandular the problem is similar to that encountered in distinguishing metastatic adenocarcinoma from mesothelioma of purely epithelioid type, which is considered next: the special techniques considered in the next section are equally applicable to the epithelial component of a sarcomatoid carcinoma or biphasic synovial sarcoma. Synovial sarcomas also stain for bcl-2 protein,[250] which is only rarely expressed in mesothelioma, and show an x:18 translocation, which is not seen in mesothelioma.

2. Epithelioid mesothelioma versus adenocarcinoma

Mucin stains afford one of the simplest and most effective means of distinguishing epithelioid mesotheliomas from carcinomas (Box 13.3). Mesotheliomas do not produce the epithelial mucins so often seen in adenocarcinomas and the periodic acid-Schiff (PAS) stain is therefore a useful first step in this differential diagnosis (Fig. 13.21). The presence of PAS-positive mucin within tumour cells or glands is generally regarded as excluding a diagnosis of mesothelioma, although rare exceptions to this are reported in which crystals of hyaluronic acid are responsible for the PAS-positivity.[113,221,251,252] PAS-positive material in mesotheliomas may also represent basement membranes rather than epithelial mucin.[253] Attention should therefore be confined to the contents of the glands or cytoplasmic vacuoles: finely granular cytoplasmic PAS-positivity should be disregarded. Diastase predigestion is essential because mesotheliomas are frequently rich in glycogen, occasionally to the extent that the tumour cells have abundant clear cytoplasm.[254]

The glycosaminoglycan hyaluronic acid is an acid mucopolysaccharide produced by both normal and neoplastic mesothelial cells. Alcian blue (pH 2.5) can be used to demonstrate its presence on the apical surface of tumour cells, and within glandular spaces and intracellular vacuoles: the staining is abolished by prior treatment with hyaluronidase, in contrast to acidic glycoproteins produced by some adenocarcinomas.[255] Attention must be confined to the epithelial component because stromal glycosaminoglycans include hyaluronic acid. Fixation in alcohol or cetyl pyridyl formalin is desirable as it preserves hyaluronic acid, which is water-soluble and may be leached out by prolonged fixation in aqueous solutions.

Mucicarmine stains both epithelial mucin and hyaluronic acid and has no place in the distinction of mesothelioma from adenocarcinoma unless hyaluronidase controls are employed.[256]

These traditional mucus stains are now widely augmented, or indeed replaced, by immunohistochemical staining (Box 13.3). Antibodies of diagnostic utility fall into two groups, those that recognise epithelial epitopes and those that recognise mesothelial characteristics. The first group includes antibodies against carcinoembryonic antigen (CEA), Leu-M1, B72.3, AUA1, BerEP4, MOC-31 and E-cadherin. Some of these reagents are not without their critics and it is best to employ a panel of such antibodies. Hyaluronic acid may account for some spuriously positive immunocytochemical results so these procedures may be worth repeating after predigestion with hyaluronidase.[256] The commonest adenocarcinoma mimicking mesothelioma is that arising in the underlying lung and antibodies specific to the

---

Box 13.3 Staining characteristics of mesothelioma and adenocarcinoma

Mesothelioma	Adenocarcinoma
Cytoplasm contains glycogen	Glycogen content is small
No diastase-resistant PAS-positive material	May contain diastase-resistant PAS-positive mucin
Alcianophilic hyaluronic acid in glands or on tumour cell surface	No hyaluronic acid within or on tumour cells
CEA, Leu M₁, BerEp4 and AUA1 negative	CEA, Leu M₁, BerEP4 and AUA1 positive
EMA positive at cell membrane	EMA positive in cytoplasm and at cell periphery
Cytokeratin 5/6, thrombomodulin and calretinin positive[a]	Cytokeratin 5/6, thrombomodulin and calretinin negative

[a]Attention should be confined to nuclear staining as cytoplasmic staining is nonspecific.

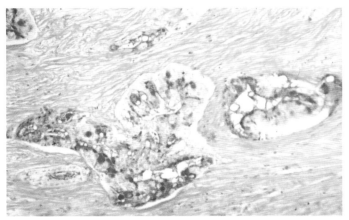

Figure 13.21   Metastatic adenocarcinoma. A diastase-controlled periodic acid Schiff stain is strongly positive, confirming that the tumour is a metastatic adenocarcinoma rather than an epithelioid mesothelioma.

of the histological types of mesothelioma presents its own diagnostic problems. A distinction has to drawn between:

1 Biphasic mesothelioma and other biphasic tumours
2 Epithelioid mesothelioma and adenocarcinoma
3 Epithelioid mesothelioma and reactive mesothelial hyperplasia
4 Sarcomatoid mesothelioma and other spindle cell tumours
5 Sarcomatoid mesothelioma and fibrosis.

These will now be considered in turn.

1. Biphasic mesothelioma versus other biphasic tumours

The distinctive biphasic pattern of the mixed type of mesothelioma presents few diagnostic problems, but pleural involvement by sarcomatoid carcinoma[245,246] or biphasic synovial sarcoma[247–249] may need to be considered, although both are rare and generally form localised rather than diffuse growths. The key to distinguishing these tumours from mesotheliomas of mixed pattern lies in their epithelioid component: if this is squamous, sarcomatoid carcinoma can be assumed, but if it

lung such as those reacting with surfactant apoprotein and TTF-1 are therefore helpful.[257,258]

Monoclonal antibodies that react with mesotheliomas but seldom with adenocarcinomas are now available and have recently been reviewed.[259] These include those directed against cytokeratin 5/6, thrombomodulin and calretinin. N-cadherin and Wilms tumour suppressor gene 1 are also promising but initial enthusiasm for HMBE1, OV632, mesothelin and CD44 hyaluronate receptor has waned. More recently MUC-4 has also been reported as being highly specific for mesothelioma.[260] With calretinin it is important to confine attention to the nuclei of the malignant cells as cytoplasmic staining is far less specific for cells of mesothelial origin (Fig. 13.22).

However, while these antibodies are relatively dependable in distinguishing mesothelioma from adenocarcinoma, they are not so dependable in relation to other carcinomas of the lung. They not infrequently stain squamous cell, small cell, large cell and giant cell carcinomas,[261,262] but most of these are distinguishable on their morphology and their expression of other epitopes such as TTF-1. Extrapulmonary carcinomas that may express these 'mesothelial' markers include transitional cell and renal cell carcinomas, the latter exceptional in also failing to express the epithelial marker CEA. Results obtained with 'mesothelial' markers therefore need to be viewed with some caution and assessed in conjunction with clinical, radiological and morphological features.[263,264] Separation of the rare clear cell type of mesothelioma[231,232] from metastatic clear cell carcinoma of the kidney can be problematical. A combination of negative Leu-M1 and positive thrombomodulin immunostaining in the former and the reverse in the latter have been reported,[265] whilst others have found calretinin more specific than thrombomodulin.[263]

In distinguishing peritoneal mesothelioma of epithelioid pattern from serous carcinoma of the ovary a similar panel of antibodies may be employed but calretinin and BerEP4 are more sensitive than thrombomodulin, cytokeratin 5/6, CEA and Leu-M1.[266]

Antigens detectable in mesotheliomas as well as other tumours include cytokeratin, epithelial membrane antigen, mesothelin, vimentin, desmin, smooth muscle actin, neuron-specific enolase, CD30, Leu 7 and NCAM (neural cell adhesion molecule). Cytokeratin and epithelial membrane antigen may be demonstrated in both adenocarcinomas and mesotheliomas but differences are evident in the intensity and distribution of staining. Thus, cytokeratin is expressed only weakly and is apical in adenocarcinomas, but is expressed strongly in mesotheliomas where it has a perinuclear distribution corresponding to that of filamentous bundles evident by electron microscopy; similarly, epithelial membrane antigen is expressed weakly both on the surface and within the cytoplasm of adenocarcinomas but strongly and on only the surface of mesothelioma cells. Cytokeratin staining is also helpful in highlighting invasion and is very helpful in distinguishing fibrous mesotheliomas from sarcomas (see below).

Electron microscopy is now less used than formerly but when the sample is small (as in cell block preparations) or the

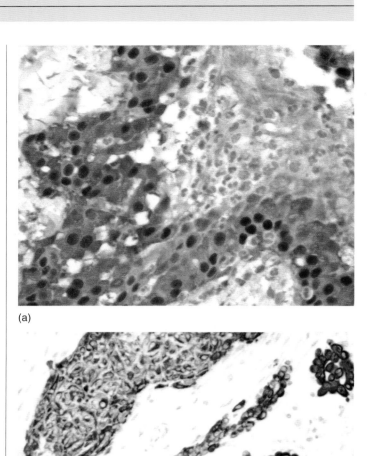

(a)

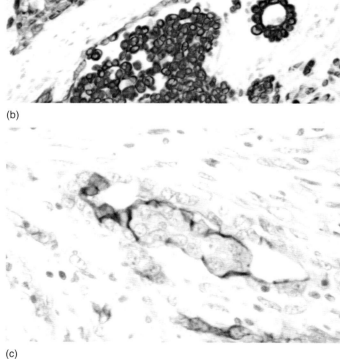

(b)

(c)

Figure 13.22 Immunohistochemistry for epithelioid mesothelioma. In contrast to metastatic adenocarcinomas, epithelioid mesotheliomas typically stain for (a) calretinin (nuclear stain), (b) cytokeratin 5/6 (cytoplasmic stain) and (c) thrombomodulin (membrane stain).

Box 13.4 Ultrastructural distinction between mesothelioma and adenocarcinoma

Mesothelioma	Adenocarcinoma
Microvilli elongated, slender and bushy without glycocalyceal bodies. May mingle with collagen fibrils	Microvilli short and stubby with glycocalyceal bodies. Generally confined to the luminal surface and seldom mingle with collagen fibrils
Apical tight junctions	Terminal bars near lumen
Long, well developed desmosomes	Short, less well developed desmosomes
Perinuclear tonofilaments	Irregularly distributed intermediate filaments
No mucin granules	May contain mucin granules
Abundant glycogen	Variable amount of glycogen
Scanty fat droplets	No fat

histological and immunohistochemical findings are of uncertain significance, it can be very helpful in distinguishing mesotheliomas from other tumours.[267,268] Although epithelioid mesotheliomas have several ultrastructural features in common with adenocarcinomas, sufficient differences may be present to enable a confident diagnosis to be made (Box 13.4).[269–273] Adenocarcinomas often contain secretory granules, which are never found in mesotheliomas. Conversely, mesotheliomas generally have long, slender, curved microvilli that give a bush-like appearance to the surface of the cells (Fig. 13.23) and differ from the short stubby microvilli of an adenocarcinoma. The long microvilli are easily recognisable by scanning electron microscopy. They cover all free surfaces of the mesothelioma cells, including both intracellular and intercellular lumina, and may come into direct contact with stromal collagen through deficiencies in the basement membrane (Fig. 13.23), a feature that is rarely encountered in carcinomas. Neither long curly microvilli nor contact between microvilli and collagen is totally specific but either of these findings is very suggestive of mesothelioma.[274] At points of contact between mesothelioma cells, well developed and often unusually long desmosomes are found. Abundant intermediate filaments (tonofilaments) form bundles that may converge on cell junctions, or more characteristically are perinuclear. Large collections of glycogen and occasional fat droplets are often evident in the cytoplasm of mesothelioma cells. Tubular structures that possibly represent crystallised proteoglycan have been identified in the rare mesotheliomas referred to above as containing hyaluronidase-resistant PAS-positive droplets.[252]

Separation of small cell anaplastic mesothelioma[222,223] from small cell carcinoma involving the pleura[275] depends upon wide sampling to identify more characteristic areas. The neuroendocrine markers chromogranin, neuron specific enolase, Leu-7 and neural cell adhesion molecule (CD56) are not specific, being found in a proportion of mesotheliomas.[233,276,277]

Flow cytometric ploidy studies have been conducted in the hope of discriminating better between carcinoma and mesothelioma. Differences are reported but these are not absolute and therefore of limited use in individual cases:

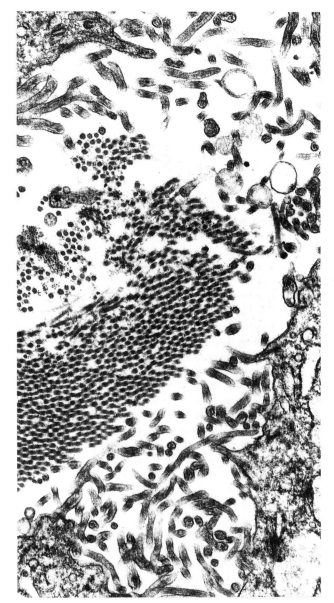

Figure 13.23 Transmission electron micrograph of an epithelial mesothelioma showing long curly microvilli intermingled with collagen. (Reproduced from Dewar et al. Pleural mesothelioma of epithelial type and pulmonary adenocarcinoma: an ultrastructural and cytochemical comparison. Journal of Pathology 1987; 152:309–316.[269] Copyright Pathological Society of Great Britain and Ireland. Reproduced by permission. Permission granted by John Wiley & Sons Ltd on behalf of PathSoc.)

47–78% of mesotheliomas are diploid whereas 85–88% of carcinomas are aneuploid.[278–280] Despite the relative lack of aneuploidy in mesotheliomas, cytogenetic studies have documented abnormal karyotypes in about three quarters of cases but no consistent abnormality has been identified.[280] However, microarray data assessing expression levels of a small number of genes as ratios has shown similar specificity to immunohistochemistry in distinguishing mesothelioma from metastatic adenocarcinoma.[281]

3. Epithelioid mesothelioma versus reactive mesothelial hyperplasia

The epithelioid pattern of mesothelioma may be simulated both by papillary hyperplasia of the surface mesothelium and by the presence of groups of hyperplastic mesothelial cells trapped in granulation tissue beneath the surface. Cellular pleomorphism and mitotic activity may be lacking in mesothelioma and there are often few other pointers to malignancy. However, mesothelial inclusions entrapped by granulation tissue differ from an invasive mesothelioma in that they are often aligned parallel to the surface because they represent the line of the former pleural surface, and they do not invade the fat underlying the parietal pleura. Invasion of fat, muscle or lung is undoubtedly the best indicator of neoplasia.[282] Caution is needed in the interpretation of non-invasive papillary proliferation of the surface mesothelium in view of the possibility that it may represent a premalignant state (see Fig. 13.14b and mesothelioma-*in-situ*[220] above). In effusions, macrophages may mimic exfoliated mesothelial cells, both reactive and malignant, but may be recognised be the inclusion of the macrophage marker CD68 in the immunohistochemical panel.

Antibodies against epithelial membrane antigen and human milk fat globule generally fail to stain benign mesothelial cells but react with malignant cells, both adenocarcinoma and mesothelioma.[250,283,284] However, many find them unhelpful in the individual case.[282] Other techniques advocated to distinguish reactive from neoplastic mesothelial cell proliferations include morphometry,[285,286] the enumeration of argyrophilic nucleolar organiser regions,[287] the identification of proliferating cell antigen expression,[288–290] the assessment of cell cycle state,[291] the immunocytochemical demonstration of P-170 glycoprotein and the p53 and bcl-2 gene products[250] and staining for telomerase reverse transcriptase (TERT).[292] These techniques need further evaluation, especially in the diagnosis of the difficult borderline lesions.

4. Sarcomatoid mesothelioma versus other spindle cell tumours

Sarcomatoid mesotheliomas may mimic a wide range of connective tissue tumours and it is necessary to consider these in the differential diagnosis, especially if the tumour is localised and there is no history of exposure to asbestos. Sarcomatoid mesotheliomas frequently express broad spectrum cytokeratins[293] and this provides strong but not infallible support for the tumour being a sarcomatoid mesothelioma rather than a sarcoma (Box 13.5),[294] and helps in the distinction of lympho-histiocytoid mesothelioma[238] from lymphoma. However, it has to be remembered that the submesothelial spindle cells of reactive pleural fibrosis also express cytokeratin;[18,295] attention should therefore be concentrated on the deeper parts of the lesion. Conversely, between 16 and 40% of fibrous mesotheliomas fail to stain for cytokeratin.[113,296] It is therefore helpful that calretinin and thrombomodulin react with some sarcomatoid as well as epithelioid mesotheliomas,[294,297] although their specificity and sensitivity in relation to primary pleural sarcomas are poorly characterised. For example calretinin often stains synovial sarcomas.[298]

The diversity of differentiation seen with mesotheliomas means that the expression of markers such as vimentin and smooth muscle actin does not exclude a diagnosis of mesothelioma, even if the tumour is cytokeratin-negative.[235,293,299,300] However, a combination of cytokeratin-negativity and CD34-positivity would favour localised fibrous tumour of the pleura (see p. 714). Epithelioid haemangioendothelioma and other vascular tumours may mimic mesothelioma both grossly and microscopically but can be distinguished by their positive endothelial markers (factor VIII-related antigen, von Willebrand factor, CD31, CD34 and *Ulex europaeus* agglutinin).[244,301–304]

Sarcomatoid mesotheliomas also need to be distinguished from a variety of epithelial spindle cell tumours, notably the pleural metastases of spindle cell carcinomas of the lung, renal carcinomas of spindle cell or eosinophilic polygonal cell type, and melanomas. The last of these differs from mesothelioma in lacking cytokeratins and staining for S-100 and HMB45 antigens. Lung markers such as surfactant apoprotein and thyroid transforming factor-1 (TTF-1) may occasionally be useful in distinguishing spindle cell carcinoma of the lung (Box 13.5) and wider sampling of many apparently monophasic sarcomatoid carcinomas of the lung reveals that they are biphasic, permitting a distinction based upon the properties of the epithelioid component, as described above. Sarcomatoid renal carcinoma may be very difficult to distinguish from mesothelioma as there is some overlap in their immunohistochemical profiles.[263,264] If a renal origin is suspected it is perhaps best to advise a non-invasive investigation of that area by computed tomography or ultrasound.[263,277] Thymomas involving the pleura may also mimic mesothelioma in their gross structure but generally retain their distinctive microscopic morphology.[305–307]

In mesotheliomas that appear purely sarcomatoid by light microscopy, electron microscopy may demonstrate the classic biphasic pattern by revealing cells with such epithelioid features as desmosomes and microvilli.[270,308,309]

Box 13.5 Immunohistochemical distinction of sarcomatoid mesothelioma, sarcoma and sarcomatoid carcinoma

	Pankeratin (%)	CK5/6	Calretinin (%)	Thrombo-modulin (%)	SMA (%)	TTF-1
Sarcomatoid mesothelioma	70	Rare	70	70	60	0/10
Sarcoma	17	Rare	17	38	58	Negative
Sarcomatoid carcinoma	90	Rare	60	40	10	Pulmonary may be positive

Adapted from Lucas et al. Sarcomatoid mesothelioma and its histological mimics: a comparative immunohistochemical study. Histopathology 2003; 42:270–279.[294] Copyright Blackwell Publishing Ltd.

5. Sarcomatoid mesothelioma versus fibrosis

Desmoplastic sarcomatoid mesotheliomas may mimic scar tissue very closely (Fig. 13.19),[310] while cellular sarcomatoid mesotheliomas may be impossible to distinguish from granulation tissue if, as is sometimes the case, they lack cellular pleomorphism and invasion is not evident in the area sampled. As submesothelial cells mature to replace lost mesothelial cells they acquire mesothelial characteristics. Thus, cytokeratin may be expressed in either reactive or neoplastic fibrous pleural lesions.[17,18,295] In the absence of invasion, features suggestive of mesothelioma include:

- an absence of the zoning usually seen in reparative processes whereby cellular granulation overlies denser scar tissue
- a storiform pattern
- necrosis
- abnormal mitoses
- cytological atypia.

Conversely, elongated capillaries aligned at right angles to the surface favour granulation tissue rather than mesothelioma.[282]

Techniques such as the enumeration of argyrophilic nucleolar organiser regions and the identification of proliferating cell and oncogene expression (see above) may eventually prove helpful but often wider sampling to identify frankly malignant foci may be the only solution. In such cases, orientation of the specimen at the time of processing may help in distinguishing the organised maturation of granulation tissue from the more disorganised growth pattern of a desmoplastic mesothelioma.

When sarcomatoid mesotheliomas invade the mediastinum the appearances may mimic those of sclerosing mediastinitis,[184] in which case cytokeratin staining may be helpful.

Desmoplastic mesothelioma is seldom so lacking in cells as the hyaline pleural plaque, which is virtually acellular (see p. 700).

Spread and prognosis of mesothelioma

Instances of mesothelioma being operable are exceptionable.[205] There is usually widespread pleural involvement at presentation. However, once the lung is surrounded, there is a period during which the tumour expands locally before metastasising. Peritoneal mesothelioma is similar, coating the abdominal viscera for some time before disseminating more widely. It is unusual for patients to present because of distant metastases.[186,187,311] Eventually however, dissemination may be widespread and should not detract from a diagnosis of mesothelioma.[312–315]

If the tumour is pleural, there is ultimately invasion of the lung and lymphatic spread to the hilar lymph nodes. Infiltration of the diaphragm results in spread to the peritoneum and upper abdominal lymph nodes, particularly the pancreaticosplenic nodes. The parietal pericardium is infiltrated and multiple deposits may develop in the opposite pleural cavity. Late in the disease, blood-borne metastases may develop in the other lung, liver, adrenals, kidneys, brain, meninges, bone,

skeletal muscle and elsewhere.[312–315] To some extent the pattern of spread and prognosis are influenced by the histological type. Epithelioid mesotheliomas tend to behave like carcinomas and spread to the regional lymph nodes whilst sarcomatoid mesotheliomas tend to behave like sarcomas and metastasise to distant sites; mixed tumours have features of both,[217,316] but these differences are by no means absolute.[313,317]

Progression of the disease is not appreciably modified by treatment. Most patients succumb within two years of diagnosis[182,217,318–320] but exceptional cases survive for more than 10 years.[321] Epithelioid mesotheliomas have a slightly better prognosis than the other histological types.[204,217,320,322–326] Evidence has been presented that mesothelioma patients without a history of asbestos exposure survive slightly longer but it is uncertain whether this is independent of histological type.[327,328] Adverse prognostic factors also include male sex, older age, advanced stage, weight loss, poor performance status[204,326,329] and the expression of proliferation markers.[330–332] Various staging systems are in use[204,326,333,334] and protocols for examining mesothelioma specimens have been established.[335] In assessing mesothelial inclusions in mediastinal lymph nodes it should be remembered that these are not always neoplastic.[336–342]

The production of autocrine growth factors by mesotheliomas would be expected to exert an adverse influence on survival, and several have now been identified, including platelet-derived growth factor, transforming growth factor-β and vascular endothelial growth factor.[343–350] Some of these mesothelioma-derived cytokines might also be involved in systemic paraneoplastic syndromes characterised by immunosuppression, thrombocytosis, cachexia, amyloidosis and hypoglycaemia.[346] The production of such cytokines implies oncogene expression in mesotheliomas, for which there is now considerable evidence.[351–353] An immediate consequence of autocrine activity would be increased mitotic activity and the production of proliferating cell nuclear antigen, both of which correlate with the degree of malignancy and may be of prognostic[289] and future therapeutic value.[354] Microarray data assessing expression levels of a small number of genes as ratios has been used to identify patients with a better prognosis.[355]

Well-differentiated papillary mesothelioma

Well-differentiated papillary mesothelioma is a rare, low-grade variant of epithelioid mesothelioma. Most examples have arisen in the peritoneum of young women but some have been pleural, predominantly affecting middle-aged or elderly patients of either sex.[356,357] Some patients give a history of asbestos exposure.[223,356,357] The tumours may be solitary but more often are multifocal. They generally grow slowly and show no histological evidence of malignancy but occasional examples pursue an aggressive course. Of 11 patients with a minimal follow-up period of 24 months, survival ranged from 36–180 months with an average of 74 months and a 10-year survival of 31%.[357]

Patients with pleural involvement present with dyspnoea due to recurrent pleural effusions. Thoracoscopy shows the pleura to be studded with firm nodules measuring less than

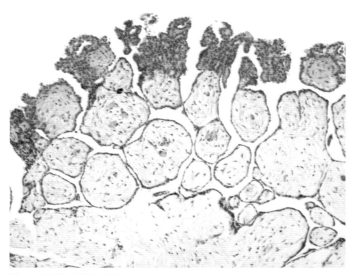

Figure 13.24 Well-differentiated papillary mesothelioma. Papillae consist of a mainly single layer of cuboidal cells covering delicate connective tissue cores.

1 cm or that there is a single arborescent tumour measuring up to 5 cm. Histology shows papillae consisting of a single layer of cuboidal cells covering a delicate connective tissue core. The surface cells have the cytochemical and ultrastructural features of an epithelioid mesothelioma, as described above (Fig. 13.24).

Multicystic mesothelioma (multicystic mesothelial proliferation)

Multicystic mesothelioma is a rare but well recognised condition of the peritoneum,[358,359] that has occasionally been described in the pleura.[360] Confusion as to its true nature has led to a plethora of names, but it is now recognised to be a reactive lesion and the term multicystic mesothelial proliferation better reflects its true nature. The prognosis is good but it is often difficult to eradicate completely and the lesion is therefore prone to recur.

Patients with peritoneal lesions are generally young adult women with a history of pelvic inflammation or surgery. Typically, multicystic lesions attached to the pelvic organs rise up into the abdomen. The patient with pleural disease was a 37-year-old woman complaining of pleuritic pain. As a child she came into contact with asbestos insulation but the condition is not thought to be related to this pollutant. A large unilateral multicystic mass continuous with the parietal pleura and tightly adherent to the visceral pleura was identified at thoracotomy: there were frequent connections between the cyst lining and the normal parietal pleura.[360]

Histologically the cysts were lined by a monolayer of flattened cells showing papillary infoldings. There was no invasive or mitotic activity. The lining cells stained with antibodies to cytokeratin and epithelial membrane antigen while staining for factor VIII-related antigen and carcinoembryonic antigen was negative. Electron microscopy confirmed the mesothelial nature of the cyst lining. Immunocytochemistry and electron microscopy are useful in distinguishing this lesion from a lymphangioma, with which it is readily confused.

Adenomatoid tumour

Adenomatoid tumours are distinctive benign mesothelial tumours that have mainly been described in the scrotum or in relation to the female generative organs. Despite the abundance of mesothelium in the pleura, adenomatoid tumours are exceptionally rare in this site, very few cases having been reported.[361] The cells are vacuolated, giving the tumours a lace-like appearance. Immunocytochemical reactions and electron microscopical appearances are those expected of a mesothelial tumour of epithelioid pattern, as described above.

Localised fibrous tumour of the pleura (solitary fibrous tumour)

This tumour was previously known as a benign or localised mesothelioma because, although there is no obvious mesothelial differentiation, early tissue culture experiments were thought to show biphasic differentiation into 'epithelial' and mesenchymal elements.[362] This may have been due to the inadvertent inclusion of normal mesothelial cells in the culture medium.[363] An alternative proposal envisages origin from subpleural mesenchyme and despite some contrary views[364,365] immunocytochemical and ultrastructural findings generally favour this theory. The tumour cells express vimentin and actin intermediate filaments but not cytokeratin or epithelial membrane antigen[18,295,366–371] and the ultrastructural features are those of fibroblasts or myofibroblasts.[70,368,371–373] Occasional microvilli and poorly formed junctions are described[366,367,372,374] but it is difficult to distinguish neoplastic mesothelial cells from inclusions of reactive mesothelium by electron microscopy.[364,375] Similarly it may be difficult to decide whether cells containing keratin intermediate filaments are an inherent part of the tumour or mere inclusions of either mesothelium or alveolar epithelium. However, the bulk of the evidence points to these cells representing entrapment of non-neoplastic elements.[376] Accordingly, the term localised fibrous tumour is preferred.

Localised fibrous tumour of the pleura differs from mesothelioma in being unrelated to asbestos exposure and in having a much better prognosis. Several hundred have now been reported.[368,372]

Clinical features

Some patients are asymptomatic but the majority complain of chest pain, cough and breathlessness. Many develop finger clubbing and hypertrophic pulmonary osteoarthropathy. Some experience hypoglycaemic episodes due to the secretion of insulin-like growth factors.[368,377–380] Recurrent pleural effusion is also recorded.[381]

Pathological features

The tumours occur with equal frequency on the left and right sides, and three to four times as many arise from the visceral

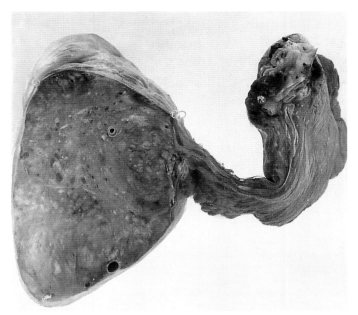

Figure 13.25 Localised fibrous tumour of the pleura, 9 cm in diameter, excised with its pedicle and a small portion of lung.

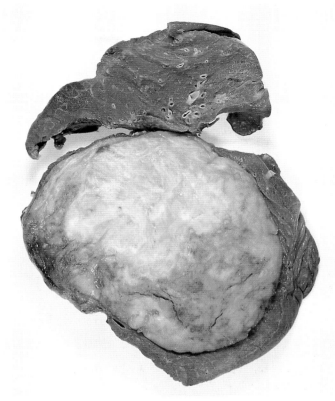

Figure 13.27 An intrapulmonary localised fibrous tumour, 12 cm in diameter. (Illustration provided by Dr W Downey, Melbourne, Australia.)

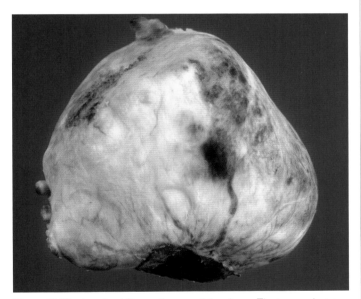

Figure 13.26 Localised fibrous tumour of the pleura. The tumour has a flattened base and is mainly encapsulated.

pleura as from the parietal pleura. Often they are attached to the surface of the lung by a pedicle and are mobile within the pleural cavity (Fig. 13.25). Tumours of the parietal pleura tend to be sessile with a broader base (Fig. 13.26). Similar tumours are wholly intrapulmonary[382–384] (Fig. 13.27), while others arise in the mediastinum[385] and more distant sites.[369,386–405] Localised fibrous tumours may also have been included in a series of invasive fibrous tumours of the trachea.[406]

Typically, localised fibrous tumours of the pleura are well circumscribed and have a smooth, often bosselated, surface covered by serosa. They may attain a weight of 2–3 kg and a diameter of 30 cm or more. The cut surface is pale grey or white, often with a whorled pattern. Small areas of softening or necrosis may be present in larger tumours and some have very vascular areas, which may become haemorrhagic.

Microscopically, the appearances are those of a low-grade spindle cell neoplasm of variable cellularity with the tumour cells dispersed in a variably hyaline collagenous stroma. The oval or spindle-shaped nuclei are fairly small and regular with finely dispersed chromatin (Fig. 13.28). In more cellular areas mitoses may be present, but they are rarely numerous. A storiform pattern, reminiscent of malignant fibrous histiocytoma, is sometimes seen. Very vascular areas may resemble haemangiopericytoma, but often the vessels have a narrow cuff of hyaline material. There may be focal, or even extensive myxoid change.[407] Liposarcomatous differentiation is recorded as an exceptional feature. At the periphery, inclusions of non-neoplastic mesothelium, bronchiolar or alveolar epithelium are frequently present. Another variable feature is the presence of microscopic irregular fissures or small cysts, lined by flattened cells. Occasionally these spaces are very conspicuous, giving a lace-like microcystic pattern (Fig. 13.29). Electron microscopy shows that their lining cells resemble the other tumour cells and lack mesothelial or epithelial features.

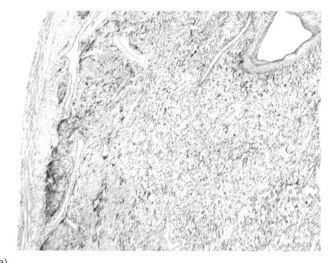

(a)

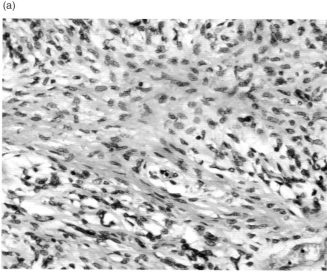

(b)

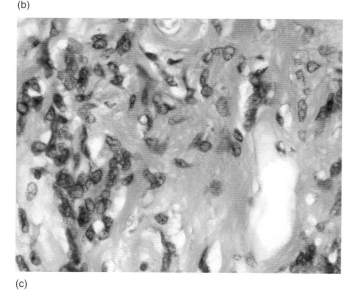

(c)

Figure 13.28 Localised fibrous tumour of the pleura. (a) The tumour is encapsulated and of variable cellularity. (b) The stroma may be myxoid or fibrous. (c) The cells are rounded or spindle-shaped and show no atypia.

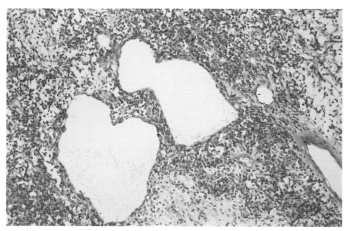

Figure 13.29 Localised fibrous tumour of the pleura of varying cellularity and showing microcystic degeneration.

Immunohistochemistry

Immunocytochemical features distinguishing localised fibrous tumour (positive reactions for vimentin and actin and negative reactions for cytokeratin or epithelial membrane antigen) have been mentioned above. In addition, positive immunostaining for CD34 is obtained in about 80% of localised fibrous tumours: this is useful in distinguishing localised fibrous tumour from mesothelioma, malignant fibrous histiocytoma and haemangiopericytoma, in all of which CD34 reactivity is limited to blood vessels.[391,408,409] However, the higher the grade of a localised fibrous tumour, the less likely is it to express CD34, and the more likely to express p53.[410] Localised fibrous tumours may be distinguished from inflammatory pseudotumours by positive staining for the p53 oncogene product,[411] and from gastrointestinal stromal tumours, to which they have been likened (both being positive for CD99) by their failure to stain for CD117.[412]

Prognosis

The prognosis following resection is generally good but in a minority, there is local recurrence and then usually a fatal outcome.[368,372,413–415] Exceptional cases present with widespread pleural dissemination.[416] Hypercellularity, pleomorphism, necrosis and excessive mitotic activity (more than four mitoses per 10 high-power fields) (Fig. 13.30) suggest that the lesion will behave aggressively[368] but the most important prognostic factor is the completeness of excision, fundamental to which is the presence or absence of a pedicle. In general, pedunculated tumours, which can be removed with their attachment, do not recur.[372,417] In a review of 360 previously reported cases it was found that 88% behaved in a benign fashion after surgical resection,[372] while in another series comprising 223 cases, 45 patients (20%) died due to invasion, recurrence or metastasis.[368] In a third series, local recurrence occurred in 6 of 40 cases and metastasis in five, and tumour size and cellularity correlated with malignancy.[413]

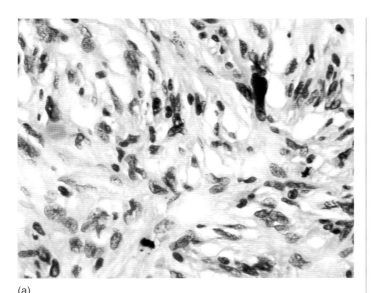

(a)

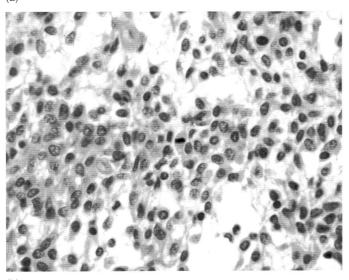

(b)

Figure 13.30 Malignant localised fibrous tumour of the pleura. (a) In places the tumour shows marked pleomorphism and mitotic activity. (b) Here, the tumour cells are more rounded, but there is still considerable cellularity and mitoses are easily seen.

Calcifying fibrous pseudotumour

Calcifying fibrous pseudotumour, as described in soft tissues, has also been reported in the pleura, peritoneum and mediastinum.[418–420] The patients with pleural tumours were young adults who were either asymptomatic or complained of chest pain. They had a plaque-like, well-circumscribed but non-encapsulated tumour of the visceral pleura. Multiple such tumours were identified in one case.[421] Microscopically, these tumours are characterised by abundant hyaline collagen containing sparse thin spindle cells and foci of psammomatous dystrophic calcification (Fig. 13.31). The nature of this lesion is uncertain but it may represent the late stage of an inflammatory

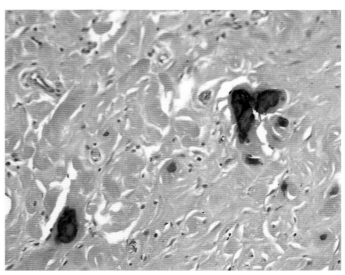

Figure 13.31 Calcifying fibrous pseudotumour of the pleura. The tumour consists of thick bundles of hyaline fibrous tissue in which there is focal psammomatous calcification. (Illustration provided by Dr A Gibbs, Penarth, UK.)

myofibroblastic tumour (see p. 609), a possibility that derives some support from the presence of sparse areas of lymphoplasmacytic infiltration, reactivity of both lesions for CD34 and factor XIIIa, and rare reports of cases showing transitional features.[422–425] Local excision appears adequate but it is suggested that if it behaves in a similar fashion to those in the soft tissues a low rate of local recurrence might be expected.[418]

Desmoplastic small round cell tumour

This is a rare tumour that typically presents with widespread abdominal involvement that is not organ-related.[426,427] It appears to be of mesothelial or submesothelial origin. A few examples arising in the pleura or lung have been reported.[428–430]

The tumour generally affects children and young adults, and has a male-to-female ratio of four. The tumours that affect the pleura do so in a diffuse manner so that the clinical, radiological and gross features all mimic mesothelioma. However, there is no association with asbestos and the histological features are quite different. Microscopy shows discrete islands of small cells set in an abundant desmoplastic stroma. The islands of tumour cells vary greatly in size and shape and are sometimes necrotic. The tumour cells are uniform but show many mitoses. They have little cytoplasm and round or oval hyperchromatic nuclei with clumped chromatin and scanty nucleoli. Pseudorosettes are present but no glands or tubules are evident by light microscopy although entrapped mesothelial islands may be seen.

Although the histological features are those of an anaplastic growth, immunocytochemistry indicates diverse differentiation, with epithelial, neuronal and myogenic expression. The most consistent immunocytochemical finding is strong focal dot-like positivity for vimentin, corresponding to a collection of intermediate filaments evident near the nucleus on electron microscopy. Other ultrastructural features include numerous desmosomes, dense-core granules and occasional gland lumina with microvilli.[431] Further positive reactions are obtained with antibodies to desmin and less consistently cytokeratin, epithelial membrane antigen, neuron-specific antigen, S-100 and glial fibrillary acidic protein. The tumour cells are negative for actin, lymphocyte markers and mesothelial markers such as cytokeratin 5/6.

The differential diagnosis is firstly from mesothelioma, which this tumour simulates in its gross form. The mixed keratin, vimentin and neuron-specific enolase expression is compatible with a mesothelioma, of which a small cell variant has been described, but the combined histological, immunocytochemical and ultrastructural features distinguish the two. There is a closer histological similarity to the malignant small cell tumour of the primitive neuroectodermal tumour series (PNETs), first described in the chest wall (see below), but the diverse differentiation towards muscle, nerve and epithelium shown by immunocytochemistry in the tumour now under discussion is wider than the purely neural differentiation of the PNETs. However, there is a close cytogenetic similarity, a t(11;22)(p13;q11 or q12) translocation nearly matching the t(11;12)(q24;q12) abnormality found in PNETs and Ewing's sarcoma. 11p13 is the locus of the Wilms tumour suppressor gene and it is notable that the desmoplastic small round cell tumour reacts with an antibody to the C-terminal region of the Wilm's tumour protein WT1, in contrast to PNETs which fail to react with this antibody.[432] The phenotype of the desmoplastic small round cell tumour is intermediate between the purely neural phenotype of the PNETs and the mixed but predominantly epithelial phenotype of a Wilm's tumour, reflecting its Ewing's/PNET and WT1 gene fusion.[433,434]

The prognosis with pleural tumours appears to be as poor as that of patients with abdominal desmoplastic small round cell tumours. Of three patients with pleural tumours, two died 15 months and 2 years, respectively after presentation and the third was alive with tumour 18 months later.[429]

Pleural lymphoma

Two unusual lymphomas are described in the pleura. One complicates pyothorax and forms a mass lesion early in its course,[435–439] whereas the other is seen in AIDS patients and is generally manifest as a pleural, pericardial or peritoneal effusion.[440–442] They have become known as *pyothorax-associated lymphoma* and *body cavity-based lymphoma*, respectively. Both are associated with Epstein–Barr virus[443] but the body cavity-based lymphoma is also associated with human herpes virus 8 and human immunodeficiency virus,[440–442,444,445] supporting the view that they are distinct entities.[446] Human herpes virus 8 was originally identified in Kaposi's sarcoma from patients with and without AIDS.[447] It is found in body cavity-based lymphoma from patients with advanced AIDS who are generally homo-

sexual and from rare HIV-negative patients.[448,449] An inflammatory effusion associated with human herpes virus 8 may represent the precursor of body cavity-based lymphoma.[450] Human herpes virus 8 is also found in multicentric Castleman's disease (see p. 657) and there are reports of patients who have developed both Castleman's disease and body cavity-based lymphoma.[451,452]

The mass lesion of the pyothorax-associated lymphoma is generally a diffuse large cell non-Hodgkin's lymphoma of B-cell phenotype, rich in reactive T cells.[437,453–456] It is suggested that immunosuppressive cytokines or growth factors produced by the inflammatory cells favour the clonal evolution of Epstein–Barr virus-infected B cells.[437,457]

The body cavity-based lymphoma is also a diffuse large cell lymphoma. Smears from the pleural fluid show round to ovoid malignant lymphoid cells with large round nuclei. Some cells have irregular or multiple nuclei. Many mitoses are evident. The cells express CD45 but neither B- nor T-cell antigens (i.e. they have a null cell phenotype).[440–442,444,445] Although this lymphoma takes the form of an effusion, a tumour mass may develop late in the course of the disease.[445]

Other primary tumours of the pleura

When considering the possibility of a primary tumour of the pleura other than mesothelioma, it must be remembered that the versatility of malignant mesothelial cells enables them to mimic many other types of primary mesenchymal tumour; for example, osteogenic sarcomatous mesotheliomas may be indistinguishable histologically from primary osteogenic sarcoma.[234] Features suggesting a non-mesothelial sarcoma include the gross appearance of a localised mass, an absence of asbestos exposure and failure to stain for cytokeratin,[458,459] but none of these features is entirely reliable. Origin from the chest wall, diaphragm, mediastinum and lung needs to be excluded. All these caveats need to be considered when evaluating reports of pleural malignant fibrous histiocytoma,[460–463] angiosarcoma,[462] liposarcoma,[464,465] rhabdomyosarcoma,[466,467] leiomyoma or leiomyosarcoma,[468–472] chondrosarcoma,[473,474] desmoid tumour[475] and malignant nerve sheath tumour.[476] However, pleural sarcomas of various type may complicate chronic pleurisy.[462]

Carcinoma

Rare instances of pleural 'epidermoid' (squamous cell) carcinoma are recorded, all of which arose in pleural cavities that showed widespread squamous change following the induction of longstanding artificial pneumothoraces.[57,477] It is possible that the squamous change represented metaplasia of the mesothelium but implantation of epidermal fragments is equally likely because numerous injections of air were required to maintain these chronic pneumothoraces. Furthermore, some cases were associated with a bronchopulmonary fistula, which also showed squamous change and malignancy and in these a bron-

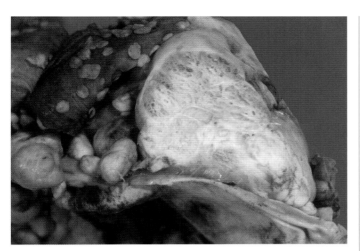

Figure 13.32 Thymoma seeding in the pleural space. A primary mediastinal thymoma adheres to the medial surface of the lung and many tumour seedlings are seen on the visceral pleura.

chogenic origin cannot be excluded. The tumours were typically well-differentiated with abundant keratinisation; although of low grade, they showed undoubted infiltrative activity with destruction of adjacent tissues. Carcinoma is also reported in association with lucite ball plombage, apparently arising in the periphery of the lung but closely associated with the lucite in the pleural cavity.[478] Primary mucoepidermoid carcinoma of the pleura is also recorded, apparently arising spontaneously.[479]

Thymoma

Thymoma has been reported in the pleura, masquerading as mesothelioma on occasion.[305–307,480,481] It is suggested that some of these tumours arise from ectopic thymic tissue in the pleura but it is always difficult to exclude seeding of the pleura from an undetected primary in the thymus (Fig. 13.32). The pleural tumours have generally resembled those encountered in the thymus, often showing the typical lobules separated by fibrous septa. However, their immunocytochemical profile may cause them to be misdiagnosed as mesotheliomas: they variably express cytokeratins 5/6 and thrombomodulin, but not calretinin.[481] A thymic nature is supported by the presence of aberrant CD20 expression in a cytokeratin positive epithelial neoplasm and the presence of an immature lymphoid population by the demonstration of CD1a, CD2 and CD99.[481]

Synovial sarcoma

Synovial sarcoma is another tumour that has been reported to arise in the pleura, usually as a localised mass but occasionally involving the pleura diffusely and so mimicking mesothelioma.[247,248,482,483] Both biphasic and monophasic spindle cell examples have been recognised, with the resemblance to mesothelioma again being seen histologically. However, subtle differences are described: synovial sarcomas are typically com-

posed of closely packed spindle cells arranged in interweaving bundles (so-called 'herringbone' pattern). The cells appear to overlap and numerous mitoses are evident, but pleomorphism is not prominent, as it is in the generally less cellular mesotheliomas. Immunohistochemical similarities include positive reactions for calretinin, epithelial membrane antigen and cytokeratin but the epithelial component stains for mucus and carcinoma markers such as BerEP4, thus permitting distinction from mesothelioma of mixed pattern, while the sarcomatous component expresses the bcl2 oncogene.[298,482] Cytogenetic analysis for the SYT-SSX transcript resulting from t(X;18)(p11;q11) chromosomal translocation is another approach to establishing the diagnosis, this being a characteristic marker of synovial sarcoma: it can be accomplished on paraffin embedded tissues by fluorescence *in situ* hybridisation.[484] Reported examples of pleural synovial sarcoma have generally been aggressive tumours, proving fatal within 3 years of initial diagnosis, although occasional localised examples appear to have been cured by surgical excision.

Vascular tumours

Vascular tumours such as angiosarcoma, epithelioid angiosarcoma and epithelioid haemangioendothelioma have been reported in the pleura, generally mimicking the diffuse distribution of a mesothelioma (see Fig. 12.3.21, p. 626).[302,303,462,485–486a] The sarcomas were particularly aggressive growths. All had morphological features typical of these tumours elsewhere in the body, including reactivity for the endothelial markers factor VIII-related antigen, CD31 and CD34.[244,301–304] Some angiosarcomas have complicated pyothoraces.[487,488]

Secondary tumours of the pleura

Pleural metastases are common in patients with malignant tumours, the most common primary neoplasms in descending order being adenocarcinomas of the breast, lung, ovary, stomach, large bowel, carcinoma of the kidney, lymphoma, various sarcomas and melanoma.[199] In many cases, the primary site is not determined during life.[199,489,490] Breast carcinoma generally first involves the parietal pleura underlying the affected breast,[491] while lung cancer more often involves the visceral pleura,[492] but at autopsy metastases generally involve both pleural surfaces.[493] Whatever the source, metastases are generally multinodular (Fig. 13.32) and commoner in the lower half of the thorax.[494] However, some peripheral adenocarcinomas of the lung, and more rarely squamous carcinomas, spread over the pleural surfaces in a manner similar to mesothelioma and it may be difficult to establish where in the lung such tumours have originated (pseudomesotheliomatous carcinoma).[240–242] Thymomas may behave similarly.[306]

In distinguishing between secondary adenocarcinoma of the pleura and mesothelioma of epithelioid type, mucus stains, immunohistochemistry and electron microscopy are all helpful.

Thymomas spreading onto the pleura should not cause any difficulty to the histopathologist, showing as they do the lobulation and mixed cellularity that is typical of these tumours. They are distinguished from pleural lymphomas by their epithelioid component staining for cytokeratin. The metastatic nature of some pleural tumours can be recognised because they carry site-specific markers that can be detected by immunocytochemistry, for example surfactant apoprotein as a marker of a pulmonary origin[495] and TTF-1 as a marker of origin in the lung or thyroid.

A pleural effusion in a patient with lung cancer does not necessarily indicate that the tumour is inoperable: other causes of a pleural effusion in these patients include secondary infection, lymphatic and venous obstruction and hypoproteinaemia. Involvement of the pleura is more likely if the effusion is blood-stained, or the lung tumour is an adenocarcinoma.[492]

Pleural splenosis

Splenosis results from the implantation of fragments of splenic tissue after traumatic rupture of this organ.[496,497] The implantation is usually on the peritoneum but if the diaphragm is also torn thoracic splenosis is a further potential complication. This may affect the left pleural cavity or pericardium. Splenosis has not been described in the right side of the chest or within the substance of either lung. The condition was first described as a chance autopsy finding in 1937 and by 1994 only 22 cases had been reported.[498,499] It is generally asymptomatic and the interval between the trauma and the diagnosis of thoracic splenosis is long (9–32 years, average 20 years). In this time the implant may grow into a large mass, which is only discovered by chance when chest radiographs are taken for some other purpose. The diagnosis is generally made when the lesion is excised and submitted for histological examination. This shows all the components of normal splenic tissue, including both red and white pulp.[500]

CHEST WALL TUMOURS

Chest wall tumours include extra-abdominal desmoid tumours (aggressive fibromatosis, sometimes developing at the site of a previous thoracotomy),[475,501–502a] elastofibroma dorsi (which particularly involves the scapular region), myositis ossificans[503] and primary tumours of muscle, fat, blood vessel, nerve sheath (Fig. 13.33) and bone.[504,504a] Bone tumours of the chest wall include multiple myeloma, chondroma, chondrosarcoma (Fig. 3.34), fibrous dysplasia and Langerhans cell histiocytosis. Of the soft tissue sarcomas of the chest wall, about half are fibrous or fibrohistiocytic (fibrosarcoma, dermatofibrosarcoma protuberans, malignant fibrous histiocytoma), while liposarcoma and nerve sheath malignancies each form 14%, 8% show muscle differentiation, 4% are vascular and 2% are synovial.[505] Some of these tumours follow radiation for breast carcinoma or Hodgkin's disease.[506] All are well described in texts devoted to skeletal and soft tissue tumours and attention here will be con-

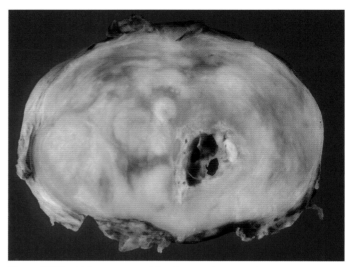

Figure 13.33 Schwannoma arising from an intercostal nerve.

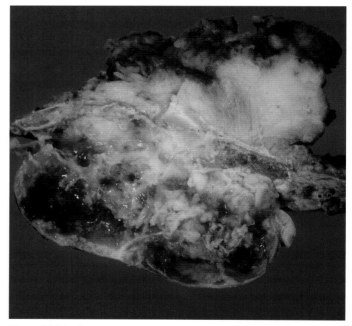

Figure 13.34 Chondrosarcoma of the sternum. This mass was predominantly deep to the anterior chest wall, but quite localised, a feature against it being a mesothelioma.

fined to two that have a particular predilection for the chest wall and a reactive condition that may be mistaken for a neoplasm.

Malignant small cell tumour of the thoracopulmonary region (Askin tumour)

First described in 1979,[507] this high-grade tumour occurs almost exclusively in the first two decades of life (average age 14 years) and 75% of patients are female. Solitary or multiple nodules occur in the chest wall, eroding the ribs and subsequently spreading to involve the pleura, pericardium, diaphragm and

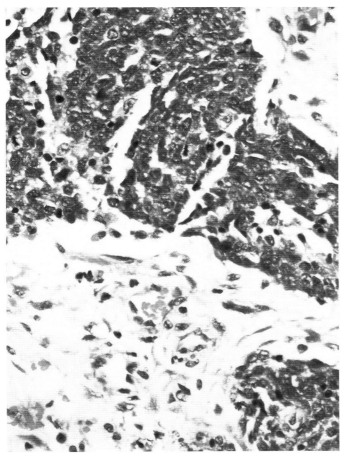

Figure 13.35 Malignant small cell tumour of the thoracopulmonary region (Askin tumour). The tumour is composed of undifferentiated, small, hyperchromatic cells.

periphery of the lung. The tumour tends to recur locally and does not disseminate widely, but the prognosis is dismal, with a 2-year survival of 38% and a 6-year survival of only 14%.[508] Rare examples develop entirely within the lung and are more amenable to surgery.[508–511]

The microscopic features are those of a malignant tumour composed of sheets of undifferentiated, small, hyperchromatic cells, which may show rosettes of radially arranged cells around a central tangle of fibrillary cytoplasmic processes (Fig. 13.35). Electron microscopy reveals dense-core neurosecretory granules, and neuroectodermal markers such as S100 protein, synaptophysin and neuron-specific enolase can be shown by immunohistochemistry, evidence that the tumour is of neural or neuroendocrine derivation.[507,512–515] Further support for this stems from the experimental induction of neuronal differentiation in Askin tumour cell lines.[516] However, the dense-core granules are scanty and the tumour fails to stain for chromogranin.[508]

Extrathoracic examples have subsequently been described and collectively they are now known as *primitive neuroectodermal tumours* (and colloquially as PNETs), of which those arising in the thoracopulmonary region comprise about a third.

Suggestions that PNETs are related to Ewing's sarcoma are supported by cytogenetic studies showing that they carry the Ewing's karyotype, a t(11;22)(q24;q12) translocation[517] and frequently express the Ewing-specific antigen MIC2 (CD99).[518–520] Malignant small cell tumour of the thoracopulmonary region also shows histological and cytogenetic similarities to the desmoplastic small round cell tumour described above, but differs in failing to react with antibodies against the Wilms tumour protein WT1.[432]

Separation of PNETs and Ewing's sarcoma from neuroblastoma is facilitated by their expression of MIC2, neuroblastomas being negative for this antigen. However, chromosomal confirmation is desirable because a small proportion of PNETs and Ewing's sarcoma are also MIC2 negative and positive reactions are obtained with occasional rhabdomyosarcomas and synovial sarcomas.[520] Separation of PNETs from lymphoblastic lymphoma may be effected by the application of lymphocyte markers.[521] Pleuropulmonary blastoma is distinguished by its location in the periphery of the lung rather than the chest wall, cystic nature and focal sarcomatous differentiation, while in doubtful cases CD99 staining and chromosomal analysis are helpful.

Mesenchymal hamartoma of the chest wall

This tumour-like malformation[522–524] is a distinctive lesion that presents at birth or soon after as an extrapleural chest wall mass with involvement of one or more ribs. It was formerly thought to be neoplastic but is now recognised to be a malformation. The few deaths that have been recorded are attributable to pressure effects on the thoracic viscera by lesions that grew to fill much of the hemithorax. Metastasis has not been observed. Former terms that are now redundant include osteochondroma, osteochondrosarcoma, chondroblastoma and mesenchymoma.

Growth may be rapid but spontaneous regression has been recorded. The lesion is usually solitary but may be multifocal or even bilateral. It generally forms a lobulated, well-circumscribed mass composed of bone, cartilage and blood-filled cysts set in a myxoid matrix. Aneurysmal bone cyst is the principal differential diagnosis but although this condition affects the young it is infrequent in the newborn and does not show the prominent cartilage seen in mesenchymal hamartoma.

Gorham's syndrome

This rare condition of unknown aetiology represents a florid proliferation of thin-walled vascular channels that predominantly involves bone and causes marked osteolysis. Underlying soft tissues may be invaded, including the lung if the disease is centred on a rib or vertebra. Respiratory function may be further impaired by thoracospinal deformity or pleural effusion.[525,526] Young adults of either sex are predominantly affected. The process may arrest spontaneously and is therefore not considered to be neoplastic, yet the histological appearances are quite alarming. The vascular channels are lined by plump atypical cells and together with evident invasive activity the appearances suggest a malignant process, either angiosarcoma or angiomatoid carcinoma, the latter condition being excluded by negative epithelial and positive endothelial markers (cytokeratin and CD34 respectively). Bilateral effusions, which may be chylous because of thoracic duct involvement, and vertebral collapse carry an adverse prognosis and may warrant radiotherapy, to which the condition has sometimes responded.

REFERENCES

Normal structure and function of the pleura

1. Barrett NR. The pleura. Thorax 1970; 25:515–524.
2. Albertine KH, Wiener-Kronish JP, Ross PJ, Staub NC. Structure, blood supply, and lymphatic vessels of the sheep's visceral pleura. Anat Rec 1982; 165:277.
3. Albertine KH, Wiener-Kronish JP, Staub NC. The structure of the parietal pleura and its relationship to pleural liquid dynamics in sheep. Anat Rec 1984; 208:401.
4. Miserocchi G. Physiology and pathophysiology of pleural fluid turnover. Eur Respir J 1997; 10:219–225.
5. Cotran RS, Karnovsky MJ. Ultrastructural studies on the permeability of the mesothelium to horseradish peroxidase. J Cell Biol 1968; 37:123–137.
6. Fedorko ME, Hirsch JG. Studies on transport of macromolecules and small particles across mesothelial cells of the mouse omentum. I. Morphologic aspects. Exp Cell Res 1971; 69:113–127.
7. Fedorko ME, Hirsch JG, Fried B. Studies of transport of macromolecules and small particles across mesothelial cells of the mouse omentum. II. Kinetic features and metabolic requirements. Exp Cell Res 1971; 69:313–323.
8. Wang N-S. The preformed stomas connecting the pleural cavity and the lymphatics in the parietal pleura. Am Rev Respir Dis 1975; 111:12–20.
9. Perira AS, Grande NR. Particle clearance from the canine pleural space into thoracic lymph nodes: an experimental study. Lymphology 1992; 25:120–128.
10. Boutin C, Dumortier P, Rey F, Viallat JR, Devuyst P. Black spots concentrate oncogenic asbestos fibers in the parietal pleura: thoracoscopic and mineralogic study. Am J Respir Crit Care Med 1996; 153:444–449.
11. Mitchev K, Dumortier P, Devuyst P. 'Black spots' and hyaline pleural plaques on the parietal pleura of 150 urban necropsy cases. Am J Surg Pathol 2002; 26:1198–1206.
12. Muller KM, Schmitz I, Konstantinidis K. Black spots of the parietal pleura: Morphology and formal pathogenesis. Respiration 2002; 69:261–267.
13. Wang N-S. The regional difference of pleural mesothelial cells in rabbits. Am Rev Respir Dis 1974; 110:623–633.
14. Andrews PM, Potter KR. The ultrastructural morphology and possible functional significance of mesothelial microvilli. Anat Rec 1973; 177:409–426.
15. Raftery AT. Regeneration of parietal and visceral peritoneum. A light microscopical study. Br J Surg 1973; 60:293–299.
16. Raftery AT. Regeneration of peritoneal and visceral peritoneum in the immature animal: a light and electron microscopical study. Br J Surg 1973; 60:969–975.
17. Bolen JW, Hammar SP, McNutt MA. Reactive and neoplastic serosal tissue. A light-microscopic, ultrastructural, and immunocytochemical study. Am J Surg Pathol 1986; 10:34–47.
18. Al-Izzi M, Thurlow NP, Corrin B. Pleural mesothelioma of connective tissue type, localized fibrous tumour of the pleura, and reactive submesothelial hyperplasia. An immunohistochemical comparison. J Pathol 1989; 158:41–44.
19. Gonzalez S, Friemann J, Muller KM, Pott F. Ultrastructure of mesothelial regeneration after intraperitoneal injection of asbestos fibres on rat omentum. Pathol Res Pract 1991; 187:931–935.
20. Ryan GB, Grobety J, Majno G. Mesothelial injury and recovery. Am J Pathol 1973; 71:93–102.
21. Whitaker D, Papadimitriou J. Mesothelial healing: morphological and kinetic investigations. J Pathol 1985; 145:159–175.
22. Mutsaers SE, Whitaker D, Papadimitriou JM. Mesothelial regeneration is not dependent on subserosal cells. J Pathol 2000; 190:86–92.
23. Eskeland G. Regeneration of parietal peritoneum in rats. A light microscopical study. Acta Path Microbiol Scand 1966; 68:355–378.
24. Herbert A. Pathogenesis of pleurisy, pleural fibrosis, and mesothelial proliferation. Thorax 1986; 41:176–189.
25. Raftery AT. Regeneration of parietal and visceral peritoneum: an electron microscopical study. J Anat 1973; 115:375–392.

Pleural effusions

26. Porcel JM, Vives M. Etiology and pleural fluid characteristics of large and massive effusions. Chest 2003; 124:978–983.
27. Waller DA, Saunders NR. Unilateral pulmonary oedema following the removal of a giant pleural tumour. Thorax 1989; 44:682–683.
28. Schwartz DR, Maroo A, Malhotra A, Kesselman H. Negative pressure pulmonary hemorrhage. Chest 1999; 115:1194–1197.
29. Light RW. Pleural effusion. N Engl J Med 2002; 346:1971–1977.
30. Gazquez I, Porcel JM, Vives M, deVera MCV, Rubio M, Rivas MC. Comparative analysis of Light's criteria and other biochemical parameters for distinguishing transudates from exudates. Resp Med 1998; 92:762–765.
31. RomeroCandeira S, Hernandez L, RomeroBrufao S, Orts D, Fernandez C, Martin C. Is it meaningful to use biochemical parameters to discriminate between transudative and exudative pleural effusions? Chest 2002; 122:1524–1529.
32. Cooper CB, Bardsley PA, Rao SS, Collins MC. Pleural effusions and pancreatico-pleural fistulae associated with asymptomatic pancreatic disease. Br J Dis Chest 1988; 82:315–320.
33. Berk JL, Keane J, Seldin DC, et al. Persistent pleural effusions in primary systemic amyloidosis – Etiology and prognosis. Chest 2003; 124:969–977.
34. Porcel JM, Vives M, Esquerda A, Salud A, Perez B, Rodriguez-Panadero F. Use of a panel of tumor markers (carcinoembryonic antigen, cancer antigen 125, carbohydrate antigen 15–3, and cytokeratin 19 fragments) in pleural fluid for the differential diagnosis of benign and malignant effusions. Chest 2004; 126:1757–1763.
35. Emerson PA. Yellow nails, lymphoedema and pleural effusions. Thorax 1966; 21:247–253.
36. Solal-Celigny P, Cormier Y, Fournier M. The yellow nail syndrome. Arch Pathol Lab Med 1983; 107:183–185.
37. Beer DJ, Pereira W, Snider GL. Pleural effusion associated with primary lymphedema – a perspective on the yellow nail syndrome. Am Rev Respir Dis 1978; 117:595–599.
38. Parry CM, Powell RJ, Johnston IDA. Yellow nails, bronchiectasis and low circulating B-cells. Respir Med 1994; 88:475–476.
39. DAlessandro A, Muzi G, Monaco A, Filiberto S, Barboni A, Abbritti G. Yellow nail syndrome: does protein leakage play a role? Eur Resp J 2001; 17:149–152.
40. Leiberman FL, Peters RL. Cirrhotic hydrothorax. Further evidence that an acquired diaphragmatic defect is at fault. Arch Intern Med 1970; 125:114–117.
41. Green A, Logan M, Medawar W, et al. The management of hydrothorax in continuous ambulatory peritoneal dialysis (CAPD). Perit Dial Int 1990; 10:271–274.
42. Roden S, Juvin K, Homasson JP, Israelbiet D. An uncommon etiology of isolated pleural effusion - The ovarian hyperstimulation syndrome. Chest 2000; 118:256–258.
43. Blankenship ME, Rowlett J, Timby JW, Roth RS, Jones RE. Giant lymph node hyperplasia (Castleman's disease) presenting with chylous pleural effusion. Chest 1997; 112: 1132–1133.
44. Hillerdal G. Chylothorax and pseudochylothorax. Eur Respir J 1997; 10:1157–1162.
45. Martinez FJ, Villanueva AG, Pickering R, Becker FS, Smith DR. Spontaneous hemothorax. Report of 6 cases and review of the literature. Medicine Baltimore 1992; 71:354–368.

46. Tatebe S, Kanazawa H, Yamazaki Y, Aoki E, Sakurai Y. Spontaneous hemopneumothorax. Ann Thorac Surg 1996; 62:1011–1015.

47. Delco F, Domenighetti G, Kauzlaric D, Donati D, Mombelli G. Spontaneous biliothorax (thoracobilia) following cholecystopleural fistula presenting as an acute respiratory insufficiency - successful removal of gallstones from the pleural space. Chest 1994; 106:961–963.

Pneumothorax

48. Gupta D, Hansell A, Nichols T, Duong T, Ayres JG, Strachan D. Epidemiology of pneumothorax in England. Thorax 2000; 55:666–671.

49. Light RW, Hamm H. Pleural disease and acquired immune deficiency syndrome. Eur Resp J 1997; 10:2638–2643.

50. Lichter I, Gwynne JF. Spontaneous pneumothorax in young subjects. A clinical and pathological study. Thorax 1971; 26:409–417.

51. Renner RR, Markarian B, Pernice NJ, Heitzman ER. The apical cap. Radiology 1974; 110: 569–573.

52. Editorial. Spontaneous pneumothorax and apical lung disease. BMJ 1971; 2:573.

53. Bense L, Eklund G, Wiman LG. Bilateral bronchial anomaly – a pathogenetic factor in spontaneous pneumothorax. Am Rev Respir Dis 1992; 146:513–516.

54. Tsukadaira A, Okubo Y, Ota M, Hotta J, Kubo K. Concurrent left-sided spontaneous penumothorax in Japanese monogerminal twins. Respiration 2001; 68:625–627.

55. Askin FB, McGann BG, Kuhn C. Reactive eosinophilic pleuritis. A lesion to be distinguished from pulmonary eosinophilic granuloma. Arch Pathol Lab Med 1977; 101:187–191.

56. Luna E, Tomashefski JF, Brown D, Clarke RE, Kleinerman J. Reactive eosinophilic pulmonary vascular infiltration in patients with spontaneous pneumothorax. Am J Surg Pathol 1994; 18:195–199.

57. Willen R, Bruce T, Dahlstroem G, Duhiel WT. Squamous epithelial carcinoma in metaplastic pleura following extrapleural pneumothorax for pulmonary tuberculosis. Virchows Arch A Pathol Anat Histopathol 1976; 370:225–231.

58. Dunnill MS. Metaplastic changes in the visceral pleura in a case of fibrocystic disease of the pancreas. J Pathol Bacteriol 1959; 77:299–302.

59. Tomashefski JF, Dahms B, Bruce M. Pleura in pneumothorax. Comparison of patients with cystic fibrosis and 'idiopathic' spontaneous pneumothorax. Arch Pathol Lab Med 1985; 109:910–916.

60. Bashir MS, Cowen PN. Mucous metaplasia of the pleura. J Clin Pathol 1992; 45:1030–1031.

61. Jackson JW, Bennett MH. Chest wall tumour following iodized talc pleurodesis. Thorax 1969; 28:788–793.

62. Lange P, Mortensen J, Groth S. Lung function 22–35 years after treatment of idiopathic spontaneous pneumothorax with talc poudrage or simple drainage. Thorax 1988; 43:559–561.

63. Bignon J. Pour et contre la pleurodese au talc. Rev Mal Resp 1995; 12:193–195.

Inflammation of the pleura (pleuritis, pleurisy)

64. Bartlett JG, Thadepalli H, Gorbach SL, Finegold SM. Bacteriology of empyema. Lancet 1974; 1:338–340.

65. Neild JE, Eykyn SJ, Phillips I. Lung abscess and empyema. Q J Med 1985; 57:875–882.

66. Brook I, Frazier EH. Aerobic and anaerobic microbiology of empyema – a retrospective review in two military hospitals. Chest 1993; 103:1502–1507.

67. Porta G, RodriguezCarballeira M, Gomez L, et al. Thoracic infection caused by Streptococcus milleri. Eur Resp J 1998; 12:357–362.

68. Chen KY, Hsueh PR, Liaw YS, Yang PC, Luh KT. A 10-year experience with bacteriology of acute thoracic empyema – Emphasis on Klebsiella pneumoniae in patients with diabetes mellitus. Chest 2000; 117:1685–1689.

69. Hindle W, Yates DAH. Pyopneumothorax complicating rheumatoid lung disease. Ann Rheum Dis 1965; 24:57–60.

70. Davies D. Pyopneumothorax in rheumatoid lung disease. Thorax 1966; 21:230–235.

71. Levine H, Metzger W, Lacera D, Kay L. Diagnosis of tuberculous pleurisy by culture of pleural biopsy specimen. Arch Intern Med 1970; 126:269–271.

72. Krakowka P, Rowinska E, Halweg H. Infection of the pleura by Aspergillus fumigatus. Thorax 1970; 25:245–253.

73. Wood JB, Watson DCT. Sputum wax-worms after plombage. Br J Dis Chest 1988; 82:321–323.

74. Weissberg D, Weissberg D. Late complications of collapse therapy for pulmonary tuberculosis. Chest 2001; 120:847–851.

75. Shepherd MP. Plombage in the 1980s. Thorax 1985; 40:328–340.

76. Joseph J, Sahn SA. Connective tissue diseases and the pleura. Chest 1993; 104:262–270.

77. Ellman P, Cudkowicz L, Elwood JS. Widespread serous membrane involvement by rheumatoid nodules. J Clin Pathol 1954; 7:239–244.

78. Gruenwald P. Visceral lesions in a case of rheumatoid arthritis. Arch Pathol 1948; 46:59–67.

79. Dodson WH, Hollingsworth JW. Pleural effusion in rheumatoid arthritis. Impaired transport of glucose. N Engl J Med 1966; 275:1337–1342.

80. Nosanchuk JS, Naylor B. A unique cytologic picture in pleural fluid from patients with rheumatoid arthritis. Am J Clin Pathol 1968; 50:330–335.

81. Engel U, Aru A, Francis D. Rheumatoid pleurisy. Acta Path Microbiol Immunol 1986; 94:53–56.

82. Anderson RJ, Hansen KK, Kuzo RS, et al. A 38-year-old woman with chronic rheumatoid arthritis and a new pleural effusion - rheumatoid pleuritis. N Engl J Med 1994; 331:1642–1647.

Non-malignant asbestos-induced pleural disease

83. Hillerdal G. Non-malignant asbestos pleural disease. Thorax 1981; 36:669–675.

84. Gibbs AR, Stephens M, Griffiths DM, Blight BJN, Pooley FD. Fibre distribution in the lungs and pleura of subjects with asbestos related diffuse pleural fibrosis. Br J Ind Med 1991; 48:762–770.

85. Gaensler EA, Kaplan AI. Asbestos pleural effusion. Ann Intern Med 1971; 74:178–191.

86. Wright PH, Hanson A, Kreel L, Capel LH. Respiratory function changes after asbestos pleurisy. Thorax 1980; 35:31–36.

87. Herbert A, Sterling GM. Lung en cuirasse: histopathology of restrictive pleurisy with asbestos exposure. Thorax 1980; 35:715.

88. Stephens M, Gibbs AR, Pooley FD, Wagner JC. Asbestos induced diffuse pleural fibrosis: pathology and mineralogy. Thorax 1987; 42: 583–588.

89. Kee ST, Gamsu G, Blanc P. Causes of pulmonary impairment in asbestos-exposed individuals with diffuse pleural thickening. Am J Respir Crit Care Med 1996; 154: 789–793.

90. Yates DH, Browne K, Stidolph PN, Neville E. Asbestos-related bilateral diffuse pleural thickening: natural history of radiographic and lung function abnormalities [see comments]. Am J Respir Crit Care Med 1996; 153:301–306.

91. Gevenois PA, Demaertelaer V, Madani A, Winant C, Sergent G. Asbestosis, pleural plaques and diffuse pleural thickening: three distinct benign responses to asbestos exposure. Eur Resp J 1998; 11:1021–1027.

92. Davies D. Asbestos related diseases without asbestosis (editorial). BMJ 1983; 287:164–165.

93. Hoffbrand BI, Goldstraw P, Hetzel MR. Fibrosing pleuritis with extrathoracic extension. J R Soc Med 1985; 78:953–954.

94. O'Brien CJ, Franks AJ. Paraplegia due to massive asbestos-related pleural and mediastinal fibrosis. Histopathology 1987; 11:541–548.

95. Buchanan DR, Johnston IDA, Kerr IH, Hetzel MR, Corrin B, Turner-Warwick M. Cryptogenic bilateral fibrosing pleuritis. Br J Dis Chest 1988; 82:186–193.

96. Azoulay E, Paugam B, Heymann MF, et al. Familial extensive idiopathic bilateral pleural fibrosis. Eur Resp J 1999; 14:971–973.

97. Frankel SK, Cool CD, Lynch DA, Brown KK. Idiopathic pleuroparenchymal fibroelastosis: description of a novel clinicopathologic entity. Chest 2004; 126:2007–2013.

98. Hillerdal G. Rounded atelectasis. Clinical experience with 74 patients. Chest 1989; 95:836–841.

99. Blesovsky A. The folded lung. Br J Dis Chest 1966; 60:19–22.

100. Stark P. Rounded atelectasis: another pulmonary pseudotumor. Am Rev Respir Dis 1982; 125:248–250.

101. Mintzer RA, Cugell DW. The association of asbestos-induced pleural disease and rounded atelectasis. Chest 1982; 81:457–460.

102. Menzies R, Fraser R. Round atelectasis. Pathologic and pathogenic features. Am J Surg Pathol 1987; 11:674–681.

103. Hourihane DO, Lessof L, Richardson PC. Hyaline and calcified pleural plaques as an index of exposure to asbestos. A study of the radiological and pathological features of 100 cases with a consideration of epidemiology. BMJ 1966; 1:1069–1074.

104. Hillerdal G. Pleural plaques in a health survey material. Scand J Respir Dis 1978; 59:257–263.

105. Roberts GH. The pathology of parietal pleural plaques. J Clin Pathol 1971; 24:348–353.

106. Langer AM, Nolan RP, Constantopoulos SH, Moutsopoulos HM. Association of Metsovo lung and pleural mesothelioma with exposure to tremolite-containing whitewash. Lancet 1987; 1:965–967.

107. Constantopoulos SH, Theodoracopoulos P, Dascalopoulos G, Saratzis N, Sideris K. Metsovo lung outside Metsovo – endemic pleural calcifications in the ophiolite belts of Greece. Chest 1991; 99:1158–1161.

108. Weiss W. Asbestos-related pleural plaques and lung cancer. Chest 1993; 103:1854–1859.

109. Andrion A, Pira E, Mollo F. Peritoneal plaques and asbestos exposure. Arch Pathol Lab Med 1983; 107:609–10.

110. Baris YI, Sahin AA, Ozesmi M, et al. An outbreak of pleural mesothelioma and chronic fibrosing pleurisy in the village of Karain/Urgup in Anatolia. Thorax 1978; 33:181–192.

111. Rosen P, Gordon P, Savino A, Melamed M. Ferruginous bodies in benign fibrous pleural plaques. Am J Clin Pathol 1973; 60:608–612.

Pleural tumours

112. Jones MA, Young RH, Scully RE. Malignant mesothelioma of the tunica vaginalis: a clinicopathologic analysis of 11 cases with review of the literature. Am J Surg Pathol 1995; 19:815–825.

113. Henderson DW, Comin CE, Hammar SP, Shilkin KB, Whitaker D. Malignant mesothelioma of the pleura: current surgical pathology. In: Corrin B, ed. Pathology of Lung Tumors. London: Churchill Livingstone; 1997:241–280.

114. Peto J, Hodgson JT, Matthews FE, Jones JR. Continuing increase in mesothelioma mortality in Britain. Lancet 1995; 345:535–539.

115. Weill H, Hughes JM, Churg AM. Changing trends in US mesothelioma incidence. Occup Environ Med 2004; 61:438–441.

116. Wagner JC, Sleggs CA, Marchand P. Diffuse pleural mesotheliomas and asbestos exposure in Northwestern Cape Province. Br J Ind Med 1960; 17:260–271.

117. Hourihane DO. The pathology of mesotheliomata and analysis of their association with asbestos exposure. Thorax 1964; 19:268–278.

118. Newhouse ML, Thompson H. Mesothelioma of pleura and peritoneum following exposure to asbestos in the London area. Br J Ind Med 1965; 2:261–269.

119. Selikoff IJ, Churg J, Hammond EC. Relation between asbestos exposure and neoplasia. N Engl J Med 1965; 272:560–565.

120. Whitwell F, Rawcliffe RM. Diffuse malignant pleural mesothelioma and asbestos exposure. Thorax 1971; 26:6–22.

121. Selikoff IJ, Hammond EC, Churg J. Carcinogenicity of amosite asbestos. Arch Env Health 1972; 25:183–186.

122. Anderson KA, Hurley WC, Hurley BT, Ohrt DW. Malignant pleural mesothelioma following radiotherapy in a 16 year old boy. Cancer 1985; 56:273–276.

123. Gilks B, Hegedus C, Freeman H, Fratkin L, Churg A. Malignant peritoneal mesothelioma after remote abdominal radiation. Cancer 1988; 61:2019–2021.

124. Hillerdal G, Berg J. Malignant mesothelioma secondary to chronic inflammation and old scars. Two new cases and review of the literature. Cancer 1985; 55:1968–1972.

125. Shannon VR, Nesbitt JC, Libshitz HI. Malignant pleural mesothelioma after radiation therapy for breast cancer – a report of two additional patients. Cancer 1995; 76:437–441.

126. Cavazza A, Travis LB, Travis WD, et al. Post-irradiation malignant mesothelioma. Cancer 1996; 77:1379–1385.

127. Neugut AI, Ahsan H, Antman KH. Incidence of malignant pleural mesothelioma after thoracic radiotherapy. Cancer 1997; 80:948–950.

128. Cicala C, Pompetti F, Carbone M. SV40 induces mesotheliomas in hamsters. Am J Pathol 1993; 142:1524–1533.

129. Carbone M, Pass HI, Rizzo P, et al. Simian virus 40-like DNA sequences in human pleural mesothelioma. Oncogene 1994; 9:1781–1790.

130. Cacciotti P, Strizzi L, Vianale G, et al. The presence of simian-virus 40 sequences in mesothelioma and mesothelial cells is associated with high levels of vascular endothelial growth factor. Am J Respir Cell Molec Biol 2002; 26:189–193.

131. Galateau-Salle F, Bidet P, Iwatsubo Y, et al. SV40-like DNA sequences in pleural mesothelioma, bronchopulmonary carcinoma, and non-malignant pulmonary diseases. J Pathol 1998; 184:252–257.

132. Mulatero C, Surentheran T, Breuer J, Rudd RM. Simian virus 40 and human pleural mesothelioma. Thorax 1999; 54:60–61.

133. Ramael M, Nagels J, Heylen H, et al. Detection of SV40 like viral DNA and viral antigens in malignant pleural mesothelioma. Eur Resp J 1999; 14:1381–1386.

134. Rizzo P, Carbone M, Fisher SG, et al. Simian virus 40 is present in most United States human mesotheliomas, but it is rarely present in non-Hodgkin's lymphoma. Chest 1999; 116:470S–473S.

135. Pilatte Y, Vivo C, Renier A, Kheuang L, Greffard A, Jaurand MC. Absence of SV40 large T-antigen expression in human mesothelioma cell lines. Am J Respir Cell Molec Biol 2000; 23:788–793.

136. Mayall F, Barratt K, Shanks J. The detection of Simian virus 40 in mesotheliomas from New Zealand and England using real time FRET probe PCR protocols. J Clin Pathol 2003; 56:728–730.

137. Huncharek M. Changing risk groups for malignant mesothelioma. Cancer 1992; 69:2704–2711.

138. Cazzadori A, Malesani F, Romeo L. Malignant pleural mesothelioma caused by nonoccupational childhood exposure to asbestos. Br J Ind Med 1992; 49:599.

139. Rey F, Viallat JR, Boutin C, et al. Les mesotheliomes environnementaux en Corse du nord-est. Rev Mal Resp 1993; 10:339–345.

140. Magnani C, Terracini B, Ivaldi C, Botta M, Mancini A, Andrion A. Pleural malignant mesothelioma and non-occupational exposure to asbestos in Casale Monferrato, Italy. Occup Environ Med 1995; 52:362–367.

141. Constantopoulos SH, Malamou-Mitsi V, Goudevenos J, Papathanasiou M, Pavlidis N, Papadimitriou C. High incidence of malignant pleural mesothelioma in neighbouring village of North-western Greece. Respiration 1987; 51:266–271.

142. Metintas S, Metintas M, Ucgun I, Oner U. Malignant mesothelioma due to environmental exposure to asbestos – Follow-up of a Turkish cohort living in a rural area. Chest 2002; 122:2224–2229.

143. Wagner JC. Mesothelioma and mineral fibres. Cancer 1986; 57:1905–1911.

144. Wagner JC, Newhouse ML, Corrin B, Rossiter CER, Griffiths DM. Correlation between fibre content of the lung and disease in east London asbestos factory workers. Br J Ind Med 1988; 45:305–308.

145. Churg A, Vedal S. Fiber burden and patterns of asbestos-related disease in workers with heavy mixed amosite and chrysotile exposure. Am J Respir Crit Care Med 1994; 150:663–669.

146. McDonald JC, Armstrong B, Case B, et al. Mesothelioma and asbestos fiber type. Evidence from lung tissue analyses. Cancer 1989; 63:1544–1547.

147. Churg A, Wright JL, Vedal S. Fiber burden and patterns of asbestos-related disease in chrysotile miners and millers. Am Rev Respir Dis 1993; 148:25–31.

148. McDonald JC, McDonald AD. The epidemiology of mesothelioma in historical context. Eur Respir J 1996; 9:1932–1942.

149. Senyigit A, Babayigit C, Gokirmak M, et al. Incidence of malignant pleural mesothelioma due to environmental asbestos fiber exposure in the southeast of Turkey. Respiration 2000; 67:610–614.

150. Wagner JC. Experimental production of mesothelial tumours of the pleura by implantation of dusts in laboratory animals. Nature 1962; 196:180–181.

151. Wagner JC, Berry G, Timbrell V. Mesotheliomata in rats after inoculation with asbestos and other materials. Br J Cancer 1973; 28:173–185.

152. Johnson NF, Edwards RE, Munday DE, Rowe N, Wagner JC. Pluripotential nature of mesotheliomata induced by inhalation of erionite in rats. Br J Exp Pathol 1984; 65:377–388.

153. Doll R. Symposium on man-made mineral fibres, Copenhagen, October 1986: overview and conclusions. Ann Occup Hyg 1987; 31:805–820.

154. Stanton MF, Layard M, Tegeris A, Miller E, May M, Kenty E. Carcinogenicity of fibrous glass: pleural response in the rat in relation to fibre dimension. J Natl Cancer Inst 1977; 58:587–603.

155. Fraire AE, Greenberg SD, Spjut HJ, et al. Effect of fibrous glass on rat pleural mesothelium histopathologic observations. Am J Respir Crit Care Med 1994; 150:521–527.

156. Kilburn KH, Powers D, Warshaw RH. Pulmonary effects of exposure to fine fibreglass - irregular opacities and small airways obstruction. Br J Ind Med 1992; 49:714–720.

157. Shannon HS, Jamieson E, Julian JA, Muir DCF. Mortality of glass filament (textile) workers. Br J Ind Med 1990; 47:533–536.

158. Hughes JM, Jones RN, Glindmeyer HW, Hammad YY, Weill H. Follow up study of workers exposed to man made mineral fibres. Br J Ind Med 1993; 50:658–667.

159. Devuyst P, Dumortier P, Swaen GMH, Pairon JC, Brochard P. Respiratory health effects of man-made vitreous (mineral) fibres. Eur Respir J 1995; 8:2149–2173.

160. Craighead JE, Richards SA, Calore JD, Fan H, Weaver DL. Genetic factors influence malignant mesothelioma development in mice. Eur Respir Rev 1993; 3:118–120.

161. Hammar SP, Bockus D, Remington F, Freidman S, Lazerte G. Familial mesothelioma: a report of two families. Hum Pathol 1989; 20:107–112.

162. Dawson A, Gibbs A, Browne K, Pooley F, Griffiths M. Familial mesothelioma – details of 17 cases with histopathologic findings and mineral analysis. Cancer 1992; 70: 1183–1187.

163. Browne K. The epidemiology of mesothelioma. J Soc Occup Med 1983; 33:190–194.

164. Lanphear BP, Buncher CR. Latent period for malignant mesothelioma of occupational origin. J Occup Med 1992; 34:718–721.

165. Yates DH. Malignant mesothelioma in south east England: clinicopathological experience of 272 cases (Correction to Vol. 52:507). Thorax 1997; 52:1018.

166. Andrion A, Bosia S, Paoletti L, et al. Malignant peritoneal mesothelioma in a 17-year-old boy with evidence of previous exposure to chrysotile and tremolite asbestos. Hum Pathol 1994; 25:617–622.

167. Brenner J, Sardillo PP, Magill CB. Malignant mesothelioma in children – report of seven cases and review of the literature. Med Pediatr Oncol 1981; 9:367–373.

168. Fraire AE, Cooper S, Greenberg SD, Buffler P, Langston C. Mesothelioma of childhood. Cancer 1988; 62:838–847.

169. Cooper SP, Fraire EA, Buffler PA, Greenberg SD, Langston C. Epidemiologic aspects of childhood mesothelioma. Pathol Immunopathol Res 1989; 8:276–286.

170. Marie LC, Lee YJ, Ho MY. Malignant mesothelioma in infancy. Arch Pathol Lab Med 1989; 113:409–410.

171. Dawson A, Gibbs AR, Pooley FD, Griffiths DM, Hoy J. Malignant mesothelioma in women. Thorax 1993; 48:269–274.

172. Browne K, Smither WJ. Asbestos-related mesothelioma: factors discriminating between pleural and peritoneal sites. Br J Ind Med 1983; 40:145–152.

173. Gross P, Harley RA, Swinburne LM, Davis JMG, Green WB. Ingested mineral fibres: do they penetrate tissues or cause cancer? Arch Env Health 1974; 29:341–347.

174. Roggli VL, Pratt PC. Numbers of asbestos bodies on iron-stained tissue sections in relation to asbestos body counts in lung tissue digests. Hum Pathol 1983; 14:355–361.

175. Roggli VL, Pratt PC, Brody AR. Asbestos content of lung tissue in asbestos associated diseases: a study of 110 cases. Br J Ind Med 1986; 43:18–28.

176. De Vuyst P, Karjalainen A, Dumortier P, et al. Guidelines for mineral fibre analyses in biological samples: report of the ERS Working Group. Eur Resp J 1998; 11:1416–1426.

177. Peterson JT, Greenberg SD, Butler PA. Non-asbestos related malignant mesothelioma. Cancer 1984; 54:951–960.

178. Gibbs AR, Jones JSP, Pooley FD, Griffiths DM, Wagner JC. Non-occupational malignant mesotheliomas. In: Bignon J, Peto J, Saracci R, eds. Non-occupational Exposure to Mineral Fibres. Lyon: International Agency for Research on Cancer; 1989:219–228.

179. Gibbs AR. Role of asbestos and other fibres in the development of diffuse malignant mesothelioma. Thorax 1990; 45:649–654.

180. Rom WN, Travis WD, Brody AR. Cellular and molecular basis of the asbestos-related diseases. Am Rev Respir Dis 1991; 143:408–422.

181. Srebro SH, Roggli VL, Samsa GP. Malignant mesothelioma associated with low pulmonary tissue asbestos burdens: a light and scanning electron microscopic analysis of 18 cases. Mod Pathol 1995; 8:614–621.

182. Yates DH, Corrin B, Stidolph PN, Browne K. Malignant mesothelioma in south east England: clinicopathological experience of 272 cases. Thorax 1997; 52:507–512.

183. Roggli VL. Quantitative and analytical studies in the diagnosis of mesothelioma. Semin Diagn Pathol 1992; 9:162–168.

184. Crotty TB, Colby TV, Gay PC, Pisani RJ. Desmoplastic malignant mesothelioma masquerading as sclerosing mediastinitis – a diagnostic dilemma. Hum Pathol 1992; 23:79–82.

185. Brenner J, Sardillo PP, Magill GB, Golbey RB. Malignant mesothelioma of the pleura. Review of 123 patients. Cancer 1982; 49:2431–2435.

186. Sussman J, Rosai J. Lymph node metastasis as the initial manifestation of malignant mesothelioma: report of six cases. Am J Surg Pathol 1990; 14:819–828.

187. Sussman J, Rosai J. Mesothelioma metastasis. Am J Surg Pathol 1991; 15:1016–1017.

188. Ohishi N, Oka T, Fukuhara T, Yotsumoto H, Yazaki Y. Extensive pulmonary metastases in malignant pleural mesothelioma: a rare clinical and radiographic presentation. Chest 1996; 110:296–298.

189. Ghosh AK, Mason DY, Spriggs AI. Immunocytochemical staining with monoclonal antibodies in cytologically 'negative' serous effusions from patients with malignant disease. J Clin Pathol 1983; 36:1150–1153.

190. Ghosh AK, Spriggs AI, Taylor-Papadimitriou J, Mason DY. Immunocytochemical staining of cells in pleural and peritoneal effusions with a panel of monoclonal antibodies. J Clin Pathol 1983; 36:1154–1164.

191. Renshaw AA, Dean BR, Antman KH, Sugarbaker DJ, Cibas ES. The role of cytologic evaluation of pleural fluid in the diagnosis of malignant mesothelioma. Chest 1997; 111:106–109.

192. Esteban JM, Yokota S, Husain S, Battifora H. Immunocytochemical profile of benign and carcinomatous effusions – a practical approach to difficult diagnosis. Am J Clin Pathol 1990; 94:698–705.

193. Singer S, Boddington MM, Hudson EA. Immunocytochemical reaction of Ca1 and HMFG2 monoclonal antibodies with cells from serous effusions. J Clin Pathol 1985; 38:180–184.

194. de Angelis M, Buley ID, Heryet A, Gray W. Immunocytochemical staining of serous effusions with the monoclonal antibody Ber-EP4. Cytopathol 1992; 3:111–117.

195. Yamashita K, Kuba T, Shinoda H, Takahashi E, Okayasu I. Detection of K-ras point mutations in the supernatants of peritoneal and pleural effusions for diagnosis complementary to cytologic examination. Am J Clin Pathol 1998; 109:704–711.

196. Chen LM, Lazcano O, Katzmann JA, Kimlinger TK, Li CY. The role of conventional cytology, immunocytochemistry, and flow cytometric DNA ploidy in the evaluation of body cavity fluids: A prospective study of 52 patients. Am J Clin Pathol 1998; 109:712–721.

197. Tao L. The cytopathology of mesothelioma. Acta Cytol 1979; 23:209–213.

198. Whitaker D, Shilkin KB. Diagnosis of pleural malignant mesothelioma in life – a practical approach. J Pathol 1984; 143:147–175.

199. Sears D, Hajdu SI. The cytologic diagnosis of malignant neoplasms in pleural and peritoneal effusions. Acta Cytol 1987; 31:85–97.

200. Roboz J, Greaves J, Silides D, Chahinian AP, Holland JF. Hyaluronic acid content of effusions as a diagnostic aid for malignant mesothelioma. Cancer Res 1985; 45:1850–1854.

201. Faravelli B, D'Amore E, Nosenzo M, Betta P-G, Donna A. Carcinoembryonic antigen in pleural effusions. Cancer 1984; 53:1194–1197.

202. Faravelli B, Nosenzo M, Razzetti A, et al. The role of concurrent determinations of pleural fluid and tissue carcinoembryonic antigen in the distinction of malignant mesothelioma from metastatic pleural malignancies. Eur J Cancer Clin Oncol 1985; 21:1083–1087.

203. Mezger J, Permanetter W, Gerbes AL, Wilmanns W, Lamerz R. Tumour associated antigens in diagnosis of serous effusions. J Clin Pathol 1988; 41:633–643.

204. Boutin C, Rey F, Gouvernet J, Viallat JR, Astoul P, Ledoray V. Thoracoscopy in pleural malignant mesothelioma – a prospective study of 188 consecutive patients. 2. prognosis and staging. Cancer 1993; 72:394–404.

205. Crotty TB, Myers JL, Katzenstein ALA, Tazelaar HD, Swensen SJ, Churg A. Localized malignant mesothelioma – a clinicopathologic and flow cytometric study. Am J Surg Pathol 1994; 18:357–363.

206. Okamura H, Kamei T, Mitsuno A, Hongo H, Sakuma N, Ishihara T. Localized malignant mesothelioma of the pleura. Pathol Int 2001; 51:654–660.

207. Erkilic S, Sari I, Tuncozgur B. Localized pleural malignant mesothelioma. Pathol Int 2001; 51:812–815.

208. Hirano H, Takeda S, Sawabata Y, et al. Localized pleural malignant mesothelioma. Pathol Int 2003; 53:616–621.

209. Asioli S, Dal Piaz G, Damiani S. Localised pleural malignant mesothelioma. Report of two cases simulating pulmonary carcinoma and review of the literature. Virchows Arch 2004; 445:206–209.

210. Denton KJ, Cotton DWK, Nakielny RA, Goepel JR. Secondary tumour deposits in needle biopsy tracks: an underestimated risk? J Clin Pathol 1990; 43:83.

211. Herbert A, Gallagher PJ. Pleural biopsy in the diagnosis of malignant mesothelioma. Thorax 1982; 37:816–821.

212. Donna A, Betta PG. Mesodermomas: a new embryological approach to primary tumours of coelomic surfaces. Histopathology 1981; 5:31–44.

213. Donna A, Betta PG. Differentiation towards cartilage and bone in a primary tumour of pleura. Further evidence in support of the concept of mesodermoma. Histopathology 1986; 10:101–108.

214. Donna A, Betta PG, Bianchi V, et al. A new insight into the histogenesis of mesodermomas - malignant mesotheliomas. Histopathology 1991; 19:239–243.

215. Attanoos RL, Gibbs AR. Pathology of malignant mesothelioma. Histopathology 1997; 30: 403–418.

216. Suzuki Y. Pathology of human malignant mesothelioma. Semin Oncol 1981; 8:268–281.

217. Law MR, Hodson ME, Heard BE. Malignant mesothelioma of the pleura: relation between histological type and clinical behaviour. Thorax 1982; 37:810–815.

218. Vangelder T, Hoogsteden HC, Vandenbroucke JP, van der Kwast TH, Planteydt HT. The influence of the diagnostic technique on the histopathological diagnosis in malignant mesothelioma. Virchows Arch A Pathol Anat Histopathol 1991; 418:315–317.

219. Klima M, Gyorkey F. Benign pleural lesions and malignant mesothelioma. Virchows Arch A Pathol Anat Histopathol 1977; 376:181–193.

220. Whitaker D, Henderson DW, Shilkin KB. The concept of mesothelioma in situ: implications for diagnosis and histogenesis. Semin Diagn Pathol 1992; 9:151–161.

221. Cook DS, Attanoos RL, Jalloh SS, Gibbs AR. 'Mucin-positive' epithelial mesothelioma of the peritoneum: an unusual diagnostic pitfall. Histopathology 2000; 37:33–36.

222. Mayall FG, Gibbs AR. The histology and immunohistochemistry of small cell mesothelioma. Histopathology 1992; 20:47–51.

223. Battifora H, McCaughey WTE. Tumors of the serosal membranes. Washington: Armed Forces Institute of Pathology, 1995.

224. Okamoto H, Matsuno Y, Noguchi M, et al. Malignant pleural mesothelioma producing human chorionic gonadotropin – report of two cases. Am J Surg Pathol 1992; 16:969–974.

225. Burdick CO. HCG positive mesothelioma. Am J Surg Pathol 1993; 17:749–750.

226. Nascimento AG, Keeney GL, Fletcher CDM. Deciduoid peritoneal mesothelioma – an unusual phenotype affecting young females. Am J Surg Pathol 1994; 18:439–445.

227. Shanks JH, Harris M, Banerjee SS, et al. Mesotheliomas with deciduoid morphology – A morphologic spectrum and a variant not confined to young females. Am J Surg Pathol 2000; 24:285–294.

227a. Henley JD, Loehrer PJ, Ulbright TM. Deciduoid mesothelioma of the pleura after radiation therapy for Hodgkin's disease presenting as a mediastinal mass. Am J Surg Pathol 2001; 25:547–548.

228. Serio G, Scattone A, Pennella A, et al. Malignant deciduoid mesothelioma of the pleura: report of two cases with long survival. Histopathology 2002; 40:348–352.

229. Shia J, Erlandson RA, Klimstra DS. Deciduoid mesothelioma: A report of 5 cases and literature review. Ultrastruct Pathol 2002; 26:355–363.

229a. Mourra N, de Chaisemartin C, Goubin-Versini I, et al. Malignant deciduoid mesothelioma: a diagnostic challenge. Arch Pathol Lab Med 2005; 129:403–406.

230. Puttagunta L, Vriend RA, Nguyen GK. Deciduoid epithelial mesothelioma of the pleura with focal rhabdoid change. Am J Surg Pathol 2000; 24:1440–1443.

231. Ordonez NG, Myhre M, Mackay B. Clear cell mesothelioma. Ultrastruct Pathol 1996; 20:331–336.

232. Dessy E, Falleni M, Braidotti P, DelCurto B, Panigalli T, Pietra GG. Unusual clear cell variant of epithelioid mesothelioma. Arch Pathol Lab Med 2001; 125:1588–1590.

233. Hurlimann J. Desmin and neural marker expression in mesothelial cells and mesotheliomas. Hum Pathol 1994; 25:753–757.

234. Yousem S, Hochholzer L. Malignant mesotheliomas with osseous and cartilaginous differentiation. Arch Pathol Lab Med 1987; 111:62–66.

235. Mayall FG, Goddard H, Gibbs AR. Intermediate filament expression in mesotheliomas – leiomyoid mesotheliomas are not uncommon. Histopathology 1992; 21:453–457.

236. Krishna J, Haqqani MT. Liposarcomatous differentiation in diffuse pleural mesothelioma. Thorax 1993; 48:409–410.

237. Chang HT, Yantiss RK, Nielsen GP, McKee GT, Mark EJ. Lipid-rich diffuse malignant mesothelioma: A case report. Hum Pathol 2000; 31:876–879.

238. Henderson DW, Attwood HD, Constance TJ, Shilkin KB, Steele RH. Lymphohistiocytoid mesothelioma: a rare lymphomatoid variant of predominantly sarcomatoid mesothelioma. Ultrastruct Pathol 1988; 12:367–384.

239. Khalidi HS, Medeiros LJ, Battifora H. Lymphohistiocytoid mesothelioma – An often misdiagnosed variant of sarcomatoid malignant mesothelioma. Am J Clin Pathol 2000; 113:649–654.

240. Harwood TR, Gracey DR, Yokoo H. Pseudomesotheliomatous carcinoma of the lung – a variant of peripheral lung cancer. Am J Clin Pathol 1976; 65:159–167.

241. Dessy E, Pietra GG. Pseudomesotheliomatous carcinoma of the lung – an immunohistochemical and ultrastructural study of three cases. Cancer 1991; 68:1747–1753.

242. Koss M, Travis W, Moran C, Hochholzer L. Pseudomesotheliomatous adenocarcinoma: a reappraisal. Semin Diagn Pathol 1992; 9:117–123.

243. Taylor DR, Page W, Hughes D, Varghese G. Metastatic renal cell carcinoma mimicking pleural mesothelioma. Thorax 1987; 42:901–902.

244. Attanoos RL, Suvarna SK, Rhead E, et al. Malignant vascular tumours of the pleura in 'asbestos' workers and endothelial differentiation in malignant mesothelioma. Thorax 2000; 55:860–863.

245. Zimmerman KG, Sobonya RE, Payne CM. Histochemical and ultrastructural features of an unusual pulmonary carcinosarcoma. Hum Pathol 1981; 12:1046–1051.

246. Mayall FG, Gibbs AR. Pleural and pulmonary carcinosarcomas. J Pathol 1992; 167:305–311.

247. Gaertner E, Zeren EH, Fleming MV, Colby TV, Travis WD. Biphasic synovial sarcomas arising in the pleural cavity: a clinicopathologic study of five cases. Am J Surg Pathol 1996; 20:36–45.

248. Jawahar DA, Vuletin JC, Gorecki P, Persechino F, Macera M, Magazeh P. Primary biphasic synovial sarcoma of the pleura. Resp Med 1997; 91:568–570.

249. Kashima T, Matsushita H, Kuroda M, et al. Biphasic synovial sarcoma of the peritoneal cavity with t(X; 18) demonstrated by reverse transcriptase polymerase chain reaction. Pathol Int 1997; 47:637–641.

250. Attanoos RL, Griffin A, Gibbs AR. The use of immunohistochemistry in distinguishing reactive from neoplastic mesothelium. A novel use for desmin and comparative evaluation with epithelial membrane antigen, p53, platelet-derived growth factor-receptor, P-glycoprotein and Bcl-2. Histopathology 2003; 43:231–238.

251. Macdougall DB, Wang SE, Zidar BL. Mucin-positive epithelial mesothelioma. Arch Pathol Lab Med 1992; 116:874–880.

252. Hammar SP, Bockus DE, Remington FL, Rohrbach KA. Mucin-positive epithelial mesotheliomas: a histochemical, immunohistochemical, and ultrastructural comparison with mucin- producing pulmonary adenocarcinomas. Ultrastruct Pathol 1996; 20:293–325.

253. Adams SA, Sherwood AJ, Smith MEF. Malignant mesothelioma: PAS-diastase positivity and inversion of polarity in intravascular tumour. Histopathology 2002; 41:260–262.

254. Ordonez NG, Mackay B. Glycogen-rich mesothelioma. Ultrastruct Pathol 1999; 23:401–406.

255. Wagner JC, Munday DE, Harington JS. Histochemical demonstration of hyaluronic acid in pleural mesothelioma. J Pathol Bacteriol 1962; 84:73–78.

256. Robb JA. Mesothelioma versus adenocarcinoma: false-positive CEA and Leu-M1 staining due to hyaluronic acid. Hum Pathol 1989; 20:400.

257. Noguchi M, Nakajima T, Hirohashi S, Akiba T, Shimosato Y. Immunohistochemical distinction of malignant mesothelioma from pulmonary adenocarcinoma with anti-surfactant apoprotein, anti-Lewis(a), and anti-Tn antibodies. Hum Pathol 1989; 20:53–57.

258. Khoor A, Whitsett JA, Stahlman MT, Olson SJ, Cagle PT. Utility of surfactant protein B precursor and thyroid transcription factor 1 in differentiating adenocarcinoma of the lung from malignant mesothelioma. Hum Pathol 1999; 30:695–700.

259. Ordonez NG. The immunohistochemical diagnosis of mesothelioma – A comparative study of epithelioid mesothelioma and lung adenocarcinoma. Am J Surg Pathol 2003; 27:1031–1051.

260. Llinares K, Escande F, Aubert S, et al. Diagnostic value of MUC4 immunostaining in distinguishing epithelial mesothelioma and lung adenocarcinoma. Mod Pathol 2004; 17:150–157.

261. Miettinen M, SarlomoRikala M. Expression of calretinin, thrombomodulin, keratin 5, and mesothelin in lung carcinomas of different types – An immunohistochemical analysis of 596 tumors in comparison with epithelioid mesotheliomas of the pleura. Am J Surg Pathol 2003; 27:150–158.

262. Attanoos RL, Gibbs AR. 'Pseudomesotheliomatous' carcinomas of the pleura: a 10-year analysis of cases from the Environmental Lung Disease Research Group, Cardiff. Histopathology 2003; 43:444–452.

263. Osborn M, Pelling N, Walker MM, Fisher C, Nicholson AG. The value of 'mesothelium-associated' antibodies in distinguishing between metastatic renal cell carcinomas and mesotheliomas. Histopathology 2002; 41:301–307.

264. Ordonez NG. The diagnostic utility of immunohistochemistry in distinguishing between mesothelioma and renal cell carcinoma: a comparative study. Hum Pathol 2004; 35:697–710.

265. Attanoos RL, Goddard H, Thomas ND, Jasani B, Gibbs AR. A comparative immunohistochemical study of malignant mesothelioma and renal cell carcinoma: the diagnostic utility of Leu-m1, Ber EP4, Tamm-Horsfall protein and thrombomodulin. Histopathology 1995; 27:361–366.

266. Attanoos RL, Webb R, Dojcinov SD, Gibbs AR. Value of mesothelial and epithelial antibodies in distinguishing diffuse peritoneal mesothelioma in females from serous papillary carcinoma of the ovary and peritoneum. Histopathology 2002; 40:237–244.

267. Comin CE, deKlerk NH, Henderson DW. Malignant mesothelioma: Current conundrums over risk estimates and whither electron microscopy for diagnosis? Ultrastruct Pathol 1997; 21:315–320.

268. Oury TD, Hammar SP, Roggli VL. Ultrastructural features of diffuse malignant mesotheliomas. Hum Pathol 1998; 29:1382–1392.

269. Dewar A, Valente M, Ring NP, Corrin B. Pleural mesothelioma of epithelial type and pulmonary adenocarcinoma: an ultrastructural and cytochemical comparison. J Pathol 1987; 152:309–316.

270. Wang N-S. Electron microscopy in the diagnosis of pleural mesotheliomas. Cancer 1973; 31:1046–1054.

271. Suzuki Y, Churg J, Kannerstein M. Ultrastructure of human malignant diffuse mesothelioma. Am J Pathol 1976; 85:241–262.

272. Warhol MJ, Hickey WF, Carson JM. Malignant mesothelioma: ultrastructural distinction from adenocarcinoma. Am J Surg Pathol 1982; 6:307–314.

273. Dardick I, Jabi M, Elliott WT, et al. Diffuse epithelial mesothelioma: a review of the ultrastructural spectrum. Ultrastruct Pathol 1987; 11:503–533.

274. Corrin B, Dewar A. Adenocarcinoma simulating mesothelioma. Ultrastruct Pathol 1996; 20:327–329.

275. Falconieri G, Zanconati F, Bussani R, Dibonito L. Small cell carcinoma of lung simulating pleural mesothelioma – report of 4 cases with autopsy confirmation. Pathol Res Pract 1995; 191:1147–1151.

276. Mayall FG, Jasani B, Gibbs AR. Immunohistochemical positivity for neuron-specific enolase and Leu-7 in malignant mesotheliomas. J Pathol 1991; 165:325–328.

277. Lantuejoul S, Laverriere MH, Sturm N, et al. NCAM (Neural cell adhesion molecules) expression in malignant mesotheliomas. Hum Pathol 2000; 31:415–421.

278. Burmer GC, Rabinovitch PS, Kulander BG, Rusch V, McNutt MA. Flow cytometric analysis of malignant pleural mesotheliomas. Hum Pathol 1989; 20:777–783.

279. Elnaggar AK, Ordonez NG, Garnsey L, Batsakis JG. Epithelioid pleural mesotheliomas and pulmonary adenocarcinomas – a comparative DNA flow cytometric study. Hum Pathol 1991; 22:972–978.

280. Sheibani K, Esteban JM, Bailey A, Battifora H, Weiss LM. Immunopathologic and molecular studies as an aid to the diagnosis of malignant mesothelioma. Hum Pathol 1992; 23:107–116.

281. Gordon GJ, Jensen RV, Hsiao LL, et al. Translation of microarray data into clinically relevant cancer diagnostic tests using gene expression ratios in lung cancer and mesothelioma. Cancer Res 2002; 62:4963–4967.

282. Churg A, Colby TV, Cagle P, et al. The separation of benign and malignant mesothelial proliferations. Am J Surg Pathol 2000; 24:1183–1200.

283. Marshall RJ, Herbert A, Braye SG, Jones DB. Use of antibodies to carcinoembryonic antigen and human milk fat globule to distinguish carcinoma, mesothelioma, and reactive mesothelium. J Clin Pathol 1984; 37:1215–1221.

284. Cury PM, Butcher DN, Corrin B, Nicholson AG. The use of histological and immunohistochemical markers to distinguish pleural malignant mesothelioma and in situ mesothelioma from reactive mesothelial hyperplasia and reactive pleural fibrosis. J Pathol 1999; 189:251–257.

285. Marchevsky AM, Gil J, Caccamo D. Computerized interactive morphometry. A study of malignant mesothelioma and mesothelial hyperplasia in pleural biopsy specimens. Arch Pathol Lab Med 1985; 109:1102–1105.

286. Bogers J, Jacobs W, Segers K, Vandaele A, Weyler J, Vanmarck E. Stereological evaluation of malignant mesothelioma versus benign pleural hyperplasia. Pathol Res Pract 1996; 192:10–14.

287. Ayres JG, Crocker JG, Skilbeck NQ. Differentiation of malignant from normal and reactive mesothelial cells by the argyrophil technique for nucleolar organiser region associated proteins. Thorax 1988; 43:366–370.

288. Soosay GN, Griffiths M, Papadaki L, Happerfield L, Bobrow L. The differential diagnosis of epithelial-type mesothelioma from adenocarcinoma and reactive mesothelial proliferation. J Pathol 1991; 163:299–305.

289. Ramael M, Jacobs W, Weyler J, et al. Proliferation in malignant mesothelioma as determined by mitosis counts and immunoreactivity for proliferating cell nuclear antigen (PCNA). J Pathol 1994; 172:247–253.

290. Bethwaite PB, Delahunt B, Holloway LJ, Thornton A. Comparison of silver-staining nucleolar organizer region (agNOR) counts and

proliferating cell nuclear antigen (PCNA) expression in reactive mesothelial hyperplasia and malignant mesothelioma. Pathology 1995; 27:1–4.

291. Sington JD, Morris LS, Nicholson AG, Coleman N. Assessment of cell cycle state may facilitate the histopathological diagnosis of malignant mesothelioma. Histopathology 2003; 42:498–502.

292. Kumaki F, Kawai T, Churg A, et al. Expression of telomerase reverse transcriptase (TERT) in malignant mesotheliomas. Am J Surg Pathol 2002; 26:365–370.

293. Blobel GA, Moll R, Franke WW, Kayser KW, Gould VE. The intermediate filament cytoskeleton of malignant mesothelioma and its diagnostic significance. Am J Pathol 1985; 121:235–247.

294. Lucas DR, Pass HI, Madan SK, et al. Sarcomatoid mesothelioma and its histological mimics: a comparative immunohistochemical study. Histopathology 2003; 42:270–279.

295. Epstein JI, Budin RE. Keratin and epithelial membrane antigen immunoreactivity in nonneoplastic fibrous pleural lesions: implications for the diagnosis of desmoplastic mesothelioma. Hum Pathol 1986; 17:514–519.

296. Mayall FG, Goddard H, Gibbs AR. The diagnostic implications of variable cytokeratin expression in mesotheliomas. J Pathol 1993; 170:165–168.

297. Attanoos RL, Dojcinov SD, Webb R, Gibbs AR. Anti-mesothelial markers in sarcomatoid mesothelioma and other spindle cell neoplasms. Histopathology 2000; 37:224–231.

298. Miettinen M, Limon J, Niezabitowski A, Lasota J. Calretinin and other mesothelioma markers in synovial sarcoma – Analysis of antigenic similarities and differences with malignant mesothelioma. Am J Surg Pathol 2001; 25:610–617.

299. Mayall FG, Gibbs AR. Leiomyoid mesotheliomas – reply. Histopathology 1993; 22:602.

300. Kung ITM, Thallas V, Spencer EJ, Wilson SM. Expression of muscle actins in diffuse mesotheliomas. Hum Pathol 1995; 26:565–570.

301. Attanoos RL, Appleton MAC, Gibbs AR. Primary sarcomas of the lung: a clinicopathological and immunohistochemical study of 14 cases. Histopathology 1996; 29:29–36.

302. Corrin B, Dewar A, Simpson CGB. Epithelioid hemangioendothelioma of the lung. Ultrastruct Pathol 1996; 20:345–347.

303. Lin BTY, Colby T, Gown AM, et al. Malignant vascular tumors of the serous membranes mimicking mesothelioma: a report of 14 cases. Am J Surg Pathol 1996; 20:1431–1439.

304. Attanoos RL, Dallimore NS, Gibbs AR. Primary epithelioid haemangioendothelioma of the peritoneum: An unusual mimic of diffuse malignant mesothelioma. Histopathology 1997; 30:375–377.

305. Payne CB, Morningstar WA, Chester EH. Thymoma of the pleura masquerading as diffuse mesothelioma. Am Rev Respir Dis 1960; 94:441–446.

306. Moran CA, Travis WD, Rosado-de-Christenson M, Koss MN, Rosai J. Thymomas presenting as pleural tumors – report of eight cases. Am J Surg Pathol 1992; 16:138–144.

307. Shih DF, Wang JS, Tseng HH, Tiao WM. Primary pleural thymoma. Arch Pathol Lab Med 1997; 121:79–82.

308. Klima M, Bossart MI. Sarcomatous type of malignant mesothelioma. Ultrastruct Pathol 1983; 4:349–358.

309. Hammar SP, Bolen JW. Sarcomatoid pleural mesothelioma. Ultrastruct Pathol 1985; 9: 337–343.

310. Cantin R, Al-Jabi M, McCaughey WTE. Desmoplastic diffuse mesothelioma. Am J Surg Pathol 1982; 6:215–222.

311. Masangkay AV, Susin M, Baker R, Ward R, Kahn E. Metastatic malignant mesothelioma presenting as colonic polyps. Hum Pathol 1997; 28:993–995.

312. Laurini RN. Diffuse pleural mesothelioma with distant bone metastasis. A case report. Acta Path Microbiol Scand Sect A 1974; 82:296–298.

313. Roberts GH. Distant visceral metastases in pleural mesothelioma. Br J Dis Chest 1976; 70:246–250.

314. Falconieri G, Grandi G, Dibonito L, Bonifaciogori D, Giarelli L. Intracranial metastases from malignant pleural mesothelioma – report of three autopsy cases and review of the literature. Arch Pathol Lab Med 1991; 115:591–595.

315. Grellner W, Staak M. Multiple skeletal muscle metastases from malignant pleural mesothelioma. Pathol Res Pract 1995; 191:456–460.

316. Adams VI, Krishnan KU, Muhm JR, Jett JR, Ilstrup DM, Bernatz PE. Diffuse malignant mesothelioma of pleura: diagnosis and survival in 92 cases. Cancer 1986; 58:1540–1551.

317. Huncharek M, Muscat J. Metastases in diffuse pleural mesothelioma: influence of histological type. Thorax 1987; 42:897–898.

318. Law MR, Gregor A, Hodson ME, Bloom HJG, Turner-Warwick M. Malignant mesothelioma of the pleura: a study of 52 treated and 64 untreated patients. Thorax 1984; 39:255–259.

319. Ribak J, Selikoff IJ. Survival of asbestos insulation workers with mesothelioma. Br J Ind Med 1992; 49:732–735.

320. Mark EJ, Shin D-H. Diffuse malignant mesothelioma of the pleura: a clinicopathological study of six patients with a prolonged symptom-free interval or extended survival after biopsy and a review of the literature of long-term survival. Virchows Arch A Pathol Anat Histopathol 1993; 422:445–451.

321. Wong CF, Fung SL, Yew WW, Fu KH. A case of malignant pleural mesothelioma with unexpectedly long survival without active treatment. Respiration 2002; 69:166–168.

322. Griffiths MH, Riddell RJ, Xipell JM. Malignant mesothelioma: a review of 35 cases with diagnosis and prognosis. Pathology 1980; 12:591–603.

323. Leigh J, Rogers AJ, Ferguson DA, Mulder HB, Ackad M, Thompson R. Lung asbestos fiber content and mesothelioma cell type, site, and survival. Cancer 1991; 68:135–141.

324. Johansson L, Linden CJ. Aspects of histopathologic subtype as a prognostic factor in 85 pleural mesotheliomas. Chest 1996; 109:109–114.

325. Beer TW, Buchanan R, Matthews AW, Stradling R, Pullinger N, Pethybridge RJ. Prognosis in malignant mesothelioma related to MIB 1 proliferation index and histological subtype. Hum Pathol 1998; 29:246–251.

326. Edwards JG, Abrams KR, Leverment JN, Spyt TJ, Waller DA, OByrne KJ. Prognostic factors for malignant mesothelioma in 142 patients: validation of CALGB and EORTC prognostic scoring systems. Thorax 2000; 55:731–735.

327. Hirsch A, Brochard P, DeCremoux H, et al. Features of asbestos-exposed and unexposed mesotheliomas. Am J Ind Med 1982; 3:413–422.

328. Law MR, Ward FG, Hodson ME, Heard BE. Evidence for longer survival for patients with pleural mesothelioma without asbestos exposure. Thorax 1983; 38:744–746.

329. Vangelder T, Damhuis RAM, Hoogsteden HC. Prognostic factors and survival in malignant pleural mesothelioma. Eur Respir J 1994; 7:1035–1038.

330. Comin CE, Anichini C, Boddi V, Novelli L, Dini S. MIB-1 proliferation index correlates with survival in pleural malignant mesothelioma. Histopathology 2000; 36:26–31.

331. Leonardo E, Zanconati F, Bonifacio D, Dibonito L. Immunohistochemical MIB-1 and p27(Kip1) as prognostic factors in pleural mesothelioma. Pathol Res Pract 2001; 197:253–256.

332. Beer TW, Shepherd P, Pullinger NC. p27 immunostaining is related to prognosis in malignant mesothelioma. Histopathology 2001; 38: 535–541.

333. Butchart EG, Ashcroft T, Barnsley WC, Holden MP. Pleuropneumonectomy in the management of diffuse malignant mesothelioma of the pleura. Thorax 1976; 31:15–24.

334. Aisner J, Boutin C, Butchart EG, et al. A proposed new international TNM staging system for malignant pleural mesothelioma. Chest 1995; 108:1122–1128.

335. Nash G, Otis CN. Protocol for the examination of specimens from patients with malignant pleural mesothelioma – A basis for checklists. Arch Pathol Lab Med 1999; 123:39–44.

336. Brooks JSJ, Livolsi VA, Pietra GG. Mesothelial cell inclusions mimicking metastatic carcinoma. Am J Clin Pathol 1990; 93:741–748.

337. Rutty GN, Lauder I. Mesothelial cell inclusions within mediastinal lymph nodes. Histopathology 1994; 25:483–487.

338. Groisman GM, Amar M, Weiner P, Zamir D. Mucicarminophilic histiocytosis (benign signet-ring cells) and hyperplastic mesothelial cells:

Two mimics of metastatic carcinoma within a single lymph node. Arch Pathol Lab Med 1998; 122:282–284.

339. Argani P, Rosai J. Hyperplastic mesothelial cells in lymph nodes: Report of six cases of a benign process that can simulate metastatic involvement by mesothelioma or carcinoma. Hum Pathol 1998; 29:339–346.

340. Nicholson AG, Graham ANJ, Pezzella F, Agneta G, Goldstraw P, Pastorino U. Does the use of immunohistochemistry to identify micrometastases provide useful information in the staging of node-negative non-small cell lung carcinomas? Lung Cancer 1997; 18:231–240.

341. Vilela DS, Garcia FMI. Embolization of mesothelial cells in lymphatics: the route to mesothelial inclusions in lymph nodes? Histopathology 1998; 33:570–575.

342. Parkash V, Vidwans M, Carter D. Benign mesothelial cells in mediastinal lymph nodes. Am J Surg Pathol 1999; 23:1264–1269.

343. Dazzi H, Thatcher N, Hasleton PS, Chatterjee AK, Lawson RAM. DNA analysis by flow cytometry in malignant pleural mesothelioma: relationship to histology and survival. J Pathol 1990; 162:51–55.

344. Donna A, Betta PG, Ribotta M, et al. Mitogenic effects of a mesothelial cell growth factor: evidence for a potential autocrine regulation of normal and malignant mesothelial cell proliferation. Int J Exp Pathol 1992; 73:193–202.

345. Ramael M, Buysse C, Vandenbossche J, Segers K, Vanmarck E. Immunoreactivity for the beta-chain of the platelet-derived growth factor receptor in malignant mesothelioma and non- neoplastic mesothelium. J Pathol 1992; 167:1–4.

346. Motoyama T, Honma T, Watanabe H, Honma S, Kumanishi T, Abe S. Interleukin 6-producing malignant mesothelioma. Virchows Arch B Cell Pathol 1993; 64:367–372.

347. Gerwin BI. Asbestos and the mesothelial cell: a molecular trail to mitogenic stimuli and suppressor gene suspects. Am J Respir Cell Mol Biol 1994; 11:507–508.

348. Fitzpatrick DR, Peroni DJ, Bielefeldt-Ohmann H. The role of growth factors and cytokines in the tumorigenesis and immunobiology of malignant mesothelioma. Am J Respir Cell Mol Biol 1995; 12:455–460.

349. Langerak AW, de Laat PAJM, van der Linden-van Beurden CAJ, et al. Expression of platelet-derived growth factor (PDGF) and PDGF receptors in human malignant mesothelioma in vitro and in vivo. J Pathol 1996; 178:151–160.

350. Strizzi L, Catalano A, Vianale G, et al. Vascular endothelial growth factor is an autocrine growth factor in human malignant mesothelioma. J Pathol 2001; 193:468–475.

351. Ramael M, Lemmens G, Eerdekens C, et al. Immunoreactivity for p53 protein in malignant mesothelioma and non-neoplastic mesothelium. J Pathol 1992; 168:371–375.

352. Ramael M, Deblier I, Eerdekens C, Lemmens G, Jacobs W, Vanmarck E. Immunohistochemical staining of RAS oncogene product in neoplastic and non-neoplastic mesothelial tissues – immunoreactivity for n-RAS and lack of immunohistochemical staining for ha-RAS and k-RAS. J Pathol 1993; 169:421–424.

353. Segers K, Ramael M, Singh SK, et al. Immunoreactivity for bcl-2 protein in malignant mesothelioma and non-neoplastic mesothelium. Virchows Arch 1994; 424:631–634.

354. Upham JW, Garlepp MJ, Musk AW, Robinson BWS. Malignant mesothelioma: new insights into tumour biology and immunology as a basis for new treatment approaches. Thorax 1995; 50:887–893.

355. Gordon GJ, Jensen RV, Hsiao LL, et al. Using gene expression ratios to predict outcome among patients with mesothelioma. J Natl Cancer Inst 2003; 95:598–605.

356. Butnor KJ, Sporn TA, Hammar SP, Roggli VL. Well-differentiated papillary mesothelioma. Am J Surg Pathol 2001; 25:1304–1309.

357. GalateauSalle F, Vignaud JM, Burke L, et al. Well-differentiated papillary mesothelioma of the pleura – A series of 24 cases. Am J Surg Pathol 2004; 28:534–540.

358. Derosa G, Donofrio V, Boscaino A, Zeppa P, Staibano S. Multicystic mesothelial proliferation – immunohistochemical, ultrastructural and DNA analysis of 5 cases. Virchows Arch A Pathol Anat Histopathol 1992; 421:379–385.

359. Sawh RN, Malpica A, Deavers MT, Liu JS, Silva EG. Benign cystic mesothelioma of the peritoneum: A clinicopathologic study of 17 cases and immunohistochemical analysis of estrogen and progesterone receptor status. Hum Pathol 2003; 34:369–374.

360. Ball NJ, Urbanski SJ, Green FHY, Kieser T. Pleural multicystic mesothelial proliferation. The so-called multicystic mesothelioma. Am J Surg Pathol 1990; 14:375–378.

361. Kaplan MA, Tazelaar HD, Hayashi T, Schroer KR, Travis WD. Adenomatoid tumors of the pleura. Am J Surg Pathol 1996; 20:1219–1223.

362. Stout AP, Murray MR. Localized pleural mesothelioma. Arch Pathol 1942; 34:951–964.

363. Alvarez-Fernandez E, Diez-Nau MD. Malignant fibrosarcomatous mesothelioma and benign pleural fibroma (localized fibrous mesothelioma) in tissue culture. Cancer 1979; 43:1658–1663.

364. Dardick I, Srigley JR, McCaughey WTE, van Nostrand AWP, Ritchie AC. Ultrastructural aspects of the histogenesis of diffuse and localized mesothelioma. Virchows Arch A Pathol Anat Histopathol 1984; 402:373–388.

365. Doucet J, Dardick I, Srigley JR, van Nostrand AWP, Bell MA, Kahn HJ. Localized fibrous tumour of serosal surfaces. Immunohistochemical and ultrastructural evidence for a type of mesothelioma. Virchows Arch A Pathol Anat Histopathol 1986; 409:349–363.

366. Said JW, Nash G, Banks-Schlegal S, Sassoon AF, Shintaku IP. Localized fibrous mesothelioma: an immunohistochemical and electron microscopic study. Hum Pathol 1984; 15:440–443.

367. Kawai T, Suzuki M. Nonmalignant tumors of the pleura. In: Chretien J, Bignon J, Hirsch A, eds. The Pleura in Health and Disease, Vol. 30 of Lung Biology in Health and Disease. NY: Marcel Dekker; 1985.

368. England DM, Hochholzer L, McCarthy MJ. Localized benign and malignant fibrous tumors of the pleura. A clinicopathologic review of 223 cases. Am J Surg Pathol 1989; 13:640–658.

369. Goodlad JR, Fletcher CDM. Solitary fibrous tumour arising at unusual sites – analysis of a series. Histopathology 1991; 19:515–522.

370. Carter D, Otis CN. Three types of spindle cell tumors of the pleura. Fibroma, sarcoma, and sarcomatoid mesothelioma. Am J Surg Pathol 1988; 12:747–753.

371. Steinetz C, Clarke R, Jacobs GH, Abdulkarim FW, Petrelli M, Tomashefski JF. Localized fibrous tumors of the pleura. Correlation of histopathological, immunohistochemical and ultrastructural features. Pathol Res Pract 1990; 186:344–357.

372. Briselli M, Mark EJ, Dickersin GR. Solitary fibrous tumors of the pleura: eight new cases and review of 360 cases in the literature. Cancer 1981; 47:2678–2689.

373. El-Naggar AK, Ro JY, Ayala AG, Ward R, Ordonez NG. Localized fibrous tumor of the serosal cavities. Immunohistochemical, electron-microscopic, and flow-cytometric DNA study. Am J Clin Pathol 1989; 92:561–565.

374. Osamura RY. Ultrastructure of localized fibrous mesothelioma of the pleura. Cancer 1977; 39:139–142.

375. Burrig K-F, Kastendieck H. Ultrastructural observations on the histogenesis of localized fibrous tumours of the pleura (benign mesothelioma). Virchows Arch A Pathol Anat Histopathol 1984; 403:413–424.

376. Keating S, Simon GT, Alexopoulou I, Kay JM. Solitary fibrous tumour of the pleura: an ultrastructural and immunohistochemical study. Thorax 1987; 42:976–979.

377. Masson EA, Macfarlane IA, Graham D, Foy P. Spontaneous hypoglycaemia due to a pleural fibroma – role of insulin like growth factors. Thorax 1991; 46:930–931.

378. Moat NE, Teale JD, Lea RE, Matthews AW. Spontaneous hypoglycaemia and pleural fibroma - role of insulin like growth factors. Thorax 1991; 46:932–933.

379. Sakamoto T, Kaneshige H, Takeshi A, Tsushima T, Hasegawa S. Localized pleural mesothelioma with elevation of high molecular weight insulin-like growth factor II and hypoglycemia. Chest 1994; 106:965–967.

380. Fukasawa Y, Takada A, Tateno M, et al. Solitary fibrous tumor of the pleura causing recurrent hypoglycemia by secretion of insulin-like growth factor II. Pathol Int 1998; 48:47–52.

381. Ulrik CS, Viskum K. Fibrous pleural tumour producing 171 litres of transudate. Eur Resp J 1998; 12:1230–1232.

382. Abrahamson JR, Friedman NB. Intrapulmonary stromal mesothelioma. J Thorac Cardiovasc Surg 1966; 51:300–306.

383. Alvarez-Fernandez E, Escalona-Zapata J. Intrapulmonary mesotheliomas: their identification by tissue culture. Virchows Arch A Pathol Anat Histopathol 1982; 395: 331–343.

384. Yousem SA, Flynn SD. Intrapulmonary localized fibrous tumor. Intraparenchymal so-called localized fibrous mesothelioma. Am J Clin Pathol 1988; 89:365–369.

385. Weidner N. Intriguing case – solitary fibrous tumor of the mediastinum. Ultrastruct Pathol 1991; 15:489–492.

386. Witkin GB, Rosai J. Solitary fibrous tumor of the upper respiratory tract – a report of six cases. Am J Surg Pathol 1991; 15:842–848.

387. Kottke-Marchant K, Hart WR, Broughan T. Localized fibrous tumor (localized fibrous mesothelioma) of the liver. Cancer 1989; 64:1096–1102.

388. Ibrahim NBN, Briggs JC, Corrin B. Double primary localized fibrous tumours of the pleura and retroperitoneum. Histopathology 1993; 22:282–284.

389. Dorfman DM, To K, Dickersin GR, Rosenberg AE, Pilch BZ. Solitary fibrous tumor of the orbit. Am J Surg Pathol 1994; 18:281–287.

390. Cameselleteijeiro J, Vareladuran J, Fonseca E, Villanueva JP, Sobrinho Simoes M. Solitary fibrous tumor of the thyroid. Am J Clin Pathol 1994; 101:535–538.

391. Hanau CA, Miettinen M. Solitary fibrous tumor: histological and immunohistochemical spectrum of benign and malignant variants presenting at different sites. Hum Pathol 1995; 26:440–449.

392. O'Connell JX, Logan PM, Beauchamp CP. Solitary fibrous tumor of the periosteum. Hum Pathol 1995; 26:460–462.

393. Suster S, Nascimento AG, Miettinen M, Sickel JZ, Moran CA. Solitary fibrous tumors of soft tissue: a clinicopathologic and immunohistochemical study of 12 cases. Am J Surg Pathol 1995; 19:1257–1266.

394. Fukunaga M, Ushigome S, Nomura K, Ishikawa E. Solitary fibrous tumor of the nasal cavity and orbit. Pathol Int 1995; 45:952–957.

395. Sciot R, Goffin J, Fossion E, Wilms G, Dom R. Solitary fibrous tumour of the orbit. Histopathology 1996; 28:188–191.

396. Ferreiro JA, Nascimento AG. Solitary fibrous tumour of the major salivary glands. Histopathology 1996; 28:261–264.

397. Barnoud R, Arvieux C, Pasquier D, Pasquier B, Letoublon C. Solitary fibrous tumour of the liver with CD34 expression. Histopathology 1996; 28:551–554.

398. Carneiro SS, Scheithauer BW, Nascimento AG, Hirose T, Davis DH. Solitary fibrous tumor of the meninges: a lesion distinct from fibrous meningioma: a clinicopathologic and immunohistochemical study. Am J Clin Pathol 1996; 106:217–224.

399. Mentzel T, Bainbridge TC, Katenkamp D. Solitary fibrous tumour: Clinicopathological, immunohistochemical, and ultrastructural analysis of 12 cases arising in soft tissues, nasal cavity and nasopharynx, urinary bladder and prostate. Virchows Archiv 1997; 430:445–453.

400. Nielsen GP, OConnell JX, Dickersin GR, Rosenberg AE. Solitary fibrous tumor of soft tissue: A report of 15 cases, including 5 malignant examples with light microscopic, immunohistochemical, and ultrastructural data. Modern Pathol 1997; 10:1028–1037.

401. Takeshima Y, Yoneda K, Sanda N, Inai K. Solitary fibrous tumor of the prostate. Pathol Int 1997; 47:713–717.

402. Chan JKC. Solitary fibrous tumour – everywhere, and a diagnosis in vogue. Histopathology 1997; 31:568–576.

403. Brunnemann RB, Ro JY, Ordonez NG, Mooney J, Elnaggar AK, Ayala AG. Extrapleural solitary fibrous tumor: A clinicopathologic study of 24 cases. Modern Pathol 1999; 12:1034–1042.

404. Hasegawa T, Matsuno Y, Shimoda T, Hasegawa F, Sano T, Hirohashi S. Extrathoracic solitary fibrous tumors: Their histological variability and potentially aggressive behavior. Hum Pathol 1999; 30:1464–1473.

405. Alawi F, Stratton D, Freedman PD. Solitary fibrous tumor of the oral soft tissues – A clinicopathologic and immunohistochemical study of 16 cases. Am J Surg Pathol 2001; 25:900–910.

406. Tan-Liu NS, Matsubara O, Grillo HC, Mark EJ. Invasive fibrous tumor of the tracheobronchial tree: clinical and pathologic study of seven cases. Hum Pathol 1989; 20:180–184.

407. Somerhausen NDA, Rubin BP, Fletcher CDM. Myxoid solitary fibrous tumor: A study of seven cases with emphasis on differential diagnosis. Modern Pathol 1999; 12:463–471.

408. van de Rijn M, Lombard CM, Rouse RV. Expression of CD34 by solitary fibrous tumors of the pleura, mediastinum, and lung. Am J Surg Pathol 1994; 18:814–820.

409. Flint A, Weiss SW. CD-34 and keratin expression distinguishes solitary fibrous tumor (fibrous mesothelioma) of pleura from desmoplastic mesothelioma. Hum Pathol 1995; 26:428–431.

410. Yokoi T, Tsuzuki T, Yatabe Y, et al. Solitary fibrous tumour: significance of p53 and CD34 immunoreactivity in its malignant transformation. Histopathology 1998; 32:423–432.

411. Ledet SC, Brown RW, Cagle PT. p53 immunostaining in the differentiation of inflammatory pseudotumor from sarcoma involving the lung. Mod Pathol 1995; 8:282–286.

412. Shidham VB, Chivukula M, Gupta D, Rao RN, Komorowski R. Immunohistochemical comparison of gastrointestinal stromal tumor and solitary fibrous tumor. Arch Pathol Lab Med 2002; 126:1189–1192.

413. Dalton WT, Zolliker AS, McCaughey WTE, Jacques J, Kannerstein M. Localised primary tumours of the pleura. Cancer 1979; 44:1465–1475.

414. Kanthan R, Torkian B. Recurrent solitary fibrous tumor of the pleura with malignant transformation. Arch Pathol Lab Med 2004; 128:460.

415. Bini A, Grazia M, Stella F, Petrella F, Bazzocchi R. Giant malignant fibrous histiocytoma of the pleura arising from solitary fibrous tumour. Thorax 2004; 59:544.

416. Zhang HQ, Lucas DR, Pass HI, Che MX. Disseminated malignant solitary fibrous tumor of the pleura. Pathol Int 2004; 54:111–115.

417. Scharifker D, Kaneko M. Localised fibrous 'mesothelioma' of pleura (submesothelial fibroma). A clinicopathologic study of 18 cases. Cancer 1979; 43:627–635.

418. Pinkard NB, Wilson RW, Lawless N, et al. Calcifying fibrous pseudotumor of pleura: a report of three cases of a newly described entity involving the pleura. Am J Clin Pathol 1996; 105:189–194.

419. Kocova L, Michal M, Sulc M, Zamecnik M. Calcifying fibrous pseudotumour of visceral peritoneum. Histopathology 1997; 31:182–184.

420. Dumont P, de Muret A, Skrobala D, Robin P, Toumieux B. Calcifying fibrous pseudotumor of the mediastinum. Ann Thorac Surg 1997; 63:543–544.

421. Mito K, Kashima K, Daa T, et al. Multiple calcifying fibrous tumors of the pleura. Virchows Arch 2005; 446:78–81.

422. VanDorpe J, Ectors N, Geboes K, DHoore A, Sciot R. Is calcifying fibrous pseudotumor a late sclerosing stage of inflammatory myofibroblastic tumor? Am J Surg Pathol 1999; 23:329–335.

423. Weynand B, Draguet AP, Bernard P, Marbaix E, Galant C. Calcifying fibrous pseudotumour: first case report in the peritoneum with immunostaining for CD34. Histopathology 1999; 34:86–87.

424. Pomplun S, Goldstraw P, Davies SE, Burke MM, Nicholson AG. Calcifying fibrous pseudotumour arising within an inflammatory pseudotumour: evidence of progression from one lesion to the other? Histopathology 2000; 37:380–382.

425. Hill KA, GonzalezCrussi F, Chou PM. Calcifying fibrous pseudotumor versus inflammatory myofibroblastic tumor: A histological and immunohistochemical comparison. Modern Pathol 2001; 14:784–790.

426. Ordonez NG. Desmoplastic small round cell tumor I: A histopathologic study of 39 cases with emphasis on unusual histological patterns. Am J Surg Pathol 1998; 22:1303–1313.

427. Ordonez NG. Desmoplastic small round cell tumor II: An ultrastructural and immunohistochemical study with emphasis on new immunohistochemical markers. Am J Surg Pathol 1998; 22:1314–1327.

428. Bian YL, Jordan AG, Rupp M, Cohn H, McLaughlin CJ, Miettinen M. Effusion cytology of desmoplastic small round cell tumor of the pleura – a case report. Acta Cytol 1993; 37:77–82.

429. Parkash V, Gerald WL, Parma A, Miettinen M, Rosai J. Desmoplastic small round cell tumor of the pleura. Am J Surg Pathol 1995; 19:659–665.

430. Syed S, Haque AK, Hawkins HK, Sorensen PHB, Cowan DF. Desmoplastic small round cell tumor of the lung. Arch Pathol Lab Med 2002; 126:1226–1228.

431. Pasquinelli G, Montanaro L, Martinelli GN. Desmoplastic small round-cell tumor: A case report on the large cell variant with immunohistochemical, ultrastructural, and molecular genetic analysis. Ultrastruct Pathol 2000; 24:333–337.

432. Hill DA, Pfeifer JD, Marley EF, et al. WT1 staining reliably differentiates desmoplastic small round cell tumor from Ewing sarcoma/primitive neuroectodermal tumor – An immunohistochemical and molecular diagnostic study. Am J Clin Pathol 2000; 114:345–353.

433. Barnoud R, Delattre O, Peoch M, et al. Desmoplastic small round cell tumor: RT-PCR analysis and immunohistochemical detection of the Wilm's tumor gene WT1. Pathol Res Pract 1998; 194:693–700.

434. Zhang PJ, Goldblum JR, Pawel BR, Fisher C, Pasha TL, Barr FG. Immunophenotype of desmoplastic small round cell tumors as detected in cases with EWS-WT1 gene fusion product. Modern Pathol 2003; 16:229–235.

435. Shuman LS, Libshutz HI. Solid pleural manifestations of lymphoma. AJR Am J Roentgenol 1984; 142:269–273.

436. Iuchi K, Ichimiya A, Akashi A, et al. Non-Hodgkin's lymphoma of the pleural cavity developing from long-standing pyothorax. Cancer 1987; 60:1771–1775.

437. Martin A, Capron F, Liguory-Brunaud M-D, Defrejacques C, Pluot M, Diebold J. Epstein-Barr virus-associated primary malignant lymphomas of the pleural cavity occurring in longstanding pleural chronic inflammation. Hum Pathol 1994; 25:1314–1318.

438. Hsu NY, Chen CY, Pan ST, Hsu CP. Pleural non-Hodgkin's lymphoma arising in a patient with a chronic pyothorax. Thorax 1996; 51:103–104.

439. Mori N, Yatabe Y, Narita M, Kobayashi T, Asai J. Pyothorax-associated lymphoma: an unusual case with biphenotypic character of T and B cells. Am J Surg Pathol 1996; 20:760–766.

440. Green I, Espiritu E, Ladanyi M, et al. Primary lymphomatous effusions in AIDS: a morphological, immunophenotypic, and molecular study. Mod Pathol 1995; 8:39–45.

441. Ansari MQ, Dawson DB, Nador R, et al. Primary body cavity-based AIDS-related lymphomas. Am J Clin Pathol 1996; 105:221–229.

442. Cesarman E, Nador RG, Aozasa K, Delsol G, Said JW, Knowles DM. Kaposi's sarcoma-associated herpesvirus in non-AIDS-related lymphomas occuring in body cavities. Am J Pathol 1996; 149:53–57.

443. Ohsawa M, Tomita Y, Kanno H, et al. Role of Epstein-Barr virus in pleural lymphomagenesis. Mod Pathol 1995; 8:848–853.

444. Cesarman E, Chang YA, Moore PS, Said JW, Knowles DM. Kaposi's sarcoma-associated herpesvirus-like DNA sequences in AIDS-related body-cavity-based lymphomas. N Engl J Med 1995; 332:1186–1191.

445. Hsi ED, Foreman KE, Duggan J, et al. Molecular and pathologic characterization of an AIDS- related body cavity-based lymphoma, including ultrastructural demonstration of human herpesvirus-8: A case report. Am J Surg Pathol 1998; 22:493–499.

446. Taniere P, Manai A, Charpentier R, et al. Pyothorax-associated lymphoma: relationship with Epstein- Barr virus, human herpes virus-8 and body cavity-based high grade lymphomas. Eur Resp J 1998; 11:779–783.

447. Moore PS, Chang YA. Detection of herpesvirus-like DNA sequences in Kaposi's sarcoma in patients with and those without HIV infection. N Engl J Med 1995; 332:1181–1185.

448. Ascoli V, Scalzo CC, Danese C, Vacca K, Pistilli A, LoCoco F. Human herpes virus-8 associated primary effusion lymphoma of the pleural cavity in HIV-negative elderly men. Eur Resp J 1999; 14:1231–1234.

449. Androulaki A, Drakos E, Hatzianastassiou D, et al. Pyothorax-associated lymphoma (PAL): a western case with marked angiocentricity and review of the literature. Histopathology 2004; 44:69–76.

450. Ascoli V, Sirianni MC, LoCoco F. Heterogeneity of Kaposi's sarcoma-associated herpesvirus (HHV-8)- positive effusions. Am J Surg Pathol 2000; 24:1036.

451. Teruya-Feldstein J, Zauber P, Setsuda JE, et al. Expression of human herpesvirus-8 oncogene and cytokine homologues in an HIV-seronegative patient with multicentric Castleman's disease and primary effusion lymphoma. Lab Invest 1998; 78:1637–1642.

452. Ascoli V, Signoretti S, Onetti-Muda A, et al. Primary effusion lymphoma in HIV-infected patients with multicentric Castleman's disease. J Pathol 2001; 193:200–209.

453. Ibuka T, Fukayama M, Hayashi Y, et al. Pyothorax-associated pleural lymphoma – a case evolving from T-cell-rich lymphoid infiltration to overt B-cell lymphoma in association with Epstein–Barr virus. Cancer 1994; 73:738–744.

454. Nakamura S, Sasajima Y, Koshikawa T, et al. Ki-1 (CD30) positive anaplastic large cell lymphoma of T-cell phenotype developing in association with longstanding tuberculous pyothorax: report of a case with detection of Epstein–Barr virus genome in the tumor cells. Hum Pathol 1995; 26:1382–1385.

455. Molinie V, Pouchot J, Navratil E, Aubert F, Vinceneux P, Barge J. Primary Epstein–Barr virus-related non-Hodgkin's lymphoma of the pleural cavity following long-standing tuberculous empyema. Arch Pathol Lab Med 1996; 120:288–291.

456. Petitjean B, Jardin F, Joly B, et al. Pyothorax-associated lymphoma – A peculiar clinicopathologic entity derived from B cells at late stage of differentiation and with occasional aberrant dual B- and T-cell phenotype. Am J Surg Pathol 2002; 26:724–732.

457. Yamato H, Ohshima K, Suzumiya J, Kikuchi M. Evidence for local immunosuppression and demonstration of c-myc amplification in pyothorax-associated lymphoma. Histopathology 2001; 39:163–171.

458. Cohn L, Hall AD. Extraosseous osteogenic sarcoma of the pleura. Ann Thorac Surg 1968; 5:545–549.

459. Reingold IM, Amromin GD. Extraosseous osteosarcoma of the lung. Cancer 1971; 28:491–498.

460. Walters KL, Martinez AJ. Malignant fibrous mesothelioma. Metastatic to brain and liver. Acta Neuropath (Berl) 1975; 33:173–177.

461. Yang H-Y, Weaver LL, Foti PR. Primary malignant fibrous histiocytoma of the pleura. Acta Cytol 1983; 27:683–687.

462. Myoui A, Aozasa K, Iuchi K, et al. Soft tissue sarcoma of the pleural cavity. Cancer 1991; 68:1550–1554.

463. Rizkalla K, Ahmad D, Garcia B, Hutton L, Novick R, Keeney GL. Primary malignant fibrous histiocytoma of the pleura a case report and review of the literature. Respir Med 1994; 88:711–714.

464. Gupta RK, Paolini FA. Liposarcoma of the pleura, report of a case with a review of the literature and views on histogenesis. Am Rev Respir Dis 1967; 95:298–304.

465. Wong WW, Pluth JR, Grado GL, Schild SE, Sanderson DR. Liposarcoma of the pleura. Mayo Clin Proc 1994; 69:882–885.

466. Duhig JT. Solitary rhabdomyosarcoma of the pleura. Report of a case with a note on the nomenclature of pleural tumours. J Thorac Surg 1969; 37:236–241.

467. Saenz NC, Ghavimi F, Gerald W, Gollamudi S, LaQuaglia MP. Chest wall rhabdomyosarcoma. Cancer 1997; 80:1513–1517.

468. Moran CA, Suster S, Koss MN. Smooth muscle tumours presenting as pleural neoplasms. Histopathology 1995; 27:227–234.

469. Gibbs AR. Smooth muscle tumours of the pleura. Histopathology 1995; 27:295–296.

470. Moran CA, Suster S, Koss MN. Smooth muscle tumours of the pleura. Histopathology 1997; 30:97–98.

471. Gibbs AR. Smooth muscle tumours of the pleura. Histopathology 1997; 30:98.

472. Proca DM, Ross P, Pratt J, Frankel WL. Smooth muscle tumor of the pleura – A case report and review of the literature. Arch Pathol Lab Med 2000; 124:1688–1692.

473. Goetz SP, Robinson RA, Landas SK. Extraskeletal myxoid chondrosarcoma of the pleura – report of a case clinically simulating mesothelioma. Am J Clin Pathol 1992; 97:498–502.

474. Luppi G, Cesinaro AM, Zoboli A, Morandi U, Piccinini L. Mesenchymal chondrosarcoma of the pleura. Eur Respir J 1996; 9:840–843.

475. Wilson RW, GallateauSalle F, Moran CA. Desmoid tumors of the pleura: A clinicopathologic mimic of localized fibrous tumor. Modern Pathol 1999; 12:9–14.

476. Ordonez NG, Tornos C. Malignant peripheral nerve sheath tumor of the pleura with epithelial and rhabdomyoblastic differentiation: Report of a case clinically simulating mesothelioma. Am J Surg Pathol 1997; 21:1515–1521.

477. Sapino A, Cavallo A, Donna A, Bussolati G. Pleural epidermoid carcinoma from displaced skin following extrapleural pneumothorax in a patient exposed to asbestos. Virchows Arch 1996; 429:173–176.

478. Harland RW, Sharma M, Rosenzweig DY. Lung carcinoma in a patient with lucite sphere plombage thoracoplasty. Chest 1993; 103:1295–1297.

479. Moran CA, Suster S. Primary mucoepidermoid carcinoma of the pleura. Am J Clin Pathol 2003; 120:381–385.

480. Fushimi H, Tanio Y, Kotoh K. Ectopic thymoma mimicking diffuse pleural mesothelioma: A case report. Hum Pathol 1998; 29:409–410.

481. Attanoos RL, GalateauSalle F, Gibbs AR, Muller S, Ghandour F, Dojcinov SD. Primary thymic epithelial tumours of the pleura mimicking malignant mesothelioma. Histopathology 2002; 41:42–49.

482. Nicholson AG, Goldstraw P, Fisher C. Synovial sarcoma of the pleura and its differentiation from other primary pleural tumours: a clinicopathological and immunohistochemical review of three cases. Histopathology 1998; 33:508–513.

483. Ng SB, Ahmed Q, Tien SL, Sivaswaren C, Lau LC. Primary pleural synovial sarcoma – A case report and review of the literature. Arch Pathol Lab Med 2003; 127:85–90.

484. Lee W, Han K, Drut RM, Harris CP, Meisner LF. Use of fluorescence in situ hybridization for retrospective detection of aneuploidy in multiple myeloma. Genes Chromosomes Cancer 1993; 7:137–143.

485. Falconieri G, Bussani R, Mirra M, Zanella M. Pseudomesotheliomatous angiosarcoma: A pleuropulmonary lesion simulating malignant pleural mesothelioma. Histopathology 1997; 30:419–424.

486. Zhang PJ, Livolsi VA, Brooks JJ. Malignant epithelioid vascular tumors of the pleura: Report of a series and literature review. Hum Pathol 2000; 31:29–34.

486a. Al Shraim M, Mahboub B, Neligan PC, et al. Primary pleural epithelioid haemangioendothelioma with metastases to the skin. A case report and literature review. J Clin Pathol 2005; 58:107–109.

487. Hattori H. Epithelioid angiosarcoma arising in the tuberculous pyothorax - Report of an autopsy case. Arch Pathol Lab Med 2001; 125:1477–1479.

488. Kimura M, Ito H, Furuta T, Tsumoto T, Hayashi S. Pyothorax-associated angiosarcoma of the pleura with metastasis to the brain. Pathol Int 2003; 53:547–551.

489. Chernow B, Sahn SA. Carcinomatous involvement of the pleura. An analysis of 96 patients. Am J Med 1977; 63:695–702.

490. Shepherd MP. Thoracic metastases. Thorax 1982; 37:366–370.

491. Canto-Armengod A. Macroscopic characteristics of pleural metastases arising from the breast and observed by diagnostic thoracoscopy. Am Rev Respir Dis 1990; 142:616–618.

492. Canto A, Ferrer G, Romagosa V, Moya J, Bernat R. Lung cancer and pleural effusion. Clinical significance and study of pleural metastatic locations. Chest 1985; 87: 649–652.

493. Meyer PC. Metastatic carcinoma of the pleura. Thorax 1966; 21: 437–440.

494. Canto A, Rivas J, Saumench J, Morera R, Moya J. Points to consider when choosing a biopsy method in cases of pleurisy of unknown origin. Chest 1983; 84:176–179.

495. Nicholson AG, McCormick CJ, Shimosato Y, Butcher DN, Sheppard MN. The value of PE-10, a monoclonal antibody against pulmonary surfactant, in distinguishing primary and metastatic lung tumours. Histopathology 1995; 27:57–60.

496. Gaines JJ, Crosby JH, Kamath MV. Diagnosis of thoracic splenosis by Tru-cut needle biopsy. Am Rev Respir Dis 1986; 133:1199–1201.

497. Cordier JF, Gamondes JP, Marx P, Heinen I, Loire R. Thoracic splenosis presenting with hemoptysis. Chest 1992; 102:626–627.

498. Shaw AFB, Shafi A. Traumatic autoplastic transplantation of splenic tissue in man with observations on the late results of splenectomy in six cases. J Pathol 1937; 45:215–235.

499. Madjar S, Weissberg D. Thoracic splenosis. Thorax 1994; 49:1020–1022.

500. Carr NJ, Turk EP. The histological features of splenosis. Histopathology 1992; 21:549–553.

Chest wall tumours

501. Kaplan J, Davidson T. Intrathoracic desmoids: report of two cases. Thorax 1986; 41:894–895.

502. Delaney TF, Shepard JO, Chakravarti A, Nielsen GP, Spiro IJ, Mark EJ. A 45-year-old woman with a thoracic mass and Pancoast's syndrome – Intrathoracic fibromatosis (Desmoid tumor). N Engl J Med 2000; 342:1814–1821.

502a. Kabiri EH, al Aziz S, el Maslout A, Benosman A. Desmoid tumors of the chest wall. Eur J Cardiothorac Surg 2001; 19:580–583.

503. Nisolle JF, Delaunois L, Trigaux JP. Myositis ossificans of the chest wall. Eur Respir J 1996; 9:178–179.

504. Gordon MS, Hajdu SI, Bains SM, Burt ME. Soft tissue sarcomas of the chest wall. Results of surgical resection. J Thorac Cardiovasc Surg 1991; 101:843–854.

504a. Gross JL, Younes RN, Haddad FJ, et al. Soft-tissue sarcomas of the chest wall: prognostic factors. Chest 2005; 127:902–908.

505. Greager JA, Patel MK, Briele HA, Walker MJ, Wood DK, Das Gupta TK. Soft tissue sarcomas of the adult thoracic wall. Cancer 1987; 59:370–373.

506. Souba WW, McKenna RJ, Meis J, Benjamin R, Raymond AK, Mountain CF. Radiation-induced sarcomas of the chest wall. Cancer 1986; 57:610–615.

507. Askin FB, Rosai J, Sibley RK, Dehner LP, McAlister WH. Malignant small cell tumor of the thoracopulmonary region in childhood. Cancer 1979; 43:2435–2452.

508. Hicks MJ, Smith JD, Carter AB, Flaitz CM, Barrish JP, Hawkins EP. Recurrent intrapulmonary malignant small cell tumor of the thoracopulmonary region with metastasis to the oral cavity: review of literature and case report. Ultrastruct Pathol 1995; 19:297–303.

509. Tsuji S, Hisaoka M, Morimitsu Y, et al. Peripheral primitive neuroectodermal tumour of the lung: report of two cases. Histopathology 1998; 33:369–374.

510. Mikami Y, Nakajima M, Hashimoto H, et al. Primary pulmonary primitive neuroectodermal tumor (PNET) – A case report. Pathol Res Pract 2001; 197:113–119.

511. Kahn AG, Avagnina A, Nazar J, Elsner B. Primitive neuroectodermal tumor of the lung. Arch Pathol Lab Med 2001; 125:397–399.

512. Gonzalez-Crussi F, Wolfson SL, Misingi K, Nakajimi T. Peripheral neuroectodermal tumors of the chest wall in childhood. Cancer 1984; 54:2519–2527.

513. Seemayer TA, Vekemans M, de Chadarevian J-P. Histological and cytogenetic findings in a malignant tumor of the chest wall and lung (Askin tumor). Virchows Arch A Pathol Anat Histopathol 1985; 408:289–296.

514. Schmidt D, Herrmann C, Jurgens H, Harms D. Malignant peripheral neuroectodermal tumor and its necessary distinction from Ewing's sarcoma – a report from the Kiel Pediatric Tumor Registry. Cancer 1991; 68:2251–2259.

515. Contesso G, Llombartbosch A, Terrier P, et al. Does malignant small round cell tumor of the thoracopulmonary region (Askin tumor) constitute a clinicopathologic entity? – an analysis of 30 cases with immunohistochemical and electron- microscopic support treated at the Institute-Gustave-Roussy. Cancer 1992; 69:1012–1020.

516. Kim MS, Kim CJ, Jung HS, et al. Fibroblast growth factor 2 induces differentiation and apoptosis of Askin tumour cells. J Pathol 2004; 202:103–112

517. Delattre O, Zucman J, Melot T, et al. The Ewing family of tumors – a subgroup of small-round-cell tumors defined by specific chimeric transcripts. N Engl J Med 1994; 331:294–299.

518. Ambros IM, Ambros PF, Strehl S, Kovar H, Gadner H, Salzer-Kuntschik M. MIC2 is a specific marker for Ewing's sarcoma and peripheral primitive neuroectodermal tumors. Cancer 1991; 67:1886–1893.

519. Nagao K, Ito H, Yoshida H, et al. Chromosomal rearrangement t(11; 22) in extraskeletal Ewing's sarcoma and primitive neuroectodermal tumour

analysed by fluorescence in situ hybridization using paraffin-embedded tissue. J Pathol 1997; 181:62–66.

520. Folpe AL, Hill CE, Parham DM, OShea PA, Weiss SW. Immunohistochemical detection of FLI-1 protein expression – A study of 132 round cell tumors with emphasis on CD99- positive mimics of Ewing's sarcoma/primitive neuroectodermal tumor. Am J Surg Pathol 2000; 24:1657–1662.

521. Lucas DR, Bentley G, Dan ME, Tabaczka P, Poulik JM, Mott MP. Ewing sarcoma vs lymphoblastic lymphoma – A comparative immunohistochemical study. Am J Clin Pathol 2001; 115:11–17.

522. Odell JM, Benjamin DR. Mesenchymal hamartoma of chest wall in infancy: natural history of two cases. Pediatr Pathol 1986; 5:135–146.

523. Cohen MC, Drut R, Garcia C, Kaschula RO. Mesenchymal hamartoma of the chest wall: a cooperative study with review of the literature. Pediatr Pathol 1992; 12:525–534.

524. SerranoEgea A, SantosBriz A, GarciaMunoz H, MartinezTello FJ. Chest wall hamartoma – Report of two cases with secondary aneurysmal bone cysts. Pathol Res Pract 2001; 197:835–839.

525. McNeil KD, Fong KM, Walker QJ, Jessup P, Zimmerman PV. Gorham's syndrome: a usually fatal cause of pleural effusion treated successfully with radiotherapy. Thorax 1996; 51:1275–1276.

526. Riantawan P, Tansupasawasdikul S, Subhannachart P. Bilateral chylothorax complicating massive osteolysis (Gorham's syndrome). Thorax 1996; 51:1277–1278.

The processing of lung specimens

While the value of cytopathology is fully acknowledged,[1–3] this book is concerned with histopathology and except for a section on bronchoalveolar lavage, consideration will be limited to specimens submitted for histology. Lung specimens are obtained by a variety of procedures and vary greatly in size (Box A.1). It is desirable that all specimens be received in the laboratory unfixed but this is best waived in the case of small biopsies because of their greater risk of drying in transit. For these specimens the clinician should be provided with small containers of fixative; for larger specimens dry containers should be provided with instructions that they should be brought to the laboratory straight away, or arrangements made for them to be inflated with formalin if there is to be undue delay. A refrigerator should be available for specimens brought to the laboratory out of hours. The various types of specimen will be dealt with in turn but consideration must first be given to laboratory safety.

HEALTH AND SAFETY ASPECTS OF HANDLING LUNG SPECIMENS

The examination of lung tissue entails two particular risks, infection and that associated with formaldehyde vapour. To minimise these, protective clothing, masks and eye shields are either desirable or (as is the case in the UK) mandatory.

It is incumbent upon the clinician to inform the pathologist if there is any possibility of the specimen being infectious but this cannot always be relied upon and it is good practice to regard all fresh tissue as being potentially infectious. It is also good practice for some fresh tissue to be sent for culture in every case and to ensure this a protocol should be established whereby one person, either the clinician or the pathologist, is responsible for this. To minimise the risk of laboratory infection, the tissue retained for histology should be immersed in formaldehyde, ideally for 72 h before it is examined,[4] but this is not generally practicable. Not infrequently, the clinical situation demands a frozen section. Then the selection of tissue must take place in a Class 1 microbiological safety cabinet and afterwards the cryostat cabinet must be fumigated with formaldehyde vapour overnight. Other specimens also need to be first

---

Box A.1 Varieties of lung specimen

Needle aspiration
Fibreoptic bronchoscopic
   Bronchial biopsy
   Transbronchial biopsy
Rigid bronchoscopic bronchial biopsy
Mediastinoscopy or mediastinotomy lymph node biopsy
Transcutaneous drill biopsy
Pleural punch biopsy
'Medical' thoracoscopy
Pleural biopsy
Thoracotomy or 'surgical' (video-assisted) thoracoscopy
   Pleural biopsy
   Wedge lung biopsy
   Segmentectomy
   Lobectomy
   Pneumonectomy
Post mortem

---

handled in a microbiological safety cabinet, either to immerse or fill them with formaldehyde. By the next day, most microbes will no longer be viable but tubercle bacilli and prions can survive much longer and continued caution is necessary.

Formaldehyde is categorised as a probable carcinogen by the International Agency for Research on Cancer.[5] Several governments have therefore stipulated maximum air-borne levels in the workplace. These levels are easily exceeded when copious amounts are used to distend lungs unless an adequately ventilated bench or cabinet is used.

NEEDLE ASPIRATION

Needle aspiration is appropriate for solid lesions such as tumours, whereas pulmonary infiltrates seldom produce satisfactory specimens if sampled by this technique. Whatever the site of the lesion within the thorax, special sampling procedures are required, namely bronchoscopy for transbronchial aspiration and radiography for transcutaneous aspiration. The pathologist is therefore seldom involved in the actual sampling procedure, which is generally undertaken by a bronchoscopist or a radiologist. As with any invasive technique the danger of tumour seeding in the needle track has to be kept in mind.[6,7]

The usual fine needles (22-gauge) produce a cell suspension that is suitable for cytological smears but the slightly wider 18-gauge needle produces a thin core of tissue that can be processed for histology,[8] especially if the needle is inserted with the aid of a spring-loaded firing device.[9–11] With this technique the aspirated material (which may be contained in the needle as much as the syringe) can be rinsed directly into the fixative as soon as practicable and processed in the laboratory in the same way as small biopsies, thus avoiding the drying artefact to which cytological smears are subject.

BRONCHIAL AND TRANSBRONCHIAL BIOPSY

Bronchoscopic biopsies may contain only bronchus, only pulmonary parenchyma or both. If the specimen floats it is more likely to contain alveoli than not but no more likely to be diagnostic or abnormal than if it sinks.[12,13] A note of the number of fragments received provides a useful check on laboratory procedures but if this information is incorporated in the report it may be disputed by bronchoscopists who have made their own count. Discrepancies are often due to the clinician counting flecks of mucus as tissue fragments. However, it is imperative that no fragment be lost in processing and to minimise this risk it is advisable that the fragments are handled just once, if at all. It is advantageous if the clinician wipes the specimens onto a small strip of filter paper and puts this into the specimen jar. Alternatively, if loose fragments are received they should be transferred with fine-toothed forceps into a capture vehicle such as tissue paper, a fine-mesh wire cage or molten agar, which when set can be further processed as if it were a button of tissue. The agar survives processing and can seen around the tissue when the slide is examined by the naked eye but is invisible when the section is examined microscopically.[14] Imprisoning the fragments in sponge is likely to cause tissue artefacts.[15,15a] Free tumour cells may remain in the fixative or other transport medium after all fragments have been removed and the sensitivity of the bronchoscopy procedure is marginally improved if the residual fluid is submitted for cytology.[16]

The largest fragments of lung obtained by transbronchial biopsy each contain about 100 alveoli. If the changes are nonspecific and few alveoli have been obtained, the paucity of lung tissue should be made clear in the report. At least three step sections should be prepared, keeping spares at each level for any special stains that might be required.[17] If no abnormalities are identified at any of these levels and tissue remains in the block, further step sections should be prepared. Many laboratories, particularly those dealing with specimens from lung transplant or otherwise immunocompromised patients, routinely examine step sections, or even serial sections through the block (see Chapter 11). In immunodeficient patients, it is advisable to stain for fungi and mycobacteria routinely as the histopathological changes may be atypical.[18]

The main indication for endoscopic biopsy is the diagnosis of bronchogenic neoplasia but transbronchial biopsy is also useful in the investigation of suspected lung infection and graft rejection. It is also often the first procedure undertaken to obtain tissue in the investigation of diffuse parenchymal disease, though more with a view to excluding sarcoidosis than diagnosing a pattern of interstitial pneumonia.

When a tumour is visible to the bronchoscopist the sensitivity of a forceps biopsy ranges between 70 and 100%.[19–21] When the tumour is not visible the diagnostic sensitivity is less and varies with the location and size of the lesion. The yield is increased if multiple specimens are obtained. One study found

Box A.2 Yield of various sampling methods in the diagnosis of peripheral lung cancer as percentages

First author	Washing	Brushing	Biopsy	All methods
Kvale[25]	13	26	37	47
McDougall[26]	36	36	49	62
Popovich[22]	–	40	70	75
Mak[27]	38	29	37	56

Box A.3 Fibreoptic biopsy: utility in various lung diseases

	Examples
Excellent for diffuse bronchial or lung disease	Sarcoidosis
	'Lymphangitis carcinomatosa'
	Amyloidosis
Good for mass lesions or patchy disease that can be targeted	Tumours
	Pneumocystis pneumonia
	Eosinophilic pneumonia
	Alveolar lipoproteinosis
May help in patchy disease that cannot be targeted	Langerhans cell histiocytosis
Poor in diseases with scanty specific features or those in which study of the lobular architecture is important to the diagnosis	Extrinsic allergic alveolitis
	Interstitial pneumonias (idiopathic pulmonary fibrosis)

that with central tumours a single biopsy succeeded in establishing the diagnosis in 92% of cases, a figure that increased to 96% if four samples were taken, but was not further improved upon with six. For peripheral tumours, positive results increased progressively from 45% through 55% and 60% to 75% when one, four, five and six samples, respectively were taken.[22] Another study evaluated the costs of diagnosing a lung tumour by four different procedures. Surgical lung biopsy was the most cost-effective, followed by bronchoscopic procedures, then fine needle aspiration and lastly sputum cytology.[23] It was concluded that sputum examination is not cost-effective except when the patient has a tumour that is evidently unresectable. However, cytology is appropriate for the evaluation of fine-needle transbronchial needle aspirates of mediastinal lymph nodes, which contributes to the staging of lung cancer. It is reported that with this technique, diagnostic yield does not plateau until seven successive samples have been examined.[24] In some circumstances, cytology and histology augment each other (Box A.2).[22,25–27] In categorising carcinomas in small specimens, a diagnosis of large cell undifferentiated carcinoma is best avoided as a subsequent resection may require a change of cell type: the phrase non-small cell carcinoma is useful in these circumstances and is quite acceptable to the clinician.[28]

In many of the diffuse parenchymal lung diseases a transbronchial biopsy is often uninformative, but it may provide an unexpected tissue diagnosis, obviating the need for more invasive procedures. Thus, in a patient suspected of having idiopathic pulmonary fibrosis, a disease in which fibreoptic specimens are seldom diagnostic, a bronchoscopic biopsy may identify unsuspected sarcoidosis or `lymphangitis carcinomatosa' and so circumvent the necessity for a surgical procedure. Indeed, these two conditions are often recognisable histologically even if an attempted transbronchial procedure samples only the bronchus. The likelihood of transbronchial biopsy giving a diagnosis in various lung diseases is shown in Box A.3.[29,30] The diseases unlikely to be identified in these small specimens are those such as idiopathic pulmonary fibrosis and extrinsic allergic alveolitis in which diagnosis depends upon their lobular distribution.[29–31] The number of fibreoptic specimens required to give diagnostic material has been studied in regard to sarcoidosis. One group found that a single biopsy provided a tissue diagnosis of sarcoidosis in 46% of cases, increasing progressively to 90% when four biopsies were taken but not appreciably increasing further thereafter.[32] On comparing the

diagnostic yield in patients with pulmonary infiltrates a diagnosis is reported to be provided by transbronchial biopsy in 59% and by open lung biopsy in 94%.[33] In the diagnosis of cryptogenic organising pneumonia, transbronchial biopsy is reported to have a sensitivity of 64% and a specificity of 86%.[34]

OPEN AND VIDEO-ASSISTED THORACOSCOPIC LUNG BIOPSIES

From the pathologist's point of view there is little difference between a biopsy obtained at thoracotomy (open biopsy)[35,36] and one obtained at video-assisted thoracoscopy.[37–40] Both give good-sized specimens and both afford the surgeon a choice of biopsy site. The optimum biopsy site often depends upon the nature of the disease being investigated. Nodules are best excised in their entirety, or if this is impracticable a wedge should be taken to include both the core of the lesion and its interface with its surroundings. Diffuse lung disease often shows a zonal difference in disease activity and it is therefore advantageous if both the upper and lower lobes are sampled. Alternatively, a site thought to show intermediate changes may be chosen. Some advise that the tip of the lingula, or indeed the tip of any lobe, should be avoided as these sites often show non-specific scarring,[41] but this is disputed.[42,43]

In many cases, the lung sample will have collapsed on removal and if fixed in this state, there will be close apposition of the alveolar walls. This makes it difficult to study the architecture of the lung and can lead to considerable misinterpretation. The lung can however be re-inflated by vacuum[44] or injection; the latter by gently instilling a little fixative into the specimen with a syringe, taking care not to over-expand the tissue.[45] Airways cannot easily be identified by eye in these peripheral lung specimens and it is sufficient to inject the fixative directly into the lung parenchyma. The only disadvantage of this procedure is that free cells may be cleared from consolidated alveoli and diagnoses such as desquamative interstitial pneumonia obscured. However, the benefits of gentle inflation-fixation outweigh this single disadvantage.

Before the specimen is fixed, thought should be given to the desirability of ancillary procedures that require unfixed or specially fixed tissue, particularly microbiological culture. Immunofluorescence microscopy and gene or chromosomal studies may also require fresh or deep-frozen tissue. However, the primary purpose of the biopsy is histopathological evaluation and it is essential that sufficient tissue remains for this. Electron microscopy requires very little tissue but has its own requirements, the most important of which is prompt fixation. Whereas light microscopy is often satisfactory despite delayed fixation this is not true of electron microscopy. If the recommended fixative (glutaraldehyde or methanol-free formaldehyde) is not available, commercial formalin is an acceptable alternative so long as fixation is rapid. Archival tissue rescued from old paraffin blocks is often satisfactory for electron microscopy if it had been fixed without delay. Rapid fixation for electron microscopy is also possible post mortem, by injecting fixative through the chest wall immediately after death; a marker dye in the fixative facilitates recognition of the injected site when autopsy is undertaken.[46] Special care should be taken against 'crush' artefact when selecting small tissue samples for electron microscopy; a new razor blade should be used for each specimen and cutting effected with a to-and-fro motion, rather than by exerting downwards pressure.

WHOLE LUNGS AND LUNG LOBES

Artefactual collapse is inevitable when a lung is removed from the chest and inflation fixation is highly desirable for these large specimens. This can be effected by having a reservoir of fixative on the top of an exhaust-ventilated cut-up cabinet and running fixative into the specimen from a height of about 25 cm via tubing that terminates in a tapering nozzle wedged into the supplying bronchus. Fixative is run in until the pleural surface is smooth. The specimen is then immersed or floated in a container of fixative overnight with a covering of lint or filter paper to prevent drying. It is not necessary to clamp the bronchus. This procedure is equally applicable in autopsy and surgical pathological practice. If the specimen needs to be examined the same day, even a few hours inflation-fixation is preferable to opening an unfixed lung. However, as with biopsies, thought should be given to the desirability of first sampling the lung for procedures that are impossible after fixation, notably culture. Whatever the type of fresh specimen, culture should always be considered before the opportunity for this is lost by fixation.

Other procedures that might be considered before either fixation or cut-up include injection of blood vessels or airways, taking care to remove as much clot or bronchial secretions as possible and afterwards excluding these as possible causes of any blockages or apparent stenoses. A coloured or radiopaque gelatine mixture (e.g. Micropaque® barium sulphate suspension 330 ml, gelatine 33 g, water 130 ml) containing thymol as a preservative may be stored for this purpose, melting the solid mix as required by immersion in warm water, but not heating it above 56° C as this would denature the gelatine (see Figs 1.34, 3.14b, pp. 20, 100).[47,48]

Radiography is also possible after fixation if the lungs are inflated with formaldehyde fume[49] or if lung slices are air-dried after being fixed with liquid formaldehyde.[50–52] Air-drying is facilitated if the fixative comprises 10 parts polyethylene glycol 400, 5 parts ethanol, 2 parts formalin and 3 parts water. However, both these procedures have been rendered largely redundant by pre-operative contrast enhanced studies that generally provide far superior images.

The choice of cut-up procedure is wide and depends upon the nature of the underlying disease. Different procedures are appropriate for studying a widespread process such as emphysema than for a localised one such as a tumour. In other circumstances it may be desirable to open the airways or the blood vessels widely, or possibly both without cutting across either. This can be achieved if the airways are opened from the hilum and the arteries from the oblique fissure.[53]

Corrosion casts of pulmonary blood vessels or airways constitute another way of demonstrating abnormalities in the lung,[54] albeit at the cost of losing all intervening tissue (see Figs 1.3, 1.9, pp. 3, 6). However, bronchial cartilage can be studied without losing the intervening tissue by rendering all but the cartilage transparent.[55]

Diffuse lung disease

To demonstrate emphysema, or other diffuse disease, sagittal slicing is customary, and for this a particularly good result can be obtained with an electric meat-slicer. Conditions such as emphysema and fibrosis can then be demonstrated more convincingly with the barium sulphate technique.[56] This requires the lung slice to be squeezed gently in a 7.5% solution of barium chloride and then for a 10% solution of sodium sulphate to be poured on, the resultant white precipitate of barium sulphate emphasising structural differences in the lung substance (see Figs 3.14b, 3.15b, 3.16b, 7.1.22, pp. 101–102, 350). Similar contrast can be achieved by fixing the lung in Bouin's solution.[57] Paper-mounted whole lung sections[58,59] provide an excellent permanent demonstration of conditions such as emphysema (see Figs 1.6, 3.14a, 3.15a, 7.1.9, 7.1.10, 7.1.12, 7.1.15, 7.1.16, pp. 5, 100, 101, 336, 337, 341, 343) but an easy alternative is to bag or laminate in plastic the thinnest slices obtainable with a meat-slicer.[60]

Lung tumours

It is often of interest to investigate the relationship of a tumour to the airways and for this, and its subsequent demonstration, the Liebow technique cannot be bettered. This entails a probe being passed down the airways to the tumour and then cutting along the line of the probe from the hilum to the pleura passing

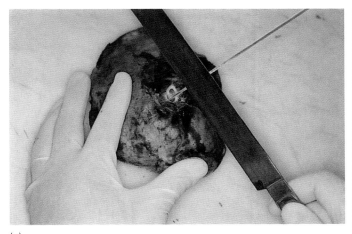

(a)

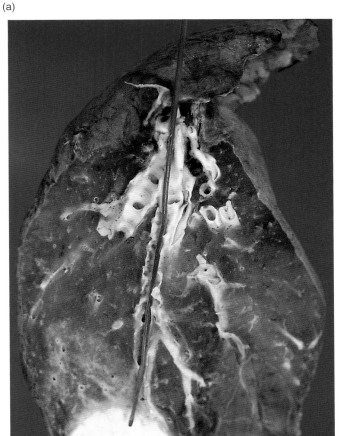

(b)

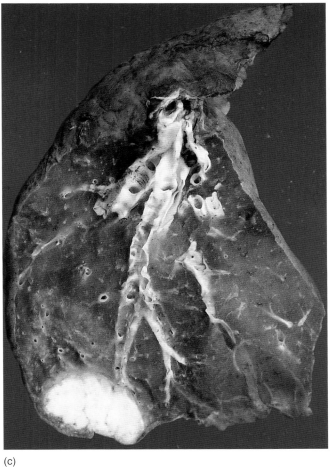

(c)

Figure A.1 Demonstration of the airways related to a lung tumour. (a) A probe is passed through the successive airways to the centre of the tumour and the lung sliced by cutting down onto the probe. (b) Cut surface of the lung showing the probe in place. (c) The same with the probe removed.

through all the successive airways leading to the tumour and the centre of the tumour itself (Fig. A.1). The fact that the plane of the cut is neither sagittal nor coronal is immaterial and is not evident when the cut surface is presented to the viewer.

In dealing with specimens excised in the treatment of lung cancer, certain information is essential for staging and to cir-

cumvent some of these points being overlooked, protocols have been produced for both carcinoma[61–66] and mesothelioma.[67] One appropriate to carcinoma is outlined in Table A.1 (copies of which can be downloaded from the Royal College of Pathologists website: *www.rcpath.org*). Particular points to be covered include:

Table A.1   A protocol for reporting lung tissue resected in the treatment of lung cancer

Specimen Type

        ☐ Right   ☐ Left

  ☐ VATS segmentectomy   ☐   VATS lobectomy

  ☐ Open segmentectomy   ☐   Open lobectomy/bi-lobectomy

  ☐ Pneumonectomy (extra-pericardial)   ☐   Pneumonectomy (intra-pericardial)

  ☐ Sleeve   ☐   Wedge resection

  ☐ Other, e.g. chest wall

Gross description

  Location of Tumour

    ☐ Main bronchus within 20 mm of carina (T3) – this will require clinical information

    ☐ Main bronchus more than 20 mm from carina (T2)

    ☐ Non-assessable

    ☐ Right upper lobe   ☐ Right middle lobe   ☐ Right lower lobe

    ☐ Left upper lobe   ☐ Left lower lobe

  Tumour size ... mm (T1 ≤30 mm or superficial tumours confined to bronchial wall, T2 > 30 mm)

  Distance from bronchial or medial resection margin . . . mm

  Extent of atelectasis/obstructive pneumonitis: ☐ None

                                       ☐ Involving hilar region but not whole lung (T2)

                                       ☐ Involving whole lung (T3)

Histology

  Histological type

    ☐ Squamous cell carcinoma   ☐ Adenocarcinoma   ☐ Bronchoalveolar cell carcinoma

    ☐ Large cell undifferentiated   ☐ Small cell carcinoma

    ☐ Mixed tumours (please specify: ....)

    ☐ Other tumour (please specify, e.g. carcinoid, etc.: ....)

  Local invasion

    ☐ Visceral pleura (T2)   ☐ Parietal pleura/chest wall (T3)   ☐ Mediastinal pleura (T3)

    ☐ Pericardium (T3)   ☐ Diaphragm (T3)

    ☐ Great vessel (aorta, central pulmonary artery or vein) (T4)   ☐ Atrium, heart (T4)

    ☐ Malignant pleural effusion (T4)   ☐ Separate tumour nodules in same lobe (T4)

  Lymph node spread

    Ipsilateral hilar/intrapulmonary (node stations 10–14)   ☐ Submitted   ☐ Involved (N1)

    Ipsilateral mediastinal (node stations 1–9)   ☐ Submitted   ☐ Involved (N2)

    Contralateral mediastinal, hilar, ipsilateral or   ☐ Submitted   ☐ Involved (N3)

      contralateral scalene, supraclavicular

  Margins

Bronchial	☐ Clear	☐ Involved	
Mediastinal	☐ Clear	☐ Involved	
Vascular	☐ Clear	☐ Involved	
Chest wall	☐ Clear	☐ Involved	

  Other Pathology

    ☐ Emphysema (moderate/severe degree)   ☐ Interstitial fibrosis; State cause (if known):

    ☐ Other (please state: ....)   ....

  Metastases

    ☐ Unknown (MX)   ☐ Absent (M0)

    ☐ Present (M1) including tumour nodules in different lobes. (please state: ....)

Pathological staging

    ☐ T   ☐ N   ☐ M (select highest stage from above data)

    Complete resection at all margins   ☐ Yes   ☐ No

Copies can be downloaded from the Royal College of Pathologists website: www.rcpath.org/resources/worddocs/dataset_lung_cancer_form_v2002.doc

- The size of the tumour, paying particular attention to those around 3 cm in size: 3 cm or less is one criterion categorising a tumour as stage T1 whereas a size greater than 3 cm places it in stage T2.
- The relation of the tumour to the pleura. Many tumours abut the pleura and it often requires histology with elastin staining[68] to ascertain whether the pleura is invaded.
- The relation of the tumour to the bronchial resection margin, giving the apparent distance of the tumour from the margin and sampling this for microscopic evidence of involvement.
- Lymph node involvement, sampling the hilar nodes in the lung specimen: extrapulmonary lymph nodes are usually submitted separately.
- The presence of other disease, particularly further tumours.
- Microscopic confirmation of the diagnosis.

It is also useful to sample lung tissue distant from, as well as distal to, the tumour, this to investigate the possibility of

Table A.2   Special stains of particular use in pulmonary pathology

Stain	Material stained	Indications
Ziehl–Neelsen	Acid–fast bacilli	Detection of mycobacteria
Grocott–Gomori methenamine silver	Fungi	Identification of fungi
Elastin van Gieson	Elastin, collagen	Assessment of vascular disease
Perl's Prussian blue	Ferric iron	Identification of haemosiderin
Periodic acid–Schiff (PAS)	Glycogen and other carbohydrates	Categorisation of clear cell tumours
		Alveolar lipoproteinosis
PAS after diastase digestion	Neutral mucin	Sub-classification of non-small cell carcinomas
		Adenocarcinoma *vs* mesothelioma
Alcian blue	Acidic mucins	Mesothelioma *vs* adenocarcinoma.
		Sub-classification of non-small carcinomas.
Congo red	Amyloid	Amyloidosis

Table A.3   Immunohistochemical markers of particular use in pulmonary pathology

Marker	Diagnostic uses
Cytokeratins	Carcinoma *vs* lymphoma and melanoma
	Sarcomatous mesothelioma *vs* sarcoma
Cytokeratin 5/6, calretinin, thrombomodulin	Epithelioid mesothelioma *vs* adenocarcinoma
Carcinoembryonic antigen	Adenocarcinoma *vs* epithelioid mesothelioma
CD56, chromogranin, synaptophysin	Neuroendocrine differentiation
TTF-1	Primary *vs* metastatic adenocarcinoma
S100	Carcinoma *vs* melanoma
	Langerhans cell histiocytosis
CD1	Langerhans cell histiocytosis
CD34	Localised fibrous tumour *vs* sarcomatoid
	mesothelioma and sarcoma
Smooth muscle actin and HMB45	Lymphangioleiomyomatosis
Leukocyte common antigen	Lymphoma *vs* carcinoma
T (CD3) and B (CD20 and CD79a) cell markers[a]	Lymphoproliferative disorders
Pneumocystis sp.	Pneumocystis pneumonia
Cytomegalovirus	Cytomegalovirus pneumonia
Legionella sp.	Legionella pneumonia

[a]Basic markers for analysis of lymphoid infiltrates. Consultation with a regional lymphoma pathology specialist is recommended for complex cases.

asbestosis having caused the tumour or other fibrosing lung diseases being present: it is embarrassing to be asked this when medicolegal proceedings have been instituted long after the specimen has been discarded if appropriate areas have not been sampled. Other points that should be described include the type of specimen (segment, lobe or whole lung), the size and weight of the specimen, the location of the tumour (segment involved) and its relation to the airways, the appearance of the tumour, and its effects on the surrounding lung, but the above are the ones the clinician will be particularly looking for, mainly to refine the preoperative staging of the tumour and thus prognosticate. It is of course customary to grade the tumour but the reproducibility of this is dubious. In resection specimens, tumour typing should adhere to the WHO classification of lung and pleural tumours.[69]

Image display

Photographs are more informative than a description and the day cannot be far off when digital images are incorporated in a computer-generated report. However, before then, photocopying is a cheap and rapid alternative to conventional photography, the flat nature of a lung slice, suitably wrapped in plastic, lending itself very well to the flat bed of a photocopier.[70]

SPECIAL MICROSCOPICAL PROCEDURES

The most useful special stains and immunohistochemical markers in pulmonary pathology are listed in Tables A.2, A.3, with more detail being provided in the relevant chapters. Molecular techniques can also be applied to tissue sections in procedures such as *in situ* hybridisation. These are finding applications in the diagnosis of infection,[71] lymphoproliferative disease[72] and the better categorisation of tumours.[73–75]

BRONCHOALVEOLAR LAVAGE (Table A.4)

This section concerns the relatively small volume lavages (up to 300 ml) that are performed with a flexible fibreoptic broncho-

Table A.4 Bronchoalveolar lavage cell counts in various lung diseases.[91]	
Disease	*Lavage cell counts*
Idiopathic pulmonary fibrosis	Neutrophil and eosinophil numbers raised
Cryptogenic organising pneumonia	Lymphocyte numbers raised; T-cell helper:suppressor ratio low; macrophages have a foamy cytoplasm
Sarcoidosis	Lymphocyte numbers and T-cell helper:suppressor ratio both raised (e.g. 40% and 4, respectively)
Extrinsic allergic alveolitis	Lymphocyte numbers very high (e.g. 65%); helper:suppressor ratio low (e.g. 0.8); mast cells present
Langerhans cell histiocytosis	Langerhans cell numbers raised
Eosinophilic pneumonia	Eosinophil numbers very high
Normal values vary between laboratories. At the Brompton Hospital, the following normal values have been established: neutrophils up to 4%, eosinophils up to 3%, lymphocytes up to 14% (60% T-cell:helper:suppressor ratio 1.8), with macrophages constituting the bulk of the remainder. Langerhans cells up to 4% in smokers (generally none in non-smokers).	

scope rather than the massive washouts (up to 30 litres) used in the treatment of alveolar lipoproteinosis (see p. 317). Small volume lavage is used in the diagnosis of several types of lung disease, infectious, neoplastic and interstitial.

The diagnosis of infection by bronchoalveolar lavage is usually the province of the microbiology department[76,77] and the histo(cyto)pathology department is more concerned with the identification of malignant cells and the enumeration of inflammatory cells.

Malignant cells may be searched for in smears or sections of the centrifuged deposit or in Cytospin® preparations in the usual way.[78] Inflammatory cell counts are informative in interstitial lung disease both in regard to pathogenesis and diagnostically, although their diagnostic specificity is probably low.[79,80] They can also be used to monitor the activity of the disease.[81] In the normal person the lavaged cells are mainly macrophages, whereas various leukocytes appear in a variety of lung diseases.[82] It follows therefore that the proportion of macrophages will diminish whenever leukocytes are also present, but total cell counts show that macrophage numbers are always increased in these circumstances. Macrophages are also more numerous in healthy smokers than in non-smokers. It is as well to bear total cell numbers in mind when considering pathogenetic mechanisms, but for diagnostic purposes attention may be concentrated on the differential cell count, performed on Geimsa-stained smears or Cytospin® preparations, augmented if required by immunocytochemical identification of lymphocyte type (B and T) and subset (T helper and suppressor), and of Langerhans cells.

The changes in cell proportions in various lung diseases are shown in Table A.4.[34,79,80,82–92] The proportions seen in lavage fluid do not necessarily represent those seen histologically, within either the air spaces or the lung as a whole.[86,93] In idiopathic pulmonary fibrosis for example, the low numbers of lymphocytes recovered by lavage does not reflect the large numbers evident histologically, perhaps because these cells are located in the interstitium rather than the air spaces. Also in idiopathic pulmonary fibrosis, lavage recovers a higher proportion of polymorphonuclear leukocytes than is evident histologically, this presumably reflecting the presence of honeycombing, the spaces of which often contain entrapped neutrophils.

Macrophages may also be harder to dislodge as whenever numbers are increased they have unusually long pseudopodia and the pseudopodia of adjacent cells intertwine. Lavage findings do not discriminate between usual interstitial pneumonia and non-specific interstitial pneumonia.[92]

Further information of diagnostic value may be obtained by studying macrophage inclusions. For example, although in many diseases the macrophages recovered by lavage contain a few Perl's-positive granules, in pulmonary haemosiderosis almost all these cells are heavily laden with such granules.[94] Similarly, in lipid pneumonia the macrophages have a foamy cytoplasm.[95]

The nature of any mineral particles present may also be identified by analytical electron microscopy (see p. 333),[96–98] but it should be noted that their presence indicates exposure rather than disease. The number of asbestos bodies in lung lavage fluid correlates with their number in lung sections,[99] but again their mere presence does not indicate that there is asbestosis.

Lavage fluid may also be examined for the characteristic proteinaceous aggregates of pulmonary alveolar lipoproteinosis (see p. 317)[100,101] and the microliths of alveolar microlithiasis (see p. 321).[102,103] Bronchoalveolar lavage is also used in the evaluation of lung transplants,[104,105] but as in many conditions the findings are best considered in conjunction with biopsy findings.[104]

Lastly, bronchoalveolar lavage is increasingly capable of providing valuable information relevant to pathogenesis, for example in identifying various inflammatory cells, cytokines and enzymes in a variety of conditions.[106–108]

REFERENCES

1. Suprun H, Pedio G, Ruttner GR. The diagnostic reliability of cytologic typing in primary lung cancer with a review of the literature. Acta Cytol 1980; 24:494–500.
2. Popp W, Rauscher H, Ritschka L, Redtenbacher S, Zwick H, Dutz W. Diagnostic sensitivity of different techniques in the diagnosis of lung tumors with the flexible fiberoptic bronchoscope – comparison of brush biopsy, imprint cytology of forceps biopsy, and histology of forceps biopsy. Cancer 1991; 67:72–75.

3. Bocking A, Klose KC, Kyll HJ, Hauptmann S. Cytologic versus histologic evaluation of needle biopsy of the lung, hilum and mediastinum – sensitivity, specificity and typing accuracy. Acta Cytol 1995; 39: 463–471.

4. Gibbs AR, Attanoos RL. Examination of lung specimens. J Clin Pathol 2000; 53:507–512.

5. International Agency for Research on Cancer. An evaluation of carcinogenic risk to humans. Overall evaluation of carcinogenicity: an updating of IARC monographs, Vols 1–42. Supplement 7. Lyons: IARC; 1987.

6. Denton KJ, Cotton DWK, Nakielny RA, Goepel JR. Secondary tumour deposits in needle biopsy tracks: an underestimated risk? J Clin Pathol 1990; 43:83.

7. Sawabata N, Ohta M, Maeda H. Fine-needle aspiration cytologic technique for lung cancer has a high potential of malignant cell spread through the tract. Chest 2000; 118:936–939.

8. Yang PC, Lee YC, Yu CJ, et al. Ultrasonographically guided biopsy of thoracic tumors – a comparison of large-bore cutting biopsy with fine-needle aspiration. Cancer 1992; 69:2553–2560.

9. Milman N. Percutaneous lung biopsy with a semi-automatic, spring-driven fine needle – preliminary results in 13 patients. Respiration 1993; 60:289–291.

10. Smyth RL, Carty H, Thomas H, van Velzen D, Heaf D. Diagnosis of interstitial lung disease by a percutaneous lung biopsy sample. Arch Dis Child 1994; 70:143–144.

11. Lohela P, Tikkakoski T, Ammala K, Strengell L, Suramo I, Repo UK. Diagnosis of diffuse lung disease by cutting needle biopsy. Acta Radiol 1994; 35:251–254.

12. Anders GT, Linville KC, Johnson JE, Blanton HM. Evaluation of the float sign for determining adequacy of specimens obtained with transbronchial biopsy. Am Rev Respir Dis 1991; 144:1406–1407.

13. Curley FJ, Johal JS, Burke ME, Fraire AE. Transbronchial lung biopsy: Can specimen quality be predicted at the time of biopsy? Chest 1998; 113:1037–1041.

14. Cook RW, Hotchkiss GR. A method for handling small tissue fragments in histopathology. Med Lab Sci 1977; 34:93–94.

15. Kepes JJ, Oswald O. Tissue artefacts caused by sponge in embedding cassettes. Am J Surg Pathol 1991; 15:810–812.

15a. Kendall DM, Gal AA. Interpretation of tissue artifacts in transbronchial lung biopsy specimens. Ann Diagn Pathol 2003, 7:20–24.

16. Rosell A, Monso E, Lores L, et al. Cytology of bronchial biopsy rinse fluid to improve the diagnostic yield for lung cancer. Eur Resp J 1998; 12:1415–1418.

17. Nagata N, Hirano H, Takayama K, Miyagawa Y, Shigematsu N. Step section preparation of transbronchial lung biopsy. Significance in the diagnosis of diffuse lung disease. Chest 1991; 100:959–962.

18. Askin FB, Katzenstein AA. Pneumocystis infection masquerading as diffuse alveolar damage. A potential source of diagnostic error. Chest 1981; 79:420–422.

19. Arroliga AC, Matthay RA. The role of bronchoscopy in lung cancer. Clin Chest Med 1993; 14:87–98.

20. Govert JA, Kopita JM, Matchar D, Kussin PS, Samuelson WM. Cost-effectiveness of collecting routine cytologic specimens during fiberoptic bronchoscopy for endoscopically visible lung tumor. Chest 1996; 109:451–456.

21. Gasparini S. Bronchoscopic biopsy techniques in the diagnosis and staging of lung cancer. Monaldi Arch Chest Dis 1997; 52:392–398.

22. Popovich J, Kvale PA, Eichenhorn MS, Radke JR, Ohorodnik JM, Fine G. Diagnostic accuracy of multiple biopsies from flexible fiberoptic bronchoscopy. A comparison of central versus peripheral carcinoma. Am Rev Respir Dis 1982; 125:521–523.

23. Goldberg-Kahn B, Healy JC, Bishop JW. The cost of diagnosis: A comparison of four different strategies in the workup of solitary radiographic lung lesions. Chest 1997; 111:870–876.

24. Chin R, McCain TW, Lucia MA, et al. Transbronchial needle aspiration in diagnosing and staging lung cancer – How many aspirates are needed? Am J Respir Crit Care Med 2002; 166:377–381.

25. Kvale PA, Bode FR, Kini S. Diagnostic accuracy in lung cancer; comparison of techniques used in association with flexible fiberoptic bronchoscopy. Chest 1976; 69:752–757.

26. Cortese DA, McDougall JC. Bronchoscopic biopsy and brushing with fluoroscopic guidance in nodular metastatic lung cancer. Chest 1981; 79:610–611.

27. Mak VH, Johnston ID, Hetzel MR, Grubb C. Value of washings and brushings at fibreoptic bronchoscopy in the diagnosis of lung cancer. Thorax 1990; 45:373–376.

28. Thomas JSJ, Lamb D, Ashcroft T, et al. How reliable is the diagnosis of lung cancer using small biopsy specimens? Report of a UKCCCR lung cancer working party. Thorax 1993; 48:1135–1139.

29. Wall CP, Gaensler EA, Carrington CB, Hayes JA. Comparison of transbronchial and open lung biopsies in chronic infiltrative lung diseases. Am Rev Respir Dis 1981; 123:280–285.

30. Johnston IDA, Gomm SA, Kalra S, Woodcock AA, Evans CC, Hind CRK. The management of cryptogenic fibrosing alveolitis in three regions of the United Kingdom. Eur Respir J 1993; 6:891–893.

31. Lacasse Y, Fraser RS, Fournier M, Cormier Y. Diagnostic accuracy of transbronchial biopsy in acute farmer's lung disease. Chest 1997; 112:1459–1465.

32. Gilman MJ, Wang K. Transbronchial lung biopsy in sarcoidosis: an approach to determine the optimal number of biopsies. Am Rev Respir Dis 1980; 122:721–724.

33. Burt ME, Flye W, Webber BL, Wesley RA. Prospective evaluation of aspiration needle, cutting needle, transbronchial and open lung biopsy in patients with pulmonary infiltrates. Ann Thorac Surg 1981; 32:146–153.

34. Poletti V, Cazzato S, Minicuci N, Zompatori M, Burzi M, Schiattone ML. The diagnostic value of bronchoalveolar lavage and transbronchial lung biopsy in cryptogenic organizing pneumonia. Eur Respir J 1996; 9:2513–2516.

35. Venn GE, Kay PH, Midwood CJ, Goldstraw P. Open lung biopsy in patients with diffuse pulmonary shadowing. Thorax 1985; 40:931–935.

36. Shah SS, Tsang V, Goldstraw P. Open lung biopsy – a safe, reliable and accurate method for diagnosis in diffuse lung disease. Respiration 1992; 59:243–246.

37. Bensard DD, McIntyre RC, Waring BJ, Simon JS. Comparison of video thoracoscopic lung biopsy to open lung biopsy in the diagnosis of interstitial lung disease. Chest 1993; 103:765–770.

38. Carnochan FM, Walker WS, Cameron EW. Efficacy of video assisted thoracoscopic lung biopsy: an historical comparison with open lung biopsy. Thorax 1994; 49:361–363.

39. Kadokura M, Colby TV, Myers JL, et al. Pathologic comparison of video-assisted thoracic surgical lung biopsy with traditional open lung biopsy. J Thorac Cardiovasc Surg 1995; 109:494–498.

40. Ravini M, Ferraro G, Barbieri B, Colombo P, Rizzato G. Changing strategies of lung biopsies in diffuse lung diseases: the impact of video-assisted thoracoscopy. Eur Resp J 1998; 11:99–103.

41. Newman SL, Michel RP, Wang NS. Lingula lung biopsy: is it representative? Am Rev Respir Dis 1985; 132:1084–1086.

42. Wetstein L. Sensitivity and specificity of lingular segmental biopsies of the lung. Chest 1986; 90:383–386.

43. Miller RR, Nelems B, Muller NL, Evans KG, Ostrow DN. Lingular and right middle lobe biopsy in the assessment of diffuse lung disease. Ann Thorac Surg 1987; 44:269–273.

44. vanKuppevelt TH, Robbesom AA, Versteeg EMM, Veerkamp JH, vanHerwaarden CLA, Dekhuijzen PNR. Restoration by vacuum inflation of original alveolar dimensions in small human lung specimens. Eur Resp J 2000; 15:771–777.

45. Churg AC. An inflation procedure for open-lung biopsies. Am J Surg Pathol 1983; 7:69–71.

46. Bachofen M, Weibel ER, Roos B. Postmortem fixation of human lungs for electron microscopy. Am Rev Respir Dis 1975; 111:247–256.

47. Reid LM. Selection of tissue for microscopic study from lungs injected with radio-opaque material. Thorax 1955; 10:197–198.

48. Hales MR, Carrington CB. A pigmented gelatin mass for vascular injection. Yale J Biol Med 1971; 43:257–270.

49. Wright BM, Slavin G, Kreel L, Callan K, Sandin B. Postmortem inflation and fixation of human lungs. A technique for pathological and radiological correlations. Thorax 1974; 29:189–194.

50. Itoh M, Tokunaga S, Asamoto H, et al. Radiologic-pathologic correlations of small lung nodules with special reference to peribronchiolar nodules. Am J Roentgenol 1978; 130:223–231.

51. Sutinen S, Paakko P, Lahti R. Post-mortem inflammation, radiography and fixation of human lungs. A method for radiological and pathological correlations and morphometric studies. Scand J Respir Dis 1979; 60:29–35.

52. Langlois SLP, Henderson DW. Radiological-pathological correlations in pulmonary disease: a simplified method for the study of post-mortem lungs. Australas Radiol 1980; 24:262–269.

53. McCulloch TA, Rutty GN. Postmortem examination of the lungs: a preservation technique for opening the bronchi and pulmonary arteries individually without transection problems. J Clin Pathol 1998; 51:163–164.

54. Liebow AA, Hales MR, Lindskog GE, Bloomer WE. Plastic demonstration of pulmonary pathology. Bull Internat Assoc Med museums 1947; 27:116–129.

55. MonforteMunoz H, Walls RL. Intrapulmonary airways visualized by staining and clearing of whole-lung sections: the transparent human lung. Modern Pathol 2004; 17:22–27.

56. Heard BE. A pathological study of emphysema of the lungs with chronic bronchitis. Thorax 1958; 13:136–149.

57. Miller RR. Bronchioloalveolar cell adenomas. Am J Surg Pathol 1990; 14:904–912.

58. Gough J, Wentworth JE. Thin sections of entire organs mounted on paper. In: Harrison CV, ed. Recent Advances in Pathology. London: Churchill; 1960:80–86.

59. Whimster WF. Rapid giant paper sections of lungs. Thorax 1969; 24:737–741.

60. Cote RA, Korthy AL, Kory RC. Laminated lung macrosections: a new dimension in the study and teaching of pulmonary pathology. Dis Chest 1963; 43:1–7.

61. Gibbs AR, Seal RME. Examination of lung specimens. J Clin Pathol 1990; 43:68–72.

62. Nash G, Hutter RVP, Henson DE. Practice protocol for the examination of specimens from patients with lung cancer. Arch Pathol Lab Med 1995; 119:695–700.

63. Myers J, Askin FB, Yousem SA. Recommendations for the reporting of resected primary lung carcinomas. Am J Clin Pathol 1995; 104:371–374.

64. Gephardt GN, Baker PB. Lung carcinoma surgical pathology report adequacy: a College of American Pathologists q-probes study of over 8300 cases from 464 institutions. Arch Pathol Lab Med 1996; 120:922–927.

65. Carter D. ASCP survey on surgical pathology: Examination of pulmonary resection and biopsy specimens. Am J Clin Pathol 1997; 108:619–624.

66. Gal AA, Marchevsky AM, Travis WD. Updated protocol for the examination of specimens from patients with carcinoma of the lung. Arch Pathol Lab Med 2003; 127:1304–1313.

67. Nash G, Otis CN. Protocol for the examination of specimens from patients with malignant pleural mesothelioma – A basis for checklists. Arch Pathol Lab Med 1999; 123:39–44.

68. Bunker ML, Raab SS, Landreneau RJ, Silverman JF. The diagnosis and significance of visceral pleural invasion in lung carcinoma – Histologic predictors and the role of elastic stains. Am J Clin Pathol 1999; 112:777–783.

69. World Health Organization. Tumours of the lung, pleura, thymus and heart. Lyons: IARC Press; 2004.

70. Olson DR. Specimen photocopying for surgical pathology reports. Am J Clin Pathol 1978; 70:94–95.

71. Unger ER, Budgeon LR, Myerson D, Brigati DJ. Viral diagnosis by in situ hybridization. Description of a rapid simplified colorimetric method. Am J Surg Pathol 1986; 10:1–8.

72. Nicholson AG, Wotherspoon AC, Diss TC, et al. Pulmonary B-cell non-Hodgkin's lymphomas. The value of immunohistochemistry and gene analysis in diagnosis. Histopathology 1995; 26:395–403.

73. Giaid A, Hamid QA, Springall DR, et al. Detection of endothelin immunoreactivity and mRNA in pulmonary tumours. J Pathol 1990; 162:15–22.

74. Hamid QA, Corrin B, Dewar A, Hoefler H, Sheppard MN. Expression of gastrin-releasing peptide (human bombesin) gene in large cell undifferentiated carcinoma of the lung. J Pathol 1990; 161:145–151.

75. Hamid Q, Corrin B, Sheppard MN, Huttner WB, Polak JM. Expression of chromogranin A mRNA in small cell carcinoma of the lung. J Pathol 1991; 163:293–297.

76. Griffiths MH, Kocjan G, Miller RF, Godfrey Faussett P. Diagnosis of pulmonary disease in human immunodeficiency virus infection: role of transbronchial biopsy and bronchoalveolar lavage. Thorax 1989; 44:554–558.

77. Baughman RP. Use of bronchoscopy in the diagnosis of infection in the immunocompromised host [editorial]. Thorax 1994; 49:3–7.

78. Poletti V, Romagna M, Allen KA, Gasponi A, Spiga L. Bronchoalveolar lavage in the diagnosis of disseminated lung tumors. Acta Cytol 1995; 39:472–477.

79. Winterbauer RH, Lammert J, Selland M, Wu R, Corley D, Springmeyer SC. Bronchoalveolar lavage cell populations in the diagnosis of sarcoidosis. Chest 1993; 104:352–361.

80. Kantrow SP, Meyer KC, Kidd P, Raghu G. The CD4/CD8 ratio in BAL fluid is highly variable in sarcoidosis. Eur Resp J 1997; 10:2716–2721.

81. Turner-Warwick M, Haslam PL. The value of serial bronchoalveolar lavages in assessing the clinical progress of patients with cryptogenic fibrosing alveolitis. Am Rev Respir Dis 1987; 135:26–34.

82. The BAL Cooperative Steering Committee. Bronchoalveolar lavage constituents in healthy individuals, idiopathic pulmonary fibrosis, and selected comparison groups. Am Rev Respir Dis 1990; 141:S169–202.

83. Reynolds HY, Fulmer JD, Kazmierowski JA, Roberts WC, Frank MM, Crystal RG. Analysis of cellular and protein content of broncho-alveolar lavage fluid from patients with idiopathic pulmonary fibrosis and chronic hypersensitivity pneumonitis. J Clin Invest 1977; 59:165–175.

84. Weinberger SE, Kelman JA, Elson NA, et al. Bronchoalveolar lavage in interstitial lung disease. Ann Intern Med 1978; 89:459–466.

85. Casolaro MA, Bernaudin J-F, Saltini C, Ferrans VJ, Crystal RG. Accumulation of Langerhans' cells on the epithelial surface of the lower respiratory tract in normal subjects in association with cigarette smoking. Am Rev Respir Dis 1988; 137: 406–411.

86. Haslam PL, Turton CWG, Heard B, et al. Bronchoalveolar lavage in pulmonary fibrosis: comparison of cells obtained with lung biopsy and clinical features. Thorax 1980; 35:9–18.

87. Haslam PL, Turton CW, Lukoszek A, et al. Bronchoalveolar lavage fluid cell counts in cryptogenic fibrosing alveolitis and their relation to therapy. Thorax 1980; 35:328–339.

88. Chollet S, Soler P, Dournovo P, Richard MS, Ferrans VJ, Basset F. Diagnosis of pulmonary histiocytosis X by immunodetection of Langerhans cells in bronchoalveolar lavage fluid. Am J Pathol 1984; 115:225–232.

88a. Danel C, Israel-biet D, Costabel U, et al. The clinical role of BAL in pulmonary histiocytosis-X. Eur Respir J 1990; 3:949–950.

89. Auerswald U, Barth J, Magnussen H. Value of CD-1-positive cells in bronchoalveolar lavage fluid for the diagnosis of pulmonary histiocytosis-X. Lung 1991; 169:305–309.

90. Costabel U, Teschler H, Guzman J. Bronchiolitis obliterans organizing pneumonia (BOOP) – the cytological and immunocytological profile of bronchoalveolar lavage. Eur Respir J 1992; 5:791–797.

90a. Danel C, Israel-biet D, Costabel U, et al. The clinical role of BAL in rave pulmonary diseases. Eur Respir Rev 1992; 2:83–88.

91. Merchant RK, Schwartz DA, Helmers RA, Dayton CS, Hunninghake GW. Bronchoalveolar lavage cellularity – the distribution in normal volunteers. Am Rev Respir Dis 1992; 146:448–453.

92. Veeraraghavan S, Latsi PI, Wells AU, et al. BAL findings in idiopathic nonspecific interstitial pneumonia and usual interstitial pneumonia. Eur Resp J 2003; 22:239–244.

93. Nagata N, Takayama K, Nikaido Y, Yokosaki Y, Kido M. Comparison of alveolar septal inflammation to bronchoalveolar lavage in interstitial lung diseases. Respiration 1996; 63:94–99.

94. Perezarellano JL, Garcia JEL, Macias MCG, Gomez FG, Lopez AJ, Decastro S. Hemosiderin-laden macrophages in bronchoalveolar lavage fluid. Acta Cytol 1992; 36:26–30.

95. Midulla F, Strappini PM, Ascoli V, et al. Bronchoalveolar lavage cell analysis in a child with chronic lipid pneumonia. Eur Resp J 1998; 11:239–242.

96. Davison AG, Haslam PL, Corrin B, et al. Interstitial lung disease and asthma in hard-metal workers: bronchoalveolar lavage, ultrastructural, and analytical findings and results of bronchial provocation tests. Thorax 1983; 38:119–128.

97. Johnson NF, Haslam PL, Dewar A, Newman-Taylor AJ, Turner-Warwick M. Identification of inorganic dust particles in bronchoalveolar lavage macrophages by energy dispersive X-ray microanalysis. Arch Environ Health 1986; 41:133–144.

98. Lusuardi M, Capelli A, Donner CF, Capelli O, Velluti G. Semi-quantitative X-ray microanalysis of bronchoalveolar lavage samples from silica-exposed and nonexposed subjects. Eur Respir J 1992; 5:798–803.

99. Karjalainen A, Piipari R, Mantyla T, et al. Asbestos bodies in bronchoalveolar lavage in relation to asbestos bodies and asbestos fibres in lung parenchyma. Eur Respir J 1996; 9:1000–1005.

100. Costello JF, Moriarty DC, Branthwaite MA, Turner-Warwick M, Corrin B. Diagnosis and management of alveolar proteinosis: the role of electron microscopy. Thorax 1975; 30:121–132.

101. Martin RJ, Coalson JJ, Rogers RM, Horton FO, Manous LE. Pulmonary alveolar proteinosis: the diagnosis by segmental lavage. Am Rev Respir Dis 1980; 121:819–825.

102. Palombini B, Da Silva Porto N, Wallau CU, Camargo JJ. Bronchopulmonary lavage in alveolar microlithiasis. Chest 1981; 80:242–243.

103. Pracyk JB, Simonson SG, Young SL, Chio AJ, Roggli VL, Piantadosi CA. Composition of lung lavage in pulmonary alveolar microlithiasis. Respiration 1996; 63:254–260.

104. Clelland C, Higenbottam T, Stewart S, et al. Bronchoalveolar lavage and transbronchial lung biopsy during acute rejection and infection in heart-lung transplant patients – studies of cell counts, lymphocyte phenotypes, and expression of HLA-DR and interleukin-2 receptor. Am Rev Respir Dis 1993; 147:1386–1392.

105. Guilinger RA, Paradis IL, Dauber JH, et al. The importance of bronchoscopy with transbronchial biopsy and bronchoalveolar lavage in the management of lung transplant recipients. Am J Respir Crit Care Med 1995; 152: 2037–2043.

106. Redington AE, Madden J, Frew AJ, et al. Transforming growth factor-beta 1 in asthma: measurement in bronchoalveolar lavage fluid. Am J Respir Crit Care Med 1997; 156:642–647.

107. Ashitani J, Mukae H, Nakazato M, et al. Elevated concentrations of defensins in bronchoalveolar lavage fluid in diffuse panbronchiolitis. Eur Resp J 1998; 11:104–111.

108. Yamanouchi H, Fujita J, Hojo S, et al. Neutrophil elastase: alpha-1-proteinase inhibitor complex in serum and bronchoalveolar lavage fluid in patients with pulmonary fibrosis. Eur Resp J 1998; 11:120–125.

INDEX

Cigars, 528
Ciliary dyskinesia, 63–5, 115
Ciliated cells, 9–10
Cirrhosis, 487, 488
    cystic fibrosis and, 69
    pulmonary hypertension and, 424
Clara cells, 12–13
    adenocarcinoma, 549
    damage by ingested chemicals, 375
    small airway disease, 102
Clear cell tumours
    benign (sugar tumour), 601, 613–15
        tuberous sclerosis and, 488, 615
    carcinoid, 585, 615
    carcinoma, 556, 615
    clear cell variant of squamous cell
        carcinoma, 544
    differential diagnosis, 556, 615, 676
    odontogenic carcinoma (metastatic), 677
Coagulopathy
    disseminated intravascular coagulation,
        139
    hypercoagulability, 406, 484
Coal pneumoconiosis, 331, 340
    compensation, 105, 342–3
    mineralogy, 340–1
    pathogenesis, 344
    pathology, 341–4
    silica and, 335, 340–1
Coal smoke and lung cancer, 529
Cobalt lung, 354
'Cobblestone' pattern in IPF, 269
Cocaine, 378–9
Coccidioidomycosis, 238–9
Coeliac disease, 486
'Coin' lesions
    cryptococcoma, 235
    solitary nodules in cancer diagnosis,
        537, 615, 671
Collagen
    diffuse alveolar damage, 137
    hyalinising granuloma, 687
    in pneumoconiosis, 336, 341
Collapsed lung, 87–8, 481
    atelectasis, 42, 87, 132
    middle lobe syndrome, 89
    treatment for tuberculosis, 695, 697–8
Collateral ventilation, 13, 88
Collecting-duct cells, 11
Colloid adenocarcinoma, 550
Community-acquired pneumonia, 174
Compensation
    asbestos-related diseases, 352, 699
    coal pneumoconiosis, 105, 342–3
Compensatory emphysema, 105
Conchoidal bodies, 322–3
    Schaumann bodies in sarcoidosis, 287
Congenital disorders, *see specific conditions*
Congestion, 401
    pneumococcal pneumonia, 177
Congo red stain, 741
Connective tissue, alveolar, 17–18
Connective tissue diseases, 471–2
    ankylosing spondylitis, 478
    Behçet's disease, 448, 479–80
    cutis laxa, 480
    Ehlers–Danlos syndrome, 480–1
    Marfan's syndrome, 481
    mixed, 478
    myositis, 478
    pleurisy and, 473, 477, 698
    pseudoxanthoma elasticum, 481
    pulmonary hypertension and, 431, 475,
        476–7, 477

relapsing polychondritis, 91–2, 479
rheumatic fever, 475
rheumatoid disease, 344, 447, 472–5, 698
Sjögren's syndrome, 479
systemic lupus erythematosus, 392, 447,
    477–8, 698
systemic sclerosis, 431, 475–7
Connective tissue tumours
    benign, 615–17
    chest wall, 720
    smooth muscle, 299, 618–19, 676–7
Constrictive bronchiolitis obliterans, 119
    autoimmune diseases, 121–2, 474–5
    drug-induced, 385
    S. androgynus, 377
Contraceptive pills, 406
COP (cryptogenic organizing pneumonia),
    307–10
COPD (chronic obstructive pulmonary
    disease), 93–4
Cor pulmonale, 432
Coronavirus, 150
Corpora amylacea, 321
Corticosteroids
    asthma, 256
    COP, 307
    eosinophilia, 461, 465
    fetal lung development, 39–40
Corynebacterium diphtheriae, 92
Corynebacterium equi, 213–14
Cotton, byssinosis, 360
Cough reflex, 88, 186, 188
Coxiella burnetii, 151, 165–6
Crack cocaine, 378
Creola bodies, 108
CREST syndrome, 431, 476
Cristobalite, 335
Crocidolite (blue asbestos), 345, 346, 702
Crohn's disease, 486–7
Crospovidone, 380
Croup, 153
Cryptococcosis (European blastomycosis),
    233–5
Cryptococcus neoformans, 233
Cryptogenic fibrosing alveolitis (CFA), *see*
    Idiopathic pulmonary fibrosis
Cryptogenic organising pneumonia
    (COP), 307–10
    lavage cell counts, 742
    terminology, 264
Cryptosporidiosis, 251
Curschmann spirals, 108
Cushing's syndrome, 540
Cutis laxa, 480
Cyanosis, 481, 482
Cylindroma (adenoid cystic carcinoma),
    591–2
Cystadenocarcinoma, 551
Cystadenoma, 594–5
Cystic adenomatoid malformation,
    congenital, 59–62, 613
Cystic carcinoma, adenoid, 591–2
Cystic fibrohistiocytic tumours, 677
Cystic fibrosis, 65–70
    lung transplants, 66, 507
    pneumonia, 67, 174
Cysticercosis, 256
Cystine storage disease, 491
Cysts
    after abscess rupture, 187
    air
        congenital, 60
        cystic fibrosis, 67
        staphylococcal pneumonia, 179, 188

bronchogenic, 52–3
in congenital lymphangiectasia, 76
hydatid, 254–5
pneumocystosis, 220–1
toxoplasmosis, 250
'worm cysts', 253–4
Cytokeratins
    carcinoma, 544, 741
        adenocarcinoma, 544, 548, 676
        large cell, 544, 555, 558
        primary vs. metastatic, 676
        small cell, 544, 555
        squamous, 676
        squamous cell, 544
    mesothelioma, 710, 712
    normal expression, 7
Cytokines
    asthma, 112, 113
    IPF, 274, 276
    leukocytes and
        eosinophils, 460
        lymphocytes, 27
        mast cells, 28, 112
    mesothelioma, 713
    pneumoconiosis, 344, 352
    sarcoidosis, 286, 288
    septic shock, 139
    tuberculosis, 196, 203
Cytomegalovirus, 159–60
    P. jiroveci and, 223
    in transplant patients, 159, 512, 517
Cytotoxicity of drugs, 385–7, 475, 521

Decidual embolism, 411
Decompression sickness, 370–1, 402
Dendritic cells, 27
Dermatomyositis, 478
Desmoplastic pattern mesothelioma, 706,
    713
Desmoplastic small round cell tumour,
    717–18
Desquamative interstitial pneumonia
    (DIP), 310–13
    childhood, 48, 311
    differential diagnosis, 273, 278, 312–13,
        315
Development, 37–40
    disorders, 48–77
Diabetes mellitus, 493–4
Dialysis, 483
Diaphragm
    congenital defects, 54, 77
    fenestrations and endometriosis, 495
Diatomaceous earth, 338–9
Diesel fumes, 529
Diet
    cancer risk, 530–1
    pulmonary hypertension, 390, 424–5
    S. androgynus poisoning, 377
    toxic oil syndrome, 376–7, 424
Dieulafoy's disease, 72
Diffuse alveolar damage (DAD)
    causes, 137–41
        cytotoxic drugs, 385
        idiopathic (AIP), 280
        parasites, 251, 256
        pollution, 358
        viruses, 140, 150, 156, 157–8
    clinical features, 131–2
    pathology, 132–7
        eosinophilic pneumonia, 463
        interstitial pneumonia, 273, 278, 280
        SARS, 157–8

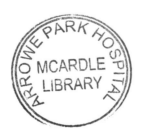